For Reference

Not to be taken from this room

W9-ASR-531

For Reference

Not to be taken from this room

ENCYCLOPEDIA
OF
HUMAN NUTRITION

ENCYCLOPEDIA
OF
HUMAN NUTRITION

Editor-in-Chief
MICHELE J. SADLER

Editors
J.J. STRAIN

BENJAMIN CABALLERO

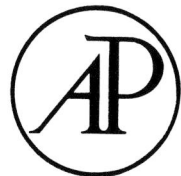

ACADEMIC PRESS
Harcourt Brace & Company Publishers
**San Diego   London   Boston   New York
Sydney   Tokyo   Toronto**

ACADEMIC PRESS
525 B Street, Suite 1900,
San Diego, CA 92101–4495, USA
http://www.apnet.com

ACADEMIC PRESS
24-28 Oval Road
London NW1 7DX, UK
http.hbuk.co.uk/ap/

Copyright © 1999 by
ACADEMIC PRESS

The following article is a US Government work in the public
domain and not subject to copyright:

Ultratrace Elements: Physiology

All rights reserved
No part of this book may be reproduced in any form, by photostat, microfilm or any other means,
without written permission from the publishers

ISBN 0-12-226694-3

A catalogue record for this Encyclopedia is available from the British Library

Access for a limited period to an on-line version of the Encyclopedia of Human Nutrition is included in
the purchase price of the print edition.
This on-line version has been uniquely and persistently identified by the Digital Object Identifier (DOI)

10.1006/0127995110

By following the link

http://dx.doi.org/10.1006/0127995110

from any Web Browser, buyers of the Encyclopedia of Human Nutrition will find instructions on how to
register for access.

Typeset by Photo·graphics, Honiton, Devon, UK.
Printed and bound in Great Britain by The Bath Press, Bath, Avon, UK.

EDITORIAL ADVISORY BOARD

EDITOR-IN-CHIEF
Michèle J Sadler
Institute of Grocery Distribution
Grange Lane, Letchmore Heath
Watford, Hertfordshire WD2 8DQ, UK

EDITORS
J J Strain
Northern Ireland Center for Diet and Health (NICHE)
University of Ulster, Coleraine
Northern Ireland BT52 1SA, UK

Benjamin Caballero
Center for Human Nutrition
Johns Hopkins University
615 North Wolfe Street
Baltimore, Maryland 21205-2179, USA

CHAIRMAN OF THE BOARD
Noel W Solomons
Center for Studies of Sensory Impairment, Aging & Metabolism
(CeSSIAM), Zone 11, Guatemala City, 01011 Guatemala

L Allen
Department of Nutrition
University of California – Davis
3113 Meyer Hall
Davis, CA 95616-8669, USA

A E Bender
2 Willow Vale
Fetcham, Leatherhead
Surrey KT22 9TE, UK

B Bistrian
Harvard Medical School
New England Deaconess Hospital
194 Pilgrim Road
Boston, MA 02215, USA

M Elia
Dunn Clinical Nutrition Centre
Hills Road, Cambridge CB2 2DH, UK

H L Greene
Slim-Fast® Foods Company
777 S. Flagler Drive
West Tower, Suite 1400
West Palm Beach, FL 33401, USA

R Grimble
Institute of Human Nutrition
University of Southampton
Southampton SO16 7PX, UK

C J K Henry
School of Biological and Molecular Sciences
Oxford Brookes University
Gipsy Lane
Headington, Oxford OX3 0BP, UK

E Jequier
Institut de Physiologie, Faculte de Medecine
University of Lausanne
7 rue du Bugnon
1005 Lausanne, Switzerland

P A Judd
Department of Nutrition and Dietetics
King's College London
Campden Hill Road
London W8 7AH, UK

Lenore Kohlmeier
Departments of Nutrition and Epidemiology
School of Public Health, CB #7400
University of North Carolina
Chapel Hill, NC 27599-7400, USA

Jun Yao Li
Department of Epidemiology, Cancer Institute
Chinese Academy of Medical Sciences, Room 1310
Building for Scientific Research, Lontan Lake,
Zuoanmenwai
Panjiayuan, Chaoyang District, PO Box 2258,
Beijing 100021
Peoples' Republic of China

D Mela
Consumer Sciences Department
Institute of Food Research
Earley Gate
Reading RG6 6BZ, UK

A O Musaiger
Food and Nutrition Programme
Bahrain Center for Studies and Research
PO Box 496
Manama, State of Bahrain

P J Nestel
Baker Medical Research Institute
PO Box 6492
Melbourne 8008, Australia

P Reeds
Children's Nutrition Research Center
Baylor College of Medicine
1100 Bates Street
Houston, Texas 77030-2600, USA

N S Scrimshaw
Food & Nutrition, Program for Human and Soc
Development
United Nations University
Charles Street Station, PO Box 500
Boston, MA 02114-0500, USA

P S Shetty
Department of Epidemiology and Public Health
London School of Hygiene and Tropical Medicine
49/51 Bedford Square
London WC1B 3DP, UK

R Uauy-Dagach
Instituto de Nutrición y Technología de los Alimentos
(INTA)
Universidad de Chile
Casilla 138-11
Santiago, Chile

B Underwood
International Union of Nutritional Sciences (IUNS)
Food and Nutrition Board
Institute of Medicine, NAS
2101 Constitution Avenue NW (FO 3049)
Washington, DC 20418, USA

D York
Pennington Biomedical Research Center
Louisiana State University
6400 Perkins Road
Baton Rouge, LA 70808-41124, USA

FOREWORD

Why an encyclopedia? The original Greek word means 'the circle of arts and sciences essential for a liberal education', and such a book was intended to embrace all knowledge. That was the aim of the famous Encyclopédie produced by Diderot and d'Alembert in the middle of the 18th century, which contributed so much to what has been called the Enlightenment. It is recorded that after all the authors had corrected the proofs of their contributions, the printer secretly cut out whatever he thought might give offence to the king, mutilated most of the best articles and burnt the manuscripts! Later, and less controversially, the word 'encyclopedia' came to be used for an exhaustive repertory of information on some particular department of knowledge. It is in this class that the present work falls.

In recent years the scope of Human Nutrition as a scientific discipline has expanded enormously. I used to think of it as an applied subject, relying on the basic sciences of physiology and biochemistry in much the same way that engineering relies on physics. That traditional relationship remains and is fundamental, but the field is now much wider. At one end of the spectrum epidemiological studies and the techniques on which they depend have played a major part in establishing the relationships between diet, nutritional status and health, and there is greater recognition of the importance of social factors. At the other end of the spectrum we are becoming increasingly aware of the genetic determinants of ways in which the body handles food and is able to resist adverse influences of the environment. Nutritionists are thus beginning to explore the genome.

In parallel with this widening of the subject there has been an increase in opportunities for training and research in nutrition, with new departments and new courses being developed in universities, medical schools and schools of public health, along with a greater involvement of schoolchildren and their teachers. Public interest in nutrition is intense and needs to be guided by sound science. Governments are realizing more and more the role that nutrition plays in the prevention of disease and the maintenance of good health, and the need to develop a nutrition policy that is integrated with policies for food production.

The appearance of this encyclopedia at the present time is therefore welcome and timely. It is as comprehensive as the present state of knowledge allows, but is not overly technical and is well supplied with suggestions for further reading. All the articles have been carefully reviewed and although some of the subjects are controversial and sensitive, the publishers have not exerted the kind of political censorship that so infuriated Diderot.

John Waterlow

J.C. Waterlow
Emeritus Professor of Human Nutrition
London School of Hygiene and Tropical Medicine
July 1998

PREFACE

The science of nutrition is a diverse and complex subject. To attempt to draw together the many different elements of this rapidly developing science into a comprehensive encyclopedia has been a particularly daunting task.

The inspiration for taking on this task and the central elements of the work were borne out of the highly acclaimed Encyclopaedia of Food Science, Food Technology and Nutrition which was published in 1993. That the content of this new work is considerably different mainly reflects the rapid developments that have occurred in nutrition since the early 1990s.

The Editors have aimed to include a balance of material of interest to many readers, including those of different nationalities where the applications of nutritional science may be very different. Those with a clinical and medical background, those with a role in producing and processing food, and those involved in applying the science to public health policy, including educating the public about the importance of sound nutrition, should find much of interest in this work.

At a time when there is a continuing increase in the general public's interest in diet and health, there is not always agreement between different groups about the advice that should be given. Moreover, topics are increasingly debated in the media at a very early stage in the scientific exploration. The public look to nutritionists for advice concerning a number of current public health problems, and this Encyclopedia should prove helpful in providing summaries of the scientific background for those who are less familiar with particular subject areas.

The extent of coverage is wide and broad-based. It includes: physiological aspects of nutrient and energy requirements by different population groups; measurement of dietary intake and nutritional status; nutrient composition of the main food groups; associations between diet, lifestyle and disease; clinical applications of nutrition to improve health; topical issues relating to the food processing industry; influences on food choice and eating behaviour; nutritional guidelines and public health policies in both developed and developing countries; international aspects of food labelling, and a range of related topics in between these key subject areas.

It has not been possible to cover every aspect of the subject in minute detail; there has been the restraint of size, and for a large work of this nature, with considerable commitment required from all of the contributors, it has been understandably difficult to ensure that every article that had been ambitiously commissioned at the outset was received. Naturally there are some gaps, but we have endeavoured to keep these to a minimum. Full guidance for further reading is given and we are satisfied that we have delivered coverage that should easily meet the requirements of most readers.

Our thanks are due to all who contributed to this project.

M.J. Sadler, J.J. Strain, B. Caballero
Editors

INTRODUCTION

"Nutrition is not a discipline to be studied but a problem to be solved". This phrase, attributed to Jean Mayer, underscores the importance of nutritional science in addressing major public health problems. The statement also epitomizes the role that nutrition plays in linking basic biomedical disciplines with operational, problem-solving activities.

Our ability to develop effective responses to major health issues can only be as good as our understanding of those issues. In the case of nutrition, that knowledge involves a staggering number of disciplines, from molecular biology to agriculture and food science, from social sciences and human behaviour to clinical medicine. Few, if any, individuals can claim to master all these disciplines but, in order for a multi-disciplinary team to communicate and be effective, each member needs to be familiar with all the relevant disciplines. Hence the need for this encyclopedia. By combining up-to-date information on fundamental nutrition science with practical, operational issues, we hope these volumes will facilitate the necessary dialogue between the many branches of modern nutrition practice.

The effects of the globalization of modern life are particularly apparent for nutrition. Food production and food availability in individual countries are highly dependent on the world market, and rapid changes in agricultural policies in a few key nations can have a major global impact on food prices and availability.

Urbanization and industrialization of developing countries are creating new, rapidly increasing nutritional problems, particularly among the urban poor, while in some cases causing significant reductions in usable land. While the declining trends in infant mortality and childhood malnutrition in many areas of the world are encouraging, the threat posed by non-communicable diseases such as obesity, diabetes, and cardiovascular diseases is increasing. Worldwide data from 1990 show that 47 per cent of deaths in the developing world were due to chronic diseases, most of them associated with unhealthy diet and lifestyle. By the year 2020, it is predicted that 67 per cent of years lost to disability (a major index of population health) in developing countries will be related to chronic non-communicable diseases. How to bring the benefits of industrialization and modern technology to large population groups while preserving their health and nutrition status will be one of the major challenges for the next decades.

In the realm of basic science, continuing discoveries of the genetic mechanisms of physiological and pathological processes are just beginning to shape the nutritional practice of the future. The contrast between deceptively simple preventive measures (such as dietary change) and sophisticated, high-tech therapies could not be sharper. And yet, there is no question that advances in molecular genetics will continue to play a major role in our understanding of nutritional disorders and in the development of novel preventive strategies, from increasing crop yields to modulating host response to illness.

This encyclopedia builds on a distinguished tradition of comprehensive, systematic information delivery, of which all Academic Press encyclopedias are excellent examples. The editors acknowledge the commitment of the authors and of the outstanding staff of the Major Reference Works division of Academic Press in enabling this encyclopedia to come to fruition. We are confident that the many authors who contributed their work are among the best that today's global nutritional science has to offer.

We trust this encyclopedia – and its electronic version – will be a valuable resource to inform and provide practical support to readers in their daily tasks, be it caring for the nutritional needs of a patient, teaching a nutrition course, advising policy makers, or communicating the science of nutrition to the general public.

GUIDE TO USE OF THE ENCYCLOPEDIA

Structure of the Encyclopedia

The material in the Encyclopedia is arranged as a series of entries in alphabetical order. Some entries comprise a single article, whilst entries on more diverse subjects consist of several articles that deal with various aspects of the topic. In the latter case the articles are arranged in a logical sequence within an entry.

To help you realize the full potential of the material in the Encyclopedia we have provided three features to help you find the topic of your choice.

1. Contents Lists

Your first point of reference will probably be the contents list. The complete contents list appearing in each volume will provide you with both the volume number and the page number of the entry. On the opening page of an entry a contents list is provided so that the full details of the articles within the entry are immediately available.

Alternatively you may choose to browse through a volume using the alphabetical order of the entries as your guide. To assist you in identifying your location within the Encyclopedia a running headline indicates the current entry and the current article within that entry.

You will find 'dummy entries' where obvious synonyms exist for entries or where we have grouped together related topics. Dummy entries appear in both the contents list and the body of the text. For example, a dummy entry appears for AIDS which directs you to HIV Disease: Nutritional Management, where the material is located.

Example

If you were attempting to locate material on Sugar via the contents list.

SUGAR *see* CARBOHYDRATES: Chemistry and Classification (including Dietary Fibre (Fiber));
   Regulation of Carbohydrate Metabolism; Requirements and Dietary Importance; GALACTOSE:
   Absorption and Metabolism; GLUCOSE: Chemistry, Dietary Sources and Glycaemic Index; Metabolism
   and Maintenance of Blood Glucose Level; Glucose Tolerance; SUCROSE: Nutritional Role, Absorption
   and Metabolism; Dietary Sucrose and Disease

At the appropriate location in the contents list, the page numbers for articles under Carbohydrates are given.

If you were trying to locate the material by browsing through the text and you looked up Sugar then the following information would be provided.

Sugar *see* **Carbohydrates**: Chemistry and Classification (including Dietary Fibre); Regulation of Carbohydrate Metabolism; Requirements and Dietary Importance. **Galactose**: Absorption and Metabolism. **Glucose**: Chemistry, Dietary Sources and Glycaemic Index; Metabolism and Maintenance of Blood Glucose Level; Glucose Tolerance. **Sucrose**: Nutritional role, Absorption and Metabolism; Dietary Sucrose and Disease.

Alternatively, if you were looking up Carbohydrates the following information would be provided.

CARBOHYDRATES

Contents
Chemistry and Classification (including Dietary Fibre)
Regulation of Carbohydrate Metabolism
Requirements and Dietary Importance
Resistant Starch and Oligosaccharides

2. Cross References

All of the articles in the Encyclopedia have been extensively cross referenced.
 The cross references, which appear at the end of an article, have been provided at three levels:

i. To indicate if a topic is discussed in greater detail elsewhere.

ANTIOXIDANTS/Diet and Antioxidant Defence.
See also: **Arthritis**: Dietary Aspects of Aetiology and Nutritional Management. **Ascorbic Acid**: Physiology, Dietary Sources and Requirements. **Cancer**: Epidemiology and Associations Between Diet and Cancer. **Carotenoids**: Chemistry, Sources and Physiology; Epidemiology. **Copper**: Physiology, Dietary Sources and Requirements. **Coronary Heart Disease**: Prevention. **Diabetes Mellitus**: Dietary Management. **Dietary Guidelines**: International Perspectives. **Folic Acid**: Physiology, Dietary Sources and Requirements. **Magnesium**: Physiology, Dietary Sources and Requirements. **Manganese**: Physiology, Dietary Sources and Requirements. **Phytochemicals**: Classification and Occurrence. **Riboflavin**: Physiology. **Selenium**: Physiology, Dietary Sources and Requirements. **Tocopherols**: Physiology. **Vitamin Supplementation**: Role. **Zinc**: Physiology.

ii. To draw the reader's attention to parallel discussions in other articles.

> **ANTIOXIDANTS/Diet and Antioxidant Defence.**
> *See also:* **Arthritis**: Dietary Aspects of Aetiology and Nutritional Management. **Ascorbic Acid**: Physiology, Dietary Sources and Requirements. **Cancer**: Epidemiology and Associations Between Diet and Cancer. **Carotenoids**: Chemistry, Sources and Physiology; Epidemiology. **Copper**: Physiology, Dietary Sources and Requirements. **Coronary Heart Disease**: Prevention. **Diabetes Mellitus**: Dietary Management. **Dietary Guidelines**: International Perspectives. **Folic Acid**: Physiology, Dietary Sources and Requirements. **Magnesium**: Physiology, Dietary Sources and Requirements. **Manganese**: Physiology, Dietary Sources and Requirements. **Phytochemicals**: Classification and Occurrence. **Riboflavin**: Physiology. **Selenium**: Physiology, Dietary Sources and Requirements. **Tocopherols**: Physiology. **Vitamin Supplementation**: Role. **Zinc**: Physiology.

iii. To indicate material that broadens the discussion.

> **ANTIOXIDANTS/Diet and Antioxidant Defence.**
> *See also:* **Arthritis**: Dietary Aspects of Aetiology and Nutritional Management. **Ascorbic Acid**: Physiology, Dietary Sources and Requirements. **Cancer**: Epidemiology and Associations Between Diet and Cancer. **Carotenoids**: Chemistry, Sources and Physiology; Epidemiology. **Copper**: Physiology, Dietary Sources and Requirements. **Coronary Heart Disease**: Prevention. **Diabetes Mellitus**: Dietary Management. **Dietary Guidelines**: International Perspectives. **Folic Acid**: Physiology, Dietary Sources and Requirements. **Magnesium**: Physiology, Dietary Sources and Requirements. **Manganese**: Physiology, Dietary Sources and Requirements. **Phytochemicals**: Classification and Occurrence. **Riboflavin**: Physiology. **Selenium**: Physiology, Dietary Sources and Requirements. **Tocopherols**: Physiology. **Vitamin Supplementation**: Role. **Zinc**: Physiology.

3. Index

The index will provide you with the volume number and page number of where the material is to be located, and the index entries differentiate between material that is a whole article, is part of an article or is data presented in a table. On the opening page of the index detailed notes are provided.

4. Colour Plates

The colour figures for each volume have been grouped together in a plate section. The location of this section is cited both in the contents list and before the *See also* list of the pertinent articles.

5. Contributors

A full list of contributors appears at the beginning of each volume.

CONTRIBUTORS

Adel Abi-Hanna
Division of Gastroenterology/Nutrition
Johns Hopkins School of Medicine
Brady 320 - 600 N. Wolfe Street
Baltimore MD 21287
USA

P B Acosta
Ross Products Division
Abbott Laboratories
625 Cleveland Avenue
Columbus OH 43215-1724
USA

J Akré
Programme of Nutrition
World Health Organization
CH-1211 Geneva 27
Switzerland

A J Alberg
Epidemiology
Johns Hopkins University
School of Hygiene and Public Health
615, North Wolfe Street, Baltimore MD 21205
USA

L Albon
Medical Unit, St Bartholemew's and the Royal London
School
of Medicine and Dentistry
Queen Mary and Westfield College
Whitechapel London E1 2AD
UK

L Allen
Department of Nutrition
University of California - Davis
3113 Meyer Hall
Davis CA 95616-8669
USA

D Alnwick
Health Section, Programme Division
UNICEF, 633 Third Avenue
TA 24A New York
NY 10017
USA

Ross Andersen
Johns Hopkins School of Medicine
Division of Geriatric Medicine and Gerontology
5501 Hopkins Bayview Circle/JHAAC 5B:81
Baltimore MD 21224
USA

D Anderson
BIBRA International
Woodmansterne Road
Carshalton
Surrey SM5 4DS
UK

J J B Anderson
University of North Carolina at Chapel Hill
Schools of Public Health & Medicine
Chapel Hill
NC 27599-7400
USA

R A Anderson
Research in Chemistry
USDA Beltsville Human Nutrition Research Center
Bldg 307, room 224
Beltsville MD 20705
USA

U Arens
British Nutrition Foundation
52-54 High Holborn
London
WC1V 6RQ
UK

M J Arnaud
Water Institute Perrier Vittel
BP 101 - 88804 Vittel Cedex
France

E W Askew
Division of Foods & Nutrition
University of Utah
Salt Lake City
UT 84112
USA

Richard L Atkinson
Medicine and Nutrition Sciences
University of Wisconsin at Madison
1415 Linden Drive, Madison
WI 53706-1571
USA

C Baldwin
Dunn Clinical Nutrition Centre
Hills Road
Cambridge
CB2 2DH
UK

D J P Barker
MRC Environmental Epidemiology Unit
Southampton General Hospital
Southampton
SO16 6YD
UK

Y A Barnett
Cancer & Ageing Research Group
Senior Lecturer in School of Biomedical Sciences
University of Ulster
Coleraine BT52 1SA
Northern Ireland UK

S Bartlett
The Johns Hopkins Bayview Medical Center
Division of Digestive Diseases
A Building, 4940 Eastern Avenue
Baltimore MD 21224
USA

C J Bates
MRC Dunn Nutrition Unit
Milton Road
Cambridge
CB4 1XJ
UK

A E Bender
2 Willow Vale
Fetcham
Leatherhead
Surrey KT22 9TE
UK

D A Bender
Department of Biochemistry & Molecular Biology
University College London
Gower Street
London WC1E 6BT
UK

I F F Benzie
Department of Nursing and Health Sciences
The Hong Kong Polytechnic University
Hung Hom
Kowloon
Hong Kong

Zulfiqar A Bhutta
Department of Paediatrics
The Aga Khan University
Stadium Road, PO Box 3500
Karachi-74800
Pakistan

J Bines
Head of Clinical Nutrition
Department of Gastroenterology and Clinical Nutrition
Royal Children's Hospital
Parkville, Victoria 3052
Australia

S A Bingham
Dunn Clinical Nutrition Centre
Hills Road
Cambridge
CB2 2DH
UK

A Bird
Institute of Food Research
Earley Gate
Whiteknights Road
Reading Berkshire RG6 6BZ
UK

George L Blackburn
Harvard Medical School
Beth Israel Deaconess Medical Center
194 Pilgrim Road
Boston MA 02115
USA

R E Blum
Channing Laboratory
181 Longwood Avenue
Boston
MA 02115
USA

J E Blundell
Biopsychology Group, Psychology Department
The University of Leeds
Leeds
LS2 9JY
UK

C Boreham
Sport and Exercise Sciences
The University of Ulster
Jordanstown
Co. Antrim BT37 0QB
Northern Ireland UK

J Brand-Miller
Department of Biochemistry
University of Sydney
NSW 2006
Australia

Ronette R Briefel
Centers for Disease Control and Prevention
National Center for Health Statistics
6525 Belcrest Road
Hyattsville, Maryland 20782
USA

H R Brunner
Division d'Hypertension et de Médecine Vasculaire
Centre Hospitalier Universitaire Vaudois
1011 Lausanne
Switzerland

A Burke
Gastroenterology Division
Dulles 3, University of Pensylvania
3400 Spruce Street
Philadelphia PA 19143
USA

V Burley
Nuffield Institute for Health
University of Leeds
Leeds LS2 9PL
UK

M L Burr
Centre for Applied Public Health Medicine
University of Wales College of Medicine
Temple of Peace and Health
Cathays Park, Cardiff CF1 3NW
Wales UK

D H Buss
5 Howard Close
Fleet, Hampshire
GU13 9ER
UK

J Buttriss
British Nutrition Foundation
High Holborn House
52-54 High Holborn
London WC1V 6RQ
UK

B Caballero
Center for Human Nutrition
Johns Hopkins University
615 North Wolfe Street
Baltimore, MA 21205-2179
USA

J E Casterline
University of California at Davis
CA, USA

A E Cathcart
Northern Ireland Centre for Diet and Health
University of Ulster, Coleraine
Co L'Derry BT52 1SA
Northern Ireland UK

Samuel Chan
BIDMC/Harvard Medical School
194 Pilgrim Road
Boston MA 02215
USA

Lawrence Cheskin
Johns Hopkins Weight Management Center
Johns Hopkins University School of Medicine
4940 Eastern Avenue
Baltimore MD 21224
USA

F S Chu
Food Research Institute
Department of Food Microbiology & Toxicology
University of Wisconsin
Madison WI 53706-1187
USA

G A Clugston
Nutrition
World Health Organisation
1211 Geneva 27
Switzerland

L Cobiac
CSIRO Human Nutrition
PO Box 10041
Gouger Street
Adelaide 5000
Australia

Miriam Coelho de Souza
Departamento de Nutrição, Universidade de Mogi das Cruzes
Av Dr Candido Xavier de Almeida Souza, 200
Mogi das Cruzes - São Paulo
CEP 08780-911
Brazil

G A Colditz
Channing Laboratory
Harvard Medical School
181 Longwood Avenue
Boston MA 02115
USA

M Collins
Muckamore Abbey Hospital
1 Abbey Road
Muckamore
Antrim BT41 4SH
Northern Ireland UK

Kim G Conner
Johns Hopkins Hospital
Children Center
600 North Wolfe Street, Brady 306
Baltimore, Maryland 21205-2179
USA

B Corridan
Department of Nutrition
University College Cork
Ireland

R Cottrell
The Sugar Bureau
Duncan House
Dolphin Square
London SW1V 3PW
UK

J Coutts
Formerly of Willink Laboratory
Royal Manchester Children's Hospital
Pendlebury
Near Manchester M27 1HA
UK

B D'Avanzo
Istituto di Ricerche Farmacologiche
Mario Negri
Via Eritrea 62
20157 Milano
Italy

G Davey
Department of Epidemiology and Population Health
London School of Hygiene and Tropical Medicine
Keppel Street
London WC1E 7HT
UK

T J David
Department of Child Health
Booth Hall Children's Hospital
Charlestown Road
Blackley Manchester M9 7AA
UK

C P Day
Department of Medicine
Floor 4 William Leech Building
The Medical School, Framlington Place
Newcastle upon Tyne NE2 4HH
UK

C P G M de Groot
Division of Human Nutrition and Epidemiology
Wageningen Agricultural University
Bomenweg 2
6703 HD Wageningen
The Netherlands

M de Onis
Programme of Nutrition
World Health Organization
1211 Geneva 27
Switzerland

S C Dennis
Bioenergetics of Exercise Research Unit
Sports Science Institute of South Africa
University of Cape Town, Boundary Road
115 Newlands 7725
South Africa

Nikhil V Dhurandhar
University of Wisconsin at Madison
1415 Linden Drive
Madison
WI 53706-1571
USA

B D Dimitrov
Department of Social Medicine
Faculty of Medicine, Higher Medical Institute
15A V Aprilov Blvd
Plovdiv 4000
Bulgaria

E Dowler
Public Health Nutrition Unit
Dept of Epidemiology and Population Health
London School of Hygiene and Tropical Medicine
Keppel Street, London WC1E 7HT
UK

J Dowsett
St Vincent's Hospital
Elm Park
Dublin 4
Ireland

A Draper
Public Health Nutrition Unit
Dept of Epidemiology & Population Health
London School of Hygiene and Tropical Medicine
Keppel Street, London WC1E 7HT
UK

H D Duncan
Department of Gastroenterology
Queen Alexandra Hospital
Southwick Hill Road
Cosham, Portsmouth PO6 3LY
UK

Jacqueline L Dupont
Department of Nutrition, Food and Movement Sciences
Florida State University
Tallahassee
FL 32306-1490
USA

Johanna T Dwyer
Tufts University School of Medicine and Nutrition
Frances Stern Nutrition Center
New England Medical Center, #783
750 Washington Street, Boston MA 02111
USA

M A Eastwood
Gastrointestinal Unit, Department of Medicine
University of Edinburgh
Western General Hospital
Edinburgh EH4 2XU
Scotland UK

J Eaton-Evans
Northern Ireland Centre for Diet and Health
University of Ulster
Coleraine
BT52 1SA
Northern Ireland UK

C Edwards
Department of Human Nutrition
University of Glasgow
Yorkhills Hospital
Glasgow G3 8SJ
UK

B Eley
Dept of Paediatrics and Child Health
University of Cape Town
Red Cross War Memorial Children's Hospital
Rondesbosch, Cape 7700
South Africa

Gloria Elfert
Johns Hopkins Diabetes Center
601 North Caroline St
Room 2008
Baltimore MD 21287-0760
USA

M Elia
Dunn Clinical Nutrition Centre
Hills Road
Cambridge
CB2 2DH
UK

L J Elsas
Division of Medical Genetics
Department of Pediatrics, Emory Uni School of Medicine
2040 Ridgewood Drive NE
Atlanta GA 30322
USA

P Emery
Department of Nutrition and Dietetics
King's College London
Campden Hill Road
Kensington London
UK

J L Ensunsa
Department of Nutrition
University of California at Davis
Meyer Hall 3rd Floor
Davis CA 95616
USA

C I Ewing
Booth Hall Children's Hospital
Manchester
M9 7AA
UK

S Fairweather-Tait
Institute of Food Research
Norwich Research Park
Colney
Norwich NR4 7UA
UK

A Fehily
Company Nutritionist
HJ Heinz Ltd
Kitt Green, Wigan
Lancashire WN5 0JL
UK

Lawrence Feinman
Mount Sinai School of Medicine
Section of Gastronenterology
Veterans Affairs Medicine Center (111D)
130 West Kingsbridge Road, Bronx NY 10468-3992
USA

A Ferro-Luzzi
Human Nutrition Unit
Via Ardeatina 546
Rome
I-00179
Italy

F Fidanza
Istituto di Scienza dell'Alimentazione
Universita degli Studi di Perugia
via S. Costanzo, CP 333
I 06100 Perugia
Italy

P Fieldhouse
Faculty of Nursing
The University of Manitoba
Winnipeg
Manitoba
Canada R3T 2N2

N Finer
Centre for Obesity Research
Luton and Dunstable Hospital NHS Trust
Luton LU4 0DZ
UK

Marta L Fiorotto
Children's Nutrition Research Center at
Baylor College of Medicine
1100 Bates
Houston, Texas 77030 - 2600
USA

Josef E Fischer
Department of Surgery
University of Cincinnati Medical Center
231 Bethesda Avenue, Cincinnati
OH 45267-0558
USA

D J Flint
Hannah Research Institute
Ayr
KA6 5HL
Scotland UK

C Ford
Human Nutrition Research Centre
University of Newcastle
Department of Biological and Nutritional Sciences
University of Newcastle upon Tyne
Newcastle upon Tyne, NE1 7RU
UK

R Fraser
Department of Obstetrics and Gynaecology
University Clinical Sciences Centre
Northern General Hospital, Herries Road
Sheffield S5 7AU
UK

R E Frisch
Harvard Center for Population and Development
Studies
9 Bow Street
Cambridge
MA 02138
USA

R Fuller
59 Ryeish Green
Reading
RG7 1ES
UK

H C Furr
Department of Nutritional Sciences
U-17, University of Connecticut
Storrs
CT 06269-4017
USA

S C Garner
Division of General Surgery
Duke University, 103A Bell Building
Box 3826 Medical Centre
Durham, NC 27710
USA

J Garrow
European Journal of Clinical Nutrition
Dial House, 93 Uxbridge Road
Rickmansworth
Hertfordshire WD3 2DQ
UK

S Gatenby
SmithKline Beecham
Consumer Healthcare
11 Stoke Poges Lane
Slough SL1 3NW
UK

J M Gaziano
Brigham and Women's Hospital
Division of Preventative Medicine
900 Commonwealth Avenue East
Boston, MA 02215-1204
USA

C Geissler
Department of Nutrition and Dietetics
Kings College London
Campden Hill Road
London W8 7AH
UK

G Gibson
Microbiology Department
Institute of Food Research
Earley Gate
Reading Berkshire RG6 6BZ
UK

T Gill
Rowett Research Institute
Greenburn Road
Bucksburn
Aberdeen AB2 9SB
Scotland UK

W S Gilmore
School of Biomedical Sciences
University of Ulster
Coleraine
BT52 1SA
Northern Ireland UK

G R Goldberg
Dunn Clinical Nutrition Centre
Hills Road
Cambridge
CB2 2DH
UK

J Gray
6 Kingswood Close
Guildford
Surrey
GU1 2SD
UK

J P Greaves
2 The Plantation
Blackheath
London
SE3 0AB
UK

S Greely
North Dakota State University
Department of Foods and Nutrition
Fargo
ND 58102
USA

C J Green
Nutricia Corporate Research
PO Box 1
2700 MA Zoetermeer
The Netherlands

J Green
Formerly of Department of Nutrition and Dietetics
Royal Marsden NHS Trust
London SW3
UK

C Greenwood
Department of Nutritional Sciences
Faculty of Medicine
University of Toronto
Toronto, Ontario, M5S 2E3
Canada

R Grimble
Institute of Human Nutrition
University of Southampton
Southampton
SO16 7PX
UK

R Gross
Deutsche Gesellschaft für
Tecnische Zusammenarbeit (GTZ) GmbH
PO Box 5180
D - 65726 Eschborn
Germany

S M Grundy
Center for Human Nutrition
University of Texas, 5323 Harry Hines Blvd
Southwestern Medical Center at Dallas
Dallas TX 75235-9052
USA

J C G Halford
Department of Psychology
University of Central Lancashire
Preston
Lancashire PR1 2HE
UK

B M Hannigan
School of Biomedical Sciences
University of Ulster
Coleraine
BT52 1SA
Northern Ireland UK

R Harding
Formerly of Nutrition, Biotechnology and Scientific
Services Unit, Food Science Division II
Ministry of Agriculture, Fisheries and Food
Ergon House, 17 Smith Square, London SW1P 3JR
UK

Edward D Harris
Department of Biochemistry and Biophysics
Texas A&M University
College Station
TX 77843-2128
USA

M Harris
UNC School of Public Health
2103 D McGarvan-Greenberg Hall
CB 7400
Chapel Hill NC 27599-7400
USA

N P Hays
USDA-Human Nutrition Research Center on Aging
Energy Metabolism Laboratory
Tufts University, 711 Washington Street
Boston MA 02111-1524
USA

C J K Henry
School of Biological and Molecular Sciences
Oxford Brookes University
Gipsy Lane
Headington, Oxford OX3 0BP
UK

J Higgs
Nutrition and Dietetic Manager
Meat and Livestock Commission
PO Box 44, Winterhill House
Snowdon Drive, Milton Keynes MK6 1AX
UK

A J Hill
Division of Psychiatry and Behavioural Sciences
School of Medicine, University of Leeds
15 Hyde Terrace
Leeds, LS2 9JT
UK

S A Hill
Southampton General Hospital
Tremona Road
Southampton
SO16 6YD
UK

G A Hitman
Medical Unit, St Bartholemew's and the Royal London
School of Medicine and Dentistry
The Royal London Hospital, Whitechapel
London E1 1BB
UK

J Hodgson
University Department of Medicine
Box X2213 GPO
Perth
WA 6000
Australia

Daniel J Hoffman
Department of Endocrine Physiology
Federal University of São Paulo, Escola Paulista de
Medicina
Rua Botucatu 862, 2 Andar
V Clementiona 04023-900, São Paulo
Brazil

M F Holick
Boston University School of Medicine
715 Albany Street
Boston
MA 02118-2394
USA

L Houghton
Ross Products Division
Abbott Laboratories
625 Cleveland Avenue
Columbus OH 43215-3453
USA

R Houston
Program Against Micronutrient Malnutrition (PAMM)
Emory University Rollins School of Public Health
and Department of International Health
1518 Clifton Road NE, Atlanta GA 30322
USA

Barbara V Howard
Medlantic Research Institute
108 Irving Street NW
Washington
DC 20010
USA

L Howard
Department of Medicine
Albany Medical College
47 New Scotland Avenue
Albany NY 12208-3479
USA

Y-S Huang
Medical Nutritional R&D
Ross Products Division, Abbott Laboratories
3300 Stelzer Road
Columbus, Ohio 43219
USA

D Hughes
The Rowett Research Institute
Greenburn Road
Bucksburn
Aberdeen AB2 9SB
Scotland UK

K F A M Hulsof
TNO Nutrition and Food Research Institute
PO Box 360
3700 AJ Zeist
The Netherlands

C Hunt
Department of Food and Nutrition
University of Huddersfield
Queensgate
Huddersfield HD1 3DH
UK

M A Hunt
Food and Drink Federation
6 Catherine Street
London WC2B 5JJ
UK

G D Hussey
Child Health Unit, Dept of Pediatrics and Child Health
University of Cape Town
46 Sawkins Road
Rondesbosch 7700
South Africa

D Hutton
Bioprocessing Limited
Medomsley Road
Consett, County Durham DH8 6SZ
UK

A A Jackson
Institute of Human Nutrition
Bassett Cres East
University of Southampton
Highfield Southampton SO16 7PX
UK

W P T James
Rowett Research Institute
Greenburn Road
Bucksburn
Aberdeen AB21 9SB
Scotland UK

Alan G Jardine
Department of Medicine and Therapeutics
University of Glasgow
Gardiner Institute
Western Infirmary
Glasgow G11 6NT
Scotland UK

David J A Jenkins
Clinical Nutrition and Risk Factor Modification Center
St Michael's Hospital
61 Queen Street East
Toronto, Ontario M5C 3E2
Canada

I Johnson
Institute of Food Research
Norwich Laboratory
Colney Lane
Norwich NR4 7UA
UK

J M Johnson
Department of Human Nutrition, Foods and Exercise
Virginia Polytechnic Institute and State University
Blacksburg
VA 24061-0426
USA

M A Johnson
Department of Foods and Nutrition
College of Family and Consumer Sciences
Dawson Hall, University of Georgia
Athens, GA 30602
USA

A M Johnstone
The Rowett Research Institute
Greenburn Road
Bucksburn
Aberdeen AB2 9SB
Scotland UK

P A Judd
Department of Nutrition and Dietetics
King's College London
Campden Hill Road
London W8 7AH
UK

S Katayama
The Fourth Department of Medicine
Saitama Medical School
38 Morohongo, Moroyama-cho
Iruma-gun, Saitama 350-0495
Japan

Festo P Kavishe
Tanzania Food and Nutrition Center
PO Box 977
Dar es Salaam
Tanzania

C L Keen
Department of Nutrition
University of California at Davis
3135 Meyer Hall, One Shields Avenue
Davis CA 95616
USA

G T Keusch
New England Medical Center
Division of Geographical Medicine/Infectious Diseases
Box 041, 750 Washington Street
Boston MA 02111
USA

A A Kielmann
Deutsche Gesellschaft für Technische
Zusammenarbeit (GTZ) GmbH
BP 26, F-83570 Cotignac, Var
France

Eric S Kilpatrick
Royal Infirmary
Oxford Road
Manchester
M13 9WL UK

J C King
Western Human Nutrition Research Center
PO Box 29997, San Francisco
CA 94129
USA

P Kirk
NICHE
School of Biomedical Sciences
University of Ulster at Coleraine
BT52 1SA
Northern Ireland

S F Kirk
Division of Public Health
Nuffield Institute of Health
71-75 Clarendon Road
Leeds LS2 9LT
UK

P Kirke
Child Health Department
The Health Research Board
73 Lower Baggot Street
Dublin 2
Ireland

C Kjolhede
Research Institute
The Mary Imogene Bassett Hospital
One Atwell Road
Cooperstown NY 13326-1394
USA

D M Klurfeld
Department of Nutrition and Food Science
Wayne State University
Detroit MI 48202
USA

G S Knight
University Department of Surgery
Auckland Hospital
Private Bag 92019
Auckland
New Zealand

Lenore Kohlmeier
Departments of Nutrition and Epidemiology
School of Public Health, CB #7400
University of North Carolina
Chapel Hill, NC 27599-7400
USA

M Kohlmeier
Department of Nutrition
University of North Carolina at Chapel Hill
McGavran-Greenberg Hall
2205A Chapel Hill
NC 27514
USA

P Kopelman
Medical Unit, St Bartholemew's and the Royal London
School of Medicine and Dentistry
Queen Mary and Westfield College
Whitechapel London E1 2AD
UK

A Kouris-Blazos
Department of Medicine
Level 5 Block E, Monash Medical Center
246 Clayton Road
Clayton Victoria
Australia 3168

Jackie Krick
Division of Nutrition
Kennedy-Krieger Institute
707 North Broadway
Baltimore MD 21205
USA

Norman I Krinsky
Department of Biochemistry
Tufts University School of Medicine
136 Harrison Avenue
Boston MA 02111-1837
USA

D Kritchevsky
Wistar Institute
3601 Spruce Street
Philadelphia PA 19104-4268
USA

C La Vecchia
Istituto di Ricerche Farmacologiche
Mario Negri
20157 Milan
Via Eritrea 62
Italy

V Lakin
The Rowett Research Institute
Greenburn Road
Bucksburn,
Aberdeen AB2 9SB
UK

A Laviano
Department of Surgery
University Hospital
SUNY Health Science Center
Syracuse, NY
USA

James B Lee
State University of New York
Buffalo
New York
USA

A R Leeds
Department of Nutrition
Kings College London
Campden Hill Road
London W8 7AH
UK

J Leiper
Department of Biomedical Sciences
University Medical School
Forester Hill
Aberdeen AB9 2ZD
Scotland UK

Claus Leitzmann
Institute of Nutrition
Justus-Liebig University
D-35392 Giessen
Wilhelmstrasse 20
Germany

A H Lichtenstein
Lipid Metabolism Laboratory
USDA Human Nutrition Research Center on Aging
Tufts University
711 Washington Street, Boston MA 02111-1524
USA

C S Lieber
Alcohol Research and Treatment Center
Veterans Affairs Medical Center (151-2)
Mount Sinai School of Medicine
130 West Kingsbridge Road, Bronx NY 10468-3904
USA

J-W Liu
Medical Nutritional R&D
Ross Products Division, Abbott Laboratories
3300 Stelzer Road
Columbus, Ohio 43219
USA

M B E Livingstone
Northern Ireland Centre for Diet and Health
University of Ulster
Coleraine
BT52 1SA
Northern Ireland UK

Michiel R H Löwik
TNO Nutrition and Food Research Institute
PO Box 360
3700 AJ Zeist
The Netherlands

M J Luetkemeier
Department of Exercise and Sport Science
300S 1850E Room 259, University of Utah
Salt Lake City
UT 84112
USA

P G Lunn
Dunn Nutrition Laboratory
Downhams Lane
Milton Road
Cambridge
UK

S R Lynch
Eastern Virginia Medical School
Hampton Veterans Affairs Medical Center
Hampton
VA 23667
USA

A MacDonald
Birmingham Children's Hospital
Steelhouse Lane
Birmingham
B4 6NH
UK

I Macdonald
University of London
Hillside
Fountain Drive
London SE19 1UP
UK

GA MacGregor
Blood Pressure Unit
Department of Medicine
St George's Hospital Medical School
Cranmer Terrace, London SW17 0RE
UK

M Malone
Albany College of Pharmacy
Albany
New York 12208
USA

J I Mann
Human Nutrition
University of Otago
PO Box 56
Dunedin
New Zealand

B Margetts
Institute of Human Nutrition
University of Southampton
Southampton General Hospital
Southampton SO16 6YD
UK

V Marks
European Institute of Health and Medical Sciences
University of Surrey, Stirling House Campus, Stirling
Road
Guildford, Surrey GU2 5RF
UK

R J Maughan
Department of Biomedical Sciences
University Medical School
Foresterhill
Aberdeen AB25 2ZD
Scotland UK

Susan McAreavey
Nutrition Services
Beth Israel Deaconess Medical Center
330 Brookline Avenue
Boston, MA 02215
USA

K C McCowen
Joslin Diabetes Center
Harvard Medical School
Boston MA 02215-5397
USA

Margaret A McDowell
Centers for Disease Control and Prevention
National Center for Health Statistics
6525 Belcrest Road
Hyattsville, Maryland 20782
USA

P McKeigue
Department of Epidemiology and Population Health
London School of Hygiene and Tropical Medicine
Keppel Street
London WC1E 7HT
UK

D McLaren
Nutritional Blindness Prevention Programme
International Centre for Eye Health
Institute of Ophthalmology, 11–43 Bath Street
London EC1V 9EL
UK

S McLaren
Faculty of Healthcare Sciences
Kingston Hill Campus
Kingston Hill, Kingston-Upon-Thames
Surrey KT2 7LB
UK

Donald J McNamara
Egg Nutrition Center
1819 H Street, NW, Suite 520
Washington DC 20006
USA

Joseph McPartlin
Department of Clinical Medicine
Trinity College, Faculty of Health Sciences
St James' Hospital
Dublin 8
Ireland

M Meguid
Department of Surgery
SUNY Health Science Center at Syracuse
750 E Adams Street
Syracuse NY 13210
USA

D Mela
Consumer Sciences Department
Institute of Food Research
Earley Gate
Reading RG6 6BZ
UK

R P Mensink
Department of Human Biology
Maastricht University
PO Box 616
6200 MD Maastricht
The Netherlands

A R Michell
Animal Health Trust
Centre for Small Animal Studies
Lanwades Park, Kentford
Suffolk CB8 7UU
UK

D J Millward
Center for Nutrition and Food Safety
School of Biological Sciences
University of Surrey, Guildford
Surrey GU2 5XH
UK

N Minaur
Royal National Hospital for Rheumatic Diseases
Upper Borough Walls
Bath BA1 1RL
UK

D M Mock
Division of Gastroenterology, Hepatology and Nutrition
Department of Pediatrics, University of Arkansas for
Medical Sciences
Arkansas Children's Hospital
800 Marshall St 512-7, Little Rock AR 72205
USA

A Ayesh Molla
Faculty of Allied Health Sciences
Kuwait University
PO Box 31470 Sulaibikaat 90805
Kuwait

A Majid Molla
Department of Pediatrics
Faculty of Medicine
Kuwait University
PO Box 24923 Safat 13110
Kuwait

J B Morgan
School of Biological Sciences
University of Surrey
Guildford
Surrey GU2 5XH
UK

T Morgan
Department of Physiology
University of Melbourne
Parkville 3052
Australia

John E Morley
Saint Louis University Health Sciences Center
Division of Geriatric Medicine
1402 S Grand Boulevard, Room M238
St Louis MO 63104-1079
USA

P A Morrisey
Department of Nutrition
University College Cork
Cork
Ireland

M Murphy
Sport and Exercise Sciences
The University of Ulster
Jordanstown
Co. Antrim BT37 0QB
Northern Ireland UK

M Stephen Murphy
Institute of Child Health
Whittal Street
Birmingham
B4 6NH
UK

Patricia Murphy-Miller
Division of Nutrition
Kennedy-Krieger Institute
707 North Broadway
Baltimore MD 21205
USA

M P Navarro
Estación Experimental del Zaidin CSIC
Departamento de Nutricion
Prof. Albereda 1
18008 Granada
Spain

M Nelson
Department of Nutrition and Dietetics
Kings College London
Campden Hill Road
London W8 7AH
UK

M C Neville
Departments of Physiology and Cell and Structural
Biology
University of Colorado
Health Science Center
4200 E 9th Avenue, Denver CO 80262-0001
USA

R Nicolosi
Center for Cardiovascular Disease Control
University of Massachusetts Lowell
Weed Hall, Rolfe St, Lowell, MA 01854
USA

F Nielsen
USDA, ARS
Grand Forks Human Nutrition Research Center
Grand Forks
ND 58202-9034
USA

C O'Brien
The Sugar Bureau
Duncan House
Dolphin Square
London SW1V 3PW
UK

K O'Brien
Johns Hopkins University
School of Hygiene and Public Health
Center for Human Nutrition
615 North Wolfe Street
Baltimore MD 21205
USA

D L O'Connor
Ross Products Division
Abbott Laboratories
625 Cleveland Avenue
Columbus OH 43215-3453
USA

M O'Neill
Northern Ireland Center for Diet and Health (NICHE)
School of Biomedical Sciences
University of Ulster, Coleraine
Co. L'Derry BT52 1SA
Northern Ireland UK

J M Ordovas
The Lipid Metabolism Laboratory
JM USDA Human Nutrition Research Center on Aging
Tufts University
Boston MA 02111
USA

L Patel
Booth Hall Children's Hospital
Manchester
M9 7AA
UK

J P Pearson
Department of Physiological Sciences
University of Newcastle
Newcastle-upon-Tyne
NE1 7RU
UK

F Pender
Queen Margaret College
Corstorphine Campus
Clewood Terrace
Edinburgh EH12 8TS
Scotland UK

J C Phillips
BIBRA International
Woodmansterne Road
Carshalton
Surrey SM5 4DS
UK

Barry M Popkin
Dept of Nutrition and Carolina Population Center
University of North Carolina, University Square
CB #8120
123 W Franklin Street
Chapel Hill, NC 27516-3997
USA

S D Poppitt
Department of Medicine
University of Auckland
Private Bag 92019
Auckland
New Zealand

E M Poskitt
Medical Research Council
Dunn Nutrition Group
Keneba
PO Box 273, Banjul
The Gambia

A D Postle
Child Health
School of Medicine
Southampton General Hospital
Southampton SO16 6YD
UK

J Pratt
Meat and Livestock Commission
PO Box 44, Winterhill House
Snowdon Drive, Milton Keynes MK6 1AX
UK

K R Price
Institute of Food Research
Norwich Laboratory, Norwich Research Park
Colney
Norwich NR4 7UA
UK

N D Priest
School of Environmental Science
Middlesex University
Bounds Green Rd
London N11 2NQ
UK

J Pryer
Public Health Nutrition Unit
Dept of Epidemiology and Population Health
London School of Hygiene and Tropical Medicine
49/51 Bedford Square, London WC1B 3DP
UK

Laura C Rall
School of Human Development and Nutritional
Sciences
University of Wisconsin
Stevens Point WI 54481-3897
USA

S Reddy
Department of Health
Skipton House
80 London Road
SE1 6LW
UK

C Reilly
10 Litchfield Close
Enstone
Chipping Norton
Oxon OX7 4LB
UK

M Rhodes
Institute of Food Research
Norwich Laboratory, Norwich Research Park
Colney
Norwich NR4 7UA
UK

R Rice
The Fish Foundation
PO Box 24
Tiverton
Devon EX16 4QQ
UK

D P Richardson
Nestle UK Ltd
St George's House
Croydon, Surrey CR9 1NR
UK

S B Roberts
USDA Human Nutrition Research Center on Aging
Energy Metabolism Laboratory
Tufts University, 711 Washington Street
Boston MA 02111-1524
USA

C L Rock
Dept of Family and Preventive Medicine
Cancer Prevention and Control Program
9500 Gilman Drive, University of California
San Diego, La Jolla, CA 92093-0901
USA

P J Rogers
Institute of Food Research
Earley Gate
Whiteknights Road
Reading RG6 6BZ
UK

Arturo R Rolla
Beth Israel Deaconess Medical Center
Harvard Medical School
110 Francis Street, Suite 2-F
Boston MA 02215
USA

J L Rombeau
Department of Surgery
Silverstein 4, University of Pennsylvania
3400 Spruce Street
Philadelphia PA 19143
USA

Pedro Rosso
Department of Pediatrics, Obstetrics and Gynecology
Facultad de Medicina
Pontificia Universidad Catolica de Chile
Casilla 114-D, Santiago
Chile

R Roubenoff
USDA Human Nutrition Research Center
Tufts University
711 Washington Street
Boston MA 02111
USA

Sharon Rubinstein
Center for Human Nutrition
Johns Hopkins University
615 North Wolfe Street
Baltimore, MA 21205-2179
USA

RDE Rumsey
Department of Biomedical Sciences
University of Sheffield
Firth Court, Western Bank
Sheffield S10 2TN
UK

C H S Ruxton
The Sugar Bureau
Duncan House
Dolphin Square
London SW1V 3PW
UK

Jose M Saavedra
Department of Pediatrics
Johns Hopkins University
School of Medicine, 300 N. Wolfe Street - Brady 320
Baltimore MD 21237
USA

Michèle J Sadler
Institute of Grocery Distribution
Grange Lane
Letchmore Heath
Watford, Hertfordshire WD2 8DQ
UK

Sofia P Salas
Department of Pediatrics, Obstetrics and Gynecology
Facultad de Medicina
Pontificia Universidad Catolica de Chile
Casilla 114-D, Santiago
Chile

M Saltmarsh
53 Blackberry Lane
Four Marks
Alton
Hants GU34 5DF
UK

J Samet
Department of Epidemiology
Johns Hopkins University
School of Hygiene and Public Health
615 North Wolfe Street
Baltimore MD 21205
USA

Patricia Queen Samour
Nutrition Services
Beth Israel Deaconess Medical Center
One Deaconess Road, Farr B
Boston, MA 02215
USA

C P Sánchez-Castillo
Department of Physiology of Nutrition
General Subdirection of Nutrition
National Institute of Nutrition "Salvador Zubirán"
Vasco de Quiroga # 15, Tlalpan 14000, Mexico DF
Mexico

Christopher D Saudek
Clinical Research Center
Osler 576, Johns Hopkins Hospital
500 North Wolfe Street
Baltimore MD 21205
USA

Sally Savidge
Division of Nutrition
Kennedy-Krieger Institute
707 North Broadway
Baltimore MD 21205
USA

G S Savige
Department of Medicine
Level 5 Block E, Monash Medical Center
246 Clayton Road
Clayton, Victoria
Australia 3168

Ana Lydia Sawaya
Department of Endocrine Physiology
Federal University of São Paulo, Escola Paulista de
Medicina
Rua Botucatu 862, 2 Andar
V Clementiona 04023-900, São Paulo
Brazil

W Schultink
Deutsche Gesellschaft fuer
Tecnische Zusammenarbeit (GTZ) GmbH
PO Box 5180
D - 65726 Eschborn
Germany

J M Scott
Department of Biochemistry
Trinity College
Dublin 2
Ireland

C J Seal
Human Nutrition Research Centre
University of Newcastle
Wellcome Research Laboratories
Royal Victoria Infirmary, Queen Victoria Road
Newcastle upon Tyne NE1 4LP
UK

C E Shaw
Royal Marsden NHS Trust
Fulham Road
London SW3
UK

D J Shaw
112 Kenwood Road
Beckenham
Kent
BR3 6RB
UK

T Sheehy
Department of Nutrition
University College Cork
Cork
Ireland

R Shepherd
Consumer Sciences Department
Institute of Food Research
Earley Gate, Whiteknights Road
Reading RG6 6BZ
UK

P S Shetty
Department of Epidemiology and Public Health
London School of Hygiene and Tropical Medicine
49/51 Bedford Square
London WC1B 3DP
UK

S M Shirreffs
Department of Biomedical Sciences
University Medical School
Foresterhill
Aberdeen AB25 2ZD
Scotland UK

D Shrimpton
Cambridge, UK

D B A Silk
Department of Gastroenterology & Nutrition
Central Middlesex Hospital NHS Trust
Acton Lane, Park Royal
London NW10 7NS
UK

H A Simmonds
Purine Research Laboratory
Guy's and St Thomas's United Medical and
Dental School
Floor 5 Thomas Guy House, Guy's Hospital
London Bridge, London SE1 9RT
UK

R J Smith
Metabolism Section
Joslin Diabetes Center
Harvard Medical School
One Joslin Place, Boston MA 02215-5397
USA

N W Solomons
Center for Studies of Sensory Impairment,
Aging and Metabolism (CeSSIAM)
Zone 11
Guatemala City
01011 Guatemala

D A T Southgate
8 Penryn Close
Norwich
Norfolk
NR4 7LY
UK

June Stevens
Departments of Nutrition and Epidemiology
UNC School of Public Health
CB 7400
Chapel Hill NC 27599-7400
USA

L Stockley
Timberland
Mill Hill
Brockweir
Near Chepstow NP6 7NN
UK

J J Strain
Northern Ireland Center for Diet and Health (NICHE)
University of Ulster, Coleraine
BT52 1SA
Northern Ireland UK

J Stubbs
The Rowett Research Institute
Greenburn Road
Bucksburn
Aberdeen AB2 9SB
Scotland UK

C Summerbell
Department of Primary Care and Population Sciences
Royal Free Hospital School of Medicine
University of London
Rowland Hill Street
London NW3 2PF UK

J F Sutcliffe
Department of Radiotherapy/Oncology
Palmerston North Hospital
Private Bag 11036
Palmerston North
New Zealand

E H M Temme
University of Leuven
Capucnenvoer 35
B-3000 Leuven
Belgium

R Tester
Department of Biological Sciences (Food Science)
Glasgow Caledonian University
Southbrae Campus, Southbrae Drive
Glasgow G13 1PP
UK

Briony Thomas
Elmers Farmhouse
Ockley
Dorking
Surrey RH5 5TQ
UK

R L Thompson
Institute of Human Nutrition
University of Southampton
Southampton General Hospital
Southampton, SO16 6YD
UK

B M Thomson
Rowett Research Institute
Grenburn Road
Bucksburn
Aberdeen AB2 9SB
Scotland UK

M Thorogood
Health Promotion Research Unit
London School of Hygiene and Tropical Medicine
Keppel Street
London WC1E 7HT
UK

D I Thurnham
Northern Ireland Centre for Diet and Health
School of Biomedical Sciences
University of Ulster, Coleraine
Co L'Derry BT52 1SA
Northern Ireland UK

D Topping
CSIRO Human Nutrition
Gate 13
Kintore Avenue
Adelaide SA 5000
Australia

Benjamin Torun
Clinical Nutrition and Metabolism
Division of Nutrition and Health
Institute of Nutrition of Central America and Panama
Apartado Postal 1188
Guatemala City
Guatemala

S U Toverud
University of North Carolina at Chapel Hill
School of Medicine
Chapel Hill
NC 27599-7455
USA

T R Trinick
Ulster Hospital
The Laboratories
Dundonald
Belfast
BT16 0RH
Northern Ireland UK

E Turley
The Northern Ireland Centre for Diet and Health
(NICHE)
Human Nutrition Research Group
University of Ulster, Coleraine BT52 1SA
Northern Ireland
UK

W H Turnbull
Centre for Nutrition and Food Research
Department of Dietetics and Nutrition
Queen Margaret College, Corstophine Campus
Clerwood Terrace, Edinburgh EH12 8TS
Scotland UK

B Underwood
International Union of Nutritional Sciences (IUNS)
Food and Nutrition Board
Institute of Medicine, NAS
2101 Constitution Avenue NW (FO 3049)
Washington DC 20418
USA

W A van Staveren
Wageningen Agricultural University
Division of Human Nutrition and Epidemiology
Bomenweg 2
6703 HD Wageningen
The Netherlands

M P Vaquero
Instituto de Nutricion y Bromatologia
CSIC-UCM, Facultad de Farmacia
Ciudad Universitaria
28040 Madrid
Spain

RG Vernon
Hannah Research Institute
Ayr
KA6 5HL
Scotland UK

M Wahlqvist
Department of Medicine
Level 5 Block E, Monash Medical Center
246 Clayton Road
Clayton Victoria
Australia 3168

Ann F Walker
Hugh Sinclair Unit of Human Nutrition
Food Science and Technology Dept, Reading University
Whiteknights Reading, PO Box 226
RG6 6AP
UK

A R P Walker
Human Biochemistry Research Unit
South African Institute for Medical Research
PO Box 1038
Johannesburg
South Africa

Donald G Weir
Department of Clinical Medicine
Trinity College Centre for Health Sciences
St James's Hospital
Dublin 8
Ireland

R W Welch
Northern Ireland Centre for Diet and Health
School of Biomedical Sciences
University of Ulster
Coleraine BT52 1SA
Northern Ireland UK

A West
Department of Food and Nutrition
University of Huddersfield
Queensgate
Huddersfield HD1 3DH
UK

K West
Johns Hopkins University
School of Hygiene and Public Health
615 North Wolfe Street
Baltimore, Maryland 21205-2179
USA

A B Williams
Department of Surgery
University of Cincinnati Medical Center
Cincinnati
OH 45267-0558
USA

D H Williamson
Metabolic Research Laboratory
Radcliffe Infirmary
Oxford
OX2 6HE
UK

D Wilmore
Brigham and Women's Hospital
Harvard Medical School
75 Francis Street
Boston MA 02115
USA

A Wilson
Department of Nutrition
University College Cork
Ireland

M-M G Wilson
Division of Geriatric Medicine
Saint Louis University Health Sciences Center
1402 South Grand Boulevard, Room M238
St Louis MO 63104-1028
USA

H Wiseman
Department of Nutrition and Dietetics
King's College London
Campden Hill Road
London W8 7AH
UK

T Wolever
Department of Nutritional Sciences
150 College Street
University of Toronto
Toronto
Canada M5S 3E2

M Wolraich
Director of the Division of Child Development
Vanderbilt University
2100 Pierce Avenue, Nashville
Tennessee 37232-3573
USA

J E Wraith
Willink Laboratory
Royal Manchester Children's Hospital
Pendlebury
Near Manchester M27 1HA
UK

Jacqueline D Wright
Centers for Disease Control and Prevention
National Center for Health Statistics
6525 Belcrest Road
Hyattsville, Maryland 20782
USA

A Wynne
Microbiology Department
Institute of Food Research
Earley Gate
Reading, Berkshire RG6 6BZ
UK

Steven H Zeisel
Department of Nutrition
University of North Carolina at Chapel Hill
2212 McGavran-Greenberg Hall
Chapel Hill, NC 27599-7400
USA

Aglaia Zellos
Division of Gastroenterology and Nutrition
Johns Hopkins School of Medicine
Brady 314 - 600 N Wolfe Street
Baltimore MD 21287
USA

S Zidenberg-Cherr
Department of Nutrition
University of California at Davis
Meyer Hall 3rd Floor
Davis CA 95616
USA

CONTENTS

VOLUME 1

VOLUME 2

G

H

I

K

L

VOLUME 3

O

P

Q

T

U

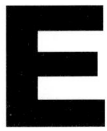

E

Eating behaviour *see* **Meal Size and Frequency**: Effect on Absorption and Metabolism.

EATING DISORDERS

Contents
Anorexia Nervosa
Bulimia Nervosa

Anorexia Nervosa

Arturo R Rolla, Harvard Medical School, Boston, Massachusetts, USA

Copyright © 1998 Academic Press

The relentless pursuit of thinness and the increasing prevalence of obesity in modern societies are the roots of the present higher prevalence of eating disorders. These eating disorders can be classified according to the interaction between the preoccupation with food and body weight, and the self-control of hunger (**Fig. 1**).

Classification of eating disorders

Obesity   Obesity can be classified as an eating disorder since, primarily or secondarily, obese patients eat inappropriately for their weight, and because obese individuals tend to suffer also from the other eating disorders.

Anorexia nervosa   Anorexia nervosa is usually seen in younger women who restrict their food intake and increase exercise, causing a voluntary, stubborn malnutrition.

Bulimia   People who cannot control their hunger over a long period of time tend to have secret bingeing episodes. This is followed by an overwhelming feeling of guilt and depression which frequently leads to self-induced vomiting. For this reason, the terms 'bulimia' (which only means binge eating) and 'self-induced vomiting' are used interchangeably (*See:* **Eating Disorders:** Bulimia Nervosa).

Anorexoid syndromes   These abnormalities are seen in individuals who can no longer control their weight by dieting and exercising and have to resort to abnormal subterfuges, such as:

* self-induced vomiting;
* ipecac abuse;

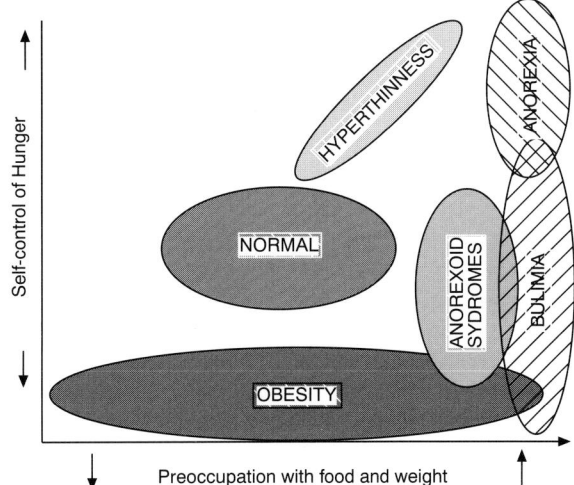

Figure 1   Classification of eating disorders based on the interaction between the preoccupation with food and body weight, and the self-control of hunger.

- laxative abuse;
- diuretic abuse;
- anorexic agents abuse;
- self-induced glycosuria in patients with insulin-dependent diabetes mellitus;
- thyroid hormone abuse;
- excessive, compulsive exercising.

Professional hyperthinness   This is a borderline condition, not necessarily pathological, in which individuals, usually with narcissistic tendencies, overvalue personal appearance and thinness as a way of obtaining professional success. It is commonly seen among models, figure skaters, ballerinas, artists, gymnasts, etc. They do not use the 'subterfuges' of the anorexoid patients; they are not socially isolated; their weight loss is not extreme; they have normal psychosexual activity; and they do not see themselves as overweight, unlike people with anorexia nervosa. For them, thinness is a mean of obtaining success, not the final goal as in anorexia nervosa.

Anorexia Nervosa

Anorexia nervosa is a serious disease with psychiatric, endocrine and nutritional connotations. It is more frequent in young women, in industrialized countries, in upper socioeconomical groups, and in recent years. Anorexia nervosa has three main components.

Psychological disturbances

Psychological disturbances are most likely to be the initial event; they result in a complex obsession characterized by the following features.

1. An intrusive body image delusion makes the patients see themselves as being overweight when they are actually severely undernourished. This leads to a pathological fear of fatness (dysmorphophobia), a chronic voluntary starvation and resistance to any external pressures to gain weight. Anorexic patients hide and dispose of food in the most ingenious ways to avoid eating.
2. An overwhelming sense of personal ineffectiveness makes anorexic patients believe that they cannot control the world around them. They continuously fear that they are going to lose their inner control. They therefore tightly control their world inside and slowly separate themselves from their social surroundings, with growing feelings of alienation and loneliness. There is no psychosexual development or interest, and no dating, unlike patients with bulimia.
3. Depression occurs which may be primary or secondary, obvious or atypical, and may or may not be amenable to treatment with psychotherapy and/or antidepressant medications.
4. Increased physical activity coexists with an apparent lack of hunger and fatigue, and is inappropriate for the degree of malnutrition and depression.

Malnutrition

Anorexia nervosa is a self-imposed starvation. The term 'anorexia' is a misnomer, since (at least initially) these patients are hungry. Anorexia nervosa is different from other forms of malnutrition because it is voluntary, resistant to nutritional treatments, accompanied by increased physical activity, without an initial organic cause (such as malignancy or surgery) and without associated infections. Because anorexia nervosa is a state of pure malnutrition without associated increased energy expenditure due to fever, immune response or tissue reconstruction, these patients have a lowered metabolic rate and do not tend to develop opportunistic infections.

The exact mechanism by which these patients are able to control their hunger is unknown. Disturbed brain serotonin activity may be implicated.

Endocrine and metabolic changes

Amenorrhoea, decreased metabolic rate, hypothermia, hypotension, bradycardia, lanugo hair, carotinodermia, leucopenia, osteoporosis, etc. are mostly secondary to the severe malnutrition and are reversible with weight gain.

Other Clinical Characteristics

Anorexia nervosa is more frequent among daughters of white, affluent, achievement-oriented families, in developed societies; it is extremely uncommon in areas of the world with poor nutrition. It tends to occur during the last years of high school or at the time of departure to college.

The patients tend to be well-behaved, perfectionists, with good academic performance. Mothers of anorexic patients have a higher incidence of obsessive-compulsive personalities, and preoccupation with diets and weight loss. Anorexic patients have done everything their mothers or families have trained them to do and, when faced with the increasing demands (and choices) of adult life, they exaggerate the only control left in their lives: *hunger*. There is an unconscious wish to revert to childhood, or to a prepubertal state, by means of undernourishing.

The onset of anorexia nervosa is usually subacute, over a period of weeks, not uncommonly after an episode of weight gain, or after somebody has made a comment about the patient being overweight. Initially it appears as an innocent attempt to lose weight, but soon thereafter it starts showing its rebellious and progressive nature. Anorexia nervosa appears in small epidemics in cities and countries, probably owing to social pressures and to imitation behaviours.

In contrast to their poor dietary intake, these patients have a paradoxical enhanced interest in nutrition and cooking. They collect recipes, read nutrition textbooks, plan a career in nutrition or cooking, or find a job in a restaurant (usually waitressing). Anorexic patients enjoy cooking and feeding the rest of the family. They know the precise energy content of all usual food and use their knowledge to select low-energy items.

When forced to eat, anorexic patients will dispose of or hide food. They use their above-average intelligence to overcome all efforts to make them gain weight. They can be very resourceful in tampering with scales (adding weights to shoes or clothing, drinking large amounts of water just before weighing, etc.), and they have the most imaginative excuses as to why they are not gaining weight. They are extremely manipulative and master the art of confusing the different members of the treating team and family in their favour and against each other.

As they lose their natural insulation (subcutaneous tissue), it is difficult for anorexic patients to maintain their body temperature. They wear layer upon layer of clothing, which also helps them to hide their malnutrition. Lack of body fat is sensed by the hypothalamus as an sufficiency of stored energy, and therefore the cycling and amplitude of gonadotrophins decrease. This leads to hypothalamic amenorrhoea, although about 30% of patients stop having menses before there is a significant weight loss. Depression may be another cause of hypothalamic amenorrhoea in these patients. Some of them will remain amenorrhoeic for several months after regaining normal weight.

In primary or classical anorexia nervosa the patients lose weight by dieting (restrictive) and exercising. These patients tend to be younger, more naive, introverted and obsessive, and they do not resort to subterfuges to lose weight. Their serum electrolytes, checked at frequent intervals, should be completely normal. Some patients find it impossible to control their hunger and start having binge episodes followed by forced vomiting (bulimia plus anorexia – 'bulimarexia') Others may start abusing laxatives or diuretics as they grow older.

There are patients in whom anorexia is secondary to an underlying, more serious psychiatric disorder such as depression, schizophrenia, hysteria or borderline personality disorder. In these cases, the course is longer and depends on the primary condition, as does its treatment. Men with anorexia nervosa are very uncommon, and in men the condition tends to be associated more often with these psychiatric problems and with homosexuality.

Physical examination

The profound weight loss and cadaveric appearance contrast with the patient's increased physical activity. While hospitalized, if allowed, these patients try to perform some of the nursing chores or even to counsel other patients. Many patients exercise secretly in their rooms, and jog or go for long walks when not supervised.

Public and axillary hair is preserved, and there is an increase in light, thin hair ('peach fuzz') on the face and neck, back, arms and thighs (lanugo hair). Patients have low body temperature and poor tolerance to cold exposure because of their malnutrition-induced lowered metabolic rate and the loss of the insulation provided by subcutaneous tissue. Layers of clothing tend to hide their cachectic appearance. Bradycardia and hypotension are common and secondary to decreased sympathetic drive due to malnutrition.

The skin is dry and has a peculiar bluish erythema over the knuckles and knees. Orange-yellow discoloration of the skin (carotinodermia), seen in palms and soles, is frequently found. It is caused, at least in part, by an increased intake of vegetables, since it may also be seen among vegetarians.

Symptoms

Symptoms are amazingly few. Most usually these patients are forced to see a physician by their families. Spontaneous complaints may be amenorrhoea, constipation, abdominal pain or distension after eating, 'fluid retention' and inability to lose weight, for which they may ask to be placed on special diets!

Laboratory Investigations

The following findings are typical:

- Mild normochromic, normocytic anaemia.
- Leucopenia with relative lymphocytosis.
- Low sedimentation rates due to low fibrinogen levels.
- Serum albumin and transferrin levels are normal, except in severe cases.
- Serum carotene and cholesterol levels are normal or slightly elevated, which helps to rule out malabsorption.

- Low normal blood glucose levels are found, with low levels of glycohaemoglobin.
- Electrolyte abnormalities, particularly low serum potassium values, occur only where there is self-induced vomiting or abuse of diuretics or laxatives.
- Low serum levels of luteinizing hormone, follicle stimulating hormone and oestradiol.
- Increased growth hormone levels with decreased levels of insulin-like growth factor I (somatomedin C) in the serum.
- Plasma renin activity and aldosterone levels may be very high in patients who abuse laxatives or diuretics (pseudo-Bartter's syndrome).
- Electrocardiography shows sinus bradycardia, flat or inverted T waves, and prolonged QT_c.
- Decreased bone density is due to decreased oestrogen and progesterone secretion, decreased calcium and vitamin D intake, protein malnutrition and increased marrow fat content of the bones. The conversion of haematopoietic to fatty marrow is related to the severity of the malnutrition and may be demonstrated with magnetic resonance imaging.

Endocrine Changes

Insulin

Low serum insulin levels occur; with increased glucagon concentration. There is a tendency to asymptomatic low blood glucose levels and a low glycohaemoglobin concentration. Fasting ketosis may be seen. The number and affinity of insulin receptors in target cells is increased, and abnormal glucose tolerance occurs due to prolonged fasting

Leptin

The adipose tissue secretes leptin; when this reaches the hypothalamus it decreases the activity of the 'hunger centre, in part by decreasing the local activity of neuropeptide Y. There is a direct correlation between the total amount of fat stores and the circulating levels of leptin. Individuals with anorexia nervosa have very low levels of leptin in blood and cerebrospinal fluid, in relation to their decreased adipose tissue. This should cause an increase in hypothalamic neuropeptide Y content and hunger, but this compensatory mechanism to maintain a normal body weight does not seem to be effective in anorexic patients.

Gonadal axis

The female hypothalamus needs to 'sense' the presence of about 14–18 kg of body fat in order to allow fertility and menstrual cycles. With lesser amounts of fat, there is a progressive regression to the prepubertal state (low, nonspiking serum gonadotrophin levels). The signal from the fat stores to the gonadal hypothalamus seems to be the levels of serum leptin. The very low levels of serum leptin, secondary to the decreased fat mass, seem to determine a decrease in luiteinizing hormone releasing hormone (LHRH) secretion. The hypothalamic, hypogonadal state of anorexia nervosa is due to the combined effects of malnutrition and the psychological disturbances on the hypothalamus. Secretion of LHRH and gonadotrophins improves as weight is regained, and leptin levels increase; but in up to one-third of these patients menses do not return immediately after nutritional rescue and weight restoration are accomplished. The decreased oestrogen secretion from the ovaries brings about a significant loss of bone mass at a critical time, which will subsequently aggravate postmenopausal osteoporosis.

In males, malnutrition seems to have a less important influence on the gonadal axis. Severe weight loss of long duration decreases serum testosterone and gonadotrophin levels, but to a lesser degree than in women. Anorexia nervosa is less frequently seen in males and seems to be associated with a high incidence of homosexuality and more severe psychiatric disturbances.

Thyroid

Thyroid stimulating hormone levels are normal but there is a delayed response to thyrotrophin releasing hormone Serum thyroxine and resin triiodothyronine (T_3) uptake (and the free thyroxine index) are normal. The level of T_3 is low owing to decreased peripheral conversion (euthyroid sick syndrome), and there is concomitant increase in reverse T_3.

The basal metabolic rate is decreased by 20–30%, and not fully corrected with T_3 replacement since it is also due to decreased sympathetic activity.

Sympathetic nervous system

There is decreased peripheral sympathetic activity, with normal adrenomedullary function. This is due to decreased ingestion of energy, and it explains the tendency to bradycardia, postural hypotension and low basal metabolic rate.

Adrenal cortex

Serum cortisol levels are slightly raised, without diurnal variation, and may not suppress with dexamethasone overnight. Urinary 17-hydroxy and 17-keto steroids are decreased by 30–50%, but urinary free cortisol may be increased. Corticotrophin releasing factor (CRF) stimulation causes a subnormal cortico-trophin rise, but a normal or supernormal serum cortisol response. Levels of CRF in the cerebrospinal fluid are elevated. These changes in the hypothalamic-pituitary-adrenal axis are very similar to those seen in untreated depression.

Growth hormone

Serum growth hormone levels are elevated in 60% of patients, particularly in the most severe cases. This is due to decreased feedback from lowered serum concentrations of insulin-like growth factor I (IGF-I). Growth hormone levels do not rise normally after L-dopa or insulin hypoglycaemia, but there may be an unexpected rise of growth hormone blood levels after stimulation with thyrotrophin releasing hormone.

Vasopressin

There is decreased capacity to concentrate urine, due at least in part to sluggish vasopressin secretion in response to osmotic stimuli. Levels of vasopressin in the cerebrospinal fluid are increased.

Bone density

Decreased oestrogen and progesterone secretion, increased levels of serum cortisol, malnutrition with protein, calcium and vitamin deficiencies, and fatty degeneration of the bone marrow lead to decreased bone density. Increased exercising does not counteract this osteopenic tendency, which affects mostly young women during the years of skeletal growth. Many of these patients do not achieve their peak bone density even after their nutritional recovery and restoration of menses, and are left with a propensity to fracture bones for the rest of their lives. The osteopenia of anorexia nervosa is mostly asymptomatic, but some of these patients may present with stress fractures (diagnosed only with bone scans) and related to their increased exercising.

Differential Diagnosis

In the majority of cases the severe and voluntary malnutrition accompanied by the typical delusion of being fat and resistance to gain weight make the diagnosis very clear. Malnutrition due to organic causes in adolescents usually has an obvious reason and the patients want to improve their nutrition. Hypothalamic tumours rarely may present with severe loss of appetite.

The differential diagnosis should include the anorexoid syndromes. In pure anorexia nervosa the weight loss is due only to restrictive eating habits and exercise. Some anorexic patients may start bingeing and inducing vomiting, in which case their condition is called 'bulimarexia'.

In some cases, anorexia nervosa is secondary to a serious, underlying psychiatric illness, with the weight loss being only an added problem. A particular diagnostic and therapeutic dilemma may occur with young women with personality disorder or chronic schizophrenia and anorexia nervosa.

Treatment

The multifaceted pathogenesis of anorexia nervosa requires an experienced team of psychiatrists, nutritionists, endocrinologists, internists or paediatricians, and nurses. *Each patient should be considered individually* since there are as many variations as there are patients. It is important to maintain communication between the different members of the team in order to present a unified front to the patient. Invariably, the patient will try to find and exploit the most minimal differences of opinion between the members of the team. Ideally, all the important decisions should be made by one central team leader. Nurses, aides and other paramedical personnel should be instructed about how to deal with the patient's behaviour and charming search for allies.

There is no specific treatment and the methods reported are, at best, controversial. The aetiology of this disorder remains unknown, and aetiological factors are probably different in each patient. It is important therefore to tailor the therapeutic approach to each patient.

Many cases of established and severe anorexia nervosa require prolonged hospitalization for psychological and nutritional rescue. Separation from parents and home environment is only part of what is to be gained from hospitalization. Administrators and health insurance companies must understand this need.

Hospitalization is indicated when there is:

- severe and rapid weight loss;
- serious metabolic or cardiovascular problems (hypokalaemia less than 2.5 mmol l^{-1}) despite oral replacement, blood urea nitrogen more than 10.6 mmol l^{-1} of urea (30 mg dl^{-1}) in the presence of normal renal function, pulse less than 45 min^{-1}, systolic blood pressure less than 70 mmHg, or a body temperature less than 36°C;
- severe depression and suicide risk;
- psychosis;
- family crisis.

Psychiatric treatment

From the outset the entire family should be interviewed to gain insight into the patient's previous behaviour, to understand the family dynamics and enlist their help in therapy. Clear simple contracts with the patient are a form of behaviour modification that is simple to carry out. Initially most daily activities and visits are curtailed and the patient is watched, particularly around mealtimes. As the patient improves, restrictions are lessened and privileges increased. Short-term goals are set from the beginning. Weight gains of 250 g daily or 1.3–1.8 kg a week are acceptable limits. Patients who accomplish these goals are rewarded by increasing levels of activity and autonomy within the hospital, as a positive reinforcement.

The general attitude of the team should be one of understanding, concern and firmness. One should try to build a trusting relationship in which the patients feel understood, but without giving them a chance to deceive. The nature and course of the illness should be clearly explained to the patient and the family. This includes the serious complications of malnutrition and the fatal outcome of severe cases. Emphasize that the goal of treatment is not to make the patient fat, but to make the patient feel better and to improve self-confidence and eating habits. Weight is only a by-product of the improvement, and 'muscle mass and protein recovery', not fat, is what has to be gained.

This firm understanding should engage the patient in a *treatment alliance* with the team. Remember that many of these patients are very polite and 'out to please you' at least superficially, and many times their initial acceptance hides deeper feelings of isolation and resentment. Psychotherapy is of help in some patients, usually accompanied by behaviour modification and family therapy.

Despite the common use of antidepressants, several double-blind trials have been inconclusive or only slightly favourable. Patients with clear manifestations of depression and the more severe cases seem to benefit more from these medications. Tricyclic antidepressants tend to increase appetite and are more suited for patients with pure anorexia nervosa. Selective serotonin reuptake inhibitors may help decrease bingeing in patients with associated bulimia. Cyproheptadine (a serotonin inhibitor that increases appetite) appeared useful in high doses (32 mg a day), and only in pure dieters.

Nutritional treatment

The psychiatric treatment is beneficial only as long as the patient's nutrition is improved. The nutritional rescue breaks down the vicious circle of the psychological consequences of starvation and makes the patient more receptive to psychotherapy. The team should be prepared to deal with the most ingenious ways to deceive. The patient should be told that because of the tendency to deceive frequently found in her illness, close supervision will be necessary at least in the beginning of the treatment. Patients should be weighed fasting in the morning, in nightgown without shoes and with the same scale, daily or at regular intervals by a nurse.

Initially, oral intake should be monitored carefully with a nurse sitting through the eating period, and for 30 min thereafter to prevent postprandial vomiting. The tray should be checked for any food not consumed. In this way, a careful energy count is obtained daily. If the energy intake is inadequate or if the patient is not gaining weight, the diet should be supplemented with low-residue, high-energy canned formulae dispensed by the nurse during medication rounds. These diet supplements should be consumed in front of the nurse. Many patients with anorexia nervosa have subclinical vitamin deficiencies and they should receive a multivitamin tablet every day.

It is not infrequent for these patients to complain of gastric distress after sudden increases in food intake; smaller and more frequent feedings and/or administration of metoclopramide or cisapride before meals may be of help. Tube feeding is poorly tolerated by most of these patients; it has connotations of a gastrointestinal 'rape'.

If severe malnutrition is present (low serum albumin and transferrin levels, anergic skin testing), parenteral hyperalimentation should be instituted from the beginning. It is recommended to start with small amounts of hyperalimentation fluid to avoid sodium and water retention (refeeding oedema) which is very distressing to the patients. The rate of hyperalimentation solution administration should be modified according to the improvement in oral intake and weight. Staff should be continuously aware of the possibility of tampering with the central lines by the patient, with the potential for air embolization, infection and bleeding. In many patients it is important to curtail all physical activity initially, to the point of confining them to absolute bed rest with only bathroom privileges. As the patient improves, the activities are progressively increased.

Oestrogen replacement is indicated to prevent the progressive decrease in bone density but it is poorly tolerated and accepted by these patients. Ideally a birth control pill with good oestrogen content should be administered.

Prognosis

The outcome of patients with anorexia nervosa, is variable; a worse outcome is associated with older age of onset, severity and duration of the illness, male sex and severe associated psychiatric disturbances. In general, 40–60% of patients achieve full nutritional and psychological recovery after 6–12 months. About 20–40% attain a borderline normal weight and existence for the rest of their lives, but with the appearance of significant stress they may revert to their previous anorexic behaviour. There is a mortality rate of 5–30% in the most severe cases, due to suicide, electrolyte imbalance, and starvation-induced myocardial damage causing intractable arrhythmias; it is rarely due to infection.

See also: **Adolescents**: Nutritional Problems. **Malnutrition**: Definition, Classification and Epidemiology; Primary Malnutrition; Secondary Malnutrition. **Obesity**: Definition, Aetiology and Assessment. **Starvation and Fasting**: Biochemical Aspects.

Further Reading

Ahima RS, Prabakaran D, Mantzoros C et al. 1996. Role of leptin in the neuroendocrine response to fasting. Nature 382:250.

Balaa MA and Drossman DA (1985) Anorexia nervosa and bulimia: the eating disorders. Disease-a-Month 31:1–52.

Garfinkel PE and Gardner DM (1982) Anorexia Nervosa, a Multidimensional Perspective. New York: Brunner/Mazel.

Garfinkel PE and Gardner DM (1987) The Role of Drug Treatments for Eating Disorders. New York: Brunner/Mazel.

Herzog DB and Copeland PM (1985) Eating disorders. New England Journal of Medicine 313:296.

Hsu LKG (1986) The treatment of anorexia nervosa. American Journal of Psychiatry 143:5.

Kennedy SH, Kaplan AS, Garfinkel PE, Rockert W, Toner B and Abbey SE (1994) Depression in anorexia nervosa and bulimia nervosa: discriminating depressive symptoms and episodes. Journal of Psychosomatic Research 38:773.

Klibanski A, Biller BM, Schoenfeld DA, Herzog DB and Saxe VC (1995) The effects of estrogen administration on trabecular bone loss in young women with anorexia nervosa. Journal of Clinical Endocrinology and Metabolism 80:898.

Mantzoros C, Flier JS, Lesem MD et al. (1997) Cerebrospinal fluid leptin in anorexia nervosa: correlation with nutritional status and potential role in resistance to weight gain. Journal of Clinical Endocrinology and Metabolism 82:1845.

Schwabe AD, moderator (1981) Anorexia nervosa. Annals of Internal Medicine 94:371.

Vande Berg BC, Malghem J, Lecouvet FE, Lambert M and Maldague BE (1996) Distribution of serouslike bone marrow changes in the lower limbs of patients with anorexia nervosa: predominant involvement of the distal extremities. American Journal of Roentgenology 166:621.

Bulimia Nervosa

A J Hill, University of Leeds, Leeds, UK

S F Kirk, Nuffield Institute of Health, Leeds, UK

Copyright © 1998 Academic Press

Episodes of ravenous overeating, referred to as compulsive eating or binge eating, have been recognized clinically since the 1950s. However, the disorder of bulimia nervosa was not formally described until 1979. This relatively recent recognition of eating disorder has two important implications. First, the clinical picture and understanding of the psychopathology has changed with time. This has led both to a refinement in the diagnostic criteria used to characterize the disorder, and to a change in reported prevalence. Second, the research base used to make judgements about development, prevalence, treatment, prognosis and prevention is smaller than that for anorexia nervosa. Quite simply, there are still many unknowns in the area of bulimia nervosa.

This article will focus on the features used to make a diagnosis of bulimia nervosa, the psychopathology and developmental course of the disorder, and the groups at risk. Specific attention will be paid to the nutritional consequences of bulimia nervosa and the ways in which dietary management is used in its treatment. Finally, long-term prognosis will be considered.

Diagnostic Criteria

The behaviour at the centre of the disorder, bingeing, has been progressively redefined. A priority has been to separate binge eating from mere indulgence and everyday overeating. Accordingly, two features of a true binge have been identified. They are, that the amount of food eaten is large, and that during eating there is a sense of loss of control.

Diagnostic schedules (such as DSM-IV and ICD-10) agree on three features that must be present in someone with bulimia nervosa. The first is the presence of the above objective and frequent binges. Second, the person must regularly use any one of a variety of extreme measures for controlling shape or weight. The most common is self-induced vomiting, but these strategies also include use of laxatives or diuretics, excessive exercise, and extreme dieting or fasting. Third, the person must show overconcern with body weight and shape. Importantly, the person should not be of low body weight, in which case a diagnosis of anorexia nervosa would be made.

The tightening of these formal diagnostic criteria has had the consequence of reducing misdiagnosis and prevalence, but has increased the numbers of those with atypical eating disorders. Failing to exhibit one or more of the key diagnostic features, such an insufficient frequency of bingeing, is classified variously as 'atypical', 'partial syndrome' or 'eating disorders not otherwise specified' (EDNOS). It is also useful to note that 'binge eating disorder' is included in DSM-IV, albeit for research purposes. The key difference from bulimia nervosa is the relative absence of the extreme compensatory behaviours that follow the binge. This group are more likely to be overweight, to be older, and to have a high level of general psychiatric symptoms.

Psychopathology

The description of body image disturbance that is central to both anorexia and bulimia nervosa has itself undergone revision. A distinction has been argued for between dissatisfaction with body shape and overvalued ideas about weight and shape. While body shape dissatisfactions are commonly found in these patients, it is their overvalued ideas about weight and shape that are the necessary diagnostic feature. In other words, concern should go beyond simply feeling fat to a point where a person's life is dominated by their feelings about body weight and shape.

If these overvalued ideas are accepted as the core psychopathology of bulimia nervosa, then the chaotic eating that typifies the condition can be seen as a behavioural consequence. Binges are often interspersed between periods of intense dieting, even fasting, themselves strategies to control weight. Purging always follows a binge and is a way of expelling the food ingested or compensating for the food energy intake. Binges are secretive, planned, often expensive, and emotionally self-destructive. Paired with purging, they are cyclical and self-perpetuating, although their frequency may wax and wane. In addition, this behaviour may have a long history before treatment is considered and clinical attention sought.

Bulimic episodes may be triggered by a variety of factors, including anxiety, boredom, tension, drinking alcohol, even tiredness. Only rarely is hunger identified as precipitating a binge, even though the individual may not have eaten for 24 h or more.

Mood disturbances are common and are part of a range of psychological and social problems characteristic of bulimia nervosa. Patients' mental state is characterized by feelings of anxiety, helplessness, failure, and self-deprecating thoughts. They are highly self-critical and feel guilty and ashamed of their lack of self-control. Low self-esteem and self-loathing are typical. A significant proportion (reported to vary from 20 to 70%) have some form of personality difficulty or disorder. This may include identity disturbance, difficulties in impulse control, and threatened or actual self-harm. However, there is still debate whether bulimia nervosa is caused by, or itself creates, these personality problems.

Aetiology

As with anorexia nervosa, the picture of development is complex and multifactorial. There is no single cause of bulimia nervosa. Rather, a variety of psychological, biological and social factors are involved in the emergence of the disorder. While aetiology is diverse, it has much in common with the forces held responsible for anorexia nervosa, and is clarified by looking at the groups of people most at risk (see below). Overall, the balance of aetiological factors is in favour of psychological and social causes, given that bulimia nervosa is a relatively new condition and has arisen at a time of profound social and cultural change, with little concurrent change in human biology.

The process of the development of eating disorders can be usefully divided into three stages. These conceptually separate the factors that predispose an individual to the disorder, precipitating events that lead to onset, and factors that perpetuate or maintain the disorder once initiated (See: **Eating Disorders**: Anorexia Nervosa). Any framework drawn up for bulimia nervosa would be very similar to that for anorexia nervosa, and therefore will not be duplicated here. This is because the aetiology of the two disorders probably has a lot in common. Indeed, up to a third of diagnosed bulimics have a pre-morbid history of anorexia. However, the relative absence of research directed to separate the developmental course of the two disorders adds to the uncertainty.

Although the aetiological picture is very similar to that for anorexia nervosa, there are a few clues to differences. One important issue is the role that affective disorder may play in predisposition. Many bulimia nervosa patients suffer from major depression sometime during their lifetime, and often concurrently with the eating disorder. Research suggests that at least a third of these have a history of depression that preceded onset, something not found in anorexia nervosa patients. A potential biological link is serotonin, and abnormalities in serotonin functioning have been identified in both bulimia nervosa and depression. Furthermore, first- and second-degree relatives of patients with an eating disorder have higher rates of affective disorder. The lifetime risk for these relatives has been found to be three times higher than for relatives of normal control patients. This family history of mood disorder is common to both anorexia and bulimia nervosa. However, a family history of substance abuse (for example alcohol) has been found in bulimia nervosa, compared with control families. What is unclear though, are the comparative rates of substance abuse in the families of other psychiatric patients, and evidence regarding why and how this might be specific to the development of bulimia.

Looking at alternative developmental pathways provides another view of aetiology. The first acknowledges a close association with anorexia nervosa. In this, dieting and progressive weight loss starts and continues during the teenage years. Despite not being overweight in the first place, weight loss is extreme and anorexia nervosa develops. After some variable period of time that person's eating control starts to break down, they binge, and control is progressively eroded. As weight approaches normal levels they fulfil all the criteria of bulimia nervosa.

A second pathway links a history of overweight, perhaps in childhood and sometimes relatively mild, to dieting and then to binge eating. A history of overweight is common to a proportion (around a third) of both anorexia and bulimia nervosa patients. Again, evidence regarding why people with a history of overweight should develop bulimia nervosa rather than anorexia is lacking. Far less common is a third pathway in which dieting does not precede the disorder. These individuals often have a range of impulse control problems of which binge eating is only one. They may not consistently fulfil all the criteria necessary for bulimia nervosa, and some may be regarded as having binge eating disorder. Clearly, these are general and rather sketchy descriptions of the precipitation of bulimia nervosa. Unfortunately, there is virtually no research evidence on what factors combine with dieting to produce an eating disorder, and on what factors are specific to bulimia nervosa.

The perspective on the perpetuation of bulimia nervosa is a cognitive one. **Fig. 1** shows the vicious circles that maintain binge eating. Four points are emphasized in explaining this to patients. First, while

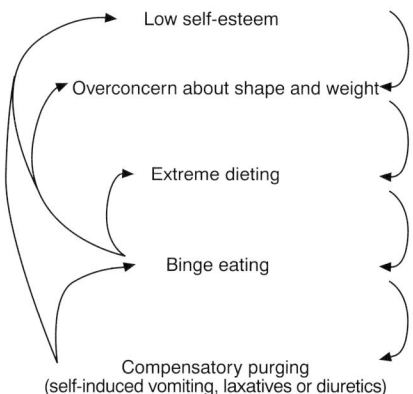

Figure 1 The cognitive view of the maintenance of bulimia nervosa (redrawn from Fairburn and Cooper, 1989).

dieting is a response to binge eating, it also maintains binge eating by both biological and psychological mechanisms. Second, compensatory purging encourages bingeing through a belief in its effectiveness at removing food for digestion. In other words, the barriers against overeating are removed since the food will not be absorbed. This is sometimes described as the reason why an individual initiated a binge–purge cycle of behaviour. Third, overconcern about body shape and weight promotes extreme dieting, and maintains the eating problem. Fourth, overconcern about shape and weight itself is commonly associated with low self-esteem and longstanding feelings of worthlessness.

Groups at Risk

Like anorexia nervosa, bulimia nervosa is far more common in women than in men. In fact, it is not possible to say with any degree of certainly what the sex ratio is, but the number of cases of male bulimia nervosa that come to clinical attention may be substantially less than the 1 in 20 reported for anorexia. Prevalence is notoriously difficult to establish for eating disorders, and for bulimia nervosa in particular. Problems in this regard include the recency of the disorder, changing diagnostic criteria, and the secrecy and non-life-threatening nature of the disorder preventing its routine appearance in clinical settings.

If women are most at risk, then how many are affected? Studies of American college students in the 1980s revealed up to 20% with bulimic symptoms. However, when such epidemiological studies are of community samples and use interviews to follow-up questionnaire surveys, the average point prevalence among young women using strict diagnostic criteria is 1000 per 100 000, or 1.0%. Clearly, in specific groups such as university students there may be more than twice this level of the disorder. Bulimia nervosa is extremely rare in girls aged under 14 and the majority of cases are recognized between the ages of 18 and 25. Cases do present clinically in women in their late 20s and 30s although they may have a long history of disordered eating.

The 'invisibility' of bulimia nervosa is demonstrated by estimates of 1-year-period prevalence rates. These are calculated by adding together figures for point prevalence and annual incidence. The 1-year-period prevalence rates for bulimia nervosa per 100 000 young women are:

In the community   1500
In primary care   170
In 'specialist' mental health care   87

These figures indicate that only 11% of the community cases of bulimia nervosa are detected, and of these only half are received by specialist services. This tiny representation of cases in specialist treatment is a combination of filtering at General Practitioner level and either a reluctance to engage in treatment or the stigma of mental health problems.

Since women are most at risk, it is reasonable to ask why. One reason is that women are far more likely to diet than men. Dieting is itself a behaviour that places individuals at risk of developing bulimia nervosa. But the motivations for dieting may be equally important. Women diet more than men for several reasons. These are bound together as a sociocultural perspective on bulimia, an approach that has become a powerful model for explaining who develops bulimia, and why. At the heart of this perspective are three issues: the importance of a thin body shape for women, the centrality of appearance in women's gender role, and the importance of appearance for societal success. The arguments and evidence to support this analysis are compelling.

The above information on prevalence indicates that the average age of someone with bulimia nervosa is older than that for anorexia. This may reflect the observation that bulimia nervosa often follows a period of anorexia or at least low weight. Developmental challenges and age-dependent life events are also seen as important. The developmental task of achieving a sense of identity during mid and late adolescence may be disrupted by relationship problems, peer or family difficulties, or events such as leaving home to go to college. The resultant erosion of self-esteem and perceived control can lead to problems with eating manifest as intensified dieting, or periods of overeating and weight gain. The disrupted pattern of eating that follows may be the early stage of the disorder.

The effect of socioeconomic status (SES) and ethnicity has yet to be properly investigated. Research suggests that non-Caucasians in Western societies are as likely to develop bulimia nervosa, and that more cases are from middle and high SES backgrounds. However, there are problems with the existing evidence in terms of referral bias (upper-class white patients are more likely to seek treatment) and assessment of the disorder. Cases of bulimia nervosa have been reported in unemployed and homeless young women in the UK.

One group that has received a lot of recent attention is those who have been abused earlier in life. Initially, it was thought that the rate of childhood sexual abuse was particularly high in patients with bulimia nervosa. While there is still debate, the available evidence suggests that women who have been sexually abused are at risk of psychological problems in general, but not bulimia nervosa in particular. The link between the eating disorder and this past experience may however be especially strong in individual cases.

Nutritional Findings

A key feature of bulimia nervosa is the extreme dietary restraint that is exhibited in between episodes of binge eating. Such behaviour has been described as 'all or nothing', so that on a good day the sufferer may describe consuming a very low energy diet, while a bad day will consist of several episodes of uncontrolled eating. This will be accompanied by the purging behaviours previously described.

During binge eating episodes, the bulimic may spend hundreds of pounds on food, selecting foods normally avoided during periods of dietary restraint which are easy to eat and subsequently remove from the body. To the bulimic, it is this overeating that is seen as the basic problem, not the dietary restraint that precedes it. Yet, it is this dietary restraint that drives the disorder. When not binge eating, it is common for sufferers to avoid eating for long periods, with 80% of bulimics reporting consumption of one meal a day or less. While restricting their intake, they will consume reduced energy foods, with a strong tendency to avoid fat and choose energy-reduced foodstuffs. It is often assumed that people with bulimia nervosa have good nutritional knowledge. Indeed, to the untrained eye, a diet history for a 'good day' consisting of foods such as wholemeal bread, lots of vegetables and fruit, and skimmed milk, can be interpreted as conforming to healthy eating guidelines. However, this is not the case. Such restrictive behaviour may fail to achieve even half the recommended energy intake and consequently may be deficient in micronutrients. The anxiety experienced through consuming diet-breaking, 'unsafe' foods leads to the individual adopting extremely restricted diets between binges. Such intakes have been found to be lower in fat and higher in protein than the intakes of controls. People with bulimia nervosa also report feeling greater anxiety and guilt after eating foods they believed to be fattening.

Purging behaviours begin as a compensatory mechanism to offset episodes of binge eating. Consequently, it is a widely held belief that they are effective methods of weight control. However, the damage done to the body by these methods far exceeds any benefits in terms of weight. Any weight loss experienced is usually related to disruption in fluid balance rather than a loss of fat tissue. Furthermore, if self-induced vomiting is adopted, binges are likely to become more frequent and severe. If vomiting is prevented, the bulimic will consume significantly less food, thus maintaining the cycle previously described. Research has shown that vomiting fails to rid the body of all the food ingested. It has been estimated that only half the contents of the stomach are removed through vomiting, although this is variable and difficult to determine. Similarly, laxatives work on the system *after* food has been digested. One classic experiment looked at the amount of food energy lost through laxative abuse and found that, despite copious diarrhoea, the amount of energy lost from the body was less than that found in the average chocolate bar.

What both laxative abuse and vomiting have in common is the depletion of fluid, leading to dehydration and electrolyte disturbances, particularly hypokalaemia (low potassium). Electrolyte disturbance has been estimated in 50% of bulimic patients. In some cases, hypoglycaemia may develop as a response to fasting or binge eating and vomiting. In extreme cases, death may occur through cardiac arrest or gastrointestinal complications, such as oesophageal or gastric rupture. Vomiting also leads to erosion of dental enamel, resulting in periodontal disease and an increased incidence of dental caries. Other effects of bulimia nervosa include menstrual irregularities, swelling of the salivary glands secondary to vomiting and reflex constipation, which occurs as a consequence of laxative abuse and dehydration. Laxative abuse has also been found to cause steatorrhoea and protein-losing enteropathy in some cases.

Some studies have shown that patients with bulimia nervosa may have lower resting energy expenditure. Studies using indirect calorimetry have found that bulimics have a measured resting energy expenditure below that predicted by standard formulae such as the Harris–Benedict equation. Bulimics also report consuming fewer kilocalories per kilogram body weight than control subjects. One explanation for this finding is that bingeing and purging may alter energy efficiency. It has been suggested that, for a normal weight bulimic woman without a history of anorexia nervosa, the difference in energy needs could be several hundred kilocalories per day less than for a peer without an eating disorder. One drawback of such studies, however, is the small number of subjects investigated and further research in this area is needed to understand more fully the mechanisms at work and to establish whether these are consistent findings. Even so, these limited findings have implications for nutritional management in bulimia nervosa, particularly in relation to the prescription of energy intakes.

Dietary Management

Dietitians are increasingly becoming involved in the treatment of bulimia nervosa. While this is best utilized within a multidisciplinary team, ideally with a psychologist or some form of psychological intervention available, it is not uncommon for dietitians to be the only professional involved. Any professional working with eating disorders should be clear about what they can address and be aware of when it is appropriate to enlist other forms of help. Thus, nutritional intervention should aim to separate food from underlying issues, leaving these to be addressed by professionals more experienced in psychological techniques. The aims of dietetic treatment are therefore:

- to establish a normal pattern of food intake;
- to encourage a nutritional intake appropriate to the individual's needs;
- to maintain a body weight within a normal range.

Dietary management of bulimia nervosa seeks to break the binge–purge cycle previously described. The individual should be informed of the problems of maintaining this cycle through dieting, and should be encouraged to stop dieting in an extreme way. They should also be educated about the damaging effects of vomiting and other purging behaviours. In some cases, this is enough to stop such behaviours. In others, this message should consistently be given to encourage them to work towards stopping these behaviours.

An important part of breaking this cycle is to get the individual to monitor their intake through completing a food diary. Completing a food diary is a valuable aspect of treatment by identifying areas of difficulty and allowing progress to be monitored as well as enabling the individual to reveal problematic thoughts and feelings at the time they are consuming food. This can then be used as the basis for planning meals to lessen anxiety around eating. In the example shown (**Table 1**), it can be seen how restricting intake earlier in the day can make the person more vulnerable to overeating later in the day. Food diaries may also include information on mood and triggers for binge eating. The trigger for the binge given in the example illustrates the effect of mood and the problems with decision-making around food that are often encountered in bulimia nervosa. Guilt for something previously eaten is often cited as a binge trigger and, together with anxiety at the time of the meal, make the bulimic individual more vulnerable to episodes of binge eating. Such issues can then be used as discussion points to identify coping strategies for preventing binges. Strategies may include planning meals in advance to lessen anxiety around meal times, not going for long periods without eating, or practising appropriate distraction techniques. Food diaries therefore provide a powerful cognitive tool to enable the individual to understand their eating behaviour more fully.

Education is essential to ensure that the individual understands why they are being asked to abandon what are essentially some of the only coping mechanisms they have. They feel anxious that by giving up the pattern of dieting, binge eating and purging they will gain excessive amounts of weight. These fears are very real and failure to address them with sensitivity can sabotage any attempts to control the disorder. This is particularly important when an individual has a history of overweight in the past. A detailed weight history should be carried out to include current, highest, lowest and ideal weights, and it should be stressed that recovery cannot be accomplished if the sufferer is trying to maintain a weight below normal. Thus, those with a pre-morbid history of obesity may have to accept that they will need to reach a weight that is higher than they would like to be. Weight stabilization should be an initial emphasis, particularly for those experiencing weight fluctuations. Initially, weight is likely to fluctuate through rehydration and repletion of glycogen stores. This effect should be explained to the individual to prevent unnecessary anxiety. They should also be discouraged from weighing themselves.

Table 1 Example of a food diary

Time	Food/drink eaten and amount	Binge/vomit/laxatives	Comment/feelings
Breakfast	Nothing	—	Not hungry
Mid morning	Cup of black coffee × 2	—	Need something to fill my stomach. Really busy at work so no time to eat
Midday 1.30 pm	2 crispbreads (dry), small tub of diet cottage cheese, 1 tomato, can of diet pop	—	Very hungry, feel as if I could eat more but mustn't
Mid afternoon	Chocolate eclair	Vomited	Someone's birthday in the office so couldn't refuse. Feel really guilty and had to be sick
Evening meal	2 dishes of blackcurrant cheesecake, a choc ice, 4 bowls of ice cream, 6 snack size chocolate bars, 5 cheese biscuits with butter and cheese, 5 slices of toast with butter and peanut butter, 2 packets of chocolate biscuits, 2 bowls of cereal, 1 packet of crisps and 1 chocolate and mint biscuit 6 glasses of water	Binge!! Vomited and took 10 laxatives	Couldn't decide what to have for tea, so started on cheesecake. Could not stop this binge at any cost. I feel terrible
During evening	—	—	
Supper	—	—	Feel so terrible and bloated. Will have to cut back tomorrow

An important goal for nutritional management is to establish the individual on a regular pattern of eating. Often, normal cues for hunger and satiety are disrupted through repeated cycles of binge and restrictive eating so encouraging a regular meal pattern also helps the sufferer to begin to identify hunger and fullness again. They should be encouraged to eat regular meals and snacks and to maintain this pattern of eating even after a binge. Each meal or snack should be based around carbohydrate, with moderate amounts of protein foods and vegetables and fruit. They should be encouraged to include non-diet foods and to include foods containing fat. It is also worth getting them to compile a list of foods normally avoided or associated only with binges and to encourage them to include these within their meal pattern, when they feel able to do so. A system of food exchanges may also be useful (see the sample meal plan in **Table 2**). The amount of food needed to meet energy needs is greater than that needed to consume sufficient nutrients. Thus, consumption of some energy dense, less nutritious food should be encouraged. A minimum intake of 6.0 MJ (1500 kcal) is usually an appropriate level to begin with, increasing to an intake corresponding to the estimated average requirement for women as recovery proceeds.

Regular monitoring of electrolytes should be carried out, particularly on individuals who use vomiting as a compensatory mechanism. The extent of monitoring will depend on the physical status of the individual but may include sodium, potassium, calcium, phosphorus, magnesium, amylase, liver function tests and an ECG. Access to medical support is therefore essential. The issue of whether to weigh a patient with bulimia nervosa remains a controversial one. It could be argued that, since the individual is often within a normal weight range, weighing creates unnecessary anxiety and should only be carried out occasionally. On the other hand, since preoccupation with weight and shape is a core feature of the disorder, it could be argued that appropriate weighing and discussion around this plays a central role in the treatment process. It is important that the sufferer and the treatment team agree at an early stage of treatment whether weighing is carried out and if so, how often and by whom.

If the bulimic is used to keeping their stomach empty, even a normal amount of food may seem excessive and may trigger the urge to vomit. They should be informed that stomach distension is a normal consequence of eating and reassured that they will get used to the feeling in time. Similarly, if someone has been abusing laxatives, they may suffer from

Table 2 Sample meal plan

Meal	Food
Breakfast	Glass of fruit juice Bowl of cereal with milk Slice of toast, spread with butter/margarine and marmalade/jam if desired
Mid morning	*Choose from exchange list*
Snack meal	Sandwiches made with 2 large slices of bread, spread with butter/margarine and filled with lean meat, egg or cheese or beans on toast, etc.
Mid afternoon	*Choose from exchange list*
Main meal	Average helping of meat, chicken, fish or vegetarian alternative Potatoes, boiled rice or pasta equivalent to 2 exchanges *Option from exchange list*
Supper	1–2 slices of toast or option from exchange list

Exchange list
1 large slice of bread or a roll, teacake or plain bun
1 small scone
2 plain biscuits or crackers
1 chocolate or cream biscuit
small bowl of breakfast cereal or porridge
2 spoons boiled rice or pasta
1 medium potato
4 spoons baked beans or tinned spaghetti
1 piece of fruit (apple, orange, pear, banana, etc.)
1 carton of yoghurt
1 glass of milk
6–8 tbs (90–120 ml) custard or rice pudding
1 packet crisps or nuts and raisins
1 average sized chocolate bar

Note: This plan deliberately does not include specific portion sizes. However, some individuals may need the reassurance of a more detailed plan. The aim is to provide a minimum of 6.25 MJ (1500 kcal). In addition to using the above to exchange foods within the meal plan, some people benefit from having an additional number of exchanges (e.g. five extra) to allow for when they are feeling more hungry and to offest binges. This also ensures an energy intake that conforms to the current estimated average requirement for women.

constipation and should be encouraged to have a reasonable fibre intake along with plenty of fluids.

Other physical complications in the nutritional management of bulimia nervosa include disturbances in fluid balance, as previously discussed. Psychologically, if an individual is encouraged to give up the coping strategies they have developed through binge eating and purging, without any alternatives being in place, there may be an escalation in other damaging behaviours, such as self-harm or abuse of alcohol. Once again, this emphasizes the importance of working within a setting providing medical and psychological support so that such issues can be addressed.

Although it is important to give positive encouragement and feedback when working with individuals with bulimia nervosa, it should also be explained that relapse is a normal occurrence and should not be viewed so negatively that the individual feels a complete failure. Education on relapse prevention should thus be an important component of any treatment programme.

Long-Term Prognosis

Once more, the relative recency of the disorder mitigates against definitive statements. However, the findings from the few outcome studies conducted show that bulimia nervosa is far from being 'intractable', as was originally suggested. About 50% of patients are asymptomatic 2 to 10 years after treatment with cognitive behaviour therapy (the most widely used and evaluated treatment procedure), although periodic post-treatment sessions may be necessary. Some types of psychotherapy may be effective, although behaviour therapy appears to have only short-lasting effects. Around 20% of patients remain persistently symptomatic, and the remainder (30%) either become 'atypical' eating disorder cases, or have a course of illness that cycles between remission and relapse. The mortality rate associated with bulimia nervosa may be higher than that in the general population.

There is uncertainty regarding prognostic indicators of treatment success. Patients with a less severe form of the disorder appear to do better in treatment. Self-help books or community-based support groups may be of particular assistance to those in whom the disorder is less fully established. Conversely, those with a history of greater obesity, in themselves pre-morbidly or in their fathers, appear to do worse. Importantly, there is no evidence that bulimia nervosa evolves over time into other psychiatric disorders, or of any persistent impairment in social functioning.

See also: **Adolescents**: Nutritional Problems. **Dental Disease**: Aetiology and Epidemiology. **Diarrhoeal (Diarrheal) Diseases**: Nutritional Factors. **Dietetics**: The Role of Dietetics in Health Care. **Eating Disorders**: Anorexia Nervosa. **Fertility**: Body Fat, Menarche and Fertility. **Hunger**: Overview.

Further Reading

American Dietetic Association (1994) Nutrition intervention in the treatment of anorexia nervosa, bulimia nervosa and binge eating. *Journal of the American Dietetic Association* **94**:902–907.

Brownell KD and Fairburn CG (eds) (1995) *Eating Disorders and Obesity: A Comprehensive Handbook*. New York: Guilford Press.

Cooper PJ (1995) *Bulimia Nervosa and Binge Eating: A Guide to Recovery*. London: Robinson.

Fairburn CG (1995) *Overcoming Binge Eating*. New York: Guilford Press.

Fairburn CG and Wilson GT (eds) (1993) *Binge Eating: Nature, Assessment, and Treatment*. New York: Guilford Press.

Fairburn CG, Norman PA, Welch SL, O'Connor ME, Doll HA and Peveler RC (1995) A prospective study of outcome in bulimia nervosa and the long-term effects of three psychological treatments. *Archives of General Psychiatry* **52**:304–312.

Fichter MM (ed.) (1990) *Bulimia Nervosa. Basic Research, Diagnosis and Therapy*. Chichester: Wiley.

Halmi KA (ed.) (1993) *Psychobiology and Treatment of Anorexia Nervosa and Bulimia Nervosa*. Washington, DC: American Psychiatric Press.

Laessle RG, Schweiger U, Daute-Herold U, Schweiger M, Fichter MM and Pirke KM (1988) Nutritional knowledge in patients with eating disorders. *International Journal of Eating Disorders* **7**:73.

Russell GFM (1979) Bulimia nervosa: an ominous variant of anorexia nervosa. *Psychological Medicine* **9**:429–448.

Stice, E. (1994) Review of the evidence for a sociocultural model of bulimia nervosa and an exploration of the mechanisms of action. *Clinical Psychology Review* **14**:633–661.

Striegel-Moore, RH, Silberstein, LR & Rodin, J (1986) Toward an understanding of risk factors for bulimia. *American Psychologist* **41**:246–263.

Walsh TB (1988) *Eating Behaviour in Eating Disorders*. Washington, DC: American Psychiatric Press.

EGGS

Nutritional Value

W H Turnbull, Centre for Nutrition and Food Research, Queen Margaret College, Edinburgh, UK

Copyright © 1998 Academic Press

Eggs have been recognized as a food source since prehistoric times and have been a highly regarded source of high-quality protein throughout the ages. There are a number of different sources of eggs but the only type of major commercial interest is chicken eggs, and all mention of 'eggs' in this chapter refers to this type of egg unless otherwise specified.

Types of Eggs and Egg Products

Apart from chicken eggs the only other types of egg consumed by humans are duck, goose and quail. They are remarkably similar to each other in nutrient composition, the only major difference being that duck, goose and quail eggs contain considerably more fat than chicken eggs.

Egg consumption in the UK has fallen slightly since 1991 (**Table 1**). Some of the possible factors accounting for the fall in egg consumption are:

1. Consumer concerns over contamination of eggs with *Salmonella enteritidis*
2. The high cholesterol content of eggs.
3. A change in breakfast eating pattern, reflecting increased consumption of breakfast cereals with reduced consumption of eggs.
4. Higher consumption of meat and ready meals in place of eggs at main meals.

There are three major egg farming systems which are of commercial importance. The most important of these is the intensive cage (battery) laying system which in 1995 accounted for 86% of egg production. This system offers a high degree of control over pro-

vision of feed and water, hygiene, environment and egg collection and is highly mechanized. The perchery (barn) system accounted for 3% of 1995 UK egg production and allows the birds slightly more freedom in an indoor environment. The free range system accounted for 11% of 1995 UK egg production and allows the birds continuous daytime access to runs with vegetation. The intensive system offers a higher production rate and standard of hygiene than the other systems, which although they offer more freedom to the birds, are associated with higher disease rates.

Eggs are sold as whole eggs in shells, and as separated yolks and whites which can be frozen or dried, processed and preserved. Frozen or dried eggs are mainly used by industry in the production of processed foods.

Macronutrient Content

Table 2 shows the macronutrient content of chicken eggs. There are no major differences in nutrient content of eggs produced by different systems although other factors can alter the composition. The age, strain and breed of the hens, individual variation between hens, feed, temperature of the environment, storage conditions and length of time stored can have effects on nutrient content. Hens produce smaller eggs at the beginning of their laying cycle; as egg size increases, the relative amount of yolk decreases. It has been established that hen age and laying season have no effect on nitrogen or total fat content of an egg.

Egg composition can be altered by the type of feed. It is quite easy to manipulate the fatty acid

Table 1 Annual egg consumption per capita in the UK

Year	No. of eggs
1991	179
1992	174
1993	169
1994	172
1995	169

Data from the British Egg Information Service.

Table 2 Macronutrient composition of raw eggs (per 100 g)

	Whole egg	Albumen	Yolk
Water (g)	75.1	88.3	51.0
Energy			
(kJ)	612	153	1402
(kcal)	147	36	339
Protein (g)	12.5	9.0	16.1
Fat (g)	10.8	Trace	30.5
Carbohydrate (g)	Trace	Trace	Trace

Data from *Milk Products and Eggs*, supplement to *The Composition of Foods*, reproduced with the permission of the Royal Society of Chemistry and the Controller of Her Majesty's Stationery Office.

composition of the egg yolk, for instance. Eggs contain only a trace of carbohydrate and this nutrient is not discussed here. The nutrient composition data given here refer to eggs produced by hens fed on commercial feed; other types of feed can result in considerable variation in nutrient composition.

Protein

Egg protein has a high biological value and is used as a reference protein, although it is now recognized that it does not possess the ideal amino acid composition for humans. Eggs contain all amino acids essential to the human body (**Table 3**). Age of the hen has a significant effect on albumen and total protein content of the egg. Eggs stored at 2°C for long periods show a significant reduction in threonine content, and this amino acid can also be reduced by cooking.

Fat, fatty acids and cholesterol

The total fat, fatty acid and cholesterol content of eggs (**Table 4**) can be significantly influenced by the type of feed given to the hen, and in some countries it is now possible to buy eggs that have had their fatty acid and cholesterol content manipulated. The major saturated fatty acids found in egg fat are $C_{16:0}$ and $C_{18:0}$, the major monounsaturated fatty acid is $C_{18:1}$ (n-9) in the *cis* configuration and the major polyunsaturated fatty acid is $C_{18:2}$ (n-6) in the *cis* configuration (**Table 5**). All other fatty acids are minor components of egg fat. Egg lipid contains a high proportion of the phospholipid lecithin. Most

Table 3 Amino acid composition of raw eggs

	Weight per 100 g		
	Whole egg (mg)	Albumen (mg)	Yolk (mg)
Ile	690	500	930
Leu	1020	730	1370
Lys	770	520	1160
Met	390	320	410
Cys	220	160	260
Phe	630	520	650
Tyr	490	360	650
Thr	630	430	900
Trp	220	160	280
Val	930	710	1110
Arg	750	490	1160
His	300	200	410
Ala	670	520	800
Asp	1320	980	1700
Glu	1480	1090	1750
Gly	370	290	440
Pro	470	360	570
Ser	970	660	1390

Data from Paul *et al.* (1979).

Table 4 Fat and cholesterol composition of raw eggs

	Weight per 100 g whole egg
Total fat (g)	6.2
Saturated fatty acids (g)	1.8
Monounsaturated fatty acids (g)	2.4
Polyunsaturated fatty acids (g)	0.9
Trans unsaturated fatty acids (g)	0.1
Other lipid (g)	1.0
Cholesterol (mg)	151

Data from Jordan M (1992) *Fatty Acids in Foods.* Unpublished report prepared by RHM Technology for the Ministry of Agriculture, Fisheries and Food.

of the phospholipid entering the human intestine undergoes hydrolysis by the digestive enzyme lecithinase so that almost all of the lecithin required by the body is produced endogenously.

Although cholesterol is not a macronutrient it is included in this section because of its relationship to dietary fat, and because eggs are one of the richest sources of dietary cholesterol. There is controversy over the effect of dietary cholesterol on plasma cholesterol levels, although it is widely accepted that saturated fat intake is the major dietary factor influencing plasma cholesterol concentration. Only about 10% of plasma cholesterol can be attributed to dietary cholesterol intake; the remaining 90% is produced endogenously by the liver. It has been proposed that some of the variation in serum cholesterol levels from one person to another may be due to differing susceptibility to dietary saturated fat and cholesterol. Other studies have shown that there are hyper- and hyporesponders to dietary cholesterol, but this may not be the case when total fat intake is low. It has been established that individuals consuming a normal healthy diet can eat one egg per day without increasing their plasma cholesterol significantly.

Energy

The weight of an average egg is approximately 60 g and its energy content is approximately 367 kJ (90 kcal). Eggs are thus a relatively low-energy food yet are of high biological value, and are often used in weight-reducing diets.

Micronutrient Content

Vitamins

Eggs are a useful source of almost all vitamins with the exception of ascorbic acid (**Table 6**). Eggs are a good dietary source of vitamin D (calciferols); the vitamin D content of eggs ranks second only to fish oils. When the skin is subjected to sunlight it can

Table 5 Fatty acid composition of eggs

Saturated fatty acids (g per 100 g TFA)		Monounsaturated fatty acids (g per 100 g TFA)		Polyunsaturated fatty acids (g per 100 g TFA)	
C14:0	0.3	C16:1 *trans*	0.7	C18:2 *trans*	0.1
C16:0	20.8	C16:1 *cis*	2.0	C18:2 *cis* n-6	14.3
C17:0	0.3	C17:1	0.4	C18:3 *cis* n-3	0.7
C18:0	7.7	C18:1 *trans*	0.3		
C20:0	0.1	C18:1 *cis* n-9	31.3		
C22:0	0.2	C18:1 *cis* iso	2.2		
C24:0	0.1	C20:1 *cis*	< 0.1		
		C22:1 *cis*	1.9		
		C24:1	0.1		
Other fatty acids not shown have analytical values < 0.05 g					

TFA, total fatty acids.
Data from Jordan M (1992) *Fatty Acids in Foods*. Unpublished report prepared by RHM Technology for the Ministry of Agriculture, Fisheries and Food.

Table 6 Vitamin composition of raw eggs

	Weight per 100 g		
	Whole egg	Albumen	Yolk
Retinol (µg)	190	0	535
Vitamin D (µg)	1.75	0	4.94
Vitamin E (mg)	1.11	0	3.11
Thiamin (mg)	0.09	0.01	0.30
Riboflavin (mg)	0.47	0.43	0.54
Niacin (mg)	0.07	0.09	0.06
Vitamin B_6 (mg)	0.12	0.02	0.30
Folate (µg)	50.0	13	130
Pantothenate (mg)	1.77	0.30	4.60
Biotin (µg)	20.0	7.0	50.0
Vitamin B_{12} (µg)	2.5	0.1	6.91

Data from *Milk Products and Eggs*, supplement to *The Composition of Foods*, reproduced with the permission of the Royal Society of Chemistry and the Controller of Her Majesty's Stationery Office.

convert 7-dehydrocholesterol to provitamin D by isomerization; the compound is then metabolized to vitamin D. Thus, the vitamin D from eggs may have a significant role to play in those individuals who receive insufficient exposure to sunlight. Some chicken feeds are fortified with vitamin D, in which case the eggs have much higher values Eggs are a good source of vitamin B_2 (riboflavin). Vitamin A (retinol) is found in significant amounts in egg yolk. The glycoprotein avidin is found in raw egg white and binds biotin, preventing its absorption. Avidin is destroyed by heat treatment and should not pose a significant problem if government recommendations to avoid the consumption of raw eggs are adhered to (see below).

Minerals

Eggs are a good source of almost all minerals with the exception of calcium (**Table 7**). They contain iron and phosphorus, although the bioavailability of the iron is low owing to the binding of iron to egg proteins. The breed of chicken significantly influences the concentration of iodine, and the age of the hen has a significant influence on the phosphorus and chloride content of the egg. The time of year of egg production has a significant effect on sodium, calcium and chloride content.

Table 7 Mineral and trace element composition of eggs

	Weight per 100 g		
	Whole egg	Albumen	Yolk
Na (mg)	140	190	50
K (mg)	130	150	120
Ca (mg)	57	5	130
Mg (mg)	12	11	15
P (mg)	200	33	500
Fe (mg)	1.9	0.1	6.1
Cu (mg)	0.08	0.02	0.15
Zn (mg)	1.3	0.1	3.9
S (mg)	180	180	170
Cl (mg)	160	170	140
Se (µg)	11	6	20
I (µg)	53	3	140

Data from *Milk Products and Eggs*, supplement to *The Composition of Foods*, reproduced with the permission of the Royal Society of Chemistry and the Controller of Her Majesty's Stationery Office.

Hygiene and Safety

The 1993 *Report on Salmonella in Eggs* produced by the UK Advisory Committee on the Microbiological Safety of Food was produced in response to consumer and government concerns about contamination of eggs by *Salmonella enteritidis*. The phage 4 type is most prevalent in the UK and eggs are a major source of infection. The illness resulting from this type of bacteria ranges from gastrointestinal symptoms to death from septicaemia in the most severe cases. Salmonellae are destroyed by heat but not by freezing or dehydration; raw or undercooked eggs are thus a potential source of infection. The contamination of eggs may be due to the contact of the organism with the shell, although it is thought that the major route of infection is via the reproductive tissue of the contaminated bird. The following recommendations were made by the Chief Medical Officer of the UK in 1993:

1. Eggs should not be eaten raw, and vulnerable groups (the elderly, the sick, infants and pregnant women) should only eat eggs that have been cooked until the white and yolk are solid.
2. Eggs should be consumed within 3 weeks of laying. Egg packs and the eggs themselves should be dated.
3. Storage temperatures of eggs during transport and retailing should remain consistent and never exceed 20°C. Once purchased, eggs should be refrigerated.
4. If recipes require eggs in raw or undercooked form, pasteurized egg should be used.

Role of Eggs in the Diet

Eggs are a valuable source of nutrients in diets where digestibility or chewing is a problem, as is sometimes the case in the elderly. In the past, egg yolks were given to infants as a source of iron, before it was realized that iron from this source has low bioavailability. There are many alternative infant foods available which are fortified with iron. Eggs fed to infants must be hard-cooked, and egg albumen should not be given to infants under the age of 9–12 months; this is because albumen can produce allergic reactions owing to its antigenic properties. Eating raw egg albumen can have toxic effects due to the protein avidin, but this protein is denatured by heat treatment.

Processed egg products are probably a major contributor to egg intake in most developed countries since the consumption of processed foods has increased considerably, and many of these foods contain egg.

There are a number of misconceptions about eggs that are worth mentioning:

- Shell colour is related to the breed of chicken and has no effect on nutrient content.
- Yolk colour is not related to nutritional value and is purely due to the xanthophyll content of the feed. Xanthophyll has no nutritional value.
- Organic eggs have the same nutrient content as eggs from battery hens.
- Raw eggs are not more digestible than cooked ones, in fact cooked eggs are more digestible.
- Eaten in moderation, eggs can make a major contribution to high-quality nutrient intake.

See also: **Cholesterol**: Sources, Absorption, Function and Metabolism; Factors Determining Blood Cholesterol Levels. **Coronary Heart Disease**: Lipid Theory of Coronary Heart Disease. **Hyperlipidaemia (Hyperlipidemia)**: Nutritional Management.

Further Reading

Advisory Committee on the Microbiological Safety of Food (1993) *Report on Salmonella in Eggs*. London: HMSO.

Burley RW and Vadehra DV (1989) *The Avian Egg: Chemistry and Biology*. New York: Wiley.

Edington JD, Geekie M, Carter R, Benfield L, Ball M and Mann J (1989) Serum lipid response to dietary cholesterol in subjects fed a low fat, high fiber diet. *American Journal of Clinical Nutrition* 50: 58–62.

Holland B, Unwin ID and Buss DH (1989) Fourth supplement to *McCance and Widdowson's The Composition of Foods*, 4th edn. Cambridge: Royal Society of Chemistry.

Katan MB, Berns MAM, Glatz JFC, Knuiman JT, Nobels A and DeVries JHM (1988) Congruence of individual responsiveness to dietary cholesterol and to saturated fat in humans. *Journal of Lipid Research* 29: 883–892.

Kline L, Meehan JJ and Sugihara TF (1965) Relation between layer egg and egg-product yields and quality. *Food Technology* 19: 114–119.

Ministry of Agriculture Fisheries and Food (1993) *National Food Survey 1992*. London: HMSO.

Paul AA, Southgate DAT and Russell J (1979) First supplement to *McCance and Widdowson's The Composition of Foods*, 3rd edn. London: HMSO.

Stadelman WJ and Cottrill OJ (1990) *Egg Science and Technology*, 3rd edn. New York: Food Products Press.

Eicosanoids *see* **Prostaglandins and Leukotrienes**: Physiology.

ELECTROLYTES

Contents
Water–Electrolyte Balance
Acid–Base Balance

Water–Electrolyte Balance

S M Shirreffs and **R J Maughan**, University
Medical School, Aberdeen, UK

Copyright © 1998 Academic Press

Body Water and Electrolytes

Humans depend on ready access to water for survival. Water is the largest component of the human body, representing approximately 45–70% of the total body mass – this corresponds to about 33–53 litres for a 75 kg man. The water content of the various tissues is maintained at a relatively constant level; as adipose tissue has a low water content (**Table 1**), the fraction of water in the body is determined largely by the fat content. The body's water can be divided into two components – the intracellular fluid and the extracellular fluid; the intracellular fluid is the major component and comprises approximately two-thirds of total body water. The extracellular fluid can be further divided into the interstitial fluid (that between the cells) and the plasma; the plasma volume represents approximately one-quarter of the extracellular fluid volume (**Table 2**).

There are numerous electrolytes and solutes dissolved within the water: an electrolyte can be defined as a compound which dissociates into ions when in solution. The major cations (positively charged electrolytes) in the body water are sodium, potassium, calcium and magnesium; the major anions (negatively charged electrolytes) are chloride and bicarbonate. Sodium is the major electrolyte present in the extracellular fluid; potassium is present in a much lower concentration (**Table 3**): within the intracellular fluid the situation is reversed, and the major electrolyte present is potassium, while sodium is found in much lower concentrations. Maintenance of the transmembrane electrical and chemical gradients is of paramount importance for maintaining the integrity of the body's cells and allowing electrical communication throughout the body.

Daily regulation of body water

The body's total body water content is normally maintained within a small window of fluctuation on a daily basis by intake of food and drink to balance the excretion of urine and other losses. Hyperhydration is corrected by an increase in urine production and hypohydration by an increase in water intake via food or drink consumption initiated by thirst. Most of our water intake is related to habit rather than thirst, but the thirst mechanism is effective at driving intake after periods of deprivation. There are also

Table 2 The body water distribution between the body fluid compartments in an adult male

	Percentage of body mass	Percentage of lean body mass	Percentage of body water
Total body water	60	72	100
Extracellular water	20	24	33
Plasma	5	6	8
Interstitium	15	18	25
Intracellular water	40	48	67

From Sawka (1990).

Table 1 Water content of various body tissues for an average 75 kg man

Tissue	Percentage water	Percentage of body mass	Water per 75 kg (l)	Percentage of total body water
Skin	72	18	9.7	22
Organs	76	7	4.0	9
Skeleton	22	15	2.5	5
Blood	83	5	3.1	7
Adipose	10	12	0.9	2
Muscle	76	43	24.5	55

From Sawka (1990).

Table 3 Ionic composition of body water compartments. The normal ranges of the plasma electrolyte compartments are shown

Ion	Plasma (mmol l^{-1})	Intracellular fluid (mmol l^{-1})
Sodium	140 (135–145)	12
Potassium	4.0 (3.5–4.6)	150
Calcium	2.4 (2.1–2.7)	4.0
Magnesium	0.8 (0.6–1.0)	34
Chloride	104 (98–107)	4
Bicarbonate	29 (21–38)	12
Inorganic phosphate	1.0 (0.7–1.6)	40

Data from Lentner (1981) and Rose (1984).

water losses via the respiratory tract, the gastrointestinal tract and the skin. The extent of these losses varies from individual to individual and is strongly influenced by environmental conditions and physical activity levels, but for a sedentary individual in a cool environment these losses generally represent only a small proportion of the total body water loss (**Table 4**).

Renal Function

As well as acting to regulate body water levels by an increase or decrease in the amount of urine produced, the kidneys are also responsible for the elimination of waste products from the body. This also influences the daily urine volume. For example, a healthy individual eating a normal diet excretes approximately 600–800 mosmol of solute per square metre of body surface area per day, amounting to about 1000–1500 mosmol per day. The kidneys can dilute urine to at least as low as 100 mosmol kg^{-1} and can concentrate it to 1200 mosmol kg^{-1}. Therefore, the daily solute load to be excreted can be accommodated in a volume ranging between approximately 500 ml and more than 13 l. To allow for waste product excretion, an obligatory minimum amount of urine must always be excreted, and this is generally in the region of 20–50 ml h^{-1}. However, in the majority of healthy individuals in most situations, the volume of urine produced and excreted is in excess of these basal levels.

Hormonal control of urine production

The volume of urine produced in a healthy individual is largely determined by circulating hormone levels, and in particular by levels of vasopressin. Vasopressin is a cyclic peptide comprising nine amino acids. It is released from the posterior pituitary gland after its transport there along the axons of neurons whose cell bodies are located in the paraventricular and supraoptic nuclei of the hypothalamus, the site of vasopressin synthesis. An increase in the rate of secretion of vasopressin results in a reduced urine production. Vasopressin acts on the renal distal tubules and collecting ducts to cause an increased permeability to water and hence an increased reabsorption of water from the filtrate. Therefore, a hyperosmotic urine can be formed and the solute load to be excreted can be accommodated in a small volume of water. A decrease in vasopressin secretion results in an increase in the volume of urine produced by causing a reduction in the permeability of the renal distal tubule and collecting ducts to water. Vasopressin secretion is largely influenced by changes in plasma osmolality: an increase in plasma osmolality results in an increased vasopressin secretion and a decrease in osmolality results in a decrease in vasopressin. The vasopressin is released rapidly in response to the stimuli and begins to act within minutes. When the secretion is inhibited, the half-life of clearance from the circulation is approximately 10 min. Therefore, changes in body fluid

Table 4 Daily water intake and output for a sedentary individual in a cool environment

Daily water loss	(ml)	Daily water intake	(ml)
Kidneys	1500	Fluid	1300
Respiratory tract	400	Food	1000
Gastrointestinal tract	200	Cellular oxidation	300
Skin	500		
Total	2600	Total	2600

Data from Åstrand and Rodahl (1986).

tonicity are rapidly translated into changes in water excretion by this tightly regulated feedback system.

In addition to plasma osmolality, other (nonosmotic) factors influencing vasopressin secretion are baroregulation, nausea and pharyngeal stimuli. A fall in blood pressure or blood volume will stimulate vasopressin release; vasopressin secretion is, however, less sensitive to these changes than to changes in osmolality. Nausea is an extremely potent stimulus to human vasopressin secretion; vasopressin levels can increase 100- to 1000-fold in response to nausea induced by various chemical agents. After a period of water deprivation followed by access to drink, vasopressin levels fall before there is any change in plasma tonicity, suggesting activation of neuronal pathways from the oropharynx.

Aldosterone, a steroid hormone, is released into the circulation after synthesis by the zona glomerulosa cells of the adrenal cortex. Its primary role, in terms of renal function, is to increase renal tubular reabsorption of sodium, and in doing so it brings about an increased excretion of potassium and, in association with vasopressin, increases water reabsorption in the distal segments of the nephron. Aldosterone causes this response by increasing the activity of the peritubular sodium-potassium pump and by increasing the permeability of the luminal membrane to both sodium and potassium. The increased luminal permeability allows potassium to move down its concentration gradient from the inside of the membrane cells into the tubule lumen. The majority of the sodium present is reabsorbed into the cell down the concentration gradient. The sodium absorption and potassium excretion are closely correlated, with a 3:2 sodium to potassium ratio. Chloride follows the sodium to maintain the electrical neutrality of the urine.

The release of aldosterone is determined by a number of factors including the renin–angiotensin system: a fall in blood or extracellular fluid volume increases renin production and, via angiotensin II, results in an increase in aldosterone secretion.

The presence in the renal filtrate of ions such as bicarbonate and sulfate, which are not reabsorbed, promotes secretion of potassium into the distal tubule of the nephron and will also result in an increased urinary loss of potassium.

Daily Sodium and Potassium Input and Output

In the UK, the average sodium intake is in the range of 1–6 g per day (approximately 50–260 mmol per day); similar molar quantities of chloride are ingested on a daily basis. When fully activated, the renal salt-conserving mechanisms can reduce the obligatory losses to as little as 1 mmol per day, but for a healthy individual living in a moderate ambient temperature salt balance can usually be achieved with an intake of less than 10 mmol per day. However, exercise, particularly in a warm environment, and diarrhoeal illness are two situations which will increase the requirement for salt to substantially greater levels. For example, an individual with a sweat sodium concentration of 50 mmol l^{-1} (see below) losing 5 litres of sweat will lose 250 mmol of sodium. If all of this sodium is lost as sodium chloride this amounts to more than 4 g. There is some evidence to suggest that hypovolaemia will increase salt appetite, and individuals with adrenal insufficiency have a much lower threshold for discriminating salt solutions.

The average potassium intake is in the region of 1–5 g (25–130 mmol) per day. Again, the renal losses are highly variable, but for a healthy individual living in a moderate ambient temperature potassium homeostasis could be achieved with an intake in the region of 20–30 mmol per day. As with sodium requirements, exercise promoting a substantial sweat loss and diarrhoeal illness may increase the requirement for potassium.

In normal circumstances the renal system is very effective at matching electrolyte losses to dietary intakes in order to maintain homeostasis. However, excessive sodium chloride intake can result in salt poisoning which can ultimately lead to death; ingestion of 4–6 tablespoons has been lethal in adults. Ingestion of a high-potassium diet will stimulate aldosterone secretion and promote adaptations in the kidney which enhance its ability to excrete the potassium load

Sweat

Eccrine sweat is a clear, watery, odourless substance whose primary function is to promote heat loss by evaporation from the skin surface. When sweat is produced, the daily water losses increase and the intake must be increased or urine production decreased accordingly if euhydration is to be maintained.

Sweat evaporation

There is a daily loss of approximately 500 ml of water through the skin; this is a true transcutaneous loss. However, when the body is exposed to a heat stress and behavioural and vasomotor mechanisms are insufficient to prevent a rise in temperature, the physiological responses generally include an increase in sweat production in an attempt to prevent hyperthermia; the high latent heat of vaporization of water makes the evaporation of sweat an effective heat loss mechanism – evaporation of 1 litre of water from the skin surface will remove 2.4 MJ (580 kcal) of heat from the body. The heat stress may be of external (environmental) origin, of internal origin due to muscular work, or a combination of the two.

In many individuals sweat rates can be in excess of $2 \, l \, h^{-1}$, especially where exercise is undertaken in a warm, humid environment, and these high sweat rates can be maintained for a number of hours. For example, body mass losses in marathon runners have been reported to range from about 1–6% (0.7–4.2 kg) at low (10°C) ambient temperatures to more than 8% (5.6 kg) in warmer conditions. However, when sweat rates are high, a significant fraction of the sweat secreted onto the skin may drip from the body and is therefore ineffective at removing heat.

Mechanism of sweat secretion

The human body has approximately 2 million sweat glands. The eccrine sweat gland consists of a single tubule, opening onto the epidermis at one end and closed at the other. The proximal half of the tubule is the secretory coil and the distal half the reabsorptive duct. The sweat secreted onto the skin is the original tubular secretion minus the substances that are reabsorbed further up the tubule; from the iso-osmotic fluid secreted by the coil most of the major electrolytes (Na^+, Cl^-, HCO_3^+, lactate) are transported out of the duct back to the extracellular fluid in excess of water. The final sweat secreted onto the skin is therefore hypotonic with respect to body fluids.

Sweat production is influenced by a number of factors; in response to thermal stress, the hypothalamic temperature and skin temperature seem to be the largest determinants.

Sweat composition

The composition of human sweat is highly variable, both between individuals and within an individual over time. However, sodium and chloride are the major electrolytes lost in sweat, with other ions being present in smaller amounts relative to the whole body status. The sweat electrolyte composition of an individual seems to be related primarily to sweat rate, but can be influenced by training status, extent of heat acclimation and diet. However, the reported range of values for sweat electrolyte composition probably reflects not only interindividual differences, but also differences in the methodology used for collection of the sweat. The latter factor may be the result of errors caused by contamination or incomplete collection of the sample, or may reflect a real difference induced by the collection procedure.

Owing to the secretion and reabsorption process involved in sweat production within the sweat gland and duct, sweat composition is influenced by sweat rate, at least within single ducts, such that a reduction in rate allows for greater reabsorption of certain electrolytes (Na^+ and Cl^-, but not K^+) from the duct, resulting in a lower concentration in the final sweat produced. There do, also, appear to be regional variations in sweat composition, as evidenced by the different values obtained when the composition of sweat obtained from different parts of the body is compared, and the values obtained by regional collection also differ from those obtained by the whole-body washdown technique. Higher electrolyte concentrations are generally observed when local sweat collection procedures are used, probably due to an alteration in composition caused by the restriction on evaporation of the sweat. Regional collection is not, therefore, appropriate when whole-body sweating is occurring and where total electrolyte or solute loss must be known. The difficulties caused by the restriction of evaporation can be overcome by using a ventilated capsule or chamber: the water in the effluent air is trapped in a cold trap, and the electrolytes recovered at the end of the study period by washing out the enclosing apparatus. This does not, however, overcome the difficulties caused by regional differences in the composition of sweat.

A selection of reported values for sweat electrolyte composition is summarized in **Table 5**.

Distribution of body water losses with sweating

The free fluid exchange between the body's fluid compartments ensures that the water content of sweat is derived from all compartments, with the distribution being influenced by sweat rate, sweat composition and total water and electrolyte loss. In one study, subjects were dehydrated by cycle exercise and heat exposure to the extent of 3%, 6% and 9% of total body water (**Fig. 1**). With a 3% body water loss, 10% of the loss was from the plasma volume, 60% from the interstitial water and 30% from the intracellular water; with a 6% body water loss, 10% was from the plasma volume, 38% from the interstitial water and 52% from the intracellular water; with a 9% body water loss, 11% was from the plasma volume, 39% from the interstitial water and 50% from the intracellular water. Therefore, at low levels of body water loss the water comes largely from the extracellular space, and as the extent of the water loss increases a greater percentage of the loss comes from the intracellular space. This picture is, of course, confused by the longer time taken to achieve the higher levels of sweat loss, as this may have resulted in some redistribution of body water.

Table 5 A selection of reported values for the mean composition of sweat with regard to the major electrolytes

	Sodium (mmol l⁻¹)	Potassium (mmol l⁻¹)	Chloride (mmol l⁻¹)	Reference
Arm bag method				
	65.7	7.9	58.7	Kleeman *et al*. 1953
	38.8	5.9	42.3	Malhotra *et al*. 1976
Patch method				
	58	5.2	63	Boisvert *et al*. 1993
	65	–	–	Kirby and Convertino 1986
Whole-body method				
	62.1	7.2	–	Armstrong *et al*. 1985a
	43.8	3.9	38.6	Costill *et al*. 1976
	49.5	4.9	46.8	Kleeman *et al*. 1953
	50.8	4.8	46.6	Shirreffs and Maughan 1997

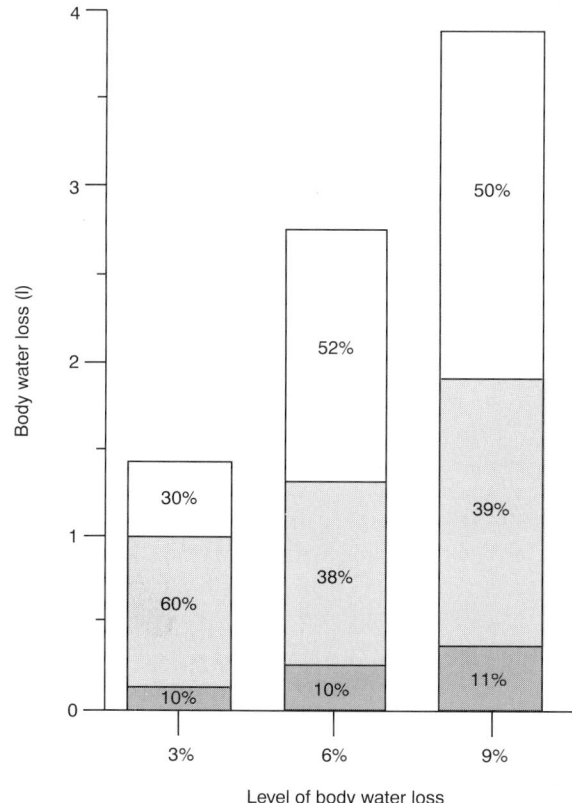

Figure 1 The division of the total body water lost with dehydration into its individual compartments. Dark shading, plasma; light shading, interstitial fluid; unshaded, intracellular fluid. Based on the data of Costill *et al*. (1976). With permission from The American Physiological Society.

Effects of a Body Water Deficit

Daily access to water is necessary to sustain life. Above this basic level, however, a body water deficit has been shown to have a negative effect on work performance; a 35% fall in the capacity to perform high-intensity exercise lasting about 7 min has been reported after a fluid loss of 2.5% of body mass by sauna exposure. In one study subjects took part in track races over 1500 m, 5000 m and 10 000 m after being dehydrated by approximately 2% of body mass with a diuretic drug (40 mg of furosemide). Compared with the subjects' performances under conditions of euhydration, finishing times were increased by 0.13 min, 1.31 min and 2.62 min respectively (**Fig. 2**), corresponding to decreases in running velocity of 3.1%, 6.7% and 6.3%.

The plasma volume decreases in association with dehydration may be of particular importance in influencing work capacity; blood flow to the muscles must be maintained at a high level during exercise to supply oxygen and substrates, but a high blood flow to the skin is also necessary to convect heat to the body surface where it can be dissipated. In a high ambient temperature, and if the blood volume has been decreased by sweat loss during prolonged exercise, there may be difficulty in meeting the requirement for a high blood flow to both these tissues. In this situation, skin blood flow is likely to be compromised, allowing central venous pressure and muscle blood flow to be maintained, but this will reduce heat loss and can cause body temperature to rise sharply.

Conclusions

In the normal healthy individual, water and electrolyte homeostasis are maintained within a relatively small window of fluctuation. Increases or decreases in dietary water and electrolyte intake are generally very efficiently matched by appropriate changes in the renal handling of the water and electrolytes.

Exercise, particularly in a warm environment, and diarrhoeal illness both have the potential to cause large water and electrolyte losses. An increased dietary intake of water and electrolytes is necessary to restore any deficit incurred.

See also: **Dehydration**: Physiological Effects and

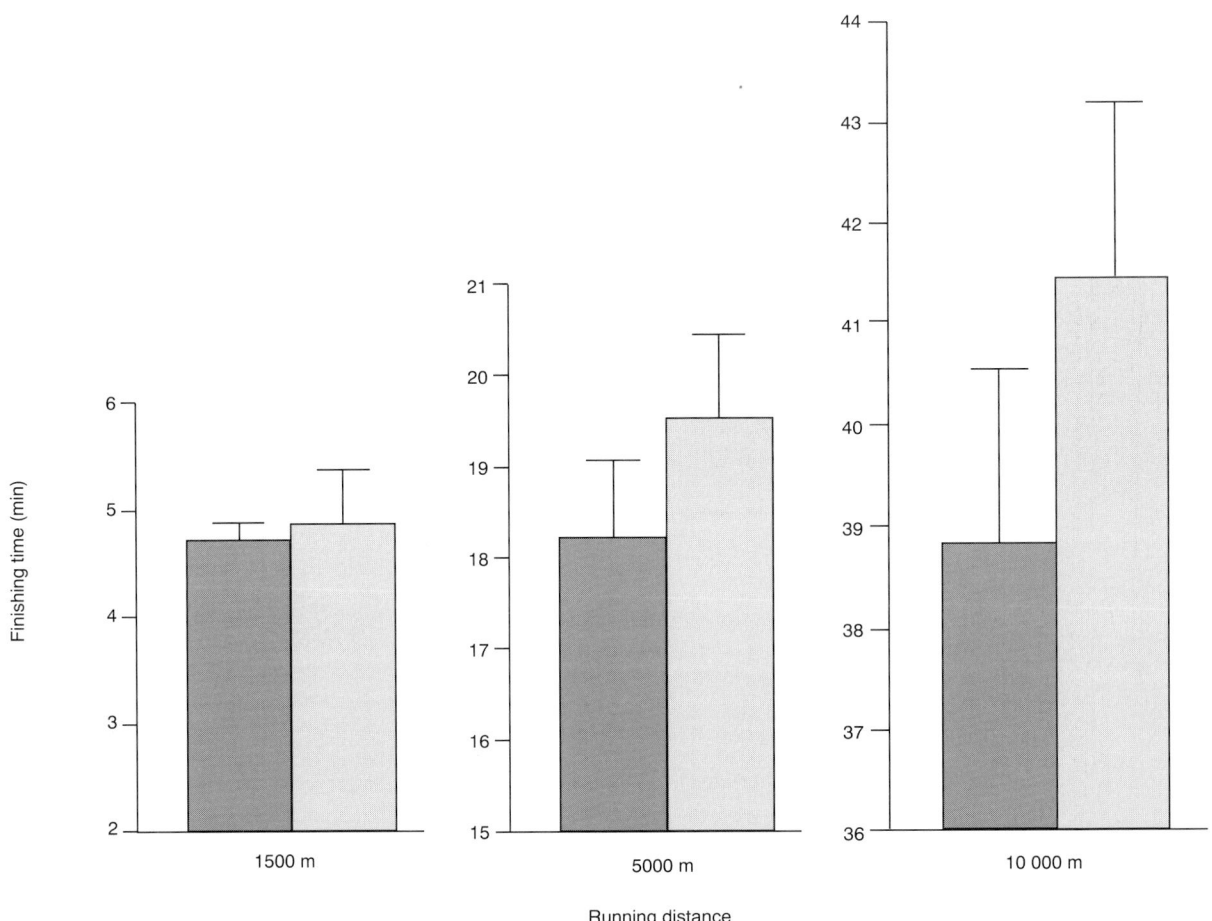

Figure 2   Finishing time in track races when euhydrated (dark shading) and when dehydrated by approximately 2% of body mass (light shading). Values are mean ± SE. Based on the data of Armstrong *et al.* (1985b).

Management. **Potassium**: Physiology, Dietary Sources and Requirements. **Renal Function and Disorders**: Nutritional Management of Renal Disorders. **Sodium**: Physiology.

Further Reading

Armstrong LE, Costill DL, Fink WJ *et al.* (1985a) Effects of dietary sodium on body and muscle potassium content during heat acclimation. *European Journal of Applied Physiology* **54**:391–397.

Armstrong LE, Costill DL and Fink WJ (1985b) Influence of diuretic-induced dehydration on competitive running performance. *Medicine and Science in Sports and Exercise* **17**:456–461.

Boisvert P, Brisson GR and Péronnet F (1993) Effect of plasma prolactin on sweat rate and sweat composition during exercise in men. *American Journal of Physiology* **264**:F816–F820.

Briggs JP, Sawaya BE and Schnermann J (1990) Disorders of salt balance. In: Kokko JP and Tannen RL (eds) *Fluids and Electrolytes*, 2nd edn, pp 70–138. Philadelphia: WB Saunders.

Costill DL (1972) Physiology of marathon running. *Journal of the American Medical Association* **221**:1024–1029.

Costill DL, Coté R and Fink W (1976) Muscle water and electrolytes following varied levels of dehydration in man. *Journal of Applied Physiology* **40**:6–11.

Engell DB, Maller O, Sawka MN, Francesconi RN, Drolet L and Young AJ (1987) Thirst and fluid intake following graded hypohydration levels in humans. *Physiology and Behaviour* **40**:229–236.

Gregory J, Foster K, Tyler H and Wiseman M (1990) *The Dietary and Nutritional Survey of British Adults*. London: HMSO.

Kirby CR and Convertino VA (1986) Plasma aldosterone and sweat sodium concentrations after exercise and heat acclimation. *Journal of Applied Physiology* **61**:967–970.

Kleeman CR, Bass DE and Quinn M (1953) The effect of an impermeable vapor barrier on electrolyte and nitrogen concentrations in sweat. *Journal of Clinical Investigation* **32**:736–745.

Lentner C, ed. (1981) *Geigy Scientific Tables*, 8th edn. Basle: Ciba-Geigy.

Malhotra MS, Sridharan K and Venkataswamy Y (1976) Potassium losses in sweat under heat stress. *Aviation, Space and Environmental Medicine* **47**:503–504.

Maughan RJ (1985) Thermoregulation and fluid balance in marathon competition at low ambient temperature. *International Journal of Sports Medicine* 6:15–19.

Rose BD (1984) *Clinical Physiology of Acid-base and Electrolyte Disorders*, 2nd edn. New York: McGraw-Hill.

Sawka MN (1990) Body fluid responses and hypohydration during exercise – heat stress. In: Pandolf KB, Sawka MN and Gonzalez RR (eds) *Human Performance Physiology and Environmental Medicine at Terrestrial Extremes*, pp 227–266. Carmel: Cooper.

Shirreffs SM and Maughan RJ (1997) Whole body sweat collection in man: an improved method with preliminary data on electrolyte content. *Journal of Applied Physiology* 82:336–341.

Sterns RH and Spital A (1990) Disorders of water balance. In: Kokko JP and Tannen RL (eds) *Fluids and Electrolytes*, 2nd edn, pp 139–194. Philadelphia: WB Saunders.

Taylor NAS (1986) Eccrine sweat glands. Adaptations to physical training and heat acclimation. *Sports Medicine* 3:387–397.

Acid–Base Balance

Alan G Jardine, University of Glasgow, UK

Eric S Kilpatrick, Royal Infirmary, Manchester, UK

Copyright © 1998 Academic Press

Maintenance of cellular and extracellular pH (hydrogen ion concentration) is essential to life, since the activity of many processes (e.g. enzyme activity) is pH-dependent. Hydrogen ions are generated by cellular metabolism (largely independent of dietary acid load) and the major role of acid–base homeostasis is to prevent acidification occurring. Blood and tissue pH are tightly regulated by the presence of buffer systems, which attenuate changes in acid load, and by the subsequent excretion of volatile acid by the lungs and fixed acids by the kidney

Definitions: Acids, Bases, Buffers

pH

The term 'pH' is an expression of hydrogen ion (H^+) concentration:

$$pH = -\log[H^+] \tag{1}$$

Blood pH is closely regulated between 7.36 and 7.44, corresponding to a hydrogen ion concentration of 37–44 nmol l^{-1} (note that pH and H^+ are inversely related).

Acids and bases

Acids are substances which dissociate to donate H^+ (eqn [2]); the 'stronger' the acid, the more readily it dissociates. The dissociation constant (pK_a) is the pH at which 50% of an acid is dissociated (at pH values greater than pK_a, more H^+ will dissociate; the lower the pK_a the 'stronger' the acid). A base is a substance which will accept a hydrogen ion. In the following text, 'fixed acid' is the term used to describe formed acid, and 'volatile acid' is used to describe the potential acid load imposed by carbon dioxide. If 'A' represents the acid, the following equation applies:

$$AH \rightleftharpoons A^- + H^+ \tag{2}$$

Buffers

Buffering is the ability of weak acids, present in excess, to accept H^+ donated from strong acids, thus reducing the changes in free H^+ concentration (and pH changes):

$$AH + Buffer^- \rightleftharpoons Buffer\text{-}H + A^- \tag{3}$$

The principal buffer system in blood is based on bicarbonate (HCO_3^-), accounting for approximately 70% of the buffering capacity. In blood, carbon dioxide (CO_2, the major product of oxidative metabolism) reacts with water, in the presence of the enzyme carbonic anhydrase, to form carbonic acid (H_2CO_3). This compound is relatively unstable and tends to dissociate (eqn [4]). The rate of formation of carbonic acid is dependent on the concentration of carbon dioxide and the rate constant of reaction 1; dissociation of carbonic acid to generate H^+ and HCO_3^- is governed by the rate constant of the reaction 2. In practice, these two reactions can be combined, and the relationship between pH ([H^+]), carbon dioxide and bicarbonate is described by a single equation – the Henderson–Hasselbach equation (eqn [5]):

$$\overset{(1)}{CO_2 + H_2O} \rightleftharpoons \overset{(2)}{H_2CO_3} \rightleftharpoons H^+ + HCO_3^- \tag{4}$$

$$pH = 6.1 + \log([HCO_3^-]/SP\text{co}_2) \tag{5}$$

pH is equal to $-\log[H^+]$; 6.1 is the value of $-\log(1/K)$, K being the equilibrium constant describing the overall equation (eqn [4]); $P\text{co}_2$ is the partial pressure of carbon dioxide; S is the solubility constant for carbon dioxide (0.225 when $P\text{co}_2$ is measured in kPa,

0.03 when CO_2 is measured in mmHg). **Table 1** shows the normal ranges for these variables in humans.

From this equation (eqn [5]) the principles of acid–base balance can be readily understood. Acidification may occur in two ways: either by the production of carbon dioxide or by the consumption of bicarbonate (as part of the buffering of fixed acid). The excretion of carbon dioxide is controlled by the lungs, and excretion of fixed acid can be accomplished only by the kidney.

Maintenance of the pH of Blood

Acid 'load'

There is one major source of 'acid'. Metabolic production of carbon dioxide represents volatile acid (being converted to H_2CO_3 in blood), about 15–20 mol of which is produced per day. The contribution from other sources is small. Only about 1 mmol of fixed (nonvolatile) acid per kg of body weight is produced per day, the major component being lactic acid produced by anaerobic metabolism. An even smaller component comes directly from the diet.

Acid or alkaline foods There are surprisingly few data on the contribution of foods to the acid burden. The major acids contained in food are citric acid (in fruit, fruit juices), acetic acid (as a preservative, pickles, vinegar), lactic acid (yogurt, fermented foods), malic acid (fruit), oxalic acid (in vegetables, which contain smaller amounts of citric and malic acids) and tartaric acid (wine). Oxalic acid precipitates in the gut to form calcium salts, excreted in the stool, and little is absorbed; the others are absorbed but quickly metabolized and they present an acid burden in the from of carbon dioxide. The largest source of fixed acid comes from dietary protein with, for example, amino acids containing sulfhydryl groups being metabolized to form sulfuric acid. The significance of this source of acid is readily demonstrated in patients taking a high-protein diet: urinary acid excretion is increased in these people. Overall,

the direct contribution of acids by foods is minimal, while that attributable to protein is in the range 20–30 mmol per day.

Alkalis are often prescribed to compensate metabolic acidosis (see below) and to neutralize gastric acidity. Milk and many milk products are also alkaline but seldom cause any disturbance unless consumed in excess (see *Metabolic alkalosis*, below).

Regulation

Blood pH is regulated at three levels: (1) buffering within the blood and tissues; (2) excretion of volatile acid by the lungs; (3) excretion of nonvolatile acid by the kidney. The processes at level 1 occur almost instantaneously, those at level 2 over minutes, and those at level 3 over many hours.

Blood Immediate buffering of an acid load (e.g. from exercising muscle) occurs in the blood. From 60% to 70% may be directly accounted for by the bicarbonate buffer system; 20–30% is dependent on binding to haemoglobin (**Fig. 1**), and the remainder includes binding to plasma proteins. Blood is in equilibrium with tissue H^+, and H^+ will pass down concentration gradients into cells in exchange for potassium ions (K^+) (and, to a lesser extent, sodium ions (Na^+) to maintain electroneutrality), or in the opposite direction depending on prevailing $[H^+]$. As a result of this, acidosis is often accompanied by increases in plasma Na^+ and K^+ – the latter being proportionately greater – and alkalosis by decreases in Na^+ and K^+. Large amounts of buffering may occur within cells and tissues, particularly bone where H^+ are buffered by calcium salts, such as apatite.

Table 1 Normal blood values

Variable	Normal range
pH	7.37–7.44
Hydrogen ions (H^+)	37–44 nmol l^{-1}
Partial pressure of carbon dioxide (P_{CO_2})	34–46 mmHg; 4.5–6.1 kPa
Bicarbonate (HCO_3^-)	24–30 mmol l^{-1}

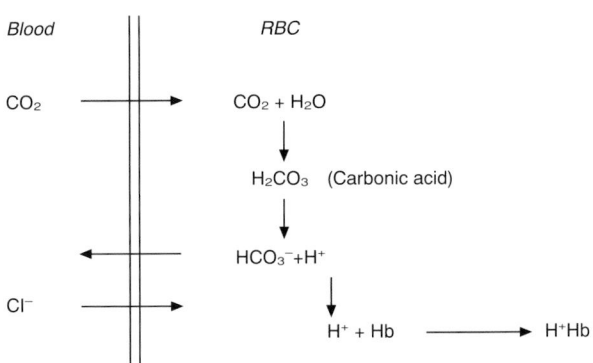

Figure 1 Diagrammatic representation of the buffering ability of the red blood cell (RBC). Carbon dioxide enters the cell and hydrogen ions (H^+) and bicarbonate (HCO_3^-) are generated by the action of carbonic anhydrase; H^+ is then buffered by haemoglobin (Hb).

Role of the Lungs and Kidneys

Lungs

The lungs excrete volatile acid (CO_2) by changes in the rate and volume of respiration. The respiratory 'drive' is regulated by respiratory centres in the brain stem which respond to changes in pH and $P\text{CO}_2$ of cerebrospinal fluid and signals from chemoreceptors in the carotid and aortic bodies that are responsive to changes in pH and $P\text{CO}_2$ of the arterial blood (increased $P\text{CO}_2$ or reduced pH cause an increase in respiration).

Kidneys

The kidneys have two major roles: the regeneration of plasma bicarbonate and the excretion of non-volatile acid (**Fig. 2**; eqn [5]). Blood is filtered in the glomeruli, and this glomerular filtrate is subsequently modified in the renal tubules. Of the total glomerular filtrate of 100–150 ml min^{-1}, more than 99% is reabsorbed to give the final urine volume of 1–2 l per day. Bicarbonate reabsorption occurs largely in the proximal tubule (Fig. 2a) by combining with H^+. Hydrogen ions pass from the renal tubular cell into the lumen of the tubule (in exchange for Na^+) where the presence of the enzyme carbonic anhydrase in the tubular brush border membrane catalyses the formation of carbon dioxide, which then diffuses back into the cell. The same enzyme present within the cell

then catalyses the regeneration of H^+ and HCO_3^-. Hydrogen ions are recycled to the tubular lumen, and HCO_3^- passes into the blood, together with Na^+ to maintain electroneutrality. The tubule cells are also exposed to plasma carbon dioxide and HCO_3^- (Fig. 2b) and, in the presence of acidosis (owing to reduced HCO_3^- or increased CO_2), will continue to generate intracellular H^+ and HCO_3^-. Hydrogen ions pass into the lumen and are buffered by other filtered buffers, notably those containing hydrogen phosphate ions (HPO_4^{2-}) and, to a lesser extent, creatinine. Strong acids (e.g. sulfuric, H_2SO_4) with low pK_a values will not dissociate in urine (pH 5–8), being excreted intact. The final mechanism by which the kidney can excrete H^+ is by the generation of ammonium (NH_4^+) by the metabolism of glutamine, a process which can be stimulated by low pH and increased $P\text{CO}_2$ (Fig. 2c).

Effects of Acid–Base Disturbance

In addition to the adaptive changes occurring, a variety of metabolic and pathophysiological changes occur in acidosis (alkalosis tends to produce milder, opposite effects). The metabolism of carbohydrates is altered: both glycolysis and gluconeogenesis are inhibited in the liver. Delivery of oxygen to tissues is increased by the reduced ability of haemoglobin to retain oxygen in an acid environment (the Bohr effect). However, the most important effects from a clinical perspective are cardiovascular: vasodilatation occurs in peripheral blood vessels and the contractility of the heart is reduced, resulting in reduced blood pressure and reduced tissue perfusion. It is these effects that exacerbate the severity of, for example, lactic acidosis in septic shock, and contribute to the high mortality in such conditions.

Abnormalities of Acid–Base Balance

Disturbances of acid–base balance are classified as either 'acidosis', indicating an excess of H^+ ions ('acidaemia', i.e. acidification of the blood), or 'alkalosis', which has the opposite definition. In practice, acidosis is a more common, serious and varied problem. Disturbances may be further classified as *respiratory*, if the primary problem is in the excretion of carbon dioxide, or *metabolic*, if the primary problem is in the excretion of fixed acid. Compensation refers to the body's response to correct a primary disturbance (e.g. the response to a primary metabolic acidosis will involve increased excretion of CO_2, i.e. respiratory compensation). If the blood pH returns to the normal reference range then the primary problem is said to be fully compensated; in general, primary

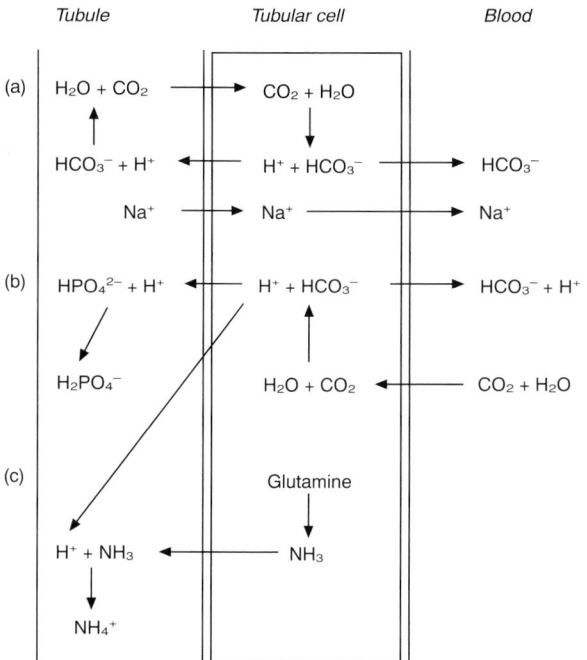

Figure 2 Diagrammatic representation of the reabsorption or bicarbonate (HCO_3^-) and the excretion of hydrogen ions (H^+) by the kidney (see text for details).

metabolic disturbances may only be partially compensated, but primary respiratory problems may be fully compensated if present for several days (**Table 2**).

Metabolic acidosis

The main causes of metabolic acidosis are excessive acid production, inappropriate loss of bicarbonate or failure to excrete acid by the kidney.

Diabetic ketoacidosis The absence of pancreatic insulin secretion in insulin-dependent diabetes causes increased plasma glucose and reduced tissue uptake and utilization of glucose. There is increased utilization of nonesterified fatty acid (NEFA) as an alternative energy source which is metabolized to acetyl coenzyme A (CoA). Under normal circumstances this substance is further metabolized in the liver via the tricarboxylic acid (TCA) cycle to carbon dioxide and water. In diabetic crises this cycle cannot fully accommodate the excess acetyl-CoA. It is instead converted to acetoacetic acid, which can be further reduced to β-hydroxybutyric acid, or decarboxylated to form acetone. These three metabolites are known as 'ketone bodies' and their accumulation results in metabolic acidosis.

Lactic acidosis Reduced tissue perfusion or tissue perfusion inadequate to meet the needs of metabolically active tissue (e.g. exercising muscle) results in an inadequate oxygen supply and change from oxidative metabolism (the end products of which are CO_2 and H_2O) to anaerobic glycolysis, resulting in lactate production. Lactate is normally further metabolized by the liver or used in the synthesis of glucose (gluconeogenesis). When the ability to metabolize lactate is exceeded, accumulation results in metabolic acidosis, which may occur in a variety of conditions,

including systemic shock, severe diabetic ketoacidosis and uraemia.

Loss of bicarbonate The secretions of the stomach are acid and are subsequently neutralized by alkaline secretions from the intestine. It follows that excessive loss of intestinal secretions by diarrhoea – and, less commonly, by vomiting of intestinal contents – leads to an inappropriate loss of bicarbonate and potentially to acidosis. Occasionally, the ureters are implanted into a loop of bowel to bypass serious bladder disease. Bowel mucosa responds to the delivery of urine rich in chloride ions (Cl^{-1}) by exchanging Cl^{-1} for HCO_3^-, resulting in excessive loss of bicarbonate.

Renal Loss of the ability to excrete acid and regenerate bicarbonate are part of the generalized loss of renal function in acute or chronic renal failure (uraemia). There is also a group of specific renal tubular defects (encompassed in the term 'renal tubular acidoses', RTA) which may be inherited or develop secondary to other renal diseases; they may occur as isolated defects or as part of generalized tubular transport abnormalities, and may affect proximal bicarbonate reabsorption (type II RTA) or distal tubular H^+ exchange (type I RTA).

Drugs and other causes Many drugs can cause metabolic acidosis, generally in overdose. The most common example is aspirin (acetylsalicylic acid). Lactic acidosis is also associated with oral hypoglycaemic agents (e.g. metformin, used in the treatment of non-insulin-dependent diabetes), paracetamol, alcohol and ethylene glycol (antifreeze) poisoning.

Compensation The body's response to metabolic acidosis is a compensatory increase in respiration to blow off excess carbon dioxide, restoring the equilibrium in the Henderson–Hasselback equation (eqn [5]). Such respiratory compensation is invariably incomplete, resulting in pH or H^+ values at, or marginally outside, the limits of the 'normal' range (Table 2). Complete compensation depends on renal excretion of excess H^+, or resolution of the underlying condition.

Treatment Treatment of metabolic acidosis is essentially that of the underlying condition: correction of tissue hypoxia in lactic acidosis; correction of fluid depletion and insulin deficiency in diabetes. Rapid correction of pH can be achieved by the administration of intravenous sodium bicarbonate if necessary. Treatment of chronic metabolic acidosis (e.g. in renal failure) can be achieved by administration

Table 2 Changes occurring in blood during acid-base disturbances, the mechanism and degree of compensation[a]

Problem	Hydrogen ions (H^+)	Bicarbonate (HCO_3^-)	Partial pressure of carbon dioxide (Pco_2)	Compensation
Metabolic				
Acidosis	↑	1°↓	2°↓	Partial
Alkalosis	↓	1°↑	2°↑	Partial
Respiratory				
Acidosis	↑	2°↑	1°↑	Complete
Alkalosis	↓	2°↓	1°↓	Complete

↑ Increase; ↓ decrease; 1°, primary; 2°, secondary.
[a]See text for details.

of oral bicarbonate to correct for inapropriate losses; in uraemia the use of a low-protein diet to ameliorate symptoms or slow progression will further reduce acid load.

Metabolic alkalosis

Metabolic alkalosis may be caused either by excessive loss of acid or by intake of alkali. The latter may be iatrogenic, e.g. excessive intake of prescribed sodium bicarbonate, or excessive intake of 'drugs' to buffer gastric acidity in peptic ulcer disease – the 'milk-alkali' syndrome. Gastric acid may also be lost by vomiting when the gastric outlet is blocked (e.g. in pyloric stenosis). Compensation is by reduced lung ventilation to increase $P\text{co}_2$ and thus balance the Henderson–Hasselbach equation (eqn [5]). Treatment is that of the underlying condition rather than administration of acid.

Respiratory acidosis

Impaired lung ventilation (which increases $P\text{co}_2$ and therefore lowers pH; see eqn [5]) may occur either acutely or chronically. Causes for this include factors affecting the neurological 'drive' (e.g. head injury, cardiac arrest, opiate and anaesthetic drugs), diseases of the respiratory muscles (e.g. poliomyelitis, Guillain-Barré syndrome) or the lungs (either acutely, e.g. pulmonary oedema and pneumonia, or chronically, e.g. chronic bronchitis and emphysema). Acutely, pH may fall dramatically to values of around 7 in situations such as cardiorespiratory arrest. With chronic conditions the pH is generally nearer normal, complete compensation occurring in the kidney with the result that high carbon dioxide levels (in the region of 50–60 mmHg) are balanced by increased plasma bicarbonate generated in the kidney (eqn [5]).

Respiratory alkalosis

Respiratory alkalosis occurs as a result of overventilation and inappropriate loss of carbon dioxide, often as part of a response to pain or hysteria. Such effects are short-lived and can be corrected by rebreathing expired air or by sedation. Alternative causes include the early phases of aspirin poisoning (where the respiratory centres are activated), hypoxia and conditions (e.g. stroke) affecting the brain stem region. These conditions are rare and long-term adaptive changes would involve the excretion of bicarbonate, but they are seldom seen.

See also: **Carbohydrates**: Regulation of Carbohydrate Metabolism. **Glucose**: Metabolism and Maintenance of Blood Glucose Level. **Renal Function and Disorders**: Nutritional Management of Renal Disorders.

Further Reading

Brenner BM and Rector FC, eds (1991) *The Kidney*. St Louis: Mosby.

Brenner BM, Coe FL and Rector FC (1987) *Renal Physiology – in Health and Disease*. Philadelphia: WB Saunders.

Bruckner PJ (1986) Water, electrolyte and hydrogen ion disorders. In: Gornall AG (ed.) *Applied Biochemistry of Clinical Disorders*, 2nd edn, pp 99–128. Philadelphia: Lippincott.

Cohen RD and Woods HF (1986) Disturbances of acid–base homeostasis. In: Weatherall DJ, Ledingham JGG and Warrell DA (eds) *Oxford Textbook of Medicine*. Oxford University Press.

Paul AA and Southgate DAT, eds. (1978) *McCance and Widdowson's The Composition of Foods*. London: HMSO.

ENERGY

Contents

Energy Requirements

P S Shetty, London School of Hygiene and Tropical Medicine, London, UK

Copyright © 1998 Academic Press

Food is required by the body for a variety of purposes. One important function is to supply energy for the biological tasks essential for the maintenance of life. Energy is also needed for all human activity in the social sphere at the community level. An adequate supply of food energy is therefore essential to maintain all functions of the body and the range of daily activities at maximum efficiency thus ensuring a healthy life for the individual in the community. Food energy requirements need to be estimated quantitatively at the level of the individual to ensure good health and at the level of the community or population for the purpose of planning food supplies, for evaluating the adequacy of current food supplies and for the detection and enumeration of those individuals within the community or population who are not achieving adequate levels of food energy intake.

Food Energy

The three principal constituents of our diet, also called the *proximate principles*, are carbohydrates, proteins and fats. Unlike other nutrients in food, carbohydrates, proteins and fats constitute the bulk of the nutrients in our daily diet and are hence referred to as 'macronutrients'. Macronutrients are the principal sources of energy in food although their relative contributions in our diet may vary. The chemical energy contained in the macronutrients in our food can be determined using a bomb calorimeter. The energy content of macronutrients determined by bomb calorimetry is referred to as *gross energy*. However, not all the gross energy in any of the macronutrients in our food is available when we eat the food. There are two important reasons for this:

1. Not all the food eaten is absorbed from the digestive tract to become available as fuel for metabolism or for use by the body. It has been estimated that, of the macronutrients from a typical Western diet, 99% of ingested carbohydrates, 92% of protein and 95% of fat are absorbed from the gut.
2. Proteins, which contain nitrogen, are not com-

pletely oxidized by the body. They are converted largely to urea and excreted in urine; the urea so lost retains about 25% of the chemical energy of the original protein that was ingested in the diet.

Energy lost to the body by nonabsorption in the gut and hence excreted in the faeces, and also that lost by excretion as nitrogenous waste products (mainly as urea) in urine, needs to be subtracted from the gross energy of food to estimate the available energy to the body. This is referred to as the *metabolizable energy* of the food. In experimental situations, the metabolizable energy intake of individuals on a mixed diet can be determined by bomb calorimetry of the ingested food and of the faeces and urine excreted following its ingestion. To simplify the determination of the metabolizable energy content of foods, Atwater estimated the metabolizable energy content of the macronutrients separately. The metabolizable energy content of the diet (or ingested food) can then be estimated from the amounts of the individual macronutrients in the diet. These values of metabolizable energy for the macronutrients are referred to as the Atwater Factors (**Table 1**).

Energy Intake

Until recent times much of the basis for estimating energy requirements was indirectly derived from data on energy intakes. The Expert Consultation of the food and Agriculture Organization (FAO), World Health Organization (WHO) and United Nations University (UNU), however, concluded that as a matter of principle estimates of energy requirements should, as far as possible, be based on estimates of energy expenditure, whether actual or desirable. The Consultation felt that determining requirements from observed intakes is largely a circular argument, since in both developed and developing countries actual intakes are not necessarily those that maintain desirable body weights or optimal levels of physical activity, and hence health in its broadest sense. However, the Consultation recognized that it is not

Table 1   Calculation of metabolizable energy contents

Macronutrient	Percentage absorbed (%)	Gross energy (kJ g⁻¹)	Digestable energy (kJ g⁻¹)	Urinary loss (kJ g⁻¹)	Metabolizable energy (kJ g⁻¹)	Atwater factor (kcal g⁻¹)
Carbohydrates						
Glucose	99	15.6	15.4	–	15.4	4
Starch	99	17.5	17.3	–	17.3	4
Protein	92	22.9	21.1	5.2	15.9	4
Fat	95	39.1	37.1	–	37.1	9
Alcohol	100	29.8	29.8	trace	29.8	7

always possible to follow this principle because adequate information on total energy expenditure may not be available in some subsections of the population such as infants and children.

In groups of healthy adults of normal weight, energy intake measurements over 7 or more days by weighed inventory techniques have been found to agree well with estimates of energy expenditure in the same group over the same period. However, the agreement between intakes and expenditure in the same individual is less consistent and convincing as compared with the agreement observed between the means of two groups for both intakes and expenditure. It is recognized that methods for the measurement of energy intake are less reliable than previously thought and that even the most careful and meticulous collection of dietary intake data is subject to bias owing to underreporting or changes in food or eating habits, or owing to random and systematic errors associated with the various techniques used for the measurement of dietary intake. This seriously undermines the representative nature of the measurement to provide a reasonably accurate estimate of an individual's habitual intake. Several studies have shown that energy intake estimates are consistently lower than estimates of energy expenditure using reliable noninvasive methods that allow the measurement of habitual energy expenditure in free-living situations. Hence it is reasonable to assume that estimates of energy intake may not reflect habitual daily intakes of energy and should not be relied upon to estimate requirements, except where data on total energy expenditure are lacking in some population subgroups such as infants and young children. Since observed energy intakes even when accurate need not reflect desirable intakes, measurements of energy expenditure are preferred as the basis for estimating requirements.

Energy Expenditure

The FAO/WHO/UNU Expert Consultation in 1985 adopted the principle of relying on estimates of energy expenditure rather than energy intake from dietary surveys to estimate the energy requirements of populations. It is generally recognized that in a group of apparently healthy and comparable individuals there is a considerable between-individual variation in habitual, total daily energy expenditure. This, however, is known not to be as large as the between-individual variation in energy intakes. Total energy expenditure (TEE) during a day is considered to be made up of three components: (1) *basal metabolic rate* (BMR) which is the largest single component of 24 h expenditure and comprises from 60%

to over 70% of TEE; (2) the *thermogenic* component, which is the excess energy expended over the basal rate owing to the physiological response following the ingestion of food or following an exposure to cold or to pharmacological agents such as caffeine, and nicotine; and (3) *physical activity* – the contribution of this component to TEE will depend on the intensity and the duration of the activity indulged in by the individual. The contribution of the level of physical activity to energy expenditure is important when assessing energy needs. Some activities are essential for an individual and the community and are generally economic activities which are life-sustaining; these are termed 'occupational' activities. Other activities, which are considered desirable for the wellbeing of the community and the health of the individual, are termed 'discretionary' activities. These include activities considered under three broad categories: optional household tasks (such as working in the home or garden), socially desirable activities (such as participation in games, religious activities, etc.) and activity for physical fitness and the promotion of health (e.g. leisure-time exercise undertaken for physical or cardiovascular fitness).

Many factors influence the total energy expenditure and hence the BMR in humans. Body size (body weight) is a major determinant, and accounts for more than half the between-subject variability in BMR. Body composition is another important determinant, since the fat and lean compartments of the body have different resting metabolisms. Sex differences in energy expenditure are largely accounted for by the differences in body composition between the sexes for the same body size. Age affects energy expenditure since the energy expended per kg of body weight declines as age increases. Diet, climate and the individual's physiological and psychological status all influence the energy expenditure of an individual, as does the administration of drugs and other pharmacological agents as well as the general health and presence of disease in an individual.

There are several methods for the measurement of energy expenditure as well as the different components of 24 h TEE. Indirect calorimetry has hitherto been the mainstay of a wide range of techniques, both in the laboratory and in the field, which have been used to measure total energy expenditure or its components in individuals. Newer techniques using stable isotopes have revolutionized the study of human energy expenditure under free-living conditions. The doubly labelled water (DLW) technique of measuring total energy expenditure permits determination of free-living energy expenditure integrated over a period of days, usually 7–20 days. This technique has contributed much to our current understanding of the energy requirements of infants, children, adolescents, adults and the elderly (men and women) as well as the additional requirements associated with physiological states such as growth, pregnancy and lactation.

BMR and PAL

Since reliable data on the measurement of habitual energy expenditure in free-living adults are limited, measures or predictions of basal metabolic rate, which constitutes 60–70% of TEE, have gained importance. The BMR of an individual can simply be defined as 'the minimal rate of energy expenditure compatible with life'. It is measured under standard conditions of immobility in the fasted state (12–14 h after a meal), in an ambient environmental temperature of between 26–30°C to avoid activation of heat-generating processes such as shivering. The rate can be quantified by direct or indirect calorimetric techniques: the former measuring the heat output directly, while the latter measures the oxygen consumption (and carbon dioxide production), which can then be appropriately converted to their energy equivalents.

It is generally recognized that in a group of apparently healthy and comparable individuals there is a considerable between-individual variation in habitual, daily TEE, and since BMR constitutes 60–70% of TEE, these between-individual variations are expected to be reflected in the BMRs. Comparisons of subjects of similar body weight and body composition show that the coefficient of variation (CV) of the between-individual variability of BMR is of the same order as that of TEE, i.e. about 12.5%. It appears that the CV of between-individual variations depends upon the variations in body size; the larger the variation in body weight among subjects, the larger the CV of TEE and hence of BMRs. Overwhelming evidence also supports the view that within-individual variations in BMR of the same subject are small and probably insignificant, even when neither the intakes nor the activity patterns of the individual are controlled. Further, analysis of data on the variations in BMR over long periods indicates that the BMR of individuals is constant over time and remains relatively constant over a period of several years, despite reasonable fluctuations in body weight, when no attempt is made to regulate either energy intake or physical activity patterns. Whether the methods used to measure BMR contribute to the variability in rates between individuals is a question that also needs to be addressed if BMR is the basis for estimating TEE using the factorial method.

Measurements of BMR involve in the first instance an estimation of the oxygen consumption of the individual, which is then converted into units of heat or energy output. In general, most investigators involved in BMR measurements use a range of techniques to estimate oxygen consumption which provide more or less the same results. Given the errors that arise as a result of the assumptions made during the conversion and final calculation of BMR (in kcal or kJ) from measures of oxygen consumption, differences in BMR between individuals or groups of individuals of the order of 5% do not have biological significance unless the methodology, the assumptions made and the calculations used to arrive at the BMR values are comparable. It can hence be assumed that given that certain stipulated minimal experimental prerequisites (such as absence of gross muscular activity, a postabsorptive state, thermoneutral environment, etc.) are strictly met in order to ensure basal levels of metabolism, then BMR measurements made between individuals or in the same individual over time are comparable.

The BMR can also be predicted with reasonable accuracy (i.e. with a coefficient of variation of 8%) in adults using predictive equations. Conventionally BMR is measured using direct or indirect calorimetry and although BMR may be accurately measured using these techniques, it is simpler, in practice, to use predictive equations. Schofield has presented gender-specific predictive equations for the following age groups: 0–3, 3–10, 10–18, 18–30, 30–60 and > 60 years. These predictive equations from the basis of the factorial approach used by the FAO/WHO/UNU report to estimate energy requirements. The BMR has thus become fundamental for estimating human energy requirements.

When total energy expenditure is expressed as a multiple of the BMR (i.e. TEE/BMR) it is referred to as the 'physical activity level' or PAL. The expression of total daily energy expenditure (or requirements) of adults as PAL (i.e. as multiples of BMR) provides a convenient way of controlling for age, sex, weight and body composition and for expressing the energy needs of a wide range of people in shorthand form. The figures derived by the 1985 Consultation were based on theoretical factorial calculations making assumptions about energy cost and duration of day-to-day activities. The PAL provides a useful means of categorizing energy requirements in a single number, taking into account differences in body size as represented by BMR. However, the value of PAL depends both on BMR and TEE, and both have errors of measurements, so that PAL is only imprecisely estimated. The CV of BMRs when actually measured is small, while the CV of BMRs predicted using the Schofield equations for a given body weight is of the order of about 8%. For TEE, the within-individual CV can be obtained from studies with repeated DLW measurements where weight, activity and physiological state have been controlled for and remained the same. Data collated from nine such studies have shown that the mean within-individual CV for 79 subjects was 8.9%, and this includes methodological error as well as variations in activity levels. Thus, the 95% confidence limits on PALs at the individual level, assuming a measured BMR and no change in body weight or physical activity level is of the order of $\pm 18.5\%$ representing about ± 0.3 PAL units on a mean PAL value of 1.65.

Energy Requirements

Nutritional requirements are estimated from our knowledge of the body's ability to absorb, store, metabolize and excrete the nutrient. The level of requirement of a nutrient can be specified as the amount required to avoid a deficiency state, to ensure normal body function and metabolism, or to achieve sufficient levels of body reserves of the nutrient. It is also essential to recognize that individuals vary in their requirements for that nutrient. Since recommendations for nutrient requirements are meant for population groups, any estimate of the requirement of a nutrient for the population group must consider this variability and attempt to cover the requirements of all, if not almost all the individuals, in this population group. This is usually done by choosing the mean + 2 standard deviations (SD) of the observed requirements in that group of individuals such that the estimate of the requirement for that nutrient covers at least 97% of that population's nutrient requirement. This estimate is often referred to as the recommended daily allowance (RDA) or recommended dietary intake (RDI). This general concept for nutritional requirements holds good for all nutrients *except* energy. Requirements for energy differ from those for other nutrients, because the consumption of more or less energy than is needed will result in body weight changes. The relatively fixed nature of each individual's requirement and the variation in requirements of a group implies that if requirements for energy are made using the same principles as for the other nutrients (i.e. mean of the group + 2 SD), then nearly all the population will exceed their individual requirements. Hence the requirement for energy is always recommended as the mean of that population group.

The FAO/WHO/UNU Expert Consultation defined the energy requirement of an individual as 'the energy intake which will balance energy expenditure when the individual has a body size and composition and level of physical activity consistent with long-term good health; and will allow for the maintenance of economically necessary and socially desirable physical activity. In children and pregnant or lactating women, the energy requirement includes the energy need associated with the deposition of tissues or the secretion of milk at rates consistent with good health'.

When an individual is maintaining a constant body weight, i.e. neither gaining nor losing weight, then the individual's energy intake must balance or be equal to the energy expenditure. Hence, in infants and children growing normally and gaining weight at an acceptable rate, energy requirements were formerly based on measures of energy intake, since data on TEE in this group were limited until the advent of the DLW technique. More recent data suggest that the energy requirements of infants and children under the age of 10 years tend to be overestimated, based on observed energy intakes compared with estimates based on TEE.

In healthy adults of normal weight estimates of energy intake have been generally found to agree well with estimates based on TEE. The currently accepted approach to estimate energy requirement in adults is to use the *factorial* method. This involves the measurement of BMR or its prediction from body weight using the age- and gender-specific equations of Schofield. Once BMR has been measured or predicted, TEE can be estimated by multiplying the BMR by the PAL value for the level of activity of the individual: light, moderate or heavy (**Table 2**). Since physical activity includes both occupational and non-occupational or socially desirable activities, provision can be made for the additional energy expended in the latter. This is essential when assessing, for example, the energy requirement of a sedentary adult in an industrialized country, where it is recommended that good health is promoted by the maintenance of optimum body weight for which a short period of physical exercise may be required,

Table 2 Average daily energy requirement of adults in occupational work classified as light, moderate or heavy, expressed as a multiple of basal metabolic rate (i.e. physical activity level, PAL)

Type of work	PAL	
	Men	Women
Light	1.55	1.56
Moderate	1.78	1.64
Heavy	2.10	1.82

in contrast with the requirement of an agricultural worker in a developing country who requires additional energy to meet the needs of socially desirable activities after habitual heavy physical activity at work. Since TEE and BMR are dependent on age, sex, body weight and the level of habitual physical activity, the energy requirements of adults would be influenced largely by these variables. The factorial method takes into consideration these variables since the BMR is measured or predicted taking age, sex and body weight into account and the PAL provides a measure of the level of habitual activity. It is thus evident that the variations in energy requirement of a group of adults in a population will be largely determined by these very same factors.

Pregnant and lactating women have additional energy needs to provide for optimum weight gain and fetal growth during pregnancy and for the production of adequate quantities of milk during lactation. The total energy needs of pregnancy have been estimated to be of the order of 335 MJ (80 000 kcal), which is equivalent to an additional energy intake averaging 1.2 MJ (285 kcal) per day throughout the 9 months of pregnancy over and above the average requirement estimated by the factorial method. This additional energy is required for the growth and development of the fetus and the other tissues such as the placenta, uterus and breasts, as well as to increase the adipose tissue stores in preparation for lactation. In well-nourished populations the weight gain during pregnancy is expected to be of the order of 12.5 kg with a median infant birthweight of 3.3 kg (with a CV of 15%). However, these additional requirements may be an overestimate in well-nourished and affluent pregnant women who may resort to possible energy-saving adjustments by reducing their levels of daily physical activity during the latter half of pregnancy, and the total requirement throughout pregnancy may be as low as 170 MJ (40 000 kcal). The incremental energy costs associated with normal lactation can be considered to be equivalent to breast milk volume × energy density of milk × conversion efficiency of dietary energy for milk secretion. In lactation, some of the additional energy requirements may be met by the adipose tissue stores laid down during a normal pregnancy. The estimated energy cost therefore needs to be reduced by the energy mobilized from the maternal adipose tissue stores and possible savings from reduced levels of maternal physical activity during the lactation period. If adequate volumes of breast milk (approximately 850 ml) are secreted per day of an estimated energy density of 3.0 kJ g^{-1} (0.72 kcal g^{-1}) with an estimated efficiency of production of 80%, the net increase in energy require-

ments for milk production is estimated at around 2.9 MJ (700 kcal) per day. Since an average woman will start lactation with a surplus of 150 MJ (36 000 kcal) of stored energy, and assuming that normal body weight and composition will be established within 6 months by utilizing this surplus, the excess energy requirements of normal lactation can be estimated to be about 2.1 MJ (500 kcal) per day. More recent recommendations for the additional energy requirements of lactation are as follows: 2.65 MJ (635 kcal) per day for 0–6 months without any fat loss or 2.00 MJ (480 kcal) per day allowing for fat loss; and 2.2 MJ (525 kcal) per day beyond 6 months for full breast-feeders or 1.2 MJ (285 kcal) per day for partial breast-feeders.

Estimates of energy requirements have both diagnostic and prescriptive applications. At the population level it is useful for nutritionists, planners and government agencies to assess the adequacy of food intakes of populations, for the identification of vulnerable groups within populations, for purposes of surveillance and monitoring and for the planning of food production and food supplies for population groups, large and small.

See also: **Energy**: Energy Balance; Measurement of Energy Intake and Expenditure. **Energy Metabolism:** Tricarboxylic Acid Cycle and Oxidative Phosphorylation. **Lactation**: Dietary Requirements. **Pregnancy**: Energy Requirements and Metabolic Adaptations.

Further Reading

IDECG (1996) Energy and protein requirements. *European Journal of Clinical Nutrition* 50:S1–197.

James WPT and Schofield EC (1990) *Human Energy Requirements*. Oxford: Oxford Medical.

World Health Organization (1985) *Energy and Protein Requirements*. Report of the joint FAO/WHO/UNU Expert Consultation. Technical Report Series 724. WHO: Geneva.

Energy Balance

Daniel J Hoffman and **Ana Lydia Sawaya**, Federal University of São Paulo, Brazil

Copyright © 1998 Academic Press

Principles of Energy Balance

Basic aspects of energy metabolism

The metabolism of nutrients (i.e. energy) in the human body is dictated by the First Law of Thermodynamics, which states that within any closed system energy is neither created nor destroyed, it simply changes form [eqn (1)].

$$\text{Energy intake} = \text{Energy output} \tag{1}$$

Energy metabolism is influenced by the amount and quality of energy in food and the cellular expenditure of energy. This emphasizes the concept that energy metabolism begins with the biochemical reactions within each and every cell. These reactions, forming the complex and wonderfully coordinated series of metabolic pathways such as the Krebs cycle, the Embden–Meyerof pathway or the electron transport chain, are the driving forces behind cellular energy metabolism.

Within each living cell these reactions serve to provide one function: to generate energy for cellular function. A corollary of this function is that these reactions must operate in such a manner as to protect the cell from energy excesses or deficits. To this end the body is able to store excess energy and utilize this stored energy during periods of energy deficits [eqn (2)].

$$\text{Energy intake} = \text{Energy output} \pm \text{Energy stored} \tag{2}$$

Energy intake is simply the ingestion of the nutrients lipids (LIP), carbohydrates (CHO) and proteins (PRO). When these components are utilized by the body during normal metabolism, along with the incorporation of molecular oxygen and water (O_2 and H_2O), the major products are carbon dioxide (CO_2), water, urea and heat (**Fig. 1**). Excess CHO is stored as glycogen (the primary CHO storage compartment of the body), with any additional unused energy converted to and stored as adipose tissue. Energy output is the energy used for reactions occurring within metabolically active cells of the body.

Energy intake

The intake of nutrients is one of the most difficult aspects of human energy metabolism to study because there are so many influences on food intake. Food intake is dependent on food availability and palatability, social and familial influences, the psychological state of the person, composition of a meal, amount and type of exercise, and possibly body composition. Nevertheless, it appears as though the fundamental controls of food intake arise from a combination of psychosocial and metabolic/physiological factors.

Cultural influences can greatly modify food intake. This is most evident when the differences in the quality of foods consumed in different countries throughout the world are considered. For example, the high-fat diet of the USA is quite different from the high-carbohydrate diet of the Mediterranean region. In addition, many social/psychological factors can greatly influence the quantity of food intake, as seen by the high prevalence of anorexia nervosa in industrialized countries. All of these factors tend to shape a person's perception of food. Thus, these outside forces modify the normal biological signals controlling food intake.

Energy output

The output of energy, energy expenditure, is made up of the energy that is used to maintain homeostatic processes and accommodate physical activity, as well as that lost as heat. The oxidation of CHO, LIP and PRO produces ATP through the reactions of the tricarboxylic acid cycle (TCA or Krebs cycle) and the electron transport system (ETS) within the cell membranes of mitochondria (**Fig. 2**). The synthesis of ATP requires oxygen at the level of the TCA and ETS in the mitochondria to generate the hydrogen gradient which drives the proton pump needed to bind inorganic phosphate (P_i) to ADP. Synthesis of 1 mole of ATP requires 75 kJ (18 kcal), and is used as a source of energy for the synthesis of DNA, PRO, glycogen, and hormones, intracellular movement of molecules, metabolism of nutrients, and the contraction of muscles.

Since the rate of ATP synthesis dictates the amount of oxygen consumed by the body during any given period of time, measurements of the volume of

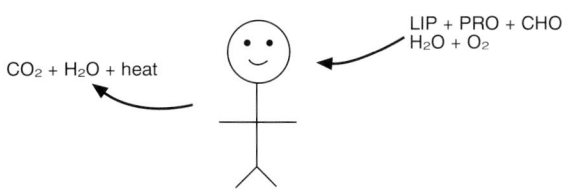

Figure 1 Major components of energy input and output.

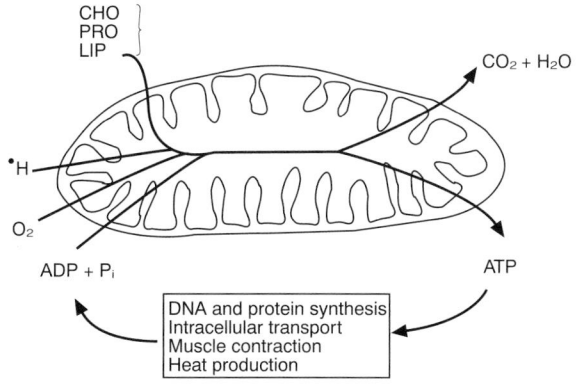

Figure 2 Mitochondrial energy expenditure with major uses of ATP.

oxygen consumed by a person reflects the energy used during a period of time. Similarly, measurements of heat produced and volume of carbon dioxide expired by a person, both products of ATP utilization, reflect energy expenditure. The majority of this activity is taking place in those cells which require a high rate of turnover, protein synthesis, membrane activity, and so on. Thus, cells of metabolically active tissues and organs (e.g. liver, brain or kidney) contribute the greatest amount of energy consumption to the total energy expenditure (TEE). Cells of metabolically less active tissues (muscle) or those with negligible activity (adipose tissue) contribute little if any to the TEE. A small amount of energy is used during cycles which provide substrates for other metabolic processes; these cycles are of great importance, but are unfortunately referred to as 'futile' cycles.

Components of total energy expenditure

The expenditure of energy can be categorized according to the principle use of the energy expended (**Fig. 3**). Thus, energy used to maintain homeostasis is referred to as the basal metabolic rate (BMR) and in adults reflects the energy used for basal functioning of metabolically active cells in the body, the lean body mass (LBM). The thermic effect of feeding (TEE) is the amount of energy expended in the process of metabolizing and storing nutrients following a meal. The amount of energy expended which is not part of either BMR or TEF is called the energy expenditure of physical activity and arousal (PA).

The contribution of each component to TEE is represented in Fig. 3. The BMR is responsible for about 60–70% of TEE. The TEF of a person accounts for 8–12% of the TEE, varying with the size and composition of the meal consumed. The PA, the most variable component between individuals, accounts for 15–30% of TEE. In addition, the proportion of TEE accounted for by each component varies depending on body composition, age, genetic make-up, diet and environment.

In rodents, there is another small but important component of energy expenditure known as facultative thermogenesis, which is created mainly by brown adipose tissue (BAT) activity. BAT is activated by the sympathetic nervous system, low environmental temperatures, meal composition and palatability, and results in thermogenesis by BAT, increasing the TEE. Conversely, warm temperatures and decrease in food intake inhibits BAT thermogenesis, lowering the TEE.

Basal metabolic rate   The BMR is generally a reflection of the amount of LBM in the body, thus it is often reported as BMR per kilogram body weight (kg BW) or per kilogram LBM (kg LBM) varying with age, gender, state of health and fitness. For example, BMR per kg BW is higher in children than in adults since children have a greater proportion of highly active tissues (brain, liver, etc.) than adults (**Fig. 4**). As a child grows and acquires more muscle and body fat, this proportion decreases along with the BMR per kg BW. This same principle applies to the elderly, who gain adipose tissue during the ageing process. The result is a very low ratio of active tissue to nonactive tissue and the overall BMR decreases. Illness can also affect BMR; burn victims have an increased BMR, stimulated by the increased activity of cells replicating to replace lost or damaged tissue.

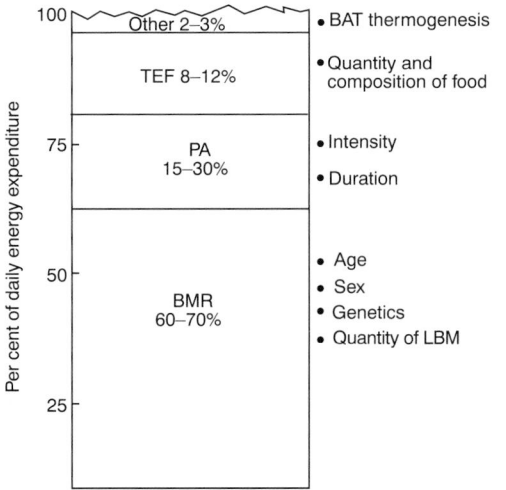

Figure 3   Components of daily energy expenditure.

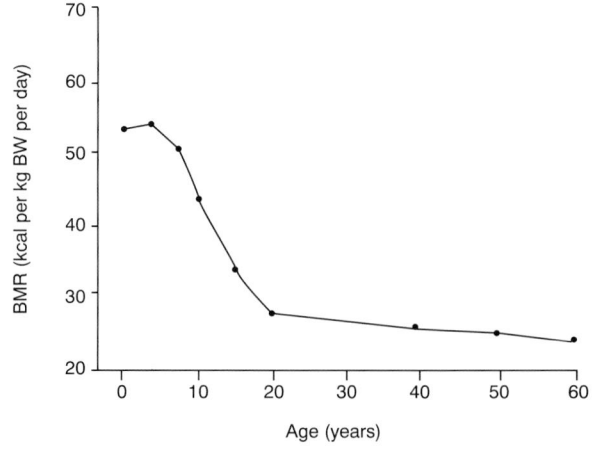

Figure 4   Changes in basal metabolic rate per kilogram body weight from birth to age 60 years.

Thermic effect of feeding This was traditionally called diet-induced thermogenesis, since the amount of heat released from an individual increases following a meal, reflecting the energy expended during metabolism of the food (**Fig. 5**). A typical study of TEF begins with a measurement of an individual's BMR. A standard test meal is provided, either delivering the same caloric load to all persons or the same number of calories per kg BW. The metabolic rate is then measured for a period of time (2–12 h postprandial) and the increase in the metabolic rate is considered the TEF. Since the 1960s great strides have been made in understanding TEF, but many questions remain unanswered and the number of factors that influence TEF is still unclear. These factors may vary from fuel mix, energy load and age to stress, timing of the meal and body composition. The main reason so much research has provided so few concrete answers is that TEF, as defined, is extremely difficult to measure. The difficulty lies in the fact that heat and carbon dioxide generated by the individual postprandially vary according to those factors mentioned above.

Still, despite the complexities and challenges in studying TEF, answers to some of the questions appear to be emerging. It may be that TEF is one of the components of TEE that promotes obesity. Obese persons tend to have a lower TEF than lean persons, resulting in less energy being expended for metabolic purposes and more energy being stored. Doubts remain concerning this idea since lean persons show a reduced TEF when their abdominal areas are insulated, mimicking the insulation provided by abdominal adipose tissue in obese persons. This suggests that the quantity of abdominal adipose tissue may influence TEF rather than the state of being obese. Also, since TEF accounts for only 10% of TEF, the variability of methods used to measure TEF may make detecting differences between individuals difficult.

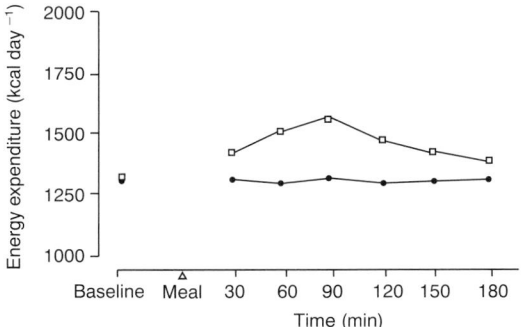

Figure 5 Energy expenditure in postprandial phase comparison with postabsorptive phase (●).

Physical activity and arousal The PA represents the amount of energy expended for exercise and for arousal (energy used by simply being awake and fidgeting normally). PA is the one controllable component of TEE, but it is also the most variable component of TEE since it depends on the condition of the person and the amount and intensity of any exercise in which he or she participates. Thus, for two persons of identical body composition (hence BMR), age and gender, the amount of PA can decide whether one person has a high or low TEE compared with the other person; the difference in TEE influenced solely by fidgeting can range from 840 to 3400 kJ day^{-1} (200 to 800 kcal day^{-1}). In addition, it is also important to consider the type, duration and intensity of exercise contributing to PA. For example, walking 3.5 km (2 miles) at a slow pace may be strenuous for one person, but it may only be a warm-up for another. However, it has been reported that, given sufficient intensity, the influence of exercise on TEE diminishes after 30 min of PA a day.

While 30 min of exercise a day may seem minimal, in the area of obesity research it has proven to be an extremely important and fundamental factor in the prevention of obesity. A strong, negative correlation between exercise and obesity exists suggesting that persons participating in little or no exercise, and thus having a minimal influence of PA on TEE, are more likely to be obese. Also, it is agreed that the decrease in exercise throughout the world, especially in developed countries, has been a major contributor to the increased worldwide prevalence of obesity.

Control of Energy Metabolism

It has been known since the 1950s that the hypothalamus is the most important region of the brain in the control of food intake and metabolism. This conclusion was drawn from several experiments which demonstrated that lesions in the hypothalamus resulted in either hyper- or hypophagia, depending on the region in which the lesions were situated. Also, electrical stimulation of different hypothalamic regions inhibited or stimulated feeding. In 1954 Stellar formulated the hypothesis that the hypothalamus contained two centres that controlled food intake: a satiety centre in the ventromedial hypothalamus and a hunger centre at the lateral hypothalamus. It is now recognized that the control of the food intake is much more complex and it is regulated in association with many other areas in the nervous system. In spite of this greater complexity, the hypothalamus is still considered to be the main region in control of food intake regulation.

According to variations in the quality and quantity

of food ingested, the body searches to regulate its metabolism in order to maintain homeostasis; the most important regulatory signal is the blood glucose levels. Homeostatic control is achieved through a series of activation/inhibition signals of the hypothalamic sympathetic and parasympathetic nervous system, and hypothalamic hormones responsible for the control of peripheral hormones and metabolism, such as corticotrophin releasing hormone (CRH), growth hormone releasing hormone (GHRH), thyroid releasing hormone (TRH), and so on.

Hypothalamic neurotransmitters

Neuropeptide Y Many substrates produced in the hypothalamus have recently been recognized as being important controllers of food intake and energy expenditure, and therefore energy balance. The most abundant peptide yet discovered in the mammalian brain is neuropeptide Y (NPY), which contains 36 amino acids and belongs to the pancreatic polypeptide family. NPY, widely expressed by neurons in the central and peripheral nervous systems as well as by adrenal medullary cells, strongly activates food intake, having its main biosynthetic site in the arcuate nucleus of the hypothalamus. Neurons that produce NPY project axons to several other hypothalamic nuclei including the paraventricular nucleus, a key brain area for the stimulation of feeding behaviour. Since daily injections of NPY in the hypothalamic paraventricular nucleus cause an increase in food intake and body weight gain in rodents, this neuropeptide is thought to be involved in both single-meal and long-term energy regulation. For example, NPY expression seems to be disturbed in genetically obese animals, since food deprivation fails to elicit significant elevation of hypothalamic preproNPY mRNA levels as it does in lean animals.

The anabolic action of NPY is also mediated by metabolic and hormonal actions favourable to the deposition of fat, including elevation in the activity of the lipoprotein lipase in white adipose tissue, enhanced lipogenesis in either liver or white adipose tissue, and increased secretion of insulin and glucocorticoids into the circulation. It is also believed that catabolic states that deplete energy stores, such as starvation and insulin-deficient diabetes, stimulate both production and release of NPY, thereby elevating anabolic processes and food intake and decreasing energy expenditure. These effects are mediated by two glucoregulatory hormones: insulin and glucocorticoids. NPY also modulates secretion of gonadotrophin releasing hormone (GnRH), cardiovascular function and sympathetic activity, and may also influence the glucocorticoid, growth hormone and thyroid axes.

Corticotrophin releasing hormone In contrast to the anabolic role of NPY, corticotrophin releasing hormone (CRH), another hypothalamic neuropeptide, is considered to be the most important catabolic stimulating substrate; CRH functions as the primary trigger of the hypothalamic–pituitary–adrenal axis. CRH contains 41 amino acids and is synthesized in the paraventricular nucleus of the hypothalamus. The actions of CRH promote a negative energy balance through the suppression of food intake, coupled with stimulation of sympathetic outflow that increases lipolysis and energy expenditure, while raising blood glucose and inhibiting the expected increase of insulin secretion. This is demonstrated by the reduction in food intake and loss of weight by chronic, central CRH administration in normal animals and genetically obese rats. CRH also works directly in opposition to the effects of NPY since inhibition of the gene expression of NPY in the arcuate nucleus is observed after CRH infusion in the brain.

In addition to these two hypothalamic neuropeptides, which are considered to be major neuroregulators of food intake and energy balance, many other molecules are believed to be involved in the control of energy balance, with either catabolic or anabolic effects, as seen in **Table 1**.

Table 1 Some candidate signalling molecules used by central effector pathways involved in the control of energy balance

	Effect on food intake	Effect on sympathetic nervous system
Catabolic		
Corticotrophin releasing hormone	⇓ ⇓	⇑ ⇑
Bombesin	⇓	⇑
Somatostatin	⇓	?
Cholecystokinin	⇓	⇑
Thyrotrophin releasing hormone	⇓	?
Calcitonin gene-related peptide	⇓	⇑
Neurotensin	⇓	⇑
Serotonin	⇓	⇑
Anabolic		
Neutropeptide Y	⇑ ⇑	⇓ ⇓
Galanin	⇑	?
β-Endorphin	⇑	⇓
Dynorphin	⇑	?
Growth hormone releasing hormone	⇑	⇓
Norepinephrine	⇑	⇓

Sympathetic nervous system

Most of the neuropeptides that control energy balance also influence autonomic activity, as shown by the stimulation and inhibition of sympathetic nervous system activity by CRH and NPY, respectively. The sympathetic nervous system controls the fate of ingested energy as it is stimulated by feeding and increases the TEF. In fact, experimental genetic obesities are often accompanied by an impaired sympathetic nervous system response to food intake and diminished regulation of body temperature, resulting in diversion of energy to fat stores.

Insulin

It has long been recognized that insulin plays an important role in the control of food intake and energy balance. Insulin can inhibit food intake after both central and systemic administration. However, this negative effect on food intake is opposed by insulin's potent anabolic stimulation in peripheral tissues. This is particularly evident in the treatment of uncontrolled insulin-dependent diabetes, where the normalization of blood glucose concentrations with insulin treatment causes weight gain despite reduced food intake. Insulin has also been shown to have an effect on the stimulation of the sympathetic nervous system and thermogenesis; TEF is partly dependent on insulin secretion. Central insulin infusion also potentiates the satiety effect of peripherally administered cholecystokinin and of centrally administered CRH. Therefore, insulin administered centrally promotes a state of negative energy balance by acting in all these above mechanisms, in opposition to insulin's potent anabolic stimulation in peripheral tissues.

Role of glucocorticoid–insulin interactions

Glucocorticoids are important components in the control of energy metabolism, as seen by their role in fat deposition and their inhibition of biosynthesis of CRH by negative feedback. Also, the ratio of glucocorticoids to insulin (G : I) may be one of the major antagonistic, long-term regulators of energy balance.

Insulin and glucocorticoids have mutually antagonistic actions in the CNS, such as the stimulation or inhibition of NPY expression in the hypothalamus by glucocorticoids or insulin, respectively. Moreover, central administration of glucocorticoids stimulates food intake whereas insulin inhibits food intake. In the periphery the G : I ratio also has important influences on energy metabolism since body weight decreases as the G : I ratio increases. Despite this relationship, the two hormones do not interact as closely in their influence on weight as they do in food intake. They appear to act in parallel, but in different target storage organs. This is seen in patients with Cushing's syndrome, who have truncal obesity and atrophied extremities while presenting with hypercortisolaemia, hyperinsulinaemia and hyperglycaemia. In fact, increased activity of glucocorticoids is associated with truncal obesity and increased waist-to-hip ratio even in patients of normal weight. Therefore, in general, one could say that elevated glucocorticoid and insulin signals redistribute body energy stores. Glucocorticoids are not seen as the primary long-term modulators of fat deposition and energy metabolism, since they respond to other factors, such as stress. Rather, they are viewed as key modulators of insulin's potency as a long-term signal, especially in the regulation of energy storage.

Glucagon

The effects of peripherally or intracerebroventricularly administered glucagon on energy metabolism are mediated by numerous and complex effects on carbohydrate, fat and protein metabolism, as well as by effects on thermogenesis, body weight and feeding. Intraparaventricular injections of glucagon increase energy expenditure, respiratory quotient and blood glucose concentration without affecting locomotor activity or 24 h food and water intake. The effect in the respiratory quotient is long-lasting and dose-dependent and more pronounced than in total energy expenditure. These findings suggest that glucagon's effect is primarily by inducing the preferential utilization of carbohydrates and sparing of fat reserves.

Thyroid hormones

The general classic effect of thyroid hormones in mammals is to increase energy expenditure and heat production. This is accomplished through the stimulation of metabolic pathways in most tissues, basically through nuclear induction of protein synthesis. For example, high levels of thyroid hormones induce lipolysis in the white adipose tissue, proteolysis in muscle, and glycogenolysis in liver. Thyroid hormones also play an essential role in facultative thermogenesis, interacting with the sympathetic nervous system at various levels, potentiating the effects of the sympathetic nervous system. The enzyme thyroxine-5′-deiodinase, which converts thyroxine to triiodothyronine, plays a central role in controlling heat production in the BAT. In general the effects of thyroid hormone in stimulating energy expenditure are long-lasting, and one single injection of thyroxine may increase basal metabolic rate for over 30 days.

Leptin

The recent discovery of the protein leptin has shed new light on the relationship between adiposity, food intake and the metabolic perturbations that may cause obesity. Leptin is a hormone secreted by adipose tissue that has been shown to have significant effects on food intake, metabolism and physical activity in rodents. Animal studies have revealed that mice with a defect in the leptin gene (*ob/ob* mice) are hyperphagic, have depressed metabolisms, and become obese quickly and easily. When *ob/ob* and wild type mice are injected with leptin there is a decrease in voluntary food intake and an increase in TEE is seen in *ob/ob* mice only. While studies are just beginning to investigate the role of leptin in humans, the use of leptin as a marker for genetic studies of obesity and as a possible treatment for obesity appear promising.

Variations in Energy Metabolism

Effect of diet on energy metabolism

Diet influences the TEE by producing an increase or decrease in the TEF following a meal, for example high-energy meals increase TEF and subsequently TEE. Recently, an hypothesis has emerged relating diet composition to energy expenditure and food intake. It suggests a stronger and more direct association between increased oxidation of CHO and PRO than LIP in response to increased dietary intake. Generally, LIP oxidation is increased only through daily exercise or an increased fat mass (i.e. increased adiposity). Also, it is well known that the body is able to store extremely large amounts of LIP while CHO and PRO stores are relatively limited. Therefore, while excess CHO and PRO are oxidized at rates which meet their intake, excess dietary LIP are more likely to be stored.

The differences in storage capabilities and oxidation rates may also relate diet composition to food intake. Since CHO stores are much smaller than LIP stores, they are more likely to be depleted sooner during periods of low CHO intake. It is hypothesized that depletion of CHO stores stimulates food intake in an effort to replace these lost stores. Thus, a high-fat diet will maintain consistently low or depleted CHO stores and a high rate of signalling which promotes food intake. Conversely, a low-fat, high-CHO diet maintains adequate CHO stores with minimal food intake signals. Thus, this hypothesis explains how a high-fat, low-CHO diet, by promoting a high intake of calories to replace CHO stores, is related to the development of obesity.

Effect of ageing on energy metabolism

As a person ages the amount of energy expended usually decreases owing to a loss of LBM and a reduction in the intensity and amount of PA. This loss of LBM is accompanied by a decrease in BMR and, since few elderly persons actively reduce their food intake, excess energy is stored as adipose tissue. In addition, it is believed that elderly persons lose the ability to control food intake. For example, children who overeat at one meal or on one day will compensate for this excess by eating less at the subsequent meal or the next day. The elderly, on the other hand, often continue to eat the excess energy for an extended period of time, gradually returning to their normal intake. Also, the elderly may have a diminished TEF which predisposes them to obesity. This presents a difficult situation for the elderly since they are likely to have many nutritional challenges, such as difficulty swallowing, eating without teeth or with dentures, loss of the sense of taste and smell, and solitary living situations. Still, with the right nutritional counselling and guidance, an elderly person can continue to eat and enjoy foods while maintaining a healthy diet and weight.

Effect of exercise on energy metabolism

Exercise has two major effects on energy expenditure: it increases fat oxidation and the ratio of LBM to fat mass. Normally fat oxidation is not increased to meet fat intake until the mass of adipose tissue has increased to a large degree. Therefore, with exercise the rate of fat oxidation is increased, preventing the increase in adipose mass. Also, as LBM increases so does the BMR and TEE, thus preventing or limiting energy storage and obesity. A second important effect of exercise is that during the later stages of aerobic exercise, glucose and glycogen are spared as the body relies primarily on LIP oxidation for energy. This increases the amount of free fatty acids in the blood and, as suggested previously, could inhibit hunger signals, thus controlling appetite.

Effect of pregnancy on energy metabolism

During pregnancy energy needs increase because of the demands placed upon the organism by the developing fetus and the state of being pregnant. FAO/WHO/UNU recommends that pregnant women consume an additional 1200 kJ (~300 kcal) daily to accommodate for the nutritional needs of the fetus, provide sufficient maternal stores, and meet the increased energy needs produced by increased body mass during pregnancy.

The major changes in energy metabolism during gestation occur during the early phases of pregnancy when fetal tissue is forming and breast tissue and fat stores are increasing. During the later months of pregnancy the majority of additional energy needs are accounted for by the maintenance of tissue produced earlier. Since the energy requirements increase during gestation it is likely that carbohydrate stores will be chronically depleted, which may result in increased hunger signals. This may account for the increased appetite of many pregnant women. Low access to quality food may mean that physical activity must be reduced or food intake increased to meet the energy needs during gestation. Conversely, adequate access to quality food may mean increased physical activity is required to avoid an excessively positive energy balance. Finally, during lactation the daily energy needs of a woman increases by 2700–3100 kJ (640–740 kcal) to accommodate milk production. These extra energy needs are generally met by utilization of the fat deposited during pregnancy, minimizing the need to increase energy intake.

Effect of obesity on energy metabolism

Obesity is defined as having a fat mass larger than what is considered healthy. The degree of obesity is best defined by the body mass index (BMI, weight in kg/(height in m)^2. Someone is generally considered to be unhealthy when their BMI exceeds 25 and are defined as obese if their BMI is greater than 30. The perturbations to normal energy balance and metab-

olism during obesity are numerous and will only be mentioned briefly.

The primary change in energy metabolism, after a person has become obese, is an increase in the TEE owing to the increased demands on the body required to carry additional weight. Since the energy intake must match the energy output an obese person must consume adequate calories to maintain the obese state. Also, it has been found that obese persons oxidize fat at a lower rate than persons of normal weight. This would explain the relative ease with which some persons are able to gain weight as adipose tissue. Obese persons also tend to have a greater resistance to insulin compared with those of normal weight. Insulin resistance, a multifactorial condition which tends to increase in severity as body fat increases, reduces glucose uptake by muscle, and thus promotes conversion of glucose to triacylglycerols and its storage in adipose tissue. From the factors described one can understand how obesity, a disease with multifactorial causes, is difficult to treat, leaving prevention as one of the best methods to reduce the prevalence of obesity.

Effect of malnutrition on energy metabolism

There is a general reduction in TEE in malnourished children as a response to reduced energy intake. The greater part is accounted for by a reduction of the

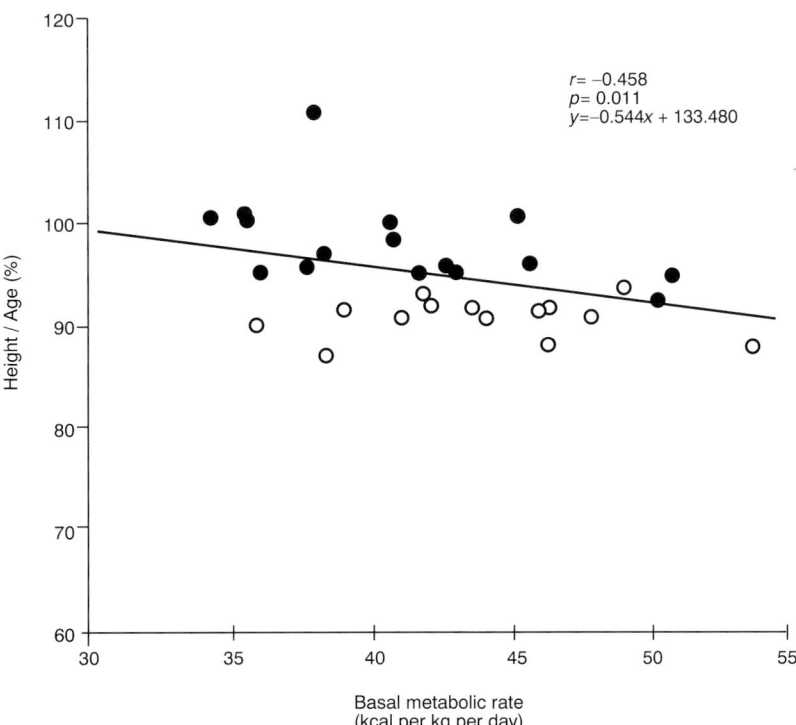

Figure 6 Basal metabolic rate according to degree of malnutrition (per cent height: age). Key: ○, stunted (malnourished); ●, nonstunted (healthy).

BMR. A yet unresolved question is why BMR is higher in malnourished children when BMR is expressed per kilogram of body weight (**Fig. 6**). One possible explanation is the fact that malnourished children have a higher ratio of more metabolically active tissue to less metabolically active tissue (e.g. increased viscera and brain and decreased muscle and fat tissue).

See also: **Adipose Tissue**: Structure, Function and Metabolism of Adipose Tissue. **Appetite**: Physiological and Neurobiological Aspects; Psychobiological and Behavioural Aspects. **Carbohydrates**: Chemistry and Classification (Including Dietary Fibre); Regulation of Carbohydrate Metabolism. **Exercise**: Physiology of Skeletal Muscle; Diet and Exercise. **Malnutrition**: Definition, Classification and Epidemiology; Primary Malnutrition; Secondary Malnutrition. **Obesity**: Definition, Aetiology and Assessment. **Older People**: Nutritional Requirements; Physiological Changes. **Pregnancy**: Energy Requirements and Metabolic Adaptations. **Protein**: Digestion and Bioavailability.

Further Reading

Bjorntrop P and Brodoff BN (eds) (1992) *Obesity*. Philadelphia: J.P. Lippincott Company.

Kinney JM and Tucker HN (eds) (1992) *Energy Metabolism: Tissue Determinants and Cellular Corollaries*. New York: Raven Press.

Waterlow JC (1992) *Protein Energy Mainutrition*. London: Edward Arnold.

Measurement of Energy Intake and Expenditure

D Hughes, Rowett Research Institute, Aberdeen, UK

M Elia, MRC Dunn Clinical Nutrition Centre, Cambridge, UK

A M Johnstone, Rowett Research Institute, Aberdeen, UK

J Stubbs, Rowett Research Institute, Aberdeen, UK

Copyright © 1998 Academic Press

Energy balance is the difference between the energy ingested and that expended and excreted over a given period of time. Thus storage is equal to energy intake (EI) minus energy expenditure (TEE). This equation is frequently simplified to give:

$$\text{energy storage} = \text{EI} - \text{TEE}$$

EI − energy lost in faeces − energy lost in urine − energy lost in combustible gas − heat produced = energy retained

Total energy expenditure (TEE) can be divided into the following components:

1. *Basal metabolic rate* (BMR) is the energy expended by an individual 10–12 hours post absorptive, lying awake in a thermoneutral environment and not subject to any physical or psychological stress. If the environment is not strictly thermoneutral or subject experiences small amounts of emotional or physical stress the term resting metabolic rate (RMR) should be used.
2. *Diet-induced thermogenesis* (DIT) is obligatory thermogenesis due to breakdown, absorption, storage and disposal of nutrients. It depends on the macronutrient content of the ingested food, meal size, time since the previous meal, nutritional status and pathological state.
3. *Energy expended in physical activity* (AEE) is the greatest source of between-person variation in human EE, except during injury, sepsis, trauma, surgery and other pathological states.

Thus:

$$\text{TEE} = \text{AEE} + \text{RMR} + \text{DIT}$$

Energy intake in mammals including humans is intermittent in nature. In humans the typical Western feeding pattern is three or four meals a day, interspersed with one or two snacks. The energy ingested can be divided into micronutrients and macronutrients. The micronutrients are of enormous importance to normal physiological functioning, but provide a quantitatively insignificant proportion of ingested energy. The macronutrients – fat, protein, carbohydrate and alcohol – are the main energy-providing substrates. Together their ingestion summates to determine EI. The expenditure of energy can also be subdivided into, and measured as, the oxidation of individual macronutrients. The difference between the intake of macronutrients on one hand, and their oxidation and loss in excreta on the other, is the balance or storage of macronutrients, and hence energy.

The importance of measuring EI and EE

The second law of thermodynamics states that energy cannot be created or destroyed but can only be transformed from one form into another. This means that solar energy is trapped at the base of ecosystems, flows through food chains and material cycles, forming the physical basis upon which biological processes are based. The concept of energy flow through ecosystems has led to a greater understanding of the manner and efficiency with which different environments and the species which occupy them function. Knowledge of the patterns of energy flow through a food chain is essential for understanding the foraging strategies and population dynamics of all species, including humans. Patterns of EI and EE form a reference for the whole of human nutrition, because it is by maintaining energy balance that body composition is maintained and functional integrity sustained. Energy flow methodology has provided a common currency which enables comparisons from the ecosystem level to that of individuals in health and disease. This energetic 'reductionism' has been criticized for its oversimplicity. However, it provides a common reference and language that forms the conceptual foundation and functional basis for understanding energy balance in human nutrition.

Obtaining precise and accurate estimates of EI and EE in human subjects of different age, sex and ethnic groups is crucial for understanding the energetic basis of human nutrition. This information is of considerable relevance to fundamental research, medical practice, public health and food policy. Research measurements of EI and EE have provided the basis upon which the energy costs of maintenance, growth and development, pregnancy and lactation have been compared and made available to public health professionals. Clinical research has made considerable advances in understanding the energy cost of disease, and how decrements in energy balance status can affect physiological function such as susceptibility to disease. This information has led to important developments for increasing the effectiveness of nutritional support in the clinical setting. Since EI and EE are fundamental to our understanding of processes and applications which maintain health or promote and limit disease, it is essential that both EI and EE are measured with precision and accuracy, under a range of conditions. In order to measure or estimate EI, it is essential to be able to estimate the energy value of the nutrients which together summate to determine the energy value of a food.

The energy value of foods and macronutrients

The majority of studies that purport to measure EI actually measure food intake and estimate EI from standard food tables, which have themselves been largely derived from the chemical analysis of foods. To appreciate the energy value of a nutrient and its impact on energy balance it is important to distinguish between its chemical energy (gross energy), the energy that the organism derives from that nutrient when it is ingested in food (metabolizable energy)

and the efficiency with which the nutrient is oxidized or stored.

Enthalpy of combustion or gross energy of foods The enthalpy of combustion (ΔH_c) values of protein, carbohydrate, fat and alcohol are given in **Table 1**. These values represent the chemical energy contained in these compounds and therefore the energy that is liberated upon complete combustion, or complete biological oxidation by the body. Carbohydrate has theoretically the lowest energy density of all of the macronutrients in purely chemical terms. This statement, however, assumes firstly that each of the macronutrients is completely digested, and secondly that each of the macronutrients is completely oxidized in the body. Neither of these assumptions is entirely correct. Do all macronutrients have the same gross energy (GE) or ΔH_c? Table 1 illustrates that they do not. Furthermore, different kinds of protein and carbohydrate can vary in their GE values. Those for different kinds of fat are more similar, although shorter-chain fats tend to have a slightly lower energy value per gram than longer-chain fats. Different proteins differ in composition to a greater extent than other macronutrients and so their heat of combustion varies considerably, ranging between 17.43 kJ g^{-1} and 21.15 kJ g^{-1} for conventional food proteins and between 17.22 kJ g^{-1} and 25.98 kJ g^{-1} for artificial amino acid mixtures. Dietary intake calculations assume an average protein composition consistent with a Western diet. The GE per gram of carbohydrate (CHO) will also vary with the chain length of the molecule. This is because di-, tri-, oligo- and polysaccharides are formed by condensation of monosaccharides. For every glycosidic bond formed a water molecule is lost and the energy density of the CHO rises. Thus, while the ΔH_c of glucose is 15.7 kJ g^{-1} that of starch or glycogen is 17.2 kJ g^{-1}. When calculating CHO energy derived from dietary intakes, total available CHOs (free sugars: glucose, fructose, galactose, sucrose, maltose, lactose and oligosaccharides) and available complex CHOs (dextrins, starch and glycogen) are often expressed as monosaccharide equivalents. It is important to note that in estimating nutrient intakes from food tables, CHO values expressed as monosaccharide equivalents can exceed 100 g per 100 g of food because the hydrolysis of di- and polysaccharides adds water to each hexose unit. Thus 100 g of starch will hydrolyse to give 110 g of monosaccharide.

Metabolizable energy of macronutrients The assumption that each of the dietary macronutrients is completely digested has been questioned in numerous metabolic balance studies in farm animals and

Table 1   Gross energy and metabolizable energy of the major macronutrients

Macronutrient	Gross energy ($kJ\,g^{-1}$)	Metabolizable energy ($kJ\,g^{-1}$)
Conventional food carbohydrate	17.5	16
Conventional food fat	37.96–40.09	37
Conventional food protein	23.61	17
Alcohol	29.67	29

subsequently in humans. Table 1 gives the *rounded* metabolizable energy (ME) values for the dietary macronutrients. The ME is the difference between the gross energy of the food ingested and that which is voided in faeces, and in the case of protein, urinary losses of the products of incomplete oxidation. The ME represents the energy available to the organism subsequent to ingestion and is naturally lower than GE. When calculating EI it is essential to use ME values and not GE (ΔH_c) values. One researcher has emphasized the limitations of using *average* ME values commonly used for human nutrients and foods, noting that (1) the ME value of a nutrient is often specific to a food and its mode of preparation; (2) the common approach of using a rounded figure predicates that the ME factors for protein, fat and CHO are constant and completely independent – they are not (for example, certain unavailable complex CHOs decrease the apparent digestion of fat); and (3) until recently these values assumed that unavailable complex carbohydrates (see below) have zero nutritive value.

Bearing these caveats in mind, it is apparent from Table 1 that using average values, the ME values of CHOs are lower than those of fats and alcohol and are lower than 'average' protein. Fat has the highest value. With the exception of proteins, all of the macronutrients can be completely metabolized to carbon dioxide and water with its attendant liberation of energy. Protein is incompletely oxidized in the body owing to the process of deamination and ureogenesis. Additional corrections have to be made to account for the urinary output of urea plus other quantitatively minor nitrogenous products which are also excreted.

Carbohydrates and proteins vary in their digestibility and hence ME values. Since protein constitutes a relatively small proportion of total EI, and CHO usually comprises the largest percentage of EI, variations in the digestibility of CHOs will contribute more to errors in the estimation of EI. The CHO fractions which are not digested in the small and large intestine are called unavailable complex CHOs (UCC). Previous estimates gave a value of zero for this undigested component of the diet; however, more recent analyses have indicated a value for (ΔH_c

of $17\,kJ\,g^{-1}$ a digestibility of 0.7 and a conversion efficiency of $0.3\,kJ$ faecal bacterial energy per kilojoule of CHO fermented, giving a ME value of $8.4\,kJ\,g^{-1}$ for mixed diets. This implies that 50% of the energy in UCC is available to humans after the process of fermentation and short-chain fatty acid absorption.

A large number of procedures for the measurement of EI and EE have been developed. **Table 2** describes methods of measuring EI, the main settings in which the measures are used, their advantages/disadvantages and examples of their use. **Table 3** gives corresponding descriptions for procedures used to measure EE.

Measurement of Energy Intake

Methods

Intake measures fall into three basic categories: (1) observational (largely qualitative); (2) quantitative estimates of intake; and (3) independent assessments of intake using biomarkers.

Observational measures   Observational measures of EI include observations made by the investigator, or more commonly observations made by the subject at the time of consumption (e.g. using a food diary) or retrospectively (e.g. 24-hour recall or food frequency questionnaire methods). Observational measures of food intake and the EI calculations made from them have limited precision, since the method of quantification involves subjective estimates on the part of the subject or the investigator. It has, however, been suggested that questionnaire and recall-based assessments of food intake disrupt the behaviour of the subject to a minimal degree and so although less precise, are more accurate in terms of the subject's 'habitual' food and EI. This assumption is only valid if errors are random (e.g. there is an equal tendency to over- or underestimate portion sizes) rather than systematic (e.g. bias towards underreporting of EI by obese subjects). It is generally recognized that random errors in observational measures of food intake are large and therefore large numbers of subjects should be used.

Table 2 Methods of measuring energy intake

Procedure	Description	Main experimental setting	Advantages	Disadvantages	Examples of use
Continuous weighing (universal eating monitor) (Quantitative)	This procedure uses concealed scales placed under a serving plate. As food is consumed from the plate the weight decrease is recorded	Laboratory	Provides highly accurate information on weight of food eaten. Provides useful information on the rate of food eaten as well as quantity	Applicable to short-term (within day) studies only. Food choice cannot be studied. Monitoring apparatus is complex and expensive	Comparative studies examining the effects of food type on food intake, intake rate, between lean and obese subjects. Such studies can include differences between solid and liquid foods
Laboratory weighing (Quantitative)	Subject is provided with a personal food store from which they can select the foods required. They are instructed to only eat food provided and to retrieve all waste (including containers and packaging). Food eaten is calculated from store depletion and waste	Laboratory	Accurate quantitative data obtained. Experimental foods can be chosen to reflect 'normally eaten' foods or specifically manipulated diets can be used to examine the effects of diet composition on energy intake	Large quantities of waste if fresh produce is used. Highly labour intensive. Selection of foods is limited to laboratory storage space	Examination of the effects of diet selection on eating behaviour and energy intake
Food dispensing machine (Quantitative)	Commercial food dispensing systems are adapted for use in a laboratory. The machine contains a variety of foods (usually snacks) from which the subject has free access. They type in a specific code to obtain their food	Laboratory. Potential use in a free-living setting by placing machine in, for example, a canteen	Data for quantity of food eaten as well as time, frequency and choice is obtained. Investigator burden lowered by automation of monitoring procedures	Computing skills required for data retrieval and analysis. Limited foods. Limited in-machine storage space	Studies that examine snacking pattern differences between different groups, for example an anorectic drug intervention on snacking energy intake
Liquid diet assessment (Quantitative)	Subject activates a peristaltic pump which can release food orally or intragastrically	Laboratory/clinical	Energy intake can be accurately monitored. Highly accurate food intake data obtained	Atypical food type and delivery procedure will affect subject's intake response. High subject burden. Very little variety with organoleptic food quality (sight, taste, texture).	Comparison of oral versus gastric functions in the short-term regulation of food intake

Continued

Table 2 Continued

Procedure	Description	Main experimental setting	Advantages	Disadvantages	Examples of use
Fixed portions (solid food unit) (Quantitative)	Food is preweighed and prepared as bite-sized snacks from which the subject selects from a covered box. These typically come in the form of small sandwiches	Laboratory	Can be used in situations where cognitive (e.g. sight) cues need to be removed from the experimental protocol. Controlled conditions, (reducing potential intake confounders) allow quantitative within-subject comparisons	Subjects need to be familiarized with the food and technique prior to the study. Atypical food type reduces the ecological validity of the resulting data	Typically used to study food variety effects on energy intake. Small groups of subjects (e.g. underweight, lean and obese) can be studied under controlled conditions.
Chemical analysis (Quantitative)	A duplicate portion of subject's food is obtained and chemically analysed. This can be: 1. Collected by subject (aliquot sampling) 2. Reproduced by investigator in the laboratory (equivalent composite) 3. Investigator collects the food and drinks retrospectively (duplicate samples)	Free-living (individual or group-based) or laboratory	Highly accurate data in terms of food composition. Fewer errors involving data transcription to nutrient	Very expensive. High investigator burden. Can be used in small populations only	Applicable to studies where a food composition table is not constructed or inadequate, so data on foods cannot easily be converted to nutrient values. This would be applicable to remote cultures consuming local foods
Weighed food records (Quantitative)	A subject or observer records the weight of all food and beverages consumed in a specified time frame	Free-living (individual or group-based)	Direct quantitative and qualitative data obtained for subjects in their natural environment. Duration variable (typically 3–7 days). Widely used and considered the 'gold standard'	Composition data less accurate for food eaten outside home. Standardization and subject training required. High subject burden. Possible change of eating habit to simplify weighing procedure	Used to study populations and individuals where accurate quantitative data are required; for example, the effect of an exercise manipulation on the food intake of subjects in their 'natural' settings
Portable electronic tape-recorded automatic weighed food record (PETRA) (Quantitative)	A specialized weighing scale with no display which automatically records verbal descriptions and weight of food eaten on analogue tapes	Free-living (individual or group-based)	As above, but also: reduces subject burden subject cannot see what they have eaten retrospectively which may affect intake	As above, but also: scales can be cumbersome. Greater risk of data loss problems if scales are incorrectly zeroed	Very useful for individuals who adjust their intake as a consequence of being aware of the quantity they are or have been eating

Table 2   Continued

Procedure	Description	Main experimental setting	Advantages	Disadvantages	Examples of use
Food diaries with estimated portion size (Observational and quantitative)	A subject, observer or investigator can record all foods and beverages consumed by a subject during a specified time period in a special diary	Free-living (individual or group-based)	Provides direct consumption data, hence omission of foods less likely than recall methods Diaries easy to construct and administer	Subjects need to be literate and motivated Quantitative data are only acquired with assumptions on portion sizes	Epidemiological studies measuring nutrient intakes of large groups simultaneously
Diet history (Observational and quantitative)	This is a three-part assessment consisting of: 1. Detailed interviews assessing general information and a 24-hour recall 2. Cross-check with a food frequency questionnaire 3. Three-day diet record	Free-living (individual or group-based)	Provides useful data on meal patterns Usual intakes over long time periods can be obtained to assess habitual consumption	Tendency to overestimate energy and nutrient intake Reliance on subject memory Indicative of relative rather than absolute data Investigator training and standardization required	Good to use in intervention studies. Diet histories at specific time periods before and after the intervention
Food balance sheets (Observational)	Statistical data bases provide demographic data on food production, import, export and stocks Food consumption can be estimated by deducting food used for nonhuman use (e.g. animal feed) and losses incurred in the food chain	Free-living (population-based)	Provides useful information on trends within populations Can be used for intercountry comparisons	Assumptions have to be made on food losses at a household level Unreported trade (bartering) is not accounted for There are significant misrecording errors at every data collection level, mainly overreporting	United Nations Food and Agriculture Organization (UN FAO) statistical division regularly publish data which can be accessed for food consumption, accounts and movement data
Universal product code (Observational)	The food retail market (e.g. supermarkets) constantly obtain data on food purchased using bar coding systems	Free-living (population-based)	Data available for specific populations within a retail catchment area Automated data collection Purchase patterns easily monitored	The information is at present commercially owned Assumptions have to be made on nonconsumed food, household size and structure This method assesses food acquisition rather than food consumption	Currently used by supermarkets to control supply depending on seasonal variations and demand. The information when made available to research bodies will have great potential power

Continued

Table 2 Continued

Procedure	Description	Main experimental setting	Advantages	Disadvantages	Examples of use
Food surveying (food account method) (Observational)	A variety of households in designated demographic regions are selected. The person responsible for food purchased in each selected household keeps a daily record of all the food entering the household during a specified time period	Free-living (household-based)	National levels of food consumption can be assessed Provides time trends Useful where individual data are hard to obtain	There is no formal measure of food waste; however, an adjustment factor of 10% is used It does not consider food eaten outside the home which may constitute a large proportion of overall consumption Cannot provide data for individuals	Large surveys such as UK National Food Survey have used this technique. This has resulted in large yearly data bases since 1950s providing data for time national time trends in food acquisition
Food surveying with larder inventory (Observational)	Identical methodology to the food account method; however, changes in food storage are also measured	Free-living (household-based)	Consumption data as well as acquisition data obtained Provides time trends Useful where individual data are hard to obtain	Higher subject burden There is no formal measure of food waste It does not consider food eaten outside the home	Used by Ministry of Agriculture, Fisheries and Food (UK) pre-1952. Subject burden was considered too high
Household food record (Observational)	Food available for consumption in a household is weighed or estimated by an investigator. Food is subdivided into portions at each meal among the family	Free-living (household-based)	Particularly applicable to households in which the majority of foods consumed are home produced Large populations can be studied at low cost Quantitatively greater accuracy than other household food measures	Data does not account for sex, age and body weight differences within households High subject burden Quantitative inaccuracies due to inconsistencies in portion size estimates	Estimation of the energy and nutrient intakes of rural nonindustrialized populations where literacy levels are low
List recall method (Observational)	For a period of time (usually one week) the main householder is asked to recall the amount and cost of foods consumed in the household	Free-living (household-based)	Information provided on food costs and financial burden of food Provides additional information on food use	Requires high subject motivation Subjects alter records due to 'health' issues Subject literacy and numeracy skills required	US food consumption surveys by the US Department of Agriculture favour this method as it is suitable to a population where most food eaten is purchased and not home-grown

Table 2 Continued

Procedure	Description	Main experimental setting	Advantages	Disadvantages	Examples of use
24-hour recall (Observational)	The subject is asked by a trained interviewer to reveal exact food intake during the previous 24 h	Free-living (individual or group-based)	Low subject burden Inexpensive Can be used in illiterate individuals Potential use in large populations	The investigator needs to be highly trained and interview protocols standardized Data do not reflect a typical intake unless repeated Great dependency on subject's memory, therefore not good with elderly or children	Used in large-scale national surveys to estimate average population food and nutrient intakes
Food frequency questionnaires (FFQ) (Observational)	The FFQ is a self-administered questionnaire to provide information on 'typical' food consumption of an individual. They generally comprise sections to include: 1. Food list 2. Frequency of consumption 3. Quantitative estimate (semiquantitative FFQs)	Free-living (individual or group-based)	Can study large numbers of subjects Questionnaire can be designed to target specific foods Provides information on dietary patterns	Difficult to construct Requires a pilot study to test effectiveness Low precision in terms of quantitative data Reliance on subjects eating similar foods during questionnaire time frame	Useful as a screening measure to decipher typical intakes before a subject is enlisted to a medical trial Also useful in rapidly assessing dietary patterns of large groups
Biological markers (Independent)	Any biochemical substance in an easily accessible biological sample that gives a predictive response to a given dietary component	Free-living (individual or group-based) or laboratory	Low subject burden. Subject can retain their normal life style Fewer errors associated with subject altering behaviour as a consequence of the measurement tool	Materials and analysis expensive Obtaining sample may be invasive, e.g. if blood sample is required Problems with loss of collection	Urinary nitrogen has shown good correlation with protein intake Urinary nitrogen (transformed into protein using a factor of 6.25) should correspond within $81 \pm 5\%$ of intake if in energy balance
Balance (factorial) method (Independent)	This method considers the basis of the energy balance equation. If energy expenditure and changes in energy stores (body composition) are measured accurately, energy intake should be equal to the sum of these	Free-living (individual or group-based) or laboratory	Reduces errors associated with behaviour modification as a consequence of measuring food intake No errors associated with conversion of food to nutrient	Can only work with accurate estimation of energy expenditure and body weight changes Minimum of 7 days needed	The use of doubly labelled water to measure energy expenditure has provided results demonstrating that energy intake is very often underreported, particularly in overweight subjects

Table 3 Methods of measuring energy expenditure

Procedure	Theoretical basis	Main experimental setting	Description	Advantages	Disadvantages	Examples of use
Whole-body direct calorimeter	Direct calorimetry	Laboratory	1. **Gradient layer** The subject resides in a chamber consisting of a heat-sensitive inner wall and thermoconstant (water-cooled) outer wall. Heat differences between the walls reflect heat production from subject 2. **Heat sink** The subject resides in a fully insulated chamber. Changes in ventilated air temperature are measured going in and out of the chamber using a water-cooled heat exchanger	Very accurate results Chamber is very responsive to changes from within Fewer assumptions related to measuring heat production directly	No information on macronutrient metabolism Very expensive system to design and maintain Expert technical assistance needed Artificial environment Electrical heat production (e.g. television) and food heat must be accounted for System needs to measure evaporative heat loss (in water vapour) also	Hardly used today but effective past use in indirect calorimetry validation
Water-cooled suit	Direct calorimetry	Laboratory	A variation on gradient layer. The subject wears a water-impermeable suit surrounded by water-filled tubes. In a constant environment heat loss is detected in the water and breath	Accurate results Easier to incorporate other variables (e.g. blood sampling) Portable system	Difficult to maintain constant environment Suit is cumbersome and restrictive Short-term investigation only	Elucidating energy expenditure differences between lean and obese subjects during exercise in a laboratory environment
Whole body	Indirect calorimetry	Laboratory	Subject resides in a ventilated airtight chamber. Chamber typically contains bed, chair, television, video. Food and urine bottles can be exchanged via a two-panel sealed hatch	Provides data on substrate metabolism High accuracy and validity Easily calibrated to maximize sensitivity	Requires extensive computing and technical skills to run Expensive instrumentation and running costs Artificial environment	As well as validation studies, this technique is ideal for within-subject comparisons lasting 1–7 days

Table 3 Continued

Procedure	Theoretical basis	Main experimental setting	Description	Advantages	Disadvantages	Examples of use
Ventilated hood	Indirect calorimetry	Laboratory, clinical	Subject lies down on a bed and is covered with a Perspex hood or tent. Samples of inspired and expired air are mechanically drawn through analysers or collected in a container for later analysis	Easy to use. Most modern systems have self-calibration function. Modern systems have all measurement apparatus contained in one unit	Modern systems are expensive. Need frequent calibration checks. Can only be used at low flow rates	Typically used to measure energy expenditure in a resting state. Favoured techniques are in resting metabolic rate or diet-induced thermogenesis measurement
Exercise testing	Indirect calorimetry	Laboratory	Subject is attached to a mask or mouthpiece (with nose clip) which is further attached to a mass flowmeter and respiratory gas analysers. Samples of air can be drawn from a mixing chamber or analysed breath by breath. Sophisticated software allows simultaneous control of exercise equipment	Can accommodate high flow rates. Relatively portable around a laboratory. Good for short-term investigation. Easy to incorporate other measures (e.g. electrocardiogram)	Poorer results at lower flow rates. Low specification gas analysers. Mouthpiece apparatus restricts breathing pattern of subject	Typically used to measure energy expenditure during exercise sessions. Also used to derive linear regression equations for heart rate vs energy expenditure
Douglas bag	Indirect calorimetry	Field or laboratory	Subjects are attached to a mouthpiece (with nose-clip) and tube which leads to a gas-impermeable bag attached to their back, typically of 100 litre volume. The bag is then emptied through a dry gas meter to measure gas volumes *post hoc*. Air samples are analysed for O_2 and/or CO_2.	The bag is relatively inexpensive. Simple to use. Produces reliable results	High subject burden, awkward and cumbersome bag. Limited storage capacity. CO_2 diffusion losses from bag. Gases need immediate analysis	Simple method to estimate energy expenditure during a short exercise bout in a laboratory or in the field

Continued

Table 3 Continued

Procedure	Theoretical basis	Main experimental setting	Description	Advantages	Disadvantages	Examples of use
Max Planck or Kofranyi–Michaelis respirometer	Indirect calorimetry	Field	This system also uses a nose-clip and mouthpiece; the subject breathes into a small (bellows) gas meter which monitors volume and small aliquots of air are continuously taken from the breath samples and stored in a butyl rubber bag	This system is smaller and far less cumbersome than containment collection systems Good relative accuracy and reproducibility Can be used over longer periods than the Douglas bag	Only average rate of gaseous consumption and/or production ($l\ min^{-1}$) can be calculated Errors during high activity Mouthpiece is uncomfortable over long periods	No longer manufactured, but still has potential use to determine average energy expenditure of individuals who are not highly physically active. Average daily expenditure can be measured by taking repeated samples throughout the day
Oxylog	Indirect calorimetry	Field	The subject is attached to a mask which is further attached to an inspiratory turbine flowmeter and lightweight polarographic oxygen electrodes at both inlet and outlet. Differences between inlet and outlet oxygen (pressure adjusted) determine energy expenditure	Lightweight and extremely portable Provides minute by minute oxygen consumption values Can be used over a range of activities Gases analysed directly	Interferes with normal activity of subject Expensive High maintenance required Not validated using adequate comparisons	Very useful in field situations to elucidate the energy cost of certain everyday physical activities (e.g. crop picking, housework)
Cosmed K2 system	Indirect calorimetry	Field	This system uses the Oxylog principle; however, the data are transmitted directly to a computer program	Sophisticated automation procedure relieves investigator burden	Very expensive Technical and computing skills required Loss of precision at low energy expenditure	A recently developed method which has become popular in submaximal and maximal exercise testing

Table 3 Continued

Procedure	Theoretical basis	Main experimental setting	Description	Advantages	Disadvantages	Examples of use
Current diary	Self-assessment	Field	A specialized diary is constructed which is broken down into specified time intervals (e.g. 5 min) over a specified period (e.g. 3 days). The subjects record their activities during each of these time intervals, typically by means of a code	Simple and inexpensive method Can be used to study large populations Numeracy and literacy requirements are low	High subject burden Lengthy analysis procedure High dependency on subject reliability and honesty Low precision and accuracy	Used in large-scale comparative studies between two populations, for example similar groups from different countries
Time-motion study	Observer assessment	Field	Similar to the diary method, but uses an observer to study a subject or group of subjects. The observer records the time and duration of activity changes throughout a specified period	Less errors due to subject reliability	High investigator burden Expensive Standardization required if many observers are to be used Low precision and accuracy	Used in groups who cannot physically record intake or withstand measurement apparatus, such as playgroup children
Retrospective recall	Interview assessment	Field	This technique uses a questionnaire and/or interview to elucidate the frequency with which a subject undergoes certain activities	Low subject burden Good qualitative tool Low cost Useful for trends between populations	Interviewer training required Reliance on subject memory Not precise or accurate	Large-scale epidemiological trials, to assess typical population activities

Continued

Table 3 Continued

Procedure	Theoretical basis	Main experimental setting	Description	Advantages	Disadvantages	Examples of use
Heart rate monitor	Linear relationship between cardiac output and energy expenditure within a range of heart rates	Field	Electrodes can be placed on the chest which transmit data to a remote unit. The data can then be stored on a storage pack attached to the subject. The Polar Sports Tester (Polar Electro, Finland) provides a much simpler method of heart rate data acquisition. A thin chest belt is worn by the subject which transmits minute by minute heart rates to a receiver worn as a watch on the wrist	Minute by minute heart rates obtainable. Data easily transferred to a computer. Polar Sports Tester has low subject burden, is discreet and can store 34 hours of information	Subjects must be individually calibrated against indirect calorimetry. Poor correlation at low energy expenditure. Posture will affect cardiac output. Has a precision and accuracy of $\pm20\%$	Excellent method to estimate energy expenditure and activity patterns in a field situation where many subjects need to be studied simultaneously
Doubly labelled water	Differences in the dilution rates of loss of hydrogen (^{2}H) and oxygen (^{18}O) isotopes from the body estimating CO_2 production	Field or laboratory	Subjects are dosed with a preweighed sample of water containing isotopes of hydrogen (^{2}H) and oxygen (^{18}O). The ^{2}H is lost from the water pools and ^{18}O is lost from the carbon dioxide and water pools. Differences between the rate of loss (disappearance) of the two isotopes reflects CO_2 production	High accuracy. Subjects can maintain normal activity. Low subject burden	High isotope and analysis costs. Minimum duration of 12–14 days (adult) or 6–7 days (children). Only mean energy expenditure over study period is obtainable. Analysis complex and expensive	Chosen method to validate other methods of energy expenditure and energy intake using the balance method over long periods (greater than 12 days)
Labelled bicarbonate	Isotopic dilution of carbon isotope (^{14}C)	Field	Subject wears a small pump which infuses labelled bicarbonate (NaH^{13}CO$_3$) into the body at a constant rate. Collected breath, blood, urine or saliva samples provide information on the extent of the isotope dilution and hence CO_2 production	Can measure day-to-day energy expenditure. Subject can be relatively mobile. Analysis is simpler than doubly labelled water. Cheaper than doubly labelled water	Some subject discomfort. Cannot be used for long periods. Theoretical limitations associated with measuring CO_2 production only in energy expenditure estimation. ^{14}C is a radioisotope	Most applicable in a clinical setting, where subjects are not highly active or are already receiving infusions. Labelled bicarbonate can be incorporated into other infused substances

Quantitative estimates of intake   Provided a subject weighs all foods eaten and food waste accurately, quantitative estimates of intake are theoretically more precise than observational measures. However, the more intrusive and quantitative a technique is, the more the normal feeding behaviour of the subject is likely to be disrupted. Substantial errors can still also accrue, for example, due to nonhomogeneity and misclassification of foods. It is becoming widely accepted that subjects often fail to record all foods eaten or alter their feeding patterns to simplify the food weighing process.

At least nine sources of error have been identified in methods used to assess dietary intake. These are errors derived from food tables, coding errors, wrong weights of food, reporting errors, variation with time, wrong frequency of consumption, change in diet, response bias and sampling bias. Most observational and quantitative methods of EI assessment given in Table 2 are subject to several of these errors. Some of these errors are considered further in **Table 4**.

Independent assessments using biomarkers   Theoretically the use of biomarkers offers an objective, independent assessment of dietary intake which is precise, accurate, unobtrusive and does not disrupt the behaviour of the subject concerned. The use of doubly labelled water to measure free-living EE is an independent means of assessing the plausibility of dietary intakes, provided both EI and EE are measured over 10 days or more. However, this approach does not measure the level of food intake, nor the composition of the food eaten. Similarly, urinary nitrogen output (derived from 24 h total urine collections) offers a means of validating protein intake, based on the fact that healthy subjects in energy balance are usually in nitrogen balance. These methods are essentially a means of verifying the validity of dietary intakes, rather than a direct means of measuring energy or nutrient intakes. The development of precise and accurate biomarkers for the assessment of energy and nutrient intakes is still in its infancy, with much work to be done before they replace more traditional measures of dietary intakes in human subjects.

It will be apparent from Table 2 that different techniques for the measurement of EI are most useful under different experimental conditions. For example, a 7-day weighed food intake measurement in a large epidemiological study would be impractical and would be unlikely to provide a reliable estimate of the habitual dietary intake of the population. Under these conditions recall methods and food fre-

quency questionnaires may give more insights into the habitual dietary intakes of a large population.

Types of study in which EI measures are used

The major study designs that rely on intake assessments can be categorized as (1) ecological/epidemiological studies; (2) intervention studies; and (3) laboratory/clinical studies.

Ecological studies   Ecological studies have the advantage of using large numbers of subjects who are in their natural setting. The ecological validity of such studies is therefore theoretically high. However, it should be borne in mind that there are a number of methodological problems associated with epidemiological and diet survey studies which must be taken into account and which inevitably weaken the conclusions derived from them. Firstly, the errors in data collection are high and are not necessarily random. A clear example of this is the systematic underreporting of EI in the obese which is discussed below. It is generally assumed that errors are random and will therefore cancel as sample size expands. Table 4 shows that this may not be the case. Moreover, as sample size increases the methods that need to be employed tend to become quantitatively less precise. Secondly, in many studies subjects are not randomly selected and the population is not therefore necessarily totally representative of the general population. Thirdly, many epidemiological studies are cross-sectional and assume that the processes influencing the phenomena under investigation are uniform over time. Clearly this is not always the case, for example patterns of food intake will change with season (Table 4). The results of diet survey and epidemiological studies should therefore be treated with some caution. More recently the phenomenon of misreporting of food and EI has received attention; this is discussed below.

Laboratory-based studies   Energy intakes can be studied with greater control in laboratory-based studies which typically use small numbers of nonrandomly selected subjects in the artificial environment of the laboratory, employing protocols and techniques which are often unfamiliar to the subject. In the laboratory, outcomes (e.g. hunger, energy and nutrient intakes) can be measured with considerable precision and accuracy and in good experimental designs there is little contamination of the protocol from extraneous influences. However, it is also important to understand the limitations of the laboratory approach when attempting to extrapolate the results of experiments conducted in the laboratory (where the signal to noise ratio may be

Table 4 Major sources of error associated with measuring energy intake

Error type	Description	Example	Methods affected	Resulting statistical error
Subject bias	Subjects modify their typical diet to include what they think they should be eating. For example, they include foods that they deem 'healthy' and omit food they view as 'unhealthy'	Subjects may report consumption of high-carbohydrate, low-fat foods owing to positive public health messages	Weighed record Food diaries 24-hour recall Diet history FFQ	Systematic
Interviewer bias	An investigator incorrectly probes the subject into a false or incomplete response with too broad or too specific questioning	Investigator or interviewer may not probe a subject to revealing that they always use butter on bread	24-hour recall Diet history FFQ (semiquantitative)	Systematic
Memory	The subject intentionally or unintentionally omits or adds food when asked to recall foods eaten. This can be particularly problematic when it comes to quantifying data	Subject may fail to report biscuits eaten with tea. Biscuits have high energy density which may cause large quantitative errors	24-hour recall Diet history FFQ	Systematic and random
Estimation of portion size	In situations where data are not directly quantified (e.g. diary methods), quantification must be retrospectively established	A 'slice of bread' can constitute anything between 20 g and 100 g depending on slice thickness, bread type, etc.	Food diaries 24-hour recall Diet history FFQ (semiquantitative only)	Systematic or random
Flat slope syndrome	This is a phenomenon within a population which causes intakes to regress towards a mean. Subjects tend to retrospectively underreport if they have eaten large quantities and overreport if they have eaten small quantities	In a study that concurrently measures the energy intake in lean and overweight individuals, significant differences between the two groups may not arise	24-hour recall Diet history FFQ (semiquantitative)	Systematic
Coding and computational	These errors are investigator-induced and are caused by inputting an incorrect data value or food code into a nutritional data base for analysis	Typing in a food code of 215 instead of 251 will analyse double cream instead of drinking yoghurt; this will overestimate energy consumption by 1586 kJ per 100 g, a 700% relative error!	Weighed record Food diaries 24-hour recall Diet history FFQ Biomarker	Generally random but can become systematic if the same mistake is repeatedly made
Inter- and intrasubject variation	Subjects' diets may vary from day to day throughout the year, thus taking a 'snapshot' of energy intake will not reflect habitual intake	If subjects record food intake on a day in which they feel unwell, they may grossly undereat relative to their normal intake	Weighed record Food diaries 24-hour recall Diet history Biomarker	Random between individuals (inter) and systematic within individuals (intra)

Table 4 Continued

Error type	Description	Example	Methods affected	Resulting statistical error
Week-day effect	Subjects consume different foods (with different energy densities) on different days of the week	Men and women have been shown to consume more food on a Sunday than on weekdays	Weighed record (less than 7 days) Food diaries (less than 7 days) 24-hour recall Diet history Biomarker	Systematic
Consecutive days	Recording intake on two consecutive days will not provide an adequate energy intake mean, since consecutive days are highly correlated compared with nonconsecutive days	Consecutive days of dietary intake may have strong autocorrelations for many subjects, i.e. one day's intake is very similar to the next	Weighed record (less than 3 days) Food diaries (less than 3 days) 24-hour recall Diet history FFQ Biomarker	Systematic
Seasonality	Subjects vary their intake depending on the time of year; this may be related to environmental temperature	Consumption of cold food (e.g. ice creams, salads) is likely to increase in the summer, and of hot food (e.g. soup) in the winter	Weighed record Food diaries 24-hour recall Diet history FFQ Biomarker	Systematic error relative to other seasons

FFQ, food frequency questionnaire.

artificially elevated) to everyday life. For instance, it is unlikely that habitual intakes could ever be measured in the laboratory.

Intervention studies   Intervention studies often represent a good compromise between the artificiality of the laboratory and the lack of control over both manipulation and measurement that occurs in epidemiological studies. Typically, subjects adhere to a given manipulation (e.g. consuming a number of low-fat foods made available *ad libitum* by the investigator) but go about their normal lives so that the impact of the manipulation (e.g. fat on feeding behaviour) can be assessed. This allows the experimental intervention to be carefully controlled without disrupting the normal routines of subjects and so enhances the ecological validity of results.

It is clear from the above considerations that the experimental setting can sometimes greatly influence the means of measurement made and the phenomenon under investigation. It is therefore appropriate to examine patterns of EI in relation to issues such as diet composition in each experimental environment. If broadly similar phenomena are apparent in each of these experimental conditions it is reasonable to accept that the phenomenon under scrutiny is robust and not an artefact of the experimental conditions themselves.

The problem of underreporting

A question inevitably arises in relation to the now numerous studies that attempt to characterize the dietary patterns of populations: to what extent do reported intakes reflect the actual dietary intakes of the subjects concerned? The recent development of new approaches which attempt to validate dietary intakes based on fundamental principles of energy balance, suggest that misreporting is particularly pronounced in Western adults, with the majority of misreporters underreporting energy and nutrient intakes. Examining the ratio of urinary nitrogen output to dietary intake can be used as a rough index of protein intake as long as totality of urine collection can also be validated using p-aminobenzoic acid (PABA). In subjects in energy and nitrogen balance the expected ratio of urinary N to dietary N is 81%. Similarly, standard regression equations can be used to estimate basal metabolic rate and multiples of these can be used to estimate physical activity levels (PAL) which identify minimum plausible levels of EE as a multiple of BMR. The energy intake can then be compared to statistically derived cutoffs which take account of the EI/PAL ratio to identify intakes below which a person of given sex, age and weight could not plausibly live a normal life style. For example it

is unlikely that any individual is able to maintain an energy intake less than a PAL of 1.2 for any significant length of time without weight loss. These approaches have been invaluable in identifying (for rejection), implausible dietary intake data, but they cannot estimate the nature and extent of misreporting (e.g. underreporting of fat or sugar intake) and do not identify a psychological tendency to misreport.

These approaches represent a critical advance in understanding that misreporting (especially underreporting) is common, may be more prevalent in women, and appears to be more prevalent as the body mass index increases. However, these approaches, based on energy balance methodology alone, do not solve the problem of misreporting and its effects on estimates of dietary intakes. It appears that significant numbers of subjects misreport in diet surveys; for example, 40% of women and 27% of men in a large-scale UK government survey were classified as underreporters of EI according to current EI/BMR cutoffs. If these data are removed from or included in the data set, patterns between dietary intake and disease prevalence (and other important outcomes) will be distorted, because either including erroneous data or analysing only those deemed not to misreport will change the relationships under scrutiny in the population.

Interestingly, with the exception of body mass index and sex, few physiological or metabolic factors are associated with misreported intakes. On the other hand, there do appear to be a number of psychological correlates of misreporting (especially underreporting) such as restraint, conscientiousness and predisposition to social norms. In order to gain a truer picture of the nature and extent of misreporting in populations, multidisciplinary projects will need to build on the approaches that have been developed to detect such discrepancies. The use of biomarkers and readily measurable psychological traits combined with data on feeding behaviour, nutrient intake and estimates of energy balance are required to derive statistical models which predict the nature and extent of misreporting in populations.

Measurement of Energy Expenditure

Methods

A number of methods for the measurement of EE are described in Table 3. While errors in the assessment of EI can arise from technical errors in dietary assessment and changes in the behaviour of the subjects, errors in the measurement of EE in the laboratory are largely of a technical nature (**Table 5**). However, only a few of the methods for measuring EE in Table

Table 5 Major sources of error associated with measuring energy expenditure

Error type	Description	Example	Methods affected	Resulting statistical error
Low accuracy	Some techniques for measuring EE do not produce values that are close to 'true' or expected values. This is a limitation of the technique used and has consequences for both the validity and reproducibility of the results	Activity diaries cannot accurately measure EE since they estimate EE using average population-based values	Heart rate monitors Self or interviewer assessment methods All field methods of indirect calorimetry	Systematic and random
Low precision (reproducibility)	Techniques for measuring EE are limited in their ability to produce the same result, even when constantly reapplied in identical environmental situations	During an exercise study the relationship between heart rate and EE will vary within an individual as body composition and fitness levels change. If the relationship is not constantly recalculated, EE estimates will be erroneous	Heart rate monitors Self or interviewer assessment methods	Random
Low measurement validity	A limitation of EE techniques is that they are not always applicable to measuring specific activities of interest	The ventilated hood is not a valid exercise EE measurement because of its low functional capacity to measure high flow rates	Subject to all methods depending on the measurement variable of interest	Systematic or random
Low ecological validity	Techniques available are inadequate at reflecting habitual or 'real life' EE. It is difficult to apply the results from these measurements to habitual situations	Whole-body calorimetry cannot be used to derive the typical daily energy expenditure of a farm worker	All methods of direct calorimetry and indirect calorimetry Labelled bicarbonate	Systematic
Low sensitivity	The sensitivity of many methods of measuring EE is that often large increases to the measured variable produce very little change to the outcome variable	During heart rate monitoring, large changes in EE as a result of anaerobic activity will not be detected in the heart rate	Self or interviewer assessment methods Heart rate monitoring	Systematic
Low specificity	Measurement techniques differ in their ability to be specific about the classification and identification of EE variables	The doubly labelled water method cannot detect a large increase in energy expenditure over a 4 h period since it can only determine average EE over 12–14 days in adults	Doubly labelled water Max Planck respirometer	Systematic

Continued

Table 5 Continued

Error type	Description	Example	Methods affected	Resulting statistical error
Calibration errors	Errors may arise as a consequence of measurement apparatus being insufficiently quantified against a known standard	In indirect calorimetry, failure to correct the gas (CO_2 and O_2) analysers relative to gases of known composition may result in a quantitative miscalculation of respiratory exchange gases	All methods of direct calorimetry and indirect calorimetry Heart rate monitor	Systematic
Analytical	Often the analysis of EE data requires complex calculations and/or sample analysis. Incorrect analysis will result in erroneous outcome data	Successful analysis of doubly labelled water urine samples are dependent on the correct use of a mass spectrometer together with an understanding of flux rate and body pool size calculation. Both of these require high technical ability	All methods of direct calorimetry and indirect calorimetry Doubly labelled water Labelled bicarbonate Heart rate monitor	Systematic or random
Investigator bias	Errors may result from poor understanding of the measurement technique and interpretation of the data	Inadequate knowledge of regression statistics or computing will result in erroneous calculations to transform heart rate into EE	All methods of direct calorimetry and indirect calorimetry Doubly labelled water Labelled bicarbonate Heart rate monitor	Systematic or random
Subject bias	Errors may result from subjects' failure to comply with the requirements of the technique used	Failure of subject to provide urine samples or misrecording the time of sampling will result in errors in the analysis of doubly labelled water urine samples	Self or interviewer assessment methods All field methods of indirect calorimetry Doubly labelled water Labelled bicarbonate Heart rate monitor	Systematic
Sample losses	Errors may result from incomplete collection of the sample required for analysis, typically heat, gas, urine or blood	Douglas bag is permeable to CO_2 and thus EE results will be miscalculated as a result of incorrect CO_2 assessment	Direct calorimetry Indirect calorimetry Doubly labelled water Labelled bicarbonate	Systematic

3 are sufficiently unobtrusive to enable measurement of the habitual free-living EE of humans, without disrupting their activity patterns and hence EE. Table 3 illustrates that there are three main approaches to the measurement of EE: (1) direct calorimetry; (2) indirect calorimetry; and (3) non-calorimetric techniques, including observational techniques (now largely disused).

Direct calorimetry The initial 'gold standard' means of EE measurement from which all other methods have been developed, direct calorimetry is a precise and accurate measure of the heat output (heat loss from the body). However, the measurement apparatus is cumbersome, has to be carefully maintained and is susceptible to environmental changes in heat transfer. The principles and assumptions of direct calorimetry and the technical details on measurement apparatus have been described meticulously by Maclean and Tobin (see Further Reading). Direct calorimetry has been instrumental in validating indirect calorimetry as the major calorimetric technique in use today.

Indirect calorimetry Although 'indirect calorimetry' sounds like an inferior version of direct calorimetry, it is actually faster, more informative and has been used as the theoretical and practical basis upon which most other forms of EE measurement have subsequently been developed and validated. In order to understand EE measurement it is therefore important to understand the principles and assumptions of indirect calorimetry.

The major principle of indirect calorimetry is the first law of thermodynamics, which states that when the chemical energy content of a system changes, the sum of all forms of energy given off or absorbed by the system must be equal to the magnitude of the changes, i.e.:

$$\Delta E = \Delta Q + \Delta W + \Delta R$$

where ΔE is the change in chemical energy, ΔQ is the heat given off, ΔW is the mechanical work performed and, ΔR is all other forms of energy given off. Where work of gaseous expansion (pressure and volume) is involved, the law may be written as

$$\Delta E - Q - (\Delta p V) - \Delta R$$

where p and V are pressure and volume respectively.

The pressure in biological systems tends to be constant within and without the system. Under these conditions we can refer to enthalpy:

$$\Delta E = \Delta H - p\Delta V - \Delta R$$

where ΔH is the change in enthalpy. Thus, if other work is neglected, the first law of thermodynamics can be applied to most biological systems:

$$\underset{\substack{\text{change in internal}\\\text{energy}}}{\Delta E} = \underset{\substack{\text{change in}\\\text{enthalpy}}}{\Delta H} - \underset{\substack{(\text{pressure} \times \text{change}\\\text{in volume})}}{(p \times \Delta V)}$$

This is of considerable relevance to the application of indirect calorimetry, because it facilitates a consideration of the second basic principle of indirect calorimetry – Hess's law of constant heat summation. This law states that the net heat released or gained (or enthalpy change) by a chain of chemical reactions is independent of the chemical pathways involved, and is dependent solely on the initial and final values or enthalpy states of the reactants and final products, respectively. As regards indirect calorimetry, this law can be reduced to the following expression: the energy produced by oxidation of food stuffs in the body is equivalent to that produced in a bomb calorimeter (chemical reaction vessel). This is true for fat and carbohydrate but not for protein.

In biological terms, the enthalpies of combustion of fuels and of formation of combustion products are not only related to initial and final states, they are stoichiometrically related to gaseous exchange. In other words, if the amounts of the many organic compounds oxidized in the body are known, the total heat produced by the subject may be calculated by summing the enthalpies of their oxidation. Conversely, if the oxygen consumed, carbon dioxide produced and other end products secreted or excreted are measured, then heat production can be calculated. This is the basis upon which indirect calorimetry is founded. The coefficients that describe the energy expended in the production of a litre of carbon dioxide and in the consumption of a litre of oxygen during the oxidation of a macronutrient are termed the 'energy equivalents' of CO_2 ($E_{eq}CO_2$) and of O_2 ($E_{eq}O_2$) respectively. These coefficients enable EE to be precisely estimated from measurements of O_2 consumption and CO_2 production. Since the $E_{eq}O_2$ is similar for most metabolic fuels (protein, CHO, fat or alcohol), O_2 consumption alone can be used to estimate EE. The same is true for CO_2 but differences in the $E_{eq}CO_2$ of different metabolic fuels add greater uncertainty if the fuel mixture being oxidized is unknown. The $E_{eq}O_2$, $E_{eq}CO_2$ and respiratory exchange ratios or respiratory quotients (RQ) for the macronutrients are given in **Table 6**.

Since the oxidation of each macronutrient has a specific gaseous exchange ratio (CO_2 produced/O_2 consumed), we can calculate the amounts of O_2 consumed and CO_2 produced as a result of the oxidation

Table 6 Standardized values for the respiratory quotient (RQ) and the energy equivalents for oxygen (E_{eq} O_2) and carbon dioxide (E_{eq} CO_2)

Macronutrient	RQ	E_{eq} O_2 (kJ l^{-1})	E_{eq} CO_2 (kJ l^{-1})
Carbohydrate	1.0	21.12	21.12
Fat	0.710	19.61	27.62
Protein[a]	0.835	19.48	23.33
Alcohol	0.667	20.33	30.49

[a]Assumes that protein is metabolized to urea, creatinine and ammonia in a 95 : 5 : 5 ratio.

of each of these fuels, *provided* we can independently measure each end product. In addition to V_{O_2} and V_{CO_2} for example, urinary nitrogen excretion can be measured as an index of protein oxidation. Under these conditions, the $E_{eq}O_2$ and $E_{eq}CO_2$ for each macronutrient and the respiratory exchange values, together with the estimation of urinary nitrogen excretion, will allow an assessment of the proportion of energy expended that is due to fat, protein and carbohydrate oxidation. In general, the number of independent measurements must be equal to the number of substrates whose oxidation rates are being estimated. The equations used to estimate energy expenditure and macronutrient oxidation can be found at the end of the article.

Total energy expenditure can be measured with great precision. Errors are unlikely to be greater than 1–2%. The errors in the estimation of EE in the oxidation of macronutrients, however, can be much greater – estimates of EE due to the oxidation of specific fuels should at best be considered to be within 5% of the true value, and the margin of error can in practice be far greater.

Indirect calorimetry therefore affords a precise and accurate means of measuring EE under standardized conditions, a means of estimating macronutrient oxidation (which summates to determine total EE) and a robust system against which other methods of assessing EE have been validated. This last point is of particular importance since, while precise and accurate, indirect calorimetry requires expensive, complex analysis systems for measurement of respiratory gases. Because of this, indirect calorimeters severely constrain the habitual EE of the subject and are not suitable to the nonlaboratory environment encountered in field studies or in the assessment of free-living EE.

Because of these constraints, considerable effort and expense have been devoted to the development of other forms of indirect calorimetry which assess EE with acceptable accuracy but do not constrain the behaviour of the subject. The development of the doubly labelled water (DLW) technique was a revolutionary step in the measurement of EE in free-living subjects. The technique is noninvasive, unobtrusive and only requires a daily aliquot (around 20 ml) of urine from the subject to be effective. The modelling and analysis of the technique are, on the other hand extremely complex. The technique is a form of indirect calorimetry since it involves calculating rates of EE from estimates of CO_2 production. Body water is enriched (relative to background) with the stable isotopes $^2H_2$ and ^{18}O. The washout kinetics are then determined for both isotopes as their concentrations decline exponentially toward natural abundance levels. The $^2H_2$ isotope (given as ^2H_2O) is assumed to label only body water; its concentration decreases as it is washed out by intake of new unlabelled water, and is lost in urine and in other excretions and secretions. On the other hand, ^{18}O in the form of water ($H_2^{18}O$) equilibrates with the bicarbonate pool via the carbonic anhydrase reaction in erythrocytes and lung tissue. Because of this ^{18}O is lost both as water and as CO_2. Thus the exponential slope for the loss of ^{18}O is steeper than that for $^2H_2$. The difference between the slopes is an indirect estimate of CO_2 production. Carbon dioxide production is related to the rate of EE via the energy equivalents of CO_2. This method allows estimates of EE over 10–20 days, or 2–3 biological half-lives of the isotopes depending on the conditions such as water turnover. Major drawbacks of the DLW method are its expense and the fact that it only gives an average estimate of EE over a period of 10–20 days.

The labelled bicarbonate method uses a constant subcutaneous microinfusion of [^{14}C]bicarbonate. The labelled bicarbonate can accumulate in cellular bicarbonate pools, fix in body tissues such as fat, or is lost in breath, kidney, faeces and urine and sweat. The losses in the sweat, faeces, kidney and any fixation in the body are considered negligible (less than 5% in a 12–36 h period), thus collected breath, blood, urine or saliva samples will provide information on the extent of the isotope dilution and hence CO_2 production. Reasonable estimates of CO_2 production can also be obtained by measuring the extent of isotopic dilution in the urea pool. Measurement of urea (in urine) is advantageous in that samples can be taken less frequently and smaller doses of ^{14}C can be administered. The measured CO_2 production together with estimated $E_{eq}CO_2$ can be used to calculate EE. Advantages of the labelled bicarbonate method are that it is cheap to use and allows day-by-day estimates of EE with a similar precision and accuracy to DLW. However, the technique uses a very low dose of radioisotope, which is technically safe but still discouraging to some potential volunteers. New developments of the technique will include use of [^{13}C] bicarbonate and possible replacement of the microinfusion with an oral bolus dose.

Heart rate monitoring has become a popular method of assessing EE owing to its ease of use and low subject burden. Indirect calorimetry is an integral part of ensuring the success of this method. Before heart rate can be extrapolated into EE, the relationship between heart rate and EE (measured by indirect calorimetry) must be established for each individual. This relationship is linear only above a certain threshold in heart rate; below this threshold heart rate becomes a poor indicator of EE, and this method is therefore unsuitable for very sedentary subjects, e.g. hospitalized patients. Heart rate monitoring is particularly useful for estimating the energy cost of exercise where collection of respiratory gases can limit the capacity to exercise and isotopic tracer methods are inapplicable.

Self or interviewer assessment methods of EE from recall are not strictly measures of EE, but more a measure of activity patterns which have been translated into estimates of EE using standard tables which give estimates for the energy cost of certain activities. The tables are derived from measures of EE during specific physical activities. The energy costs are expressed as multiples of BMR and are referred to as physical activity levels, and are specific for a whole range of activities. Many of the errors in these assessments are similar to those affecting dietary intake assessments. For example, tabulated values may differ from the actual EE of the study population for a given activity, or subjects may misreport their activities. However, for a number of situations such as historical comparisons in establishing secular trends in physical activity, these are the only data available.

Types of study in which EE measures are used

As with measurements of EI, techniques for the measurement of EE are often chosen on the basis of the research objective and the environment in which the study is conducted. For example, the constrained environment of a whole-body calorimeter will not provide the investigator with information on the habitual EE of a subject. Measurement techniques are also practically constrained to particular environments; for example the Oxylog (see Table 3), although useful in field situations, cannot be used to estimate the energy cost of water-borne activities, and labelled bicarbonate could not be used to measure EE in 1000 schoolchildren over a 7-day period.

The major study designs that employ EE assessments are similar to those previously discussed for EI assessment (ecological/population studies, laboratory studies and intervention studies). However, the majority of EE measurement methods are limited to the laboratory and small-scale ecological studies. It is unfeasible to conduct accurate EE measurements in large-scale epidemiological studies. Methods available to ecological studies such as DLW or heart rate monitoring are generally constrained to smaller subsets of large study populations; large-scale ecological or epidemiological studies typically use qualitative or semiquantitative self-reported diaries and questionnaires which lack quantitative precision, accuracy and sensitivity.

Studies that are able to incorporate independent measures of EI, EE and energy stores (often by using body weight over periods in excess of 7 days) provide the most valuable insights into factors that exert important influences on energy balance. This approach has been invaluable in estimating the extent of misreporting of dietary intakes. By demonstrating that misreporting is systematically greater in obese subjects, energy balance assessments have refuted the notion that the obese require a lower EI to maintain a higher body weight than lean, subjects. Similarly, meticulous measures of the components of the energy balance equation have shown that the elevated EE often associated with disease and trauma is countered by a decreased EE due to lower levels of physical activity. The negative energy balance often associated with disease is therefore likely to include a genuine suppression of appetite.

Future Developments in Measuring EI and EE

Measurements of dietary intakes and of EE in human subjects have been in operation for over a century. It may be asked whether there is any more progress to be made in these related fields. It is important to emphasize that despite a century of data collection in these areas, we are still extremely ignorant of the processes controlling energy balance in humans. Much of this ignorance rests on the technical and behavioural limitations of the many methods used to measure EI and EE. Only in the last few years has a precise and accurate measure of free-living EE been available in the form of DLW and labelled bicarbonate, methods. This in turn has allowed estimates of the plausibility of dietary intake reports. The results of these assessments have been depressing, since they suggest that a significant proportion of subjects in most dietary surveys misreport EI, with a systematic bias towards underreporting. There is therefore a great deal of work to be done in these areas. The measurement of EI and EE will remain important fields of endeavour for a number of years to come.

An area of critical importance for improving estimates of EI is the validation of EI and nutrient intake measures in studies that attempt to assess the dietary intakes of free-living populations. In order to do so it will be necessary to gain a better understanding of who tends to misreport and what foods tend to be misreported. Rather than identify and exclude misreporters in the population it is necessary to identify and model the misreporting so that it can be corrected for, in order to obtain more accurate estimates of dietary intake patterns. If the nature and extent of misreporting can be modelled, correction factors may be derived which will facilitate more accurate assessments of dietary intakes in populations and hence improve our understanding of the relationship between diet and disease. The importance of this area cannot be overemphasized, because if the data derived from epidemiological studies are distorted then so too are our conclusions relating to the effects of diet on the aetiology of noninfectious disease. The development of economically feasible biomarkers that independently assess the EI or the intake of specific nutrients with acceptable precision and accuracy will represent a considerable advance in the measurement of EI and its constituents.

One particular development, related to the measurement of EE, which may greatly assist in the validation of dietary intakes and our understanding of energy and nutrient balance would be the development of free-living indirect calorimetry. With the development of the labelled bicarbonate method daily EE can now be measured in free-living subjects. Collection of total urine samples allows protein oxidation to be estimated, and as discussed above, has been instrumental in validating the plausibility of dietary intakes. A biomarker for fat or carbohydrate oxidation would effectively facilitate free-living indirect calorimetry and open up a whole field of investigation into the effects of activity, environment, growth, development, pregnancy and lactation and diseases on whole-body substrate metabolism. Furthermore, since in most free-living subjects protein and carbohydrate oxidation tends to match their intake, the extent and composition of misreported EIs could be assessed. These developments would not solve the problems of altered feeding behaviour by subjects when they are studied, although unobtrusive use of biomarkers may have less effect on feeding behaviour than overt self-recorded intakes.

Stable isotopes are becoming useful tools to quantify the turnover of a number of micronutrients, trace elements and amino acids. A number of techniques exist for the determination of amino acid flux and protein turnover. These approaches are highly specialized, often invasive and require extensive use of high-resolution mass spectrometry in analysis of isotopic enrichments. Researchers have noted that more comprehensive models are needed to develop plausible physiological models of the metabolism of amino acids and proteins and their interactions; the same arguments can be made for a number of other isotopic techniques which have been developed to assess bioavailability, metabolic function and flux of micronutrients or minerals. Unfortunately, since there are a limited number of stable isotopes in use (^{2}H, ^{13}C, ^{15}N and ^{18}O being the most common), the flux of only a few nutrients can be determined in any one subject at any one time. However, as new techniques are developed and current approaches refined, the knowledge gained in one area is often exploited in another, which should assist in the growth of biomarkers and tracers to estimate flux of energy and its constituents through the body in health and disease.

A further area that has been touched upon only briefly above is the measurement of EE and substrate metabolism in specific organs. Arteriovenous difference studies, novel imaging techniques and isotopic tracer methods are leading to considerable advances in our understanding of the interorgan flux of energy nutrients in health and in disease. The majority of these measurements are necessarily made in the clinical setting. It is not impossible that in the future, the measurement of energy and nutrient flux on a whole-body and organ-specific basis may become possible in free-living subjects. The rapid pace of developments in the measurement of energy and nutrient flux in the last few years hints at possible progress in the measurement of EI and EE which would reveal new dimensions to our understanding of energy and nutrient flux in human health and disease.

See Colour plate 1.

See also: **Energy**: Energy Requirements; Energy Balance.

Further Reading

Bigham SA (1987) The dietary assessment of individuals; methods, accuracy, new techniques and recommendations. *Nutrition Abstracts and Reviews* 57:705–742.

Black A, Goldberg G, Jebb S, Livingstone M, Cole T and Prentice A (1991) Critical evaluation of energy intake data using fundamental principles of energy physiology: 2. evaluating the results of published surveys. *European Journal of Clinical Nutrition* 45:583–599.

Blaxter K (1987) *Energy Metabolism in Animals and Man.* Cambridge University Press.

Dubois CF (1954) Energy metabolism. *Annual Review of Physiology* 16:125–134.

Elia M (1991) The estimation of short-term energy expenditure by the labelled bicarbonate method. In: Whitehead RG and Prentice A (eds) *New Techniques in Nutrition Research*, pp 208–232. New York: Academic Press.

Elia M and Livesey G (1992) Energy expenditure and fuel selection in biological systems: the theory and practice of calculations based on indirect calorimetry and tracer methods. In: Simopoulos AP (ed.) *Control of Eating, Energy Expenditure and the Bioenergetics of Obesity*, pp 68–131. Basel: Karger.

Hill AJ, Rogers PJ and Blundell JE (1995) Techniques for the experimental measurement of human eating behaviour and food-intake – a practical guide. *International Journal of Obesity* 19:361–375.

Holland B, Welch AA, Unwin ID, Buss DH, Paul AA and Southgate DAT (1991) *McCance and Widdowson's The Composition of Foods*, 5th edn. Cambridge Royal Society of Chemistry.

James W and Schofield E (1990) *Human Energy Requirements*. Oxford University Press.

Livesey G (1992) The energy values of dietary fibre and sugar alcohols in man. *Nutrition Research Reviews* 5:61–84.

Margatroyd P, Shetty P and Prentice A (1993) Techniques for the measurement of human energy expenditure: a practical guide. *International Journal of Obesity* 17:549–568.

McLean JA and Tolbin G (1987) *Animal and Human Calorimetry*. Cambridge University Press.

Prentice AM, ed. (1990) *The Doubly Labelled Water Method for Measuring Energy Expenditure: Technical Recommendations for Use in Humans*. A consensus report by the IDECG Working group. Vienna: International Atomic Energy Agency.

Spurr G, Prentice A, Murgatroyd P, Goldberg G, Reina J and Christman N (1988) Energy expenditure from minute-by-minute heart rate recording: comparison with indirect calorimetry. *American Journal of Clinical Nutrition* 48:552–559.

Equations for calculating energy expenditure

$$EE \text{ (kJ)} = 15.913 \, V_{O_2} + 5.207 \, V_{CO_2} - 4.464 \, N_u \quad [1]$$

$$EE \text{ (kJ)} = 15.818 \, V_{O_2} + 5.176 \, V_{CO_2} \quad [2]$$

where V_{O_2} is the volume of oxygen in litres, V_{CO_2} is the volume of carbon dioxide in litres and N_u is the total urinary nitrogen in grams. Equation [2] assumes that protein accounts for 15% of energy expenditure.

These equations can be extended to accommodate alcohol and glycerol oxidation, hydrogen, free glycerol (different from glycerol in triacylglycerol), hydroxybutyrate, acetoacetate and acetone production.

Equations for estimation of substrate utilization in a subject consuming a normal diet (no alcohol)

1. A single gram of urinary nitrogen corresponds to 116 kJ. Given the $E_{eq}O_2$ for protein (Table 6) this will equate to 5.95 litres of oxygen (116/19.48 = 5.95). The RQ for a standard dietary protein is 0.835 (see Table 6).
2. Multiplication of urinary nitrogen (in grams) by 5.95 (l) will give the oxygen consumption as a result of protein oxidation. Multiplying the resulting value by the RQ (0.835) gives the carbon dioxide production in litres as a result of protein oxidation. The energy associated with protein oxidation is calculated by multiplying the weight (in grams) of urinary nitrogen by 116 kJ.
3. The oxygen consumption and carbon dioxide production derived from fat and carbohydrate oxidation together are calculated by deducting the values in step 2 from total measured oxygen and carbon dioxide.
4. The energy associated with fat and carbohydrate oxidation can be derived using equation [1] above.
5. Percentage energy expenditure from carbohydrate oxidation can then be calculated using the following equation:

$$E\%_{carb} = \frac{2112 \, (RQ - 0.71)}{21.12 \, (RQ - 0.71) + 19.61 \, (1 - RQ)}$$

Note: The values in this equation are based on the $E_{eq}O_2$ and $E_{eq}CO_2$ for fat and carbohydrate (Table 6).

6. Multiplying the percentage (step 5) by the result of step 4 (energy associated with fat and carbohydrate oxidation) will deduce the energy (kJ) associated with carbohydrate oxidation.
7. Deducting the result of step 6 (% energy from carbohydrate oxidation) from step 4 (total energy expenditure from fat and carbohydrate oxidation) allows the calculation of energy expenditure from fat oxidation.

If a fourth substrate (e.g. alcohol) is involved in this oxidation mixture then one can still calculate the contribution of each substrate provided that the quantities metabolized and the end products are known.

Worked example

The energy expenditure for a human subject was measured in a whole-body calorimeter over 24 h. During a specific 4 h period this subject produced 166 litres of O_2, 140 litres of CO_2 and 3 g urinary nitrogen.

What is the energy expenditure if this subject is consuming a normal diet and not consuming alcohol? Give the energy expenditure attributable to each of the macronutrients fat, carbohydrate and protein.

Total energy expenditure – eqn [1]

$15.913 \times 166 + 5.207 \times 140 - 4.464 \times 3$
$= 2641.56 + 728.98 - 13.39$
$= 3357 \text{ kJ}$

Energy expenditure attributable to each of the macronutrients

1. Oxygen consumed in protein oxidation:
   $3 \times 5.95 = \textbf{17.85 litres}$
2. Carbon dioxide produced in protein oxidation:
   $17.85 \times 0.835 = \textbf{14.90 litres}$
3. Energy associated with protein oxidation:
   $3 \times 116 = \textbf{348 kJ}$
4. Oxygen consumed from fat and carbohydrate oxidation: $166 - 17.85 = \textbf{148.15 litres}$
5. Carbon dioxide produced from fat and carbohydrate oxidation: $140 - 14.90 = \textbf{125.10 litres}$

6. Energy expenditure from fat and carbohydrate oxidation:
   $(15.913 \times 148.15) + (5.207 \times 125.10)$
   $= 2357.51 + 651.40 = \textbf{3008.91 kJ}$

7. RQ = 140/166 = **0.84**
8. Percentage energy expenditure from carbohydrate oxidation:

$$\frac{2112\,(0.84 - 0.71)}{21.12\,(0.84 - 0.71) + 19.61\,(1 - 0.84)} = \textbf{46.667\%}$$

9. Therefore energy expenditure from carbohydrate oxidation:

   $3008.91 \times 0.46667 = \textbf{1404.17 kJ}$

10. Therefore energy expenditure from fat oxidation:

    $3008.91 - 1404.17 = \textbf{1604.74 kJ}$

11. Total energy expenditure (sum of steps 3 + 8 + 10) = **3357 kJ**

ENERGY METABOLISM

Tricarboxylic Acid Cycle and Oxidative Phosphorylation

Sharon Rubinstein, Johns Hopkins University, Baltimore, Maryland, USA

Copyright © 1998 Academic Press

Energy is essential for life; food is the fuel through which the body obtains its energy. The reactions involved in the process of obtaining and spending energy are known as energy metabolism. The energy in foods is chemical energy, which is converted by the body to mechanical, electrical or heat energy to perform necessary biological functions.

Metabolism

Metabolism is defined as the series of physico-chemical reactions that take place in cells with the purpose of synthesizing, converting, utilizing and catabolizing substrates. Most reactions of human metabolism are performed by enzymes, protein molecules highly adapted and regulated. Many reactions also require cofactors or coenzymes, most commonly vitamin molecules.

The energy in foods becomes available after metabolism in the form of carbohydrate, fat or protein (amino acids). After adjustment for net absorption and urinary losses, the energy value of these substrates is estimated as 4 kcal g^{-1} for carbohydrate, 4 kcal g^{-1} for protein and 9 kcal g^{-1} for fat (16.8 kJ g^{-1}, 16.8 kJ g^{-1} and 37.8 kJ g^{-1} respectively).

The chemical reactions that occur in the body can be divided into anabolic and catabolic reactions. In anabolic reactions, energy is used to bind the basic units from energy-yielding nutrients (glucose, glycerol, fatty acids and amino acids) to build larger compounds. In catabolic reactions the opposite occurs: larger molecules are broken down to form smaller compounds. While in anabolic reactions energy is used, in catabolic reactions energy is released. The energy released during catabolic reactions can radiate away as heat, can be captured in another chemical bond, or both. Coupled reactions are those in which the energy released from the breakdown of one compound is used to build a new compound.

ATP

Adenosine triphosphate (ATP) is a form of energy storage used by cells (**Fig. 1**). Body cells make ATP to help meet their energy requirements. The way in which cells use the energy stored in ATP is by splitting the molecule into adenosine diphosphate (ADP) and a molecule of phosphate (P). Splitting the ADP into adenosine monophosphate (AMP) and a molecule of phosphate can release additional energy.

Adenosine triphosphate is the only form of energy that can be used directly by the cells; energy released as heat is lost and cannot be used. It is a very stable compound that requires an enzyme to break its bonds to release energy.

Metabolism of Energy-yielding Compounds

Glucose

The 3-carbon compound pyruvate and the 2-carbon compound acetyl-CoA are essential in energy metabolism. Glucose can be made from pyruvate but not from acetyl-CoA; as a result, only compounds that can be converted to pyruvate can be used to make glucose.

Glucose is the major form of carbohydrate fuel substrate. It is also a preferential energy substrate for the brain, the renal cortex and red blood cells. The first step is the metabolic breakdown of glucose to pyruvate known as glycolysis, which takes place in the cytosol of the cell. During glycolysis, the 6-carbon glucose is split into two molecules of the 3-carbon compound pyruvate. The two molecules of pyruvate then enter a sequence of reactions that include the tricarboxylic acid (TCA) cycle and the electron transport chain. During these reactions, the molecules of pyruvate continue to break down and release most of their energy, which is used to form ATP. Glycolysis begins with the phosphorylation of the glucose molecule, a step that consumes two molecules of ATP. However, during the conversion of

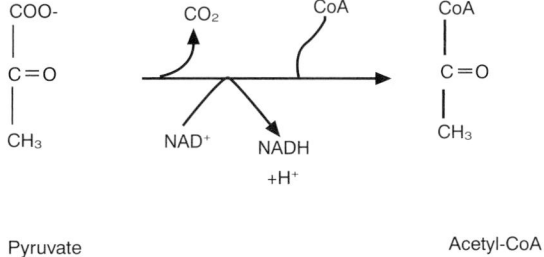

Figure 2 Conversion of pyruvate to acetyl-CoA, a critical junction in energy metabolism, linking glycolysis, the tricarboxylic acid cycle and fatty acid synthesis.

glucose to pyruvate, four molecules of ATP are generated, resulting in a net production of two molecules of ATP. The breakdown of glucose to pyruvate also releases four hydrogen molecules and four electrons, which are attached to a molecule of nicotinamide adenine dinucleotide (NAD^+), to form NADH and yield further energy.

In order to enter the TCA cycle, pyruvate is converted to acetyl-CoA by the action of pyruvate decarboxylase, with release of carbon dioxide. Coenzyme A is then attached to the acetate moiety, forming acetyl-CoA. This irreversible metabolic step releases two hydrogen molecules, converting NAD^+ to NADH + H^+ (**Fig. 2**). The conversion of pyruvate to acetyl-CoA is an oxygen-dependent step, and cannot proceed at low oxygen concentrations. In that situation,

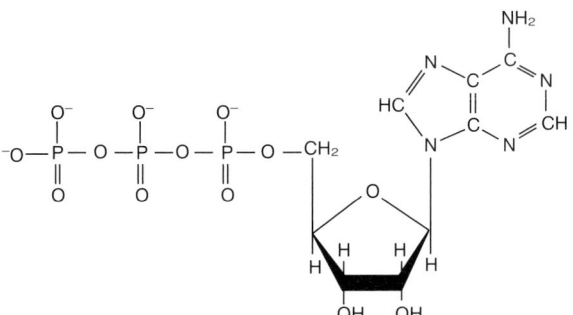

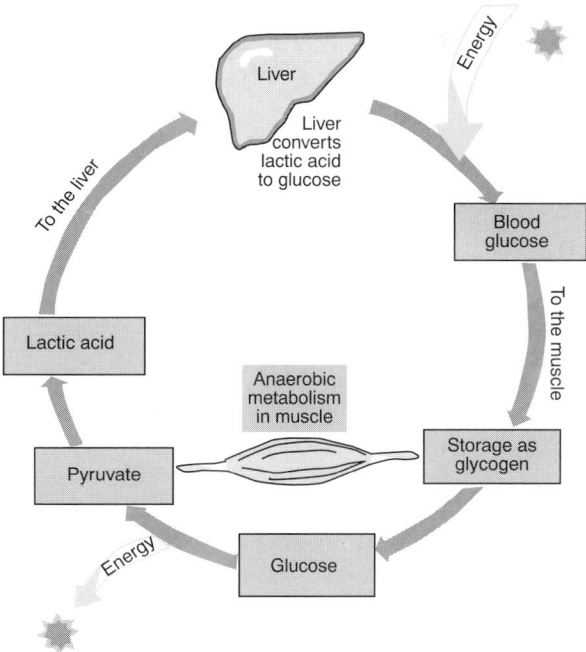

Figure 3 The Cori cycle, an important route for the removal of lactic acid produced during anaerobic glucose utilization in peripheral tissues and for gluconeogenesis in the liver. From Whitney and Rolfes (1993).

Figure 1 Structure of adenosine triphosphate (ATP).

pyruvate is converted to lactic acid. This 3-carbon compound may be further metabolized by the liver via the Cori cycle (**Fig. 3**) with *de novo* generation of glucose.

The subsequent metabolic fate of the pyruvate-derived acetyl-CoA will depend on the energy status of the cell. If immediate release of energy is required, the acetyl-CoA will enter the TCA cycle, where it will release a greater amount of energy compared with glycolysis. If energy fuel is not needed immediately, acetyl-CoA enters the fatty acid synthesis pathway, and energy is eventually stored as fatty acids in adipose tissue.

Fat

Dietary fat is distributed primarily as triacylglycerols. Upon entering the tissues, fatty acids are released and the glycerol moiety becomes available for further metabolism as well. Glycerol enters the glycolytic pathway as a 3-carbon compound, and its carbon skeleton eventually yields pyruvate. It can also follow the reverse direction, and contribute to glucose synthesis. Fatty acid oxidation is a complex sequence of reactions, in which 2-carbon sections of the fatty acid chain are removed sequentially.

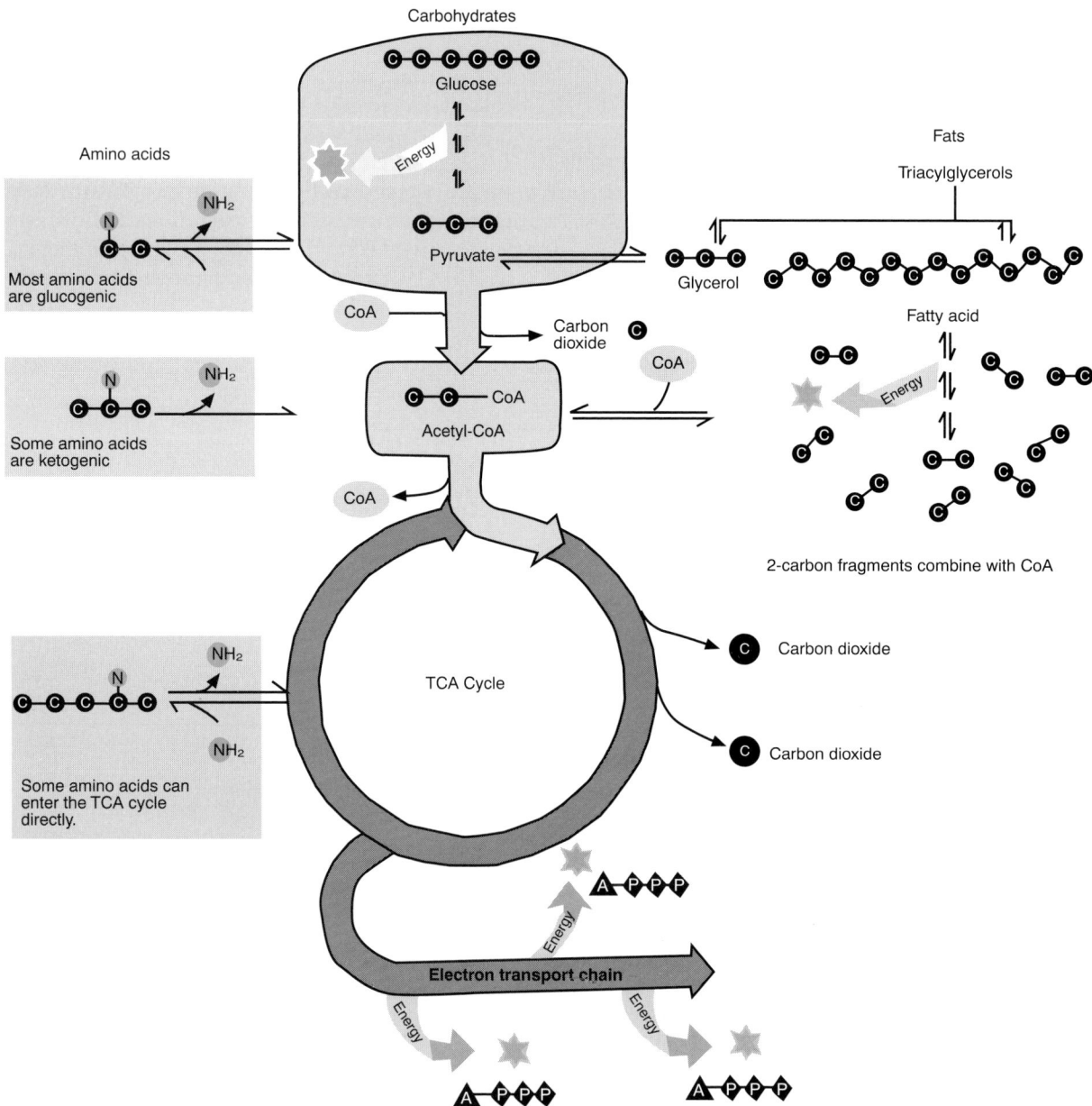

Figure 4 Overview of energy metabolism. From Whitney and Rolfes (1993). TCA, tricarboxylic acid cycle.

Amino acids

Certain amino acids are 'glucogenic', i.e. they can be used to synthesize glucose. After the amino group is removed from the molecule, glucogenic amino acids are converted to pyruvate and can follow the same fate as this compound. The ketogenic amino acids contribute their carbon skeleton to the synthesis of acetyl-CoA. **Fig. 4** summarizes the common path of these energy-producing reactions.

The tricarboxylic acid cycle

The TCA cycle is also known as the citric acid cycle and the Krebs cycle, in honour of Hans Krebs, the biochemist who discovered it. The cycle is an extraordinarily ingenious sequence of reactions, which, while primarily designed to convert the carbon skeleton of acetyl-CoA into carbon dioxide, also permits the entry of different compounds at several steps. The cycle is regulated primarily by the energy state

of the cell, which in turn determines how much acetyl-CoA will be shifted to the cycle instead of to fatty acid synthesis. As the carbon skeleton is oxidized, hydrogen atoms and their electrons are released and enter the electron transport chain. As previously described by Whitney and Rolfes (1993), the steps of the TCA cycle (**Fig. 5**) are as follows:

1. Acetyl-CoA enters the cycle to form citrate by combining with oxaloacetate. The CoA moiety is lost in this step.
2. A molecule of water enters the cycle to help rearrange the atoms of citrate to form isocitrate. A molecule of water is also lost at this step.
3. A molecule of NAD^+ reacts with isocitrate by removing two molecules of hydrogen and two electrons to form $NADH + H^+$. One carbon is combined with two molecules of oxygen and released as carbon dioxide. After this reaction, isocitrate is converted into the 5-carbon compound α-ketoglutarate.

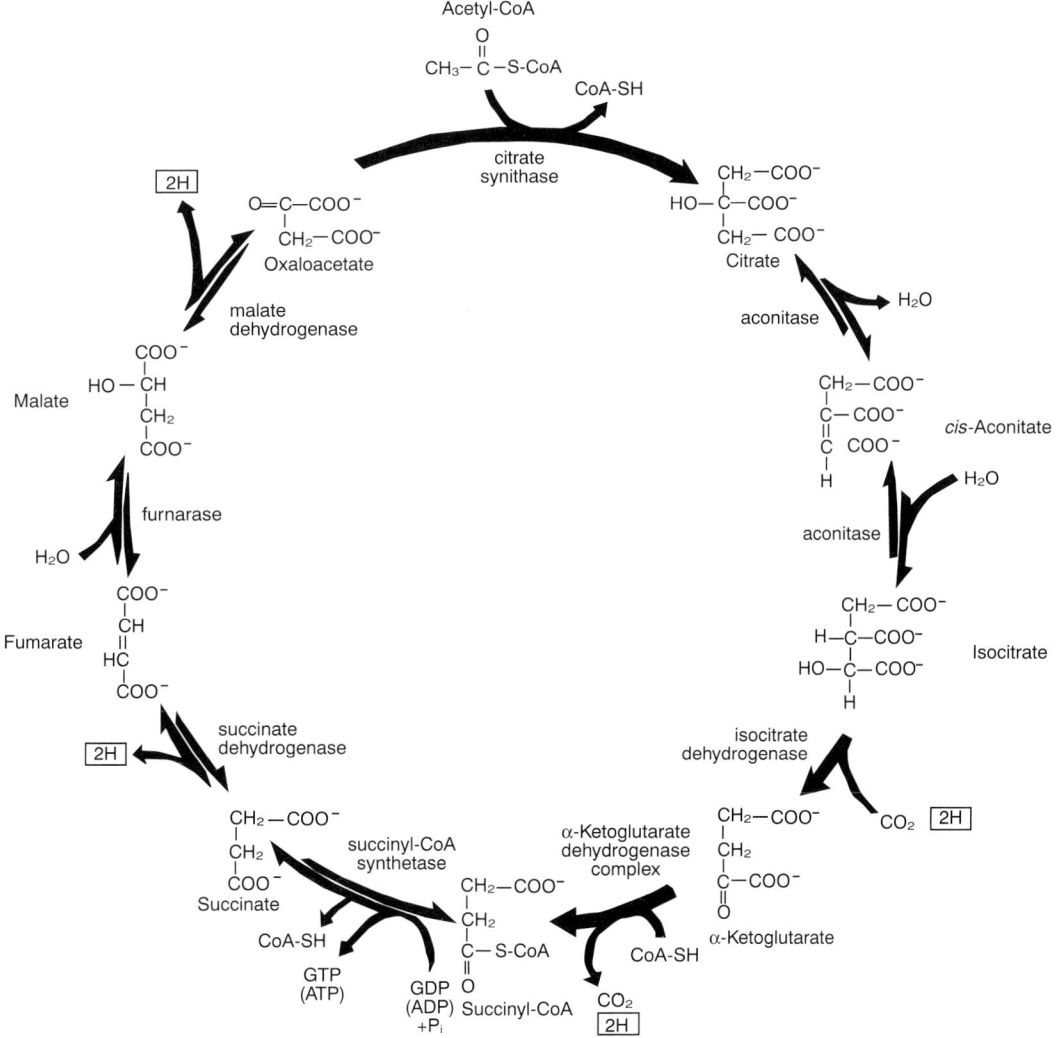

Figure 5   Tricarboxylic acid cycle. From Lehninger, Nelson and Cox (1993).

4. Alpha-ketoglutarate interacts with a molecule of CoA and a molecule of NAD^+. In this reaction, one carbon and two oxygen molecules are again released as carbon dioxide and two hydrogen molecules are removed and attached to NAD^+ to form $NADH + H^+$. The four remaining carbons are attached to the molecule of CoA to form succinyl-CoA.
5. Succnily-CoA goes through a series of reactions to form succinate in which a molecule of water is involved. The CoA is lost and a molecule of guanosine diphosphate (GDP) and one phosphate (P) are combined to form the high-energy compound guanosine triphosphate (GTP), which is comparable to ATP.
6. Two hydrogen molecules (with their associated energy) are released from succinate and transferred to an electron-hydrogen receiver molecule called flavin adenine dinucleotide (FAD). The result is the formation of $FADH_2$ and fumarate.
7. A molecule of water interacts with fumarate to form malate.
8. A molecule of NAD^+ reacts with malate by attaching itself to two molecules of hydrogen (with their associated energy) to form $NADH + H^+$. The remaining product is a 4-carbon compound, oxaloacetate, which reacts with acetyl-CoA to restart the cycle.

Each time a hydrogen atom is removed from one of the molecules in the TCA cycle, it takes with it a pair of electrons. Furthermore, the energy from this chemical bond is captured in the compound to which the hydrogen became attached. In the TCA cycle, energy is transferred to other compounds in steps 3, 4, 6 and 8, and stored in GTP in step 5. As a result, three molecules of $NADH + H^+$, one $FADH_2$ and one GTP are obtained, which contain energy originally found in acetyl-CoA. For the resulting energy to end up in ATP molecules, an additional step is required: the electrons must enter the electron transport chain.

The electron transport chain

As implied by its name, the chain consists of a series of reactions among electron carrier molecules. As each electron is transferred from carrier to carrier, it releases energy in the form of heat and ATP. The chain ends with the formation of a molecule of water, which is achieved when the low-energy electrons are donated to a molecule of oxygen. At this point, it is impossible for the cell to extract any more energy from it. Thus, the end point of the electron transport chain is the formation of ATP and water.

Since oxygen is required, oxidative phosphorylation often occurs in these reactions. During oxidat-ive phosphorylation, a molecule of phosphate (P) is attached to an ADP to form ATP. This reaction is an example of a coupled reaction. Each energy-carrying molecule yields a different number of ATP molecules depending on the step in which it enters the electron transport chain. This process has been previously illustrated by Whitney and Rolfes (1993) by following the trail of a molecule of $NADH + H^+$ (**Fig. 6**).

1. NADH reacts with a flavoprotein losing its electrons and its hydrogen molecules. The result is NAD^+ and a reduced flavoprotein. Energy is lost as heat.
2. The reduced flavoprotein transfers its electrons to a molecule called coenzyme Q. In this step, some energy is lost as heat but also ATP is formed in a coupled reaction by bonding ADP + P.
3. Coenzyme Q passes the electrons to cytochrome b and again some energy is lost as heat.
4. Cytochrome b passes the electrons to cytochrome c in a coupled reaction resulting in the formation of a molecule of ATP.

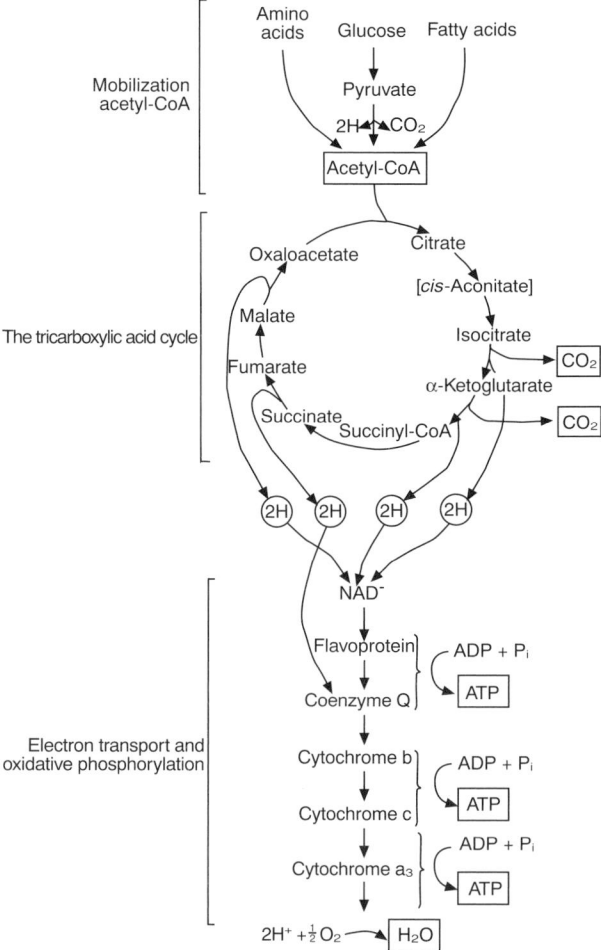

Figure 6   The electron transport chain. From Lehninger (1975).

5. Cytochrome *c* transfers its electrons to cytochrome *a*, which transfers them with its hydrogen molecules to an atom of oxygen to form water. Another molecule of ATP is formed through a coupled reaction.

For each molecule of NADH that enters the electron transport chain, three molecules of ATP are formed. Each molecule of $FADH_2$ only yields two molecules of ATP because its electrons enter the chain at coenzyme Q. Guanosine triphosphate does not enter the chain but yields one molecule of ATP by giving its energy directly to ADP in a simple phosphorylation reaction.

The complete oxidation of one molecule of glucose yields 38–40 molecules of ATP. Because two ATP molecules are needed to phosphorylate glucose and initiate the glycolytic path, the net yield is 36–38 molecules of ATP for each molecule of glucose.

See also: **Amino Acids**: Metabolism. **Fatty Acids**: Metabolism. **Glucose**: Metabolism and Maintenance of Blood Glucose Level.

Further Reading

Lehninger AL (1989) *Biochemistry*. New York: Worth.
Linder MC (1991) *Nutritional Biochemistry and Metabolism*. New York: Appleton & Lange.
Wardlaw GM and Insel PM (1993) Metabolism. In: *Perspectives in Nutrition*, pp 205–229. St Louis, Missouri: Mosby.
Whitney EN and Rolfes SR (1993) Metabolism: Transformations and Interactions. In: *Understanding Nutrition*, 6th edition, pp 205–232. St. Paul, Minnesota: West Publishing.

EPIDEMIOLOGICAL STUDIES

Role and Interpretation

M L Burr, University of Wales College of Medicine, Cardiff, UK

Copyright © 1998 Academic Press

Epidemiological methods address populations by means of ecological, cross-sectional, case–control and cohort studies, together with randomized trials. They provide information about health status and the causation of disease. Each method has its own limitations; cohort studies and randomized trials are the most valuable but are also the most difficult.

Aims of Epidemiological Studies

Epidemiology is the study of the distribution and determinants of health-related states or events in populations. Nutritional epidemiology examines the nutritional status of groups and shows how nutritional factors are related to various indices of health within the population under consideration. Its aims and objectives can be summarized as follows.

Describing populations

Ascertaining the nutritional status of an individual forms an important part of the assessment of that person's state of health. Similarly, the nutritional status of a defined population needs to be investigated if that population's state of health is to be understood. The nutritional epidemiologist is interested in (for example) the average values and distributions of nutrient intakes, height, body mass index and serum concentrations of biochemical variables. Questions to be addressed might include: what is the prevalence of obesity in this population? In which groups does it most often occur?

Uncovering need

One important purpose in investigating a population is to assess the amount of unmet need. For example, is there any evidence of malnutrition in an area, and if so, in which sections of the population? This kind of information is very useful in the planning and management of health services. We may have to decide whether another dietitian should be employed in the community, and it would be helpful to know where the needs are greatest.

Monitoring progress

Repeated epidemiological studies provide information about trends over time. Suppose we have set up a programme to tackle nutritional deficiency among the children of an ethnic minority group, and want to know whether we are succeeding. Only by conducting repeated surveys in this group can we learn whether we are improving their nutritional status.

Investigating the whole spectrum and natural history of disease

Studies of diseases tend to be based on patients who attend hospital, who are likely to have more severe disease, so that little information is obtained about its milder forms. A survey of general practitioners' patients known to have the disease – for example, diabetes – will give a broader picture, but if we want to study the whole spectrum of diabetes we should ideally conduct a survey in the community. Epidemiology can further assist our understanding of diabetes if we follow up a group of newly diagnosed diabetic patients and discover how the disease progresses over time and what factors predict and modify the outcome.

Investigating causation

Epidemiological techniques have been particularly helpful in elucidating the causes of diseases. Most diseases do not have a single cause that operates in every case; there are usually several factors that combine to increase or decrease the risk. Studies of groups of people will reveal what factors are associated positively or negatively with the disease, and randomized trials (if feasible) will show whether altering one factor leads to a corresponding change in outcome.

Evaluating treatment

In exactly the same way, epidemiology investigates the effectiveness of treatment, particularly for conditions that do not always take the same course. By following up groups of patients who have received different types of treatment, preferably allocated at random, we can compare the advantages and disadvantages (including side effects) of alternative methods of management.

Methodology

Epidemiologists use certain techniques which are suitable for a wide variety of applications. The main techniques are outlined below, with examples of their use in nutritional research.

Ecological studies

In an ecological study, the unit of analysis is a population or group of people rather than the individual. It is used in comparing published data from different geographical areas to relate potential determinants of health (e.g. per capita consumption of various foods) and mortality rates. For example, **Fig. 1** relates the annual consumption of wine (in litres per head, using a logarithmic scale) in 18 countries with the death rates from ischaemic heart disease in men aged 55–64 years in those countries. There is a clear negative relationship, in that the more wine is drunk per head of population, the lower is the death rate from ischaemic heart disease.

The ecological study is the only available approach when data exist for populations but not for individuals. There are circumstances when it is also suitable for the analysis of data that relate to individuals. If serum cholesterol has been measured in random samples of the population in several countries, we can compare the average cholesterol levels in those countries with the national death rates from heart disease to see if they are related. In this case we have individual data on one variable but not on the other, so we are restricted to an ecological analysis. Even when individual data are available for both variables, however, an ecological approach may still be

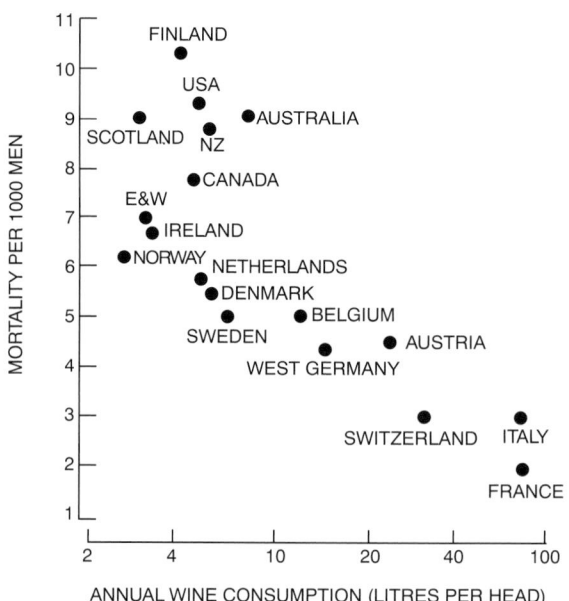

Figure 1   Relationship between ischaemic heart disease mortality in men aged 55–64 years and wine consumption. E&W, England and Wales; NZ, New Zealand. From St Leger *et al.* (1979).

preferable. **Fig. 2** summarizes data from surveys in 24 communities, relating mean sodium intake (estimated in various ways) to mean blood pressure. Since the sodium intakes and blood pressures were measured in the same people, it would be perfectly possible to examine their relationship in the individuals; however, the sodium intake of any one person can vary widely from day to day, so that the intake estimated on a single occasion (e.g. by 24 h urine collection) gives very little indication of that person's usual intake. The blood pressure is also liable to fluctuate within each individual. By examining the average values we find out whether communities that habitually eat more salt have higher blood pressures than those that eat less, which seems to be the case (at least for the undeveloped populations), whereas analyses of individual data seldom show any association.

The ecological approach is also useful in examining trends over time and in comparing various sets of people, such as distinctive ethnic or religious groups and migrants. There are important limitations in this method, however, which are discussed below.

Cross-sectional surveys

The simplest epidemiological method is the cross-sectional survey, which takes a 'snapshot' of a population or group at one point in time. The object may be to describe the population, to establish the prevalence of some disease within it, or to ascertain whether certain variables are related to each other. Examples include surveys of height and weight, of dietary intake, and of biochemical indices such as serum cholesterol. If the survey involves medical history and special tests for disease, it may be possible to show (for instance) whether heart disease is associated with short stature and a high cholesterol level. If the intention is to describe a large population, a random sample is usually chosen to provide sufficient subjects to represent the community.

Case–control studies

The case–control study is a convenient way of investigating causation. It usually involves the comparison of representative cases of a disease, drawn from a defined population, with persons drawn from the same population who are free from that disease. If we suspect that a certain disease is to some extent caused by one food and prevented by another, we can take a dietary history from people with and without the disease ('cases' and 'controls' respectively) and see whether their diets differ in the expected directions. The controls should resemble the cases apart from the disease. This can be ensured by matching each case with a control who is of the same age, sex, area of residence, etc., and drawn from a suitable set of people (e.g. the same general practitioner's list); alternatively, we can use a group of people who are broadly similar to the group of cases, and make statistical adjustments in the analysis for any differences between them. Sometimes it is convenient to use patients with other diseases for the control group, but we then have to be careful that the factors we are investigating are not associated positively or negatively with the control conditions. It is also important to ensure, as far as possible, that the dietary history is taken from the two groups in a similar manner so as to avoid bias.

The broad design of the case–control study is illustrated in **Fig. 3**. This method has several advantages: it can be carried out fairly quickly, it can easily be repeated in other populations, and it is suitable for investigating rare conditions. If the same associations emerge from case–control studies carried out in

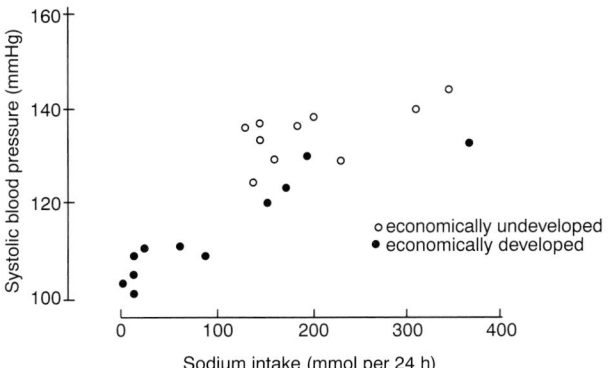

Figure 2 Average systolic blood pressures and sodium intakes in persons aged 40–49 years in different populations. Open circles, economically undeveloped countries; solid circles, economically developed countries. From Law *et al.* (1991).

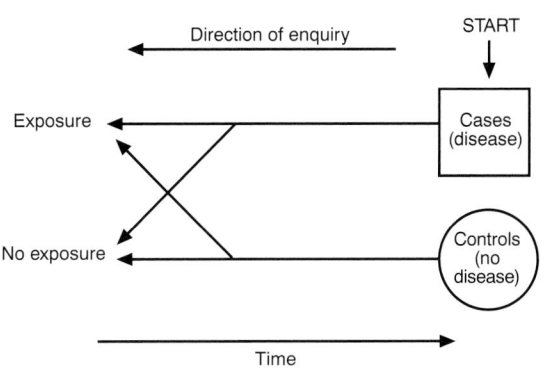

Figure 3 Design of case–control studies.

many diverse conditions, one can be fairly confident that they are genuine. For example, case–control studies of stomach cancer in numerous countries show a negative relationship with fruit consumption, suggesting that fruit protects against this disease.

Cohort studies

A cohort is a group of persons defined at the start of a period of time and followed up over that period. Cohort studies are useful in a variety of ways. They reveal the incidence of disease as distinct from its prevalence: for this purpose, the group is selected so as to be initially free from the disease in question, and cases of the disease are ascertained within the cohort during or at the end of the follow-up period. Valuable information about causation is revealed if potentially relevant factors are recorded at the start, and much of our knowledge of the relationship between diet and disease has been obtained in this way. One example is the protective effect of a moderate intake of alcohol against ischaemic heart disease, producing a J-shaped curve for the relationship between alcohol intake and all-cause mortality (**Fig. 4**). Other uses of the cohort study include enquiry into the predictive significance of various indices (e.g. do obese children become obese adults?), the natural history of a given disease (e.g. what proportion of newly diagnosed diabetic patients acquire complications?) and the outcomes of different methods of treatment. For some of these purposes the cohort will comprise patients rather than population samples, but the principle is the same.

Cohort studies are usually prospective, in that baseline observations are made at the start, and the follow-up period coincides with the time between setting up and completing the study. The advantage of this approach is that the investigators can decide what are the important variables, both as baseline characteristics (e.g. diet, body mass index, plasma ascorbate) and as end points (e.g. heart attacks, strokes, deaths), and ensure that they are monitored and recorded with the desired degree of precision. Occasionally it is possible to identify a cohort at some point in the past, when relevant baseline observations were recorded, and follow it up to the present time. This method (the historical cohort study) depends on the existence and preservation of suitable records, so it requires an element of luck, but when it is possible it greatly reduces the duration of the study. Examples include the follow-up of people whose birth and placental weights were recorded, to see whether these measurements predict blood pressure and heart disease in later life. The general design of cohort studies is illustrated in **Fig. 5**.

A hybrid method, combining the case–control and cohort approaches, is the nested case–control study. This involves detecting cases of a disease that have occurred during the follow-up of a cohort, matching them with persons who have remained free from the disease, and comparing them with respect to data deriving from the start of the study. An example is the use of deep-frozen stored samples of serum taken from a cohort; when cases of disease occur, their samples are identified and analysed for some component of interest, together with samples from matched controls. This combines the precision of the cohort study with the efficiency of the case–control analysis.

Randomized controlled trials

The most convincing evidence on causation comes from the randomized controlled trial. In its simplest form, this involves identifying suitable people who agree to participate, and then dividing them into two groups by random allocation. Those in one group are subjected to an intervention (e.g. the issue of a vitamin supplement) and the effect is monitored by comparing appropriate outcome measures in the two

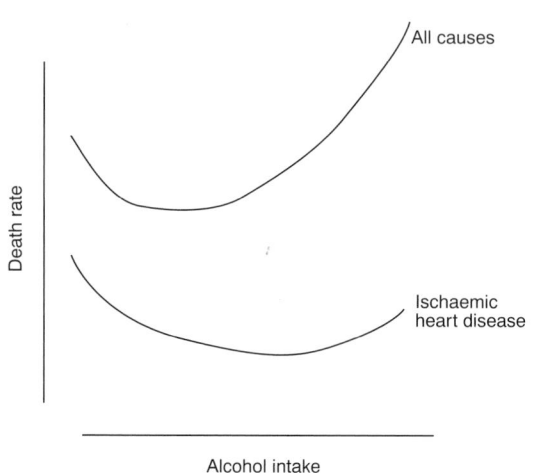

Figure 4   Relationship between alcohol intake and mortality.

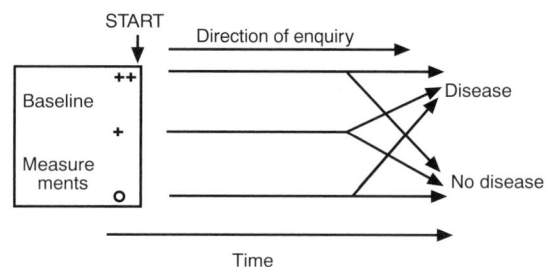

Figure 5   Design of cohort studies.

groups. In this way it is possible to detect the effect of altering a single factor, and by using a randomized design we can avoid much of the bias that attends other epidemiological methods.

The double-blind trial is the ideal way of minimizing bias. Here, the subjects are given either the active intervention or a matching placebo (usually as capsules of identical appearance), so that neither they nor the observers know which is which. This is not usually feasible in dietary trials, so a single-blind method is then adopted, the allocation of the subjects being unknown by the observer who records the outcome measures. If the end points are physiological variables that are measured in everybody, the trial can be conducted in (say) 150 subjects over 6 weeks; for example, if we are examining the effect of reducing saturated fat intake on serum cholesterol. However, if we want to detect an effect on the course of a disease (e.g. to see whether we can reduce the risk of recurrent heart attack), we must embark on a very much larger and longer trial.

There are certain variants of randomized trials that are suitable in different situations. The parallel design is the simplest: the subjects are randomly allocated into two or more groups; each group receives a different form of dietary advice or supplement for the duration of the trial, at the end of which the groups are compared in respect of the relevant end points. A factorial design is more complex, and examines the effect of two or more interventions singly and in combination: the subjects are randomized into sufficient subgroups for every combination to be accommodated. The advantage of this design is twofold. Interactions between the interventions are detectable, and in the absence of interactions the trial can be analysed for each factor separately, so in effect two or more trials take place simultaneously in the same subjects. **Fig. 6** shows the results of one such trial, in which three interventions (advice to eat less saturated fat, more cereal fibre or more fatty fish) were randomly applied in eight com-

binations (including a subgroup that received no specific advice) among 2033 men recovering from myocardial infarction. There was no clear effect of advice concerning fat or fibre, but the men advised to eat more fish had a 29% lower 2-year mortality than the other men. In the absence of any interaction between the interventions, it is legitimate to compare all the men advised to eat fish with all those not so advised, since equal proportions had received advice on the other dietary factors.

The crossover design is another type of trial. Here, the subjects are randomly allocated to two groups; one of these receives the advice or supplements until a specified period has elapsed, when measurements of the end points are made. The groups are then transposed so that the intervention is now applied to the subjects who had been the controls, and, after the same interval as before, the end points are measured again. This design is economical in that all subjects receive the intervention and are their own controls, although it is suitable only for short-term studies. **Fig. 7** summarizes these various trial designs.

Limitations

Since epidemiology purports to provide information about populations, the first limitation to be considered is the extent to which the data do not truly represent the population in question. When a survey is conducted, the subjects are usually selected from a source (the 'sampling frame') that is thought to comprise the whole population eligible for study and to which the results will refer. The sampling frame may be the electoral roll (for surveys of adults), general practitioners' lists, or a school register. These sources rapidly become out of date and are liable to miss certain types of people (e.g. those who move house or are of no settled abode), and to that extent the survey will not represent the whole population. Furthermore, when the sample has been drawn, not everyone selected will agree or be able to participate. Nonresponders tend to be different from responders (who are usually healthier), so that a low response rate implies that the findings probably do not represent the population as a whole.

The issue of representativeness takes a different form in the case of randomized controlled trials. Here the findings may be internally valid – i.e. the results really do show that the intervention had a certain effect in the group studied – yet they may not represent what would have happened in the general population, to which they are intended to apply. People who agree to participate in a trial tend to be different from those who do not (the 'healthy volunteer' effect), and the more that is required of

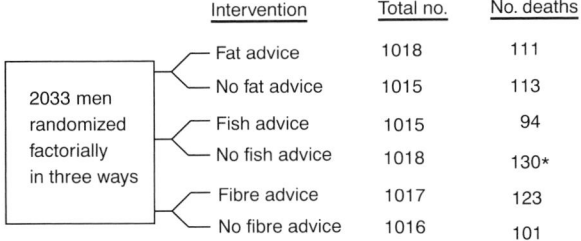

Intervention	Total no.	No. deaths
Fat advice	1018	111
No fat advice	1015	113
Fish advice	1015	94
No fish advice	1018	130*
Fibre advice	1017	123
No fibre advice	1016	101

2033 men randomized factorially in three ways

Figure 6 Results of randomized trial of the effects of dietary advice on fat, fish and fibre in post-infarct men. From Burr *et al.* (1989). *P < 0.05.

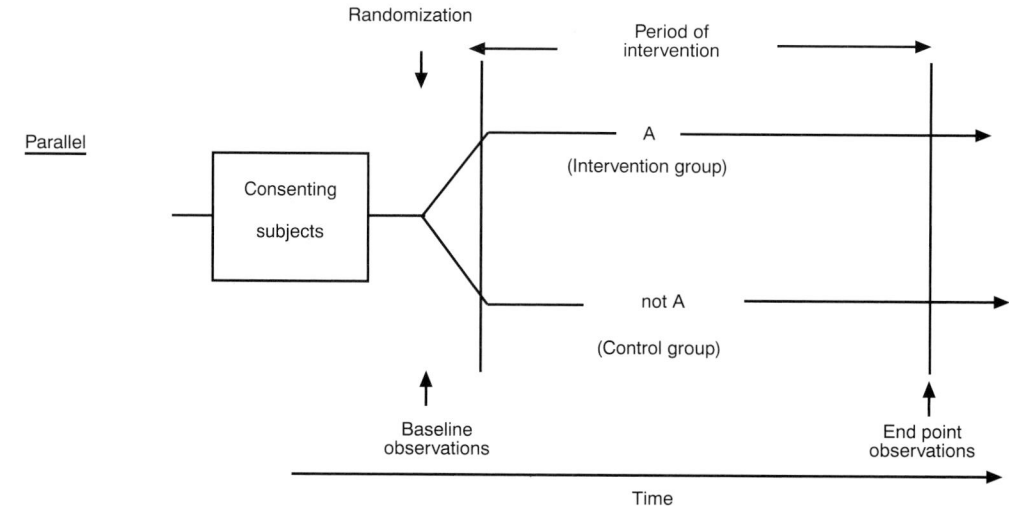

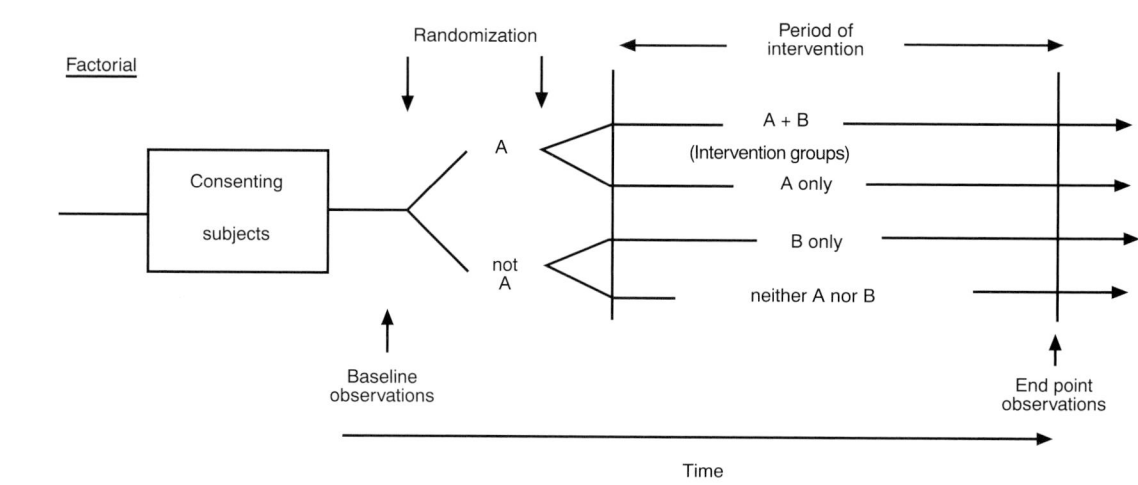

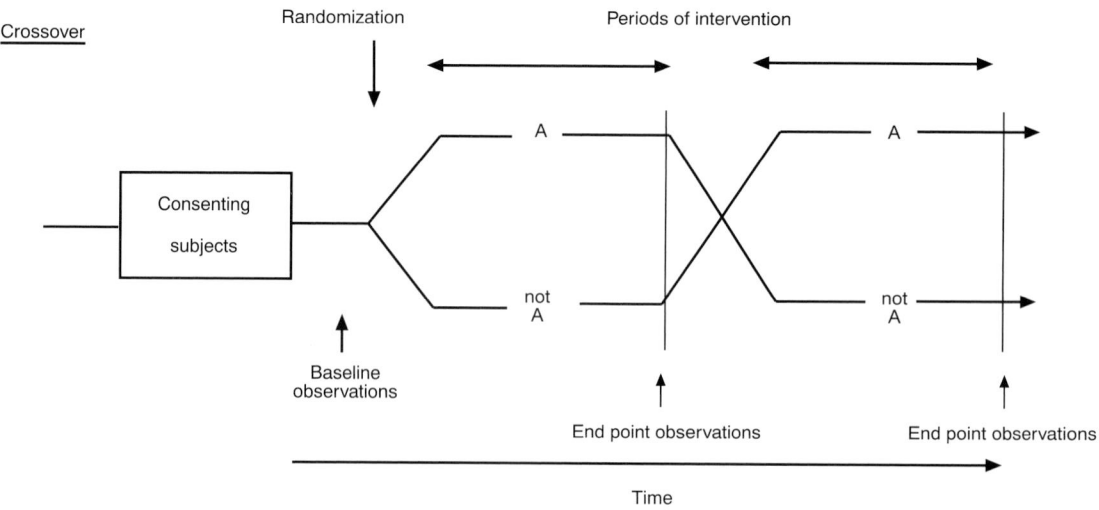

Figure 7 Design of different types of randomized trials.

participants the less representative they are likely to be.

Observational studies have the important limitation that association does not necessarily imply causation. Alcohol is associated with lung cancer because of its association with cigarette smoking, the true cause of the disease. This 'confounding' effect is particularly difficult to deal with in ecological studies because so many associated factors distinguish the way of life of each population under consideration. It is all too easy to attribute a difference in disease pattern to the wrong factor (the 'ecological fallacy'), owing to inability to control adequately for one factor in relation to another. Cross-sectional surveys do not reveal which of two associated variables came first: if obese people take less exercise than others, is that a cause or a consequence of their obesity? The limitations of the case–control approach include the inaccuracy of information obtained retrospectively (especially dietary information), and the possibility that a difference between cases and controls is due to a peculiarity of the latter rather than the former. Cohort studies usually take many years to yield their results, which may be invalidated if subjects cannot be traced; furthermore, they are unsuitable for the study of uncommon diseases.

Randomized trials have other limitations. They are difficult to conduct, especially if the end point is disease incidence. Compliance is never perfect, particularly in dietary trials, in which unforeseen covariations may occur (if people are told to avoid butter they may stop eating bread). A choice may have to be made between a 'laboratory' study (in which exact quantities of nutrients are taken by highly selected volunteers) and a 'real-life' study (which shows what actually happens in the community).

Interpretation of Data

Objectives

In evaluating published data (or in analysing one's own), the first consideration is the purpose of the study. What hypothesis is being tested? Was the study design suitable? Beware the hypothesis that was generated by the findings but is presented as though it were thought of first.

Subjects

How were the subjects identified and what population do they represent? Are we given sufficient information about exclusion criteria and other details? What was the response rate? Consider the possibility of selection bias – in a case–control study the controls are less motivated than the cases, so those who agree to participate may be somewhat unrepresentative.

Data

How were the data collected? What checks were there on validity? Look out for possibilities of bias, both in the exposure and the outcome measures. Patients suffering from a disease may remember details that would be forgotten by healthy controls. Interviewers may unconsciously ask questions in different ways if they know whether subjects are cases or controls, or whether they were exposed to the suspected causal factor.

Analysis

First consider whether the analysis is appropriate to the material. Has proper account been taken of potential confounders? Are the basic data given in sufficient detail? In a randomized trial, what are we told about the dropouts, and is the analysis by 'intention to treat' (the only way of avoiding dropout bias)? If the trial showed no difference between two interventions, the confidence interval will show how large an effect might have been missed.

Conclusions

Do the authors spell out the limitations of the study? Are their conclusions warranted by the results? If an association has been demonstrated, is it likely to be causal, as judged by such criteria as strength of association, dose response, temporality (the exposure preceding the disease) and biological plausibility? How do the findings fit in with those of other workers? It is reassuring if studies of different designs and in different countries have consistent results; nevertheless, there is often a possibility of publication bias in favour of studies with positive findings. The techniques of systematic review (a methodical search for all published and unpublished studies addressing a given issue) and meta-analysis (combining the results of studies conducted in similar ways) provide much firmer conclusions than can be drawn from any one study.

The Concept of Risk Factors

A risk factor is some personal characteristic (whether inherited, acquired by exposure or an aspect of behaviour) that is positively associated with the risk of acquiring a disease. The term is often used to denote any attribute that is associated with an adverse health outcome, whether it is known to be causal or not; thus the plasma homocysteine concentration is related to the risk of acquiring cardiovascular disease, but it is not yet certain whether homocysteine is part of the causal chain or merely a marker for something else. Causal risk factors may or may not be open to modification.

The investigation of risk factors illustrates the whole range of epidemiological methods. Clinical, ecological and cross-sectional studies draw attention to associations between the disease of interest and certain variables. Case–control studies confirm the relationships and give some indication of their relative importance. The cohort study demonstrates that the risk factor precedes the onset of the disease and enables the size of its effect to be calculated – i.e. by how much does the incidence of the disease rise (absolutely or proportionately) for a given increase in the risk factor? A randomized trial (if feasible) shows whether reducing the risk factor produces a reduction in incidence and of what size. At each stage, statistical adjustment for other possible risk factors shows whether they have independent effects.

The identification of risk factors has been useful in several ways. If a risk factor turns out to be causal and can be modified, prevention becomes a real possibility. Even if it is not modifiable, it enables high-risk individuals to be identified so that their risks can be reduced in other ways. For example, people with a strong family history of heart disease (a nonmodifiable risk factor) can be given lipid-lowering treatment at a lower serum cholesterol level than others. Whether a risk factor is directly causal or not, its identification and investigation are likely to lead to a better understanding of the disease.

Progression of Epidemiological Research

Experience shows the value of cohort studies in identifying risk factors, and of randomized trials in showing how to prevent disease. In order to reduce the duration of these studies they need to be large, and this can be achieved by using several centres. International collaboration has the further advantage of broadening the population base, so that risk factors may emerge that would be less obvious within one country. The incidence of most diseases varies widely between different countries; if we knew how to bring down the highest rates to those of the more fortunate populations we could prevent a great deal of suffering.

It is particularly desirable to monitor populations that are undergoing rapid change, as many are at present, particularly in developing countries. Where new eating habits and life styles are appearing, we have an opportunity to study their effects in communities that have not yet adapted to them. It is to be hoped that nutritionists and epidemiologists will collaborate to make use of these opportunities.

Acknowledgments

We gratefully acknowledge permission by The Lancet to reproduce Fig. 1 and the BMJ for Fig. 2.

See also: **Alcohol**: Disease Risk and Beneficial Effects. **Coronary Heart Disease**: Aetiology. **Fetal Origins of Disease**: Fetal Development and Later Disease.

Further Reading

Beaglehole R, Bonita R and Kjellström T (1993) *Basic Epidemiology*. Geneva: World Health Organization.

Burr ML, Fehily AM, Gilbert JF *et al.* (1989) Effects of changes in fat, fish and fibre intakes on death and myocardial reinfarction: diet and reinfarction trial (DART). *Lancet* **ii**:757–761.

Friedman GD (1987) *Primer of Epidemiology*, 3rd edn. New York: McGraw-Hill.

Last JM, ed. (1995) *A Dictionary of Epidemiology*, 3rd edn. Oxford University Press.

Law MR, Frost CD and Wald NJ (1991) By how much does dietary salt reduction lower blood pressure? I – Analysis of observational data among populations. *British Medical Journal* **302**:811–815.

Margetts BM and Nelson M, eds (1997) *Design Concepts in Nutritional Epidemiology*, 2nd edn. Oxford University Press.

St Leger AS, Cochrane AL and Moore F (1979) Factors associated with cardiac mortality in developed countries with particular reference to the consumption of wine. *Lancet* **i**:1017–1020.

EXERCISE

Contents
Physiology of Skeletal Muscle
Diet and Exercise
Beneficial Effects

Physiology of Skeletal Muscle

S C Dennis, University of Cape Town, South
Africa

Copyright © 1998 Academic Press

In humans, there are three main types of muscle: smooth, heart and skeletal. Smooth muscles lack the striations of other muscles and are extremely diverse. They are involved in functions such as gut motility and blood pressure. Heart muscles pump blood around the body. Skeletal muscles are responsible for posture and movement, and their physiology is described below.

Skeletal Muscle Organization

Whereas smooth and cardiac muscles contract spontaneously and are regulated by hormones and nerves from the subconscious regions of the brain, skeletal muscle fibres are under voluntary control. With the exception of certain reflexes, skeletal muscle fibres contract only when electrical impulses are transmitted from the motor cortex of the brain to the muscle via the spinal and motor nerves.

Motor units

When signals to contract are sent along motor nerves that stimulate 5–15 muscle fibres, tension is adjusted in small increments and movements are precise. However, when signals to contract are delivered to the muscle by motor nerves that stimulate several hundred muscle fibres, large increases in tension lead to strong, but less precise, contractions. Information on the tension of the muscle and its length is relayed back to the central nervous system from the Golgi tendon organs and the muscle spindles. The absence of feedback from the Golgi tendon organs on the tension of a muscle contracted in a shortened position leads to a muscle cramp. A failure to set the muscle spindle to the desired length (for example in a child learning to walk) results in clumsy movements that need to be corrected by adjusting the number of motor units activated.

Muscle fibre types

Skeletal muscle contraction is usually initiated by the recruitment of small to intermediate motor units. Small to intermediate motor units are comprised of either red slow-twitch (type I) or red fast-twitch (type IIa) muscle fibres. Type I and IIa muscle fibres are relatively resistant to fatigue. They contain a red oxygen-transport protein called myoglobin and obtain most of their energy for contraction from oxidative metabolism in structures called mitochondria.

In contrast, large motor units comprise white fast-twitch (type IIb) muscle fibres, which contain little myoglobin and few mitochondria. Energy for type IIb muscle fibre contractions comes from a massive 1000-fold acceleration of an oxygen-independent pathway that can only maintain maximum force development for around 20 s. These white muscle fibres are designed to power escape reactions. They are only recruited when either the signal to contract is prolonged, as occurs in the slow lifting of a heavy weight, or the frequency of the signal to contract is consciously increased to elicit an explosive movement.

Skeletal Muscle Ultrastructure

Microscopic examinations of cross-sections of skeletal muscle show that types I, IIa and IIb fibres are arranged in parallel and are randomly mixed. Ratios of types I: IIa: IIb fibres are genetically determined and range from around 40% : 50% : 10% to 80% : 15% : 5%.

Myofibril arrangement

Within a muscle fibre, there are hundreds and thousands of smaller parallel fibres known as myofibrils. Surrounding each myofibril is a lattice-like network of sarcoplasmic reticulum longitudinal tubules. The sarcoplasmic reticulum initiates and terminates contraction. Interspersed among the myofibrils of type I and IIa fibres are mitochondria that provide energy for contraction in the form of adenosine triphosphate (ATP). Among the mitochondria are carbohydrate and fat fuels, stored as glycogen granules and triacylglycerol droplets.

Lateral 'striations' of skeletal muscle result from myofibrils being composed of a series of repeated units known as sarcomeres. Sarcomeres are separated by Z discs, which pass from myofibril to myofibril. Between the Z discs are light I bands on either side of a central, dark A band.

Myofilament arrangement

The I and A bands of the sarcomere result from a partial interdigitation of yet smaller parallel fibres, the thin and thick myofilaments. Thin myofilaments are attached to the Z discs and form the I bands. Thick myofilaments create the central A band.

Within the A band, there are around 1500 thick myofilaments surrounded by hexagonal arrays of twice that number of thin myofilaments. Thick myofilaments are anchored by a very large protein (titan) and a lattice network of proteins at the centre of the sarcomere. Thin myofilaments are kept in position by their interdigitation with the thick myofilaments and their attachment to the Z discs.

Skeletal Muscle Contractile Proteins

When muscles contract, thin myofilaments slide between thick myofilaments and shorten the sarcomeres by pulling the Z discs closer together. Sarcomeres shorten whenever the thick and thin myofilaments interact.

Myosin

Thick myofilaments are composed of around 300 spirally arranged protein molecules called myosin. Each myosin molecule forms a fibrous, rigid 'coiled coil' in what are known as the 'tail' and 'neck' regions, and then splits into a pair of globular heads. Hinges at either end of the neck region allow the myosin heads to protrude from the thick myofilaments and rotate freely during the cross-bridge cycling with the thin myofilaments (described below).

Actin

Thin myofilaments are composed of a double helical filament of actin protein molecules. On each actin molecule are sites to which myosin heads will bind. In noncontracting muscles, these myosin-binding sites are blocked by a protein called tropomyosin, which has a structure similar to that of the myosin tail.

Tropomyosin–troponin complex

Tropomyosin molecules attach to the troponin complexes that occur every 40 nm along the thin myofilaments. Troponin complexes contain three proteins:

troponin I, troponin T and troponin C. Troponin I anchors the complex to the thin myofilament, troponin T attaches to tropomyosin and troponin C binds calcium ions. Increases in cytoplasmic calcium ion concentrations lead to muscle contraction.

Skeletal Muscle Electromechanical Coupling

Signals to contract are delivered to the midpoints of muscle cells by a motor nerve. As the nerve enters the muscle, it branches into a number of nerve endings that come to lie in troughs on the surface of each of the muscle cells of the motor unit.

Neuromuscular transmission

When a wave of electrical excitation arrives at a motor nerve ending, a small influx of Ca^{2+} into the nerve causes around 300 vesicles to fuse with the nerve cell membrane. These vesicles release acetylcholine which diffuses across a 20–30 nm cleft and binds to receptors on the underlying muscle cell membrane. Within the 1–2 ms before the acetylcholine is broken down, its binding opens receptor-operated channels that allow positively charged sodium ions (Na^+) to flow into the electronegative interior of the muscle cell.

Entry of Na^+ decreases the negative electrical potential across the muscle cell membrane to a threshold at which voltage-gated Na^+ channels open. A rapid influx of Na^+ causes the inside of the cell to become transiently positive for 1–2 ms before the Na^+ channels close and voltage-gated potassium (K^+) channels open. A rapid efflux of K^+ returns the interior of the muscle cell to its resting electronegative state.

Electrical conduction along muscle cells

With the transient depolarization of the muscle cell membrane at the neuromuscular junction, positively charged ions outside the muscle and negatively charged ions inside the muscle are electrostatically attracted into the region of depolarization. This migration of ions decreases the electrical potential across the adjacent regions of the muscle cell membrane and sets off further voltage-activated Na^+ influx. In this manner, waves of depolarization are propagated outwards from the centre of the motor unit towards each end of the muscle fibres as an 'all or none' response.

Waves of depolarization descend from the surface of the muscle cell to the myofibrils via transverse T tubules. These tubules are invaginations of the muscle cell membrane that enter the muscle cell at the junctions between the thick and thin myofilaments. On either side of the T tubules, structures known as foot processes attach the T tubule to the cisternae or 'chests' of the sarcoplasmic reticulum.

Voltage-dependent sarcoplasmic reticulum Ca²⁺ release

Foot processes are composed of four proteins which transiently alter their shape with each wave of T tubule membrane depolarization. A change in the shape of the foot processes opens Ca^{2+} release channels in the cisternae of the sarcoplasmic reticulum. Release of Ca^{2+} from the cisternae of the sarcoplasmic reticulum exceeds the rate at which Ca^{2+} is pumped back into the network of longitudinal sarcoplasmic reticulum tubules that surround each myofibril. Depending on the frequency of the waves of T tubule membrane depolarization, 'free' cytoplasmic Ca^{2+} concentrations in the muscle rise from around 0.1 μatom l^{-1} to 1–10 μatom l^{-1}.

Calcium ion activation of thin myofilaments

Increased cytoplasmic Ca^{2+} concentrations cause the ion to bind to troponin C. When this occurs, a change in the shape of the troponin complex rotates the tropomyosin into the grooves between the double helical actin myofilaments and exposes the binding sites for the myosin heads.

Cross-bridge cycling

Once there is a persistent Ca^{2+} 'activation' of the thin myofilaments of a sarcomere, the approximately 300 myosin heads of the thick myofilaments begin repeated attachments and detachments with the actin of the thin myofilaments. This 'cross-bridge cycling' steadily pulls the thin myofilaments and their attached Z discs towards the centre of the sarcomere and a continuous shortening of millions of sarcomeres in series leads to muscle contraction.

Energy for cross-bridge cycling comes from the binding of ATP to the myosin head. This binding cocks the myosin head, like the trigger of a gun, at a 'strained' 90° angle to the thick myofilament. At this angle, the bound ATP is cleaved by the myosin head to adenosine diphosphate (ADP) and inorganic phosphate (P_i). That cleavage of ATP creates an actin-binding site on the myosin head. Attachment of the myosin head to actin then leads to a release of P_i that causes the 'strained' 90° myosin head to move to an 'unstrained' 45° angle to the thick myofilament. This movement pulls the thin myofilament and the attached Z disc around 12 nm towards the centre of the sarcomere. At full excursion, the ADP is then replaced by ATP that causes a rapid detachment

from the actin and a return of the myosin head to a 'strained' 90° angle.

Muscle Movement

Muscle contraction is analogous to a man pulling in a rope attached to increasingly heavy weights. As the weight on the rope becomes heavier, less of his time is spent in changing hands and more is spent in slowly hauling in the rope. For the same reason, the slowest step in muscle contraction depends on the load opposing the movement of the myosin heads to their 45° state.

Maximum shortening velocity

When a muscle contracts rapidly against a near-zero load, less than 5% of the myosin heads are attached at any one time. Maximum shortening velocity is therefore limited by the rate at which the myosin heads can hydrolyse ATP to recreate an actin binding site. Since fast-twitch motor units hydrolyse ATP at more than twice the rate of slow-twitch motor units, muscles with a high proportion of fast-twitch fibres can contract more rapidly against a minimal load than muscles with mainly slow-twitch fibres.

Maximum power output

A high proportion of fast-twitch muscle fibres is also advantageous for maximum power output. Maximum power output occurs when the product of the muscle shortening velocity and the load is optimized. The optimization is achieved by adjusting the number of motor units recruited so that each contracts against around one third of its maximum load. Under these circumstances, roughly 20% of the myosin heads are attached. Thus, maximum power outputs are also largely determined by the rate at which myosin heads can hydrolyse ATP to recreate binding sites for actin.

Maximum load

In contrast, further increases in the loads opposing shortening shift the control of contraction away from the rate of ATP hydrolysis towards the speed at which the myosin heads can detach from the actin filament. Once all of the available myosin heads have to be attached in order to restrain (or lower) a maximum load, the size of the load is more a function of muscle mass than of muscle fibre-type composition.

Energy for Muscle Movement

Whenever a muscle contracts, the ATP hydrolysed by the myosin heads has to be immediately resynthesized in order to provide ATP for cross-bridge detachments. In rapidly working muscles, ATP molecules can turnover every few seconds.

Creatine phosphate hydrolysis

As ATP is hydrolysed by myosin ATPase activity, it is locally re-synthesized by the transfer of phosphate from creatine phosphate to ADP. Because the resultant creatine is present in more than 100-fold higher concentrations than the approximately 10 $\mu mol\ l^{-1}$ concentration of ADP in the cytoplasm, it is the creatine rather than the ADP that diffuses back to the mitochondria. At the mitochondria, creatine is rephosphorylated to creatine phosphate at the expense of ATP and it is creatine phosphate that 'shuttles' energy from the sites of production to the sites of consumption. Creatine phosphate is not a 'reservoir' of chemical energy, as is commonly supposed. Net creatine phosphate hydrolysis can sustain maximal contractile activity for only about 4 s.

Oxygen-independent glycogen utilization

An accelerated resynthesis of ATP decreases creatine phosphate concentrations and increases inorganic phosphate concentrations. At the same time, small percentage reductions in the concentrations of ATP (in $mmol\ l^{-1}$) are amplified into much larger percentage increases in the concentrations (in $\mu mol\ l^{-1}$) of adenosine monophosphate (AMP) by a condensation of two ADP molecules to form one ATP molecule and one AMP molecule. Falls in creatine phosphate concentration and rises in P_i and AMP concentrations act in concert to stimulate ATP resynthesis from a breakdown of muscle glycogen. Muscle glycogen breakdown is also promoted by rises in Ca^{2+} concentrations during contractions. Increases in Ca^{2+} concentration lead to an interconversion of the glycogen phosphorylase enzyme from a less active 'b' form to a more active 'a' form. Glycogen phosphorylase 'b' to 'a' conversion is particularly rapid when a need to escape is anticipated and rises in circulating adrenaline concentrations stimulate the intramuscular production of cyclic AMP.

Because it takes time for muscle blood flow to increase at the start of exercise, almost all of the ATP for a 10–20 s sprint is generated from an accelerated conversion of glycogen to lactate. The metabolic pathway leading to lactate formation is called oxygen-independent glycolysis and is especially important in the white fast-twitch (type IIb) muscle fibres that power escape reactions. Type IIb muscle fibres generate ATP for contraction by a massive, 1000-fold increase in the conversion of glycogen to lactate. Such a large acceleration of oxygen-independent glycolysis is achieved by decreases in creatine phosphate concentration and rises in P_i and

AMP concentrations. These changes in metabolite concentrations activate a forward reaction catalysed by the enzyme phosphofructokinase and inhibit a reverse reaction catalysed by fructose diphosphatase. Fructose diphosphatase is unique to type IIb muscle fibres and its presence allows rates of glycogen utilization to be increased from around 0.05 μmol to 60 μmol hexose equivalent min^{-1} per gram fresh weight during intense muscle activity.

Since the glycogen content of untrained human muscle is approximately 80 μmol hexose equivalent per gram fresh weight, oxygen-independent glycolysis could theoretically provide enough energy for around 80 s of maximum activity. In practice, however, hydrogen ion (H^+) accumulation decreases intramuscular pH from approximately 7.1 to 6.5, and that limits the duration of near-maximum power output to around 20 s.

When ATP is resynthesized by glycolysis, rather than by mitochondrial oxidative phosphorylation or net creatine phosphate hydrolysis, the hydrogen ions produced by the breakdown of ATP^{2-} to ADP^-, P_i^{2-} and H^+ are not reconsumed. Contrary to general belief, hydrogen ions do not come from lactic acid production. When ATP formation is taken into consideration and the electrical charges of the reactants and products of the glycolytic pathway at intracellular pH are balanced, the conversion of glycogen to lactate actually consumes a hydrogen ion:

$$Glycogen + 3ADP^- + 3\ P_i^{2-} + H^+$$
$$\Rightarrow 2\ lactate^- + 3ATP^{2-}$$

Lactate formation is more a consequence of than a cause of metabolic acidosis. Muscles 'dump fuel' in the form of lactate in order to remove hydrogen ions by a H^+ + lactate ion coefflux.

Once intracellular H^+ concentrations rise, however, further acidification by glycolytic ATP turnover is prevented by a slowing of muscle contraction. Accumulating H^+ combines with P_i^{2-} from creatine phosphate breakdown to form P_i^{-1} ions, which inhibit P_i^{-1} release from the myosin heads. This metabolite-induced mechanical arrest during intense exercise ensures that muscle ATP concentrations cannot fall below the levels required for cross-bridge detachments. Muscle ATP concentrations only fall below the levels required for cross-bridge detachments after death, leading to rigor mortis.

Oxygen-dependent metabolism

Rapid oxygen-independent glycolysis is not used for endurance exercise. For sustained physical activity, the hydrogen ions arising from the hydrolysis of the ATP generated by glycolysis have to enter the mitochondria together with pyruvate ions and this means that most of the ATP must be derived from mitochondrial oxidative phosphorylation.

The major fuels for mitochondrial oxidative phosphorylation in the more fatigue-resistant type I and IIa muscle fibres are muscle glycogen, plasma glucose, plasma lactate and circulating fatty acids. Utilization of these fuels is regulated by the return of ADP to the mitochondria from the myofibrils by the creatine phosphate shuttle. Unless ADP is available for rephosphorylation, a mitochondrial pathway that transports H^+ and electrons (e^-) from carbohydrate and fat breakdown to oxygen does not proceed. Thus, muscle metabolism is controlled by the demand for energy rather than the supply of fuel.

Fuel supply only limits muscle metabolism when increasing rates of fat oxidation fail to compensate for the decreasing rates of carbohydrate oxidation over time. Because the rate of ATP production from fat oxidation is approximately 50% slower than from carbohydrate oxidation, no more than 40% of the energy can come from fat oxidation during exercise at, say, 80% of maximum sustained power output. At this marathon running pace, exercise intensity has to be decreased when rates of carbohydrate oxidation fall below around 3 g min^{-1} so that more energy can come from fat.

Rises in plasma glucose oxidation also fail to compensate for muscle glycogen depletion during prolonged exercise. Rates of plasma glucose oxidation are limited to approximately 1 g min^{-1}. Thus, exercise intensity also has to be decreased when the direct and indirect (via lactate) oxidation of muscle glycogen falls below around 2 g min^{-1}. For this reason, it is important for endurance athletes to start exercise with an adequate muscle glycogen content. They should also ingest carbohydrate during exercise. Postprandial liver glycogen stores of around 135 g are sufficient to sustain exercise at around 80% of maximum effort for only 2–3 h. Once the rates of liver glycogen conversion to plasma glucose no longer match rates of plasma glucose oxidation, hypoglycaemia leads to a lack of coordination, an inability to concentrate and ultimately collapse.

See Colour Plate 2.

See also: **Carbohydrates**: Regulation of Carbohydrate Metabolism. **Electrolytes**: Acid-Base Balance. **Energy Metabolism**: Tricarboxylic Acid Cycle and Oxidative Phosphorylation. **Exercise**: Diet and Exercise. **Glucose**: Metabolism and Maintenance of Blood Glucose Level.

Further Reading

Dennis SC, Noakes TD and Hawley JA (1997) Nutritional strategies to minimise fatigue during prolonged exercise: fluid, electrolyte and energy replacement. *Journal of Sports Science*:305–313.

Guyton AC (1976) *Textbook of Medical Physiology*. Philadelphia: WB Saunders.

Newsholme EA and Leech AR (1983) *Biochemistry for the Medical Sciences*. Chichester: John Wiley.

Peachy LD, Adrian RH and Geiger SR (1983) *Handbook of Physiology*, section 10. Bethesda: American Physiological Society.

Diet and Exercise

R J Maughan, University Medical School, Aberdeen, UK

Copyright © 1998 Academic Press

Introduction

Exercise has an impact on nutritional requirements, increasing the total energy demand and also influencing the requirement for some specific nutrients. Conversely, energy and nutrient supply can influence an individual's capacity to perform occupational or recreational physical activity. It is now well recognized that the ability to perform exercise will be impaired if the diet is inadequate, although the concept of dietary inadequacy may be quite different for the physically active individual compared with the sedentary population. Exercise performance may be improved by manipulation of the amount, type and timing of food intake, but we still have an incomplete understanding of how best to control diet to optimize sports performance. The elite athlete is predisposed to success by genetic endowment and has undergone the most rigorous training. Nutritional intervention will not turn the average individual into an Olympic champion, but where other things are equal it may make the difference between success and failure. It is not surprising, therefore, that sportsmen and sportswomen generally are concerned about their diet, although this concern is not always matched by a knowledge of basic nutrition. Although some of the dietary practices followed by athletes in pursuit of success are sound, many are of no benefit – other than possibly by a placebo effect – and some may even be harmful. As in other areas of nutrition, the sale of dietary supplements and the use of controversial dietary practices are often encouraged by those who stand to gain financially. No recent figures are available for the sales of nutritional products to athletes, but the market is substantial.

Two distinct aspects of nutrition for the competitive athlete must be considered. The first is the diet in training, which must be consumed on a daily basis for a large part of the year, and must allow the athlete to sustain an intensive training programme. The second is the dietary preparation for the demands of competition. Considering the range of activities encompassed by the term 'sport' and the variation in the characteristics of the individuals taking part, it is not surprising that the nutritional requirements and recommendations vary. For noncompetitive activities, and for the individual who exercises for recreational and health reasons, the daily diet forms part of a lifestyle which may be quite different from that of the competitive athlete, but the same nutritional implications of exercise participation apply, albeit to a different degree. Similar considerations apply to occupational physical activity, and many people in the developing world face problems of a need for hard manual labour coupled with a limited availability of food, but these problems are less amenable to solution.

Nutrition for Training

Energy balance

The primary need for the diet of the athlete in training is to meet the additional nutrient requirement imposed by the training load. All physical activity increases the metabolic rate above the resting level, and impact on energy balance will depend on the intensity, duration and frequency of training. In sports involving prolonged strenuous exercise on a regular basis, participation has a significant effect on energy balance. The rate of energy turnover during running or cycling, for example, may be 15–20 times the resting rate, and such levels of activity may be sustained for several hours by trained athletes. In these events, the rate of energy expenditure is roughly proportional to speed, and the total energy expenditure is determined primarily by the total distance covered. In walking or running, where body mass has to be lifted against gravity, the total energy expenditure is strongly influenced by body mass, but this is much less of a factor in cycling or swimming.

At very low speeds, the energy cost of walking is less than that of jogging, because of the smaller vertical displacements of the centre of mass. As velocity increases, however, the cost of walking increases faster than that of running, and at speeds in excess of about 6–7 km h^{-1}, running is less energetically demanding than jogging. As a rough approximation, the energy cost of walking or jogging is about 4.2 kJ per kg per km (1 kcal per kg per km). The approximate energy cost of some different types of locomotion is shown in **Table 1**, but there may be large differences between individuals in the energy cost of even simple activities such as running.

After exercise, the metabolic rate falls rapidly, but there is evidence to suggest that it may remain above the resting level for at least 12 and possibly up to 24 h if the exercise is prolonged and close to the maximum intensity that can be sustained. This may apply to the distance runner, cyclist or swimmer engaged in hard training, but it is unlikely that metabolic rate remains elevated for long periods after more moderate exercise. For the recreational exerciser, however, the cumulative effect of even small elevations in metabolic rate may be important over the longer term. There may also be a potentiation of the thermogenic response to meals consumed in the postexercise period, adding to the total energy cost associated with a bout of exercise.

If body mass and performance levels are to be maintained, the increased rate of energy expenditure must be matched by an increase in energy intake. Available data for most athletes suggest that they are in energy balance within the limits of the techniques used for measuring intake and expenditure. This is to be expected as a chronic deficit in energy intake would lead to a progressive loss of body mass. However, data for women engaged in sports where a low body mass, and especially a low body fat content, are important, including events such as gymnastics, distance running and ballet, consistently show a lower than expected energy intake. There is no obvious physiological explanation for this finding other

Table 1 Energy cost of covering a fixed distance of 1 km in different types of locomotion. These figures are approximate, and there may be a large difference between individuals

	Energy cost (kcal per kg per km)	Energy cost (kJ per kg per km)
Walking (6 km h^{-1})	0.8	3.4
Running (20 km h^{-1})	1.1	4.5
Cycling (20 km h^{-1})	0.2	0.9
Cycling (40 km h^{-1})	0.4	1.7
Swimming (3.6 km h^{-1}, freestyle)	2.7	11.2
Swimming (3.6 km h^{-1}, butterfly)	5.0	21.0

1 kcal = 4.2 kJ.

than methodological errors in the calculation of energy intake and expenditure, but it seems odd that these should apply specifically to this group of athletes. Many of these women do, however, have a very low body fat content: a body fat content of less than 10% is not uncommon in female long distance runners.

Investigations into the effects of exercise upon appetite and the regulation of food intake are complicated by a number of confounding factors and by the difficulties of making reliable measurements. The common perception is that exercise stimulates appetite, leading to an increase in total energy intake equivalent to the energy expended during the exercise period. It is nonetheless clear that a programme of regular activity, combined with some restriction of energy intake, is a crucial part of any effective weight loss programme. The acute depression of appetite that follows high-intensity exercise is generally of short duration. Short-term suppression of the subjective sensation of hunger without an effect on overall daily energy intake has also been reported after moderate exercise lasting 30 min.

Protein requirements

Athletes engaged in strength and power events have traditionally been concerned with achieving a high dietary protein intake in the belief that this is necessary for muscle hypertrophy. An inadequate dietary protein intake will inevitably lead to loss of muscle mass, and may limit the repair and recovery process. This will eventually compromise training, but there is no evidence from controlled laboratory studies to support the idea that excess dietary protein will drive the system in favour of protein synthesis. Protein consumed in excess of the requirement for growth and tissue repair will simply be used as a substrate for oxidative metabolism, either directly or as a precursor of glucose, and the excess nitrogen will be lost in the urine. This, however, does not mean that athletes in training do not have a higher protein require-

ment than their sedentary counterparts, as exercise, whether it is long distance running, aerobics or weight training, will cause an increased protein oxidation compared with the resting state.

The fractional contribution of protein oxidation to energy production during the exercise period may decrease to about 5% of the total energy requirement, compared with about 10–15% (i.e. the normal fraction of protein in the diet) at rest, but the absolute rate of protein degradation is increased during exercise. This leads to an increase in the minimum daily protein requirement, and an intake of about 1.4–1.7 g kg^{-1} body mass is recommended for athletes in training, compared with the recommended intake of about 0.8–1.0 g kg^{-1} for the sedentary population. This amount will be provided if a normal mixed diet adequate to meet the increased energy expenditure is consumed (**Table 2**). In spite of this, however, many athletes ingest large quantities of protein-containing foods and expensive protein supplements; daily protein intakes of up to 400 g are not unknown in some sports. It is often stated that disposal of the excess nitrogen may pose a problem if renal function is compromised, but there does not appear to be any evidence that excessive protein intake among athletes is damaging to health. Although high protein intakes are common among athletes, the recommended diet for athletes may even contain a lower than normal proportion of protein on account of the increased total energy intake (Table 2).

Carbohydrate and fat metabolism

The energy requirements of training are largely met by oxidation of fat and carbohydrate: these may be derived from the diet or from the body's endogenous stores. The higher the intensity of exercise, the greater the reliance on carbohydrate as a fuel. At an exercise intensity corresponding to about 50% of an individual's maximum oxygen uptake (Vo_2max), approximately two-thirds of the total

Table 2 Dietary protein intake for diets varying in quantity and composition for athletes with body weights of 50 and 80 kg

Daily energy intake				
(kcal) *(MJ)*		*Protein content* *(% energy)*	*Protein intake* *(g per day)*	*Intake (50 kg athlete)* *(g per day)*	*Intake (80 kg athlete)* *(g per day)*
2000	8.4	10%	50	1.0	0.6
2000	8.4	15%	75	1.5	0.9
3000	12.6	10%	75	1.5	0.9
3000	12.6	15%	113	2.3	1.4
4000	16.8	10%	100	2.0	1.3
4000	16.8	15%	150	3.0	1.9
5000	21.0	10%	125	2.5	1.6
5000	21.0	15%	188	3.8	2.4

energy requirement is met by fat oxidation, with carbohydrate oxidation supplying about one-third. If the exercise intensity is increased to about 75% of Vo_2max the total energy expenditure is increased, and carbohydrate is now the major fuel. This pattern of fuel utilization is largely determined by the metabolic characteristics of the muscle fibre types and their recruitment patterns. If carbohydrate is not available, or is available in only a limited amount, the intensity of the exercise must be reduced to a level where the energy requirement can be met by fat oxidation. In very high intensity exercise, type 2 muscle fibres are recruited, and a large fraction of the energy demand is met by anaerobic metabolism, with a heavy reliance on anaerobic glycolysis. This results in rapid conversion of the muscle glycogen stores to lactate, much of which is then oxidized by other tissues. It has been estimated that as much as 16% of the glycogen store of the quadriceps was used in a single 6 s treadmill sprint at maximum power output. Sprinters or games players whose training consists of multiple short sprints may therefore deplete their muscle glycogen stores to an even greater extent than the endurance athlete.

The primary need, therefore, is for the carbohydrate intake to be sufficient to enable the training load to be sustained at the high level necessary to produce a response. During each strenuous training session, substantial depletion of the glycogen stores in the exercising muscles and in the liver takes place. If this carbohydrate reserve is not replenished before the next training session, the training intensity must be reduced, leading to corresponding decrements in the adaptive response. Any athlete training hard on a daily basis can readily observe this; if a low-carbohydrate diet, consisting mostly of fat and protein, is consumed after a day's training, it will be difficult to repeat the same training load on the following day.

Feeding a high-fat, low-carbohydrate diet for prolonged periods has been shown to increase the capacity of muscle to oxidize fat and hence improve endurance capacity in the rat, but may not be effective in man, although there have been rather few long-term studies in man. Similarly short-term fasting increases endurance capacity in the rat, but results in a decreased exercise tolerance in man. It is generally recommended therefore, that the training diet should be high in carbohydrate, with a mixture of complex carbohydrates and simple sugars. This suggestion conforms with the recommendations of various Government expert committees that carbohydrates provide at least 50% of dietary energy intake. It has been shown that a high-carbohydrate diet (70% of energy intake as carbohydrate) enabled runners who were training for 2 h per day to maintain muscle glycogen levels, whereas if the carbohydrate content was only 40%, a progressive fall in muscle glycogen content was observed. Although it has been common practice to express dietary recommendations for dietary carbohydrate as a percentage of total energy intake, there is a growing realization that the carbohydrate requirement is an absolute, determined primarily by the total training load and by body mass. Where the total energy intake is restricted, this will inevitably represent a high fraction of total energy intake. However, where a high volume of training is performed, with much of it inevitably at moderate intensity, there must be a high total energy intake, and the carbohydrate intake, while high in absolute terms, may represent a smaller fraction of total energy intake. A dietary carbohydrate intake of 500–600 g day^{-1} may be necessary to ensure adequate glycogen resynthesis when training on a daily basis: for athletes with high body weight, the daily requirement may exceed 1000 g. These high levels of intake are difficult to achieve without consuming large amounts of simple sugars: most athletes find that they can only satisfy the requirement for carbohydrate by eating confectionery and sweet snacks between, or even instead of, meals.

Micronutrients and dietary supplements

With regular strenuous training, there must be an increased total food intake to match the increased energy expenditure, except where a loss of body mass is required. Provided that a reasonably normal diet is consumed, this will supply more than adequate amounts of protein, minerals, vitamins and other dietary requirements. Many surveys show that some athletes consume amounts of vitamins and minerals that are less than those deemed desirable, and this is taken as evidence that the intake is inadequate to meet the need. The methodology used to assess dietary intake, and the basis for the establishment of requirements, are both questionable in many of these studies, however, and biochemical assessment of micronutrient status is seldom carried out. Where metabolic markers have been measured, they generally fail to confirm the presence of any deficiency, with the possible exceptions of iron and calcium as discussed below.

There is currently much interest in the role of a number of nutrients in maintaining health and functional capacity in intensively trained athletes. Much of this interest centres on the antioxidants, including vitamins A, C and E. There are also suggestions that supplementation with the amino acid glutamine may help to maintain the integrity of the immune system, which may be compromised as a result of over-training. At present, however, there is insufficient evidence to suggest that specific supplementation with any of these dietary components is necessary to maintain health or that it will improve performance. A daily diet which may be considered inadequate in terms of nutrient density for a sedentary individual consuming 4 MJ (~1000 kcal) may meet the requirements of an athlete taking 12–15 MJ. Indeed, without resorting to sweets, snacks and convenience foods, such a high intake may be difficult to achieve. There is, however, no evidence that this pattern of eating is harmful; for the individual who has to fit an exercise programme into a busy day, it is inevitable that changes to eating patterns must be made, but these need not compromise the quality of the diet. When the energy expenditure is very high, carbohydrate-rich drinks and snacks become an essential part of the diet, even though their use is discouraged in the sedentary population because of their low micronutrient density.

The only exceptions to the generalization about micronutrient supplements may be iron and, in the case of very active women, calcium. It is normal to find low circulating haemoglobin levels in highly trained endurance athletes, but the total red cell mass is usually increased and the low haemoglobin concentration is the result of the dilutional effect of a disproportionately large increase in plasma volume. This may be considered to be an adaptation to the trained state, but the possibility of a real anaemia should not be discounted. Hard training may result in an increased iron requirement and exercise tolerance will be impaired in the presence of anaemia. Low serum folate and serum ferritin levels are not associated with impaired performance, however, and correction of these deficiencies does not influence indices of fitness in trained athletes.

Moderate exercise has been reported to increase bone mineral density in women, and this may be a significant benefit of exercise for most women. Sustained hard training, however, may reduce circulating oestrogen levels and hence accelerate bone loss, and this is clearly undesirable. Apart from the possible long-term consequence, there may be an increased susceptibility to stress fractures and to traumatic fracture. For all women, but especially for these athletes, an adequate calcium intake should be ensured, although calcium supplements themselves will not reverse bone loss while oestrogen levels remain low. Reduction of the training load and restoration of normal menstrual function is generally associated with a gain of bone mass.

In recent years, the use of creatine as a dietary supplement has become popular among strength and power athletes, and more recently its use has become widespread amongst games players. A few days of high creatine intake (about 20 g per day, compared with the normal intake from foods of about 1 g per day) results in an increased total creatine content in skeletal muscle. Of this, about 70% is in the form of creatine phosphate. The increase is largest among those with a low initial muscle creatine content; this group includes many vegetarians, whose normal diet is almost free of creatine. Laboratory studies have shown significant improvements in the ability to perform high-intensity exercise, especially where multiple bouts of exercise lasting a few seconds are repeated with short recovery periods, and this may allow higher intensity training to be performed. Although an acute gain in body mass of 1–2 kg seems to be normally associated with supplementation, there are anecdotal reports of increases of 5 kg or more.

Nutrition for Competition

There is no doubt that the ability to perform prolonged exercise can be substantially modified by dietary intake in the pre-exercise period, and this becomes important for the individual aiming to produce peak performance on a specific day. The pre-exercise period can conveniently be divided into two phases – the few days prior to the exercise task, and the day of exercise itself.

Dietary manipulation to increase muscle glycogen content in the few days prior to exercise has been extensively recommended for endurance athletes following observations that these procedures were effective in increasing endurance capacity in cycle ergometer exercise lasting about 1.5–2 h. The suggested procedure was to deplete muscle glycogen by prolonged exercise about 1 week prior to competition and to prevent resynthesis by consuming a low-carbohydrate diet for 2–3 days before changing to a high-carbohydrate diet for the last 3 days during which little or no exercise was performed. This procedure can double the muscle glycogen content and is effective in increasing cycling or running capacity, measured as the time for which a given workload can be sustained. There is now a considerable amount of evidence that it is not necessary to include the low-carbohydrate glycogen depletion phase of the diet for endurance athletes. All that is necessary is to reduce the training load over the last few days before competition and simultaneously to maintain or slightly increase the dietary carbohydrate intake. This avoids many of the problems associated with the more extreme forms of the diet. Although an increased pre-competition muscle glycogen content is undoubtedly beneficial, there is a faster rate of muscle glycogen utilization when the glycogen content itself is increased, thus nullifying some of the advantage gained. Attempts to spare the limited glycogen stores by ingestion of caffeine to stimulate fat mobilization and oxidation have met with mixed success.

Consumption of a high-carbohydrate diet in the days prior to competition may also benefit competitors in games such as rugby, soccer or hockey, although it appears not to be usual for these players to pay attention to this aspect of their diet. It has been shown that players starting a soccer game with low muscle glycogen content did less running, and much less running at high speed, than those players who began the game with a normal muscle glycogen content. It is common for players to have one game in midweek as well as one at the weekend, and it is likely that full restoration of the muscle glycogen content will not occur between games unless a conscious effort is made to achieve a high carbohydrate intake. This glycogen-loading procedure is generally restricted to use by athletes engaged in endurance events, but there is some evidence that the muscle glycogen content may influence performance even in events lasting only a few minutes. A high muscle glycogen content may be particularly important when repeated sprints at near maximum speed have to be made: at major athletics championships, the sprinter who competes in the 100 and 200 m as well as in the relay may be required to run as many as eight or nine races within a rather short space of time, perhaps with a protracted warm-up before each. Short-term high-intensity exercise may also be improved by ingestion of alkaline salts prior to exercise to enhance the buffering of the protons produced by anaerobic glycolysis.

There is scope for nutritional intervention during competition only when the duration of events is sufficient to allow absorption of drinks or foods ingested and where the rules of the sport permit. The primary aims must be to ingest a source of energy, usually in the form of carbohydrate, and fluid for replacement of water lost as sweat, but the balance between these two aims will be influenced by a number of factors. It has also been shown that the effects of supplying water and carbohydrate are independent and additive. High rates of sweat secretion are necessary during hard exercise in order to limit the rise in body temperature which would otherwise occur. If the exercise is prolonged, this leads to progressive dehydration and loss of electrolytes. Fatigue towards the end of a prolonged event may result as much from the effects of dehydration as from substrate depletion. It is often reported that exercise performance is impaired when an individual is dehydrated by as little as 2% of body weight, and that

losses in excess of 5% of body weight can decrease the capacity for work by about 30%. It seems likely, however, that even smaller losses of body water will have a negative effect. Sprint athletes are generally less concerned about the effects of dehydration than are the endurance athletes, but the capacity to perform high-intensity exercise that results in exhaustion within only a few minutes has been shown to be reduced by as much as 45% by prior prolonged exercise that resulted in a loss of water corresponding to only 2.5% of body weight. Smaller, but substantial, reductions in performance occurred after administration of diuretics or after sweat loss in a sauna. Although there is little opportunity for sweat loss during sprint events, these athletes may lose substantial amounts of sweat during training and during warm-up prior to competition. Athletes normally resident in temperate zones who travel to hot climates are likely to experience chronic dehydration, often without being conscious of this.

The composition of drinks to be taken during exercise should be chosen to suit individual circumstances. During exercise in the cold, fluid replacement may not be necessary as sweat rates will be low, but there is still a need to supply additional glucose to the exercising muscles. Although consumption of a high-carbohydrate diet in the days prior to exercise should reduce the need for carbohydrate ingestion during exercise in events lasting less than about 2 h, it is not always possible to achieve this; competition on successive days, for example, may prevent adequate glycogen replacement between exercise periods. In this situation, more concentrated glucose drinks are to be preferred. These will provide more glucose, thus supplementing the limited glycogen stores in the muscles and liver without overloading the body with fluid. In many sports there is little provision for fluid replacement: participants in games such as football or hockey can lose large amounts of fluid, but opportunities for replacement are restricted and many players will drink only during the half-time interval. The major limitation to intake in many situations is the reluctance of the athlete to ingest large volumes and the failure to practise drinking strategies during training. These difficulties have led some competitors in events where large sweat losses are incurred to resort to the use of intravenous fluid replacement. This practice has been used at the half-time interval in hockey games and in prolonged events such as the decathlon and the modern pentathlon.

In the postexercise period, replacement of fluid and electrolytes can usually be achieved through the normal dietary intake. If there is a need to ensure adequate replacement before exercise is repeated, then extra fluids should be taken and additional salt (sodium chloride) might usefully be added to food. Restoration of fluid balance requires replacement of the electrolytes lost in sweat as well as the water. Where training sessions or competitions are close together with limited opportunities for consumption of solid food, drinks should contain relatively high sodium concentrations (perhaps as much as 50–60 mmol l^{-1}) and should also contain sufficient carbohydrate to replenish liver and muscle glycogen stores. The other major electrolytes, particularly potassium, magnesium and calcium, are present in abundance in fruit and fruit juices. Mineral supplements are not normally necessary.

See also: **Calcium**: Physiology. **Carbohydrates**: Chemistry and Classification (Including Dietary Fibre); Regulation of Carbohydrate Metabolism. **Dehydration**: Physiological Effects and Management. **Electrolytes**: Water-Electrolyte Balance; Acid-Base Balance. **Energy**: Energy Balance. **Exercise**: Physiology of Skeletal Muscle; Beneficial Effects. **Iron**: Physiology, Dietary Sources and Requirements. **Protein**: Requirements and Role in Diet. **Vitamin Supplementation**: Role.

Further Reading

Bahr R (1992) Excess postexercise oxygen consumption – magnitude, mechanisms and practical implications. *Acta Physiologica Scandinavica* **144** (supplement 605):1–70.

Below PR, Mora Rodriguez R, Gonzalez-Alonso J and Coyle EF (1994) Fluid and carbohydrate ingestion independently improve performance during 1 h of intense cycling. *Medicine and Science in Sports and Exercise* **27**:200–210.

Bergstrom L and Hultman E (1967) A study of the glycogen metabolism during exercise in man. *Scandinavian Journal of Clinical and Laboratory Investigation* **19**:218–228.

Boobis LH (1987) Metabolic aspects of fatigue during sprinting. In: Macleod D *et al.* (eds) *Exercise: Benefits, Limits and Adaptations*, pp 116–140. London: Spon.

Brouns F, Saris WHM, Stroecken J, Beckers E, Thijssen R, Rehrer NJ and ten Hoor F (1989) Eating, drinking and cycling. A controlled Tour de France simulation study. *International Journal of Sports Medicine* **10**:S41–S48.

Clarkson PM (1991) Minerals: exercise performance and supplementation. *Journal of Sports Science* **9** (special issue):91–116.

Costill DL and Miller JM (1980) Nutrition for endurance sport: Carbohydrate and fluid balance. *International Journal of Sports Medicine* **1**:2–14.

Coyle EF (1991) Timing and method of increased carbohydrate intake to cope with heavy training, competition and recovery. *Journal of Sports Sciences* **9** (special issue):29–52.

Dohm GL (1986) Protein as a fuel for endurance exercise. *Exercise and Sport Science Reviews* **14**:143–173.

Drinkwater BL, Nilson K, Ott S and Chestnet CH (1986) Bone mineral density after resumption of menses in amenorrheic athletes. *Journal of the American Medical Association* **256**:380–382.

Eichner ER (1986) The anemias of athletes. *Physician and Sportsmedicine* **14**:122–130.

Hultman E and Nilsson LH (1971) Liver glycogen in man. *Advances in Experimental Biology and Medicine* **11**:143–151.

King NA and Blundell JE (1995) High-fat foods overcome the energy expenditure due to exercise after cycling and running. *European Journal of Clinical Nutrition* **49**: 114–123.

Lemon PWR (1991) Effect of exercise on protein requirements. *Journal of Sports Sciences* **9** (special issue):53–70.

Maughan RJ and Greenhaff PL (1991) High intensity exercise and acid–base balance: the influence of diet and induced metabolic alkalosis on performance. In: Brouns F (ed.) *Advances in Nutrition and Top Sport*, pp 147–165. Basel: Karger.

Maughan RJ (1991) Fluid and electrolyte loss and replacement in exercise. *Journal of Sports Sciences* **9**:117–142.

Murray R (1987) The effects of consuming carbohydrate-electrolyte beverages on gastric emptying and fluid absorption during and following exercise. *Sports Medicine* **4**:322–351.

Williams MH (1985) *Nutritional Aspects of Human Physical and Athletic Performance*. Springfield: Charles C Thomas.

Beneficial Effects

C Boreham and **M Murphy**, University of Ulster at Jordanstown, Northern Ireland, UK

Copyright © 1998 Academic Press

Introduction

This article examines the roles that physical activity, exercise and fitness may play in the regulation of energy balance, and in the aetiology of major diseases such as coronary heart disease, cancer and osteoporosis. First, it is necessary to define some important terms:

- *Physical activity*: any bodily movement produced by skeletal muscles that results in energy expenditure.
- *Exercise* (often used interchangeably with 'physical activity'): physical activity that is regular, planned and structured with the aim of improving or maintaining one or more aspects of physical fitness.

- *Physical fitness*: a set of outcomes or traits relating to the ability to perform physical activity.

Exercise and Energy Balance

Energy balance occurs when the total energy expenditure of an individual equals that individual's total energy intake from the diet. If intake exceeds expenditure the result is an increase in the storage of energy as body fat. If intake is below expenditure body energy content or body fat decreases.

In humans, energy is expended in three ways: in maintaining the physiological functions of the body at rest, often termed the 'basal metabolic rate' (BMR); in ingesting food and digesting and assimilating nutrients, or the thermic effect of food (TEF); and finally in skeletal muscular contractions involved in spontaneous physical activity or planned exercise. Of these three components, the energy expenditure associated with physical activity and exercise is the factor that accounts for the greatest variability between individuals (**Table 1**). In addition, energy expenditure through physical activity is the only component that may be reasonably controlled by an individual, and therefore may represent an appropriate method for altering energy balance. Physical activity is estimated to make up between 5% and 40% of daily energy expenditure depending on the activity habits of the individual, with BMR and TEF accounting for 60–75% and 10–15% respectively.

Aside from its direct independent effect on daily energy expenditure, recent evidence suggests that exercise may also alter BMR, TEF and the energy expenditure caused by spontaneous physical activity.

Energy expenditure during exercise

The magnitude of energy expenditure during exercise is dependent upon several factors including the mode, intensity and duration of exercise, as well as the body mass of the individual.

When determining the metabolic cost of weight-bearing physical activity, energy expenditure needs to be expressed in relation to body size, since a small person will expend less energy performing a given activity (e.g. walking up a flight of stairs) than a larger person performing the same activity. Therefore to calculate the energy cost of a given activity it is necessary to know the energy cost in kilojoules or kilocalories per kilogram of body weight. The term 'metabolic equivalent' (MET) may also be used to indicate the ratio of the rate of energy expenditure during a given activity to the BMR. An example illustrates how the MET is used to quantify energy expenditure during exercise. If an individual with a body mass of 70 kg expends 300 kJ (70 kcal) per hour at rest (BMR), and walking at a speed of 5.6 km h^{-1} requires 1200 kJ (280 kcal) per hour, the energy cost of the activity is 4 MET four times the BMR of the individual. Since body size is a determinant of both BMR and the energy expenditure during exercise, a heavier individual will have a higher BMR but will still require 4 times this level of expenditure (or 4 METs) to walk at the same speed. **Table 2** indicates the energy cost in METs of many popular types of exercise.

Energy expenditure after exercise

As well as the additional energy consumed during an exercise bout, several researchers have found that

Table 1   Estimated daily energy expenditure (approximate) for individuals of different age, weight, gender and level of activity. Values are based on estimated average requirements from a report in 1991 by the UK Committee on Medical Aspects of Food Policy. Dietary reference values are for food energy and nutrients for the UK

	Estimated daily energy expenditure	
Status	*kcal*	*MJ*
Infant, male, age 3 months, body weight 6 kg	760	3.2
Child, male, age 4 years, body weight 17 kg	1520	6.4
Teenager, male, age 13 years, body weight 46 kg	2200	9.2
Sedentary female[b]	1950	8.1
Sedentary male[a]	2500	10.2
Female[b] – moderately active	2200	9.2
Male[a] – moderately active	3000	12.5
Female[b] – very active	2500	10.4
Male[a] – very active	3200	13.3

[a]Based on male aged 25 years, body weight 70 kg.
[b]Based on female aged 25 years, mass 60 kg.

Table 2 Energy costs of popular physical activities

Activity	Intensity	MET
Walking	6.4 km h^{-1}	4
Running	10.8 km h^{-1}	11
Cycling	20.9 km h^{-1}	8
Swimming	Front crawl (moderate)	8
Tennis	Singles	8
Aerobics	Moderate	6

Adapted from Ainsworth et al. (1993).
MET, metabolic equivalent.

energy expenditure remains elevated for a period following exercise. However, conclusions regarding the magnitude and duration of this postexercise elevation in energy expenditure have been equivocal. Studies have found an increase in energy expenditure in the postexercise period varying in from 5 kcal (21 kJ) to 130 kcal (546 kJ), with some suggesting that this additional energy expenditure lasts a few minutes, and others suggesting that the elevated metabolic rate persists for up to 24 h. The divergence in the findings may be accounted for by the various modes, durations and intensities of exercise employed in the studies as well as the methods used for measuring alterations in energy expenditure and the confounding effects of food ingestion during the recovery period. In addition, alterations in postexercise energy consumption may exhibit intraindividual variations according to the fitness level of subjects. Several mechanisms underlying this increased energy expenditure during the postexercise period have been postulated, including the energy cost of replenishing fuel stores, the cost of dissipating by-products of ATP resynthesis, restoration of cellular homeostatis and the futile cycling of energy substrates. The magnitude of this increase may be related to the intensity and duration of exercise, with longer or more strenuous activity creating a greater perturbation to homeostasis and therefore causing greater energy expenditure in restoring the body to its preexercise condition.

Effects of exercise training on BMR

Aside from the transient increase in energy expenditure in the period immediately following exercise, several researchers have examined the chronic effect of exercise on BMR. Although findings are far from consistent, some investigators have found that regular exercise causes a persistent augmentation in BMR. The mechanism for effect has yet to be confirmed, but it has been hypothesized that this increase may be due to the high energy turnover associated with the elevated levels of energy intake and expenditure typical of trained individuals.

Effects of exercise on the thermic effect of food

The TEF is largely dictated by the composition and energy content of the meal as well as by the individual's body composition. However, some studies have indicated that pre- or postprandial exercise may enhance the TEF. In addition to this acute effect of exercise, regular training may alter the TEF. In men the thermic effect of a meal is lower in highly trained compared with untrained individuals. In one study, moderate levels of fitness were associated with a greater increase in the TEF than either high or low fitness levels (**Fig. 1**). It is possible that very high or very low levels of fitness may decrease the thermic effect possibly by adaptive mechanisms such as a lower insulin or lower noradrenaline response to feeding. Interestingly, no equivalent effect has been found in women. Studies with monozygotic twins also suggest a strong genetic factor controlling whether exercise has such an effect.

Effect of exercise on energy expenditure in spontaneous physical activity

In addition to the energy expenditure during planned exercise, other skeletal muscle contraction associated with spontaneous physical activity (including fidgeting) incurs an energy cost. Research indicates that the quantity of energy expended in spontaneous physical activity is highly variable between individuals. Recent studies show that in addition to its effect on BMR, participation in a planned exercise programme increases the energy expenditure of an individual during nonexercising time.

Physiological Adaptations to Exercise Training

Aside from alterations in energy balance, regular

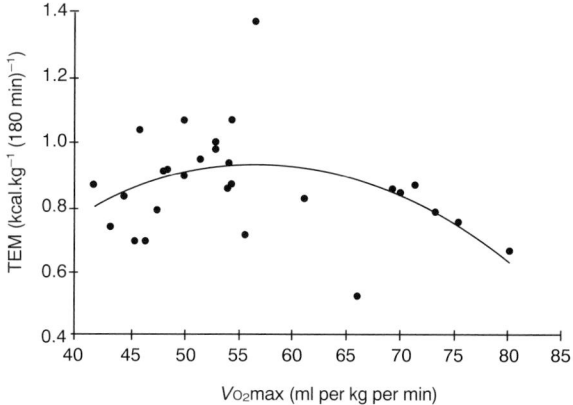

Figure 1 The curvilinear relationship between aerobic capacity (V_{O_2}max) and the thermic effect of a test meal (TEM) in 28 non-obese subjects. From Poehlman (1989), with permission.

exercise brings about many physiological adaptations. The human body is remarkably plastic in response to the increased metabolic demands of exercise training (overload), with many adaptations occurring that enable the body to function more efficiently. The nature and magnitude of these changes are dependent upon the volume (duration and frequency), intensity and type of exercise performed. For this reason the physiological adaptation to training is classified according to the nature of the exercise undertaken.

It is important to remember two principles when considering the physiological adaptations to exercise training. Firstly, there is a degree of intraindividual variation in response to exercise training which may be attributed in part to hereditary factors. Secondly, while exercise training will cause adaptation, the removal of this stimulus will result in a reversal of adaptation, or 'detraining'.

Adaptations to submaximal or endurance exercise training

Submaximal exercise generally refers to an intensity of exercise that requires less than an individual's maximal oxygen uptake. Submaximal exercise challenges the body to deliver and utilize an increased amount of oxygen in the resynthesis of adenosine triphosphate (ATP). With training, changes occur that increase the body's ability to utilize oxygen. For simplicity, the adaptations to submaximal exercise training are considered according to the site at which they occur.

Central adaptations   Central adaptations to regular submaximal exercise include alterations in the morphology and function of the heart and circulatory systems which allow greater delivery of oxygen to the working muscle. The pulmonary system in healthy individuals does not provide a significant limitation to exercise, and therefore little alteration in the lung volumes, respiratory rate or pulmonary ventilation and diffusion occurs as a result of training. Modest cardiac hypertrophy, characterized by an increase in left ventricular volume, occurs in response to training. This adaptation allows an increase in stroke volume, leading to a reduction in heart rate at rest and during submaximal workloads, and an increased cardiac output during maximal workloads. Finally, an increase in total plasma volume and an increase in the total amount of haemoglobin have been observed in response to submaximal endurance training.

Peripheral adaptations   Peripheral adaptations refer principally to changes in the structure and function of skeletal muscle which enhance its ability to use oxygen to produce energy aerobically. As a result of endurance training there is an increase in blood supply to the working muscle. This is achieved by an increased capillarization in trained muscles, greater vasodilatation in existing muscle capillaries and a more effective redistribution of cardiac output to the working muscle. An increase in the activity of aerobic enzymes and an increased mitochondrial volume density (from 4% to 8% approximately) within trained muscle has been noted. This is coupled with increased glycogen storage within the muscle and increased fat mobilization, allowing a higher rate of aerobic ATP resynthesis from free fatty acids and glucose.

Adaptations to high-intensity exercise and strength training

High-intensity exercise requires energy utilization rates that exceed the oxidative capabilities of the muscle. Activities such as sprinting require the anaerobic resynthesis of ATP to produce and maintain high levels of muscular force, and are therefore limited in duration. Strength training also relies heavily on anaerobic energy sources and requires high force production by specific muscle groups.

The main alterations that occur in response to regular high-intensity exercise or strength training are improvements in the structure and function of the neuromuscular system which allow more efficient production of the forces required for these activities, and an enhanced ability to produce the energy required through anaerobic processes.

Neuromuscular adaptations   The initial improvements in performance which occur with high-intensity exercise training are largely a result of improved coordination of the nervous system. Increased nervous system activation, more efficient neuromuscular recruitment patterns and a decrease in inhibitory reflexes allow the individual to produce greater levels of force. The maximum force a muscle can exert is largely determined by its cross-sectional area. In addition to the neural adaptations, strength training stimulates an increase in muscle size. This hypertrophy occurs preferentially in fast twitch muscle fibres and is brought about by increased protein synthesis in response to resistance training. The degree to which muscle hypertrophy occurs is dependent upon many factors including sex and body type. Although some researchers have suggested that strength training may increase the number of muscle cells (hyperplasia), the results of these studies are still far from conclusive.

Since both high-intensity and strength training rely

largely on anaerobic processes for energy production, adaptative alterations in oxygen delivery and utilization, such as increased capillarization or mitochondrial mass of muscle cells are relatively minor.

Metabolic adaptations   In addition to the neuromuscular alterations that occur with high-intensity and strength training, several metabolic adaptations improve the ability of the muscle to resynthesize ATP from anaerobic sources. Intramuscular stores of the anaerobic energy intermediates such as creatine phosphate (CP) and glycogen increase after a period of maximal training. The activity of enzymes involved in anaerobic production of energy such as creatine kinase and myokinase is also increased.

The Role of Exercise and Fitness in Coronary Heart Disease

Coronary heart disease (CHD) has a multifactorial aetiology, and major 'biological' risk factors include elevated concentrations of blood total and low-density lipoprotein (LDL) cholesterol, reduced concentration of high-density lipoprotein (HDL) cholesterol, high blood pressure, diabetes mellitus and obesity. In addition, 'behavioural' risk factors for CHD include cigarette smoking, a poor diet, and low levels of physical activity and physical fitness associated with the modern, predominantly sedentary way of living. Among these risk factors, a sedentary life style is by far the most prevalent according to figures for both the USA and England (**Fig. 2**).

Scientific verification of a link between an indolent life style and CHD has been forthcoming since the 1950s, with the publication of over a hundred large-scale epidemiological studies investigating the relationships between physical activity and cardiovascular health. These studies have produced consistently compelling evidence that regular physical activity can protect against CHD (**Fig. 3**). Pooled data and meta-analyses of the 'better' studies indicate that the risk of death from CHD doubles in individuals who are physically inactive in comparison with their more active counterparts. Relationships between aerobic fitness and CHD appear even stronger, with reported age-adjusted relative risks of approximately 8.0 for both sexes, when the least fit quintile of a study population is compared with the most fit quintile. For both physical activity and fitness, adjustment for a wide range of other risk factors only slightly weakens these associations, suggesting independent relationships.

A common weakness of such studies is that they have often relied upon a single measurement of fitness or activity at baseline, with subsequent follow-up for mortality within the cohort. With such a design, it is difficult to discount the possibility that genetic or other confounding factors are influential in the observed relationship between physical activity, fitness and mortality. A further weakness in single baseline studies is that subsequent changes in activity or fitness during the follow-up are not monitored, even though they may affect the risk of mortality.

Two large-scale prospective studies overcame these deficiencies by examining the effects of *changes* in physical activity and fitness on mortality. One study reported on the relationship of changes in physical activity and other life style characteristics to CHD mortality in 10 269 alumni of Harvard University. Changes in life style over a period of 11–15 years were evaluated on the basis of questionnaire

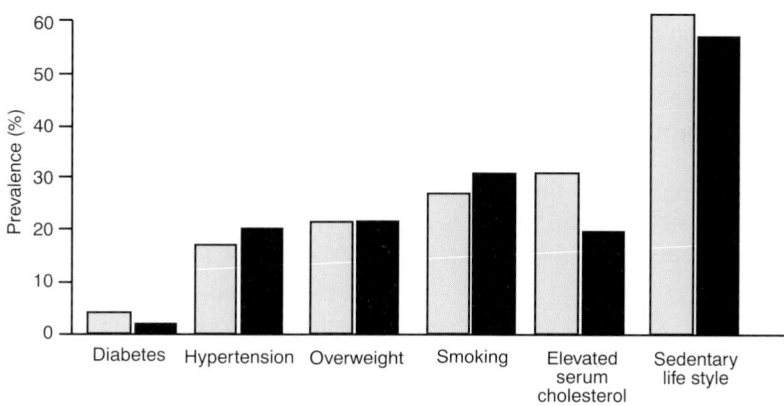

Figure 2   Estimates of the prevalence (%) of selected risk factors for coronary heart disease. Figures for the USA are taken from the Centers for Disease Control study reported in 1990 (shaded bars) and for England from the 1991 Health Survey (solid bars). In both studies a sedentary life style was taken as 'no physical activity' or irregular physical activity (i.e. fewer than three times per week and/or less than 20 min per session). From Killoran AJ, Fentem P and Caspersen C, eds (1994) *Moving On: International Perspectives on Promoting Physical Activity*, London: Health Education Authority, with permission.

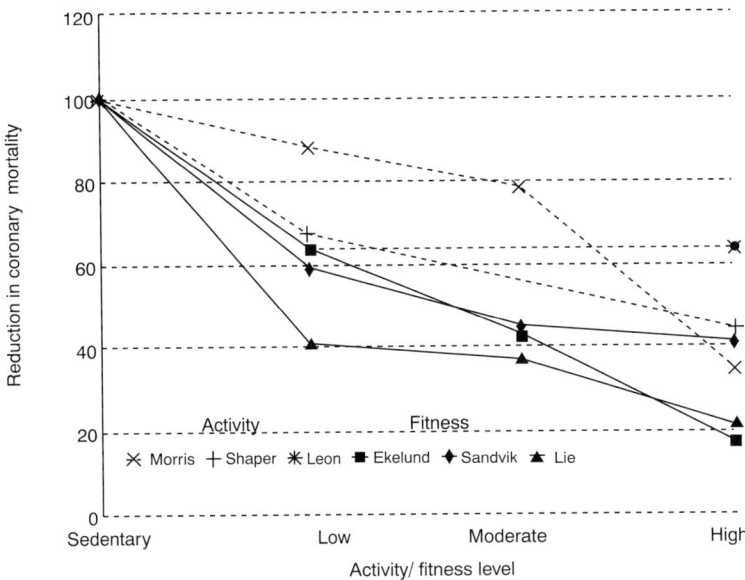

Figure 3 Summary of the results from six studies in which fitness level was determined (three studies) or activity level assessed by questionnaire (three studies) in individual populations. Follow-up was generally 7–9 years except in Sandvik's study, which had a 16-year follow-up. The 'low level' group for each study represented in this figure was the activity/fitness level next to the least active/fit group. The 'high level' represents the group that was the most active/fit for the particular study. If the study participants were grouped by quintile, the 'moderate' group is the average of the third and fourth quintiles. From Killoran AJ, Fentem P and Caspersen C, eds (1994) *Moving On. International Perspective on Promoting Physical Activity*, London: Health Education Authority, with permission.

information, and subsequent mortality was assessed over an 8-year period (**Fig. 4**). In men who were initially sedentary but started participating in moderately vigorous sports (intensity of 4.5 MET or greater), there was a 41% reduced risk of CHD compared with those who remained sedentary. This reduction was comparable to that experienced by men who stopped smoking. The second study examined changes in physical fitness and their effects on mortality. In this study of 9777 men, two clinical examinations (including treadmill tests of aerobic fitness) were administered approximately 5 years apart, with a mean follow-up of 5.1 years after the second examination to assess mortality. Results showed that men who improved their fitness (by moving out of the least fit quintile) reduced their aged-adjusted CHD mortality by 52% compared with their peers who remained unfit. Furthermore, such changes in fitness proved to be the most effective in reducing all-cause mortality, when compared with changes in other health risk factors (**Fig. 5**).

Mechanisms of effect

Exercise appears to reduce the risk of CHD through both direct and indirect mechanisms. Regularly performed physical activity may reduce the vulnerability of the myocardium to fatal ventricular arrhythmia, and reduce myocardial oxygen requirements. Aerobic training also increases coronary vascular trans-

port capacity via structural adaptations and altered control of vascular resistance. Risk of thrombus formation may also be reduced with regular exercise through its effects on blood clotting and fibrinolytic mechanisms. Regular endurance exercise may also improve the serum lipid profile (particularly in favour of an increased ratio of HDL to total cholesterol levels) and have beneficial effects on adipose tissue lipolysis and distribution.

Exercise prescription

For protection against CHD and other diseases associated with inactivity, exercise needs to be habitual, predominantly aerobic in nature and current. Evidence from work carried out on British civil servants suggests that to be cardioprotective, exercise should be moderately vigorous, using at least 7.5 kcal min^{-1} (31.4 kJ min^{-1}) or 6 MET (equivalent to walking at about 4.8 km h^{-1} up a slope of 1 in 20) and performed at least twice weekly. However, other studies have indicated that lower intensity activity is also effective as long as the total accumulated exercise energy expenditure is greater than approximately 8.4 MJ (2000 kcal) per week.

Recommendations from the US Surgeon General suggest that everyone over the age of 2 years should accumulate 30 min or more of at least moderate-intensity physical activity on most – preferably all – days of the week. Such activity may embrace

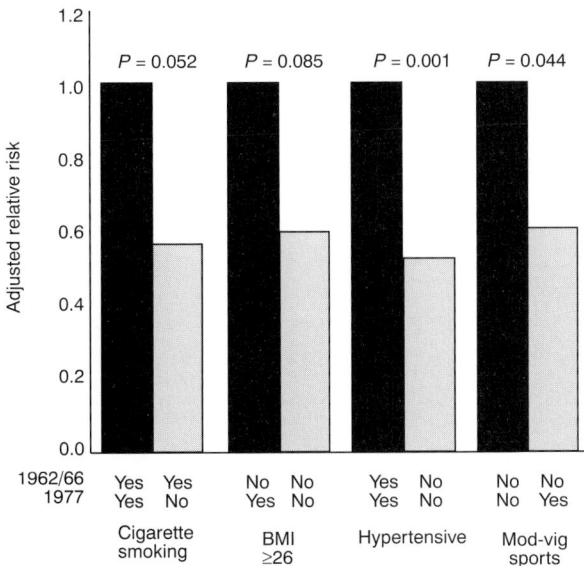

Life- style characteristics in 1962/66 and 1977

Figure 4 Adjusted relative risks (each relative risk is adjusted for age and all other variables in the figure) for coronary heart disease mortality by changes in life-style characteristics. The solid bars represent men who had unfavourable characteristics at baseline (in 1962 or 1966) and at follow-up (in 1977). The shaded bars show the adjusted relative risks for men who made favourable changes on the variable of interest between baseline and follow-up. There were 10 269 men in the cohort, with 130 deaths from coronary heart disease. The relative risk is adjusted for age and other factors in the figure; BMI, body mass index; Mod-vig, moderately vigorous. Data from Paffenbarger *et al.* (1993). Reprinted with permission from Blair SN *Research Quarterly for Exercise and Sport* 64(4):365–376. Copyright 1993 by the American Alliance for Health, Physical Education, Recreation and Dance, 1900 Association Drive, Reston, Va 20191.

everyday tasks such as stair-climbing and walking, recreational physical activities and more formal aerobic exercise programmes and sports. Intermittent or shorter bouts of activity (of at least 10 min duration) may be accumulated throughout the day to confer similar benefits to single, continuous 30 min bouts of exercise. A consistent finding is that previous exercise that has been abandoned confers no benefit (**Table 3**).

Desirable aerobic fitness levels have also been described for women (maximal aerobic power of approximately 9 MET, 32.5 ml per kg per min) and men (10 MET, 35 ml per kg per min) (**Fig. 6**).

Table 3 History of vigorous sports in men reporting none currently in 1976 and the incidence of coronary heart disease, 1976–86. The subjects were male executive-grade civil servants aged 45–64 years on entry

	Incidence of CHD	
Vigorous sports	No. of cases	Rates per 1000 man-years[a]
Played none previously	128	5.7
Played up to 25 years of age	27	4.1
Played up to 30 years of age	54	6.4
Played up to 40 years of age	92	5.7
Played past 40 years of age	112	6.2

From Morris JN (1994) Exercise in the prevention of coronary heart disease: today's best buy in public health. *Medicine and Science in Sports and Exercise* 26(7): 810, with permission.
[a]Age-standardized rates.

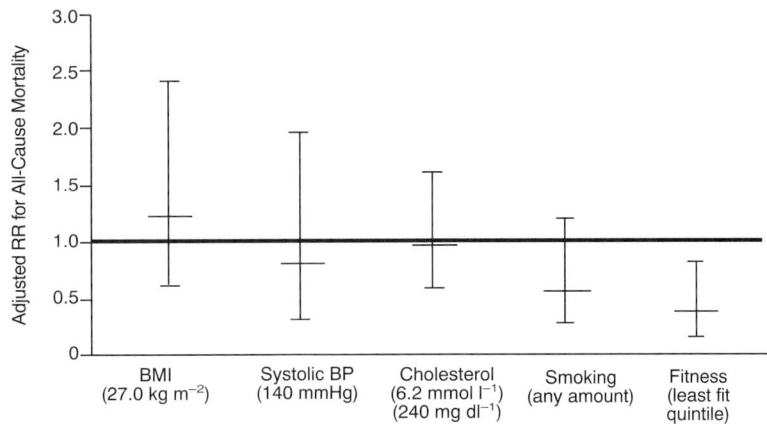

Figure 5 Relative risks (adjusted for age, family history of coronary heart disease, health status, baseline values, and changes for all variables in the figure, and interval in years between examinations) of all-cause mortality by favourable changes in risk factors between first and subsequent examinations. The analyses were for men at risk on each particular variable at the first examination. Cutoff points designating high risk are given parenthetically at the bottom of the figure. The number of men at high risk (and the number of deaths) for each characteristic were as follows: body mass index (BMI), 2691 (66); systolic blood pressure (BP), 1013 (55); cholesterol, 2212 (79); cigarette smoking, 1609 (45); and physical fitness, 1015 (56). RR, relative risk. Reproduced from Blair *et al.* (1995), with permission, American Medical Association.

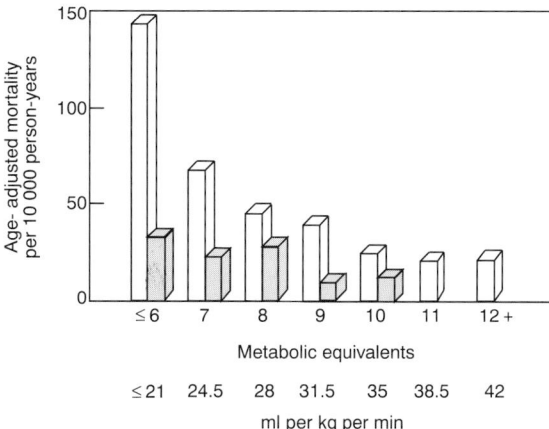

Figure 6 Age-adjusted, all-cause mortality rates per 10 000 person-years of follow-up by physical fitness categories in 3120 women (shaded bars) and 10 224 men. Physical fitness categories are expressed here as maximal metabolic equivalents (work metabolic rate/BMR) achieved during the maximal treadmill exercise test. One metabolic equivalent equals 3.5 ml per kg per min. The estimated maximal oxygen uptake for each category is shown also. Reproduced from Blair SN *et al.* (1989) Physical fitness and all-cause mortality. A prospective study of healthy men and women. *Journal of the American Medical Association* 262:2395–2401, with permission.

The Role of Exercise in the Aetiology of Other Diseases

Obesity

Obesity is defined as an excess of adipose tissue. This condition plays a central role in the development of diabetes mellitus, and confers an increased risk for CHD, high blood pressure, osteoarthritis, dyslipoproteinaemia, various cancers and all-cause mortality. The prevalence of obesity in the UK has risen dramatically since the 1970s (**Fig. 7**), in parallel with a fall in daily energy expenditure of about 3.3 MJ (800 kcal).

Based on the principles of energy balance, such circumstantial evidence indicates that physical inactivity may promote the development of obesity in humans. However, confirmatory data are scarce, particularly from well-designed prospective studies. One large-scale national study in the USA evaluated the relationship of physical activity to weight gain over a 10-year follow-up of 3515 men and 5810 women. Individuals who were sedentary at both baseline and follow-up were much more likely – relative risk 2.3 (95% confidence interval, 0.9 to 5.8) in men and 7.1 (CI, 2.2 to 23.3) in women – to experience considerable weight gain (>13 kg) than subjects who were active at both examinations. Other similar studies support these findings.

Difficulties are encountered in interpreting results from intervention studies investigating the effects of

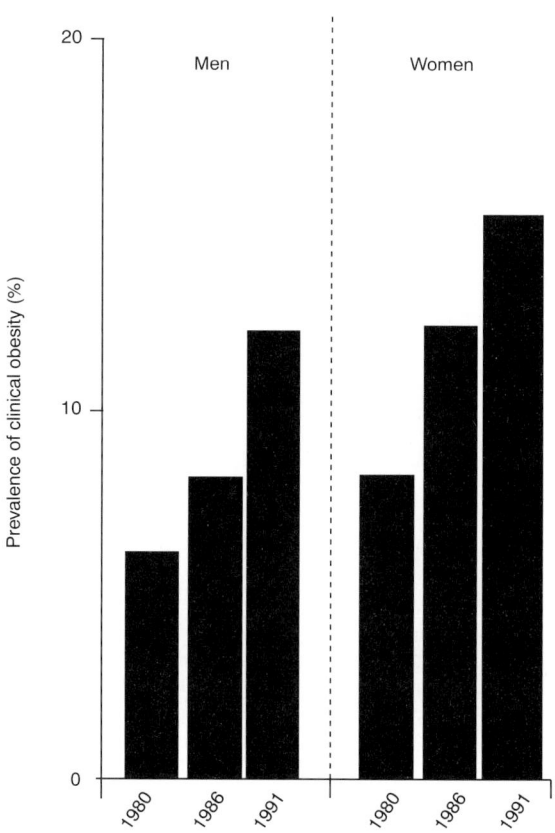

Figure 7   Prevalence of clinical obesity (body mass index > 30) in England. Source: Office of Population Censuses and Surveys. From Prentice AM and Jebb SA (1995) Obesity in Britain: gluttony or sloth? *British Medical Journal* 311:437–439, with permission.

exercise and/or diet on body weight, body composition and BMR (the latter being the single greatest component of total energy expenditure). Both energy intake and physical activity are notoriously difficult to quantify accurately, as is body fat status and distribution. Methodological differences between studies, a lack of control for possible confounding factors and the fact that weight loss leads to enhancement of metabolic economy (owing to reductions in BMR, energy cost of physical activity and TEF) further complicate matters. Nevertheless, exercise probably helps to protect fat-free mass while promoting the loss of fat mass, but does not appear to prevent the decline in BMR during weight loss. Similarly, long-term physical activity has minimal effects on BMR beyond its effect on lean body mass. While studies have shown that exercise alone can reduce body weight, the rate and amount of weight loss is less than can be achieved through dieting alone.

Although the combination of exercise and dieting might be expected to improve weight loss, most data show only a slightly greater loss (2–3 kg). When the total daily energy deficit is kept constant, diet, exercise, and diet plus exercise all result in similar weight loss, but the inclusion of exercise generally results in greater fat loss and an increased lean tissue mass.

Osteoporosis

Osteoporosis-related fractures represent a public health concern of major proportions. Once established, osteoporosis may be irreversible, emphasizing the need for primary prevention strategies based on minimizing bone loss and maximizing peak bone mass. Nearly half the variation in bone mineral density (BMD) may be attributable to nongenetic factors. Behavioural factors of importance include diet, smoking and the amount and type of habitual physical activity. These factors may be particularly influential during adolescence when (depending on site) up to 90% of adult bone mineral content may be deposited, prior to the attainment of peak bone mass in the third decade of life.

Several studies on the relation of physical activity to bone mineral density have now been conducted, allowing a few conclusions to be drawn. Clearly, bone responds positively to the mechanical stresses of exercise. Regular physical activity is likely to boost peak bone mass in young women, probably slows the decline in BMD in middle-aged and older women, and may increase BMD in patients with established osteoporosis. More research is required to clarify the type and amount of exercise that is most effective in promoting bone health, although current evidence favours relatively high-impact exercise such as Volleyball and basketball. It is also unclear how physical activity and other intervention strategies such as calcium supplementation and oestrogen replacement therapy interact to promote bone health.

In addition to its osteogenic effects, exercise may also promote better coordination, balance and ambulatory muscle strength, thus minimizing the risk of falling. The reported reduced risk of fracture (relative risk 0.41 in men and 0.76 in women) in active individuals compared with sedentary ones is likely to result from these combined direct and indirect effects of physical activity.

Cancer

In general, data relating to associations between physical activity and breast, endometrial, ovarian, prostate and testicular cancers are inconclusive at present, although the suggestion that activity in adolescence and young adulthood may provide subsequent protection against breast cancer is worthy of further study. To date the only clear evidence in this field comes from epidemiological studies relating a reduced risk of cancer of the colon to both occupational and leisure-time physical activity. One such study investigated 17 148 Harvard alumni, who were assessed for physical activity at two points, 10–15 years apart. Those who were highly active (exercise energy expenditure at least 10.5 MJ (2500 kcal) a week) at both assessments displayed half the risk of developing colon cancer of those who were relatively inactive, expending no more than 4.2 MJ (1000 kcal) a week. Interestingly, higher levels of physical activity at one assessment but not at both were not associated with lower cancer risk, suggesting that consistently higher levels of activity may be necessary to provide a measure of protection. Possible biological mechanisms for this association include exercise-induced alteration of local prostaglandin synthesis (particularly prostaglandin $F_{2\alpha}$) and a decreased gastrointestinal transit time – the latter possibly decreasing the duration of contact between the colonic mucosa and potential carcinogens.

See also: **Body Composition**: Determination and Physiological Significance. **Bone**: Composition, Metabolism and Bone Growth. **Cancer**: Epidemiology and Associations Between Diet and Cancer; Epidemiology of Colorectal Cancer. **Carbohydrates**: Regulation of Carbohydrate Metabolism. **Coronary Heart Disease**: Lipid Theory of Coronary Heart Disease; Haemostatic Factors and Coronary Heart Disease; Aetiology; Prevention. **Energy**: Energy Requirements; Energy Balance; Measurement of Energy Intake and Expenditure. **Epidemiological Studies**: Role and Interpretation. **Exercise**: Physiology of Skeletal Muscle; Diet and Exercise. **Infants**: Nutritional Requirements. **Obesity**: Definition, Aetiology and Assessment; Early Obesity and Prognosis; Fat Distribution; Treatment; Prevention; Complications of Obesity. **Older People**: Nutritionally Related Problems. **Osteoporosis**: Aetiology; Treatment and Prevention. **Weight Management**: Approaches; Weight Cycling.

Further Reading

Ainsworth BE, Haskell WL, Leon AS *et al.* (1993) Compendium of physical activities: classification of energy costs of human physical activities. *Medicine and Science in Sports and Exercise* 25(1):71–80.

Blair SN (1993) Physical activity, physical fitness and health. *Research Quarterly for Exercise and Sport* 64(4):365–376.

Blair SN, Kohl HW and Gordon NF (1992) How much physical activity is good for health? *Annual Review of Public Health* 13:99–126.

Blair SN, Kohl HW, Barlow CE, Paffenbarger RS, Gibbons LW and Macera C (1995) Changes in physical fitness and all-cause mortality. A prospective study of healthy and unhealthy men. *Journal of the American Medical Association* 273:1093–1098.

Bouchard C, Shephard RJ, Stephens T, eds (1994) *Physical Activity, Fitness and Health. International Proceedings and Consensus Statement.* Champaign, IL: Human Kinetics.

Hardman AE (1996) Exercise in the prevention of atherosclerotic, metabolic and hypertensive diseases: a review. *Journal of Sports Sciences* 14:201–218.

Paffenbarger RS, Hyde RT, Wing AL, Lee I-M, Jung DL and Kampert JB (1993) The association of changes in physical activity level and other lifestyle characteristics with mortality among men. *New England Journal of Medicine* 328:538–545.

Poehlman ET (1989) A review: exercise and its influence on resting energy metabolism in man. *Medicine and Science in Sports and Exercise* 21(5):515–525.

Poehlman ET, Melby CL and Goran MI (1991) The impact of exercise and diet restriction on daily energy expenditure. *Sports Medicine* 11(2):78–101.

US Department of Health and Human Services (1996) *Physical Activity and Health: A Report of the Surgeon General.* Atlanta: US Department of Health and Human Services, Centres for Disease Control and Prevention, National Centre for Chronic Disease Prevention and Health Promotion.

FAMINE

Population Responses

K West, Johns Hopkins University, Baltimore, Maryland, USA

Copyright © 1998 Academic Press

Famines in History

Famine has afflicted humankind, shaping its demography and history from antiquity. Records of famine in ancient Egypt during the third millennium BC are depicted in bas-relief on the causeway of the pyramid of Unas in Saqqura. Biblical accounts of famine in Egypt during the second millennium BC (Middle Kingdom) describe the devastation wrought on the land and society and the means by which Joseph predicted and attempted to minimize its consequences. The fall of the Roman Empire followed repeated food shortages and famines from 500 BC to AD 500. China experienced 1829 famines, or about 13 per year in different areas, from 108 BC to AD 29. The ranks of the Crusades in the eleventh and twelfth centuries swelled in response to assurance of food. The storming of the Bastille and the French Revolution followed decades of rising flour and bread prices which had caused widespread hunger and hardship.

Recurrent famine motivated the European settling of the New World. The Great Irish Famine in the 1840s caused 1.5 million deaths and an equal number of migrations, mostly to America. Decades of Russian famines following crop failures in the late nineteenth century resulted in waves of immigration to the USA. Famine helped usher in the Bolshevik Revolution. Multiple famines throughout nineteenth century China reportedly led to over 50 million deaths. However, possibly the worst single famine in human history occurred in China in 1959–60, during which up to 30 million people reportedly perished, unknown to the rest of the world, following the policy failures of the 'Great Leap Forward'. Famine was notorious on the Indian subcontinent through the mid twentieth century, but recurred only once in the latter half of the century, in Bangladesh in 1974–5. Famine-free decades in India since the Great Bengal Famine in 1943 have been attributed, in part, to the country's democratic process and flourishing free press.

Famines in the late twentieth century have inflicted heavy losses of human and animal life in Africa, especially in the Horn (i.e. Ethiopia, Somalia and the Sudan). These increasingly complex famines have resulted from deteriorating crop production, failures in development and commerce, the impact of repressive regimes, civil unrest and war. At least one regime's demise, that of Emperor Haile Selassie in 1974, followed famine. Tragically, these recent famines occurred at a time in human history when our understanding of the causes and consequences of famine and our global ability to prevent it, monitor its antecedents and intervene to avert starvation have never been greater.

Definitions of Famine

Definitions of famine vary but all contain the necessary elements of widespread starvation with dramatically increased mortality. More comprehensive descriptions include elements of time-dependency (e.g. sudden collapse in food available for consumption), causation (e.g. due to a natural calamity or war), class (e.g. affecting certain groups more than others) or other population responses (e.g. accompanied by epidemics of disease or massive migrations). All formal definitions tend to lack precision yet they clearly distinguish famine from other aspects of deprivation, such as chronic food insecurity, extreme poverty, high prevalence of wasting malnutrition and mortality which characterize many regions of the developing world. Nor can single definitions capture the vast array of indigenous responses, particularly by those affected at local levels, to survive famine. Irrespective of definition, famine is catastrophic, distinct and a human tragedy of unparalleled proportion. In virtually every famine, infants, young children and women endure the greatest risk of starvation.

Causes of Famine

There can be many factors that, individually, rarely lead to famine but may contribute to its risk in a population or region. Commonly ascribed causes of famine include chronic and acute failures in food security, rising food demands imposed by rapid population growth, failure in demand for food through loss of 'entitlement', failure in governance with respect to development, assuring democratic freedoms, peace and law and order, and failure in providing relief in a timely, adequate and effective manner to mitigate massive migrations and numbers of famine-related deaths.

A severe, widespread decline in food availability has classically been considered to be the single most important cause of famine. A gradual deterioration in food production or aggregate food availability for local consumption, owing to drought or other factors (e.g. conflict, excessive reliance on cash or export crops) can precondition a population or region to famine. The situation is made worse by high population growth.

Despite an intuitive link of famine to acute food shortage, the relationship between the quantity of food in a region and probability of widespread starvation is highly variable. In fact, many well-documented famines have occurred in the presence of ample national food supplies. The Great Irish Famine from 1844 to 1847 was triggered by a potato blight that stripped the country of the only staple that Irish peasantry could afford to grow on their small parcels of land. Peasants who did grow other staple grains had to sell them to pay rent to landlords. However, during these same years, there were substantial exports of wheat, barley, oats and animal products by landowners to English markets. Food did not enter the local Irish markets because the peasants lacked effective demand.

The Great Bengal Famine of 1943, during which about 1.5 million people died, was originally considered to be due to a shortage in rice supply. However, an analysis years later by Amartya Sen showed that the famine occurred in a year during which rice production in Bengal was only 5% lower than the average of the previous five years. It was also a year when most economic indicators of Bengal were showing a wartime 'boom' in growth. Rural food stocks, however, were being procured by the government to support military needs and to subsidize rations for civil servants in Calcutta, thus driving up the price of rice in rural areas. This practice, coupled with a boat blockade that was imposed for defence reasons along the Bay of Bengal, left low-paid members of the wage-earning rural classes (agricultural workers, day labourers, artisans and fishermen) unable to acquire enough food for their own survival. Sen reasoned that their 'entitlement', which represents a net ability to exchange one's personal 'endowment' (money, services, goods, etc.) for food, had collapsed, leaving 1.5 million people to face death from starvation and disease.

In Bangladesh, an estimated 100 000 people died in a famine in 1974–5 that followed an unusually severe flood. During the years leading up to the famine there were events that brought the country to a highly vulnerable state, including a devastating cyclone and tidal wave, a civil war that led to the country's independence, and a series of partial crop failures, all superimposed on preexisting high burdens of malnutrition, disease and underdevelopment. The flood in the middle of 1974 was expected to destroy much of the major *aman* rice to be harvested a few months later. In anticipation of an impending rice shortage, rural traders began to hoard grains in early September of that year, causing rice prices to spike across the country's rural markets in a contagious pattern (**Fig. 1**). Rice remained at about double its normal price for months thereafter, even after it became evident that the speculated poor rice harvest was, in fact, a normal one. Thus, total and per capita aggregate grain supplies in Bangladesh remained at about average levels throughout the famine. Local area food deficits and hoarding of grains by traders led to the observed points of inflection in the price of rice throughout the country that caused the entitlements of rural wage earners to collapse, initiating a famine that resulted in extremely high mortality and massive migrations to urban centres in search of relief.

Aggregate food shortage has appeared to play a more variable and, at times, prominent role in recent famines in sub-Saharan Africa and the eastern Horn of Africa. In these countries large tracts of land are drought-prone, average annual rainfall has been declining since the 1930s, and robust, indigenous farming and animal husbandry practices have been weakened as increased agricultural land has been used for growing export crops. In the Ethiopian famine of 1972–5, in which over 100 000 people died, national crop production dropped to only about 7% below normal levels, a decline that (as in Bengal in 1943 and 1974) would not have been expected to trigger a famine. However, crop production had been

severely below normal in Wollo Province, where the famine began. Although the famine subsequently spread to other areas of the country, a reluctance by the government to formally recognize the famine and excessive delays in mobilizing and targeting food aid within the country (whether from national or international stocks) were deemed responsible for unleashing a famine that, based on national stocks, should have been averted.

Famines during 1982–5 in Ethiopia and in the Sudan appeared to be more closely tied to gradual declines in national food security during the preceding decade. These trends were exacerbated by repressive governments enacting targeted, famine-promotive rather than preventive policies, resulting in civil wars and severely deteriorating economic conditions that were compounded by weak international food aid responses. These famines, and a more recent famine in Somalia in the early 1990s, serve to highlight the rapid emergence of military conflict as a precipitating cause of famine. With significant transfers of weaponry to rogue vigilante groups in Somalia and increased deployments of land mines in other settings in recent years, war, civil violence and lawlessness also pose a major hindrance to the effective provision of short-term relief during the acute phase of famine and to subsequent economic recovery.

The occurrence of famine, and the responses mounted by communities and governments to famine risk, can be depicted in an epidemiologic framework (**Fig. 2**). The multiple conditions, events and population characteristics described above may be viewed as individual components that may combine, often with a precipitating event, to form a 'sufficient cause' of famine. As a population or a vulnerable segment begins to be affected by famine, certain points of

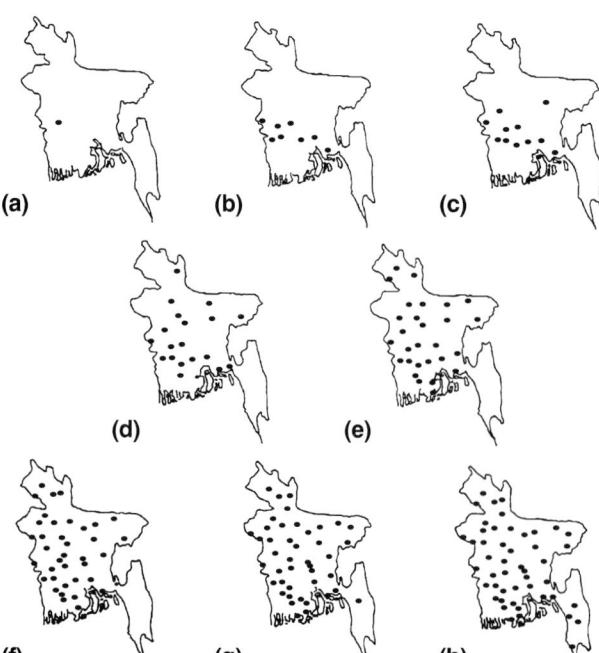

Figure 1 Consecutive maps of a contagious spread of spikes in the price of rice in local markets throughout rural Bangladesh from late August 1974 (a) through the end of October 1974 (h), during the period of a flood-associated famine which killed about 100 000 persons.

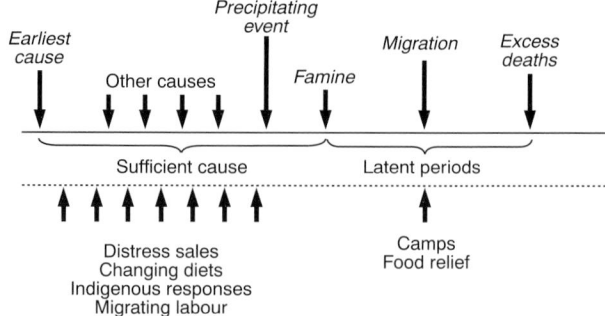

Figure 2 Individual or component causes leading to a sufficient cause that precipitates famine, and the responses to famine. Famine may be latent or delayed from external view until migrations or excess deaths occur. Early responses may mitigate or delay famine. Government relief is often a late response to famine.

inflection occur such as the spikes in grain prices, collapse in the ratios of livestock to grain, migrations and excess deaths. Coping mechanisms exhibited by individual households and communities may prevent the formation of a sufficient cause of famine, or forestall its occurrence. Typically, in cultures where famine risk is high, government responses are late and in the form of relief.

Coping Strategies

In most cultures where food shortages are routine and the threat of famine periodic, there exist numerous indigenous responses that enable the local populace to cope, protect their entitlement and minimize the threat to their survival as terms of exchange for food become less favourable (**Fig. 3**). A first line of responses may be viewed as insurance against uncertainty; these are activities that minimize the loss of endowment such as restructuring the farming system, or pastoral practices that insulate against drought-induced shortages. Examples include planting more robust crops, dispersing crops across a wider area, staggering plantings, or increasing livestock diversity and mobility. Food preservation practices and dietary changes to include 'famine foods' can initially increase the size and diversity of the food base. As the terms of exchange become more threatening, coping mechanisms may increasingly cost households their endowment. These responses include working longer and at different jobs for lower wages, migrating far from home to find marginal work in distant areas, reducing meal frequency and nutritional quality, and consuming the next planting's seeds. Household assets such as pots, utensils, watches and small animals are increasingly sold, as eventually are larger assets such as bullock carts,

draught animals and property. An indicator of severe entitlement loss in a community is the ratio of livestock to grain prices in local markets. Normally this ratio reflects the superior value of livestock compared with grain. However, it may invert as the cost of grain and feeding animals and the level of animal wasting all continue to rise, such that at a peak of famine vulnerability, large numbers of animals may be sold at very low prices relative to the costs of grain.

As household and community entitlement erodes owing to deteriorating conditions of exchange and losses in endowment, destitution and the likelihood of starvation become more likely. As prices of food in markets reach points of inflection, so too does the probability of entitlement collapse, risk of starvation and mass migration from rural areas to urban centres in search of famine relief. **Fig. 4** depicts a hypothetical shift in distribution of starving individuals in a population facing a nonuniform increasing risk of famine. Within extremely poor societies, a certain proportion of individuals deal routinely with the threat of starvation (top panel). During periods of high or repeated stress, such as that attending prolonged drought, coping mechanisms protect most vulnerable groups from starvation. In the severe distress of famine, entitlement has collapsed for those who are most vulnerable, leaving large numbers of persons at risk of starvation, migration or death.

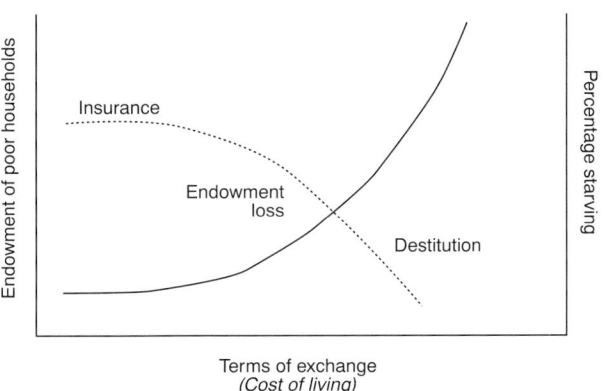

Figure 3 Collapse in entitlement: as endowment of the poor (.....) decreases toward a state of destitution with increasingly severe (costly) terms of exchange for food, the risk of starvation (——) and famine increases.

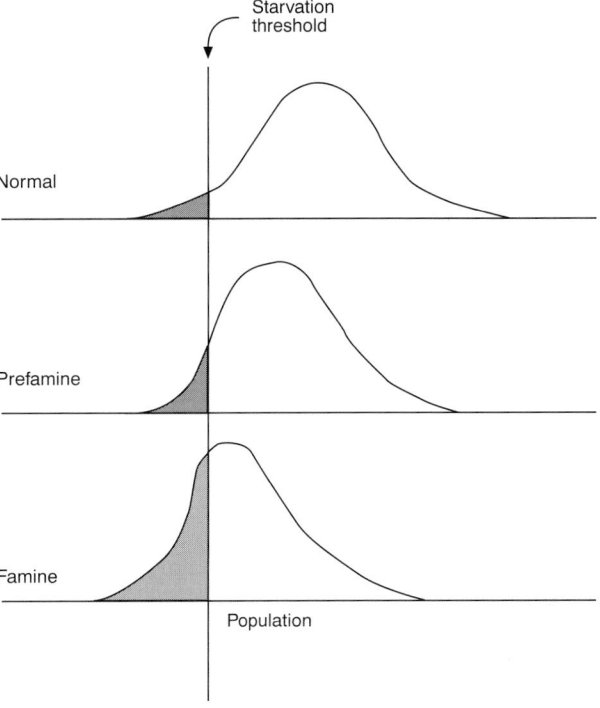

Figure 4 Shifting of a population toward starvation with increasingly severe prefamine and famine conditions.

However, not all individuals starve. Some segments of society lose little or no economic ground, and some may benefit considerably from the plight of others who must sell property or other assets, or borrow thereby incurring future indebtedness to avoid starvation during famine. Still other segments, particularly those trading in famine relief goods and services, stand to gain large profits throughout the famine and recovery periods.

Government and International Responses

Government responses to famine can be classified as preventive, preemptive and relief-oriented or lagged. At times, government actions may provoke or promote famine in war-torn areas.

Preventive action relates to setting and enacting a development agenda that recognizes high-risk areas of the country and seeks to strengthen the productivity and wellbeing of famine-vulnerable population groups in these areas. Measures taken can include boosting infrastructural, commercial, education, agricultural and other inputs to improve long-term economic conditions.

Preemptive government policies are directed toward relieving a prefamine condition once it becomes apparent. Setting up famine early warning systems that monitor climatic, agricultural, population mobility, economic and nutritional indicators is considered preemptive in that such information is intended to identify high-risk trends so that corrective action can be taken long before famine becomes imminent. Normally, early warning surveillance is only possible in high-risk countries with significant international assistance. An example is a government making large purchases of food on the international market and releasing the commodities through ration shops, food-for-work and other programmes that do not disrupt the local food economy but rather stabilize local market grain prices to prevent speculation throughout the period of high risk.

Lagged or relief-oriented responses comprise emergency responses to acute and enormous need that typically are enacted after famine begins and its harsh consequences already evident in a population. These actions, usually in coordination with major international relief and donor agencies, are typically intended to relieve acute suffering and death and promote the rehabilitation of those masses who have survived to migrate, and reach encampments. By definition, lagged responses represent policy failure for governments intending to minimize the destruction, malnutrition and mortality of famine.

See also: **Refugees**: Nutritional Management. **United Nations Children's Fund**: History and Role. **World Health Organization**: Role.

Further Reading

Aykroyd WR (1974) *The Conquest of Famine*. London: Chatto & Windus.

Cahill GF Jr (1978) Famine symposium – physiology of acute starvation in man. *Ecology of Food and Nutrition* 6:221–230.

Dreze J and Sen A, eds. (1990) *The Political Economy of Hunger: Famine Prevention*, vol. 2. Wider Studies in Developmental Economics. Oxford: Clarendon Press.

Keys A, Henschel A, Michelson O and Taylor HL (1950) *The Biology of Human Starvation*. Minneapolis: Univ. of Minnesota.

Newman LF, ed. (1992) *Hunger in History: Food Shortage, Poverty and Deprivation*. Oxford: Blackwell.

Ravallion M (1997) Famines and economics. *Journal of Economic Literature* 35:1205–1242.

Rothman K (1986) *Modern Epidemiology*, pp 7–21. Boston: Little, Brown.

Scrimshaw NS (1987) The phenomenon of famine. *Annual Review of Nutrition* 7:1–21.

Seaman J and Holt J (1980) Markets and famines in the third world. *Disasters* 4(3):283–297.

Sen A (1977) Starvation and exchange entitlements: a general approach and its application to the great Bengal famine. *Cambridge Journal of Economics* 1:33–59.

Sevoy RE (1986) *Famine in Peasant Societies*. New York: Greenwood.

The Bible. *Genesis* 47:4–26.

Yip R (1997) Famine. In: Noji EK (ed.) *Public Health Consequences of Disasters*, pp 305–335. Oxford, UK: Oxford University Press.

Fat-soluble Vitamins *see* **Cholecalciferol and Ergocalciferol**: Physiology, Dietary Sources and Requirements. **Retinol**: Physiology. **Tocopherols**: Physiology. **Vitamin K**: Physiology.

Fat stores *see* **Adipose Tissue**: Structure, Function and Metabolism of Adipose Tissue.

Fats *see* **Fatty Acids**: Metabolism; Health Effects of Saturated Fatty Acids; Health Effects of Monounsaturated Fatty Acids; Health Effects of n-6 Polyunsaturated Fatty Acids; Health Effects of n-3 Polyunsaturated Fatty Acids; Health Effects of *trans* Fatty Acids. **Lipids**: Chemistry and Classification; Composition and Role of Phospholipids in the Body.

FATS AND OILS

Nutritional Value

Jacqueline L Dupont, Florida State University, Florida, USA

Copyright © 1998 Academic Press

Fats and oils are generally called lipids and are defined as substances that are insoluble in water but soluble in organic solvents. In foods, the most abundant form of fats and oils is triacylglycerols. Other lipids are sterols (cholesterol and phytosterols), phospholipids and sphingolipids, vitamins A, D, E and K, and some waxes and other complex lipid substances in small amounts. The nutritional value of fats and oils depends upon their abundance and type in foods, their bioavailability through digestion, absorption and transport, and their unique functional properties.

Physiological functions of lipids are diverse and vital to life and health. They provide structural integrity for all tissues, contribute energy for metabolism, physical activity and storage, and are the necessary precursors for hormones. The steroid hormones are derived from cholesterol, either from the diet or by biosynthesis. The eicosanoids are derived from essential fatty acids. Reproduction, growth, development and neural function all depend on appropriate supplies of lipids.

Nomenclature, Physical and Chemical Properties

Lipids

Because lipids are predominately hydrocarbons, they are nonpolar and thus insoluble in water. When they have polar groups such as those in fatty acids, phospholipids, sphingolipids, and bile acids they become increasingly water-soluble with the ratio of polar groups to hydrocarbon structure. The occurrence of polar (hydrophilic) and nonpolar (hydrophobic) groups in the same molecule makes them amphipathic. This property is important for such functions as membrane components and interfaces between hydrophobic and hydrophilic compounds.

Fatty acids

In foods, fatty acids are present mostly as triacylglycerols (**Fig. 1**). They are distributed among the three carbons of the glycerol molecule in distinct configurations determined by their biosynthesis in plants or animals. They may be short-chain (4–6 carbons), medium-chain (8–12 carbons), long-chain (14–18 carbons) or very long-chain (20 carbons and longer). The short-chain fatty acids are water-soluble and volatile at usual ambient temperatures. Each group with different chain length is metabolized differently. Fatty acids may be saturated, i.e. having no double bonds (each carbon has a hydrogen at every possible bond), or unsaturated. There are three families of unsaturated fatty acids: n-3 (also referred to as omega-3), n-6 and n-9. The number stands for the position of the double bond nearest the methyl terminal end (*n*th carbon) of the chain. Humans and other animals can introduce a double bond into the ninth position of a saturated fatty acid, so the n-9 series is not essential in the diet. No desaturase can act between the C-9 and the methyl terminal carbon

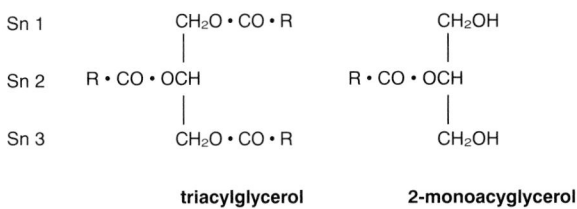

Figure 1 Acylglycerols showing stereospecific numbering.

in animals, thus n-6 and n-3 fatty acids are dietary essentials (**Fig. 2**).

Fats and oils in foods are predominantly 18 carbons long or less. Plant oils contain di- and triunsaturated C_{18} fatty acids of the n-6 and n-3 families, and both plant and animal fats contain C_{16} and C_{18} saturated and monounsaturated (n-9) fatty acids. Food products from land animals contain very small amounts of 20:4 n-6, 22:4 n-6 and 22:5 n-6 (**Table 1**). Those from aquatic animals contain 20:5 n-3 and 22:6 n-3. Some plants have seed oils that contain short- and medium-chain saturated fatty acids.

Unsaturated vegetable oils may be partially hydrogenated to produce more solid fats. During the process a mixture of *cis* and *trans* isomers (**Fig. 3**) of monounsaturated fatty acids are formed from hydrogenation of linolenate. Hydrogenated oils are used in margarines and shortenings and the hydrogenation is desirable to reduce fatty acids susceptible to oxidative rancidity and to produce a cooking fat with desirable properties.

Sterols

Cholesterol is present almost exclusively in animal foods. Phytosterols are found in plants. Cholesterol is required for many functions but is not required in the diet because it is synthesized in humans to meet all needs. The sterol hydrocarbon ring structure makes the molecule extremely hydrophobic and rigid. This characteristic is important in sterol function in membranes and nerve tissues. Free cholesterol (not esterified with a fatty acid) provides the nonpolar insulation for nerve transmission and constitutes 10% of the dry weight of total lipids in adult brain, most of which is myelin. Plant sterols exert effects on digestion and absorption of cholesterol as described in relation to cardiovascular disease. The storage form of cholesterol in human tissues is cholesteryl ester. Free cholesterol can cross membranes by chemical means, whereas esterified cholesterol must be hydrolysed to cross membranes.

Cholesterol is required as the precursor for synthesis of bile acids (or salts, depending on the pH). Bile acids are amphipaths having the sterol ring structure and a carboxyl group conjugated with glycine or taurine to provide a strongly polar domain. They act as specific detergents in many metabolic processes.

Phospholipids and sphingolipids

Foods are not major sources of these complex structures although they are present in plants (especially oilseeds) and animal products. Their essential precursors are derived from the diet, and regulation of their vital functions is complex. Most phospholipids are derivatives of glycerol, with fatty acids on the sn1 and sn2 positions and phosphorylcholine, phosphorylethanolamine, phosphorylserine or phosphorylinositol on the sn3 position. The phospholipids are major functional components of membranes and are integral components of many cell signalling circuits.

Sphingolipids are synthesized in the body and include ceramides, cerebrosides, sulfated glycolipids, gangliosides and sphingomyelin. They are important as structural parts of cells and also perform many vital functions. Their regulation by diet is not direct, and is a topic of intensive investigation, especially in relation to brain function.

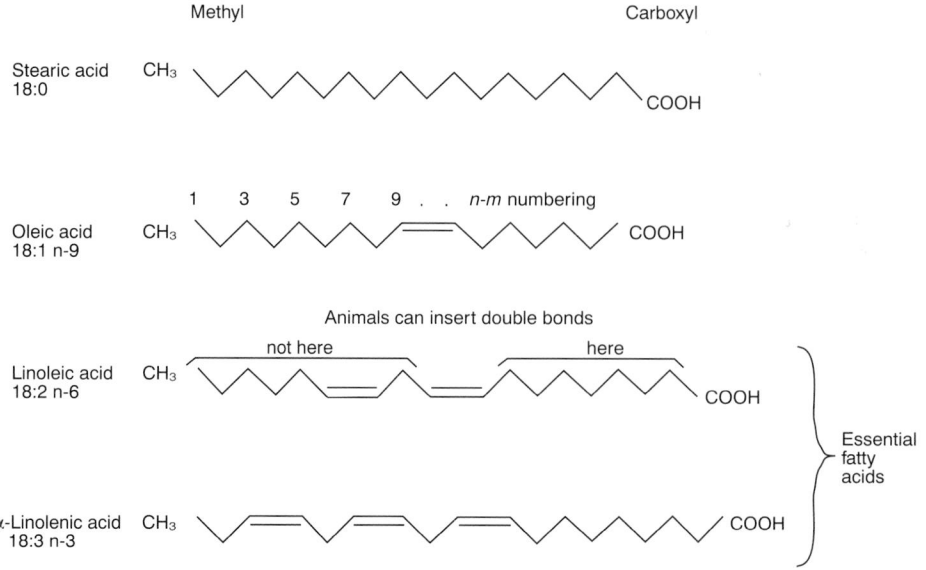

Figure 2 Fatty acids. From FAO (1994) with permission.

Table 1 Some fatty acids in food fats and oils

Symbol	Systematic name	Common name	Typical source
Saturated fatty acids			
4:0	Butanoic	Butyric	Butterfat
6:0	Hexanoic	Caproic	Butterfat
8:0	Octanoic	Caprylic	Coconut oil
10:0	Decanoic	Capric	Coconut oil
12:0	Dodecanoic	Lauric	Coconut
14:0	Tetradecanoic	Myristic	Butterfat, coconut oil
16:0	Hexadecanoic	Palmitic	Most fats and oils
18:0	Octadecanoic	Stearic	Most fats and oils
20:0	Eicosanoic	Arachidic	Lard, peanut oil
22:0	Docosanoic	Behenic	Peanut oil
24:0	Tetracosanoic	Lignoceric	
Unsaturated fatty acids			
10:1 n-1	9-Decenoic	Caproleic	Butterfat
12:1 n-3	9-Dodecenoic	Lauroleic	Butterfat
14:1 n-5	9-Tetradecenoic	Myristoleic	Butterfat
16:1 n-7t	*trans*-Hexadecenoic	Palmitelaidic	HVO
16:1 n-7	9-Hexadecenoic	Palmitoleic	Fish oils
18:1 n-9	9-Octadecenoic	Oleic	Most fats and oils
18:1 n-9t	*trans*-Octadecenoic	Elaidic	Butterfat, beef fat, HVO
18:1 n-7	11-Octadecenoic	Vaccenic	Butterfat, beef fat
18:2 n-6	9,12-Octadecadienoic	Linoleic	Most vegetable oils
18:3 n-6	6,9,12-Octadecatrienoic	Gamma-linolenic	Evening primrose oil, borage oil
18:3 n-3	9,12,15-Octadecatrienoic	Alpha-linolenic	Soyabean and canola (rapeseed) oils, meat
20:1 n-11	9-Eicosaenoic	Gadoleic	Fish oils
20:1 n-9	11-Eicosaenoic	Gondoic	Rapeseed oil
20:3 n-6	8,11,14-Eicosatrienoic	Dihomogamma-linolenic	
20:4 n-6	5,8,11,14-Eicosatetraenoic	Arachidonic	Meat
20:5 n-3	5,8,11,14,17-Eicosapentaenoic	EPA, timnodonic	Fish oils
22:1 n-9	13-Docosaenoic	Erucic	
22:4 n-6	7,10,13,16-Docosatetraenoic	Adrenic	Brain
22:5 n-3	7,10,13,16,19-Docosapentaenoic		Brain
22:5 n-6	4,7,10,13,16-Docosapentaenoic	DPA, Clupanodonic	Brain
22:6 n-3	7,10,13,16,19-Docosahexaenoic	DHA, cervonic	Fish oils, brain

HVO, hydrogenated vegetable oil.

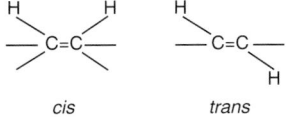

Figure 3 Structure of *cis* and *trans* double bonds.

Substances associated with fats and oils

Vitamins A and D are found predominantly in butterfat and fish oils. Vegetable oils contain vitamin E. Vitamin K is a lipid, but fats and oils are not good dietary sources of it. Vitamin E is an especially important constituent of oils because the oils contain polyunsaturated fatty acids that are susceptible to oxidation. Vitamin E is the principal fat-soluble antioxidant in the body. Soya bean, corn, cottonseed and canola (rapeseed) oils are the major sources. Vitamin E is the term for an assortment of tocopherols that have different potencies as biological antioxidants. Alpha-tocopherol is the most active, and beta and gamma forms are present in substantial quantities in foods.

Meat, poultry and fish provide fat in the diet but also contribute protein, vitamins and minerals. Of high importance is their content of vitamin B_{12}. Nuts are another source of fat in the diet and contribute important amounts of vitamins and minerals, such as folate, zinc, copper and manganese.

Food Sources of Lipids

Information on nutrient composition of food is available in most countries and via United Nations materials. Tables 2–7 provide information on some nutrients, particularly fatty acids, vitamins A and E and sterols obtained from the US Department of

Agriculture, Agricultural Research Service and may be accessed from the Nutrient Data Laboratory Home Page, http://www.nal.usda.gov/fnic/foodcomp.

Most foods contain some fat. The exceptions are fruits and vegetables that contain a large proportion of water. The most visible of fats and oils in the diet are in spreads, salad dressing and sauces. The composition of vegetable oils used to prepare such foods is given in **Table 2**. The composition of examples of spreads, salad dressings and sauces is given in **Table 3**.

Dairy products are major sources of many important nutrients, including fat. The content of some nutrients, including vitamins A and E and fatty acids, in dairy products is given in **Table 4**. Fish provides the essential fatty acids of the n-3 series as well as many other nutrients (**Table 5**). The composition of fats used for cooking and meat and poultry is provided in **Table 6**.

Nuts and some seeds are sources of fat and contain many other trace nutrients in important quantities. Some information about nuts, soya beans and sunflower seeds is given in **Table 7**.

Digestion, Absorption and Transport

For food to have nutritional value it must be digested and the products of digestion distributed to their sites of utilization. Most food fats and oils are triacylglycerols, but the digestion and absorption of the other lipid components is essential to nutrition in a number of ways. The daily food consumption in the Western diet yields about 100 g triacylglycerol, 4–6 g phospholipid and 300–500 g cholesterol. Fat digestion begins in the mouth. Chewing releases fat from other food components and lingual lipase begins hydrolysis of triacylglycerols.

In the stomach, lingual lipase continues action on triacylglycerols to yield diacylglycerols and free fatty acids. Short- and medium-chain fatty acids are the preferred substrates and these are absorbed from the stomach. Most of the triacylglycerols enter the duodenum where they come in contact with pancreatic lipase, bile salts and lecithin from the bile (**Fig. 4**). Pancreatic lipase, colipase and bile acids are needed to allow fat droplets to be hydrolysed to free fatty acids and monoacylglycerols. These are solubilized in mixed micelles that diffuse through the aqueous interface with the mucosa and then enter the mucosal cells by monomolecular diffusion. In normal people dietary fat is almost completely absorbed. The saturated fatty acids are least absorbed, but approximately 90% of 18:0 is absorbed. Disorders of bile acids, lipases or intestinal mucosal disease will lead to malabsorption with excretion of undigested lipids in the faeces.

Phospholipids are hydrolysed by pancreatic phospholipase A2, with release of a free fatty acid and lysophospholipid (i.e. lysophosphatidylcholine) which diffuse into the mucosal cells. The components are reassembled into phospholipids. Cholesterol is usually in free form in the gut but if esterified can be hydrolysed by a pancreatic cholesterol esterase. About 50–60% of cholesterol is absorbed.

For lipids to be transported in the aqueous medium of the blood they must be combined with a surface coat of proteins (apolipoproteins) and polar lipids (phospholipids and free cholesterol). In the mucosal cells, triacylglycerols are reassembled and incorporated into lipoproteins called chylomicrons, which are secreted into lymph. Chylomicrons are large lipoproteins having triacylglycerols as the core. The main apoprotein of chylomicrons is apolipoprotein B-48, a large hydrophobic protein. The surface coat contains apo C-II, apo C-III, apo Es, apo A-I and apo A-IV in small amounts. These proteins serve as binding sites for further metabolism of the particles. Chylomicrons are secreted into the intestinal lymph where they pass through the thoracic duct into the systemic circulation. In the peripheral circulation chylomicrons come into contact with lipoprotein lipase, an enzyme located on the endothelial surface of capillaries. Lipoprotein lipase is synthesized in adipose tissue and skeletal muscle and then migrates to the capillaries. Apoprotein C-II acts as the activator for interaction between the chylomicron and the lipase. At the endothelial cell surface the lipase hydrolyses triacylglycerols of chylomicrons and free fatty acids are released. A process similar to that in the intestine occurs and fatty acids are taken up by the adipose cells for storage as triacylglycerols or by skeletal muscle cells for use for energy. Some of the free fatty acids bind to albumin and remain in the systemic circulation.

This process is repeated until most of the triacylglycerols are hydrolysed and the chylomicron is a smaller particle called a remnant. The chylomicron remnant contains all the cholesteryl esters and some triacylglycerols in its core. The apo B-48 on the remnant surface binds to a site on a liver cell and by a process involving apo E the remnant is internalized. Two receptors on the liver cell bind to different forms of apo E to effect remnant uptake. Genetic defects in any of the chylomicron apoproteins lead to failure to clear chylomicrons from the blood and hyperlipidaemia occurs.

Table 2 Fatty acid, vitamin E and phytosterol composition of vegetable oils

	SFA	MUFA	PUFA	10:0	12:0	14:0	16:0	18:0	16:1	18:1	20:1	18:2	18:3	Vitamin E	Phytosterols
Almond	8.2	69.9	17.4	0	0	0	6.5	1.7	0.6	69.4	0	17.4	0	8.66	266
Apricot kernel	6.3	60	29.3	0	0	0	5.8	0.5	0	29.3	0	0	0	0	266
Avocado	11.56	70.55	13.49	0	0	0	10.9	0.66	2.66	67.89	0	12.53	0.96	NA	NA
Babassu (1)	81.2	11.4	1.6	5.5	43.5	15	8.2	2.8	0	11.4	0	1.6	0	20.95	95
Canola (2)	7.1	58.9	29.6	0	0	0	4	1.8	0.2	56.1	1.7	20.3	9.3	20.95	NA
Cocoa butter	59.7	32.9	3	0	0	0.1	25.4	33.2	0.2	32.6	0	2.8	0.1	NA	201
Coconut (3)	86.5	5.8	1.8	6	44.6	16.8	8.2	1.8	0	5.8	0	1.8	0	0.28	86
Corn	12.7	24.2	58.7	0	0	0	10.9	1.8	0	24.2	0	58	0.7	21.11	968
Cotton seed (4)	25.9	17.8	51.9	0	0	0.8	22.7	2.3	0.8	17	0	51.5	0.2	38.26	324
Grape seed	9.6	16.1	69.9	0	0	0.1	6.7	2.7	0.3	15.8	0	69.6	0.1	NA	180
Hazelnut	7.4	78	10.2	0	0	0.1	5.2	2	0.2	77.8	0	10.1	0	NA	120
Mustard (5)	11.58	59.19	21.23	0	0	1.39	3.75	1.12	0.22	11.61	6.19	15.33	5.9	NA	NA
Oat	19.62	35.11	40.87	0	0.39	0.24	16.67	1.05	0.2	34.9	0	39.08	1.79	14.4	221
Olive	13.5	73.7	8.4	0	0	0	11	2.2	0.8	72.5	0.3	7.9	0.6	12.4	NA
Palm	49.3	37	9.3	0	0.1	1	43.5	4.3	0.3	36.6	0.1	9.1	0.2	21.76	95
Palm kernel (6)	81.5	11.4	1.6	3.7	47	16.4	8.1	2.8	0	11.4	0	1.6	0	3.81	95
Peanut (7)	16.9	46.2	32	0	0	0.1	9.5	2.2	0.1	44.8	1.3	32	0	12.92	207
Rice bran	19.7	39.3	35	0	0	0.7	16.9	1.6	0.2	39.1	0	33.4	1.6	NA	1190
Safflower															
Linoleic over 70%	9.1	12.1	74.5	0	0	0.1	6.2	2.2	0.4	11.7	0	74.1	0.4	43.06	444
Oleic over 70% (8)	6.1	75.3	14.2	0	0	0	4.8	1.3	0	75.3	0	14.2	0	34.4	444
Sesame	14.2	39.7	41.7	0	0	0	8.9	4.8	0.2	39.3	0.2	41.3	0.3	4.09	865
Sheanut	46.6	44	5.2	0.2	1.3	0.1	4.4	38.8	0.1	43.5	0	4.9	0.3	NA	357
Soybean	14.4	23.3	57.9	0	0	0.1	10.3	3.8	0.2	22.8	0.2	51	6.8	18.19	250
Soybean, hyd	14.9	43	37.6	0	0	0.1	9.8	5	0.4	42.5	0	34.9	2.6	18.19	132
Sunflower															
Linoleic over 60%	10.3	19.5	65.7	0	0	0	5.9	4.5	0	19.5	0	65.7	0	50.58	100
Linoleic under 60%	10.1	45.4	40.1	0	0	0	5.4	3.5	0.2	45.3	0	39.8	0.2	NA	100
Linoleic over 70%	9.75	83.59	3.8	0	0	0	3.68	4.32	0	82.63	0.96	3.61	0.19	NA	NA
Linoleic hyd	13	46.2	36.4	0	0	0	7.1	5.5	0	46	0	35.3	0.9	51	10
Tea seed	21.1	51.5	23	0	0.1	0.1	17.5	3.1	0.5	49.9	1	22.2	0.7	NA	102
Tomato seed	19.7	22.8	53.1	0	0	0.2	15	4.4	0.5	21.9	0	50.8	2.3	NA	100
Walnut	9.1	22.8	63.3	0	0	0	7	2	0.1	22.2	0.4	52.9	10.4	3.22	176
Wheat germ	18.8	15.1	61.7	0	0	0.1	16.6	0.5	0.5	14.6	0	54.8	6.9	192.44	553

Data from US Department of Agriculture, Agricultural Research Service (1997).
Units: fatty acid contents are given in g per 100 g; vitamin E contents are in mg α-tocopherol units per 100 g; phytosterols are in mg per 100 g.
HYD, hydrogenated; MUFA, monounsaturated fatty acids; NA, not available; PUFA, polyunsaturated fatty acids; SFA, saturated fatty acids.

Table 3   Selected nutrients in some spreads, salad dressings, and sauces (values per 100 g portion)

	Water (g)	Protein (g)	Fat (g)	Carbohydrate (g)[a]	Vitamin A (RE)	Vitamin E (mg)[b]	SFA (g)	MUFA (g)	PUFA (g)
Spreads									
Magarine, regular	15.5	0.9	80.5	0.9	799	12.8	15.8	35.8	25.4
Margarine, soft	16.2	0.8	80.4	0.5	799	12	13.8	28.5	34.6
Margarine-like spreads									
60% fat	37	0.6	60.8	0	799	9.01	12.8	31.5	13.8
40% fat	58.1	0.5	38.8	0.4	799	2.32	7.7	15.7	13.8
Salad dressings									
Blue or Roquefort cheese	32.3	4.8	52.3	7.4	66	9.3	9.9	12.3	27.8
French	38.1	0.6	41	17.5	130	8.42	9.5	8	21.7
Italian	38.4	0.7	48.3	10.2	78	10.36	7	11.2	28
Mayonnaise									
Soya bean oil	15.3	1.1	79.4	2.7	84	11.79	11.8	22.7	41.3
Imitation	62.7	0.3	19.2	16	0	6.43	3.3	4.5	10.6
Mayonnaise type	39.9	0.9	33.4	23.9	84	4	4.9	9	18
Thousand Island	46.1	0.9	35.7	15.2	96	1.14	6	8.3	19.8
Vinegar and oil	47.4	0	50.1	2.5	0	8.8	9.1	14.8	24.1
Sauces									
Cheese	70.5	6.71	13.29	6.83	63	0.32	6.01	3.82	2.6
White	74.89	3.84	10.63	9.17	55	1.36	2.85	4.42	2.86

[a]By difference.
[b]Alpha-tocopherol equivalents.
MUFA, monounsaturated fatty acids; PUFA, polyunsaturated fatty acids; RE, retinol equivalents; SFA, saturated fatty acids.

Use of Fat for Energy

Fat from the diet is primarily used for energy. Some fat is synthesized from carbohydrate and protein as they are metabolized in the liver. Only if there is little fat and a large proportion of carbohydrate is fat synthesized for storage. The fatty acids released from chylomicrons and very low-density lipoprotein (VLDL) in adipose tissue are activated by forming coenzyme A derivatives and transferred to glycerol 3-phosphate to form triacylglycerol. The glycerol is derived from glucose metabolism and cannot be recycled in the adipocyte. Triacylglycerols are stored in adipocytes as globules of fat. The fatty acid composition of adipose tissue is an indicator of past dietary fat consumption, especially in relation to fatty acids only available from food.

To be made available for energy use, fatty acids are released from adipose tissue by action of a hormone-sensitive lipase. The lipase is activated by adrenaline, glucagon and adrenocorticotrophic hormone. The hormones stimulate adenylate cyclase which acts to increase cellular levels of cyclic adenosine monophosphate, which in turn stimulates protein kinase that phosphorylates the lipase, activating it. Fatty acids are released into the circulation where they bind to albumin. Skeletal muscle is the major organ that uses fatty acids for energy, but all tissues except brain and kidney are capable of oxidizing fatty acids

for energy. Fatty acids are continually used by resting muscle, whereas glucose is the preferred substrate for acute muscle activity. Fatty acids are oxidized in mitochondria. First they are activated by coenzyme A at the mitochondrial outer membrane, then the coenzyme A is replaced by carnitine to effect membrane translocation; then the carnitine is replaced by CoA on the inner membrane. Within the mitochondria fatty acids are metabolized by a process called beta-oxidation in which 2-carbon units are progressively removed as acetyl-CoA which enters the Krebs tricarboxylic acid cycle. The fatty acid oxidation enzyme complex binds the fatty acid and releases all the acetyl units with no intermediate chain length products. Instead of entering the Krebs cycle two units of acetyl-CoA may condense to form acetoacetate and β-hydroxybutyrate; these must be transferred to the liver for use for energy.

Fat in the diet yields 9 kcal (37.7 kJ) per gram. This value is called the Atwater factor for energy, and approximates the energy value taking into account the heat of combustion and digestibility. Because fat yields 9 kcal g^{-1} and protein and carbohydrate yield 4 kcal g^{-1} (16.8 kJ g^{-1}), the amount of fat in the diet determines the energy density of the diet. The more fat, the greater the energy per gram of food. In some population groups, fat in the diet is limited and there is a concern for adequacy of energy

Table 4   Selected nutrients in some dairy products (values per 100 g portion)

	Water (g)	Protein (g)	Fat (g)	Carbohydrate (g)[a]	Vitamin A (RE)	Vitamin E (mg)[b]	SFA (g)	MUFA (g)	PUFA (g)
Butter	15.87	0.85	81.11	0.06	754	1.58	50.49	23.43	3.01
Cream, fluid									
Heavy whipping	57.71	2.05	37	2.79	421	0.63	23.03	10.69	1.37
Half and half	80.57	2.96	11.5	4.3	107	0.11	7.16	3.32	0.43
Light	73.75	2.7	19.31	3.66	182	0.15	12.02	5.58	0.72
Sour, cultured	70.95	3.16	20.96	4.27	195	0.57	13.05	6.05	0.78
Substitute, lauric acid oil	77.27	1	9.97	11.38	9	0	9.3	0.11	0.003
Substitute, hyd vegetable oil, soya protein	77.27	1	9.97	11.38	9	1.62	1.94	7.55	0.027
Substitute, powdered	2.21	4.79	35.48	54.88	20	0.27	32.52	0.97	0.014
Cheeses									
Blue	42.41	21.4	28.74	2.34	228	0.64	18.67	7.78	0.8
Brie	48.42	20.75	27.68	0.45	182	0.66	17.41	8.01	0.83
Camembert	51.8	19.8	24.26	0.46	252	0.66	15.26	7.02	0.72
Cheddar	36.75	24.9	33.14	1.28	278	0.36	21.09	4.01	0.94
Cream	53.75	7.55	34.87	2.66	382	0.94	21.97	9.84	1.26
Cottage, creamed	78.96	12.49	4.51	2.68	48	0.12	2.85	1.28	0.14
Edam	41.56	24.99	27.8	1.43	253	0.75	17.57	8.12	0.66
Feta	55.22	14.21	21.28	4.09	128	0.03	14.95	4.62	0.59
Goat	45.52	21.58	29.84	2.54	400	0.65	20.64	6.81	0.71
Mexican, Anejo	38.06	21.44	29.98	4.63	63	0.1	19.03	8.53	0.9
Mozzarella									
Whole milk	54.14	19.42	21.6	2.22	241	0.35	13.15	6.57	0.76
Part skim milk	53.78	24.26	15.92	2.77	177	0.43	10.11	4.51	0.47
Neufchatel	62.21	9.96	23.43	2.94	1134	300	14.8	6.77	0.65
Parmesan	29.16	35.75	25.83	3.22	149	0.8	16.41	7.52	0.57
Port Salut	45.45	23.78	28.2	0.57	372	0.5	16.69	9.34	0.73
Ricotta, part skim	74.41	11.39	7.91	5.14	113	0.21	4.93	2.31	0.26
Swiss	37.21	28.43	27.45	3.38	253	0.5	17.78	7.27	0.97

[a]By difference; [b]Alpha-tocopherol equivalents.
Hyd, hydrogenated; MUFA, monounsaturated fatty acids; PUFA, polyunsaturated fatty acids; RE, retinol equivalent; SFA, saturated fatty acids.

intake. The Food and Agriculture Organization (FAO) and World Health Organization (WHO) of the United Nations have issued recommendations that for most adults at least 15% of the dietary energy should come from fat, but women of reproductive age should consume at least 20% of dietary energy as fat. It is important for people with diets providing only 15% energy from fat to assure ample availability of total food to avoid energy deficits. Infants receive 50–60% of energy from fat via breast milk. Infant formulae are recommended to contain as much, and after weaning until 2 years of age, children should receive 30–40% of energy from fat.

People consuming diets with high energy density have a greater chance for overconsumption of energy than those with lower-fat diets. Imbalance of energy consumption with expenditure results in change in body fat stores. A positive imbalance results in obesity. Active individuals are recommended to have up to 35% of energy as fat and sedentary individuals should not consume more than 30% of energy from fat.

Health Factors of Fats and Oils

Essential fatty acids

In addition to provision of energy, fats and oils in the diet have specific beneficial and harmful aspects. Some fatty acids are classified as 'essential fatty acids' because they cannot be synthesized by the human body and are necessary for vital functions. These are the n-6 and n-3 families. The FAO/WHO recommendations are for linoleic acid (n-6) to provide 4–10% of energy. Linolenic acid (n-3) should provide 0.5–4% of energy as a 0.1–0.4 ratio of n-3 to n-6.

Vitamin E

Vitamin E acts in the body as a scavenger of free

Table 5 Selected nutrients in fish (values per 100 g portion)

	Water (g)	Protein (g)	Fat (g)	Vitamin A (RE)	Vitamin E (mg)[a]	SFA (g)	16:1 (g)	18:1 (g)	20:1 (g)	22:1 (g)	18:2 (g)	18:3 (g)	18:4 (g)	20:4 (g)	20:5 (g)	22:5 (g)	22:6 (g)	Cholesterol (mg)
Anchovy, European, canned in oil	50.3	28.89	9.71	21	5	2.2	0.59	2.94	0.009	0.163	0.362	0.017	0.078	0.01	0.763	0.041	1.292	85
Catfish, farmed	71.58	18.72	8.02	50	15	1.79	0.292	3.738	0.106	0	1.029	0.082	0.016	0.041	0.049	0	0.128	64
Catfish, wild	80.36	16.38	2.82	15	0.6	0.722	0.176	0.594	0.021	0.008	0.101	0.071	0.013	0.149	0.13	0.1	0.234	58
Cod, Atlantic	75.92	22.83	0.86	14	0.3	0.168	0.021	0.078	0.019	0.004	0.006	0.001	0.001	0.028	0.004	0.013	0.154	55
Flatfish (flounder and sole spp.)	73.16	24.16	1.53	38	1.89	0.363	0.236	0.154	0.035	0.02	0.014	0.016	0	0.048	0.243	0.046	0.258	68
Haddock	74.25	24.24	0.93	63	19	0.167	0.022	0.086	0.013	0.029	0.012	0.003	0.004	0.029	0.076	0.024	0.162	74
Halibut	71.69	26.69	2.94	54	1.09	0.417	0.209	0.463	0.159	0.131	0.038	0.083	0.05	0.178	0.091	0.121	0.374	41
Mackerel, Atlantic	53.27	23.85	17.81	180	54	4.176	0.534	1.202	1.598	2.498	0.147	0.113	0	0.051	0.504	0.106	0.699	75
Mullet	70.52	24.81	4.86	141	42	1.431	0.177	0.196	0	0	0.094	0	0	0.097	0.18	0.092	0.148	63
Ocean perch	72.69	23.88	2.09	46	14	0.313	0.11	0.265	0.128	0.294	0.036	0.073	0.031	0.005	0.103	0.029	0.271	54
Salmon																		
Atlantic, farmed	64.75	22.1	12.35	50	15	2.504	0.767	2.046	1.368	0	0.666	0.113	0.184	1.273	0.69	0	1.457	63
Pink, canned	68.81	19.78	6.05	17	1.35	1.535	0.466	1.068	0.272	0.018	0.058	0.058	0.135	0.077	0.845	0.048	0.806	55
Sockeye	61.84	27.31	10.97	209	63	1.917	0.321	1.338	0.922	0.664	0.113	0.062	0	0.03	0.53	0.132	0.7	87
Sardine, Atlantic, canned in oil	59.61	24.62	11.45	67	0.3	1.528	0.22	2.145	0.423	1.081	3.543	0.498	0.125	0	0.473	0	0.509	142
Seatrout	71.91	21.46	4.63	115	35	1.293	0.464	0.602	0.064	0	0.088	0.005	0.01	0.247	0.211	0.097	0.265	106
Snapper, mixed spp.	70.35	26.3	1.72	115	35	0.365	0.048	0.123	0	0	0.025	0	0	0.044	0.048	0.022	0.273	47
Swordfish	68.75	25.39	5.14	137	41	1.406	0.322	1.392	0.156	0.11	-0.037	0.238	0	0.087	0.138	0	0.681	50
Trout, rainbow																		
Farmed	67.53	24.27	7.2	287	86	2.105	0.319	1.427	0.326	0	0.949	0.082	0.068	0.036	0.334	0	0.82	68
Mixed spp.	63.36	26.63	8.47	63	19	1.47	0.899	1.847	0.359	1.064	0.224	0.199	0.082	0.242	0.259	0.235	0.677	74
Tuna, bluefin	59.09	29.91	6.28	756	NA	1.612	0.208	1.185	0.355	0.304	0.068	0	0.05	0.055	0.363	0.16	1.141	49
Whitefish, mixed spp.	65.09	24.47	7.51	131	39	1.162	0.667	1.727	0.133	0.032	0.349	0.235	0.064	0.286	0.406	0.209	1.206	77
Whiting, mixed spp.	74.71	23.48	1.69	114	34	0.4	0.121	0.277	0.027	0.02	0.02	0.013	0	0.02	0.283	0.017	0.235	84

[a]Alpha-tocopherol equivalents.
RE, retinol equivalents; SFA, saturated fatty acids.

Table 6 Selected nutrients in cooking fat, meat, and poultry

	Water (g)	Protein (g)	Fat (g)	SFA (g)	16:1 (g)	18:1 (g)	20:1 (g)	18:2 (g)	18:3 (g)	20:4 (g)	Cholesterol (mg)
Cooking fats											
Beef tallow	0	0	100	49.8	4.2	36	0.3	3.1	0.6	0	109
Chicken fat	0.2	0	99.8	29.8	5.7	37.3	1.1	19.5	1	0.1	85
Goose fat	0.2	0	99.8	27.7	2.8	53.5	0.1	9.8	0.5	0	100
Mutton tallow	0	0	100	47.3	2.3	37.6	0	5.5	2.3	0	102
Lard (pork fat)	0	0	100	39.2	2.7	41.2	1	10.2	1	0	95
Shortening, soya bean and cottonseed, hyd	0	0	100	25	0	44.5	0	24.5	1.6	0	0
Shortening, soya bean and palm, hyd	0	0	100	30.42	50.97	0	0	13.6	0.604	0	0
Meat and poultry											
Beef, rib, lean only	57.44	26.34	13.81	5.62	0.53	5.15	0.01	0.38	0.05	0.05	77
Chicken, meat only	63.79	28.93	7.41	2.04	0.35	2.22	0.04	1.37	0.07	0.11	89
Duckling, Pekin; breast meat only	68.25	27.6	2.5	0.578	0.066	0.792	0.01	0.302	0.012	0.064	143
Lamb, loin, lean only	60.98	29.99	9.73	3.48	0.29	3.95	0	0.52	0.06	0.06	95
Pork, loin, lean only	60.72	28.57	9.8	3.64	0.32	4	0.09	0.68	0.02	0.04	79

Hyd, hydrogenated; SFA, saturated fatty acids.

Table 7 Selected nutrients in nuts, soya beans and sunflower seeds

	Water (g)	Protein (g)	Fat (g)	Carbohydrate (g)[a]	Vitamin E (mg)[b]	SFA (g)	16:1 (g)	18:1 (g)	20:1 (g)	18:2 (g)	18:3 (g)
Almonds	3.08	20.39	57.67	15.88	5.55	5.466	0.336	36.752	0.055	11.591	0.413
Cashew nuts, oil roasted	3.91	16.15	48.21	28.52	1.56	9.526	0.331	27.886	0.144	7.968	0.167
Filberts or hazelnuts, oil roasted	1.2	14.25	63.6	19.15	23.92	4.675	0.214	49.379	0.099	5.922	0.154
Macadamia nuts, oil roasted	1.67	7.26	76.52	12.9	0.41	11.456	16.567	42.725	1.087	1.319	0
Peanuts, oil roasted	1.95	26.35	49.3	18.93	7.41	6.843	0.009	23.788	0.662	15.576	0.003
Pecans, oil roasted	4.2	6.95	71.2	16.05	13	5.7	0.326	43.338	0.489	16.824	0.713
Soya beans, green, cooked	68.6	12.35	6.4	11.05	0.01	0.74	0.01	1.188	2.657	0.354	
Sunflower seeds, oil roasted	2.6	21.36	57.45	14.73	50.27	6.02	0.057	10.843	0.055	37.818	0.08

[a]By difference. [b]Alpha-tocopherol equivalents.

radicals. Free radicals are formed when a hydrogen is removed from a carbon, usually the carbon between the two double bonds of polyunsaturated fatty acids. Other free radicals are normally formed by cellular enzyme systems, mitochondrial electron transport and exposure to environmental factors. Vitamin E is a primary factor in the defence system because it is lipid-soluble and thus can protect cell membranes. The tocopherol molecule reacts with a free radical, forming the tocopheroxyl radical which can be reduced back to tocopherol by either vitamin C or glutathione.

Vitamin E protects against heavy metals and ozone from the environment and hepatotoxins that generate free radicals. It is important for normal immune function. People with low vitamin E intake and plasma levels have an increased risk for some types of cancer as shown by epidemiological studies. Supplementation with vitamin E has not been shown to date to reduce cancer risk. Vitamin E and other

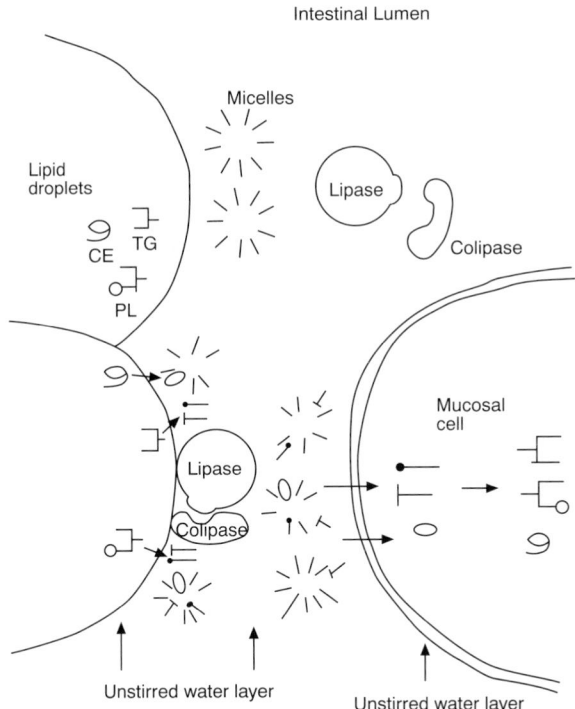

Figure 4 Digestion and absorption of dietary fat. Bile micelles prevent access of pancreatic lipase to lipid droplets by adhering to their surface; colipase has a high affinity for the lipid droplets and complexes with lipase to allow hydrolysis of triacylglycerols; hydrolysed fatty acids and monoacylglycerols are made water-soluble by incorporation into micelles and there cross the unstirred water layer where the fatty acids enter the mucosal cells by monomolecular diffusion. Fatty acids are then reesterified to triacylglycerols, phospholipids and cholesteryl esters. From Dupont (1990) with permission.

antioxidants seem to protect against oxidation of low-density lipoprotein (LDL), thus possibly protecting against coronary artery disease. Vitamin E is needed for normal development of the neuromuscular system and functioning of the retina. The production of neurotransmitters in the nervous system generates a large amount of free radicals and vitamin E seems to be an essential agent to prevent oxidative damage to mitochondria and axonal membranes. The recommended consumption of vitamin E is dependent on the form; α-tocopherol is the most bioactive, with β-tocopherol having 25–50% bioactivity, γ-tocopherol having 10–35%, and α-tocotrienol having about 30%. One international unit of vitamin E is defined as the activity of 1 mg of R,R,R-α-tocopherol. The recommended dietary allowance in the USA is 10 mg of α-tocopherol equivalents for adult men, 8 mg for women and 3 mg for infants, increasing to 7 mg for children 7–10 years old. During pregnancy 10 mg per day is recommended, and 12 mg is recommended for lactation. Increasing the amount of polyunsaturated fatty acids in the diet increases the vitamin E requirement. About 0.4 mg of α-tocopherol for each gram of polyunsaturated fatty acid, has been suggested to be adequate for adults.

Obesity

Life insurance statistics from the USA indicate that excess weight is associated with higher mortality rates. If body weight is 10% above average it is accompanied by an 11% increase in mortality for men and 7% for women; 20% excess weight increases excess mortality to 20% for men and 10% for women. These indications of risk do not suggest cause and effect; rather that obesity is associated with some defect in a mechanism related to cardiac function, or a disorder of lipid or glucose metabolism. The *Dietary Guidelines for Americans* recommend that people attain a desirable weight by regulation of food intake and achieving adequate physical activity. As fat contributes twice the energy of protein and carbohydrate, it must be carefully monitored in weight control programmes.

Diabetes mellitus

Excessive weight gain and overweight are major nutritional factors that increase the risk of developing non-insulin-dependent diabetes mellitus (NIDDM). An indication of the degree of risk is the body mass index (weight in kilograms divided by the square of stature in metres). In individuals with a

BMI of 20 or less NIDDM is rare, but it is increased 8-fold in those with a BMI of 35 as compared with 25. There is some indication from epidemiological studies that higher intakes of dietary fat or weight associated with it may be a factor in the onset of NIDDM. Reduction of risk of NIDDM is dependent on maintaining an appropriate body weight.

Coronary heart disease

The amount and composition of dietary fat are major determinants of serum cholesterol levels, particularly LDL. In populations there is a continuous association between serum cholesterol levels and coronary heart disease death rates. Populations with relatively high intakes of fat, especially animal fat and cholesterol, have relatively high serum cholesterol levels and higher mortality rates than populations with less fat in the diet. In general, compared with carbohydrates, saturated fatty acids elevate serum cholesterol, concentration, polyunsaturated fatty acids (linoleate) lower it and monounsaturated fatty acids have no statistically significant effect. Palmitic acid is the major saturated fatty acid in most diets, and palmitic, lauric and myristic acids are considered to be the most hypercholesterolaemic fatty acids. *Trans* fatty acids have about the same effect on serum cholesterol as do saturated fatty acids.

Compared with carbohydrate or saturated fatty acids, linoleate causes reduction of serum cholesterol concentration. Dietary linoleate is reflected in adipose tissue concentration of linoleate. Linoleate content of adipose tissue has been shown to have an inverse correlation with the incidence of myocardial infarction. Fish oils contain the very long-chain n-3 fatty acids eicosapentaenoic acid (EPA) and docosahexaenoic acid (DHA). The consumption of fish with high levels of these fatty acids seems to have a protective effect against coronary heart disease. Recommendations to reduce the risk of heart disease include consumption of no more than 30% of energy as fat, with saturated fat contributing no more than 10% of energy. Polyunsaturated fat should contribute up to 10% of energy and monounsaturated fat should replace saturated fat and carbohydrate when possible.

The recommendations for moderate fat consumption by adults are not applicable to children under 5 years old, as this is a period of rapid growth, and low-fat, high-bulk diets may cause toddlers to feel full before they have ingested sufficient energy for their needs.

Cancer

Cancer of the breast and colon show a positive correlation with fat consumption in studies comparing populations of different countries. A combined analysis of 12 case–control studies indicated an association between fat intake and breast cancer in postmenopausal women. When data are adjusted for energy intake, the association with dietary fat is less evident. Epidemiological and case–control studies involve estimates of current diets and do not address the consequences of life long exposure to a low- or high-fat diet. The association of some tumours with obesity suggests that the effects of high-fat diets may be partially explained by positive energy balance. International studies indicate that over a range of consumption of linoleate of 4–8% of energy there seems to be no relation to breast cancer. The dietary guidelines applicable to heart disease seem to be suitable for reduction of cancer risk.

See Colour Plate 3.

See also: **Cancer**: Epidemiology and Associations Between Diet and Cancer; Epidemiology of Breast Cancer. **Coronary Heart Disease**: Lipid Theory of Coronary Heart Disease; Prevention. **Dietary Guidelines**: International Perspectives. **Fatty Acids**: Health Effects of Saturated Fatty Acids. **Infants**: Nutritional Requirements. **Lipoproteins**: Physiology. **Obesity**: Treatment; Prevention.

Further Reading

Carstea ED, Morris JS, Coleman KG *et al.* (1997) Niemann-Pick C1 disease gene: homology to mediators of cholesterol homeostasis. *Science* 277: 228–231.

Dupont J (1990) Lipids. In: Brown M (ed.) *Present Knowledge in Nutrition*, 6th edn, pp 56–66. New York: ILSI Press.

FAO (1994) *Fats and Oils in Human Nutrition*. FAO Food and Nutrition Paper 57. Rome: FAO.

Grundy SM (1996) Dietary fat. In: Ziegler EE and Filer LJ (eds) *Present Knowledge in Nutrition*, 7th edn, pp 44–57. Washington: ILSI Press.

Hopkins PN (1992) Effects of dietary cholesterol on serum cholesterol: a meta-analysis and review. *American Journal of Clinical Nutrition* 55: 1060–1070.

Jones PJH (1997) Regulation of cholesterol biosynthesis by diet in humans. *American Journal of Clinical Nutrition* 66: 438–446.

Sokol RJ (1996) Vitamin E. In: Ziegler EE and Filer LJ (eds) *Present Knowledge in Nutrition*, 7th edn, pp 130–136. Washington: ILSI Press.

US Department of Agriculture, Agricultural Research Service (1997) USDA Nutrient Database for Standard Reference, Release 11-1. Nutrient Data Laboratory Home Page http://www.nal.usda.gov/fnic/foodcomp.

FATTY ACIDS

Contents
Metabolism
Health Effects of Saturated Fatty Acids
Health Effects of Monounsaturated Fatty Acids
Health Effects of n-6 Polyunsaturated Fatty Acids
Health Effects of n-3 Polyunsaturated Fatty Acids
Health Effects of *trans* Fatty Acids

Metabolism

Y-S Huang and **J-W Liu**, Ross Products Division, Columbus, Ohio, USA

Copyright © 1998 Academic Press

In the human body, water constitutes more than 75% of the total weight, and the rest is made of organic and inorganic compounds. Fat (including triacylglycerols, phospholipids, steroids, etc.) is the most abundant of these compounds, constituting approximately 15% of the body weight (or equivalent to 10 kg of a 70 kg person). The major building block of fats is fatty acid. A fatty acid is composed of a nonpolar hydrocarbon chain, varying in length from 2 to 30 carbon atoms, with a terminal carboxylic group, $CH_3-(CH_2)_n-COOH$.

Classification

There are two approaches to the classification of fatty acids:

- Based on chain length, fatty acids are classified as short-chain (4–6 carbon atoms), medium-chain (8–12 carbons) and long-chain (14 or more carbons).
- Fatty acids can also be classified according to the degree of unsaturation. Each carbon atom has four bonding sites. Two sites in each carbon atom are used for chain formation. When the remaining bonding sites in each of the carbon atoms except the one in the carboxyl group are all bonded to hydrogen atoms, the acid is a saturated fatty acid (SFA). When two adjacent carbons are bonded to only two hydrogen atoms, an ethylenic double bond is formed, and the acid is unsaturated. If there is only one double bond in the chain, the acid is called a monounsaturated fatty acid (MUFA). When there is more than one double bond, it is called a polyunsaturated fatty acid (PUFA) (**Fig. 1**).

Unsaturated fatty acids can be further subdivided in two ways:

- Geometric configuration: the unsaturated fatty acids can be grouped into *cis* and *trans* fatty acids based on their geometric configuration. The *cis* fatty acids are those with two hydrogen atoms on the same side of the molecule as follows:

$$\begin{array}{ccc} H & & H \\ | & & | \\ -C & = & C- \end{array}$$

- while *trans* fatty acids are those with hydrogen atoms on opposite sides of the molecule.

$$\begin{array}{ccc} H & & \\ | & & \\ -C & = & C- \\ & & | \\ & & H \end{array}$$

- Natural unsaturated fatty acids are mostly in the *cis* form in relation to the ethylenic double bond. The double bonds are methylene-interrupted and are of the *cis* configuration. The *trans* fatty acids are formed when unsaturated vegetable oils are partially hydrogenated to make margarines and shortenings. In the process, the double bond of the

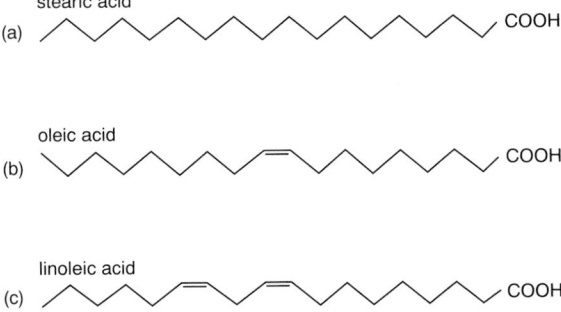

Figure 1 Three different types of fatty acids according to the degree of unsaturation: (a) saturated – stearic acid; (b) monounsaturated – oleic acid; (c) polyunsaturated – linoleic acid.

unsaturated fatty acids is converted from the more prevalent *cis* formation to a *trans* double bond. These processed vegetable fats may contain 5–30% of the *trans* isomers. The *trans* type of fatty acids are also formed in the rumen of cattle, and make up about 5% of dairy and beef fats. The average consumption of *trans* fatty acids in the USA is 2–4% of the daily energy intake, or 8% of the fat. The average daily intake per person is about 8–12 g.

- Position of double bond: although some unsaturated fatty acids are identical in terms of carbon chain length, number of double bonds and geometrical configuration, they could still be different if their double bonds are located at different positions on the carbon chain. Unsaturated fatty acids which differ only in the position of double bond are positional isomers. For example, linolenic acid (18:3) has two positional isomers: α and γ. The three double bonds of α-linolenic acid are located at positions 9, 12 and 15, while those of γ-linolenic acid are at positions 6, 9 and 12 (**Fig. 2**). More practical notations for the two positional isomers are 18:3 n-3 for α-linolenic acid and 18:3 n-6 for γ-linolenic acid. The use of shorthand names for unsaturated fatty acids is discussed below.

Nomenclature

Trivial and systematic chemical names

Many trivial names of fatty acids are derived from their sources. For example, caproic, caprylic and capric acids are from milk fat of goats (of the genus *Capra*), lauric acid is derived from laurel oil, palm oil is rich in palmitic acid, linseed oil is rich in linoleic and linolenic acids. Other names reflect the structure: stearic acid, which has 18 carbon atoms, is called *octadecanoic* acid; oleic acid, which has 18 carbon atoms and a double bond, is called *octadecaenoic* acid, whereas linoleic acid, which has 18 car-

bon atoms and two double bonds, is called *octadecadienoic* acid (**Table 1**).

Shorthand names

For convenience, fatty acids are generally expressed in shorthand notations. The position of the first unsaturated bond from the methyl end of the carbon chain is specified by 'n' or by omega (ω), the last letter of the Greek alphabet. Most of the natural unsaturated fatty acids fall into three major families, namely n-3, n-6 and n-9 (**Fig. 3**). For example, 18:1 n-9 is oleic acid, where the number before the colon indicates the total number of carbons (18 carbons), the number immediately after the colon represents the number of unsaturated bonds (one double bond) and the n-9 indicates that the first double bond is located at the ninth carbon atom from the methyl end (Table 1).

If the positions and configurations of the double bonds are important for discussions, the position of double bonds in the fatty acid chain is denoted by a prefix indicating the position of the double bonds starting from the carboxyl carbon as the carbon atom number 1. For example, *cis*-9, *cis*-12-18:2 represents a fatty acid with 18 carbon atoms and two double bonds (in the *cis* configuration) located at 9 and 12 positions from the carboxyl carbon atom (Table 1).

Physical Properties

For saturated fatty acids, the longer the chain, the higher is the melting point. When fatty acids with same carbon number are compared, the greater the number of double bonds, the lower is the melting point. However, *trans* fatty acids are in many ways similar to saturated fatty acids; they have higher melting points than the corresponding acids with *cis* configurations.

Occurrence in Nature

Fatty acids in nature are seldom free. They are generally esterified into either triacylglycerols (frequently referred to as 'triglycerides' in literature for the more general reader) for storage, or into phospholipids which are important structural components of cell membranes. In mammals, fatty acids are continuously exchanged between structural and storage pools via the bloodstream. The storage fat may be derived from fat in the diet, or synthesized by tissues such as adipose tissue, mammary glands or liver from simple sugars originating from the dietary carbohydrates. When the amount of fat in the diet is high, the endogenous synthetic activity of the tissues is

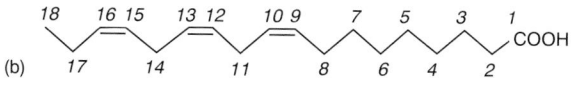

Figure 2 The two positional isomers of linolenic acid (18:3): (a) γ-linolenic acid (*cis*-6, *cis*-9, *cis*-12-octadecatrienoic acid); (b) α-linolenic acid (*cis*-9, *cis*-12, *cis*-15-octadecatrienoic acid).

Table 1 Nomenclature of fatty acids

Trivial name	Systematic name	Shorthand notation	Chemical formula
Saturated			
Caproic	hexanoic	6:0	$C_6H_{12}O_2$
Caprylic	octanoic	8:0	$C_8H_{16}O_2$
Capric	decanoic	10:0	$C_{10}H_{20}O_2$
Lauric	dodecanoic	12:0	$C_{12}H_{24}O_2$
Myristic	tetradecanoic	14:0	$C_{14}H_{28}O_2$
Palmitic	hexadecanoic	16:0	$C_{16}H_{32}O_2$
Stearic	octadecanoic	18:0	$C_{18}H_{36}O_2$
Arachidic	eicosanoic	20:0	$C_{20}H_{40}O_2$
Behenic	docosanoic	22:0	$C_{22}H_{44}O_2$
Lignoceric	tetracosanoic	24:0	$C_{24}H_{48}O_2$
Monounsaturated			
Palmitoleic	*cis*-9-hexadecenoic	16:1 n-7	$C_{16}H_{30}O_2$
Oleic	*cis*-9-octadecenoic	18:1 n-9	$C_{18}H_{34}O_2$
Gadoleic	*cis*-11-eicosenoic	20:1 n-9	$C_{20}H_{38}O_2$
Erucic	*cis*-13-docosenoic	22:1 n-9	$C_{22}H_{42}O_2$
Cetoleic	*cis*-11-docosenoic	22:1 n-11	$C_{22}H_{42}O_2$
Nervonic	*cis*-15-tetracosenoic	24:1 n-9	$C_{24}H_{46}O_2$
Elaidic	*trans*-9-octadecenoic	t18:1 n-9	$C_{18}H_{34}O_2$
Polyunsaturated			
n-9 family:			
Mead	all *cis*-5,8,11-eicosatrienoic	20:3 n-9	$C_{20}H_{34}O_2$
n-6 family:			
Linoleic	*cis,cis*-9,12-octadecadienoic	18:2 n-6	$C_{18}H_{32}O_2$
γ-Linolenic (GLA)	all *cis*-6,9,12-octadecatrienoic	18:3 n-6	$C_{18}H_{30}O_2$
Dihomo-γ-linolenic (DGLA)	all *cis*-8,11,14-eicosatrienoic	20:3 n-6	$C_{20}H_{34}O_2$
Arachidonic (AA)	all *cis*-5,8,11,14-eicosatetraenoic	20:4 n-6	$C_{20}H_{32}O_2$
Adrenic	all *cis*-7,10,13,16-docosatetraenoic	22:4 n-6	$C_{22}H_{36}O_2$
Osmond	all *cis*-4,7,10,13,16-docosapentaenoic	22:5 n-6	$C_{22}H_{34}O_2$
n-3 family:			
α-Linolenic	all *cis*-9,12,15-octadecatrienoic	18:3 n-3	$C_{18}H_{30}O_2$
Stearidonic	all *cis*-6,9,12,15-octadecatetraenoic	18:4 n-3	$C_{18}H_{28}O_2$
Timnodonic	all *cis*-5,8,11,14,17-eicosapentaenoic (EPA)	20:5 n-3	$C_{20}H_{30}O_2$
Clupanodonic	all *cis*-7,10,13,16,19-docosapentaenoic	22:5 n-3	$C_{22}H_{34}O_2$
Cervonic	all *cis*-4,7,10,13,16,19-docosahexaenoic (DHA)	22:6 n-3	$C_{22}H_{32}O_2$

suppressed. The composition of storage fat is influenced by the fatty acid composition of the diet. On the other hand, when there is little fat in the diet, the composition of storage fat is dependent mainly on the characteristic synthetic activity of the tissue.

Beta-oxidation

Fatty acid β-oxidation is a step-by-step breakdown process by which cells release and utilize the energy contained in fatty acids. The β-oxidation is carried out in the mitochondrial matrix in tissues such as heart and skeletal muscles. In these tissues, a fatty acid is shortened by two carbons as a result of a cleavage between the α-carbon and β-carbon in the chain. Prior to the metabolism, fatty acids present in the cytosol are activated to their corresponding acyl thioesters by acyl-CoA synthases specific to the length of the substrate, short-chain, medium-chain or long-chain acyl-CoA:

Fatty acid + ATP + CoA-SH →
    acyl-CoA + AMP + PP$_i$

The enzymes of β-oxidation are located in the mitochondrial matrix. However, the inner mitochondrial membrane is not permeable to medium-chain (C_{12}–C_{14}) and long-chain (C_{16}–C_{24}) fatty acyl-CoA;

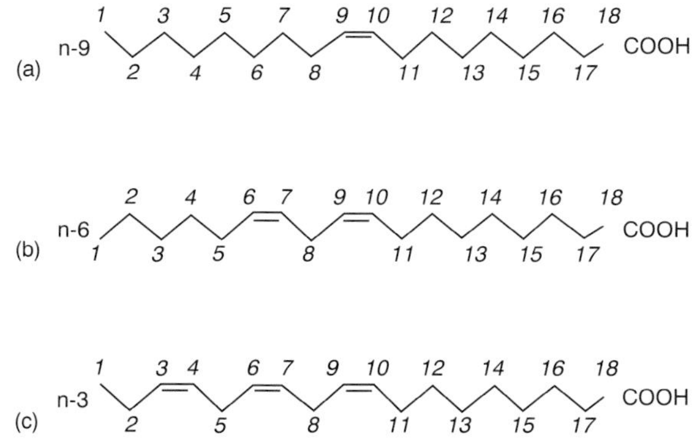

Figure 3 The three major families (n-9, n-6 and n-3) of unsaturated fatty acids: (a) oleic acid (18:1 n-9); (b) linoleic acid (18:2 n-6); (c) linolenic acid (18:3 n-3).

these fatty acyl thioesters therefore cannot directly penetrate this membrane but are carried across it by the carnitine-dependent transfer mechanism (**Fig. 4**).

After entering the mitochondrial matrix, fatty acid thioesters (R-$(CH_2)_n$-CO-S-CoA) are degraded in a stepwise fashion. First, the β and γ carbon atoms of the fatty acid undergo dehydrogenation, hydration and further dehydrogenation to form a β-ketoacyl-CoA, which is then cleaved to give a two-carbon fragment, acetyl-CoA (CH_3-CO-S-CoA) and an acyl-CoA molecule (R-$(CH_2)_{n-2}$-CO-S-CoA). The acyl-CoA molecule, which is two carbon atoms shorter than the original molecule, will enter the cycle again and proceed through the next round of oxidation

reactions (**Fig. 5**). In general, the rate of oxidation decreases with increasing fatty acid chain length.

The β-oxidation of unsaturated fatty acids is similar to that of saturated fatty acids except that it stops when an intermediate acyl-CoA containing a *cis* double bond between β and γ carbons is formed. The unsaturated acyl-CoA is converted to the regular *trans* α,β-unsaturated intermediate by two auxiliary enzymes (isomerase and epimerase) in the mitochondrial matrix, and is again a substrate for the β-oxidation enzymes. Evidence indicates that SFAs are oxidized more slowly than unsaturated fatty acids.

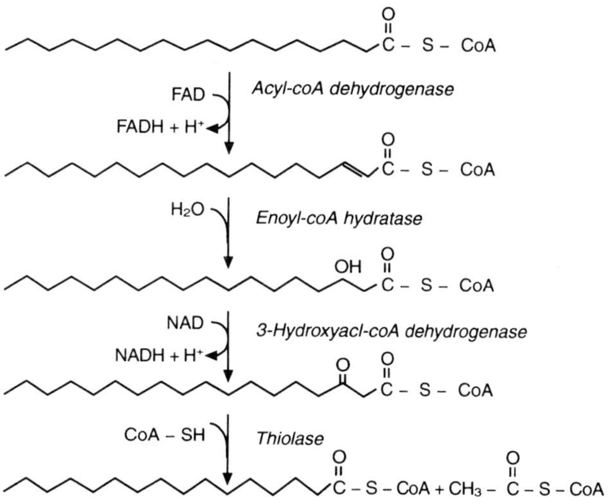

Figure 5 The stepwise β-oxidation of fatty acyl-CoA in the mitochondrial matrix to produce acetyl-CoA fragments.

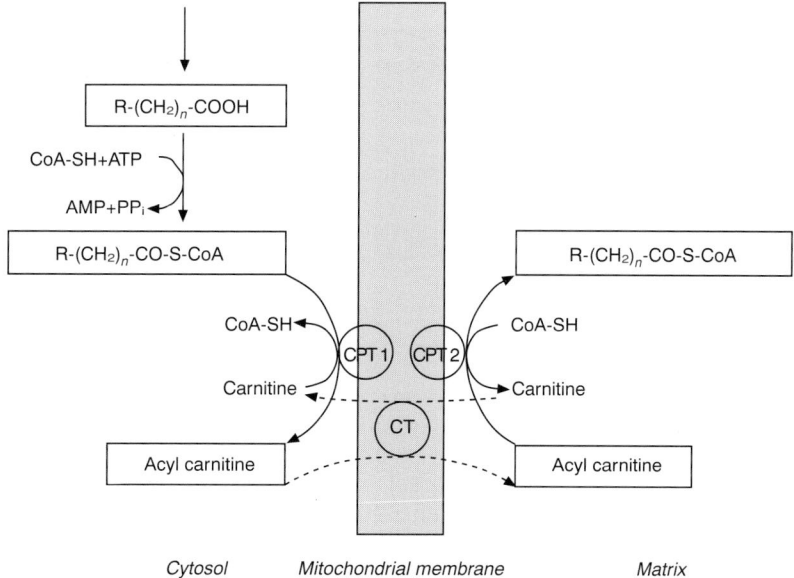

Figure 4 Carnitine-dependent translocation of fatty acids across the inner mitochondrial membrane. CPT1, outer carnitine palmitoyltransferase 1; CPT2, inner carnitine palmitoyltransferase II; CT, carnitine:acylcarnitine translocase.

Beta-oxidation can also take place in peroxisomes which are prevalent in liver and kidney. They are responsible for shortening long-chain (22-carbon) fatty acids such as erucic acid (22:1 n-9) and docosahexaenoic acid (22:6 n-3). The shortening of long-chain fatty acid by a β-oxidation process is sometimes called 'retroconversion'.

The function of fatty acid oxidation is to generate metabolic energy. Overall, the total oxidation of one molecule of fatty acyl-CoA generates approximately $(17n/2 - 5)$ ATP, where n represents the number of carbons in each fatty acid. On average, each fatty acid provides 37 kJ g^{-1} (9 kcal g^{-1}).

Synthesis of Fatty Acids

All animals can synthesize saturated fatty acids from carbohydrates and proteins, and can also introduce double bonds to the fatty acid carbon chain. Fatty acid synthesis begins from the generation of acetyl-CoA. The acetyl-CoA may be derived from pyruvate oxidation, fatty acid β-oxidation or the degradation of amino acids. However, generation of acetyl-CoA occurs in the mitochondrial matrix, whereas utilization of acetyl-CoA for fatty acid synthesis is in the cytoplasm. Since acetyl-CoA cannot cross the inner mitochondrial membrane, the transfer of the intramitochondrial acetyl-CoA to its utilization site (the cytoplasm) is achieved by an alternative transport system. The acetyl-CoA is first condensed with oxaloacetate to form citrate by citrate synthase. Citrate can then cross the membrane into the cytosol, where it is cleaved to produce oxaloacetate and acetyl-CoA (**Fig. 6**).

In cytosol, the *de novo* synthesis of fatty acids is catalysed by the multiple enzyme complex, fatty acid synthase. First of all, malonyl-CoA (HOOC-CH$_2$-CO-S-CoA) is derived from acetyl-CoA by acetyl-CoA carboxylase. This enzyme, which is subject to hormonal regulation, controls the overall rate of fatty acid synthesis. Both acetyl-CoA and malonyl-CoA are bound to a sulfhydryl group (–SH) of the acyl carrier protein (ACP) to form acetyl-S-ACP and malonyl-S-ACP, respectively. The role of ACP in fatty acid synthesis is analogous to that of coenzyme A in mitochondrial fatty acid oxidation. A molecule of acetyl-ACP is then condensed with a malonyl-S-ACP molecule to form acetoacetyl-S-ACP (CH$_2$-CO-CH$_2$-CO-S-ACP). This reaction is followed in sequence by hydrogenation, dehydration and another hydrogenation (**Fig. 7**), producing a four-carbon butyryl-ACP derivative (CH$_3$-CH$_2$-CH$_2$-CO-S-ACP).

The same reactions proceed to the next round where butyryl-S-ACP replaces the CH$_3$-CO-S-ACP. Each synthetic cycle requires one additional molecule of malonyl-CoA, and produces a fatty acyl-S-ACP derivative two carbon atoms longer than the previous one. After the cycle is repeated seven times, the end product is palmitoyl-S-ACP. Palmitic acid may be further elongated to form stearic acid or other long-chain fatty acids through the action of the malonyl-CoA dependent elongation systems located in the endoplasmic reticulum or in mitochondrial membranes.

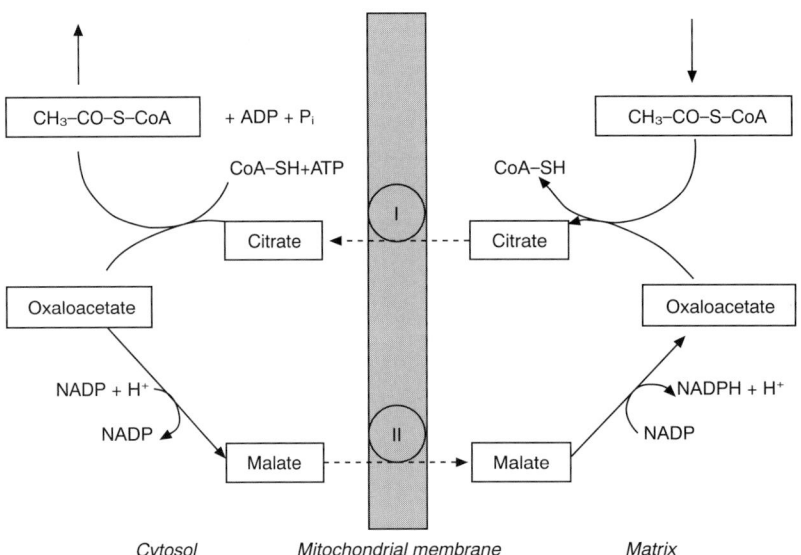

Figure 6 The transfer of acetyl-CoA across the inner membrane to the cytosol. I, tricarboxylate and II, dicarboxylate transport systems.

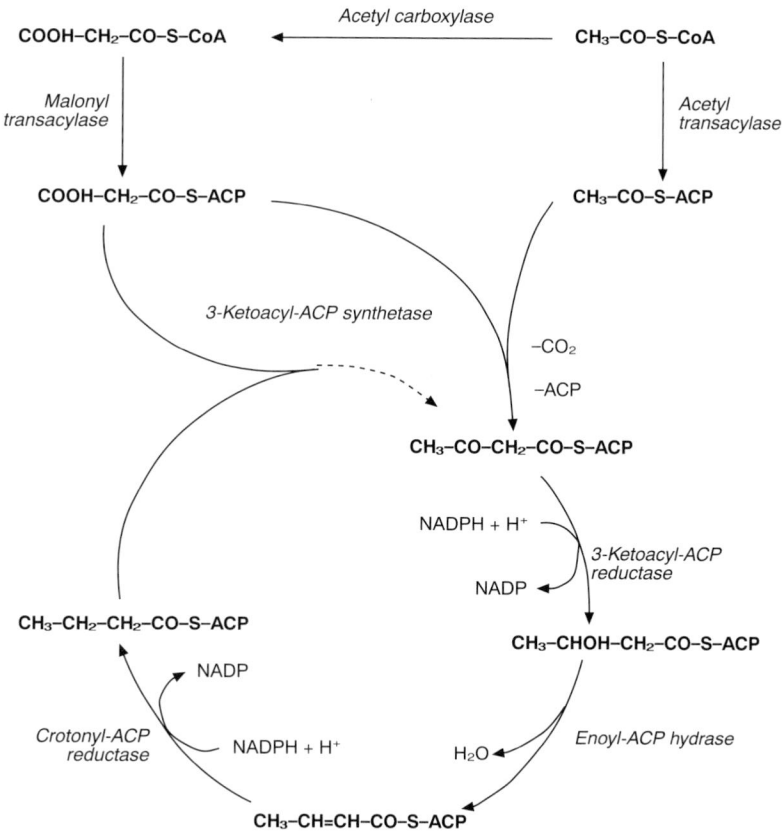

Figure 7 The *de novo* synthesis of fatty acid catalysed by the multiple enzyme complex (fatty acid synthase) in cytosol.

Metabolism of Short-chain Fatty Acids

Short-chain fatty acids (SCFAs), also called volatile fatty acids, are produced predominantly in the proximal colon by microbial fermentation of dietary polysaccharides. The chain ranges in length from one to six carbons. The major SCFAs include acetic (CH_3-COOH), propionic (CH_3-CH_2-COOH) and butyric acids (CH_3-CH_2-CH_2-COOH). In the free acid form SCFAs are highly soluble in the aqueous phase and diffuse freely across the mucosa of the digestive tract to enter the venous blood, and are therefore absorbed rapidly by the human jejunum, colon and rectum. The daily production of SCFAs is estimated to be 200–500 mmol, mostly acetate. Increasing dietary intake of fibre has been shown to increase faecal SCFA output. A significant amount of SCFAs in the form of triacylglycerols can be found in cow's milk. They can be digested readily, because human gastric juice contains lipolytic activity specific for short-chain and medium-chain triacylglycerols.

Butyrate and (at a lower rate) propionate can be converted to acetate, which may be subsequently metabolized to carbon dioxide and provide energy for the gastric epithelium. By entering the tricarboxylic acid cycle via succinyl-CoA propionate can also be metabolized to carbon dioxide. In the large intestine, acetic and butyric acids are precursors of ketone bodies (acetoacetate and D-β-hydroxybutyrate). Acetate can also serve as a precursor of other higher lipids, e.g. free and esterified cholesterol, and long-chain fatty acids in the gastrointestinal mucosa. On the other hand, propionate may reduce serum cholesterol through inhibition of HMG-CoA reductase, the rate-limiting step for cholesterol synthesis.

Production of Ketone Bodies

Acetyl-CoA formed during fatty acid oxidation is ultimately metabolized to carbon dioxide and water by two different pathways: either through the citric acid cycle or via the formation of ketone bodies. The liver is the main organ producing ketone bodies.

In mitochondria, two molecules of acetyl-CoA are condensed to form one molecule of acetoacetyl-CoA, which is conjugated with another molecule of acetyl-CoA to form 3-hydroxyl-3-methylglutaryl-CoA (HMG-CoA, $COOH$-CH_2-$C(CH_3)(OH)$-CH_2-CO-S-CoA). The HMG-CoA molecule is then cleaved to yield a molecule each of acetyl-CoA and free acetoacetate. Some of the free acetoacetate may be dehydrogenated to 3-hydroxybutyrate. Both acetoacetate and 3-hydroxybutyrate can readily diffuse into the blood; they are taken up by extrahepatic tissues, where 3-hydroxybutyrate is reoxidized to acetoacetate, which is then converted to form acetoacetyl-CoA, followed by cleavage to yield two molecules of acetyl-CoA. The latter then enters the citric acid cycle for complete oxidation (**Fig. 8**). By forming ketone bodies, the liver can deliver energy via the blood to extrahepatic tissues. For example, the brain obtains energy normally from glucose, but can shift to using ketone bodies when glucose is in short supply, as in starvation, or when it is not readily available, as in diabetes.

Function

The biological roles of dietary fatty acids include the following:

1. *Source of energy*: fat is a principal source of energy. When dietary energy is low, as in starvation or strenuous exercise, fatty acids are mobilized from adipose tissue to meet the needs for energy. In heart and skeletal muscles, free fatty acids are activated to acyl-CoA and transported to mitochondria, where they are oxidized to acetyl-CoA. The newly formed acetyl-CoA then enters the Krebs citric acid cycle and results in the production of ATP for muscular activity.
2. *Components of cell membranes*: phospholipids are the major components of cell membranes, where they are present as a biomolecular sheet with fatty acid chains in the interior of a bilayer. The physical properties of a cell membrane are modulated by the fatty acid composition of phospholipids. The presence of double bonds in the chains bends the fatty acid molecule, causing it to occupy more space than saturated fatty acids. Thus, unsaturated fatty acids take up more space and pack less well together in the bilayer of cell membrane. This in turn increases the membrane fluidity. Through their effects on the lipid phase and interactions with membrane proteins, fatty acids can modulate cell membrane function.
3. *Precursors of biologically active metabolites, such as eicosanoids*: some of the 20-carbon polyunsaturated fatty acids can generate locally a complex group of highly biologically active, short-lived compounds, such as prostaglandins, thromboxanes and leukotrienes. Even at very low concentrations, these compounds exert a wide range of profound physiological functions.
4. *Carrier of fat-soluble vitamins*: in addition to being a source of energy and building blocks for many tissues, fatty acids are important carriers of fat-soluble vitamins such as A, D, E and K during their absorption by the small intestine.
5. *Organoleptic properties*: dietary fats provide flavour in foods. Short-chain fatty acids such as

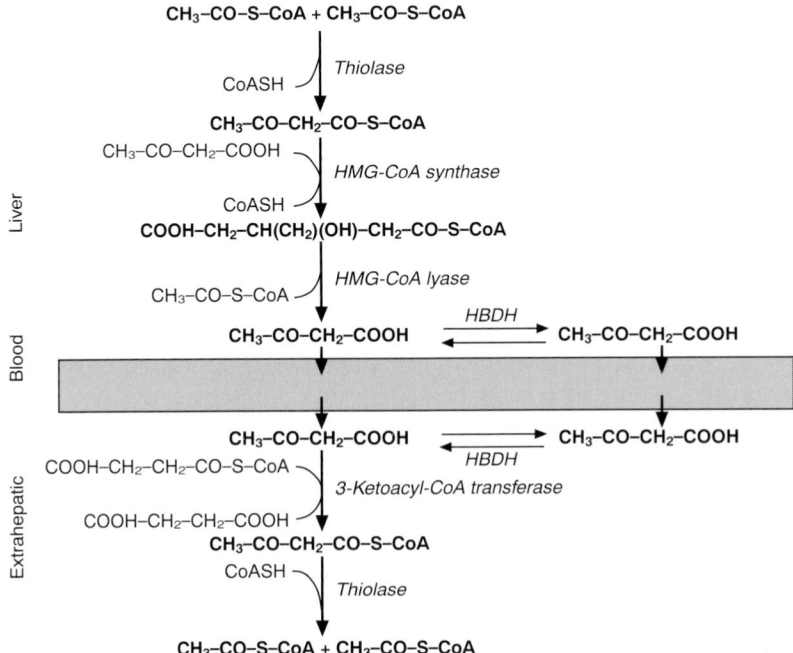

Figure 8 The hepatic synthesis of ketone bodies from acetyl-CoA and the transport of ketone bodies through the blood to extrahepatic tissues. In extrahepatic tissues, ketone bodies are converted back to acetyl-CoA which then enters the citric acid cycle to generate energy. HBDH, hydroxybutyrate dehydrogenase; HMG-CoA, 3-hydroxy-3-methylglutaryl-coenzyme A.

acetic acid and propionic acid are used as preservatives. In their free forms, short-chain and medium-chain fatty acids usually have strong odours. The long-chain fatty acids in the diets when digested promote the feeling of satiety.

Dietary Fat and Nutrition

Since the beginning of the twentieth century, the amount of fat in the diet has been increasing. Although much of the fat is from animal sources, the use of vegetable fat is increasing. Thus, the fat intake is changing from the saturated to more unsaturated diets. There are reports demonstrating the varying atherogenic effects of different fatty acids: for example, saturated fatty acids have been shown to be atherogenic; n-6 polyunsaturated fatty acids have a hypocholesterolaemic effect; the n-3 polyunsaturated fatty acids have hypolipidaemic and antithrombotic effects; and the monounsaturated fatty acids have certain beneficial effects on plasma cholesterol levels. More recently, the *trans* fatty acids have also been shown to be atherogenic. There are also reports relating increasing dietary intake of fat, particularly the polyunsaturated fatty acids, to carcinogenesis. However, evidence suggests that this effect may be attributed to a deficiency of antioxidant, as it is known that increasing the intake of PUFA (which is more readily oxidized) increases the requirement for antioxidant. How much fat and what type of fat should be taken by individuals are subjects of controversy. It has been recommended that for healthy people, moderation in fat intake should be the rule of thumb.

Effect of Other Nutrients of Fatty Acid Biosynthesis

Dietary carbohydrate can be converted into fatty acids by way of glycolysis to form pyruvate, which is then decarboxylated to form acetyl-CoA. The acetyl-CoA thus formed is available for fatty acid synthesis as acyl primer or as an elongating C_2 unit after carboxylation to malonyl-CoA. This process is regulated by nutritional (fed or fasting) and hormonal (e.g. insulin deficiency) states. Evidence also indicates that fatty acid synthesis can be modified by the presence of various metabolites. For example, citrate increases fatty acid synthesis, whereas the end product of fatty acid synthesis such as long-chain acyl-CoA derivatives inhibits the process.

See also: **Carbohydrates**: Regulation of Carbohydrate Metabolism. **Coronary Heart Disease**: Lipid Theory of Coronary Heart Disease; Haemostatic Factors and Coronary Heart Disease; Aetiology; Prevention. **Energy**

Metabolism: Tricarboxylic Acid Cycle and Oxidative Phosphorylation. **Ketosis**: Biochemical and Dietary Aspects. **Prostaglandins and Leukotrienes**: Physiology. **Starvation and Fasting**: Biochemical Aspects.

Further Reading

Bugaut M (1987) Occurrence, absorption and metabolism of short chain fatty acids in the digestive tract of mammals. *Comparative Biochemistry and Physiology* 86B:439–472.

Gunstone FD, Harwood JL and Padley FB (eds) (1994) *The Lipid Handbook*, 2nd edn. London: Chapman & Hall.

McGarry JD and Foster DW (1980) Regulation of hepatic fatty acid oxidation and ketone body production. *Annual Review of Biochemistry* 49:395–420.

Numa S ed. (1984) *Fatty Acid Metabolism and Its Regulation*. New York: Elsevier.

Potter BJ, Sorrentino D and Berk PD (1989) Mechanisms of cellular uptake of free fatty acids. *Annual Review of Nutrition* 9:253–270.

Schulz H (1991) Beta oxidation of fatty acids. *Biochimica Biophysica Acta* 1081:109–120.

Vance DE and Vance JE, eds (1985) *Biochemistry of Lipids and Membrane*. Don Mills: Benjamin/Cummings.

Health Effects of Saturated Fatty Acids

E H M Temme, University of Leuven, Belgium

Ronald P Mensink, Maastricht University, The Netherlands

Copyright © 1998 Academic Press

Fats and oils always consist of a mixture of fatty acids, although one or two fatty acids are usually predominant. **Table 1** shows the fatty acid composition of some edible fats rich in saturated fatty acids. In the Western diet, palmitic acid ($C_{16:0}$) is the major saturated fatty acid in the diet. A smaller proportion comes from stearic acid ($C_{18:0}$), followed by myristic acid ($C_{14:0}$), lauric acid ($C_{12:0}$) and short-chain and medium-chain fatty acids (MCFA)($C_{10:0}$ or less).

When discussing the effects of the total saturated fat content of diets, this class of fatty acids has to be compared with some other component of the diet that provides a similar amount of energy (isoenergetic or 'isocaloric'). Otherwise, three variables are being introduced: changes in total dietary energy intake, changes in body weight, and changes in dietary (saturated) fatty acid content. Normally, an isoenergetic amount from carbohydrates or from another fatty acid is used for comparisons.

Table 1 Composition of fats rich in saturated fatty acids

	$\leq C_{10:0}$	$C_{12:0}$	$C_{14:0}$	$C_{16:0}$	$C_{18:0}$	$C_{18:1}$	$C_{18:2}$	$C_{18:3}$	Other
	Weight per 100 g of total fatty acids (g)								
Butter fat	9	3	17	25	13	27	3	1	2
Palm kernel fat	8	50	16	8	2	14	2		
Coconut fat	15	48	17	8	3	7	2		
Palm oil			1	45	5	39	9		1
Beef fat			3	26	22	38	2	1	8
Pork fat (lard)			2	25	12	44	10	1	6
Cocoa butter				26	35	35	3		1

Cholesterol Metabolism

Lipoproteins and their associated apoproteins are strong predictors of the risk of coronary heart disease (CHD). Concentrations of total cholesterol, low-density lipoproteins (LDL) and apoprotein B are positively correlated with CHD risk; high-density lipoprotein (HDL) and apoprotein AI concentrations are negatively correlated. Controlled dietary trials have demonstrated that serum lipid and lipoprotein levels are affected by the total saturated fat content and the type of saturated fatty acid in the diet.

Total saturated fat content of diets

Using statistical techniques, results from independent experiments have been combined to develop equations that estimate the mean change in serum lipoprotein levels for a group of subjects when carbo-

hydrates are replaced by an isoenergetic amount of a mixture of saturated fatty acids. The predicted changes for total LDL and HDL cholesterol, and triacylglycerols are shown in **Fig. 1**. Each bar represents the predicted change in the concentration of that particular lipid or lipoprotein when 10% of the daily energy intake from carbohydrates is replaced by a particular fatty acid class. For a group of adults with an energy intake of 10 MJ daily, 10% of energy is provided by about 60 g of carbohydrates or 27 g of fatty acids.

A mixture of saturated fatty acids strongly elevates serum total cholesterol levels. It was predicted that when 10% of dietary energy provided by carbohydrates was exchanged for a mixture of saturated fatty acids, serum total cholesterol concentrations would increase by 0.39 mmol l^{-1}. This increase in total cholesterol level will result from a rise in both

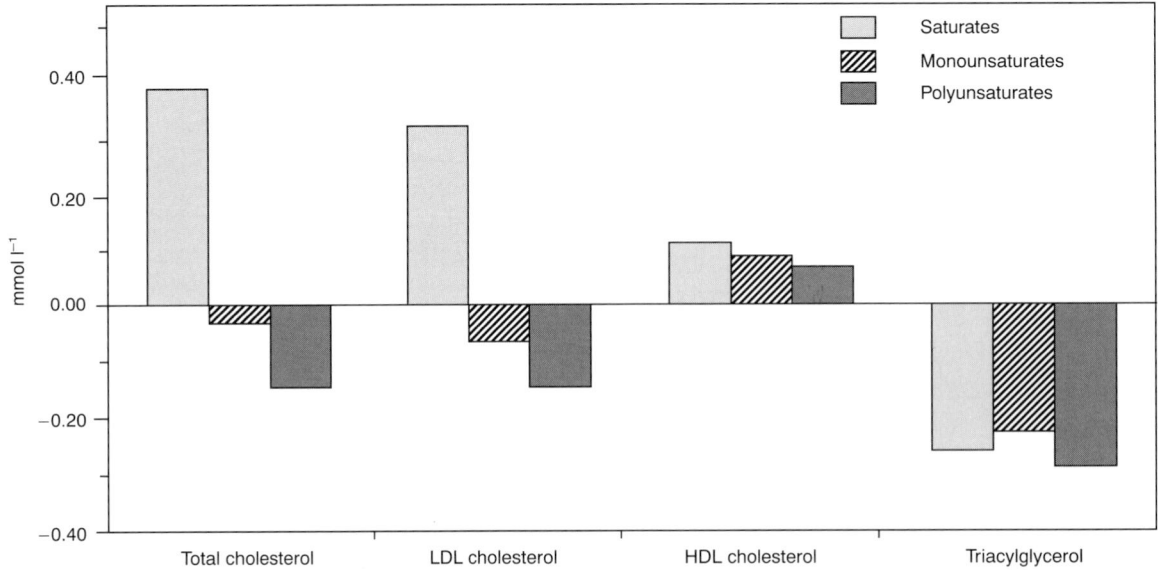

Figure 1 Predicted changes in serum lipids and lipoproteins when 10% of energy from dietary carbohydrates is replaced by an isoenergetic amount of saturated fatty acids or unsaturated fatty acids. Adapted from Mensink and Katan (1992).

LDL and HDL cholesterol concentrations. Saturated fatty acids will also lower fasting triacylglycerol concentrations compared with carbohydrates. Besides affecting LDL and HDL cholesterol concentrations, a mixture of saturated fatty acids also changes the concentrations of their associated apoproteins. In general, strong associations are observed between changes in LDL cholesterol and changes in apo-B, and between changes in HDL cholesterol and apo-AI.

The figure also shows that total and LDL cholesterol concentrations decrease when saturated fatty acids are replaced by unsaturated fatty acids. In addition, slight decreases of HDL cholesterol concentrations are then predicted.

Effects of specific saturated fatty acids

Cocoa butter has been shown to raise total cholesterol concentrations to a lesser extent than palm oil. This difference in the serum cholesterol-raising potency of two fats high in saturated fatty acids (see Table 1) showed that not all saturated fatty acids have equal effects on cholesterol concentrations. **Fig. 2** illustrates the effects of MCFA and lauric, myristic, palmitic and stearic acids on LDL and HDL cholesterol concentrations.

Palm kernel and coconut fat contain relatively high levels of lauric acid, and both of these fats raise total cholesterol levels. This cholesterol-raising effect, however, can also be ascribed to myristic acid which is also present, because the levels of these two saturated fatty acids in natural fats are strongly corre-

lated. To circumvent this problem, synthetic fats with high levels of lauric acid have also been examined. Results on the effects of lauric acid, however, are not in agreement with each other. One experiment with a lauric acid-rich synthetic fat found that, relative to oleic acid, lauric acid raised total and LDL cholesterol levels less than did palmitic acid. However, in another study using natural fats, lauric acid increased total and LDL cholesterol levels more than did palmitic acid. Concentrations of HDL cholesterol in both experiments were highest with diets rich in lauric acid. Of the saturates, myristic acid may have the strongest potency to increase serum total and LDL cholesterol concentrations and also HDL cholesterol concentrations.

Scientists are not unanimous about the cholesterol-raising properties of palmitic acid, the major dietary saturated fatty acid. Many studies have indicated that, compared with carbohydrates, palmitic acid raises serum total and LDL cholesterol levels, but has less effect on HDL cholesterol (Fig. 2). However, a few studies indicated that palmitic acid may *not* raise total and LDL cholesterol concentrations compared with carbohydrates. It has been proposed that this negative finding is only present when the linoleic acid content of the diet is adequate (6–7% of energy). It is hypothesized that the increased hepatic apo-B100 production caused by palmitic acid, and the consequent elevation of concentrations of serum very low-density lipoproteins (VLDL) and LDL particles, are counteracted by an increased uptake of LDL particles by the LDL receptor which is upregulated by linoleic

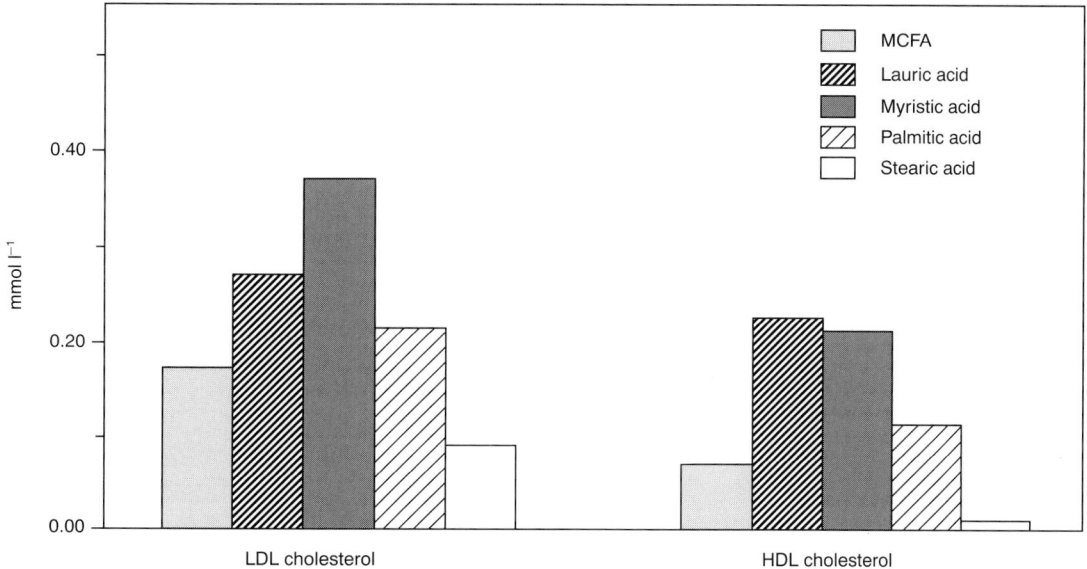

Figure 2 Overview of the effects of particular saturated fatty acids on serum LDL and HDL cholesterol concentrations when 10% of energy from dietary carbohydrates is replaced by an isoenergetic amount of particular saturated fatty acids. The values in most studies were obtained by direct comparison with oleic acid.

acid. To explain the discrepancy with other studies, it has been suggested that in some situations, such as hypercholesterolaemia or obesity, linoleic acid is unable to increase LDL receptor activity sufficiently to neutralize the cholesterol-raising effects of palmitic acid. This theory, however, awaits confirmation, and for now it seems justified to classify palmitic acid as a cholesterol-raising saturated fatty acid.

Stearic acid, a major fatty acid in cocoa butter, does not raise total, LDL and HDL cholesterol levels compared with carbohydrates. Also, MCFA have been reported not to raise LDL and HDL cholesterol concentrations compared with carbohydrates, but data are limited. Like carbohydrates, diets containing large amounts of MCFA increase fasting triacylglycerol concentrations compared with the other saturated fatty acids. However, such diets are the sole energy source only in parenteral or enteral nutrition, or in sports drinks. Other saturated fatty acids have not been reported to raise triacylglycerol concentrations compared with each other, but lower triacylglycerol concentrations compared with carbohydrates.

Platelet Aggregation

Increased platelet aggregation may be an important marker for the occurrence of cardiovascular disease, and platelet aggregation *in vitro* can be modified by different types of fatty acids. However, reports of research on this topic are confusing because of the many methods used to measure aggregation. All measurements have their limitations, and it is not known whether measurement *in vitro* of platelet aggregation reflects the reality of platelet reactivity *in vivo*.

Many methods are available to measure platelet aggregation *in vitro*. First, the blood sample is treated with an anticoagulant to avoid clotting of the blood in the test tube or in the aggregometer; many different anticoagulants are used, which all differ in their mechanism of action. Secondly, platelet aggregation can be measured in whole blood, in platelet-rich plasma or (to remove the influence of the plasma constituents) in a washed platelet sample. Finally, the platelet aggregation reaction in the aggregometer can be initiated with many different compounds, such as collagen, ADP, arachidonic acid and thrombin. Platelet aggregation can also be studied by measuring the stable metabolites of the proaggregatory thromboxane A_2 (TxA_2), thromboxane B_2 (TxB_2), or the stable metabolite of the antiaggregatory prostaglandin (prostacyclin: PGI_2), 6-keto-$PGF_{1\alpha}$.

Total saturated fat content of diets

Platelet aggregation and clotting activity of plasma were studied in British and French farmers, who were classified according to their intake of saturated fatty acids. A positive correlation was observed between thrombin-induced aggregation of platelet-rich plasma and the intake of saturated fatty acids. Aggregation induced by ADP or collagen, however, did not correlate with dietary saturated fat intake. In a follow-up study, a group of farmers consuming high-fat diets were asked to replace dairy fat in their diets with a special margarine rich in polyunsaturated fatty acids. Besides lowering the intake of saturated fatty acids, this intervention also resulted in a lower intake of total fat. A control group of farmers did not change their diets. After this intervention the thrombin-induced aggregation of platelet-rich plasma decreased when saturated fat intake decreased. Aggregation induced by ADP, however, increased in the intervention group. From these studies, it is not clear whether the fatty acid composition of the diets or the total fatty acid content is responsible for the changes in platelet aggregation. Furthermore, it is not clear if one should favour increased or decreased platelet aggregation after decreasing the saturated fat content of diets. Saturated fatty acids from milk fat have also been compared with unsaturated fatty acids from sunflower and rapeseed oils. Aggregation induced by ADP or collagen in platelet-rich plasma was lower with the milk fat diet than with either oil.

One of the mechanisms affecting platelet aggregation is alteration of the proportion of arachidonic acid in the platelet phospholipids. Arachidonic acid is a substrate for the production of the proaggregatory TxA_2 and the antiaggregatory PGI_2, and the balance between these two eicosanoids affects the degree of platelet activation. The proportion of arachidonic acid in membranes can be modified through changes in dietary fatty acid composition. Diets rich in saturated fatty acids increase the arachidonic acid content of the platelet phospholipids, but this is also dependent on the particular saturated fatty acid consumed (see below).

Diets rich in saturated fatty acids have also been associated with a lower ratio of cholesterol to phospholipid in platelet membranes, which may affect receptor activity and platelet aggregation. However, these mechanisms have been described from studies *in vitro* and on animals and have not adequately been confirmed in human studies.

Effects of specific saturated fatty acids

Diets rich in coconut fat have been reported to raise TxB_2 and lower $6\text{-keto-PGF}_{1\alpha}$ concentrations in collagen-activated plasma compared with diets rich in palm or olive oils, indicating a less favourable eicosanoid profile. The main saturated fatty acids of coconut fat – lauric and myristic acid – did not, however, change collagen-induced aggregation in whole-blood samples compared with a diet rich in oleic acid. Also, diets rich in MCFA or palmitic acid did not change collagen-induced aggregation in whole-blood samples. Compared with a diet rich in a mixture of saturated fatty acids, a stearic acid diet increased collagen-induced aggregation in platelet-rich plasma. In addition, a decreased proportion of arachidonic acid in platelet phospholipids was demonstrated after a cocoa butter diet compared with a diet rich in butterfat. Changes in eicosanoid metabolite concentrations in urine, however, were not observed after either diet. These results are conflicting and it is debatable whether measurement *in vitro* of platelet aggregation truly reflects the situation *in vivo*.

Coagulation and Fibrinolysis

Processes involved in thrombus formation include not only those required for the formation of a stable thrombus (platelet aggregation and blood clotting), but also a mechanism to dissolve the thrombus (fibrinolysis). Long-term prospective epidemiological studies have reported that in healthy men factor VII coagulant activity (factor VIIc) and fibrinogen concentrations were higher in subjects who developed cardiovascular diseases at a later stage of the study. Factor VIIc in particular was associated with an increased risk of dying from cardiovascular disease. A high concentration of plasminogen activator inhibitor type 1 (PAI-1) indicates impaired fibrinolytic capacity of the plasma and is associated with increased risk of occurrence of coronary events.

Saturated fatty acids can affect the plasma activity of some of these coagulation and fibrinolytic factors and thus the prethrombotic state of the blood. However, the effects of saturated fatty acids on coagulation and fibrinolytic factors in humans, unlike effects on cholesterol concentrations, have received little attention, and few well-controlled human studies have been reported. Also, regression equations derived from meta-analysis, which predict the effects on coagulation and fibrinolytic factors of different fatty acid classes compared with those of carbohydrates, do not exist. Therefore, the reference fatty acid is dependent on the experiment discussed.

In the epidemiological studies that have found associations between CHD risk and factors involved in thrombogenesis or atherogenesis, subjects were mostly fasted. Also, the effects of saturated fatty acids on cholesterol metabolism, platelet aggregation, and coagulation and fibrinolysis have been studied mainly in fasted subjects. It should be noted, however, that concentrations of some coagulation factors (for example, factor VIIc) and fibrinolytic factors change after a meal.

Total saturated fat content of diets

Coagulation   Results of studies on the effects of low-fat diets compared with high-fat diets provide some insight into the effects of decreasing the saturated fat content of diets. However, in these studies multiple changes are introduced which makes interpretation of results difficult.

Decreased factor VIIc levels were demonstrated in subjects on low-fat diets compared with those on high-fat diets, in both short-term (several weeks) and longer-term dietary experiments. In these studies, the low-fat diet provided smaller quantities of both saturated and unsaturated fatty acids and more fibre than the high-fat diet. The results of a short-term study are shown in **Fig. 3**(a). In another study investigating low-fat and high-fat diets, factor VIIc levels did not change (Fig. 3(b)). In the second study the low-fat diet provided smaller amounts of unsaturated fatty acids than the high-fat diet, but both diets contained comparable amounts of saturated fatty acids and fibre. The combined results suggest that, apart from a possible effect of dietary fibre, saturates increase factor VII levels compared with carbohydrates. This is supported by studies of specific saturated fatty acids which indicate that those with 12–16 carbon atoms raise factor VII levels (see below). However, the hypothesis that factor VII levels are increased by saturates is contradicted by the observation that replacing polyunsaturates with saturates does not elevate factor VIIc levels, or does so only slightly. Effects on factor VII of mixtures of saturated fatty acids are therefore still inconclusive. Additional clotting factors, fibrinogen concentrations and markers of *in vivo* coagulation (for example, prothrombin fragment 1+2) might have provided more information on the effect of saturates on blood coagulation, but were not measured in most experiments.

Fibrinolysis   Effects of low-fat and high-fat diets on the fibrinolytic capacity of the blood have also been studied. A similar problem, as stated before, is that multiple changes were introduced within a single experiment. Results of longer-term and shorter-term studies with dietary changes of total fat (decrease of saturated and unsaturated fatty acids content) and increased fibre content indicate beneficially increased

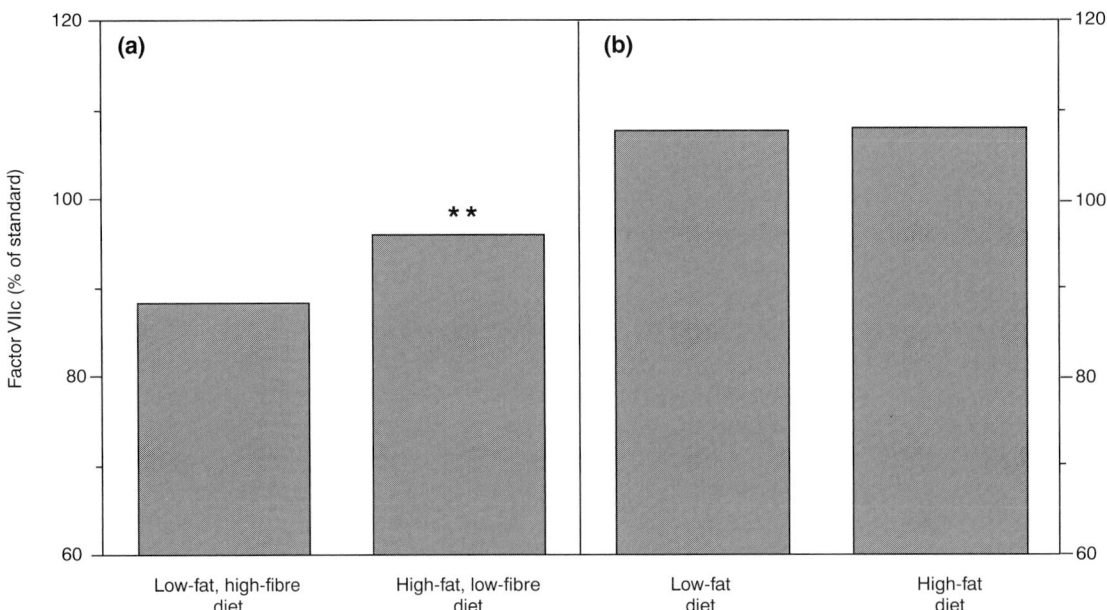

Figure 3 (a) Factor VIIc activity after 2 weeks on a low-fat, high-fibre diet or a high-fat, low-fibre diet; (b) effects of low-fat and high-fat diets with similar fibre contents and almost similar saturated fatty acid contents. **, $P < 0.01$, significantly different from the low-fat, high-fibre diet. Data from (a) Marckmann *et al.* (1994) *American Journal of Clinical Nutrition* **59**:935–939, (b) Marckmann *et al.* (1992) *Arteriosclerosis and Thrombosis* **12**:201–205.

euglobulin fibrinolytic capacity of the blood. The results of the short-term study are depicted in **Fig. 4**(a). This study also reported a decrease in tissue plasminogen activator (tPA) activity after the high-fat, low-fibre diet. However, when the saturated fatty acid and fibre content of two diets were almost identical and only the unsaturated fatty acid content was changed, no significant differences of fibrinolytic capacity were observed (Fig. 4(b)).

Little is known about the relative effects on

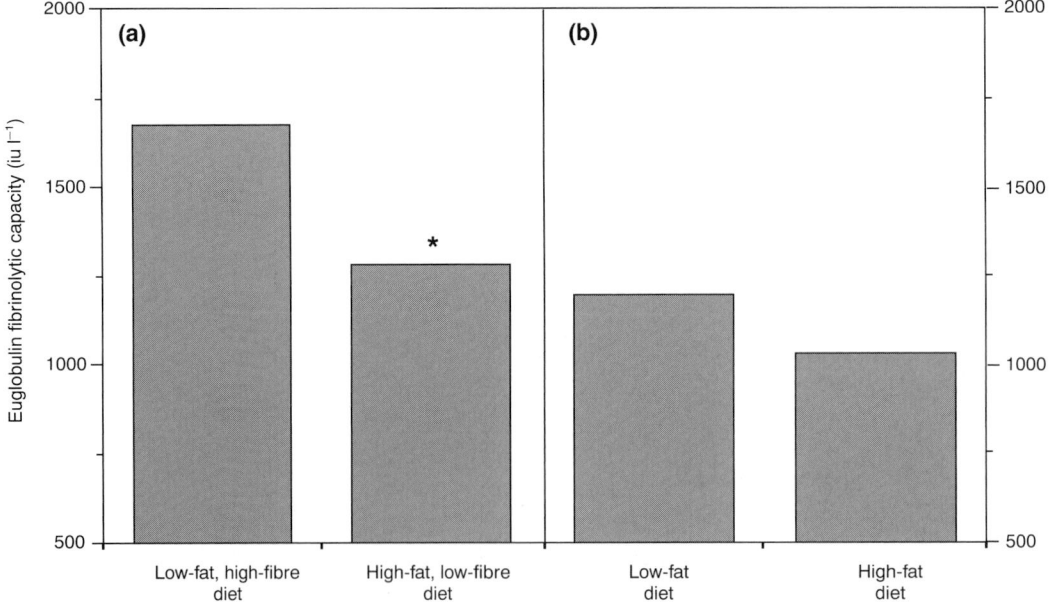

Figure 4 (a) Euglobulin fibrinolytic activity after 2 weeks on low-fat, high-fibre or high-fat, low-fibre diets; (b) effects of low-fat and high-fat diets, with similar fibre contents and almost similar saturated fatty acid contents. * $P < 0.02$, significantly different from the low-fat, high-fibre diet. Data from (a) Marckmann *et al.* (1994) *American Journal of Clinical Nutrition* **59**: 935–939, (b) Marckmann *et al.* (1992) *Arteriosclerosis and Thrombosis* **12**: 201–205.

fibrinolytic capacity of saturated fatty acids compared with unsaturated fatty acids. Euglobulin clot lysis time and concentrations of tPA and PAI-1 have not been studied in the experiments with diets that exchanged saturates for polyunsaturated fatty acids. Recently, it has been reported that diets rich in butterfat decreased PAI-1 activity compared with a diet rich in partially hydrogenated soyabean oil, but whether this is because of changes in the saturated acid or the *trans* fatty acid content is not clear from this study.

As for coagulation factors, the findings on the fibrinolytic effects of saturates are still inconclusive and need to be confirmed by more specific assays, measuring the activities of the separate fibrinolytic factors such as tPA and PAI-1.

Effects of specific saturated fatty acids

Coagulation   The interest in the effects of particular fatty acids on coagulation and fibrinolytic factors has increased since the observation that different saturated fatty acids raise serum lipids and lipoproteins in different ways (see section on cholesterol metabolism above). Effects on total factor VII activity of MCFA and of lauric, myristic, palmitic and stearic acids compared with oleic acid are shown in **Fig. 5**. The results indicate that the dietary saturated fatty acids that raise serum total and LDL cholesterol concentrations also increase factor VII activity. Stearic acid and MCFA, however, do not raise factor VII activity in the fasting state.

Diets rich in lauric plus myristic acids compared

with a diet rich in stearic acid also increase concentrations of other vitamin K-dependent coagulation proteins. In addition, this mixture of saturated fatty acids raised F_{1+2} concentrations, indicating increased *in vivo* turnover of prothrombin to thrombin. This agreed with a study in rabbits where increased F_{1+2} concentrations were indeed associated with increased hepatic synthesis of vitamin K-dependent clotting factors.

Diets rich in certain saturated fatty acids (lauric acid and palmitic acid) and also diets rich in butter fat have been reported to raise fibrinogen concentrations, but increases were small and results await confirmation.

Postprandially, increased factor VIIc concentrations have been demonstrated after consumption of diets rich in fat compared with fat-free meals. The response is stronger when more fat is consumed, but this occurs regardless of whether the fat is high in saturated or unsaturated fatty acids. Only meals with unrealistically high amounts of MCFA have been reported not to change factor VIIc levels in comparison with a meal providing a similar amount of olive oil.

Fibrinolysis   Increased PAI-1 activity of a palmitic acid-rich diet has been observed compared with diets enriched with oleic acid, indicating impaired fibrinolytic capacity of the plasma. However, this was not confirmed by other experiments on the effects of particular saturated fatty acids (including palmitic acid), which did not indicate changes in

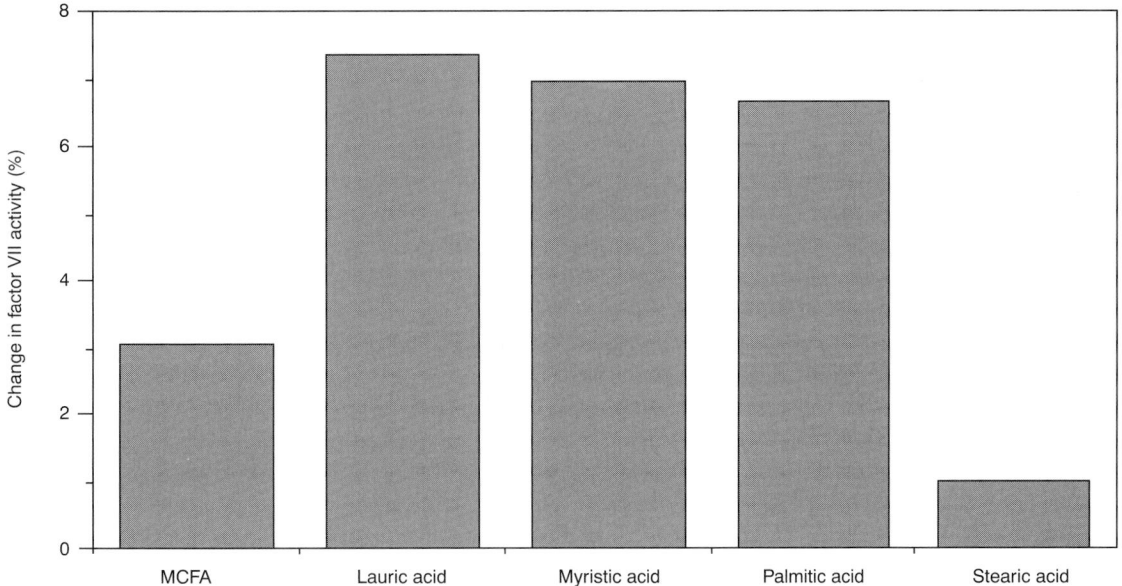

Figure 5   Effects of particular saturated fatty acids on factor VII activity. Data from Temme EHM *et al.*, unpublished results, and from Bladbjerg *et al.* (1995) *Thrombosis and Haemostasis* **2**: 239–242.

fibrinolytic capacity of the blood, measured as tPA, PAI-1 activity or antigen concentrations of tPA and PAI-1.

Conclusion

Saturated fatty acids as a group affect factors involved in cholesterol metabolism. Relative to the carbohydrate content of the diet, a decrease in saturated fat content induces a favourable decrease in serum total and LDL cholesterol concentrations, but unfavourably reduces HDL cholesterol concentrations. Both increasing and decreasing effects of saturates on platelet aggregation have been observed, as well as absence of effect, so results are inconsistent and difficult to interpret. Whether the beneficial effect of a diet low in saturated fat on the prethrombotic state of blood depends on the dietary fibre content is still unclear.

Of the saturated fatty acids, myristic acid and probably lauric acid have the strongest potency to raise total and LDL cholesterol concentrations. In addition, both of these saturated fatty acids raise HDL cholesterol levels. Palmitic acid raises total and LDL cholesterol levels compared with carbohydrates but is less potent than lauric and myristic acids. Stearic acid does not raise LDL and HDL cholesterol concentrations compared with carbohydrates. Lauric, myristic and palmitic acids increase factor VII activity in a similar way, whereas the effects of MCFA and stearic acid seem limited.

See also: **Cholesterol**: Sources, Absorption, Function and Metabolism; Factors Determining Blood Cholesterol Levels. **Coronary Heart Disease**: Lipid Theory of Coronary Heart Disease; Haemostatic Factors and Coronary Heart Disease; Aetiology; Prevention. **Fats and Oils**: Nutritional Value. **Fatty Acids**: Metabolism. **Lipids**: Chemistry and Classification. **Lipoproteins**: Physiology. **Obesity**: Definition, Aetiology and Assessment; Early Obesity and Prognosis; Fat Distribution; Treatment; Prevention; Complications of Obesity.

Further Reading

Hamsten A (1993) The hemostatic system and coronary heart disease. *Thrombosis Research* 70:1–38.

Heemskerk JWM, Vossen RCRM and van Dam-Mieras MCE (1996) Polyunsaturated fatty acids and function of platelets and endothelial cells. *Current Opinion in Lipidology* 7:24–29.

Khosla P and Sundram K (1996) Effects of dietary fatty acid composition on plasma cholesterol. *Progress in Lipid Research* 35:93–132.

Kris-Etherton PM, Krummel D, Russel ME *et al.* (1988) The effect of diet on plasma lipids, lipoproteins, and coronary heart disease. *Journal of the American Dietetic Association* 88:1373–1400.

Marckmann P, Sandstrom B and Jespersen J (1992) Fasting blood coagulation and fibrinolysis of young adults unchanged by reduction in dietary fat content. *Arteriosclerosis and Thrombosis* 12:201–205.

Marckmann P, Sandstrom B and Jespersen J (1994) Low-fat, high-fiber diet favorably affects several independent risk markers of ischemic heart disease: observations on blood lipids, coagulation, and fibrinolysis from a trial of middle-aged Danes. *American Journal of Clinical Nutrition* 59:935–939.

Mennen LI, Schouten EG, Grobbee DE and Kluft C (1996) Coagulation factor VII, dietary fat and blood lipids: a review. *Thrombosis and Haemostasis* 76:492–499.

Mensink RP and Katan MB (1992) Effect of dietary fatty acids on serum lipids and lipoproteins. *Arteriosclerosis and Thrombosis* 12:911–919.

Mensink RP, Temme EHM and Hornstra G (1994) Dietary saturated and *trans* fatty acids and lipoprotein metabolism. *Annals of Medicine* 26:461–464.

Mutanen M and Freese R (1996) Polyunsaturated fatty acids and platelet aggregation. *Current Opinion in Lipidology* 7:14–19.

Nordøy A and Goodnight SH (1990) Dietary lipids and thrombosis. *Arteriosclerosis* 10:149–163.

Health Effects of Monounsaturated Fatty Acids

P Kirk, University of Ulster, Coleraine, UK

Copyright © 1998 Academic Press

Fatty acids are described according to two characteristics: chain length and degree of saturation with hydrogen. Monounsaturated fatty acids (MUFA) have, as the name suggests, only one unsaturated bond attached to the carbon chain. This double bond is fixed in nature and is positioned on the ninth carbon counting from the methyl (omega) end of the fatty acid chain. Four of these MUFA are found in significant quantities in food, the most common being oleic acid ($C_{18:1}$) (**Fig. 1**). This n-9 fatty acid is capable of being synthesized by animals, including humans, but is predominantly incorporated via the diet. While butter and animal fats contain only small amounts of 18:1, olive oil is a rich source. Olive oil, which composes up to 70% of the fat intake in Mediterranean diets, is postulated to be effective in

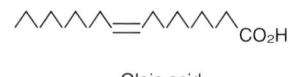

Oleic acid

Figure 1 Structure of oleic acid, $C_{18:1}$.

decreasing the risk of certain chronic diseases. These include such diseases as coronary heart disease, cancers and inflammatory disorders, particularly rheumatoid arthritis.

Cholesterol Metabolism

Cholesterol metabolism is of fundamental biological importance. All vertebrates require cholesterol as a precursor for bile acids and hormones including corticosteroids, sex steroids and vitamin D. The amount of cholesterol found in tissues greatly exceeds the requirement for production of these hormones and bile acids, and the bulk of this excess is associated with cell membrane structure where it is believed to modulate the physical state of phospholipid bilayers.

Cholesterol circulates in plasma as a component of lipoproteins. There are several distinct classes of plasma lipoprotein which differ in several respects, including type of apolipoprotein and relative content of triacylglycerol and cholesterol.

Cholesterol transport

Chylomicron remnants deliver dietary cholesterol to the liver. It is then incorporated into very low-density lipoproteins (VLDL) which are secreted in plasma. The very low-density lipoproteins acquire cholesteryl esters and apolipoprotein E (apo E) from high-density lipoproteins (HDL) to produce intermediate-density lipoproteins (IDL), which are rapidly taken up by the liver or are further catabolized into low-density lipoproteins (LDL). These cholesterol-rich LDL particles are catabolized only slowly in human plasma and are therefore present at relatively high concentrations. Elimination of cholesterol from these extrahepatic cells is achieved by the delivery of cholesterol from cell membranes to plasma HDL in the first step of a pathway known as reverse cholesterol transport. This process allows for esterification of cholesterol and its delivery back to the liver.

LDL, HDL and atherosclerosis

Membrane function is compromised if it contains either too much or too little cholesterol. Epidemiological studies have classified raised plasma cholesterol levels as a risk factor for atherosclerosis and it is one of the more important predictors of coronary heart disease (CHD). Elevated plasma cholesterol concentration (hypercholesterolaemia) is associated with an increased concentration of LDL, owing to either an increased rate of LDL formation or a decrease in the rate at which they are cleared from plasma, and usually a decreased concentration of

HDL. Numerous dietary intervention studies have aimed to prevent both CHD and reduce total mortality, but almost all have been ineffective.

MUFA and CHD

Many of the trials conducted concentrated on the substitution of polyunsaturated vegetable oils for saturated fat from animal sources and on decreasing the amount of dietary cholesterol. These studies followed the reasoning that fats rich in saturated fatty acids (SFA) raised plasma cholesterol mainly by increasing plasma LDL cholesterol levels, and oils rich in polyunsaturated fatty acids (PUFA) lowered plasma cholesterol mainly by decreasing LDL cholesterol. The MUFA were first considered neutral in regard to their influence on plasma cholesterol, but more recent findings suggest a decrease in total LDL cholesterol concentration following substitution of SFA by MUFA. Moreover, clinical trials have also shown that a MUFA-rich diet does not decrease HDL concentrations, the lipoprotein inversely correlated with CHD.

Although important links exist between cholesterol metabolism and aspects of cell function, other complicating factors must be considered. Cholesterol metabolism is sensitive to the inflammatory response, which accompanies most pathological events. Tumour necrosis factor (TNF) reduces LDL and HDL cholesterol levels and inhibits lipoprotein lipase, resulting in a fall in cholesterol and an increase in triacylglycerol levels. These changes may be perpetuated beyond the acute phase if an inflammatory process is present. Cholesterol metabolism is also sensitive to genetic and environmental factors which may have independent effects on noncardiovascular disease. As a consequence, the relationship between cholesterol levels and the presence or absence of a disease state must be interpreted with caution.

Atherogenesis and Endothelial Dysfunction

Atherosclerosis can be considered as a chronic inflammatory disease which slowly progresses over a period of decades before clinical symptoms become manifest. The atherogenic process comprises interactions between multiple cell types which initiate a cascade of events involving alterations in vascular production of autocoids, cytokines and growth factors. The endothelium, because of its location between blood and the vascular wall, has been implicated in the atherogenic process from the initial stages.

Function of endothelial cells

Owing to the strategic location of the endothelium, it is able to perform many different functions. In addition to acting as a protective barrier, endothelial cells have been shown to play important roles in control of homeostasis, capillary transport and, more importantly, in regulation of the tone of underlying vascular smooth muscle. The endothelium evokes relaxation of these muscle cells, allowing vasodilation via the chemical factor endothelium-derived relaxing factor (EDRF), which has been identified as nitric oxide (NO). The EDRF or NO is vital for maintaining the vasodilatory capacity of vascular muscle and also controls levels of platelet function and monocyte adhesion. Any endothelial injury or dysfunction could therefore be an important factor in atherosclerosis.

Endothelial dysfunction

Decrease in the production, release or action of NO may lead to enhanced expression of adhesion molecules and chemotactic factors at the endothelial surface. The exact nature of endothelial dysfunction is unknown, although possibilities include a decreased expression of NO synthase, imbalance between the production of endothelium-derived constricting and relaxing factors, production of an endogenous NO synthase inhibitor and overproduction of oxygen-derived free radicals including O_2^-. The release of the free radical O_2^- from smooth muscle cells is believed to be responsible for the oxidation of LDL cholesterol. Raised cholesterol levels and – more importantly – increased levels of oxidatively modified LDL cholesterol (OxLDL) are considered to be among the most powerful inhibitors of normal endothelial function, and hence contribute to the process of atherogenesis.

Lipid peroxidation and atherosclerosis

Lipid peroxidation apparently plays a major role in the pathology of atherosclerosis. Atherosclerosis, which is usually a precondition for CHD, is a degenerative process leading to the accumulation of a variable mixture of substances including lipid in the endothelium of the arteries. This disease is characterized by the formation of a fatty streak and the accumulation of cells loaded with lipid: the foam cells. These cells are believed to arise from white blood cell-derived macrophages or arterial smooth muscle cells. Most of the lipid in the foam cells is in the form of LDL particles. Although research has determined that LDL receptors are responsible for the uptake of LDL by cells, the arterial uptake of LDL, which leads to development of foam cells,

occurs by a different pathway. It is only when the LDL particles have undergone oxidative modification that they are available for uptake by macrophages via the scavenger receptor. During the course of oxidative modification, LDL cholesterol acquires various biological properties not present in native LDL that make it a potentially important mediator, promoting atherogenesis. The LDL, once oxidized, becomes cytotoxic and causes local cellular damage to the endothelium. This process, which enhances LDL uptake to generate foam cells, is considered one of the earliest events in atherogenesis (**Fig. 2**).

MUFA and atherogenesis

Studies have looked at the oxidizability *in vitro* of LDL using nonphysiological oxidizing conditions to evaluate the susceptibility of LDL to oxidation and hence its atherogenic potential. It is well known that modification of LDL is inhibited by various antioxidants commonly present within plasma LDL particles. More recent studies, however, indicate that raising the ratio of $C_{18:1}$ to $C_{18:2}$ (linoleic acid) may also reduce the susceptibility of LDL to oxidation. The LDL is particularly vulnerable to peroxidation once PUFA forms part of the lipoprotein fraction of cell membranes, as these fatty acids have reactive double bonds in their structure. The MUFA are much less easily oxidized as they have only one double bond. This property may confer a protective effect against CHD by generating LDL particles more resistant to oxidation. Further protection may be afforded from MUFA as they do not lower HDL lipoprotein. It is postulated that oxidized HDL, in contrast to oxidized LDL, is not avidly taken up by macrophages, but instead inhibits the modification of LDL, thereby substantially decreasing oxidized LDL cellular uptake.

Oxidation of LDL cholesterol is, therefore, clearly linked to damage to the endothelium and hence to

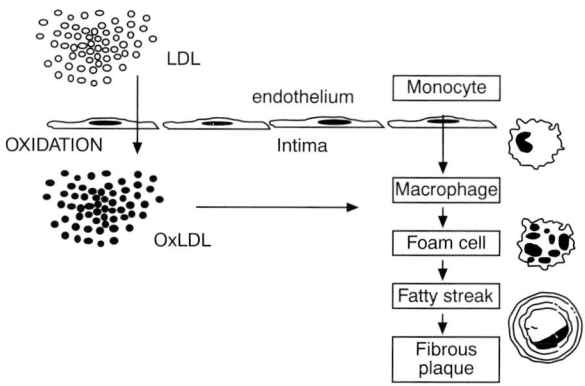

Figure 2 The role of oxidized LDL (OxLDL) in formation of foam cells. From Ashwell (1993).

the process of atherogenesis. It has, however, more far-reaching effects, as it has also been linked to activation and aggregation of platelets. This process is involved in the production of occlusive thrombosis, which contributes significantly to the fibrous atherosclerotic plaque.

Thrombosis and Fibrinolysis

The importance of thrombosis in causing heart disease is receiving increasing attention. Thrombosis, in contrast to atherosclerosis, is an acute event resulting in the formation of a thrombus or blood clot, which is an aggregate of fibrin, platelets and red cells. Blood clotting or coagulation is an important process as it is responsible for repairing tissues after injury. Under normal physiological conditions, a blood clot forms at the site of injury. Platelets are attracted to the damaged tissue and adhere to the surface. They are then activated to release substances which attract more platelets, allowing platelet aggregation, and triggering coagulation mechanisms.

The coagulation cascade

The process of blood coagulation involves two pathways: the extrinsic and intrinsic pathways (**Fig. 3**). The cascade is dependent on a series of separate clotting factors, each of which act as a catalyst for the next step in the system. The process results in the formation of insoluble fibrin from the soluble protein fibrinogen. This then interacts with a number of blood components, including red blood cells, to form the thrombus. Any damage to the endothelium, therefore, causes platelet aggregation and adherence to the lining of the blood vessels walls, thereby triggering the coagulation cascade. An imbalance of this process, by increasing the rate of thrombus formation, could increase the risk of CHD, and data have shown that levels of factor VII and fibrinogen are particularly important in balancing the coagulation cascade.

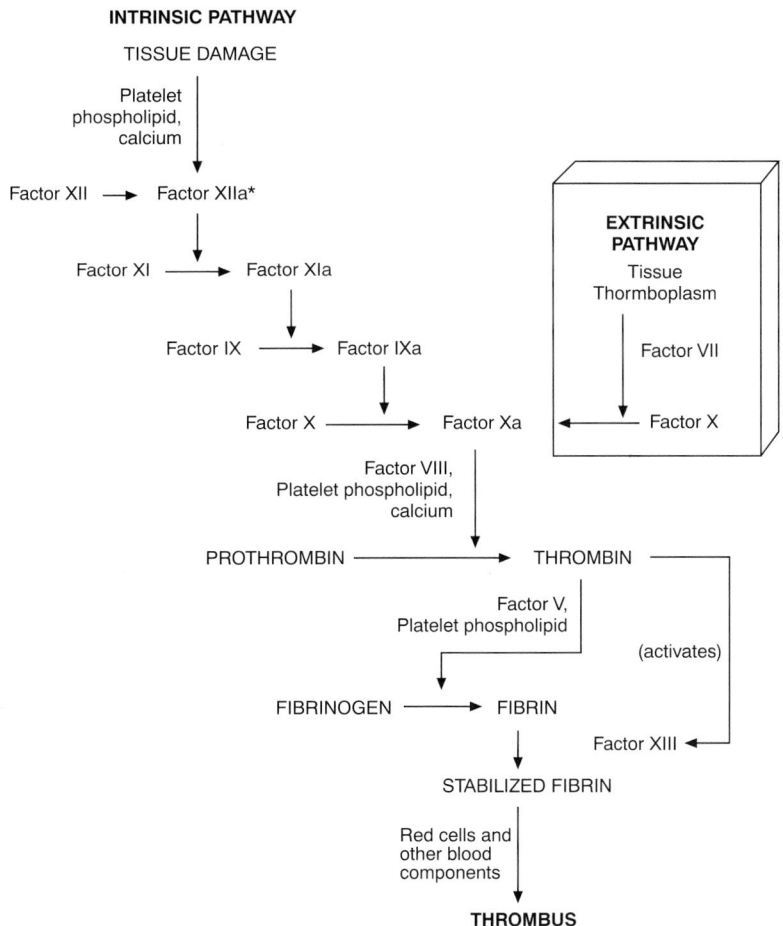

Figure 3 The coagulation cascade; a, active. From Buttriss JL and Gray J (1992) *Coronary Heart Disease II, Fact File 8*. London: National Dairy Council. Copyright National Dairy Council.

Factor VII and fibrinogen

There is accumulating evidence the factor VII is involved in arterial thrombosis and atherogenesis. The physiology of the factor VII system is intricate, not least since it can potentially exist in several forms. Activation of factor VIIc is generally achieved by tissue factor, and initiates blood coagulation by subsequent activation of factors IX and X. It has been further suggested that tissue factor associated with the lipoproteins LDL and VLDL, but not HDL, may possibly generate factor VIIc activity, and a direct relationship is believed to exist between the level of factor VII complex in plasma and the dietary influence on plasma triacylglycerol concentration.

Several mechanisms have been suggested whereby an increase in plasma fibrinogen concentration may be linked to CHD. These include the involvement of fibrinogen and fibrin in the evolution of the atheromatous plaque through fibrin deposition and in platelet aggregation through its impact on blood viscosity, which in turn is related to the risk of thrombosis. A mechanism exists to dissolve the thrombus by the breakdown or lysis of the fibrin meshwork (fibrinolysis). Plasminogen, which is generated by plasmin, is the zymosan which ultimately effects fibrinolysis. Failure of the mechanism to activate will cause obstruction of blood vessels and prevent normal blood supply.

Fibrinolysis

Investigators have shown that a decrease in the release of tissue plasminogen activator (tPA), and an elevation of plasminogen activator inhibitor 1 (PAI-1) will reduce fibrinolytic function. It has emerged that triacylglycerol-rich lipoproteins stimulate PAI-1 secretion from endothelial cells, and furthermore it has been shown that OxLDL induces secretion, whereas native LDL has no detectable effect. Lipoprotein (a) (Lp(a)) has also been linked with a decrease in fibrinolysis. Lp(a) is a LDL-like particle consisting of the protein apo(a). It is believed that apo(a) competes with plasminogen and plasmin for binding to fibrin, thus interfering with fibrinolysis; LDL and Lp(a) may represent, therefore, an important link between thrombotic and lipid mechanisms in atherogenesis.

MUFA and thrombosis

Results from animal studies have shown an elevation of platelet activation and hence greater risk of thrombosis as a result of feeding saturated fat. Platelet aggregation thresholds, however, decrease when total fat intake is decreased or when dairy and animal fats are partially replaced with vegetable oils rich in PUFA. These studies failed, however, to keep the intakes of SFA and total fat constant. More recent work has shown that, in fact, diets high in PUFA significantly increase platelet aggregation in animals, compared with MUFA-rich diets. The changes in fatty acid composition may affect blood clotting because the increase in PUFA allows for oxidation of LDL. As previously mentioned, OxLDL is cytotoxic and this can cause endothelial damage leading to the activation of platelets, generation of factor VII and hence thrombus formation. Increased dietary intakes of MUFA may also increase the rate of fibrinolysis by lowering levels of LDL cholesterol and reducing the susceptibility of LDL to oxidation, and thereby affecting both PAI-1 secretion and apo(a) activity.

It must be noted that both atherosclerosis and thrombosis are triggered by inflammation, and evidence suggests that several haemostatic factors other than the glycoprotein fibrinogen not only have an important role in thrombotic events but are also recognized as potentially important CHD risk factors.

Inflammation and Oxidative Damage

Many diseases that have an inflammatory basis such as cancer, sepsis and chronic inflammatory diseases like rheumatoid arthritis (RA) have symptoms mediated by pro-inflammatory mediators named cytokines. These mediators, which include interleukins (IL) 1–8, tumour necrosis factors (TNF) and interferons, are essential for protection from invading bodies. They act by producing a situation in which immune cells are attracted to the inflammatory site and are activated. An inflammatory stimulus, such as tissue damage incurred by trauma or invasion of tissue by bacteria or viruses, induces production of IL-1, IL-6 and TNF from a range of immune cells, including phagocytic leucocytes, and T and B lymphocytes. Once induced, IL-6, IL-1 and TNF further induce each other's production, and leading to a cascade of cytokines, which are capable of producing metabolic and immune effects. Inflammatory stimuli also bring about the activation of neutrophils to release free radicals, which enhance the production of TNF and other cytokines. Overproduction of these pro-inflammatory mediators may, therefore, allow excessive release of reactive oxygen species into extracellular fluid to damage its macromolecular components.

Oxidative damage

Free radicals are any species capable of an independent existence that contain one or more unpaired electrons. Reactive Oxygen Species (ROS) is a collective term, referring not only to oxygen-centred radicals such as superoxide (O_2^-) and the hydroxy radical ($\cdot OH$), but also to hydrogen peroxide (H_2O_2), ozone (O_3) and singlet oxygen ($^1O_2$). These are produced as the by-products of normal metabolism and, as such, are highly reactive in chemical terms. In order to become more stable chemically, the free radical reacts with other molecules by either donating or taking an electron, in either case leaving behind another unstable molecule, and hence this becomes a chain reaction. So, although oxygen is essential for life, in certain circumstances it may also be toxic. Damage caused by ROS to cellular target sites includes oxidative damage to proteins, membranes (lipid and proteins) and to DNA. Polyunsaturated fatty acids are particularly vulnerable to ROS attack because they have unstable double bonds in their structure. This process is termed 'lipid peroxidation'; because PUFA are an essential part of the phospholipid fraction of cell membranes, uncontrolled lipid peroxidation can lead to considerable cellular damage. The balance of MUFA in cell membranes is also critical to cell function, but as already noted, MUFA are far less vulnerable to lipid peroxidation.

MUFA and inflammation

Oxidative damage by ROS to DNA and lipids contributes significantly to the aetiology of cancer and atherosclerosis. A decrease in production of pro-inflammatory mediators would, therefore, be beneficial by decreasing the release of ROS. Diminishing the production of cytokines is also believed to improve the symptoms of RA. It has been suggested that olive oil may have antiinflammatory properties as it can reduce the production of these pro-inflammatory mediators. Although few studies have been carried out on the benefits of olive oil on symptoms of inflammation, it is possible that olive oil produces a similar effect to fish oil. Fish oils and butter have both been shown to reverse the pro-inflammatory effects of one cytokine, TNF. Further research, where $C_{18:1}$ was added to a diet containing coconut oil, resulted in responses to TNF that were similar to those seen in animals fed butter. It was assumed that as the antiinflammatory effects of butter appeared to be owing to its 18:1 content, olive oil should be more antiinflammatory. This was put to the test, and while both butter and olive oil reduced the extent of a number of symptoms of inflammation, olive oil showed a greater potency than butter. From this, it can be concluded that dietary factors such as olive oil may play a significant protective role in the development severity of RA.

Carcinogenesis

Cancer is second only to CHD as a cause of death in Western countries. Cancer in humans is a multistep disease process in which a single cell can develop from an otherwise normal tissue into a malignancy that can eventually destroy the organism. Carcinogenesis is believed to proceed through three distinct stages. Initiation is brought about when carcinogens mutate a single cell. This mutation provides a growth advantage and cells rapidly proliferate during the second stage, promotion. Tumour promotion produces relatively benign growths that can be converted into cancer in the third stage, malignant conversion. While the causes of cancer are not known with certainty, both initiation and conversion require some form of genetic alteration, and ROS and other free radicals have long been known to be mutagenic (**Fig. 4**).

Oxidation and cancer

Although PUFA are the most reactive of substrates for ROS attack leading to lipid peroxidation, interest is centring on the detection of oxidized nucleic acids as an indicator of prooxidant conditions. It has been indicated that significant oxidative damage occurs *in vitro* and contributes to the aetiology of cancer. It has become apparent that many genotoxic agents act through the common mechanism of oxidative damage to DNA. Oxidative processes may be responsible for initiating carcinogenic changes via DNA oxidative damage and may also act as tumour promoters, modulating the expression of genes that regulate cell differentiation and growth and act synergistically with the initiators. Animal studies have indicated diets containing high levels of $C_{18:2}$ as strong promoters of tumours and this may be as a result of increased oxidative stress. The fact that MUFA are much less readily oxidized may therefore confer a protective effect against carcinogenesis.

Immune function and cancer

The diet is believed to play an important role in the onset of carcinogenesis and there are a number of carcinogens present in food, including mycotoxins, polycyclic hydrocarbons and pesticides. Associations have been made between dietary fat intake and morbidity and mortality from breast and colon cancer. Another possible mechanism for the proposed protective effects against cancer of olive oil compared with sunflower oil involve diet-induced alterations in host immune responses. Both the type and concentration of dietary fats have been reported to influence immune status in several animal models. The PUFA $C_{18:2}$ is necessary for T cell-mediated immunity, but

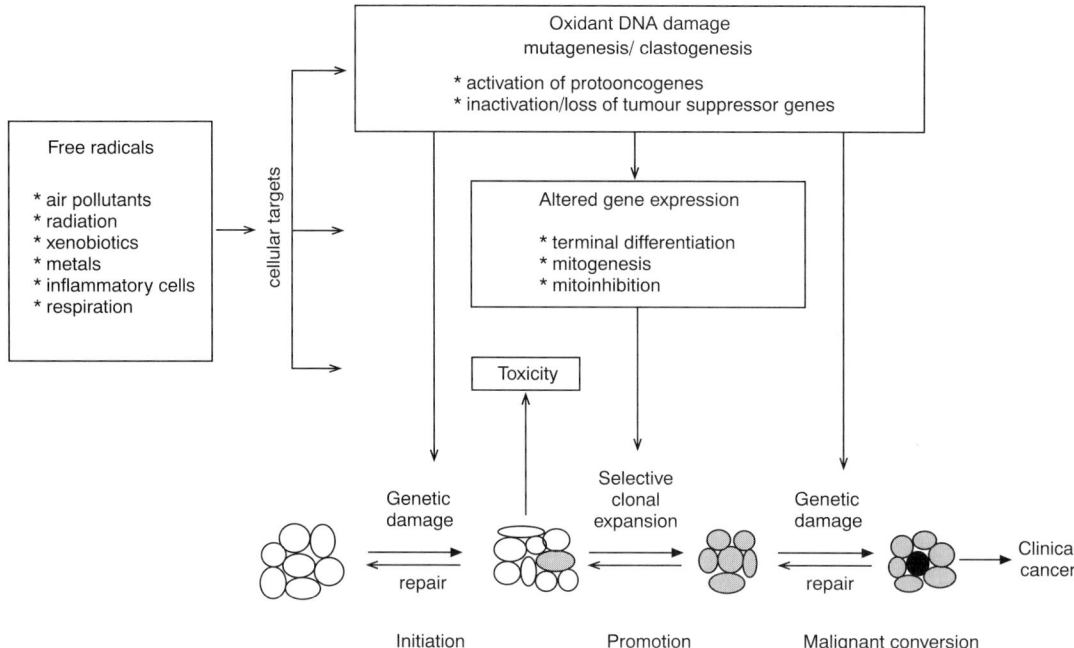

Figure 4   The role of oxidants in multistage carcinogenesis. From Guyton and Kensler (1993).

high intakes will suppress immune function and may therefore increase the risk of cancer. Furthermore, comparisons between the effects of diets rich in $C_{18:2}$ and $C_{18:1}$ on varying indicators of immune function in mice have shown that while dietary $C_{18:2}$ predisposed animals to suppression of certain T cell-mediated reactions, diets rich in $C_{18:1}$ did not. MUFA may therefore have a significant effect in humans against cancer, by lowering the risk of suppression of T cell activity.

Other Physiological Effects

Because many, sometimes competing, mechanisms appear to mediate the relation between intake of MUFA and CHD incidence, no single surrogate biochemical or physiological response can predict with confidence the effect of a particular dietary pattern. For this reason examination of the relation between specific dietary factors and CHD incidence itself are particularly valuable because such studies integrate the effects of all known and unknown mechanisms. The extremely low rates of CHD in countries with high consumption of olive oil, for instance, suggests the benefits of substituting this fat for other fats. This kind of analysis has been expanded further by noting that MUFA intake is inversely associated to total mortality as well as CHD. Some effects may well be because of the amount of antioxidant vitamins olive oil contains. Vegetable oils are the most important source of α-tocopherol in most diets, and olive oil contains about 12 mg per 100 g. Evidence indicates

that α-tocopherol functions as a free radical scavenger to protect cellular membranes from oxidative destruction. Oxidative stress has been linked to an increased risk of many chronic diseases, including atherosclerosis, cancer and inflammatory disorders. Other injuries such as cataract and reperfusion injury are also associated with an increase in oxidative stress and a decrease in antioxidant activity.

A large body of evidence suggests a beneficial effect of MUFA in the diet. Although much remains to be learned about the mechanisms by which $C_{18:1}$ acts, it is believed to lower risks of CHD, several common cancers, cataracts and other inflammatory disorders. It is suggested, therefore, that consuming MUFA, for instance in the form of olive oil as used widely in the Mediterranean diet, is likely to enhance long-term health.

See also: **Antioxidants**: Diet and Antioxidant Defence. **Arthritis**: Dietary Aspects of Aetiology and Nutritional Management. **Cancer**: Epidemiology and Associations Between Diet and Cancer; Epidemiology of Breast Cancer. **Cholesterol**: Sources, Absorption, Function and Metabolism; Factors Determining Blood Cholesterol Levels. **Coronary Heart Disease**: Lipid Theory of Coronary Heart Disease; Haemostatic Factors and Coronary Heart Disease; Aetiology; Prevention. **Cytokines**: Nutritional Aspects. **Dairy Products**: Nutritional Value. **Fats and Oils**: Nutritional Value. **Fatty Acids**: Metabolism; Health Effects of Saturated Fatty Acids; Health Effects of n-6 Polyunsaturated Fatty Acids; Health Effects of n-3 Polyunsaturated Fatty Acids; Health Effects of *trans* Fatty

Acids. **Immunity**: Physiological Aspects. **Lipids**: Chemistry and Classification. **Lipoproteins**: Physiology.

Further Reading

Ashwell M (1993) *Diet and Heart Disease – A Round Table of Factors*. London: British Nutrition Foundation.

Barter P (1994) Cholesterol and cardiovascular disease: basic science. *Australia and New Zealand Journal of Medicine* 24:83–88.

Besler HT and Grimble RF (1993) Modulation of the response of rats to endotoxin by butter and olive and corn oil. *Proceedings of the Nutrition Society* 52:68A.

Cerutti PA (1985) Prooxidant states and tumor promotion. *Science* 227:375–381.

Daae LW, Kierulf P, Landass S and Urdal P (1993) Cardiovascular risk factors: interactive effects of lipid, coagulation, and fibrinolysis. *Scandinavian Journal of Clinical Laboratory Investigation*. 532(15):19–27.

Dunnigan MG (1993) The problem with cholesterol. No light at the end of the tunnel. *British Medical Journal* 306:1355–1356.

Ernst E (1993) The role of fibrinogen as a cardiovascular risk factor. *Atherosclerosis* 100:1–12.

Guyton KZ and Kensler TW (1993) Oxidative mechanisms in carcinogenesis. *British Medical Bulletin* 49:523–544.

Halliwell B (1989) Tell me about free radicals, doctor: a review. *Journal of the Royal Society of Medicine* 82:747–752.

Hannigan BM (1994) Diet and immune function. *British Journal of Biomedical Science* 51:252–259.

Hoff HF and O'Neil J (1991) Lesion-derived low density lipoprotein and oxidized low density lipoprotein share a lability for aggregation, leading to enhanced macrophage degradation. *Arteriosclerosis and Thrombosis* 11:1209–1222.

Linos A, Kaklamanis E and Kontomerkos A (1991) The effect of olive oil and fish consumption on rheumatoid arthritis – a case control study. *Scandinavian Journal of Rheumatology* 20:419–426.

Mensink RP and Katan MB (1989) An epidemiological and an experimental study on the effect of olive oil on total serum and HDL cholesterol in healthy volunteers. *European Journal of Clinical Nutrition* 43(supplement 2):43–48.

Morel DW, Dicorleto PE and Chisolm GM (1984) Endothelial and smooth muscle cells alter low density lipoprotein *in vitro* by free radical oxidation. *Arteriosclerosis* 4:357–364.

National Dairy Council (1992) *Coronary Heart Disease*. Fact File No. 8. London: NDC.

Visioli F and Galli C (1995) Natural antioxidants and prevention of coronary heart disease: the potential role of olive oil and its minor constituents. *Nutrition Metabolism and Cardiovascular Disease* 5:306–314.

Health Effects of n-6 Polyunsaturated Fatty Acids

J Hodgson, University Department of Medicine, Perth, Western Australia

Mark L Wahlqvist, Monash Medical Centre, Victoria, Australia

Copyright © 1998 Academic Press

Presented in this article is a summary of several of the major fields of research on the health effects of n-6 polyunsaturated fatty acids (PUFAs). The first sections focus on the effects of n-6 PUFAs on cardiovascular disease (CVD) and its major risk factors. The main topics discussed are cholesterol and lipoprotein metabolism, lipoprotein oxidation, and atherosclerosis and CVD. A presentation of the roles of n-6 PUFAs in endothelial function, thrombosis and inflammation, including a brief discussion of eicosanoids, then follows. Finally, the potential involvement of n-6 fatty acids in carcinogenesis and relationships with various cancers are discussed.

Structure and Function of n-6 Fatty Acids

The n-6 fatty acids are a class of polyunsaturated fatty acids (PUFAs) with two or more *cis*-unsaturated centres separated from each other by one methyl group, and having the first unsaturated centre six carbon atoms from the methyl end of the molecule. The general formula of n-6 fatty acids is $CH_3(CH_2)_4(CH=CHCH_2)_x(CH_2)_yCOOH$, where $x = 2–5$. Linoleic acid (*cis*-9, *cis*-12-octadecaenoic acid, 18:2n-6) serves as a precursor of a family of n-6 fatty acids formed by chain elongation and desaturation in which the n-6 terminal is retained. Enzymes involved in elongation and desaturation are common to the n-6 and n-3 series of fatty acids. In addition, metabolic roles and functions of these two series of fatty acids are often related.

Fatty acids from the n-6 and n-3 series are classed as essential fatty acids (EFA). The two most important n-6 EFAs, with respect to biological functions in animals, are 18:2n-6 and arachidonic acid (*cis*-5, *cis*-8, *cis*-11, *cis*-14-eicosatetraenoic acid, 20:4n-6). 20:4n-6 can be derived by chain elongation and desaturation of 18:2n-6, or directly from dietary sources.

The functions of n-6 EFAs can be broadly grouped into two main areas. First, they are incorporated into the cell membrane phospholipids in humans where they have an important structural and functional role. Clinical indications of EFA deficiency are suggestive of impaired membrane function. Second, 20:4n-6 serves as a major precursor for eicosanoids, which are hormone-like compounds with wide ranging activities.

Cholesterol and Lipoprotein Metabolism

Cholesterol is the most common animal sterol. It occurs only in foods of animal origin, but can also be biosynthesized by humans, so no dietary requirement has been established. Cholesterol plays a vital role in cell membranes, and serves as a precursor for bile acids, adrenal hormones, sex hormones and vitamin D_3.

A major interest in cholesterol metabolism has been in relation to atherosclerosis and cardiovascular disease (CVD). Between-population studies have shown positive associations between blood total cholesterol concentrations and CVD risk. In addition, lowering of blood cholesterol concentrations can reduce cardiovascular mortality. Furthermore, cholesterol accumulation in the arterial wall is recognized as an early event in the development of atherosclerosis. Cholesterol circulates in blood as part of lipoprotein particles. The metabolism of these particles plays a role in the development and progression of atherosclerosis and CVD.

n-6 Fatty acids and the lipoproteins

The major classes of lipoproteins circulating in human plasma are chylomicrons, very low-density lipoproteins (VLDL), low-density lipoproteins (LDL) and high-density lipoproteins (HDL). High fasting plasma concentrations of LDL cholesterol and triglycerides – predominantly circulating as part of VLDL – and low plasma concentrations of HDL cholesterol are associated with increased risk of CVD. Dietary fatty acids can influence lipoprotein metabolism, and therefore have the potential to influence atherosclerosis and CVD risk. Most studies examining the effects of n-6 PUFAs on cholesterol metabolism have focused on 18:2n-6, the major dietary n-6 fatty acid.

In the fasting state LDL is the major cholesterol-carrying lipoprotein in human plasma. Higher plasma concentrations of LDL cholesterol are associated with an increased risk of CVD. The mechanisms through which raised plasma LDL cholesterol concentrations increase CVD risk are not entirely understood, but oxidative modification of LDL is thought to be involved. Furthermore, it is now established that lowering LDL cholesterol reduces the risk of CVD. An increase in 18:2n-6 intake results in a

lowering of plasma LDL cholesterol concentrations, and therefore has the potential to reduce CVD risk. These effects may not be linear over the entire range of 18:2n-6 intake, and most of the benefits appear to be gained by moving from lower (<2% of energy) to moderate (~ 4–5% of energy) intakes. In addition, it is worthy of note that the effects of dietary n-6 PUFAs are less than half that of lowering dietary saturated fatty acids. Therefore if total fat intake is maintained, the LDL cholesterol-lowering effects of increasing n-6 PUFA intake are greatly enhanced if saturated fatty acid intake is decreased.

HDL cholesterol is inversely associated with CVD risk. The mechanism by which HDL reduces CVD risk remains to be established, but there is evidence that HDL participates in reverse cholesterol transport and reduces cholesterol accumulation in the arterial wall. Intakes of 18:2n-6 within the normal ranges of intakes in most populations do not appear to alter HDL cholesterol concentrations. However, very high intakes – above 12% of energy – can lower HDL cholesterol concentrations.

Although LDL is the major cholesterol-carrying lipoprotein in the fasting state, over a 24 h period chylomicrons are also major cholesterol-carrying lipoproteins. Raised concentrations of chylomicron remnant particles are suggested to be a risk factor for CVD, and may be a major contributor to the deposition of lipid, and cholesterol in particular, into the arterial wall (thought to be an early event in the development of atherosclerosis). Studies that have assessed the effect of fatty acid composition of the diet on remnant clearance are limited and have been difficult to interpret. Results of some studies suggest that PUFAs may improve clearance. However, in general, the fatty acid composition of the diet does not appear to be a major factor influencing remnant clearance. It is therefore unlikely that the n-6 fatty acid composition of the diet can greatly influence remnant clearance. Nevertheless, there may be more subtle influences of n-6 and other fatty acids on remnant metabolism.

Lipoprotein Oxidation

Oxidative damage to cells and tissues is thought to play a role in the development of chronic diseases including atherosclerotic CVD. Increasing evidence suggests that oxidative modification of LDL, and possibly other lipoproteins, is involved in atherogenesis. n-6 PUFAs enhance the susceptibility of LDL to oxidation *in vitro*, when compared with monounsaturated fatty acids. However, these findings do not provide evidence for a direct link between LDL n-6 fatty acid composition, LDL oxidation, and atherosclerosis. Other factors, such as the presence of antioxidants, may influence *in vivo* oxidation. The dietary source of n-6 PUFAs, and the overall diet, may therefore be determinants of the ultimate susceptibility of LDL to oxidative damage.

Atherosclerosis and Cardiovascular Disease

Alterations to the normal structure and function of the vasculature is the major factor involved in the development and progression of CVD. Atherosclerosis is a disease characterized by degenerative changes, deposition of cholesterol, proliferation of smooth muscle cells and fibrosis. Resulting atheromatous plaques cause narrowing of arteries and increase the likelihood of occlusion. This process occurring in coronary arteries can result in myocardial infarction and death.

n-6 Fatty acids and cardiovascular disease

When exploring the influence of n-6 PUFAs on atherosclerosis it is useful to examine relationships between n-6 PUFA intake and rates of CVD within and between populations. Natural human experiments of high intakes of n-6 PUFAs are the Israelis, Taiwanese and !Kung bushmen in the African Kalahari desert. The contribution of n-6 PUFAs to total energy intake has been estimated to be around 10% in the Israelis and Taiwanese and about 30% in the !Kung bushmen. Rates of CVD are low in the Taiwanese, where the dietary n-6 PUFAs are obtained mainly from soya bean oil, and estimated to be very low in the !Kung bushmen, where the dietary n-6 PUFAs were obtained mainly from the monongo fruit and nut. In the Taiwanese the Soya bean oil is refined, but is accompanied by a diet rich in antioxidant polyphenols, notably from Chinese oolong tea, fruits and vegetables, and in the !Kung bushmen the oil is unrefined. There is, however, a high prevalence of CVD in the Israeli population, where n-6 PUFAs are obtained largely from refined sources. These observations suggest that a high n-6 PUFA intake is compatible with low risk of CVD, but this may not be the case where n-6 fatty acids are consumed against a background diet low in antioxidants.

It is also useful to explore relationships between n-6 PUFA intake and CVD end points such as angina, myocardial infarction and coronary heart disease death. Atherosclerosis is implicated in CVD end points but can be more difficult to measure. A higher intake of 18:2n-6, which can be determined either by direct assessment of dietary intake or by measurement of 18:2n-6 in adipose tissue (which provides a good estimate of long-term intake), has

been associated with a reduced risk of heart disease – angina, myocardial infarction or sudden death. However, studies which have used end points of structural changes in the arteries, possibly relating more to atherosclerosis, are not suggestive of a benefit of higher 18:2n-6 intake. Several factors may need to be considered in the interpretation of these results. The effect of 18:2n-6 on atherosclerosis and CVD may depend upon the background intake levels in the population being studied. Relationships observed may also relate to intake of other foods from which 18:2n-6 derives. Observed relationships may be due to other dietary factors related to 18:2n-6 intake. Finally, 18:2n-6 may be protective against CVD events due to beneficial effects on endothelial function, thrombosis and arrhythmia rather than the development of atherosclerosis. Therefore, although a low intake of 18:2n-6 is associated with an increased risk of heart disease, a causative relationship has not been proven.

n-6 Fatty acids and cardiovascular disease risk factors

Two of the major established risk factors for atherosclerosis and CVD are hypertension and hypercholesterolaemia or dyslipidaemia. n-6 fatty acids have the potential to influence atherosclerosis and CVD via effects on these major risk factors. The effects of n-6 PUFAs on lipoprotein and cholesterol metabolism have been discussed.

The possible effects of dietary fatty acids on blood pressure have been explored in population studies and dietary intervention trials. With the exception of studies comparing vegetarian and nonvegetarian populations, from which there is a suggestion of a blood pressure-lowering effect of diets high in PUFAs, including 18:2n-6, and lower in saturated fatty acids, the results of most within- and between-population studies have generally not found significant associations. The results of intervention studies suggest that n-6 fatty acids, 18:2n-6 in particular, may be responsible for a small blood pressure-lowering effect. However, these studies are also inconsistent, with several failing to find a significant blood pressure-lowering effect.

Endothelial Function

Functional changes in the vasculature also influence CVD, and many of these changes are related to endothelial function. The vascular endothelium is a single layer of epithelial cells lining blood vessels which has several important functions including regulation of vascular tone, coagulation and fibrinolysis. Endothelial cells form a monolayer between smooth muscle cells of the arterial wall and circulating blood cells. In response to circulating and mechanical signals, the vascular endothelium modulates contraction and proliferation of smooth muscle cells, platelet adhesion and aggregation, coagulation and monocyte adhesion through the release of various mediators including many eicosanoids. There is multiple and close interaction between the endothelial cells and circulating cells. The vascular endothelium is involved in the development of atherosclerosis, but is also thought to precede clinically apparent atherosclerotic disease; its function is adversely influenced by atherosclerosis. The vascular endothelium is also important in the control of thrombosis.

Studies in humans reveal associations between endothelial dysfunction and established risk factors for CVD. Dyslipidaemia, hypertension and perhaps other factors may induce changes in endothelial cell structure and function leading to atherosclerosis, increasing thrombotic tendency and further deterioration in endothelial function. It has also been shown that endothelial dysfunction can be reversed with cholesterol-lowering therapy. It is not clear whether lowering of blood pressure can reverse endothelial dysfunction. The effects of changes in n-6 PUFA intake on endothelial dysfunction have not been assessed.

The fatty acid composition of the membrane phospholipids of endothelial cells can be altered by feeding of dietary fatty acids. It appears that the membrane fatty acid composition can be extensively changed without influencing the overall general functioning of the cells. However, membrane composition does influence cellular reactions in which the fatty acids are involved. Therefore, although the effects of changes in n-6 fatty acid intake on endothelial function are not clearly understood, there is the potential for changes in n-6 PUFA intake to influence endothelial function via effects on membrane composition and eicosanoid production.

Eicosanoids: Roles in Endothelial Function, Thrombosis and Inflammation

One of the most important group of compounds which mediate endothelial function, thrombosis and inflammation are the eicosanoids. Eicosanoids is the common name given the metabolic products of 20-carbon PUFAs. The main eicosanoid precursor is 20:4n-6. The other major eicosanoid precursor fatty acids are dihomo-γ-linolenic acid (20:3n-6), which can also be derived from 18:2n-6, and eicosapentaenoic acid (20:5n-3). These fatty acids can be metabolized via three major enzymatic pathways, namely cyclooxygenases, lipoxygenases and cytochrome P-

450, giving rise to prostaglandins, leukotrienes and 5-, 12- and 15-hydroxyeicosatetraenoic acids and oxygenated metabolites, respectively. These eicosanoids have a diverse range of biological activities including effects on vasomotor tone, platelet aggregation and inflammatory processes.

Many of the eicosanoids derived from 20:4n-6 have potent pro-thrombotic and pro-inflammatory activity. Eicosanoids derived from the n-3 precursor generally have reduced biological activity, and are less pro-thrombotic and pro-inflammatory compared with the n-6 derived analogues. Eicosanoid production is generally tightly controlled through homeostatic mechanisms. However, when the system is disturbed in some way, such as with endothelial dysfunction, atherosclerosis and plaque rupture, and various thrombotic and inflammatory conditions, the balance of eicosanoids can be altered.

Prostaglandins and leukotrienes

The prostaglandins have a central role in the regulation of platelet aggregation and vascular tone. Two of the major prostaglandins derived from 20:4n-6 are thromboxane A_2, produced in platelets, and prostacyclin I_2, produced in endothelial cells. Thromboxane A_2 promotes platelet aggregation and blood vessel constriction, while prostacyclin I_2 has the opposite effects. An increase in availability of 20:5n-3 can decrease thromboxane A_2 and increase thromboxane A_3, while prostacyclin I_2 is unaffected and prostacyclin I_3 formation is stimulated. Thromboxane A_3 has little or no physiological activity and prostacyclin I_3 has similar activity to prostacyclin I_2. The net result is a shift in the thromboxane/prostacyclin balance towards a reduced pro-thrombotic state.

Leukotriene B_4 is a potent inflammatory mediator. Leukotriene B_4 is produced by neutrophils from 20:4n-6 at the site of injury, and is a powerful chemotactic factor responsible for attracting neutrophils to the site of injury. Leukotriene B_5, which is produced from 20:5n-3, has significantly lower biological activity. Therefore an increased availability of 20:5n-3 has the potential to result in a reduced pro-inflammatory state.

Fatty acid intake and eicosanoids

The proportional concentrations of the eicosanoid precursor fatty acids both circulating and in tissues depends upon dietary intake. 20:3n-6 and 20:4n-6 can be obtained from animal meat and fat, and by desaturation and chain elongation of 18:2n-6. The major dietary source of 20:5n-3 is fish. 20:5n-3 can also be obtained indirectly from 18:3n-3, although desaturation and chain elongation of 18:3n-3 appears to be a less important pathway.

Only the free form of the fatty acid precursors of eicosanoids can be converted into the biologically active metabolites. The amount of precursor free fatty acids in the cytoplasm and circulating is usually low and so, too, is the basal eicosanoid formation. Basal eicosanoid formation may depend upon dietary and adipose tissue fatty acid composition. The amount of eicosanoid precursor free fatty acid is also controlled by incorporation and release from cellular phospholipids. Which eicosanoids are produced during stimulated synthesis may depend upon membrane fatty acid composition. Dietary fatty acid composition therefore has the potential to affect basal and stimulated synthesis of eicosanoids and influence endothelial function, thrombosis and inflammation.

Thrombosis

Fatty acids can influence the processes involved in thrombosis through effects on the activity and function of endothelial cells, platelets and other blood cells. These effects can be mediated by alterations in eicosanoid metabolism. Studies examining the effect of dietary fatty acids on thrombosis indicate that an increase in n-3 fatty acid intake has the potential to increase vasodilation and inhibit platelet aggregation. In addition, epidemiological studies indicate that an increase in n-3 fatty acids can reduce the risk of thrombosis. It is not clear if the major factor influencing these functions is the absolute increase in n-3 fatty acids, or the relative proportions of n-6 and n-3 eicosanoid precursors. It is possible that an increased n-3 fatty acid intake is more beneficial in populations consuming small amounts of fish, the major dietary source. A similar benefit may be obtained in populations with low intakes of 18:2n-6. Inverse associations between adipose tissue 18:2n-6 and heart disease have been observed in such populations.

The role of platelets in thrombosis is established, and the influence of fatty acid intake on platelet function has been the subject of research. Platelets take part in thrombosis by adhering to and aggregating on the site of injury. Platelet reactivity and increased platelet activation may increase the risk of thrombosis. Because it is difficult to measure platelet reactivity *in vivo*, the main method used in platelet studies has been the *in vitro* aggregation test. The results of these studies are difficult to interpret. *In vitro* studies indicate that 18:2n-6 is antithrombotic, but there is no good evidence that a high 18:2n-6 diet in humans decreases platelet aggregation, and some studies have found increased aggregation with high 18:2n-6 diets. The effects of an increased 20:4n-6 intake in humans on platelet aggregation is also not

clear. One of the main difficulties in interpreting these studies is the unresolved issue as to how the *in vitro* aggregation test reflects platelet function *in vivo*.

Inflammation

Inflammatory processes are generally tightly controlled. However, a number of inflammatory conditions may be influenced by n-6, as well as by n-3, fatty acids. These conditions include inflammatory arthritis, dermatological conditions such as psoriasis and atopic dermatitis, chronic inflammatory bowel disease, autoimmune diseases and bronchial asthma. In relation to these conditions most of the research focus has been on the disease suppressive roles of n-3 fatty acids. Much of the evidence, which at this time is very limited, for a role of n-6 PUFAs in inflammatory conditions is from nutritional epidemiology rather than from intervention studies. To suppress a disease with candidate n-3 fatty acids is more acceptable than to risk exacerbating it with n-6 fatty acids.

Although epidemiological and intervention studies indicate that n-3 fatty acids have the potential to suppress inflammatory conditions, and n-6 fatty acids have the potential to exacerbate these conditions, it is not clear if absolute or relative intake of n-6 and n-3 fatty acids is more important, or if both can influence inflammatory processes. The effects of changes in n-6 fatty acid intake on inflammatory processes may depend upon the background dietary fatty acid intake, as well as proportional and absolute intake of n-3 fatty acids.

Carcinogenesis

There has been much controversy as to whether total fat intake or type of fat influences the risk of developing various cancers. The main cancers in question have been breast, prostate, colorectal and skin (melanoma and squamous cell carcinoma). Much of the research focus has been on total fat and saturated fat intake. Epidemiological studies suggest a positive association between total and saturated fat intake and risk of different cancers.

Much of the epidemiological research focus on the role of fat in carcinogenesis has been on breast cancer. For breast cancer, the results of between-population studies suggest a positive association between cancer rates and total fat intake. Results of within-population studies, particularly those conducted in North American populations, have not been consistent with this suggestion. However it may be possible that lower intakes of fat than that found in North

American populations may be necessary for a protective effect of low fat intake to be observed. An intake of total fat of less than 20% of energy, as it has been in several Asian populations such as China and Japan, may be necessary. In addition, low fat intake may need to be accompanied by nutritional protective factors for its benefits to be evident. Generally, where total fat is the issue, the major fat ingested, and therefore incriminated, is saturated animal fat.

There has also been some interest in the role of other fatty acid classes in carcinogenesis. The n-6 PUFAs promote tumorogenesis and tumour cell proliferation indirectly by increasing the synthesis of particular eicosanoids. The long-chain n-3 PUFAs suppress tumorogenesis and tumour cell proliferation by similar mechanisms. Increasing dietary n-6 PUFA intake may therefore enhance tumour development. Population studies, however, have generally failed to find a relationship between 18:2n-6 and risk of various cancers. In addition, studies which have examined the role of n-6 fatty acids in skin cancer indicate that, if anything, 18:2n-6 is protective.

Although experimental studies point to a link between n-6 PUFAs and carcinogenesis, there is by no means a clear relationship in humans. A possible explanation for the lack of a relationship with cancer risk in humans is that n-6 PUFA intake is often accompanied by factors which may be protective against tumour development. Examples of possible protective factors include vitamin E, tocotrienols and a wide variety of polyphenols including flavonoids and isoflavonoids. The more unrefined the dietary source of 18:2n-6, the more likely it is to contain factors protective against tumour development, and indeed other disease processes. These dietary interactions would seem most important in assessing the place of any fat in carcinogenesis.

Conclusions

Diets low in n-6 fatty acids, principally 18:2n-6, appear to be related to an increased risk of CVD. The results of studies examining the effects of 18:2n-6 on risk factors for atherosclerosis and CVD are consistent with this observation. They suggest that an increase in n-6 PUFA intake from a low to a moderate intake level, in conjunction with decreases in total and saturated fat intake, may beneficially influence lipoprotein metabolism, lower blood pressure, and reduce CVD risk. Observations in populations with high n-6 PUFA intake indicate that high intakes of n-6 fatty acids (>10%) can occur together with low rates of CVD and possibly also cancer. However, where antioxidant composition of the diet is low, there is the potential for increased risk of both

CVD and particular cancers. An increased susceptibility of PUFAs to oxidative damage, particularly in the presence of low concentrations of protective antioxidants, may be an important factor involved. The source of n-6 PUFAs in the diet – refined versus unrefined – and background diet of the individual and population may therefore be important determinants of whether high n-6 fatty acid intake increases or decreases risk of CVD and cancer.

In relation to eicosanoid metabolism and possible effects on endothelial function, thrombosis and inflammation, available evidence suggests that beneficial effects can be obtained with n-3 fatty acids derived mainly from fish. Although eicosanoids derived from the n-6 fatty acids are more pro-inflammatory and pro-thrombotic than those derived from the n-3 precursor, effects of altering n-6 PUFA intake on these processes are not clearly understood.

See also: **Cancer**: Epidemiology and Associations Between Diet and Cancer. **Cholesterol**: Sources, Absorption, Function and Metabolism. **Coronary Heart Disease**: Lipid Theory of Coronary Heart Disease. **Fatty Acids**: Health Effects of n-3 Polyunsaturated Fatty Acids. **Prostaglandins and Leukotrienes**: Physiology.

Further Reading

Grundy SM (1996) Dietary fat. In: Ziegler EE and Filer Jr LJ (eds) *Present Knowledge in Nutrition*, 7th edn, pp 44–57. Washington, DC:ILSI Press.

Henning B, Toborek M, Alvarado Cader A and Decker EA (1994) Nutrition, endothelial cell metabolism and atherosclerosis. *Critical Reviews in Food Science and Nutrition* 34:253–282.

Hodgson JM and Puddey IB (1996) Diet and the control of dyslipidaemia. *Modern Medicine of Australia*, March: 58–64.

Hodgson JM, Wahlqvist ML, Boxall, JA and Balazs NDH (1995) Can linoleic acid contribute to coronary artery disease? *American Journal of Clinical Nutrition* 58:228–234.

Hodgson JM, Wahlqvist ML and Hsu-Hage B (1995) Diet, hyperlipidaemia and cardiovascular disease. *Asia Pacific Journal of Clinical Nutrition* 4:304–313.

Horrobin DF (ed.) (1990) *Omega-6 Essential Fatty Acids: Pathophysiology and Roles in Clinical Medicine*. New York: Wiley-Liss.

Innis SM (1996) Essential dietary lipids. In: Ziegler EE and Filer Jr LJ (eds) *Present Knowledge in Nutrition*, 7th edn, pp 58–66. Washington, DC:ILSI Press.

Jones GP (1997) Fats. In: Wahlqvist ML (ed.) *Food and Nutrition, Australia, Asia and the Pacific*, pp 205–214. Sydney: Allen and Unwin.

Knapp HR (1997) Dietary fatty acids in human thrombosis and hemostasis. *American Journal of Clinical Nutrition* 65 (supplement 5): 1687S–1698S.

Kohlmeier L, Simonsen N and Mottus K (1995) Dietary modifiers of carcinogenesis. *Environmental Health Perspectives* **103** (supplement 18):177–184.

Lyu LC, Shieh MJ, Posner BM, Ordovas JM, Dwyer JT, Lichtenstein AH, Cupples LA, Dallal GE, Wilson PW, Schaefer EJ (1994) Relationship between dietary intake, lipoproteins and apolipoproteins in Taipei and Framingham. *American Journal of Clinical Nutrition* **60**:765–774.

Mensink R and Connor W (eds) (1996) Nutrition. *Current Opinion in Lipidology* **7**:1–53.

Miccozzi MS and Moon TE (1992) *Macronutrients: Investigating Their Role in Cancer.* New York: Marcel Decker Inc.

National Health and Medical Research Council (1992) *The role of polyunsaturated fats in the Australian diet: report of the NHMRC working party.* Canberra: Australian Government Publishing Service.

Salem N, Simopoulos AP, Galli, Lagarde M and Knapp HR (eds) (1996) Fatty acids and lipids from cell biology to human disease: Proceedings of the 2nd International Congress of the International Society for the Study of Fatty Acids and Lipids. *Lipids* **31** (supplement).

Truswell AS (1977) Diet and nutrition of hunter gatherers. *Ciba Foundation Symposium*:213–221.

Vane JR, Anggard EE and Botting RM (1990) Regulatory functions of the vascular endothelium. *New England Journal of Medicine* **323**:27–36.

Wahlqvist ML (1993) Nutritional factors in carcinogenesis. *Asia Pacific Journal of Clinical Nutrition* **2**:141–148.

Yam D, Eliraz A and Berry EM (1996) Diet and disease – the Israeli paradox: possible dangers of a high omega-6 polyunsaturated fatty acid diet. *Israeli Journal of Medical Sciences* **32**:1134–1143.

Health Effects of n-3 Polyunsaturated Fatty Acids

B Corridan and **A Wilson**, University College Cork, Ireland

Copyright © 1998 Academic Press

Cross-cultural comparisons have shown that the incidence of autoimmune disorders, inflammatory disorders and coronary heart disease (CHD) is low amongst Japanese and Inuit populations compared with Europeans. The diets of these populations are characterized by high fish intakes (100–400 g fish per day). This suggests that n-3 polyunsaturated fatty acid (PUFA) consumption may have a protective role against these types of disease. This has been supported by prospective epidemiological studies in Europe and the USA, in which persistent evidence indicates that death from coronary heart disease is more unusual in men who eat some fish than in men who do not. A controlled intervention trial with n-3 PUFA in the secondary prevention of myocardial infarction (MI) indicated that fatty fish or fish oil reduced mortality in men by approximately 29%. Intervention trials also indicate that n-3 PUFA may have beneficial therapeutic effects in inflammatory disorders such as Crohn's disease.

Cholesterol Metabolism

Effects of n-3 PUFA on plasma lipid levels

Numerous studies have documented the beneficial effects of lowering cholesterol levels in patients with established CHD. In addition, a coronary prevention study in the west of Scotland provided further evidence that cholesterol reduction is effective in the primary prevention of CHD in middle-aged men with hypercholesterolaemia. In 1989, a review of 41 supplementation studies demonstrated that n-3 PUFA had little effect on plasma total cholesterol and low-density lipoprotein (LDL) cholesterol levels. This has been confirmed by several subsequent investigations involving normolipidaemic and hyperlipidaemic subjects. However, many investigators have reported increases in plasma and LDL cholesterol levels when humans were supplemented with doses of 1.5–2 g of n-3 PUFA. This increase in LDL cholesterol concentration in response to n-3 PUFA supplementation may be due to an increased conversion of very low-density lipoprotein (VLDL) to LDL particles. In contrast, reductions in total and LDL cholesterol levels have been reported at high doses of n-3 PUFA (24 g). The reported variability in the effects of n-3 PUFA on total and LDL cholesterol levels may be attributable to the lipid status of the individual, the particular n-3 PUFA supplement administered, or the composition of the diet. The conflicting findings may be partly due to different effects in normolipidaemic and hyperlipidaemic patients. Studies that used large doses of n-3 PUFA may be testing the effect of a change in fat quality and in the polyunsaturated to saturated fat (P : S) ratio rather than the specific influences of n-3 PUFA. Meta-analysis showed that administration of n-3 PUFA concomitant with maintenance of a constant level of dietary saturated fat resulted in a 10% increase in LDL cholesterol. Some studies may not acknowledge that removal of saturated fat from the diet lowers LDL cholesterol levels, regardless of the oil that replaces it. In addition, the relationship between n-3 PUFA and total cholesterol levels may be modulated by the percentage energy derived from dietary fat. This point was illustrated in a study in which n-3 PUFA increased total cholesterol levels compared with control 40% fat diets; 30% fat diets with or without fish oil were equally efficacious in reducing total cholesterol levels. Animal studies have shown that C22:6 n-3 is the most effective and C20:5 n-3 is intermediate to C18:3 n-3 in reducing plasma cholesterol concentrations. A human study in which oils with different C20:5 n-3 to C22:6 n-3 ratios were supplemented, has also indicated that oils rich in C22:6 n-3 were more potent in lowering LDL cholesterol levels.

High-density lipoprotein (HDL) particles are involved in reverse cholesterol transport (**Fig. 1**). High concentrations of HDL cholesterol are associated with reduced risk of CHD morbidity and mortality. Variable effects of n-3 PUFA administration on total HDL cholesterol levels were noted in normolipidaemic and hyperlipidaemic volunteers. Possibly n-3 PUFA exerts differential effects on HDL subfractions. The major apolipoproteins of HDL are apo A-I and apo A-II. HDL$_2$ particles mainly contain only apo A-I, whereas HDL$_3$ contain both apo A-I and apo A-II. Because HDL$_2$ is generally considered to be more antiatherogenic, an increase in the HDL$_2$ to HDL$_3$ ratio is associated with a reduction in coronary artery disease risk. Several studies have demonstrated that HDL$_2$ cholesterol concentration increase following n-3 PUFA supplementation of normolipidaemic and hyperlipidaemic volunteers. Data on the effects of dietary n-3 PUFA on the concentration of HDL$_3$ cholesterol are, however, conflicting. Increases in the ratios of HDL$_2$ to HDL$_3$

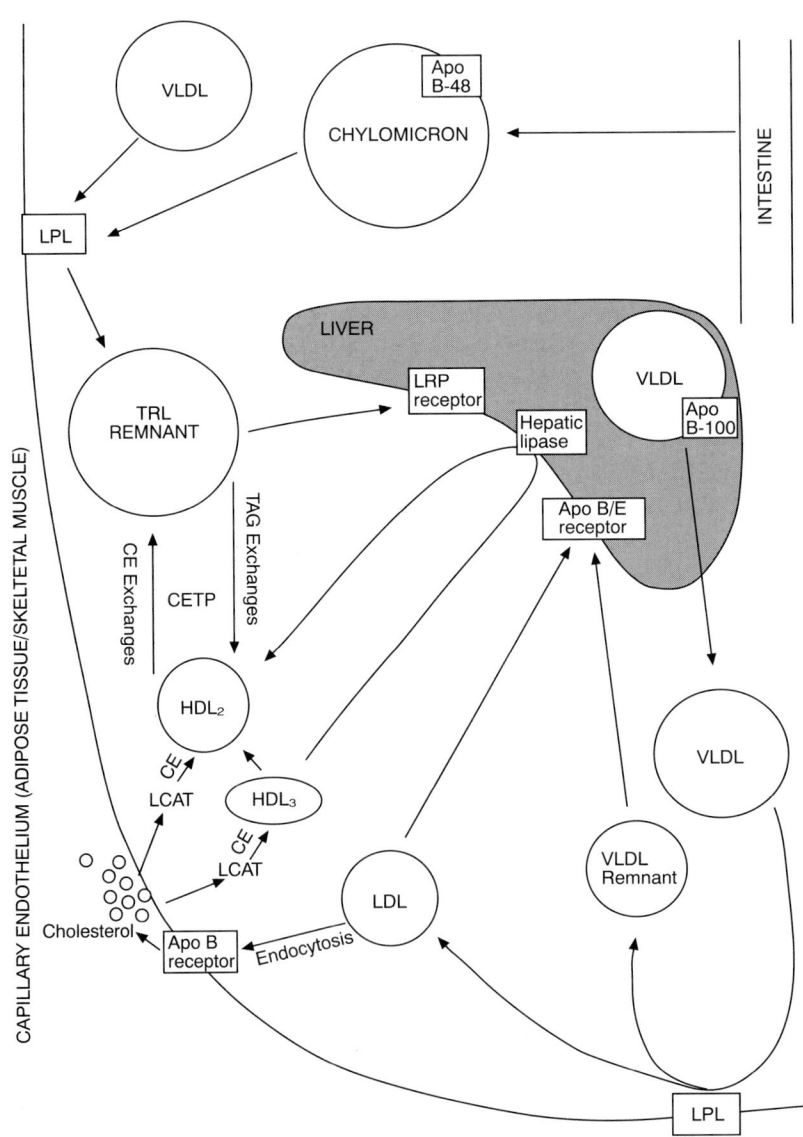

Figure 1　Metabolism of lipoproteins. CE, cholesteryl ester; CETP, cholesteryl ester transfer protein; HDL, high-density lipoprotein; LCAT, lecithin: cholesterol acyltransferase; LDL, low-density lipoprotein; LPL, lipoprotein lipase; LRP, LDL receptor-related protein; TAG, triacylglycerol; TRL, triacylglycerol-rich lipoprotein; VLDL, very low-density lipoprotein.

cholesterol and apo A-I to apo A-II have been reported following n-3 PUFA supplementation.

In many prospective studies, plasma triacylglycerol concentration emerged as a strong risk factor for CHD in univariate analysis, but multivariate analysis tended to diminish this association. However, it is now established that raised plasma triacylglycerol, in association with raised LDL cholesterol or lowered HDL cholesterol concentrations, contributes independently to CHD risk. Reductions in plasma triacylglycerol levels have been confirmed in many studies of normolipidaemic and hyperlipidaemic volunteers, where the minimum daily dose of n-3 PUFA was 2.4 g. Several studies have noted a significant dose–response effect of n-3 PUFA supplementation (range 1.3–9 g per day) on plasma triacylglycerol levels. A trend towards decreased triacylglycerol levels, not only in plasma but also in chylomicron, LDL and HDL fractions, has also been observed in response to n-3 PUFA. An inhibition of hepatic fatty acid synthesis by n-3 PUFA and impaired triacylglycerol synthesis (including VLDL assembly and secretion) are among some of the mechanisms proposed for the plasma triacylglycerol lowering effect of n-3 PUFA. Studies comparing the effects of flaxseed oil (rich in C18:3 n-3) with fish oils (rich in C20:5 n-3 and C22:6 n-3) indicated that fish oil lowered plasma triacylglycerol concentrations whereas flaxseed oil did not. In addition, administration of C22:6 n-3 on its own indicates that it is an effective hypotriacylglycerolaemic agent.

Effects of n-3 PUFA on lipoprotein interactions

Postprandial changes in lipoproteins have become increasingly important because accumulating evidence suggests that delayed clearance of postprandial triacylglycerol-rich lipoproteins (TRL), namely intestine-derived chylomicrons and liver-derived VLDL, increase atherogenic risk. The postabsorptive concentration of triacylglycerols in plasma is an important determinant of the magnitude and duration of the postprandial triacylglycerol response. Administration of n-3 PUFA decreases fasting plasma triacylglycerol concentrations and this affects the postprandial response. In addition, the magnitude of the postprandial lipidaemic response is itself directly diminished by dietary n-3 PUFA, when consumed regularly. The effects of n-3 PUFA may be due to reduced intestinal absorption, decreased synthesis of hepatic VLDL or increased catabolism of TRL. However, postprandial studies in humans and studies of lymph-duct cannulated animals indicate that absorption of n-3 PUFA is similar to that of other fatty acids. This has been demonstrated with free fatty acid, ethyl ester and triacylglycerol formu-

lations of n-3 PUFA. Whether decreased absorption could account for the lower lipidaemic response following n-3 PUFA supplementation has yet to be resolved. Alternatively, reduced TRL production or secretion could attenuate postprandial lipaemia. It has also been proposed that the synthesis of chylomicrons in enterocytes may be reduced by n-3 PUFA by mechanisms analogous to the reduction in hepatic VLDL triacylglycerol production. Studies *in vitro* using Hep G2 cells incubated with C20:5 n-3 have demonstrated reduced VLDL output. Increased catabolism of TRL postprandially is another mechanism by which the postprandial response may be diminished. However, the most likely reason is diminished competition from VLDL remnants for the removal of chylomicron remnants. The metabolism of VLDL exerts a major influence on the heterogeneity of LDL particle size and composition, with positive associations observed between plasma concentrations of small VLDL and dense LDL.

Lipoprotein lipase (LPL) is the major enzyme responsible for the hydrolysis of triacylglycerol molecules present in circulating lipoproteins and regulates the extent and duration of postprandial lipidaemia. It is generally accepted that larger TRL particles have a greater affinity for LPL than the smaller, denser VLDL particles, with LPL appearing to hydrolyse larger TRL more effectively than smaller particles. However, the more rapid clearance of chylomicrons compared with VLDL may in fact be a function of capillary size. The effect of n-3 PUFA on LPL activity is equivocal. Cross-sectional studies have implicated TRL as the major contributor to atherosclerosis and indicate that more dense VLDL subclasses are associated with its progression. A reduction in the concentration of large VLDL particles and an increase in the small VLDL particles with a concomitant decrease in the mean diameter of VLDL have been reported in response to n-3 PUFA supplementation.

Cross-sectional studies of mildly hypertriacylglycerolaemic patients have consistently found an association between small dense LDL and coronary artery disease. It has been suggested that LPL activity and the response of TRL to fat intake are major determinants in LDL heterogeneity. Positive associations were observed between the integrated postprandial responses of small chylomicron remnants and small VLDL and the plasma concentration of dense LDL. These findings point towards the importance of postprandial lipoproteins for the regulation of LDL particle size and composition. Supplementation with n-3 PUFA has been shown to have several effects on the structural and compositional properties of lipoprotein particles; these include a decrease in the ratio of LDL cholesterol to apo B; a decrease in LDL size and a decrease in the cholesteryl ester content of the LDL particle (although both of these have been disputed); an enrichment of LDL with n-3 PUFA; and an increase in the relative mobility of the acyl chain within the lipoprotein particles, which has implications for fluidity of the particle, conformation of the apo B and metabolism of the LDL particle. On the basis of an inverse association between LDL cholesteryl ester content and LDL fractional catabolic rate and a reduced affinity of n-3 PUFA for the LDL receptor, it has been proposed that alterations in LDL composition are the primary determinants of reduced LDL clearance in monkeys given supplementary n-3 PUFA. In addition, n-3 PUFA may also directly affect the LDL receptor, as suggested by studies in rats demonstrating reduced affinity of the receptor for LDL following n-3 PUFA supplementation. Cellular studies *in vitro* have also demonstrated that there is decreased receptor binding following incubation with n-3 PUFA and LDL receptor expression may be reduced simultaneously.

High triacylglycerol levels combined with low HDL cholesterol levels are associated with an increased risk of coronary artery disease. In humans, cholesteryl ester transfer protein (CETP) diverts cholesterol ester from HDL to TRL in gram quantities per day in exchange for triacylglycerols. Therefore, the increase in triacylglycerol concentrations that occurs postprandially may influence HDL metabolism. It has been suggested that HDL cholesterol concentration may represent a surrogate for inefficient metabolism of triacylglycerol. It has been shown that n-3 PUFA reduces CETP and possibly lecithin : cholesterol acyltransferase (LCAT) activities. These effects of n-3 PUFA may have adverse consequences for reverse cholesterol transport, but alternatively may be beneficial, by reducing the amount of cholesteryl ester available for transfer to atherogenic apo B-containing lipoproteins.

Inflammation

Experimental and clinical studies have shown that the immune response can be modulated by nutritional interventions with n-3 PUFA supplements. Alterations include changes in the production of immunological mediators (cytokines, prostanoids) and lymphocyte proliferation in response to mitogens (**Table 1**).

Effects of n-3 PUFA on leucocyte function

Data from studies *in vitro* and *in vivo* indicate that lymphocyte proliferation is reduced in response to n-3 PUFA. However, this effect may be modulated by factors such as composition of the diet and longevity. Supplementation with n-3 PUFA reduces the mitogenic response in older women but not in younger ones. Providing n-3 PUFA in the form of a low-fat fish diet reduces lymphocyte proliferation compared with normal or low-fat only diets, and may also affect the distribution of lymphocyte subsets. Consumption of a low-fat diet rich in n-3 PUFA resulted in lower proportions of helper T cells and a higher proportion of cytotoxic T cells. Furthermore, the proliferation of monocytic cell lines can be inhibited by the addition of n-3 PUFA, and it has been reported that C22:6 n-3 can suppress human antigen-presenting cell function *in vitro*. It has also been shown that n-3 PUFA modulates the chemotactic activities of neutrophils and monocytes in humans. Cell surface expression of major histocompatibility complex (MHC) class II molecules is a prerequisite for the antigen-presenting function of mononuclear phagocytes. Dietary supplementation with n-3 PUFA inhibits the intensity of expression of MHC class II antigens in human monocytes and this represents a potential mechanism by which n-3 PUFA could suppress cell-mediated responses.

Effects of n-3 PUFA on cell adhesion

Adhesion molecules are cell surface proteins involved in the binding of cells – usually leucocytes – to each other, to endothelial cells or to the extracellular matrix. The interactions and responses initiated by binding of these to their receptors or ligands are important in the mediation of inflammatory and immune reactions. Animal studies have shown that the level of expression of the adhesion molecules – intercellular adhesion molecule 1 (ICAM-1) and leucocyte function associated antigen 1 (LFA-1) – are reduced by 33% and 20% respectively in mitogen-stimulated splenic lymphocytes of animals fed a diet enriched with n-3 PUFA. This finding of reduced expression of ICAM-1 and LFA-1 has also been observed in monocytes isolated from human volunteers supplemented with n-3 PUFA. These observations suggest that n-3 PUFA may affect the movement of lymphocytes and monocytes between body compartments and perhaps into areas of inflammatory activity.

Effects of n-3 PUFA on eicosanoids

The production of eicosanoids is initiated by particular stimuli, e.g. cytokines, reactive oxygen species (ROS) and thrombin, in a cell-specific manner. Once produced, the eicosanoids are themselves able to modify the response to the stimulus. The fatty acids C22:6 n-3 and C20:5 n-3 competitively inhibit the oxygenation of C20:4 n-6 by cyclooxygenase. In

Table 1 Modulatory effects of n-3 PUFA on mediators of inflammation

Immune mediator	Produced mainly by	Main effects	Modulation of effects by n-3 PUFA
TXA_2	Platelets	Stimulates platelet aggregation Constricts blood vessels	Reduces TXA_2 synthesis Results in production of the less active TXA_3
PGI_2	Endothelial cells	Powerful inhibitor of platelet aggregation Promotes vasodilation	Results in production of the equipotent PGI_3
PGE_2	Macrophages	Suppresses T lymphocyte proliferation Suppresses IL-2 production Inhibits TNF-α synthesis Inhibits IL-1β synthesis Mediates interaction of macrophages with other cells	Reduces PGE_2 production
LTB_4	Leucocytes	Chemotactic for neutrophils Increases degranulation of platelets Increases adherence of polymorphonuclear cells to receptor cells Enhances IL-1 production by macrophages Enhances IFN-γ production by lymphocytes	Inhibits LTB_4 synthesis Results in production of the less active LTB_5
IL-2	Lymphocytes	Promotes proliferation of all T and B cells	Inhibits IL-2 production
IFN-γ	Lymphocytes	Activates macrophages Promotes growth and differentiation of B-cells Downregulates macrophage scavenger receptor type I isoform expression	Inhibits IFN-γ production
IL-1	Macrophages (oxidized LDL stimulates IL-1 synthesis)	Stimulates fibroblast proliferation Stimulates PGE_2 production Increases leucocyte adhesion to endothelial cells Primes polymorphonuclear cells to facilitate ROS production Induces adhesion molecule expression, e.g. ICAM-1 and VCAM	Reduces IL-1 synthesis
TNF	Macrophages (oxidized LDL stimulates TNF synthesis)	Acts synergistically with IL-1 Primes PMNs to facilitate ROS production Downregulates macrophage scavenger receptor expression	Reduces TNF synthesis
MHC class II expression	Activated leucocytes	Involved in antigen presentation to T helper cells	Decreases level and intensity of expression of MHC class II
Adhesion molecules	Expressed on leucocytes, endothelial cells and platelets	Adherence and migratin of cells	Reduces expression of VCAM-1, ICAM-1, LFA-1 and E-selectin

ICAM, intercellular adhesion molecule; IFN, interferon; IL, interleukin; LFA, leucocyte function-associated antigen; LT, leukotriene; MHC, major histocompatibility complex; PG, prostaglandin; PMN, polymorphonuclear leucocyte; ROS, reactive oxygen species; TNF, tumour necrosis factor; TX, thromboxane; VCAM, vascular cell adhesion molecule.

addition, C20:5 n-3 (but not C22:6 n-3) acts as a substrate for both cyclooxygenase and lipoxygenase. Ingestion of n-3 PUFA decreases membrane C20:4 n-6 levels and consequently reduces the capacity for eicosanoid synthesis from C20:4 n-6 (**Fig. 2**).

A large body of evidence supports the hypothesis that many of the effects of n-3 PUFA on the immune system are mediated by changes in the production of eicosanoids. Dietary supplementation with n-3 PUFA leads to the formation of the less biologically active leukotriene (LT) B_5 at the expense of the pro-inflammatory LTB_4. Thromboxane (TX) A_2 synthesis by mononuclear cells, which is involved in platelet aggregation and blood vessel constriction, is reduced in volunteers supplemented with n-3 PUFA. In addition, urinary excretion of TXB_2 metabolites and collagen-induced TXB_2 synthesis in platelets are also reduced in volunteers on salmon-rich diets.

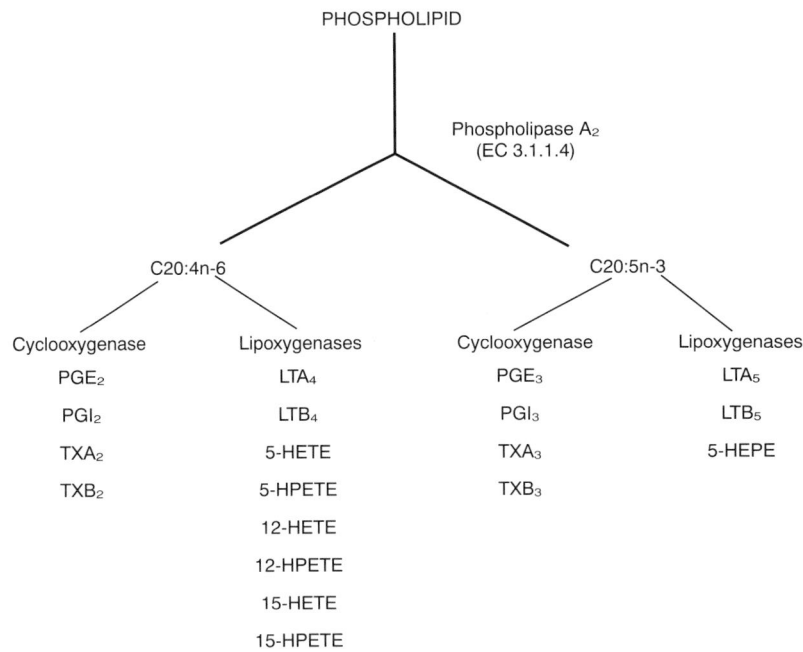

Figure 2 Pathways of eicosanoid synthesis from n-3 PUFA and n-6 PUFA. 5-HEPE, hydroxypentaenoic acid; 5-HETE, hydroxytetraenoic acid; 5-HPETE, hydroperoxyeicosatetraenoic acid; LT, leukotriene; PG, prostaglandin; TX, thromboxane.

Prostaglandin (PG) E_2 production is consistently reported to decline following n-3 PUFA supplementation. Prostaglandin E_2 inhibits the production of the pro-inflammatory mediators interleukin (IL) 1 and tumour necrosis factor (TNF) by macrophages, IL-2 production and lymphocyte proliferation, and modulates the expression of MHC class II receptors by macrophages. The production of many cytokines is also decreased in response to n-3 PUFA supplementation, indicating that the modulation of cytokine production proceeds by PGE_2-independent as well as PGE_2-dependent pathways.

Effects of n-3 PUFA on cytokines

Cytokines are synthesized by activated cells of the immune system and enhance the proliferation and differentiation of other cells in response to immune stimulation. Individual cytokines such as IL-1β have been shown to modulate arterial cell functions, such as induction of cell adhesion molecule expression. Alternatively, IL-1β and TNF-α can act by priming polymorphonuclear cells to facilitate ROS production. Therapeutic strategies that inhibit the production of these cytokines could prove useful in regulating the inflammatory response. Both *in vitro* and *in vivo*, studies have shown that n-3 PUFA can directly inhibit the synthesis of pro-inflammatory cytokines such as IL-1 and TNF-α by human mononuclear cells, independently of eicosanoid regulation. n-3 PUFA could also indirectly inhibit IL-1β and TNF-α production by inhibition of LTB_4 production.

IL-2 is produced by activated T cells and has a variety of immunological functions, notably the proliferation and maturation of activated T cells. Eicosanoids have differential effects on IL-2 expression. Reduced LTB_4, but conversely increased PGE_2, suppress IL-2 production. Production of IL-2 by stimulated peripheral blood mononuclear cells is decreased in humans supplemented with n-3 PUFA. There are three possible mechanisms by which n-3 PUFA can effect reductions in IL-2: (1) directly, by suppression of IL-2 synthesis at the transcriptional level; (2) indirectly, by suppression by LTB_4; or (3) by reduction of IL-1 concentrations.

The modulatory properties of n-3 PUFA on immune cell function, adhesion and eicosanoid and cytokine production have encouraged their therapeutic application in the treatment of a number of inflammatory diseases. These diseases include rheumatoid arthritis, psoriasis, inflammatory bowel disease, atopic dermatitis, systemic lupus erythematosus and multiple sclerosis. A number of trials of supplementation with n-3 PUFA in inflammatory conditions such as rheumatoid arthritis and psoriasis consistently showed significant biochemical changes in response to supplementation. However, symptomatic improvements did not always ensue, with more modest clinical benefits generally reported. Several studies have reported beneficial clinical effects of n-3 PUFA on inflammatory bowel disease, but the results have been equivocal. It has also been suggested that the clinical benefit from treatment with n-3 PUFA is confined to ulcerative colitis and that n-3 PUFA supplementation is without effect in Crohn's disease. A recent definitive study has shown that supplementation with n-3 PUFA for 1 year in a placebo-controlled trial resulted in a reduced relapse rate in Crohn's disease. Apart from the larger samples size and the long period of intervention, another distinguishing feature of this study was the provision of n-3 PUFA in the form of an enteric-coated concentrate. This indicates that n-3 PUFA is clinically beneficial in inflammatory bowel disease and that the formulation may determine its efficacy *in vivo*.

Oxidative Damage

Tissue damage is accompanied by increased amounts of prostaglandins, cytokines and ROS. Reactive oxygen species are generated by activated phagocytic cells, and can oxidize lipids and induce cytotoxicity. Measures that decrease ROS production may consequently reduce the ability of phagocytic cells to contribute to inflammatory processes. Genes encoding adhesion molecules and chemokines are regulated through antioxidant-sensitive mechanisms. Furthermore the ROS, superoxide, stimulates IL-1 release from monocytes. Therefore, strategies for reducing ROS could also reduce cytokine and adhesion molecule expression. Dietary n-3 PUFA supplementation has been shown to decrease superoxide production and chemiluminescence in phagocytic cells. The formation of the ROS species OCl— is catalysed by myeloperoxidase, which is an index of inflammatory activity. Supplementation with n-3 PUFA has also been shown to reduce plasma myeloperoxidase levels.

There is concern that n-3 PUFA may induce oxidative damage. However, if n-3 PUFA were exerting oxidative stress *in vivo*, one might expect antioxidant systems to be depleted or upregulated in response to the stress. There is little evidence to suggest that antioxidant defences are challenged, as several studies have demonstrated that n-3 PUFA supplementation does not affect plasma tocopherol levels, and the effects on antioxidant enzymes are contradictory. Both increased and unaltered levels of glutathione peroxidase (EC 1.11.1.9) enzyme activity have been observed in response to fish oil supplementation.

Effects of n-3 PUFA on oxidative LDL

Several studies indicate that the oxidative modification of LDL plays an important role in the initiation and progression of atherosclerotic lesions. Oxidized LDL differs greatly from native LDL and is recognized by macrophage scavenger receptors which are not subject to downregulation. There is

concern that elevation of n-3 PUFA may result in the formation of undesirable concentrations in LDL, breakdown products, such as aldehydes, thereby increasing the susceptibility of LDL to oxidative modification (**Fig. 3**).

Several studies in which oxidative modification of LDL was stimulated *in vitro*, by incubation with copper, have demonstrated that LDL from animals or humans receiving n-3 PUFA supplements is more susceptible to oxidative damage. A major criticism of this finding is that *in vitro* methods, used to stimulate oxidative modification of LDL, may have limited physiological relevance. This view is supported by animal studies in which n-3 PUFA diets increased the susceptibility of LDL to copper-stimulated oxidation compared with n-6 PUFA diets. However, the extent of atherosclerotic lesion development was similar in all the test groups (rabbits and swine). It is possible that if n-3 PUFA-enriched LDL is oxidized more easily *in vivo*, the other effects of n-3 PUFA such as reduced expression of adhesion molecules, reduced chemotaxis of monocytes and reduced IL-1β and TNF-α production by mononuclear cells, may blunt the capacity of oxidized LDL to promote atherosclerosis. Additionally, alterations in the structure and composition of LDL in response to n-3 PUFA, e.g. increased motional freedom of the fatty acyl chains in LDL, may diminish the potential for increased susceptibility of LDL to oxidative modification.

Oxidized LDL is undoubtedly important in atherosclerosis. However, the role of LDL fatty acid and antioxidant composition in this process may have been overemphasized. The protective effects of the antioxidant nutrients, tocopherol and carotenes, in atherosclerosis may not act through the inhibition of LDL oxidation. It has been proposed that these nutrients affect the interaction of oxidized LDL with endothelial and smooth muscle cells through protein kinase C modulation. This could imply that the role of fatty acid composition may also have been overestimated, and thus n-3 PUFA may not profoundly influence the susceptibility of LDL to oxidative modification *in vivo*.

Atherogenesis and Endothelial Dysfunction

Effects of n-3 PUFA on atherogenesis

Oxidatively modified LDL is central to the development of atherosclerosis and mediates development of atherosclerosis through the following mechanisms, which are potentially modulated by n-3 PUFA:

1. Oxidized LDL can induce IL-12 expression in monocytes; IL-12 selectively induces the Th1

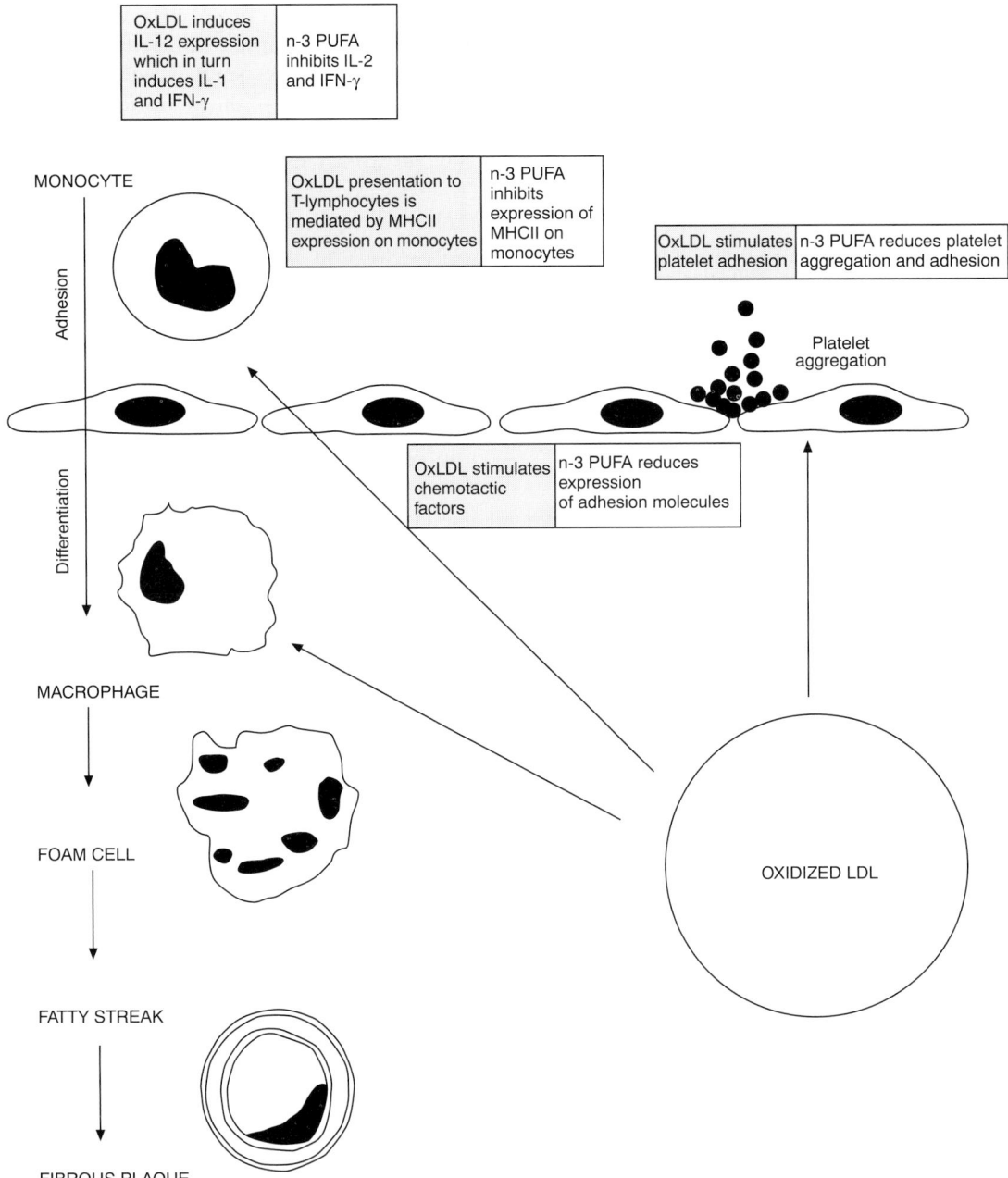

Figure 3 Potential mechanisms by which n-3 PUFA could modulate effects of oxidized LDL (OxLDL). IL, interleukin; IFN, interferon; MHCII, major histocompatibility complex class II.

cytokine pattern which is characterized by IL-2 and interferon γ (IFN-γ). Strong expression of mRNA for IFN-γ has been demonstrated in atherosclerotic plaques. The inhibitory effect of n-3 PUFA on IL-2 and IFN-γ has been outlined previously (Table 1).

2. Atherosclerotic plaques contain T helper cells (CD4+) immunospecific for oxidized LDL. The response of the oxidatively modified LDL-specific T cells is dependent on the presence of autologous antigen-presenting monocytes and is blocked by antibodies to MHC class II molecules; n-3 PUFA can inhibit the expression of MHC class II molecules on monocytes.

3. Oxidized LDL stimulates P selectin-mediated leucocyte adhesion to endothelial cells. As discussed above, n-3 PUFA may inhibit the expression of adhesion molecules.

A large number of growth factors, cytokines and vasoregulatory molecules participate in the development of atherosclerotic lesions. The ability of n-3

PUFA to control the expression of genes encoding these molecules, and to target specific cell types, provides opportunities to induce the regression and possibly prevent the formation of lesions. Several animal studies have demonstrated that n-3 PUFA exert protective effects against the progression of atherosclerosis, compared with saturated fat or n-6 PUFA diets. Furthermore, dietary n-6 PUFA resulted in less coronary artery atherosclerosis in monkeys, compared with MUFA or saturated fat. Administration of n-3 PUFA could inhibit the development of atherosclerosis by decreasing the levels of atherogenic lipoproteins, by increasing HDL_2 or by mediating factors which are independent of plasma lipid concentrations.

Effects of n-3 PUFA on endothelial dysfunction

The vascular endothelium plays numerous physiological roles, including:

1. The provision of a non-thrombogenic, non-adherent permeability barrier.
2. Maintenance of vascular tone by release of small molecules such as nitric oxide, prostacyclin (PGI_2) and endothelin, which modulate vasodilation and vasoconstriction respectively.
3. Formation and secretion of growth regulatory molecules and cytokines.
4. Modification of lipoproteins as they are transported into the artery wall.

Endothelial dysfunction promotes vasospasm and thrombosis, and probably plays an important role in the processes of atherosclerosis and restenosis.

It has been shown that n-3 PUFA reduces platelet adhesion at the functional level (by platelet adhesion on glass beads). At the molecular level, adhesion molecules have a primary role in the recruitment of platelets to injured vessels. This process involves various pathways culminating in firm adhesion (depending on the level of shear stress). The initial events that lead to platelet adhesion are followed by further platelet recruitment (aggregation) to form a haemostatic plug or a pathologic thrombus. Supplementation with n-3 PUFA has been shown to reduce platelet aggregation; however, the relevance of this functional finding *in vivo* is questionable. PgI_2 generated in the endothelium has antiplatelet aggregation and vasodilator actions, whereas TXA_2 generated by platelets from the same precursors induces platelet aggregation and vasoconstriction. The 3-series prostanoids derived from n-3 PUFA result in the production of PGI_3, which is equipotent to PGI_2, and TXA_3, which is less biologically active than TXA_2. It has been shown that n-3 PUFA tends to decrease platelet adhesion *in vitro* to a greater extent than platelet aggregation.

Local leucocyte recruitment and adhesion to the vessel wall is an early step in atherogenesis. Factors that modulate the expression of endothelial leucocyte adhesion molecules and other endothelial cytokines may be important in modulating lesion formation. As discussed above, n-3 PUFA has been shown to reduce expression of both members of the integrin family and the immunoglobulin superfamily of adhesion molecules.

Effects of n-3 PUFA on hypertension and arrhythmia

In the presence of hypertension and atherosclerosis, endothelial function is often impaired. It was found that n-3 PUFA lowered blood pressure in normotensive and hypertensive subjects in some, but not all, intervention trials. A meta-analysis of the effects of dietary fish oil supplementation on blood pressure reported a dose-dependent benefit, most pronounced in hypertensive patients with concomitant hypercholesterolaemia or atherosclerosis. Dietary supplementation with fish oil did not change mean blood pressure in subjects who ate fish three or more times per week as part of their usual diet, or in those who had a baseline concentration of plasma phospholipid n-3 PUFA above 175.1 mg l^{-1}. There are several possible mechanisms by which n-3 PUFA may affect blood pressure: these include changes in membrane fluidity (which in turn produce alterations in ion transport via effects on second messengers), PGE_2 and PGI_2 production, nitric oxide production and ion transport systems.

Cardiac arrhythmia precipitates myocardial infarction which may result in sudden cardiac death. In a secondary prevention trial, subjects advised to eat fatty fish or take fish oil supplements had a 29% reduction in 2-year all-cause mortality compared with controls. These findings need to be confirmed by adequately designed and controlled intervention trials. However, the beneficial effect of the increased n-3 PUFA consumption was apparent early in the intervention, and suggested that modulation of ventricular fibrillation during acute MI was the mechanism responsible. Diets rich in n-3 PUFA exert beneficial effects on cardiac function and the incorporation of n-3 PUFA into cardiac membrane phospholipid has been reported to reduce ventricular fibrillation induced by myocardial ischaemia. The basis for dietary lipid modification of arrhythmogenesis has not yet been identified with certainty. Alterations in cellular calcium concentration can contribute significantly to abnormalities in both impulse generation and impulse conduction in myocardial ischaemia. The changes in membrane fluidity and function effected by n-3 PUFA supplementation may influence calcium entry or removal and thereby affect cardiac function. An alternative mechanism may be the changes effected by n-3 PUFA on myocardial production of eicosanoids. The n-3 PUFA alterations in cardiac eicosanoid production, in particular the inhibition of TXA_2 production, is likely to be of significant pathophysiological benefit, as TXA_2 has been implicated in myocardial ischaemia, arrhythmogenesis and myocardial injury.

Thrombosis and Fibrinolysis

The coagulation cascade involves activation of a series of intermediates including factor VII, thrombin and fibrinogen, which ultimately leads to the formation of the fibrin clot (**Fig. 4**). Formation of fibrin thrombi on plaques is a determining factor in the growth of atherosclerotic lesions and the appearance of clinical manifestations. The role of fibrinogen as a primary cardiovascular risk factor is well established and has been demonstrated in a number of prospective epidemiological studies of healthy individuals and CHD patients. High levels of factor VII coagulant activity are also associated with an increased risk of coronary events. Plasma factor VIIc is positively correlated with serum triacylglycerol concentrations and is increased in type IIb and type IV hyperlipidaemic subjects. The correlation between factor VII and lipids may be explained by the binding of factor VII with TRL particles. Dietary intervention studies that have resulted in lowering serum triacylglycerol levels have also observed a simultaneous improvement in fibrinolytic activity. Therefore, n-3 PUFA may directly or indirectly modulate the levels of factor VII and fibrinogen. However, several studies have failed to observe reductions in either factor

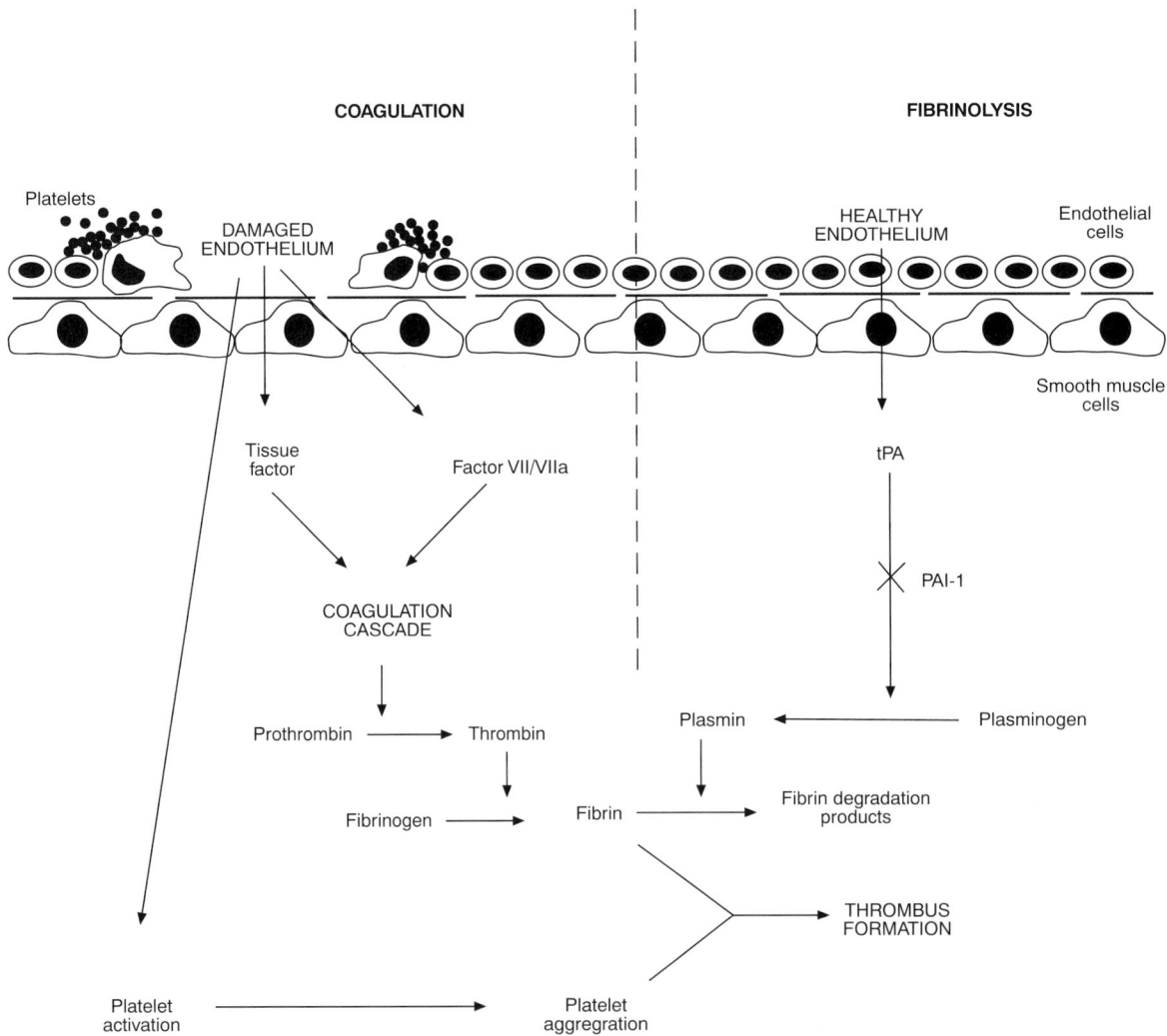

Figure 4 Haemostatic pathways of coagulation and fibrinolysis. PAI-1, plasminogen activator inhibitor 1; tPA, tissue plasminogen activator.

VII or fibrinogen levels following n-3 PUFA supplementation, although this finding has been inconsistently observed.

Several recent clinical and epidemiological studies have indicated that plasminogen activator inhibitor (PAI), responsible for reduced fibrinolytic activity, is a risk factor for CHD. Elevated PAI plasma concentrations have also been found in patients with elevated triacylglycerol concentrations. There is no clear explanation for the association between PAI and triacylglycerol, but VLDL has been shown to induce the synthesis and release of PAI by endothelial cells *in vitro*. Administration of diets rich in n-3 PUFA may cause an increase in PAI levels in both healthy individuals and diabetic patients, but reductions or no effect on PAI activity have also been documented. The importance of n-3 PUFA in regulating coagulation and fibrinolytic pathways remains to be determined.

Carcinogenesis

Data from the Multiple Risk Factor Intervention Trial indicate that a high ratio of n-3 to n-6 PUFA is protective against cancer mortality. The incidence of cancer is low in Inuit populations on their traditional diet and suggests that n-3 PUFA can be exploited as a possible anticancer agent. The n-3 PUFA may induce cytotoxic actions by augmenting the generation of ROS and the lipid peroxidation process in tumour cells, but not in normal cells. In addition, n-3 PUFA and its products can modulate immune response, augment the respiratory burst of neutrophils and the generation of ROS by macrophages. It has been shown that n-3 PUFA has antitumour effects in animal models, e.g. n-3 PUFA suppresses growth of tumour transplants in mice.

Other Physiological Effects

The fatty acids C20:5 n-3 and C22:6 n-3 have distinct roles *in vivo*, with C22:6 n-3 characteristically incorporated into membrane phospholipid structures and C20:5 n-3 acting as an eicosanoid precursor. The divergent metabolism of C20:5 n-3 and C22:6 n-3 is suggested by a number of observations in human and animal studies, including the higher level of C22:6 n-3 than C20:5 n-3 in various tissues; the preferential incorporation of C22:6 n-3 over C20:5 n-3 into adipose tissue; the preferential mobilization of C20:5 n-3 from adipose tissue; and the more rapid return to baseline of C20:5 n-3 in supplementation studies with a washout design.

The fatty acid C22:6 n-3 may comprise as much as 30–40% of the fatty acids in some phospholipids of human rod outer-segment membranes and is known to be important to normal visual function. The presence of C22:6 n-3 in nonmyelin membranes in the brain indicates that it is also essential to normal central nervous system function and learning behaviour. The pathway by which developing brain normally acquires C22:6 n-3 remains unclear. Several studies have shown that the brain and eye contain all the enzymes necessary for synthesis of C22:6 n-3 from the essential fatty acid C18:3 n-3. Synthesis of C22:6 n-3 requires adequate activity of the fatty acid desaturase enzymes, adequate dietary intake of C18:3 n-3, and an appropriate balance of C18:2 n-6 to C18:3 n-3. Conversion of C18:3 n-3 to C22:6 n-3 has been shown to occur in both term and preterm infants. It is not certain, however, if the rate of C22:6 n-3 synthesis is sufficient to meet the tissue needs of young infants, and in particular those of preterm infants. It is recommended that C22:6 n-3 be included in the diets of preterm infants: firstly, the fetal accumulation of C22:6 n-3 that normally occurs between the 26th and the 40th week of gestation may not take place; and secondly, preterm infants may be unable to form C22:6 n-3 in sufficient quantities from C18:3 n-3 provided by soya oil based formula products. In term infants, the role of C22:6 n-3 is not as firmly established, but the levels of C22:6 n-3 in brain cortical phospholipids are reported to be higher in breast-fed than in formula-fed infants. The presence of 0.2–0.4% C22:6 n-3 in mature breast milk may serve as a rationale for its addition to term infant formula feeds, provided the amounts do not exceed those of human milk. However, a multicentre parallel group study in the USA comparing term infants fed breast milk with those fed formulae containing 1.9–4.7% C18:3 n-3 but devoid of C22:6 n-3, observed no differences in growth and looking acuity among the groups at 3 months of age.

Insulin sensitivity and glucose homeostasis have been variously reported to improve, be unaltered, transiently worsen, or deteriorate in individuals with insulin-dependent diabetes mellitus given n-3 PUFA. In healthy non-diabetic subjects n-3 PUFA supplementation has been shown to cause a decrease in C peptide excretion, which is a marker for insulin production. In contrast, a study of the long-term metabolic effects of n-3 PUFA in patients with coronary artery disease did not result in any discernible effects on glucose homeostasis as assessed by glucose, insulin and C peptide levels.

Conclusions

The effects of n-3 PUFA have been well characterized and have resulted in the use of these compounds in the prevention of CHD. n-3 PUFA may also be useful therapeutic agents in the treatment of inflammation disorders such as Chrohn's disease.

The formulation of n-3 PUFA is an important issue, as functional foods containing n-3 PUFA are becoming increasingly available. Natural sources of fish oils usually contain approximately 30% n-3 PUFA, but more concentrated reesterified triacylglycerols and ethyl ester formulations (comprising of up to 85% n-3 PUFA) are also available. Concentrates of n-3 PUFA offer the advantages of higher concentrations of n-3 PUFA and lower concentrations of cholesterol and saturated fat per capsule. However, there has been concern that ethyl esters and reesterified triacylglycerols with altered intramolecular structure may not have the same biological effects as natural sources. Nevertheless, the balance of data from long-term and well-controlled short-term studies suggests that concentrates can be as effective as fish oil preparations in raising the levels of n-3 PUFA in plasma, and effecting measurable changes in lipid profiles and platelet aggregation.

The appropriate level of n-3 PUFA intake may be determined by the health or disease status of the individual. In inflammatory diseases, higher doses may be appropriate: e.g. 2.7 g n-3 PUFA per day was found to be effective in preventing relapse in Crohn's disease. However, the levels required for effective reductions in CHD risk may be more modest. A secondary prevention trial in MI survivors indicated that consumption of 2.3 g of C20:5 n-3 per week (equivalent to 200–400 g of fatty fish) reduced the subsequent risk of death from MI. These data indicate that reductions in risk factors for CHD can be achieved with levels equivalent to an intake of two fish per week. Public health recommendations advise an increase in consumption of long-chain n-3 PUFA to levels of 1.5 g per week, through weekly consumption of oily fish. Epidemiological data suggest that increases beyond this modest level are unlikely to reduce coronary events substantially. In conclusion, the current consensus is that n-3 PUFA are integral component of a healthy diet and may play a part in the prevention of many diseases.

See also: **Antioxidants**: Diet and Antioxidant Defence; Intervention Studies. **Arthritis**: Dietary Aspects of Aetiology and Nutritional Management. **Brain and Nervous System**: Biology, Metabolism and Nutritional Requirements. **Cancer**: Epidemiology and Associations Between Diet and Cancer; Diet in Cancer Treatment. **Cholesterol**: Factors Determining Blood Cholesterol Levels. **Coronary Heart Disease**: Lipid Theory of Coronary Heart Disease; Haemostatic Factors and Coronary Heart Disease; Aetiology; Prevention. **Cytokines**: Nutritional Aspects. **Diabetes Mellitus**: Dietary Management; Secondary Complications and Their Prevention. **Dietary Guidelines**: International Perspectives. **Fatty Acids**: Metabolism; Health Effects of Saturated Fatty Acids; Health Effects of Monounsaturated Fatty Acids; Health Effects of n-6 Polyunsaturated Fatty Acids; Health Effects of *trans* Fatty Acids. **Fish**: Nutritional Value. **Functional Foods**: Definition and Potential for Nutritional Role. **Health Foods**: Dietary Supplements - Micronutrients. **Hyperlipidaemia (Hyperlipidemia)**: Nutritional Management. **Hypertension**: Nutritional Management. **Infants**: Milk-feeding and Weaning; Low-birthweight and Preterm Infants. **Lipids**: Chemistry and Classification; Composition and Role of Phospholipids in the Body. **Lipoproteins**: Physiology. **Prostaglandins and Leukotrienes**: Physiology.

Further Reading

Abbey M, Clifton P, Kestin M, Belling B and Nestel PJ (1990) Effect of fish oil on lipoproteins, lecithin: cholesterol acyltransferase, and lipid transfer protein activity in humans. *Arteriosclerosis* 10:85–94.

Ascherio A, Rimm EB, Stampfer MJ, Giovannucci EL and Willett WC (1995) Dietary intake of marine n-3 fatty acids, fish intake, and the risk of coronary disease among men. *New England Journal of Medicine* 332:977–982.

Belluzzi A, Brignola C, Campieri M, Pera A, Boschi S and Migliolli M (1996) Effect of an enteric-coated fish-oil preparation on relapses in Crohn's disease. *New England Journal of Medicine* 334:1557–1560.

British Nutrition Foundation (1992) *Unsaturated Fatty Acids. Nutritional and Physiological Significance.* London: Chapman & Hall.

Burr ML, Fehily AM, Gilbert JF *et al.* (1989) Effects of changes in fat, fish and fibre intakes on death and myocardial reinfarction: diet and reinfarction trial (DART). *Lancet* ii:757–761.

Calder PC (1996) Immunomodulatory and anti-inflammatory effects of n-3 polyunsaturated fatty acids. *Proceedings of the Nutrition Society* 55:737–774.

Daviglus ML, Stamler J, Orencia AJ, Dyer AR, Liu K, Greenland P, Walsh MK, Morris D and Shekelle RB (1997) Fish consumption and the 30-year risk of fatal myocardial infarction. *New England Journal of Medicine* 336:1046–1053.

Department of Health (1994) *Nutritional Aspects of Cardiovascular Disease.* Report on Health and Social Subjects 46. London: HMSO.

Endres S, Ghorbani R, Kelley VE *et al.* (1989) The effect of dietary supplementation with n-3 polyunsaturated fatty acids on the synthesis of interleukin-1 and tumour necrosis factor by mononuclear cells. *New England Journal of Medicine* 320:265–271.

Eritsland J, Arnesen H, Seljeflot I and Hostmark AT (1994) Long-term metabolic effects on n-3 polyunsaturated fatty acids in patients with coronary artery disease. *American Journal of Clinical Nutrition* **61**:831–836.

Frenette PS and Wagner DD (1996) Adhesion molecules – Part II: Blood vessels and blood cells. *New England Journal of Medicine* **335**:43–45.

Harris WS (1989) Fish oils and plasma lipid and lipoprotein metabolism in humans: a critical review. *Journal of Lipid Research* **30**:785–807.

Karpe F, Tornvall P, Olivecrona T, Steiner G, Carlson LA and Hamsten A (1993) Composition of human low density lipoprotein: effects of postprandial triglyceride-rich lipoproteins, lipoprotein lipase, hepatic lipase and cholesteryl ester transfer protein. *Atherosclerosis* **98**:33–49.

Keaney JF, Guo Y, Cunningham D, Shwaery GT, Xu A and Vita JA (1996) Vascular incorporation of α-tocopherol prevents endothelial dysfunction due to oxidised LDL by inhibiting protein kinase C stimulation. *Journal of Clinical Investigation* **98**:386–394.

Kromhout D (1993) Epidemiological aspects of fish in the diet. *Proceedings of the Nutrition Society* **52**:437–439.

Roche HM and Gibney MJ (1995) Postprandial triacylglycerolaemia – nutritional implications. *Progress in Lipid Research* **34**:249–266.

Sanders TAB (1993) Marine oils: metabolic effects and role in human nutrition. *Proceedings of the Nutrition Society* **52**:457–472.

Whitman SC, Fish JR, Rand ML and Rogers KA (1994) n-3 Fatty acid incorporation into LDL particles renders them more susceptible to oxidation *in vitro* but not necessarily more artherogenic *in vivo*. *Arteriosclerosis and Thrombosis* **14**:1170–1176.

Health Effects of *trans* Fatty Acids

M J Sadler, IGD, Watford, UK

Copyright © 1998 Academic Press

Chemistry

The *trans* fatty acids are unsaturated fatty acids that contain one or more ethylenic double bonds in the *trans* geometrical configuration, i.e. on opposite sides of the carbon chain (**Fig. 1**). The *trans* bond is more thermodynamically stable than the *cis* bond, and is therefore less chemically reactive.

Trans bonds have minimal effect on the conformation of the carbon chain such that their physical properties more closely resemble those of saturated fatty acids than of *cis* unsaturated fatty acids. The

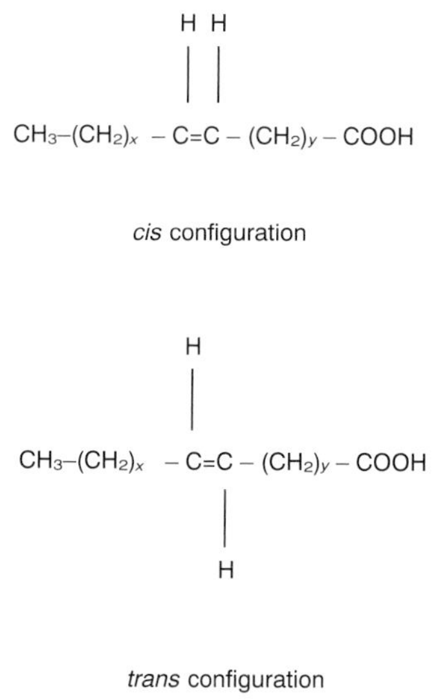

Figure 1 The *trans* and *cis* configurations of unsaturated bonds. Reproduced with kind permission of the British Nutrition Foundation.

conformation remains linear, compared with *cis* fatty acids, which are kinked (**Fig. 2**). Hence, *trans* isomers can pack together more closely than their *cis* counterparts.

Trans fatty acids have higher melting points than their *cis* counterparts, while saturated fatty acids have higher melting points than both *trans* and *cis* fatty acids. For example, the melting points of C_{18} fatty acids are 69.6°C for stearic acid (18:0), 44.8°C for elaidic acid (*trans*-18:1), and 13.2°C for oleic acid (*cis*-18:1). The relative proportion of these different types of fatty acids influences the physical properties of cooking fats and their suitability for different uses in the food processing industry.

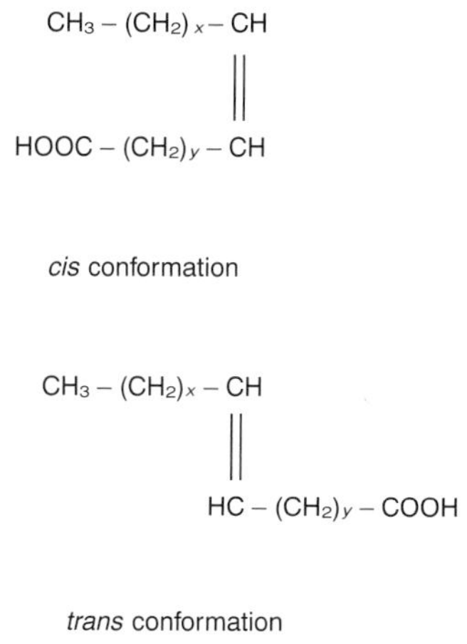

Figure 2 Conformation of the carbon chain with *trans* and *cis* bonds. Reproduced with kind permission of the British Nutrition Foundation.

In addition to geometrical isomerism (*cis* and *trans*), unsaturated fatty acids also exhibit positional isomerism, where the double bonds can occur in different positions along the chain in fatty acids which have identical chemical formulae. As with *cis* fatty acids, *trans* fatty acids also occur as mixtures of positional isomers.

Occurrence

Trans fatty acids present in the diet arise from two origins. The first is from bacterial biohydrogenation in the forestomach of ruminants, which is the source of *trans* fatty acids present in mutton and beef fats. These are present at a concentration of 2–9% of bovine fat. *Trans*-11-octadecenoic acid is the main isomer produced although *trans*-9- and *trans*-10-octadecenoic acid are also produced. Thus, *trans* fatty acids occur in nature and cannot be considered to be foreign substances.

The second origin is from the industrial catalytic hydrogenation of liquid oils (mainly of vegetable origin, but also of fish oils). This produces solid fats and partially hydrogenated oils and is undertaken to increase the thermal stability of liquid oils and to alter their physical properties. The margarines, spreads, shortenings and frying oils produced are thus more useful in the food processing industry than liquid oils. Chemically, a range of *trans* isomers is produced that, for vegetable oils containing predominantly C_{18} unsaturated fatty acids, is qualitatively similar to those produced by biohydrogenation, although the relative proportions of the isomers may differ. Use of fish oils containing a high proportion of very long-chain (C_{20} and C_{22}) fatty acids with up to six double bonds produces more complex mixtures of *trans*, *cis* and positional isomers. However, the use of hydrogenated fish oils in food processing is declining, owing to a general fall in edible oil prices and to consumer preference for products based on vegetable oils.

Analysis

Methods available for the estimation of total *trans* unsaturation and to determine individual *trans* fatty acids are outlined in **Table 1**. At present there is no one simple and accurate method suitable for both research applications and for use in the food industry. In dietary studies data for *trans* fatty acid intake are generally expressed as the sum of the fatty acids containing *trans* double bonds, and there is generally no differentiation between the different isomers.

A report from the British Nutrition Foundation (BNF) in 1995 highlighted concerns over the vari-ations in estimations of *trans* fatty acid concentrations in some food products provided by different analytical techniques. A thorough review of the available analytical techniques was called for.

Sources and Intakes

The main sources of *trans* fatty acids in the UK diet are cereal-based products (providing 27% of total *trans* fatty acid intake), margarines, spreads and frying oils (22%), meat and meat products (18%), and milk, butter and cheese (16%). In the USA, the main sources of intake are baked goods (28%), fried foods (25%), margarine, spreads and shortenings (25%), savoury snacks (10%), milk and butter (9%).

Typical ranges of *trans* fatty acids in foods are shown in **Table 2**. *Trans* isomers of $C_{18:1}$ (elaidic acid) are the most common *trans* fatty acids, accounting for 65% of the total *trans* fatty acids in the UK diet.

Intakes of *trans* fatty acids are difficult to assess because of:

- analytical inaccuracies;
- difficulties of obtaining reliable information about food intake.

A number of countries have attempted to assess intakes of *trans* fatty acids (**Table 3**). Reliable intake data are available for the UK, based on a 7-day weighed intake of foods eaten both inside and outside the home, for 2000 adults aged 16–64 years (Table 3). Data from the UK National Food Survey, which does not include food eaten outside the home, shows a steady decline in intake of *trans* fatty acids from 5.6 g per person per day in 1980 to 4.8 g in 1992. In the UK *trans* fatty acids account for approximately 6% of dietary fat, and in the USA for approximately 7–8% of dietary fat. Estimates of *trans* fatty acid intake are likely to show a downward trend because of:

- improved analytical techniques which give lower but more accurate values for the *trans* fatty acid content of foods;
- the availability of values for *trans* fatty acids in a wider range of foods which allows more accurate estimation of intakes;
- the reformulation of some products which has led to a reduction in the concentration of *trans* fatty acids in recent years.

Advances in food technology that are enabling a gradual reduction in the *trans* fatty acid content include:

1. refinements in hydrogenation processing con-

Table 1 Analytical methods for *trans* fatty acids

General method	Determines	Advantages	Disadvantages
Infrared (IR) absorption spectrometry	Total *trans* unsaturation	Inexpensive; reliable results provided concentrations of *trans* isomers exceed 5%; can analyse intact lipids	Unreliable results if concentrations of *trans* isomers less than 5%; interpretive difficulties – need to apply correction factors
Fourier transform IR spectroscopy	Total *trans* unsaturation	Reliable results if concentrations of *trans* isomers less than 2%	Does not distinguish between two esters each with one *trans* bond or between one ester with two *trans* bonds and one with none
Gas–liquid chromatography (GLC)	Individual *trans* fatty acids		Presence of unidentified compounds can give false estimates of *trans* fatty content
Argentation – GLC	Individual *trans* fatty acids	Saturated, monounsaturated and diunsaturated fatty acids can be resolved	Method is time-consuming
Capillary column GLC	Individual *trans* fatty acids which can be summated to give total *trans* unsaturation	Accurate resolution of fatty acid esters including *cis* and *trans* isomers	Great skill required for preparing columns and interpretation of chromatograms
High-performance liquid chromatography	Individual *trans* fatty acids	*cis,cis*-, and *trans,trans*-dienoic fatty acids can be separated	
Nuclear magnetic resonance (NMR)	Individual *trans* fatty acids	Intact lipids can be analysed; can identify *trans*-diene isomers by use of proton (^{1}H) NMR	Equipment is costly; more use as a research tool than for general analysis

ditions which will enable the reduction and in the future, the elimination of *trans* fatty acids;

2. the interesterification (rearrangement of fatty acids within and between triacylglycerols) of liquid oils with solid fats;

3. the future genetic modification of oils.

Physiology of *trans* Fatty Acids

Extensive reviews of the health effects of *trans* fatty acids conducted in the 1980s found no evidence for any adverse effects of *trans* fatty acids on growth, longevity, reproduction or the occurrence of disease, including cancer, from studies conducted in experimental animals.

Digestion, absorption and metabolism

Trans fatty acids are present in the diet in esterified form, mainly in triacylglycerols but those from ruminant sources may also be present in phospholipids.

Before absorption into the body, triacylglycerols must be digested by pancreatic lipase in the upper small intestine. There is no evidence of differences in the hydrolysis and absorption of *trans* fatty acids, in comparison with that of *cis* fatty acids. *Trans* fatty acids are transported from the intestine mainly in chylomicrons, but some are also incorporated into cholesteryl esters and phospholipids.

Trans fatty acids are incorporated into the lipids of most tissues of the body, and are present in all the major classes of complex lipids. The positional distribution of *trans* fatty acids tends to show more similarity to that of saturated fatty acids than to that of the corresponding *cis* fatty acids. Some selectivity between tissues results in an uneven distribution of *trans* fatty acids throughout the body.

Trans fatty acids occur mainly in positions 1 and 3 of triacylglycerols, the predominant lipids in adipose tissue. The concentration of *trans* fatty acids in adipose tissue is approximately proportional to long-

Table 2 Typical content of *trans* fatty acids in a range of foods

Food	Content of trans *fatty acids per 100 g product (g)*
Butter	3.6
Soft margarine, not high in PUFA	9.1
Soft margarine, high in PUFA	5.2
Hard margarine	12.4
Low-fat spread, not high in PUFA	4.5
Low-fat spread, high in PUFA	2.5
Blended vegetable oil	1.1
Vegetable oil (sunflower, safflower, soya, sesame)	0
Commercial blended oil	6.7
Potato crisps	0.2
Wholewheat crisps	0.2
Low-fat crisps	0.3
Beefburger, 100% beef frozen, fried or grilled	0.8
Sausage, pork, fried	0.1
Sausage roll, flaky pastry	6.3
Hamburger in bun with cheese, take-away	0.5
Biscuits, cheese-flavoured	0.2
Biscuits, chocolate, full coated	3.4
Chocolate cake and butter icing	7.1
Chips, old potatoes, fresh, fried in commercial blended oil	0.7
Chips, frozen, fine cut, fried in commercial blended oil	0.7

Reproduced with kind permission of the British Nutrition Foundation.
PUFA, polyunsaturated fatty acids. *Trans* fatty acid methyl esters were determined by capillary gas chromatography.

Table 3 Estimated intakes of *trans* fatty acids in various countries

Country	Estimated daily intake of total trans *fatty acids (g)*	Year published and basis for estimation
UK	5.6 (men) 4.0 (women)	1990: 7-day weighed intake undertaken in 1986–7 including food eaten outside the home
USA	8.1 3.8	1991: availability data 1994: food frequency questionnaire
Denmark	5.0	1995: availability data
Finland	1.9	1992: duplicate diets
Spain	2.0–3.0	1993: calculated from food consumption data
Norway	8.0	1993: food frequency questionnaire

term dietary intake, and determination of the concentrations in storage fat is one method used to estimate *trans* fatty acid intake. However, this is not entirely straightforward as variation has been reported in the composition of adipose tissue obtained from different sites and depths, and factors that influence adipose tissue turnover rates such as dieting and exercise are also complicating factors. *Trans*-18:1 isomers account for approximately 70% of the *trans* fatty acids found in adipose tissue, and *trans*-18:2 isomers (*trans,trans*; *trans,cis*; and *cis,trans*) account for about 20%.

In heart, liver and brain, *trans* fatty acids occur mainly in membrane phospholipids. The position of the double bond as well as the conformation of the carbon chain may determine the pattern of *trans*

fatty acid esterification in phospholipids, but there is evidence that *trans*-18:1 fatty acids are preferentially incorporated into position 1 of the phosphoacylglycerols, as are saturated fatty acids; in contrast, oleic acid is randomly distributed.

The turnover of *trans* fatty acids parallels that of other types of fatty acids in the body, and *trans* fatty acids are readily removed from the tissues for oxidation. Studies in which human subjects were fed labelled carbon-13 isotope, have demonstrated that the whole-body oxidation rate for *trans*-18:1 is similar to that for *cis*-18:1. *Trans* fatty acids are a minor component of tissue lipids, and their concentrations in tissues are much lower than their concentrations in the diet. However, research has focused on C_{18} *trans* fatty acids, and more studies are needed to investigate the effects of very long-chain *trans* fatty acids derived from the hydrogenation of fish oils.

Interactions with metabolism of essential fatty acids

From experiments mainly with laboratory animals, it has been demonstrated that relatively high intakes of *trans* fatty acids in the diet in conjunction with marginal intakes of essential fatty acids (less than 2% dietary energy from linoleic acid), can lead to the presence of Mead acid (*cis*-5,8,11-20:3) in tissue lipids, and an increase in the ratio of 20:3 n-9 to 20:4 n-6. This has been interpreted to suggest early signs of essential fatty acid deficiency, with potentially increased requirements for essential fatty acids. Mead acid can accumulate in the presence of linoleic acid, if large amounts of nonessential fatty acids are also present. Two mechanisms have been suggested to explain these observations in relation to intake of *trans* fatty acids:

- that *trans* fatty acids may compete with linoleic acid in metabolic pathways;
- that *trans* fatty acids may inhibit enzymes involved in elongation and further desaturation of linoleic acid.

The consensus is that the significance of Mead acid production in humans has not been established, and further research is needed in this area. It is unlikely that a competitive effect between polyunsaturated fatty acids (PUFA) and *trans* fatty acids would arise, because of the relatively high intakes of linoleic acid in people freely selecting their own diets. Also, as there is a large body pool of linoleic acid available for conversion to long-chain PUFA, it is unlikely that the *trans* fatty acids in the body would interfere even at relatively low ratios of dietary linoleic acid to *trans* fatty acids. The appearance of Mead acid is not specifically induced by *trans* fatty acids, and experiments in animals have not demonstrated any adverse health effects of its production.

Effect of *trans* fatty acids on plasma lipoproteins

Raised plasma concentrations of low-density lipoprotein (LDL) are considered to be a risk factor for coronary heart disease (CHD); in contrast, reduced concentrations of high-density lipoprotein (HDL) are considered to increase risk. It therefore follows that to help protect against CHD, diets should ideally help to maintain plasma concentrations of HDL cholesterol and to lower those of LDL cholesterol. Dietary factors that raise LDL and lower HDL concentrations would be considered to be undesirable in this context.

Several trials have evaluated the effects of C_{18}

trans monounsaturated fatty acids on plasma lipoproteins (**Fig. 3**). The results have been relatively consistent, and the following general conclusions have been drawn from these studies:

- C_{18} monounsaturated *trans* fatty acids raise LDL cholesterol concentration; the cholesterol-raising effect is similar in magnitude to that of the cholesterol-raising saturated fatty acids, i.e. myristic (14:0) and palmitic (16:0) acids;
- C_{18} monounsaturated *trans* fatty acids decrease HDL cholesterol concentration; this is in contrast to saturated fatty acids which produce a small rise in HDL levels;
- in comparison with the effects of oleic and linoleic fatty acids, C_{18} monounsaturated *trans* fatty acids raise LDL cholesterol and lower HDL cholesterol levels.

It has been calculated that *theoretically*, each 1% increase in energy from *trans* fatty acids (18:1) in place of oleic acid (*cis*-18:1) would raise plasma LDL concentration by 0.040 mmol l^{-1} (an approximately 1% increase based on average UK plasma cholesterol concentration); HDL would be decreased by 0.013 mmol l^{-1} (a 1% decrease).

The 1995 BNF Task Force calculated that, in the UK, replacing 2% energy from *trans* fatty acids with 2% energy from oleic acid would reduce mean plasma LDL cholesterol concentration by 0.08 mmol l^{-1}; plasma HDL concentration would rise by 0.026 mmol l^{-1}, and the HDL ratio would fall from 3.92 to 3.77. From estimates of the effect of

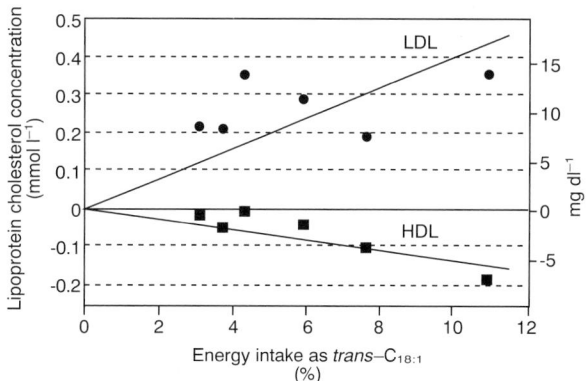

Figure 3 Effects of monounsaturated C_{18} *trans* fatty acids on lipoprotein cholesterol concentrations relative to oleic acid (*cis*-$C_{18:1}$). Data are derived from six dietary comparisons between *trans* and *cis* monounsaturated fatty acids; differences between diets in fatty acids other than *trans* and *cis* monounsaturated fatty acids were adjusted for by using regression coefficients from a meta-analysis of 27 controlled trials. The regression lines were forced through the origin because a zero change in intake will produce a zero change in lipoprotein concentrations. From Zock *et al.* (1995), reproduced with kind permission of the *American Journal of Clinical Nutrition*.

Rincker Memorial Library-Concordia

changes in LDL and HDL concentrations on CHD risk, this was predicted to reduce the risk of CHD by 5–15%. In comparison, replacing *trans* fatty acids with either saturated fatty acids or carbohydrate would decrease risk by up to 8%.

The influence of *trans* fatty acids on plasma lipoproteins in relation to CHD risk would thus appear to be more unfavourable than that of saturated fatty acids, as determined by the effect on the ratio of LDL to HDL cholesterol. However, the overall magnitude of the effect would be dependent on the relative intakes of *trans* fatty acids and saturated fatty acids. In the UK *trans* fatty acids contribute about 2% of dietary energy, in contrast to saturated fatty acids which contribute about 15% dietary energy, and this needs to be considered when formulating dietary advice. The Task Force also estimated, on the same basis, that a reduction of 6% in energy from saturated fatty acids would decrease risk by 37%.

However, these conclusions of the adverse effect of *trans* fatty acid on plasma lipoprotein concentrations are not universally accepted. It has been commented that some trials used an inappropriate basis for comparison of the different diets and did not always control for other fatty acids that are known to influence blood cholesterol levels.

Several studies have suggested that *trans* fatty acids raise the plasma concentration of lipoprotein(a), particularly in individuals with already raised levels. Lipoprotein(a) has been suggested to be an independent risk marker for CHD, although this is not universally accepted.

Atherosclerosis and haemostasis

Despite the reported effects of *trans* fatty acids on blood lipoproteins, experiments with laboratory animals have not provided evidence that dietary *trans* fatty acids are associated with the development of experimental atherosclerosis, provided that the diet contains adequate levels of linoleic acid. Similarly, there is no evidence that *trans* fatty acids raise blood pressure, or affect the blood coagulation system. However, there has been no thorough evaluation of the effect of *trans* fatty acids on the coagulation system, and this is an area worthy of investigation.

The Role of *trans* Fatty Acids in Coronary Heart Disease

A number of epidemiological studies have suggested an association between *trans* fatty acids and CHD.

Case–control studies

A study by Ascherio in 1994 demonstrated that in subjects who had suffered acute myocardial infarction (AMI), past intake of *trans* fatty acids, assessed from a food frequency questionnaire, was associated with increased risk. *Trans* fatty acid intake per day in the top quintile was 6.5 g compared with 1.7 g in the lowest quintile. After adjusting for age, energy intake and sex, relative risk of a first AMI for the highest compared with the lowest quintile was 2.44 (95% confidence interval, 1.42 to 4.10). However, there was not a clear dose–response relationship.

A case–control study of sudden cardiac death found that higher concentrations of *trans* isomers of linoleic acid in adipose tissue, compared with lower concentrations, were associated with increased risk of sudden death. After controlling for smoking and making an allowance for social class, this relationship became insignificant.

A multicentre study in eight European countries plus Israel found that the risk of AMI was not significantly different across quartiles of the concentration of *trans*-18:1 fatty acids in adipose tissue, the multivariate odds ratio being 0.97 (95% confidence interval, 0.56 to 1.67) for the highest compared with the lowest quartiles. However, there were significant differences within countries. In Norway and Finland, relative risk was significantly increased in the highest compared with the lowest quartiles, but in Russia and Spain relative risk was significantly decreased in these groups. Exclusion from the multicentre analysis of the Spanish centres, which had particularly low intakes of *trans* fatty acids, resulted in a tendency to increased risk of AMI in the highest quartiles of *trans*-18:1 concentration. However, the trend was not statistically significant, and adjustment for confounding factors had no effect on the results.

A prospective study

The relationship between *trans* fatty acid intake and subsequent CHD events was investigated in approximately 85 000 US nurses (the Nurses Health Study). *Trans* fatty acid intake was calculated from food frequency questionnaires for women who had been diagnosed free from CHD, stroke, diabetes and hypercholesterolaemia. The subjects were followed up for 8 years and CHD events were recorded. The relative risk of CHD in the highest compared with the lowest quintile was 1.5 (95% confidence interval, 1.12 to 2.0), after adjustment for age, energy intake, social class and smoking. However, there was no clear dose–response relationship between the highest and the lowest intake groups. The intake of *trans* fatty acids in the top quintile was 3.2% dietary energy compared with 1.3% in the lowest quintile.

It has been commented on that the benefit predicted by the authors, that individuals in the top quintile of intake could halve their risk of myocardial infarction by reducing their intake of *trans* fatty acids to that of the lowest quintile, seems a large effect in view of the small difference in intakes between these groups (3.3 g). The changes in plasma lipoprotein cholesterol concentrations that would be predicted to occur as a result of lowering *trans* fatty acid intake would not explain all of the observed increase in risk. Also, the study was carried out in a selected population of women and it is unclear that the findings are applicable to the whole population or to other population groups.

Cancer

Although there is much evidence concerning the effect of different intakes of different types of fats on experimental carcinogenesis, data for *trans* fatty acids are limited and are hampered by confounding due to the lack of a suitable control diet.

Studies using different tumour models in mice and rats have shown no effect of *trans* fatty acids on tumour development. Increasing the intake of *trans* fatty acids, in place of *cis* fatty acids, has not demonstrated an adverse outcome with regard to cancer risk. In humans, there is little to suggest that *trans* fatty acids are adversely related to cancer risk at any of the major cancer sites. Early studies did not generally find that *trans* fatty acids were an important risk factor for malignant or benign breast disease. One study did report an association between the incidence of cancer of the colon, breast and prostate and the use of industrially hydrogenated vegetable fats in the USA; however, other known risk factors were not allowed for.

Cancer of the breast

Some epidemiological evidence suggests that total fat intake may be related to increased risk of cancer of the breast, although this is by no means conclusive. There is no strong evidence that intake of *trans* fatty acids *per se* is related to increased risk of breast cancer and many studies have not reported examining this relationship. A study in which adipose tissue concentrations of *trans*-18:1 fatty acids were assessed in 380 women with breast cancer at various stages and in controls, revealed no consistent pattern of association. A similar, smaller study suggested an increased risk with higher body stores of *trans* fatty acids, but it was concluded that any such association may be modified by adipose tissue concentrations of polyunsaturated fatty acids.

Cancer of the colon

Epidemiological data from the Nurses Health Study suggested a link between intake of meat and meat products and colon cancer. The data indicated that high intakes of total, animal, saturated and monounsaturated fat were associated with increased risk. Consuming beef, pork or lamb as a main dish was positively associated with risk; though beef and lamb contain *trans* fatty acids, there was no evidence that high intakes of *trans* fatty acids increased risk. The Health Professionals Follow-up Study (a prospective study in male health professionals of parallel design to the Nurses Health Study) found similar dietary associations for colon cancer risk, with no suggestion of any link with intake of *trans* fatty acids.

Prostate cancer

Dietary associations with risk of prostate cancer were also assessed from the Health Professionals Follow-up Study. High intakes of total, saturated, monounsaturated fatty acids and of α-linolenic acid were associated with increased risk, whereas high intakes of saturated fatty acids and linoleic acid were found to be protective. Intake of *trans* fatty acids was not found to be associated with risk of prostate cancer.

Dietary Guidelines

The details of population dietary guidelines for the quality and quantity of fat intake differ between countries. However, in consideration of prevention of CHD, dietary guidelines generally reflect advice to reduce average total fat intakes to 30–35% dietary energy, and to lower saturated fat intakes to approximately 10% of dietary energy. Though the effect of *trans* fatty acids on the plasma LDL/HDL ratio is less favourable than that of saturated fatty acids, dietary advice needs to reflect the relative intakes of these two types of fatty acids. Since the contribution of saturated fat intake to dietary energy is approximately 5–7 times higher than that of *trans* fatty acids, advice on *trans* fatty acids should not assume more importance than advice to lower saturated fatty acids. However, because of the unfavourable effect of *trans* fatty acids on plasma lipoprotein concentrations, the 1995 BNF Task Force report concluded that the average intake of *trans* fatty acids in the UK diet (2% of energy) should not rise, and that dietary advice should continue to focus on reducing intake of saturated fatty acids as a priority.

Extreme consumers of *trans* fatty acids may be at greater risk, and individuals with high intakes may benefit from advice to lower their intake. It has been calculated that lowering total fat and increasing carbohydrate intake (which reduces plasma HDL cholesterol) will have minimal effect on risk of CHD. Substituting *cis* unsaturated fatty acids for saturated and *trans* fatty acids would be predicted to have a greater impact. For individuals at risk of CHD, high intakes of *trans* fatty acids would appear to be undesirable. To follow dietary guidelines to reduce intake of *trans* fatty acids. consumers need to be informed about the relative levels of different types of fatty acids in food products. Nutritional labelling of *trans* fatty acids would thus be important. In Europe there is no requirement as yet to label *trans* fatty acids, although some manufacturers have chosen to provide this information.

It has been suggested that *trans* fatty acids should be included with saturated fatty acids for labelling purposes. However, labelling information is currently provided on a chemical basis, whereas this suggestion would imply a change to providing information on a physiological basis. However, it is advisable for food manufacturers to think in terms of the total amount of *trans* and saturated fatty acids present in a food product. If the decision is made to lower the levels of *trans* fatty acids, this should not be accompanied by an increase in the level of saturated fatty acids.

Conclusions

There is some evidence to suggest that *trans* fatty acids may have adverse effects on plasma lipoproteins, that would be predicted to increase risk of CHD, although further evidence supporting adverse health outcomes is required. It would be impossible to eliminate *trans* fatty acids from the diet as they occur naturally in beef, mutton and dairy products. However, developing technologies will enable the *trans* fatty acid content of foods to be reduced, but this should not be at the expense of increasing the content of saturated fatty acids. Public health advice should continue to focus on reducing saturated fatty acids, but labelling information on *trans* fatty acids may be helpful for informed consumers.

See also: **Cancer**: Epidemiology and Associations Between Diet and Cancer; Epidemiology of Breast Cancer. **Cholesterol**: Factors Determining Blood Cholesterol Levels. **Coronary Heart Disease**: Lipid Theory of Coronary Heart Disease; Aetiology. **Dairy Products**: Nutritional Value. **Dietary Guidelines**: International Perspectives. **Dietary Intake Measurement**: Methodology; Validation.

Dietary Surveys: Surveys of National Food Intake; Surveys of Food Intake in Groups and Individuals. **Epidemiological Studies**: Role and Interpretation. **Food Composition Data**: Compilation, Uses and Limitations. **Food Processing**: Nutritional Influences. **Hyperlipidaemia (Hyperlipidemia)**: Nutritional Management. **Lipids**: Chemistry and Classification; Composition and Role of Phospholipids in the Body. **Lipoproteins**: Physiology. **Meat, Poultry and Meat Products**: Nutritional Value. **Nutritional Labelling**: European Perspectives. **Socioeconomic Status**: Relationship with Diet and Nutritional Status.

Further Reading

AIN/ASCN (1996) Position paper on *trans* fatty acids. *American Journal of Clinical Nutrition* 63:663–670.

Aro AV, Kardinal AFM, Salminen I *et al.* (1995) Adipose tissue isomeric *trans* fatty acids and the risk of myocardial infarction in different countries: the EURAMIC study. *Lancet* 345:273–278.

Ascherio A, Hennekens CH, Buring JE *et al.* (1994) *Trans* fatty acids intake and risk of myocardial infarction. *Circulation* 89:94–101.

Berger KG (1996) *Lipids and Nutrition: Current Hot Topics*. Bridgwater: PJ Barnes.

British Nutrition Foundation (1995) *Trans Fatty Acids*. Report of the British Nutrition Foundation Task Force. London: BNF.

Giovannucci E, Rimm E, Colditz GA *et al.* (1993) A prospective study of dietary fat and risk of prostate cancer. *Journal of the National Cancer Institute* 85:1571–1579.

Giovannucci E, Rimm EB, Stampfer MJ *et al.* (1994) Intake of fat, meat and fiber in relation to risk of colon cancer in men. *Cancer Research* 54:2390–2397.

Gurr MI (1996) Dietary fatty acids with *trans* unsaturation. *Nutrition Research Reviews* 9:259–279.

International Life Sciences Institute (1995) *Trans* fatty acids and coronary heart disease risk. Report of the expert panel on *trans* fatty acids and coronary heart disease. *American Journal of Clinical Nutrition* 62:655S–707S.

Ip C and Marshall JR (1996) Trans fatty acids and cancer. *Nutrition Reviews* 54:138–145.

Mensink RP and Katan MB (1990) Effect of dietary fatty acids on high density and low density lipoprotein levels in healthy subjects. *New England Journal of Medicine* 323:439–444.

Willett WC, Stampfer MJ, Manson JE *et al.* (1993) Intake of *trans* fatty acids and risk of coronary heart disease among women. *Lancet* 341:581–585.

Zock PL, Katan MB and Mensink RP (1995) Dietary *trans* fatty acids and lipoprotein cholesterol. *American Journal of Clinical Nutrition* 61:617.

FERTILITY

Body Fat, Menarche and Fertility

R E Frisch, Harvard Center for Population and Development Studies, Massachusetts, USA

Copyright © 1998 Academic Press

Women who are underweight, or too lean, because of injudicious dieting, excessive athletic activity or both, experience disruption of their reproductive ability. It is now well documented that moderate weight loss, in the range of 10–15% of normal weight for height, unassociated with anorexia nervosa (where weight loss is in the range of 30% below ideal weight), results in amenorrhoea due to hypothalamic dysfunction. Weight loss in this moderate range is equivalent to a loss of one-third of body fat. If the excessive leanness occurs before menarche, menarche may be delayed until as late as the age of 19–20 years. Under special medical circumstances, normal menarche and ovulatory cycles can be delayed until after the age of 30 years.

In addition to these disruptive effects of weight loss and athletic activity on the menstrual cycle, women who exercise moderately or who are regaining weight into the normal range may have a menstrual cycle that appears to be normal, but which actually has a shortened luteal phase or is anovulatory. All of these partial or total disruptions of reproductive ability are usually reversible, after varying periods of time, following weight gain, decreased athletic training or both.

Excessive fatness is also associated with infertility in women; fertility is restored by loss of weight. Too little or too much fat are thus both associated with infertility. It is hypothesized that these associations are causal, and that the high percentage of body fat, 26–28% in women after completion of growth, is necessary for, and may influence, reproduction directly.

The hypothesis led to the prediction of minimum or threshold weights for height for the onset and maintenance of regular ovulatory menstrual cycles. These weights have been found to be useful clinically as target weights for the restoration of ovulatory cycles in cases of amenorrhoea due to weight loss. Both the absolute and relative amounts of fat are important, since the lean mass and the fat must be in a particular absolute range as well as a relative range, i.e. the woman must be big enough to reproduce successfully.

Why Fat? The Energy Cost of Reproduction

A human pregnancy and lactation each have a high energy cost: a pregnancy requires about 336 MJ (74 000 kcal) over and above normal metabolic requirements. Lactation requires about 2.5 MJ (600 kcal) a day. In premodern times lactation was an essential part of reproduction.

While the reproductive system is slowly maturing during growth, the body changes in composition, as well as in size and proportions. Direct measurements of body water of girls from birth to completion of growth at ages 16–18 years show a continuous decline in the proportion of body water, because girls have a large relative increase in body fat (**Fig. 1**). This decrease is particularly rapid during the adolescent growth spurt in height and weight, which precedes menarche.

At the completion of growth, between age 16–18 years, the body of a well-nourished woman contains about 26–28% fat and about 52% water, whereas the body of a man at completion of growth contains about 14% fat and 61% water. A young girl and boy of the same height and weight (**Table 1**) differ markedly in the percentages of body water and fat. The main function of the 16 kg of stored female fat,

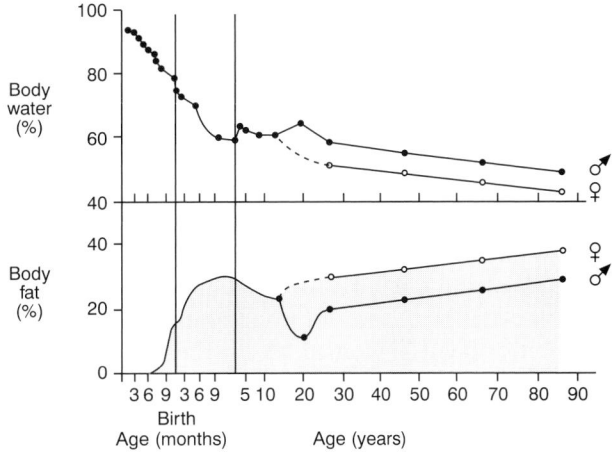

Figure 1 Changes in body water as percentage of body weight throughout the life span, and corresponding changes in the percentage of body fat. Adapted from Friis-Hansen (1965).

Table 1 Total body water as percentage of body weight: an index of fatness. Comparison of an 18-year-old girl and a 15-year-old boy of the same height and weight

Variable	Girl	Boy
Height (cm)	165.0	165.0
Weight (kg)	57.0	57.0
Total body water (l)	29.5	36.0
Lean body weight (kg)	41.0	50.0
Fat (kg)	16.0	7.0
Fat/body weight (%)	28.0	12.0
Total body water/body weight (%)	51.8	63.0

Lean body weight = total body water/0.72.
Fatness/body weight % = 100 − [(total body water/body wt %)/0.72].

which is equivalent to over 600 MJ (144 000 kcal), may be to be provide energy for a pregnancy and for about 3 months lactation. In prehistoric times when the food supply was scarce or fluctuated seasonally, stored fat would have been necessary for successful reproduction. Fat is the most labile component of body weight. Body fat therefore would reflect environmental changes in food supplies more rapidly than other tissues.

Body weight and infant survival

Infant survival is correlated with birthweight, and birthweight is correlated with the prepregnancy weight of the mother and, independently, her weight gain during pregnancy. From a teleologic and evolutionary view, it is economical to hypothesize that the physical ability to deliver a viable infant and the hypothalamic control of reproduction are synchronized. Adipose tissue may be the synchronizer.

How Adipose Tissue May Regulate Female Reproduction

There are at least four mechanisms already known by which adipose tissue may directly affect ovulation and the menstrual cycle, and hence fertility:

1. Adipose tissue is a significant extragonadal source of oestrogen. Conversion of androgen to oestrogen takes place in the adipose tissue of the breast and abdomen, the omentum and the fatty marrow of the long bones. This conversion accounts for roughly a third of the circulating oestrogen of premenopausal women, and is the main source of oestrogen in postmenopausal women. Men also convert androgen into oestrogen in body fat.
2. Body weight, hence fatness, influences the direction of oestrogen metabolism to more potent or less potent forms. Very thin women have an increase in the 2-hydroxylated form of oestrogen,

which is relatively inactive and has little affinity for the oestrogen receptor. Lean women athletes also have an increase in the 2-hydroxylated form of oestrogen. In contrast, obese women metabolize less of the 2-hydroxylated form and have a relative increase in the 16-hydroxylated form, which has potent oestrogenic activity.
3. Obese women and young girls who are relatively fatter have a diminished capacity for oestrogen to bind to serum sex hormone-binding globulin (SHBG); this results in an elevated percentage of free serum oestradiol. Since SHBG regulates the availability of oestradiol to the brain and other target tissues, the changes in the proportion of body fat to lean mass may influence reproductive performance through the intermediate effects of SHBG.
4. The adipose tissue of obese women stores steroid hormones.

Changes in relative fatness may also affect reproductive ability indirectly through disturbance of the regulation of body temperature and energy balance by the hypothalamus. Very lean women, both anorexic and nonanorexic, display abnormalities of temperature regulation, in addition to delayed response, or lack of response, to exogenous luteinizing hormone releasing hormone.

Hypothalamic Dysfunction, Gonadotrophin Secretion and Weight Loss

It is now known that the amenorrhoea of underweight and excessively lean women is due to hypothalamic dysfunction. Hypothalamic dysfunction has been implicated also in the amenorrhoea of athletes. Consistent with the view that this type of amenorrhoea is adaptive, the pituitary-ovarian axis is apparently intact, and functions when exogenous gonadotrophin releasing hormone (GnRH) is given in pulsatile form or in a bolus.

Women with this type of hypothalamic amenorrhoea have both quantitative and qualitative changes in the secretion of the gonadotrophins – luteinizing hormone (LH) and follicle stimulating hormone (FSH) – and of oestrogen:

1. Levels of LH, FSH and oestradiol levels are low.
2. The secretion of LH and the response to GnRH are reduced in direct correlation with the amount of weight loss.
3. Underweight patients respond to exogenous GnRH with a pattern of secretion similar to that of prepubertal children; the FSH response is

greater than the LH response. The return of LH responsiveness is correlated with weight gain.

4. The maturity of the 24 h LH secretory pattern and body weight are related; weight loss results in an age-inappropriate secretory pattern resembling that of prepubertal or early pubertal children. Weight gain restores the postmenarcheal secretory pattern.

5. A reduced response or absence of response to clomiphene is correlated with the degree of the loss of body weight and hence of fat. A normal response occurs after weight gain to the normal range.

Supportive of the view that this type of hypothalamic amenorrhea is adaptive are the findings of one study that women in whom ovulation had been induced had a higher risk of babies who were small for dates, and this risk was greatest (54%) in those who were underweight. The authors of this study concluded that the most suitable treatment for infertility secondary to weight-related amenorrhoea is dietary, rather than induction of ovulation.

The Physiological Basis of Reproductive Ability

Weight at menarche

The idea that relative fatness is important for female reproductive ability followed findings that the events of the adolescent growth spurt, particularly menarche in girls, were closely related to an *average* critical body weight. This result was unexpected for human beings, although it was well known for rats and monkeys that puberty (defined by vaginal opening, or more precisely, by first oestrus) was more closely related to body weight than to chronological age.

In the USA, the mean weight at menarche for girls was 47.8 ± 0.5 kg, at the mean height of 158.5 ± 0.5 cm and at the mean age of 12.9 ± 0.1 years. This mean age included girls from Denver, who had a slightly later age of menarche than the sea-level populations, owing to the slowing effect of altitude on prenatal and postnatal weight growth.

The secular trend towards an earlier age of menarche

Even before analysing the meaning of the critical weight for an individual girl, the idea that menarche is associated with a critical weight for a population explained simply many observations associated with early or late menarche. Observations of earlier menarche are associated with attaining the critical weight more quickly. The most important example is the secular (long-term) trend to an earlier menarche of about 3–4 months per decade in Europe in the last 100 years (**Fig. 2**). Our explanation is that children are bigger sooner; therefore girls on average reach 46–47 kg, the mean weight at menarche of US and many European populations, more quickly. Theoretically the secular trend should end when the weight of children of successive cohorts remains the same

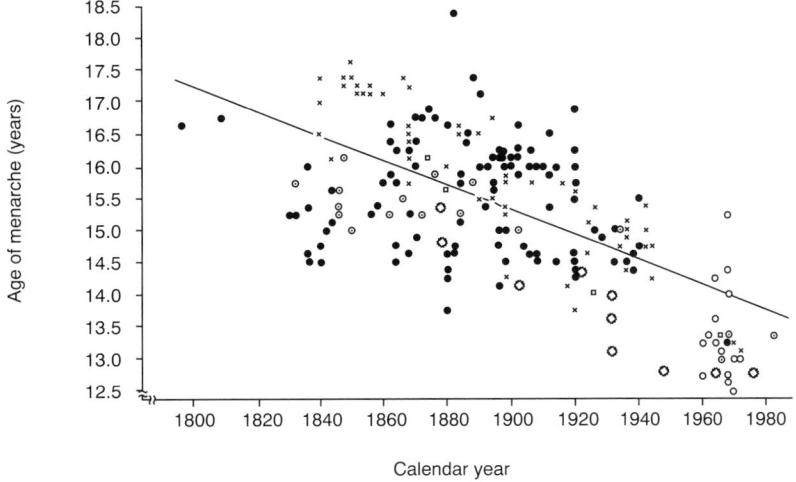

Figure 2 Mean or median age of menarche as a function of calendar year from 1790 to 1980. The symbols refer to England ⊙, France ●, Germany ⊗, Holland □, Scandinavia (Denmark, Finland, Norway and Sweden) ×; Belgium, Czechoslovakia, Hungary, Italy, Poland (rural), Romania (urban and rural), Russia (15.2 years at an altitude of 2500 m and 14.4 years at 700 m), Spain and Switzerland, all labelled ○; and the USA ✿ (data not included in the regression line). Twenty-seven points were identical and do not appear on the graph. The regression line of course cannot be extended indefinitely. The age of menarche has already levelled off in some European countries, as it has in the USA. From Wyshak and Frisch (1982) with permission from the *New England Journal of Medicine*.

because of the attainment of maximum nutrition and child care; this now has happened in the USA.

Conversely, a late menarche is associated with body weight growth that is slower prenatally, postnatally or both, so that the average critical weight is reached at a later age: malnutrition delays menarche; twins have later menarche than do singletons of the same population; and high altitude delays menarche.

Components of weight at menarche

Individual girls have menarche at varied weights and heights. To make the notion of a critical weight meaningful for an individual girl, the components of body weight at menarche were analysed. We investigated body composition at menarche because total body water (TW) and lean body weight (LBW, TW/0.72) are more closely correlated with metabolic rate than is body weight, since they represent the metabolic mass as a first approximation. Metabolic rate was considered to be an important clue, since G.C. Kennedy hypothesized a food intake-lipostat-metabolic signal to explain his elegant findings on weight and puberty in the rat.

The greatest change in estimated body composition of both early- and late-maturing girls during the adolescent growth spurt was a large increase in body fat, from about 5 kg to 11 kg, a 120% increase, compared with a 44% increase in lean body weight. There was thus a change in the ratio of lean body weight to fat from 5:1 at initiation of the spurt to 3:1 at menarche. The shortest, lightest girls at menarche had a smaller absolute amount of fat, 8.9 ± 0.4 kg, compared with the tallest, heaviest girls, 12.3 ± 0.6 kg (the mean of all subjects was 11.5 ± 0.3 kg). However, both extreme groups have about 22% of their body weight as fat at menarche as do all subjects, and the ratio of lean body weight to fat of both groups is in the range of 3:1, as it is in all subjects.

Since adipose tissue can convert androgens to oestrogens, the relative degree of fatness can be directly related to the quantity of circulating oestrogen. The biological effectiveness of the oestrogen is also related to body weight. Rate of fat gain therefore is a neat mechanism for relating rate of growth, nutrition and physical work to the energy requirements for reproduction.

Fatness as a determinant of minimal weights for menstrual cycles

As shown in Table 1 and Fig. 1, total body water as a percentage of body weight is an index of fatness. This index in each of the same 181 girls followed from menarche to the completion of growth at ages 16–18 years provided a method of determining a minimal weight for height necessary for menarche in primary amenorrhoea and for the resumption of normal, ovulatory cycles in cases of secondary amenorrhoea, when the amenorrhoea was due to undernutrition or intensive exercise. These weights have been found useful in the evaluation and treatment of patients with primary or secondary amenorrhoea due to weight loss.

Percentiles of total body water/body weight, which are percentiles of fatness, were made at menarche and for the same 181 girls at age 18 years, the age at which body composition stabilized. Patients with amenorrhoea due to weight loss, other possible causes having been excluded, were studied in relation to the weights indicated by the diagonal percentile lines of total water/body weight percent (**Fig. 3**). It was found that 56.1% of total water/body weight the 10th percentile at age 18 years (equivalent to about 22% fat of body weight), indicated a minimal weight for height necessary for the restoration and maintenance of menstrual cycles. For example, a 20-year-old woman whose height is 165 cm (65 in) should weigh at least 49 kg (108 lb) before menstrual cycles would be expected to resume (Fig. 3).

The weights at which menstrual cycles ceased or resumed in postmenarcheal patients age 16 years and older were about 10% greater than the minimal weights for the same height observed at menarche (**Fig. 4**). The explanation was that both early- and late-maturing girls gain an average of 4.5 kg of fat from menarche to age 18 years. Almost all of this gain is achieved by age 16 years, when mean fat is 15.7 ± 0.3 kg, 27% of body weight. At age 18 years mean fat is 16.0 ± 0.3 kg, 28% of the mean body weight of 57.1 ± 0.6 kg. Reflecting this increase in fatness, the total water/body weight percent decreases from 55.1 ± 0.2% at menarche (12.9 ± 0.1 years in this sample) to 52.1 ± 0.2% (standard deviation 3.0) at age 18 years.

Because girls are less fat at menarche than when they achieve stable reproductive ability, the minimal weight for onset of menstrual cycles in cases of primary amenorrhoea due to undernutrition or exercise is indicated by the 10th percentile of fractional body water at menarche, 59.8% which is equivalent to about 17% of body weight as fat. For example, a 15-year-old girl whose completed height is 165 cm (65 in) should weigh at least 43.6 kg (96 lb) before menstrual cycles can be expected to begin (Fig. 4).

The minimum weights indicated in Fig. 4 would be used also for girls who become amenorrhoeic as a result of weight loss shortly after menarche, as is often found in cases of anorexia nervosa in adolescent girls.

The absolute and relative increase in fatness from

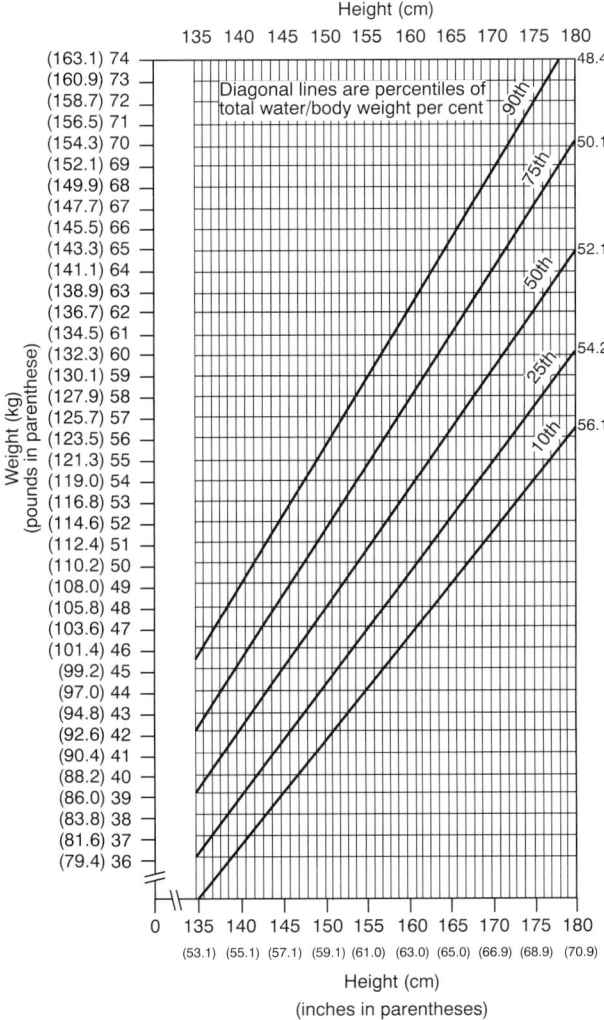

Figure 3 The minimal weight necessary for a particular height for restoration of menstrual cycles is indicated on the weight scale by the 10th percentile diagonal line of total water/body weight per cent, 56.1%, as it crosses the vertical height line. For example, a 20-year-old woman whose height is 165 cm (65 in) should weigh at least 49 kg (108 lb) before menstrual cycles would be expected to resume. Adapted from Frisch and McArthur (1974) with permission from *Science*.

menarche to ages 16–18 years coincides with the period of adolescent subfecundity. During this time there is still rapid growth of the uterus, the ovaries and the oviducts.

Other factors such as emotional stress affect the maintenance or onset of menstrual cycles. Therefore, menstrual cycles may cease without weight loss and may not resume in some subjects even though the minimum weight for height has been achieved. Also, these standards apply as yet only to Caucasian US females and European females, since different races have different critical weights at menarche and it is not yet known whether the different critical weights represent the same critical body composition of fatness.

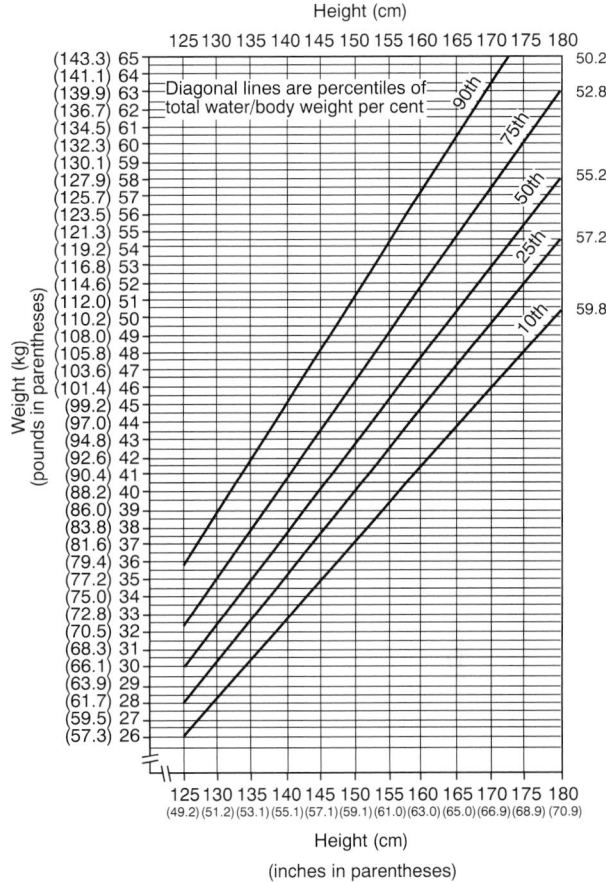

Figure 4 The minimal weight necessary for a particular height for onset of menstrual cycles is indicated on the weight scale by the 10th percentile diagonal line of total water/body weight per cent, 59.8%, as it crosses the vertical height lines. The height growth of girls must be completed, or approaching completion. For example, a 15-year-old girl whose completed height is 165 cm (65 in) should weigh at least 43.6 kg (96 lb) before menstrual cycles can be expected to start. Adapted from Frisch and McArthur (1974) with permission from *Science*.

Since the prediction of the minimum weights for height is based on total water/body weight percent (not fat to body weight percent) successful prediction may be related to the ratio of lean mass to fat, which is normally about 3:1 at menarche and 2.5:1 at the completion of growth at age 18 years. No prediction can as yet be made above the threshold weight for a particular height.

Physical Exercise, Delayed Menarche and Amenorrhoea

Does intense exercise cause delayed menarche and amenorrohea of athletes, or do late maturers choose to be athletes and dancers? We found that the mean age of menarche of 38 college swimmers and runners was 13.9 ± 0.3 years, significantly later ($P < 0.001$) than that of the general population, 12.8 ± 0.05 years, in accord with other reports. However, the mean menarcheal age of the 18 athletes whose training began *before* menarche was 15.1 ± 0.5 years, whereas the mean menarcheal age of the 20 athletes whose training began after their menarche was 12.8 ± 0.2 years ($P < 0.001$). The latter mean age was similar to that of the college controls, 12.7 ± 0.4 years, and the general population. Therefore, training, not preselection, is the delaying factor. Each year of premenarcheal training delayed menarche by 5 months (0.4 year). This suggests that one constructive way to reduce the incidence of teenage pregnancy would be to have girls join teams at ages 8–9 years and maintain regular moderate exercise. Such a programme might reduce the risk of serious diseases of women in later life as is presented below.

Training also directly affected the regularity of the menstrual cycles during the training year. Of the premenarche-trained athletes, only 17% had regular cycles; 61% were irregular and 22% were amenorrhoeic. In contrast, 60% of the postmenarche-trained athletes were regular, 40% were irregular and none were amenorrhoeic. However, during intense training, the incidence of oligomenorrhoea and amenorrhoea increased in both groups.

As other workers have found, plasma gonadotrophins and oestrogen levels were in the low-normal range in this study for the athletes with irregular cycles or amenorrhoea. Progesterone was at follicular phase level. Thyroid hormones, however, were in the normal range. These athletes had increased muscularity and decreased adiposity, compared with nonathletes. The explanation of their menstrual disturbances may therefore be the same as for dieting, nonathletic women: too little fat in relation to the lean mass. Some of the swimmers and track and field athletes were above average weight for height. A raised lean mass to fat ratio may nevertheless have caused their menstrual problems, because their body weight represented a greater amount of muscle and less adipose tissue than the same weight of a nonathletic woman.

Psychologic stress and changes in weight

The psychologic stress of competition, which may increase the secretion of adrenal corticosteroids and catecholamines, thus affecting the hypothalamic control of gonadotrophins, may also be involved; but stress does not seem to be the main factor in many individuals.

Nutrition and Male Reproduction

Undernutrition delays the onset of sexual maturation in boys in a similar way to the delaying effect of undernutrition on menarche. Undernutrition and weight loss in men also affect their reproductive ability. The sequence of effects, however, is different from that in the female. In men loss of libido is the first effect of a decrease in energy intake and subsequent weight loss. Continued energy reduction and weight loss result in a loss of prostate fluid, and decreases of sperm motility and sperm longevity, in that order. Sperm production ceases when weight loss is in the range of 25% of normal body weight. Refeeding results in a restoration of function in the reverse order of loss.

Effects of exercise on men

Men marathon runners have recently been shown to have decreased hypothalamic GnRH secretion. Also reported are changes in serum testosterone levels with weight loss in wrestlers, a reduction in serum testosterone and prolactin levels in male distance runners, and changes in reproductive function and development in relation to physical activity.

Nutrition, Physical Work and Natural Fertility

The effects of hard physical work and nutrition on reproductive ability, set forth above, suggested that differences in the fertility of populations, historically and today, may be explained by a direct pathway from food intake to fertility (**Fig. 5**), in addition to the classic Malthusian pathway through mortality. Charles Darwin described this common-sense direct relationship between food supplies and fertility, observing that:

1. Domestic animals that have regular, plentiful food without working to get it are more fertile than the corresponding wild animals.
2. 'Hard living retards the period at which animals conceive'.
3. The amount of food affects the fertility of the same individual.
4. It is difficult to fatten a cow that is lactating.

All of Darwin's dicta apply to human beings.

The paradox of rapid population growth in undernourished populations

In many historical populations with slow population growth, poor couples living together to the end of their reproductive lives had only 6–7 living births. Most poor couples in many developing countries today also only have 6–7 living births during their reproductive life span. This total fertility rate is far below the human maximum of 11–12 children observed among well-nourished couples not using

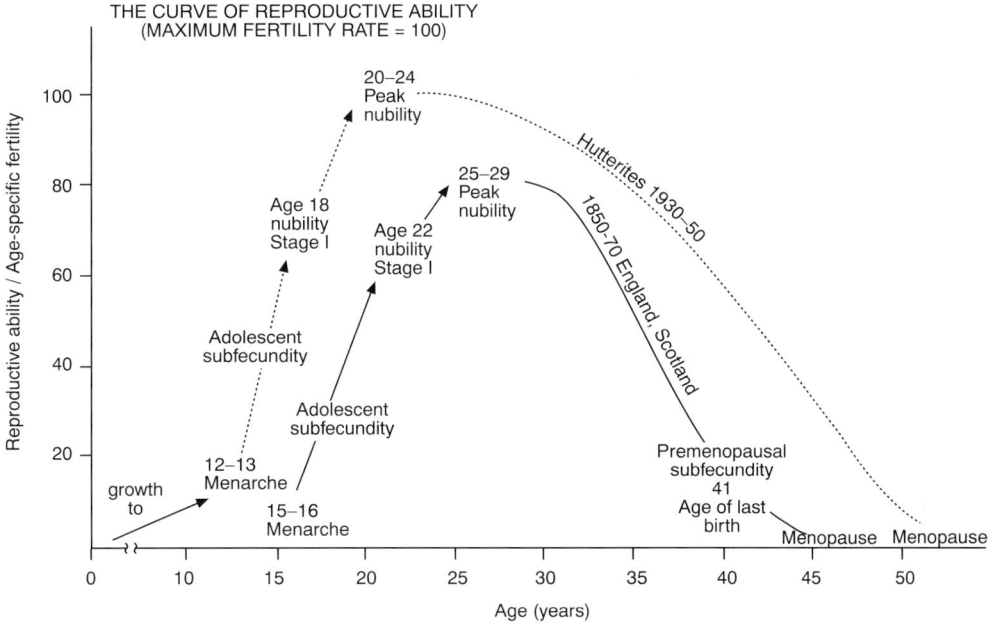

THE CURVE OF REPRODUCTIVE ABILITY
(MAXIMUM FERTILITY RATE = 100)

Figure 5 The mid-nineteenth century curve of female reproductive ability (variation of the rate of childbearing with age) compared with that of the well-nourished, modern Hutterites who do not use contraception. The Hutterite fertility curve (broken line) results in an average of 10–12 children; the 1850–70 fertility curve (solid line) in about 6–8 children. From Frisch (1978) with permission from *Science*.

contraception, such as the Hutterites. However, six children per couple today in developing countries results in a very rapid rate of population growth because of decreased mortality rates, resulting from the necessary introduction of modern public health procedures. The difference between the birth rate per 1000 and the death rate per 1000, which gives the percentage growth rate, is now as high as 2–4%. Populations growing at 2%, 3% and 4% double in 35 years, 23 years and 18 years, respectively.

British data from the mid-nineteenth century on growth rates, food intake, age-specific fertility, sterility, and ages of menarche and menopause show that females who grew relatively slowly to maturity, completing height growth at ages 20–21 years (instead of 16–18 years as in well-nourished contemporary populations) also differed from well-nourished females in each event of the reproductive span: menarche was later, for example, 15.0–16.0 years, compared with 12.8 years; adolescent sterility was longer, and the age of peak nubility was later; the levels of specific fertility were lower; pregnancy wastage was higher; the duration of lactational amenorrhoea was longer; the birth interval was therefore longer; and the age of menopause was earlier, preceded by a more rapid period of perimenopausal decline (Fig. 5). Thus, the slower, submaximal growth of women to maturity is subsequently associated with a shortened and less efficient reproductive span. The differences in the

rate of physical growth of women and men result not only in a displacement of the age-specific fertility curve in time, but in a difference in the ultimate level: the faster the growth of the females and males, the earlier and more efficient the reproductive ability.

Recent endocrinological data show that undernourished women have a longer lactational amenorrhoea than do well-nourished women. The amount of suckling is not the only factor, as has been suggested in explaining reduced natural fertility. In addition, age of menarche and the other events of the reproductive span, which are known to be affected by the nutritional state, are pertinent to overall fertility.

Long-term regular exercise lowers the risk of sex hormone-sensitive cancers

The amenorrhoea and delayed menarche of athletes raise the question: are there differences in the long-term reproductive health of athletes with moderate training compared with nonathletes?

A study of 5398 college alumnae ages 20–80 years, of whom 2622 were former athletes and 2776 were nonathletes, showed that the former athletes had a significantly lower lifetime occurrence of breast cancer and cancers of the reproductive system compared with the nonathletes. Over 82.4% of these former college athletes began their training in high school or earlier, compared with 24.9% of the nonathletes. The analysis controlled for potential confounding factors including age, age of menarche, age of first birth, smoking and cancer family history. The relative risk (RR) for nonathletes compared with athletes for cancers of the reproductive system was 2.53, 95% confidence limits (CL) 1.17 to 5.47 (**Fig. 6**). The RR for breast cancer was 1.86 (95% CL, 1.00 to 3.47). The former college athletes were leaner in every age group compared to the nonathletes.

Although one can only speculate at present as to the reasons for the lower risk, the most likely explanation is that long term, the former athletes had lower levels of oestrogen because they were leaner, and more oestrogen was metabolized to the nonpotent catechol oestrogens. Also, the former athletes may have consumed diets lower in fat and saturated fat. Such diets shift the pattern of oestrogen metabolism toward the less active catechol oestrogens.

The lower risk of breast cancer observed among the former college athletes is in accord with the hypothesis that regular, ovulatory menstrual cycles would be expected to *increase* the risk of breast cancer. Compared with the nonathletes, the former college athletes also had a lower lifetime occurrence (prevalence) of benign tumours of the breast and reproductive system, a lower prevalence of diabetes, particularly after age 40 years, and no greater risk of bone fractures, including risk of wrist and hip fractures, in the menopausal period.

These data indicate that long-term exercise, which was not at Olympic or marathon level but moderate and regular, reduces the risk of sex hormone-sensitive cancers, and the risk of diabetes for women in later life. Recent data showing moderate exercise also reduces the risk of nonreproductive system cancers suggest that other factors, such as changes in immunosurveillance, may also be involved.

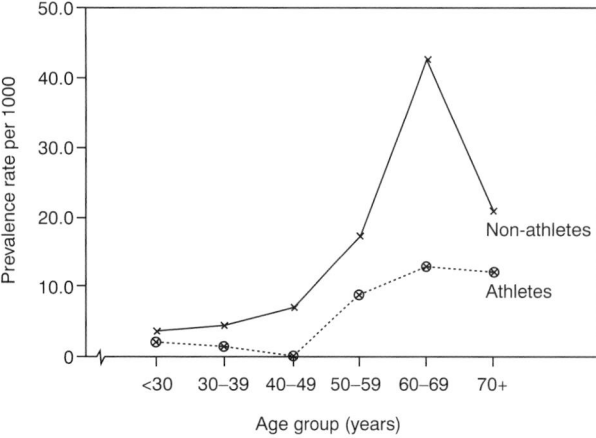

Figure 6 Prevalence rate of cancers of the reproductive system for athletes (circles) and nonathletes (crosses) by age group. From Frisch *et al.* (1985) with permission from the *British Journal of Cancer*.

Magnetic resonance imaging to determine body fat of athletes and controls

Using magnetic resonance imaging for direct quantification of body fat showed that athletes who did not differ in body weight from nonathletes, actually had 30–40% less fat than the nonathletes. Muscles are heavy (80% water) so the body weight of an athlete does not necessarily indicate body composition. Athletes had a more sensitive insulin response to a glucose tolerance test compared with controls. The insulin area under the curve of athletes and controls was significantly related to their total fat as a percentage of total volume, determined by magnetic resonance imaging.

Athletes with menstrual disorders had significantly decreased subcutaneous and internal fat, overall and at all regional sites, compared with controls. The extent of oestradiol 2-hydroxylation to 2-hydroxyoestrone, determined by radiometric analysis, was significantly ($P = 0.005$) inversely related to total fat as a percentage of total volume and to subcutaneous fat as a percentage of total volume ($P = 0.004$) overall and at each of the regional fat depots. This inverse relationship may be a determinant of the anovulatory cycles and amenorrhoea of excessively lean women by a feedback to the hypothalamus, since 2-hydroxyoestrone is antioestrogenic.

In accord with these relations on fatness and fertility are the recent findings on the *obese* gene that adipose tissue produces a protein hormone, leptin, which has receptors in the hypothalamus. Leptin controls appetite and energy metabolism and thus acts as a 'lipostat' regulating body fat storage.

See also: **Cancer**: Epidemiology of Breast Cancer. **Exercise**: Physiology of Skeletal Muscle; Diet and Exercise; Beneficial Effects. **Growth and Development**: Physiological Aspects. **Infants**: Low-birthweight and Preterm Infants. **Obesity**: Definition, Aetiology and Assessment; Complications of Obesity. **Pregnancy**: Energy Requirements and Metabolic Adaptations; Nutrient Requirements; Appropriate Maternal Weight Gain; Safe Diet for Pregnancy; Role of Placenta in Nutrient Transfer; Preconception Nutrition and Prevention of Neural Tube Defects; Pre-eclampsia and Diet.

Further Reading

Chehab FF, Mounzih K, Ronghva L and Lim ME (1997) Early onset of reproductive function in normal female mice treated with leptin. *Science* 275:88–90.

Friis-Hansen B (1965) Hydrometry of growth and aging. In: Brozek J (ed.) *Human Body Composition*, vol. 7, Symposia of the Society for the Study of Human Biology, pp 191–209. Oxford: Pergamon Press.

Frisch RE (1978) Population, food intake and fertility. *Science* **199**:22–30.

Frisch RE (1981) What's below the surface? *New England Journal of Medicine* **305**:1019–1020.

Frisch RE (1985) Fatness, menarche and female fertility. *Perspectives in Biology and Medicine* **28**:611–633.

Frisch RE, ed. (1990) *Adipose Tissue and Reproduction*, Basel: Karger.

Frisch RE and McArthur JW (1974) Menstrual cycles: fatness as a determinant of minimum weight for height necessary for their maintenance or onset. *Science* **185**:949–951.

Frisch RE, Wyshak G and Vincent L (1980) Delayed menarche and amenorrhea of ballet dancers. *New England Journal of Medicine* **303**:17–19.

Frisch RE, Wyshak G, Albright NL *et al.* (1985) Lower prevalence of breast cancer and cancers of the reproductive system among former college athletes compared to non-athletes. *British Journal of Cancer* **52**:885–891.

Frisch RE, Snow RC, Johnson L, Gerard B, Barbieri R and Rosen B (1993) Magnetic resonance imaging of overall and regional body fat, estrogen metabolism and ovulation of athletes compared to controls. *Journal of Clinical Endocrinology and Metabolism* **77**:441–477.

Vigersky RA, Andersen AE, Thompson RH *et al.* (1977) Hypothalamic dysfunction in secondary amenorrhea associated with simple weight loss. *New England Journal of Medicine* **297**:1141–1145.

Wyshak G and Frisch RE (1982) Evidence for a secular trend in age of menarche. *New England Journal of Medicine* **306**:1033–1035.

FETAL ORIGINS OF DISEASE

Fetal Development and Later Disease

D J P Barker, University of Southampton, UK

Copyright © 1998 Academic Press

Many human fetuses have to adapt to a limited supply of nutrients and in doing so they permanently change their physiology and metabolism. These 'programmed' changes may be the origins of a number of diseases in later life, including coronary heart disease and the related disorders stroke, diabetes and hypertension.

Programming

During embryonic life, that is during the 8 weeks after conception, the basic form of the human baby is laid down in miniature. The 5-week-old embryo does not contain a description of the person to whom it will give rise; rather, it contains in its genes a generative programme for making a person, a programme that has been likened to a recipe. As development proceeds, the destiny of cells becomes determined by their surroundings, by the position they come to occupy in the body, by the signals they receive from neighbouring cells, and hence by the genes that become activated.

The body does not increase greatly in size during embryonic life, but in the fetal period – from 9 weeks after conception onwards – there begins the phase of rapid growth which continues until after birth. Growth does not simply expand the miniature human being; through differences in growth rates of different parts of the body, it moulds the baby's form. The diversity of size and form of babies born after normal pregnancies is remarkable. Studies of the birthweights of relatives have led to the conclusion that variation in size at birth is essentially determined by the intrauterine environment rather than the fetal genome.

The main feature of fetal growth is cell division. The tissues of the body grow during periods of rapid cell division; the timing of these differs for different tissues. The kidney, for example, has a period of rapid cell division in the weeks immediately before birth. Growth depends on the availability of nutrients and oxygen, and the main adaptation of the fetus to lack of these essentials is to slow its rate of cell division.

Cell division slows either as a direct effect of undernutrition on the cell or through altered concentrations of growth factors or hormones, of which insulin and growth hormone are particularly important. Even brief periods of undernutrition may permanently reduce the numbers of cells in particular organs. This is one of the mechanisms by which undernutrition may permanently change or 'programme' the body. Other lasting 'memories' of undernutrition include change in the distribution of cell types, in hormonal feedback, in metabolic activity and in organ structure. It is not in question that the human body can be programmed by undernutrition. Rickets has for a long while served as a demonstration that undernutrition at a critical stage of early life leads to persisting changes in structure. What is new is the realization that some of the body's 'memories' of early undernutrition become translated into pathological states and thereby determine disease in later life.

Animal studies

One of the earliest demonstrations of programming was that showing the lifelong effects of early exposure to sex hormones on sexual physiology. A female rat injected with the male hormone testosterone on the fifth day after birth develops normally until puberty, but fails to ovulate or show normal patterns of female sexual behaviour thereafter. The release of gonad stimulating hormones from the hypothalamus in the brain has been irreversibly altered from the cyclical female pattern of release to the tonic male pattern. If the same injection of testosterone is given when the animal is 20 days old it has no effect. Thus there is a critical period at which the animal's sexual physiology is sensitive and can be permanently changed. Numerous animal experiments such as this have shown that hormones, undernutrition and other influences that affect development during sensitive periods of early life can programme persisting changes in structure and in metabolic, hormonal and immune functions, some of which are known to be important in disease.

Epidemiological Evidence

The main focus for research into coronary heart disease, the commonest cause of death in the Western world, has been the life styles of men and women. Inappropriate behaviours – a high-fat diet, cigarette smoking, becoming obese – have been implicated. Adult life styles, however, fail to explain much about the geography of the disease, its trends over time, and why one person dies from coronary heart disease while another does not.

In the search for a new model for coronary heart disease an important clue, suggesting that it might originate *in utero*, came from studies of death rates among babies in Britain during the early years of the twentieth century. Death during infancy was remarkably common in those days. In 1917 the Bishop of London remarked 'while nine soldiers died every hour in 1915, twelve babies died every hour, so that it was much more dangerous to be a baby than a soldier'. The usual certified cause of death in newborn babies was low birthweight. Death rates in the newborn differed considerably between one part of Britain and another, being highest in some of the northern industrial towns and the poorer rural areas in the north and west. This geographical pattern in death rates closely resembles today's large variations in death rates from coronary heart disease, variations which form one aspect of the continuing north-south divide in health in the UK. A conclusion suggested by this observation was that low rates of growth before birth are linked to the development of coronary heart disease in adult life. The suggestion that events in childhood influence the pathogenesis of coronary heart disease was not new. A focus on intrauterine life, however, offered a new point of departure for research.

In the UK, early epidemiological studies to pursue this were based on the simple strategy of examining individual men and women, in middle and late life, whose size at birth was recorded. The records on which these studies were based came to light as a result of the UK Medical Research Council's systematic search of the archives and records offices of Britain – a search which led to the discovery of three important collections of birth records, in Hertfordshire, Preston and Sheffield. In Hertfordshire the Lady Inspector of Midwives from 1905 onwards, Margaret Burnside, had recruited an army of trained nurses to attend women in childbirth and to advise mothers on how to keep their babies healthy. Throughout the county when women gave birth they were attended by a midwife. The baby was weighed at birth and again at 1 year. These weights were recorded in ledgers.

A total of 15 726 men and women born in Hertfordshire during 1911–1930 were traced from birth to the present day. Death rates from coronary heart disease among them fell progressively from those who weighed less than 2.5 kg (5.5 lb) at birth to those who weighed 4.31 kg (9.5 lb) (**Table 1**). Another study, in Sheffield, showed that it was babies who were small because they failed to grow, rather than small because they were born prematurely, who were at increased risk of coronary heart disease. A subsequent study of 80 000 nurses in the USA showed a similar 2-fold fall in risk of coronary heart disease between those with low birthweight and those with high birthweight.

Examination of men and women who were still living in the Hertfordshire study showed that these trends in coronary heart disease with birthweight were paralleled by similar trends in two disorders, hypertension and diabetes mellitus, that are associated with the disease. **Table 2** shows the steep fall in prevalence of adult onset diabetes mellitus, or its

Table 1 Death rates from coronary heart disease among 15 726 men and women according to birthweight

Birthweight		Standardized mortality ratio	No. of deaths
(lb)	(kg)		
≤5.5	≤2.50	100	57
6.5	2.95	81	137
7.5	3.41	80	298
8.5	3.86	74	289
9.5	4.31	55	103
>9.5	>4.31	65	57
Total		74	941
P value for trend		< 0.0001	

Table 2 Prevalence of non-insulin-dependent diabetes mellitus and impaired glucose tolerance in men aged 59–70 years

Birthweight		No. of men	Percentage with impaired glucose tolerance or diabetes	Odds ratio adjusted for body mass index (95% confidence interval)
(lb)	(kg)			
≤5.5	≤2.50	20	40	6.6 (1.5 to 28)
6.5	2.95	47	34	4.8 (1.3 to 17)
7.5	3.41	104	31	4.6 (1.4 to 16)
8.5	3.86	117	22	2.6 (0.8 to 8.9)
9.5	4.31	54	13	1.4 (0.3 to 5.6)
> 9.5	> 4.31	28	14	1.0
Total		370	25	

preclinical state impaired glucose tolerance, between men who were small at birth and men who were large at birth. This finding has been confirmed in both men and women in two other studies in Britain, in two studies in the USA, and in a study in Sweden.

One hypothesis to explain such findings is that people who were exposed to an adverse environment *in utero* and failed to grow, continued to be exposed to an adverse environment in childhood and adult life, and it is this later adverse environment that produces the effects attributed to programming *in utero*. There is, however, little evidence to support this argument. Rather, associations between birthweight and later disease are found in each social group, and are independent of adult behaviours such as smoking and becoming obese. Variations in disease rates associated with birthweight are large and strongly statistically significant. They are being replicated in different populations around the world, and are supported by animal experiments. It is reasonable to conclude that influences that lead to low growth rates *in utero* also determine later coronary heart disease.

Adult life-style does, however, add to intrauterine effects. The highest prevalences of non-insulin-dependent diabetes mellitus and impaired glucose tolerance, for example, are seen in people who were small at birth but obese as adults. Around the world,

communities with high prevalences of diabetes generally conform to this pattern. They include peoples such as the Ethiopian Jews airlifted to Israel, or Indian people who migrate to Britain, whose fetal growth was poor but who subsequently became affluent and obese in their adult life. The reason why people who had low growth rates *in utero* are unable to withstand the stress of becoming obese as adults may be explained by evidence from studies (of humans and animals) that their poor fetal growth resulted in a reduced number of pancreatic cells and hence a reduced capacity to make insulin; however, there is stronger evidence that they became resistant to the effects of insulin.

Disproportionate size at birth

In the early years of the twentieth century a new record form came into use in maternity hospitals in Britain. Known as the 'Queen Charlotte form', it required measurements of the newborn baby's head circumference and length at birth as well as its weight. These measurements allow thin and short babies to be distinguished. The Hertfordshire study showed that low birthweight was associated with the 'insulin resistance' syndrome (**Table 3**) – a common disorder in adult life in which impaired glucose tolerance, raised blood pressure and disturbed lipid metabolism coincide in the same patient.

Table 3 Prevalence of the insulin resistance syndrome in men aged 59–70 years according to birthweight

Birthweight		Total no. of men	Percentage with insulin resistance syndrome	Odds ratio adjusted for body mass index (95% confidence interval)
(lb)	(kg)			
≤5.5	≤2.50	20	30	18 (2.6 to 118)
6.5	2.95	54	19	8.4 (1.5 to 49)
7.5	3.41	114	17	8.5 (1.5 to 46)
8.5	3.86	123	12	4.9 (0.9 to 27)
9.5	4.31	64	6	2.2 (0.13 to 14)
>9.5	>4.31	32	6	1.0
Total		407	14	

Biochemically the syndrome is characterized by raised serum insulin concentrations, and it leads to coronary heart disease. Studies in Preston where the Queen Charlotte term was used showed that it is specifically thinness at birth, measured by a low ponderal index (birthweight/length^3), that is associated with resistance to insulin and its associated disorders in later life.

Mechanisms of Programming

Muscle growth *in utero*

In fetal life insulin has a key role in stimulating cell division. The thin newborn baby lacks skeletal muscle, as well as fat. It is thought that at some point in mid to late gestation the thin neonate became undernourished, and in response its muscles became resistant to insulin. Growth of its muscle was therefore sacrificed but the brain, which does not require insulin to utilize glucose, was spared. Persisting resistance to insulin through childhood into adult life impairs the response to a glucose challenge, because muscle is the main peripheral site of insulin action. Studies using magnetic resonance spectroscopy show that adults who were thin at birth have reduced rates of glycolysis in their muscles. It is unclear how this is linked to insulin resistance, but further research into muscle metabolism of people who were thin at birth

may lead to a new understanding of insulin resistance.

Liver growth *in utero*

Studies have shown that the neonates who have a short body in relation to the size of their head (although within the normal range of birthweight) have persisting disturbances of cholesterol metabolism and blood coagulation. Disproportion in body length relative to head size is thought to result from undernutrition in late gestation. The fetus uses an adaptive response present in mammals and diverts oxygenated blood away from the trunk to sustain the brain. One of the organs whose growth is prejudiced by this is the liver, and two of the liver's regulatory functions, cholesterol metabolism and blood clotting, seem to be permanently perturbed. Disturbance of cholesterol metabolism and blood clotting are both important features of coronary heart disease.

A small abdominal circumference at birth, reflecting small liver size, predicts raised serum low-density lipoprotein cholesterol concentrations, a major coronary risk factor. The difference in serum cholesterol concentrations between people who had small abdominal circumferences at birth and those who had large circumferences (**Table 4**) is equivalent to around 30% difference in risk of coronary heart disease. The findings for plasma fibrinogen

Table 4 Mean serum cholesterol concentrations according to abdominal circumference at birth in men and women aged 50–53 years

Abdominal circumference		No. of people	Total cholesterol (mmol l^{-1})	Low-density lipoprotein cholesterol (mmol l^{-1})
(inches)	(cm)			
≤11.5	≤29.2	53	6.7	4.5
12.0	30.5	43	6.9	4.6
12.5	31.8	31	6.8	4.4
13.0	33.0	45	6.2	4.0
>13.0	>33.0	45	6.1	4.0
Total		217	6.5	4.3
P value adjusted for gestational age of regression			0.003	0.007

concentrations, a measure of blood coagulability, are of similar size.

In keeping with these associations, a small abdominal circumference at birth is also associated with raised death rates from coronary heart disease. This, however, is only seen in babies of below average weight. In large babies the trend is reversed, so that it is the large baby with the large abdominal circumference who is at increased risk. This kind of baby is known to result from a pregnancy in which the mother develops diabetes. The fetus is exposed to abnormally high concentrations of glucose and is therefore, in a sense, overnourished. In these babies the abdomen enlarges rapidly in late gestation. It seems that accelerated as well as reduced liver growth in late gestation are linked to later coronary heart disease.

Experiments on rats have shown how undernutrition may permanently alter the way the liver metabolizes glucose. A low-protein diet in gestation was followed by permanent changes in the activity of two enzymes – one of which, phosphoenolpyruvate carboxykinase (PEPCK), is part of the process by which glucose is synthesized, while the other, glucokinase, acts in the utilization of glucose. A low-protein diet in gestation permanently changes the balance of activity in favour of glucose synthesis, even if it is followed by normal protein intake after birth. A low-protein diet after birth has no effect. The enzyme PEPCK is largely made in the cells around the portal veins of the liver, while glucokinase is made in the cells around the hepatic vein. An interpretation of these findings, therefore, is that undernutrition reprogrammes the zonal structure of the liver, enhancing the development of periportal cells in relation to the perivenous cells. The findings are of particular interest because they show clearly that undernutrition after birth has no effect.

Growth in infancy

In late gestation rates of cell division fall and growth slows. After birth, growth mainly consists of the development and enlargement of existing cells rather than addition of new ones. Babies who are short at birth, with reduced abdominal circumferences, tend to grow slowly after birth. Low rates of infant weight gain are highly predictive of coronary heart disease among men. In the Hertfordshire study, men who were small at 1 year old were three times more likely to develop or die from coronary heart disease than those who were large, an association that does not depend on the way in which the infants were fed (**Fig. 1**). Low weight gain during infancy is also followed by hypertrophy of the left ventricle in adult life, which predicts coronary heart disease independently

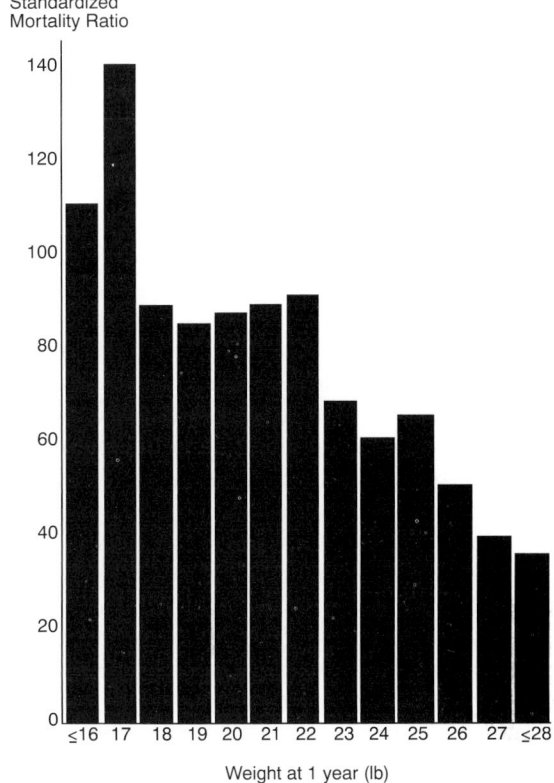

Figure 1 Mortality from coronary heart disease in 8175 men born during the period 1911–1930 according to weight at 1 year of age.

of the systemic blood pressure. One possible explanation is that, in the short baby, the structure of the heart is permanently changed by the adaptive responses that occurred before birth. Redistribution of blood flow in favour of the brain increases left ventricular output and peripheral resistance and may therefore lead to muscular hypertrophy.

Thin and short babies are two forms of disproportionate baby, whose growth was restricted at different stages of gestation and in whom different tissues, muscle and liver, were sacrificed to sustain the brain. Perhaps the origins of coronary heart disease partly lie in the large size of the human brain, in comparison with that of other mammals. Adaptive responses that protect the brain do so at exaggerated costs to other tissues.

Proportionate small size at birth

Some babies are proportionately small; their length, head size and weight are reduced in the same proportion. Such babies are thought to have established a slow trajectory of growth in early gestation which they were able to sustain throughout late gestation and thereby avoided becoming disproportionate. Early slowing of the growth trajectory is a major adaptation to undernutrition because it reduces the subsequent demand for nutrients. We know little about what sets the early growth trajectory in humans or when in embryonic or early fetal life it is set. It may be hormonally controlled. Experiments in sheep have shown that progesterone given to the ewe after mating resets the trajectory upwards and leads to the birth of giant lambs.

Little is known about proportionately small babies, except that they develop raised blood pressure. Persisting elevation of blood pressure through childhood and into adult life seems to follow interference with growth at any stage of gestation, since it is seen in people who were small, thin or short babies. **Table 5** shows the progressive fall in blood pressure with increasing birthweight among men and women in Hertfordshire. There have been similar findings in 23 other studies of men, women and children. The mechanisms underlying these associations between reduced fetal growth and raised blood pressure may depend on the stage of gestation when they are initiated. One possible mechanism is changes in vascular structure, with persisting loss of elasticity. People who were small at birth have been found to have reduced compliance in their large arteries as adults, possibly the result of lesser deposition of the scleroprotein elastin in their arterial walls *in utero*. Reduced compliance will increase pulse pressure. Another mechanism may be the effects of glucocorticoid hormones. In animals modest glucocorticoid excess retards intrauterine growth and programmes raised blood pressure. Such an excess may occur either from fetoplacental stress or from deficiency in the normal placental enzyme barrier which protects the fetus from its mother's glucocorticoids. An enzyme deficiency of this kind can be produced experimentally by undernourishing pregnant rats, which also causes persisting elevation of the offspring's blood pressure from 9 weeks of age onwards.

The placenta

At an early stage of development an embryo comprises two groups of cells, the inner and outer cell masses. The outer cell mass does not give rise to any structures in the embryo itself but develops into the placenta. It is from the inner cell mass that we have our origins. Experiments in animals suggest that the distribution of cells between the two groups is influenced by nutrition and hormones. In sheep, undernutrition in early pregnancy will lead to placental enlargement, thought to be an adaptation to extract more nutrients. This will only occur, however, if the ewe was well nourished before mating – one of many pointers to the importance to the fetus of the mother's nutritional plane before conception. There is evidence that placental enlargement may also be an adaptive response in humans. Ultrasound studies in humans show that at around 18 weeks fetuses of a given size already have a range of placental volumes; and we know that mothers who are anaemic, who exercise heavily in pregnancy or who live at altitude have babies with large placentas.

Observations suggest that expansion of the placenta is another fetal adaptation that exacts a long-term price. The blood pressures of a group of men and women in Preston in the UK were measured and are shown in **Table 6** according to their birthweights and placental weight. As expected, pressures fell with increasing birthweight. At any birthweight, however, pressures rose as placental weight increased; so that the highest pressures were in people who, in fetal life, allocated a greater proportion of their resources to placental development rather than to their own growth. Other studies have shown that placental enlargement is followed in adult life not only by elevated blood pressure, but by impaired glucose tolerance, disordered blood coagulation and death from coronary heart disease. Placental enlargement therefore seems a general marker of fetal undernutrition

Table 5 Mean systolic pressure in men and women aged 60–71 years according to birthweight

Birthweight		Systolic blood pressure, adjusted for sex (mmHg)	No. of subjects
(lb)	(kg)		
5.5	2.50	168	54
6.5	2.95	165	174
7.5	3.41	165	403
8.5	3.86	164	342
9.5	4.31	160	183
> 9.5	> 4.31	163	72
Total		164	1228
Standard deviation		25	
P value for trend		0.02	

Table 6   Mean systolic blood pressure (mmHg) of men and women aged 46–54 years, born after 38 completed weeks of gestation, according to placental weight and birthweight

Birthweight pounds (kg)	Placental weight pounds (kg)				
	≤ 1.0 (0.45)	− 1.25 (0.57)	− 1.5 (0.68)	> 1.5 (0.068)	All
6.5 (2.95)	149 (24)	152 (46)	151 (18)	167 (6)	152 (94)
7.5 (3.41)	139 (16)	148 (63)	146 (35)	159 (23)	148 (137)
> 7.5 (3.41)	131 (3)	143 (23)	148 (30)	153 (40)	149 (96)
Total	144 (43)	148 (132)	148 (83)	156 (69)	149 (327)

Figures in brackets are numbers of subjects. Values of P for trend with birthweight = 0.04, for trend with placental weight = 0.002.

and its consequences rather than a specific marker of later hypertension. **Table 7** shows the raised death rates from coronary heart disease associated with a high ratio of placental weight to birthweight, among a group of men born in Sheffield. The distribution of death rates is U-shaped, however, both high and low ratios of placental weight to birthweight being associated with raised rates.

Time Trends in Coronary Heart Disease

Coronary heart disease was rare in Britain at the beginning of the twentieth century, and having risen rapidly to become the commonest cause of death, it is now declining. Such rapid changes cannot be genetically determined; neither it seems can they be explained by coincident alterations in the life styles of adults. Could they result from changes during development? An important difference between fetal growth rates worldwide is that proportionate growth retardation is common in the less industrialized countries while disproportionate growth retardation prevails in Westernized countries. Perhaps coronary heart disease occurs in populations at a stage of nutrition between chronic maternal malnutrition, with early downregulation of fetal growth, and nutrition at a plane that allows adequate fetal nutrition through gestation.

Fetal undernutrition

A study in south India, where the incidence of coronary heart disease is rising rapidly, has shown the disease is associated with small size at birth. Fetal growth is remarkably restricted in Indian populations, the mean birthweight in this study being 2.7 kg. Importantly, it was the small babies born to mothers who themselves had low body weight who were most at risk of coronary heart disease. This association with mothers' weight is another indication that the associations between small size at birth and later disease reflect fetal undernutrition, itself a result of low maternal dietary intakes and nutrient stores and inadequate transport of nutrients to the placenta and transfer across it. Other direct evidence of the importance of nutrition comes from a UK study where imbalances in mothers' intakes of carbohydrate and protein during pregnancy were found to be related to their offspring's blood pressure 40 years later.

Twins

Because twins are growth-retarded it is sometimes suggested that they must have an increased risk of coronary heart disease. Twins are, however, heterogeneous, a mixture of proportionately and disproportionately small babies. Depending therefore on

Table 7   Death rates from coronary heart disease among 3108 men according to the ratio of placental weight to birthweight

Placental weight to birthweight ratio	Standardized mortality ratio	No. of deaths
≤ 15.0	107	57
17.5	92	77
19.0	78	46
21.5	103	78
> 21.5	130	83
Total	99	341

which predominates a group of twins may have low or high rates of coronary heart disease. Studies of the long-term effects of retarded growth due to twinning are, however, of interest apart from this issue, and a number of such studies are in progress.

Conclusions

The search for the environmental causes of coronary heart disease has hitherto focused on a 'destructive' model in which influences acting in adult life, such as smoking and obesity, hasten ageing processes – the formation of atheroma, rise in blood pressure and loss of the ability to metabolize glucose. The observations described above, however, suggest that coronary heart disease may originate during fetal development. We know surprisingly little about how the nutrition of human mothers influences that of their fetuses – much less than is known in domestic animals. We need to discover how maternal nutrition, body composition and hormonal profile interact to establish the fetal growth trajectory in early gestation, and to sustain the growth of the fetus thereafter.

It seems that many, if not all, human fetuses have to adapt to a limited availability of nutrients and oxygen. These adaptations programme the body's physiology, metabolism and structure. We need to know more about them: what they are, what induces them, how they leave a lasting mark upon the body, and how they give rise to the diseases of later life.

See Colour Plate 4.

See also: **Coronary Heart Disease**: Aetiology. **Diabetes Mellitus**: Aetiology and Epidemiology. **Insulin Resistance**: Aetiology and Association with Disease.

Further Reading

Barker DJP (1994) *Mothers, Babies and Disease in Later Life.* London: BMJ Publishing.

Barker DJP and Osmond C (1986) Infant mortality, childhood nutrition, and ischaemic heart disease in England and Wales. *Lancet* i:1077–1081.

Barker DJP, Winter PD, Osmond C, Margetts B and Simmonds SJ (1989) Weight in infancy and death from ischaemic heart disease. *Lancet* ii:577–580.

Barker DJP, Gluckman PD, Godfrey KM, Harding JE, Owens JA and Robinson JS (1993) Fetal nutrition and cardiovascular disease in adult life. *Lancet* 341:938–941.

Edwards CRW, Benediktsson R, Lindsay RS and Seckl JR (1993) Dysfunction of placental glucocorticoid barrier: link between fetal environment and adult hypertension? *Lancet* 341:355–357.

Gluckman P and Harding J (1992) The regulation of fetal growth. In: Hernandez M and Argente J (eds) *Human Growth: Basic and Clinical Aspects*, pp 253–259. Amsterdam: Elsevier.

Hales CN and Barker DJP (1992) Type 2 (non-insulin-dependent) diabetes mellitus: the thrifty phenotype hypothesis. *Diabetologia* 35:595–601.

Lucas A (1991) Programming by early nutrition in man. In: Bock GR and Whelan J (eds) *The Childhood Environment and Adult Disease*, pp 38–55. Chichester: Wiley.

McCance RA and Widdowson EM (1974) The determinants of growth and form. *Proceedings of the Royal Society (London) Biol* 185:1–17.

Morton NE (1955) The inheritance of human birthweight. *Annals of Human Genetics* 20:123–134.

Robinson JS, Owens JA, DeBarro T, Lok F and Chidzanja S (1994) Maternal nutrition and fetal growth. In: Ward RHT, Smith SK and Donnai D (eds) *Early Fetal Growth and Development*. London: RCOG Press.

Stein CE, Fall CHD, Kumaran K, Osmond C, Cox V and Barker DJP (1996) Fetal growth and coronary heart disease in South India. *Lancet* 348:1269–1273.

Wheeler T, Sollero C, Alderman S, Landen J, Anthony F and Osmond C (1994) Relation between maternal haemoglobin and placental hormone concentrations in early pregnancy. *Lancet* 343:511–513.

Wolpert L (1991) *The Triumph of the Embryo*. Oxford University Press.

Fibre *see* **Dietary Fibre**: Physiological Effects and Effects on Absorption; Potential Role in the Aetiology of Disease; Role in Nutritional Management of Disease.

FISH

Nutritional Value

R Rice, The Fish Foundation, Tiverton, Devon

Copyright © 1998 Academic Press

This article covers the wider nutritional aspects of fish, including the types of fish and shellfish that are important in the human diet, their nutritional composition, the problem of toxins in seafoods, and a perspective on the significance of seafoods in the human diet.

Types of Seafood

The foods we derive from the aquatic environment fall broadly into two major categories: fish and shellfish. The marine mammals, such as whales, dolphins, seals and porpoises, do not constitute a major food source except for a few communities, and are not considered further in this article.

Fish

The distinction between freshwater and saltwater fish has little nutritional significance. Of more importance is the division of fishes into those with bones and those without – the cartilaginous fish. The latter includes sharks, skate, rays and dogfish. Dogfish (also known as huss or rock salmon) and skate are moderately popular in the UK, accounting for around 2% of fresh fish landings. The remaining 98% (excluding shellfish) consist of bony fish; this group is split into two, on the basis of feeding habits.

Demersal fish   Just over half of all UK fresh fish landings are of demersal fish: They comprise the 'white' fish, the low-fat fish. Demersal fish feed deep in the water or even on the sea bed, and catching technology is adapted to this. Cod, haddock, plaice and whiting make up 65% of this group, with sole, saithe or coley, ling and monkfish being important members of the rest.

Pelagic fish   Pelagic fish feed more in the surface layers of the water (though at different stages of the breeding cycle, some pelagic fish can temporarily become demersal). The pelagic fish are primarily those with higher levels of lipid in the flesh, giving them nonwhite flesh. The major members of this group are herring and mackerel, which make up over 90% of fresh pelagic landings in the UK. Sprats, pilchards (mature sardines) and tuna are also sometimes landed in the UK. Nutritionally, salmon and trout are probably closer to this group than any other. As these are mainly farmed fish, there are few reliable published figures to indicate production or consumption levels, but both are significant contributors to fish intake.

Shellfish

The term 'shellfish' is used to describe not only creatures with obvious shells, but also other marine lifeforms without apparent shells, such as squid and octopus. There are two groups of shellfish of importance in human food: the molluscsa and the arthropods.

Molluscs include bivalves (with a two-piece shell) such as oysters, mussels and scallops, and univalves with a one-piece shell such as whelks, limpets and cockles. The cephalopods such as squid, cuttlefish and octopus are also univalves.

The arthropods of relevance to human nutrition comprise the crustaceans, a group which includes lobster, prawns, shrimps, crayfish and crabs.

Macronutrient Content

Fish

Demersal fish provide 80–90% of their energy content in the form of protein. Lipid levels are 0–2 g per 100 g. Carbohydrate is virtually absent from all bony fish commonly eaten. Levels of protein in pelagic fish are similar to those in demersal fish (**Table 1**), but higher lipid levels of 5–15 g per 100 g mean that a smaller proportion of food energy is derived from protein when pelagic fish are eaten. A corollary of this is that overall food energy intake is higher from pelagic fish than from demersal fish. The higher lipid level in pelagic fish is the reason they are often referred to as fatty fish, oily fish or oil-rich fish.

Protein   The major proteins in fish are actin and myosin, which combine in muscle to form actomyosin. Albumins are also present. The amino acid composition of fish protein is such that it can provide the sole source of protein for humans, as a consequence of the presence and extent of the essential amino acids it contains. The actual amino acid pattern is comparable with that of other proteins of high

Table 1 Macronutrient content (g per 100 g edible food) of major cartilaginous and bony fish

Type of seafood (raw unless specified)	Water (g)	Protein (g)	Lipid (g)	Energy (kcal)	Engery (kJ)
Huss/Dogfish	68.3	16.6	9.7	154	641
Skate	80.7	15.1	0.4	64	272
Cod	80.8	18.3	0.7	80	337
Haddock	79.4	19.0	0.6	81	345
Plaice	79.5	16.7	1.4	79	336
Whiting	80.7	18.7	0.7	81	344
Sole	81.2	17.4	1.5	83	351
Saithe/Coley	80.2	18.3	1.0	82	348
Ling	79.3	18.8	0.7	82	346
Monkfish	83.8	15.7	0.4	66	282
Herring	68.0	17.8	13.2	190	791
Mackerel	64.0	18.7	16.1	220	914
Sprat	69.3	17.0	9.9	162	678
Pilchard/Sardine	67.7	20.6	9.2	165	691
Tuna	70.4	23.7	4.6	136	573
Salmon	67.2	20.2	11.0	180	750
Trout (Rainbow)	76.7	19.6	5.2	125	526

Source: Holland B, Brown J and Buss DH (1993) *Fish and Fish Products*: the third supplement to *McCance and Widdowson's The Composition of Foods* (5th edition). London: HMSO.

biological value, such as beef, egg or milk protein. The amount of connective tissue in fish and shellfish muscle is relatively low. The connective tissue softens and dissolves more readily when heated compared with the connective tissue of land animals, and is readily hydrolysed by digestive enzymes. It is therefore easy to chew and digest when cooked.

Lipid The lipid content of seafoods is primarily in the form of triacylglycerols, and is the area of most interest nutritionally, since seafoods are the only major source of certain long-chain polyunsaturated fatty acids (PUFA). The level of lipid in fish flesh varies widely, not only between different species, but also within the same species depending on season, feeding grounds, water salinity and other factors. Demersal fish in general do not have a great deal of lipid in their flesh. Lipid stores in these fish are found in the liver, in the lining of the peritoneum, and/or immediately under the skin. Some, such as halibut, store part of their lipid in the liver, and part in muscle. Pelagic fish store lipid in head and muscle tissue.

In general, fish do not feed when they are spawning, in spite of higher nutritional demands at this time. Their nutrient supply is thus provided by body stores, and as a result, the level of lipid falls steadily as spawning progresses. Thus as salmon head upstream into freshwater rivers during the early months of the year to their spawning grounds, flesh lipid content can be as high as 13 g per 100 g. As the salmon journey upriver they do not feed, so that by the time of spawning, around November, the lipid level may be as low as 5 g per 100 g. After spawning,

the lipid level continues to fall, and by the time the fish dies, the level may be below 1 g per 100 g. Herring show a more seasonal variation in lipid level. From an overwinter low of 3–4 g per 100 g in April, the level rises within a few weeks to as much as 20 g per 100 g. Feeding begins to diminish as the autumn spawning season approaches, so the lipid level begins to drop to around 10–15 g per 100 g. During winter, lower sea temperatures and a scarcity of food cause the level to continue falling. When lipid is drawn from muscle reserves, it is replaced by water, so that the total mass of the fish remains much the same. The muscle water content therefore rises, and this makes the flesh weak and accounts for the poor eating quality of spawning fish.

The high liver lipid content (which can exceed 50% of wet weight) of species in the family Gadidae, such as cod, saithe or coley and haddock, is exploited to produce cod liver oil, a rich source of n-3 long-chain PUFA as well as vitamins A and D. Fish liver oils are also produced from ling, shark, huss, halibut and tuna. The livers are removed at the time of evisceration of the fish, and processed to separate the oil. This can be simple steam cooking to obtain the highest quality medicinal oil, with various other techniques used to extract the residual oil which, being of poorer quality, is used for veterinary or industrial purposes. Though cod liver oil is still a popular product, the annual level of production now is around 20 000 tonnes, down considerably from the 70 000–80 000 tonnes in the first half of the twentieth century.

Table 2 Impact of processing on the macronutrient content of certain fish

Type of fish (100 g as eaten)	Water (g)	Protein (g)	Lipid (g)	Energy (kcal)	Energy (kJ)
Haddock (steamed)	78.3	20.9	0.6	89	378
Smoked Haddock	71.6	23.3	0.9	101	429
Herring (grilled)	63.9	20.1	11.2	181	756
Kipper	61.2	17.5	17.7	229	952
Mackerel (grilled)	58.6	20.8	17.3	239	994
Mackerel (smoked)	47.1	18.9	30.9	354	1465
Salmon (steamed)	64.5	21.8	11.9	194	812
Salmon (smoked)	64.9	25.4	4.5	142	598
Tuna (raw, fresh or frozen)	70.6	23.7	4.6	136	573
Tuna (canned in brine)	74.6	23.5	0.6	99	422

Source: Holland B, Brown J and Buss DH (1993) *Fish and Fish Products*: the third supplement to *McCance and Widdowson's The Composition of Foods* (5th edition). London: HMSO.

Effect of processing By and large, processing does not have a major impact on the macronutrient content of bony fish. Dehydration potentially has the biggest effect, but this is not practised commercially to any great extent in the UK. Smoking of fish results in partial dehydration, as does brining which usually accompanies the smoking process. The partial removal of moisture, leads to consequent increases in the proportions of the macronutrients. Lack of care (resulting in excessive temperatures) in smoking can cause loss of lipid from herring, mackerel and salmon. **Table 2** compares the macronutrient content of unprocessed and processed fish. The parts of the carcase used for producing smoked salmon have a lower lipid level than the carcase as a whole, so the product has a lower lipid content than unprocessed salmon, in spite of having lost some water in the smoking process. Since salmon are only fairly lightly smoked, the loss of moisture is not great.

Canning and freezing do not have much impact on macronutrient content, except in the case of tuna. Since tuna is a large fish, it is customarily cooked before being packed in the can for final processing. During this initial cooking process, some lipid is lost. A more important loss of lipid occurs when the lighter-coloured (low lipid) meat is selectively used for canning. This is done for reasons of consumer preference, since the high-lipid dark meat has a deep brown-red colour, which is unacceptable to consumers.

Shellfish

The macronutrient content of different types of shellfish (**Table 3**) is much more variable than that of fish, though true comparison is difficult, since analytical data are not available on all species in the same state (e.g. some data are available for cooked forms only). Generally speaking, protein levels are a little lower and lipid levels a little higher than in the demersal fish. Small amounts of carbohydrate (primarily

Table 3 Macronutrient content (g per 100 g edible food) of shellfish

Type of seafood (raw unless specified)	Water (g)	Protein (g)	Lipid (g)	Carbohydrate (g)	Energy (g)	Energy (g)
Oyster	85.7	10.8	1.3	2.7	65	275
Mussel	80.9	12.1	1.8	2.5	74	312
Scallop (steamed)	73.1	23.2	1.4	3.4	118	501
Whelk (boiled)	73.9	19.5	1.2	tr	89	376
Cockle	83.0	12.0	0.6	tr	53	226
Squid	80.5	15.4	1.7	1.2	81	344
Cuttlefish	80.8	16.1	0.7	0	71	300
Octopus	82.1	17.9	1.3	tr	83	352
Lobster	74.3	22.1	1.6	tr	103	435
Prawn	79.2	17.6	0.6	0	76	321
Shrimp (boiled)	62.5	23.8	2.4	tr	117	493
Crayfish	83.8	14.9	0.8	0	67	283
Crab (boiled)	71.0	19.5	5.5	tr	128	535

tr = trace amounts only; r = data not available.
Source: Holland B, Brown J and Buss DH (1993) *Fish and Fish Products*: the third supplement to *McCance & Widdowson's The Composition of Foods* (5th edition). London: HMSO.

glycogen) are found in some shellfish. Shrimp and crab are notable for a relatively high level of lipid (2.5–5.5 g per 100 g), and oysters and scallops for a significant amount of carbohydrate (2.7–3.4 g per 100 g).

Fatty Acids

Biochemical Structure

Polyunsaturated fatty acids (PUFA) are characterized by the presence of two or more methylene interrupted double bonds. The metabolic fate of PUFA depends on the position of the first double bond with respect to the terminal methyl group, since mammalian systems in general lack the enzymes necessary to alter the configuration of this part of the molecule. Polyunsaturated fatty acids can be elongated, desaturated, shortened or converted to other bioactive molecules such as prostaglandins or leukotrienes. However, no matter what changes may be brought about in the biochemical structure of the molecule, the section between the terminal methyl end and the first double bond remains unaltered.

Essential Fatty Acids

There are three 'families' of PUFA that are important in human nutrition; they differ in the position of the first double bond counting from the methyl (or omega) end of the chain. These three families are known as the n-3, n-6 and n-9 families (also known as the omega-3, omega-6 and omega-9 families) (**Fig. 1**).

The n-9 family is only of significance when there is an insufficiency of either or both of the other two families, which are essential to human health and must be supplied in the diet. When adequate amounts of n-6 or n-3 PUFA are not available, the body compensates by producing n-9 PUFA to take the place of the essential n-3 or n-6 PUFA. Though the n-9 derivatives can substitute to a certain extent, they are not as effective as the n-3 or n-6 derivatives, and this may eventually lead to adverse health effects. The main value of the n-9 PUFA is thought to be as a marker for dietary insufficiency of the essential PUFA.

Long-chain n-3 PUFA

Fish and seafood from cold waters characteristically and uniquely contain significant quantities of long-chain n-3 PUFA (*See:* **Fatty Acids**: Health Effects of n-3 Polyunsaturated Fatty Acids). Though there is some evidence that fish can elongate and desaturate the shorter-chain n-3 PUFA, current opinion is that most of the long-chain n-3 PUFA is formed in the microscopic algae, plankton and planktonic crustacea at the base of the marine food chain. These fatty acids

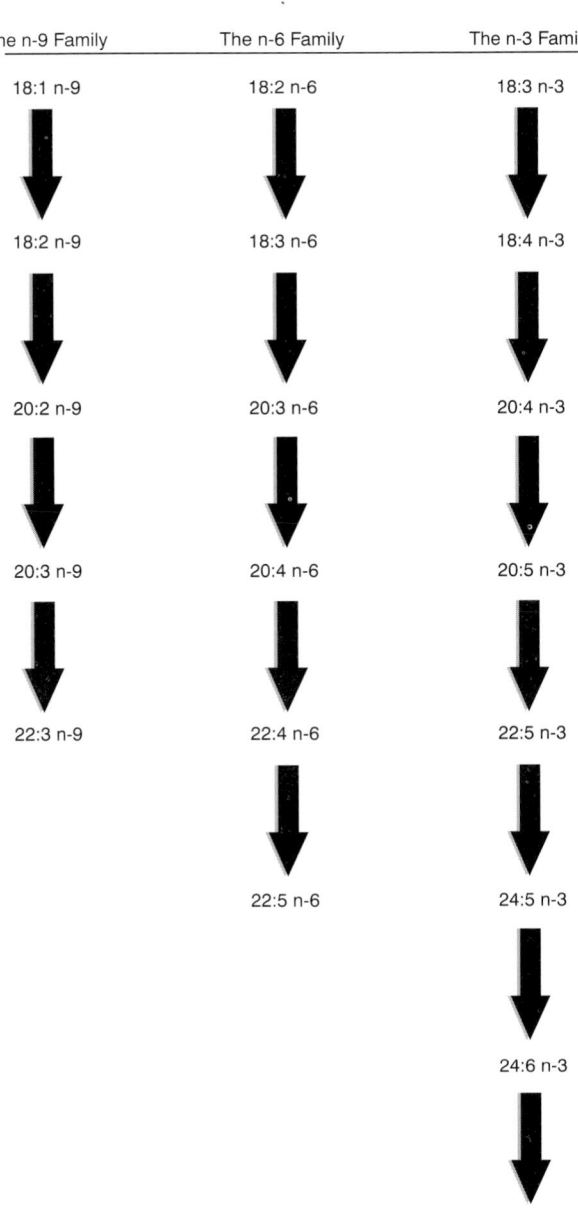

Figure 1 The three families of dietary polyunsaturates and their metabolic conversions.

pass up the food chain into the higher fish, and ultimately to humans. There are three significant members of the n-3 family, all with 20 or more carbon atoms, and all with five or more double bonds.

Eicosapentaenoic acid (20:5 n-3) The most widely researched of the long-chain PUFA is all *cis*-5,8,11,14,17-eicosapentaenoic acid (20:5 n-3), usually referred to as EPA, but also sometimes called timnodonic acid. It is capable of being elongated to all *cis*-7,10,13,16,19-docosapentaenoic acid (22:5 n-3) which in turn can be converted to all *cis*-4,7,10,13,16,19-docosahexaenoic acid (22:6 n-

3), usually called DHA, but sometimes also known as clupadonic or cervonic acid. Eicosapentaenoic acid is also capable of being metabolized to a range of biologically active substances referred to generically as eicosanoids. Prostaglandins and leukotrienes are important members of this group. They are locally produced, powerful regulators of biological activity. A parallel series of eicosanoids can also be produced from all *cis*-5,8,11,14-eicosatetraenoic acid (20:4 n-6), usually called arachidonic acid (AA), which tends to have even more potent biological activity.

Since the n-6 family tends to predominate in human food, by a factor of eight times or more, compared with the n-3 family, most eicosanoids produced by the human body tend to be of the n-6 type. Increasing the dietary intake of n-3 PUFA alters this balance, and this is thought to be one mechanism for the beneficial health effects of n-3 PUFA from seafoods (*See:* **Fatty Acids**: Health Effects of n-3 Polyunsaturated Fatty Acids).

Docosahexaenoic acid (22:6 n-3)   The second most abundant long-chain n-3 PUFA is 22:6 n-3, docosahexaenoic acid (DHA). It is the most abundant n-3 PUFA in certain fish such as tuna. It is not thought capable of being metabolized directly to eicosanoids, but since it can be retroconverted to EPA, it is possible that a high DHA intake could also affect the eicosanoid balance.

The most significant aspect of DHA for human nutrition is its role as a major structural component of brain, nerve and retinal membranes. In these membranes it can form up to 60% of the PUFA present, and research suggests that functional abnormalities may result from depletion of DHA levels in membranes. This acid plays a unique role in the building of these tissues in the fetus, and such is its importance, especially during the first few months of life, that breast milk supplies 0.1–0.4% of fatty acids as DHA, while there is almost no EPA present in breast milk. The concentration of DHA in breast milk can be augmented by maternal dietary intake of fish and fish oils, but the EPA level does not vary much.

Minor polyunsaturated fatty acids   All *cis*-7,10,13,16,19-docosapentaenoic acid (22:5 n-3) sometimes called clupanodonic acid, is a minor component of most fish, present to the extent of 1–3% of the total fatty acids. Little is known of any specific physiological effects of this PUFA although it is in principle capable of being converted either to 20:5 n-3, or to 22:6 n-6, and as such could augment the available supplies of either.

All *cis*-5,8,11,14-eicosatetraenoic acid, (20:4 n-6) is a minor component of some fish lipids. Fish from tropical waters can have significant amounts of 20:4 n-6, but analytical information is not readily available. Small amounts of short-chain n-3 PUFA are also present in fish lipids, chiefly the all *cis*-9,12,15-octadecatrienoic acid (18:3 n-3) α-linolenic acid, and all *cis*-6,9,12,15-octadecatetraenoic acid (18:4 n-3) stearidonic acid, but the amounts rarely exceed 0.1–0.2% of all fatty acids.

Variation in n-3 content

The pattern of individual PUFA in fish can be a characteristic of the species, though in practice, the potential variations which can occur make it difficult to draw conclusions based on this alone. The geographic location of the feeding grounds, water temperature, water salinity, stage of breeding cycle, and the season of the year are all factors that can and do complicate this issue. **Table 4** gives typical values for the three major n-3 PUFAs and total lipid content in a number of major fish species.

Micronutrient Content

Vitamins

Certain types of fish and shellfish are well known as sources of the fat-soluble vitamins A and D; they also can provide significant amounts of some of the B vitamins. **Table 5** provides details of the vitamin content of selected fish and shellfish. Vitamin A in the form of retinol is found in large amounts in huss and oysters, as well as in the oil-rich fish such as sprats, herring and mackerel. Eating 100 g of these seafoods would provide around 10–15% of the UK adult reference nutrient intake (RNI) for retinol. The oil-rich pelagic fish are excellent dietary sources of vitamin D_3 (cholecalciferol). Though there is no accepted adult RNI for vitamin D, using a value of 10 μg (as may be required for older adults) the oil-rich fish provide 50–200% of such a level per 100 g.

The fish liver oils have much higher levels of the fat-soluble vitamins, and have been used as dietary supplements for over 200 years. The actual levels vary considerably, but halibut liver oil (for example) may contain up to 5000 μg of retinol per gram of oil and up to 120 μg of cholecalciferol. Such levels would be toxic to humans if ingested regularly. Cod liver oil provides generally lower levels, around 100–150 μg of retinol and 1–2 μg of cholecalciferol per gram of oil. Oil used for capsule production tends to be somewhat higher in vitamin concentration, and one capsule (containing 350–500 mg of oil) supplies 100% of the adult RNI for vitamin A. Vitamin E is present in significant amounts in many seafoods, providing around 10–20% of the average daily

Table 4   Omega-3 polyunsaturate fatty acid content (g per 100 g edible portion) of selected fish and shellfish

Type of fish (raw unless specified)	Lipid content	20:5 w-3	22:5 w-3	22:6 w-3	Total w-3
Huss/Dogfish	9.7	0.8*	0.2	1.4	2.5
Skate	0.4	0.0	0.0	0.1	0.1
Oyster	1.3	0.2	tr	0.2	0.5
Squid	1.7	0.1	tr	0.3	0.5
Lobster	1.6	0.2	tr	0.1	0.3
Crab	5.5	0.5	0.1	0.5	1.2
Saithe/Coley	1.0	0.0	0.0	0.2	0.2
Mussel	1.8	0.3	tr	0.1	0.5
Shrimp (boiled)	2.4	0.4	tr	0.3	0.8
Herring	13.2	0.8	0.1	1.0	2.0
Mackerel	16.1	0.7	0.1	1.1	2.0
Sprat	9.9	0.9	0.1	1.3	2.4
Pilchard/Sardine	9.2	0.9	0.1	1.1	2.2
Tuna	4.6	0.3	0.1	1.1	1.6
Salmon	11.0	0.5	0.4	1.3	2.3
Trout (Rainbow)	5.2	0.2	0.1	0.8	1.2
Cod Liver Oil	100.0	9.0	1.0	9.0	20.0

*Shown in source as 20:4 n-6, but assumed to be a printer's error.
tr = trace amounts only; r = data not available.
Source: Holland B, Brown J and Buss DH (1993) *Fish and Fish Products*: the third supplement to *McCance and Widdowson's The Composition of Foods* (5th edition). London: HMSO.

Table 5   Vitamin content of selected fish and shellfish (per 100 g raw edible portion unless otherwise specified)

Type of fish or shellfish	Vitamin A (μg)	Vitamin D (μg)	Vitamin E (mg)	Thiamin (mg)	Riboflavin (mg)	Vitamin B6 (mg)	Vitamin B12 (μg)
Huss/Dogfish	94	n	n	0.07	0.08	0.21	n
Cod	2	tr	0.44	0.04	0.05	0.18	1
Haddock	tr	tr	0.39	0.04	0.07	0.39	1
Plaice	tr	tr	n	0.20	0.19	0.30	1
Herring	44	19.0	0.76	0.01	0.26	0.44	13
Mackerel	45	5.0	0.43	0.14	0.29	0.41	8
Sprat	60	13.0	0.51	tr	0.20	0.27	7
Pilchard	n	11.0	0.29	tr	0.22	0.39	11
Tuna	26	7.2	n	0.10	0.13	0.38	4
Salmon (Atlantic)	13	8.0	1.91	0.23	0.13	0.75	4
Trout (Rainbow)	49	10.6	0.71	0.20	0.11	0.34	5
Oyster	75	1.0	0.85	0.15	0.19	0.16	17
Mussel	n	tr	0.74	tr	0.35	0.08	19
Lobster (boiled)	tr	tr	1.47	0.08	0.05	0.08	3
Crab	tr	tr	n	0.07	0.86	0.16	tr
Shrimp (boiled)	n	tr	n	0.01	0.01	0.08	3
Prawn	tr	tr	2.85	0.04	0.12	0.05	7

tr = trace amounts only; r = data not available.
Source: Holland B, Brown J and Buss DH (1993) *Fish and Fish Products*; the third supplement to *McCance and Widdowson's The Composition of Foods* (5th edition). London: HMSO.

vitamin E intake of 5–10 mg in a 100 g portion. Since vitamin E requirement is related to the intake of PUFA, it may be considered that the vitamin E present in seafoods is in general sufficient to provide for the additional vitamin E needs that the PUFA content in seafood imposes. However, there is little or no contribution to the vitamin E needs imposed by other dietary sources of PUFA.

Of the water-soluble vitamins, seafoods generally provide little or no vitamin C. The B vitamins are represented to varying extents, with the supply of thiamin, riboflavin and pyridoxine being most significant nutritionally. Consumption of 100 g of most seafoods will supply 10% or more of the adult RNI for these nutrients. Seafoods are especially rich in vitamin B_{12}, supplying 100% or more of the adult RNI in 100 g.

Minerals

Seafoods are better known, nutritionally, for the dietary minerals they supply than for the vitamins – in particular iodine and selenium, which are present in higher concentrations than in many other non-marine foods (**Table 6**).

In general, the balance between sodium and potassium is favourable in fish, with ratios ranging from 1 : 2 to 1 : 10 shellfish contain more sodium, so the ratio is not so favourable. Shrimp, oysters, lobster and crab contain more sodium than potassium. The high sodium content for shrimp reported in Table 6 is probably due to cooking the shrimp in seawater, which would contribute a substantial amount of sodium. However, most shrimps are purchased ready cooked, and will presumably have comparable high sodium levels.

Calcium levels are not high in most seafoods, though sprats, sardines, oysters and shrimps are exceptions, supplying 10–20% of the adult RNI per 100 g. Canned salmon contains softened bones, and when these are eaten with the fish the level of calcium supplied rises to 300 mg per 100 g, almost half of the adult RNI for calcium. Iron levels are not high in seafoods, but since the iron is easily absorbed, especially from white fish, it is a valuable dietary source. The level of iron in molluscs (oysters, mussels) is similar to that in red meat. Zinc is also especially rich in the molluscs, in particular oysters. The reputed aphrodisiac qualities of oysters are commonly attributed to the high level of zinc, although they have not been studied in controlled trials. The adult RNI for zinc is 9.5 mg, and 100 g of most shellfish contributes around 30–50% of this; for fish, the contribution is closer to 5–10%. Seafood is the richest source of iodine in the normal diet, and one or two seafood meals per week will supply an average of 100–200 µg per day, enough to meet the adult RNI of 140 µg. Few other commonly eaten foods can match this. The same can be said of selenium, though the variation is greater. Seafoods supply 20–60 µg selenium per 100 g, with the exception of lobster, which contains 130 µg selenium per 100 g. The adult RNI for selenium is 75 µg and 100 g of many seafoods will make a significant contribution to this. Cereal and meat sources of selenium provide about 10–12 µg per 100 g, considerably less than most seafoods.

Minor components

Though not nutrients in the classic sense of the word, the sterols present in seafoods are important nutritionally. Cholesterol is the best known, but the content is generally not as significant as once thought; what was once identified as cholesterol is now known to include other plant-derived sterols, or phytosterols. There is no doubt that crustaceans contain high levels of cholesterol. Prawns in particular contain about 195 mg of cholesterol per 100 g meat. In the context of a recommended maximum cholesterol intake of 300–600 mg per day, this is significant, though it is still less than the cholesterol contained in a chicken's egg (250 mg per egg). Shrimp meat contains about 130 mg cholesterol per

Table 6   Mineral content of selected fish and shellfish (mg per 100 g raw edible portion unless otherwise specified)

Type of seafood	Sodium	Potassium	Calcium	Iron	Zinc	Iodine (µg)	Selenium (µg)
Huss/Dogfish	120	290	8	0.9	0.4	n	55
Cod	60	340	9	0.1	0.4	110	28
Haddock	67	360	14	0.1	0.4	250	27
Plaice	123	280	45	0.3	0.5	33	37
Herring	123	320	60	1.2	0.9	29	35
Mackerel	63	290	11	0.8	0.6	140	30
Sprat	200	320	97	1.1	1.7	64	10
Pilchard/Sardine	120	360	84	1.4	1.0	29	34
Tuna	47	400	16	1.3	0.7	30	57
Salmon (Atlantic)	45	360	21	0.8	1.0	76	24
Trout (Rainbow)	45	420	18	0.3	0.5	13	18
Oyster	510	260	140	5.7	59.2	60	23
Mussel	290	320	38	5.8	2.5	140	51
Lobster (boiled)	330	260	62	0.8	2.5	100	130
Crab	420	250	n	1.6	5.5	n	17
Shrimp (boiled)	3840	400	320	1.8	2.3	100	46
Prawn	190	330	79	1.6	1.5	21	16

n = data not available.
Source: Holland B, Brown J and Buss DH (1993) *Fish and Fish Products*; the third supplement to *McCance and Widdowson's The Composition of Foods* (5th edition). London: HMSO.

100 g, while crab and lobster meat contains 50–100 mg per 100 g. At one stage it was thought that molluscs also contained high cholesterol levels, but in fact this was due to an analytical error. Cholesterol is present in molluscs, but a high proportion of the sterols present are now known to be phytosterols. Cholesterol levels in molluscs range from 40–60 mg in mussels, scallops and oysters to 150–200 mg in cuttlefish and squid. Phytosterols, though not widely studied, are considered to be beneficial in the diet, since they interfere with the absorption of cholesterol.

Toxins and Contaminants

The presence of minor amounts of substances that can adversely affect human health can act as a deterrent to eating seafoods, though in most instances the actual risk of suffering ill effects from the tiny amounts commonly present is far outweighed by the benefits accruing from the dietary value of the seafood. However, there are exceptions to this general rule.

Natural toxins

Natural toxins present from time to time in certain types of fish are considered to originate lower down in the food chain, most often in the microscopic plants that form the base of the food chain. Very few examples of this type of problem arise in the UK, the most prominent problem being diarrhetic shellfish poisoning which occasionally occurs. Monitoring procedures carried out by government agencies provide a satisfactory level of protection for the public. Local and/or regional fisheries are closed if such a problem is detected by the routine sampling and testing programme. The source of the toxins is thought to be dinoflagellates such as *Dinophysis fortii* or *D. acuminata*, which are consumed by mussels and scallops. The symptoms include diarrhoea, nausea, vomiting and abdominal pain. The duration is usually only a few days, and the condition is not generally life-threatening.

Different diatoms and plankton around the world can cause different symptoms, but the basic mechanism is the same: the toxin is formed by an organism at the base of the food chain, and is subsequently passed up the food chain and concentrated in the seafoods that humans eventually eat. Thus ciguatera poisoning, amnesic shellfish poisoning, paralytic shellfish poisoning and neurotoxic shellfish poisoning are all variants of the same problem, with differing (generally low) mortality. The incidence of each type of poisoning is not large, and sampling and testing programmes are in force where the problem is likely to be common. The most likely cause of an outbreak is from seafoods harvested by the consumer, rather than from seafoods acquired commercially. The most severe form of natural toxic contamination occurs in the puffer fish, *Arothon hispidus*. The toxin is concentrated in the liver and viscera of the fish, and can be substantially removed by careful preparation. Fugu (Puffer fish) restaurants are common in Japan, where licensed puffer fish chefs prepare the delicacy with great care. Even so, fugu poisoning remains a major cause of fatal food intoxications in Japan, accounting for 20–100 deaths every year.

Toxins arising from poor storage

The most common type of intoxication arising from poor storage is that due to the development of high levels of histamine. This results in a type of poisoning termed 'scombroid poisoning', because it was originally associated with scombroid fish such as tuna and mackerel, though now it is known to affect other types of fish as well. The symptoms are generally mild and short-lived, and include nausea, vomiting, diarrhoea, abdominal cramp, headache and palpitations. Tingling, burning and localized inflammation can also occur. The symptoms are the result of ingesting histamine, a substance that is in turn produced by the action of the enzyme histidine decarboxylase acting on the histidine naturally present in fish. The source of the histidine decarboxylase is bacterial growth resulting from storage at temperatures higher than recommended for safe storage. Thus any fish that appear to be the subject of excessive bacterial growth should be rejected as human food. Normally a poor smell or appearance is sufficient to ensure that such fish do not reach the table. The level of free histamine can be measured and is used as an objective indicator of bacterial spoilage. A level of 20 mg per 100 g is indicative of poor storage conditions, and a level above 50 mg per 100 g is considered to represent a toxic dose.

Contaminants

Seafood may be contaminated not only by synthetic compounds such as polychlorinated biphenyls (PCBs) and dioxins, but also by heavy metals and by sewage containing viruses and bacteria. Problems with sewage contamination are easily avoidable, since thorough cooking will destroy any microorganisms. Freezing also greatly reduces the viability of any contaminant organisms, though the protection is not as complete as with cooking. Effective sewage treatment, and careful siting of outfalls and harvesting areas, also reduce the likelihood of a problem.

The problem of contamination with heavy metals and synthetic chemicals of various kinds is not so easily solved, requiring as it does international cooperation, since the seas and oceans are subject to contamination from outside national boundaries, and indeed from airborne sources also.

Heavy metals Lead, mercury and cadmium are the most serious of these contaminants. Lead arises from the manufacture of storage batteries, ammunition, solder and other industrial processes, as well as from its use in 'antiknock' additives in petrol. Virtually all of these sources are now in decline, and surveys show that marine lead contamination is falling. Extensive surveys in the USA have shown that the general level of lead in edible fish rarely exceeds the acceptable daily intake of 0.429 mg defined by the Food and Drug Administration (FDA). Children and developing fetuses are most sensitive to the toxic effects of lead contamination, and care should be exercised in giving children or pregnant women fish or shellfish that are likely to be heavily contaminated with lead or other heavy metals. Fish from freshwater sources, estuarine seafoods and seafoods from near-coastal waters in areas of high industrial activity are best avoided for these groups. For adults, both the absorption of lead and its toxicity are much less.

Cadmium in the marine food chain is derived from paint pigments, sewage sludge dumping, fertilizer manufacture, electroplating activities and mining run-off waters. It is a particular problem in crustacea and molluscs because it is selectively accumulated in these organisms as a result of binding to metallothionine ligands. Kidney damage is the most common outcome of cadmium toxicity. Levels of 0.05–0.07 mg per day are considered acceptable, though smokers may have lower tolerances because of the cadmium they absorb from cigarette smoke. Surveys in the USA show cadmium levels in edible marine fish samples to be generally below this level, though fish from estuaries and coastal regions with high industrial activity are likely to have somewhat higher levels.

Mercury, like lead, is potentially a problem for fetuses and young children. The brain and the kidneys are the most vulnerable organs, and severe exposure can lead to tremors, seizures, paraesthesia and kidney failure. Inorganic mercury is not especially toxic (indeed it was used widely in the past by physicians as a medicine), but once converted to the organic form of methylmercury, it is much more toxic. An intake of 0.2 mg per day is considered acceptable for adults, and surveys in the USA of fish and shellfish have shown levels around one-tenth of this. An extensive survey of mothers and babies in the Seychelles examined the relationship between maternal exposure to mercury from seafood, and birth and developmental outcomes. With one minor exception (a subjective measure of physical activity in boys), the investigators were unable to show any significant harmful effects from the exposure resulting from frequent (median intake 10 times a week) fish intake by these women. They concluded that the infants examined in the programme were no different from those they examined normally in the USA.

Synthetic contaminants Certain synthetic substances that enter the marine environment are extremely persistent, and can accumulate in the marine food chain. Polychlorobiphenyls, dioxins, polycyclic aromatic hydrocarbons (PAHs) and organochlorine pesticides are the most problematic. Similar considerations apply to most foods eaten by humans, whether marine or terrestrial in origin. That these contaminants are toxic is not seriously questioned, although debate is taking place about the health significance of the extremely low levels that are capable of being detected by sophisticated modern analytical equipment. Determining the health risks associated with eating foods contaminated with low levels of these substances is extremely difficult. Tests on animals are of uncertain significance to human exposure, as are tests on model systems or cell culture systems. While there is no doubt that the presence of these substances is not desirable, it is clear that effective and concerted international action is necessary to deal with the problem. Some progress in this direction has already been made, though much still remains to be done. At present, the only generally agreed risk to health arises from the consumption of freshwater fish from inland lakes. Such bodies of water are especially prone to contamination by persistent chemicals, and lack the cleansing and diluting action of oceanic water exchange to keep levels low. Avoidance of seafood from estuarine waters may also be advisable.

The Role of Seafood in the Diet

Seafood and the nutrients it supplies have played a crucial role in the evolution of *Homo sapiens*, and evidence is accumulating that the relevance of these foods to modern human society is just as great. It is the presence in certain seafoods of long-chain n-3 PUFA that makes them so important to human nutrition. Brain neuronal membranes and retinal rod cells are richly endowed with the long-chain n-3 PUFA DHA (22:6 n-3). Experts in mammalian evolution have hypothesized that the extent of brain development in different species of mammals was in part dependant on the dietary supply of n-3 PUFA available to the species at the time. Thus those species with good access to the long-chain n-3 PUFA are hypothesized to have evolved a larger and more complex brain and nervous system, which enabled them to compete more effectively with other, less well-developed species. Much of human evolution seems to have occurred at the edge of water, thus providing a rich supply of n-3 PUFA.

Evidence accumulated in the 1980s and 1990s is leading to the view that the dietary supply of PUFA may be having an adverse effect on social behaviour in Western democracies. Research has shown that the dietary supply of long-chain n-3 PUFA can affect eyesight and brain development in infants. Studies have indicated superior problem solving ability in 9-month-old babies fed on a formula supplemented with long-chain n-3 PUFA. Preliminary results indicate a beneficial impact of dietary EPA and DHA supplementation on certain aspects of dyslexia in children as well as on the negative behavioural aspects of schizophrenia and extraggression (i.e. aggression directed towards others) in adults. Indirect data suggest that a low dietary n-3 supply may be a factor in hyperactivity and dyspraxia in children, and depression in adults. These ideas are as yet largely unproved and further research is required in this area. However, the link between dietary DHA supply and brain DHA level is already well established. Preliminary evidence that dietary PUFA could affect brain structure – and hence brain function – has been reported, providing a theoretical framework for these ideas.

Two temporal changes have led to this scenario. Fish consumption has fallen in the UK since the 1950s, and eating habits have changed to favour the white, low-lipid fish over the oil-rich fish. Thus the overall intake of long-chain n-3 PUFA from fish has fallen. This would normally not be important, since humans can in principle convert the α-linolenic (n-3) acid found in green vegetables and certain vegetable oils into the long-chain versions EPA and DHA. This conversion process is not very efficient, and is subject to competitive inhibition from n-6 PUFA. In evolutionary times, estimates of human n-3/n-6 intakes have suggested a ratio close to 1. In such a situation, it is not unreasonable to expect that α-linolenic acid could be converted to EPA and DHA. Modern diets supply 7, 8 or even 10 times more n-6 than n-3, and at these levels it is conceivable that conversion of α-linolenic acid will not occur at a sufficient rate. Thus the supply of DHA available to maintain brain levels may be inadequate, contributing to the increasing prevalence of the problems outlined above.

Of more immediate significance is the beneficial impact of the dietary long-chain n-3 PUFA on risk of death from coronary heart disease. A 29% reduction in risk of death from a second heart attack (secondary prevention) has been observed in an intervention study in which a group of 1000 men consumed two portions of oil-rich fish a week (200–400 g) or 1 g of n-3 PUFA daily in the form of capsules. This level of risk reduction is comparable to that achievable with orthodox pharmacological intervention. So far only this one study has investigated the effect of additional long-chain n-3 fatty acid intake on coronary heart disease mortality. However, there is a a vast body of clinical and laboratory data indicating beneficial changes in established coronary disease risk factors when long-chain n-3 intake is increased. A number of epidemiological studies support this finding, and suggest that long-chain n-3 PUFA also has a role in primary prevention. The role of n-3 PUFA in inflammatory diseases is also well established (*See:* **Fatty Acids**: Health Effects of n-3 Polyunsaturated Fatty Acids).

Per capita UK fish and shellfish intake in the 1990s averages 175 g per week, down from nearly 300 g per week at the end of World War II. The 1994 report of the UK government Committee on Medical Aspects of Food Policy (COMA) on Nutritional Aspects of Cardiovascular Disease recognized the dietary value of the long-chain n-3 PUFA; it was recommended that fish intake should be doubled, and that oil-rich fish should be eaten at least once each week. The beneficial role of fish in the diet needs no more endorsement than that.

See Colour Plate 5.

See also: **Coronary Heart Disease**: Prevention. **Fatty Acids**: Health Effects of n-3 Polyunsaturated Fatty Acids. **Pregnancy**: Nutrient Requirements.

Further Reading

Ahmed FE (1991) *Seafood Safety*. Washington: National Academy Press.
Barker TC and Yudkin J (1971) *Fish In Britain*. University of London.
Burgess GHO, Cutting CL, Lovern JA and Waterman JJ (1965) *Fish Handling and Processing*. London: HMSO.
COMA (1994) *Nutritional Aspects of Cardiovascular Disease*. Report no. 46. London: HMSO.
Davidson S, Passmore R, Brock JF and Truswell AS (1979) *Human Nutrition and Dietetics*. Edinburgh: Churchill Livingstone.
Groom H and Ashwell M (1993) *Nutritional Aspects of Fish*. BNF Briefing Paper 10. London: BNF.
Gunstone FD (1967) *An Introduction to the Chemistry*

and Biochemistry of Fatty Acids and their Glycerides. London: Chapman & Hall.

Holland B, Brown J and Buss DH (1993) *Fish and Fish Products.* Third supplement to *McCance & Widdowson's The Composition of Foods,* 5th edn. London: HMSO.

National Food Survey (1990) London: HMSO.

National Food Survey (1994) London: HMSO.

Nettleton JA (1995) *Omega-3 Fatty Acids and Health.* New York: Chapman & Hall.

Myers GJ, Marsh DO. Cox C *et al.* (1996) A pilot neuro-developmental study of Seychellois children following *in utero* exposure to methylmercury from a maternal fish diet. *Neurotoxicology* 16(4): 629–638.

Paul AA and Southgate DAT (1978) *McCance & Widdowson's The Composition of Foods,* 4th edn. London: HMSO.

Windsor M and Barlow S (1981) *Introduction to Fishery By-products.* Farnham: Fishing News Books.

Flavonoids *see* **Phytochemicals**: Classification and Occurrence; Epidemiological Factors.

Fluoride *see* **Dental Disease**: Aetiology and Epidemiology. **Ultratrace Elements**: Physiology.

Folate *see* **Folic Acid**: Physiology, Dietary Sources and Requirements.

FOLIC ACID

Physiology, Dietary Sources and Requirements

Joseph McPartlin, Donald G Weir and **J M Scott**, Trinity College, Dublin, Ireland

Copyright © 1998 Academic Press

Folic acid was initially distinguished from vitamin B_{12} as a dietary antianaemia factor by Wills in the 1930s. The subsequent chemical isolation of folic acid and its role as a cofactor in one-carbon metabolism led to the elucidation of deficiency diseases at the molecular level. The term 'folate' includes the entire group of folate vitamin forms, i.e. the naturally occurring folylpolyglutamates found in food, and folic acid (pteroylglutamic acid), the synthetic form of the vitamin added to dietary supplements and to fortified foods. 'Folate' is thus the general term used to include any form of the vitamin irrespective of the state of reduction, type of substitution or degree of polyglutamylation.

Folate functions metabolically as an enzyme cofactor in the synthesis of nucleic acids and amino acids. Deficiency of the vitamin leads to impaired cell replication and other metabolic alterations particularly related to methionine synthesis. The similar clinical manifestations of cobalamin deficiency and folate deficiency underline the metabolic interrelationship between the two vitamins. Folate deficiency alone, manifested clinically as megaloblastic anaemia, is the most common vitamin deficiency in developed countries. An improvement in folate status at the population level is likely, however, with the introduction of food fortification as a result of findings that folic acid supplementation reduces the incidence of neural tube defects and potentially reduces the risk of cardiovascular disease.

An integrated approach to the treatment of folate disorders and a comprehension of the advantages as well as the drawbacks of various supplementation programmes currently under consideration require an understanding of folic acid physiology and biochemistry.

Physiology and Biochemistry

Chemistry and biochemical functions

Folic acid consists of a pterin moiety linked via a

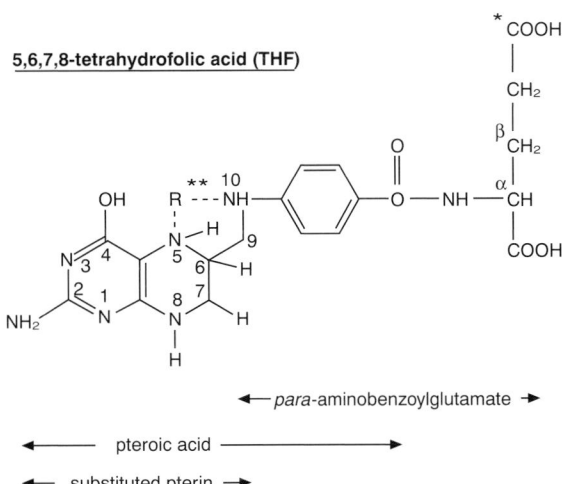

5,6,7,8-tetrahydrofolic acid (THF)

←— *para*-aminobenzoylglutamate —→

←——————— pteroic acid ———————→

←— substituted pterin —→

Figure 1 Structure of 5,6,7,8-tetrahydrofolate (THF) compounds. In tetrahydrofolic acid, R = H; other substituents are listed in Table 1. *Site of attachment of extra glutamate residues; **hatched line indicates the N5 and/or N10 site of attachment of one-carbon units.

methylene group to a *para*-aminobenzoylglutamate moiety. Folic acid is the synthetic form of the vitamin, metabolic activity requiring reduction to the tetrahydrofolate (THF) derivative (**Fig. 1**), the addition of a chain of glutamate residues in γ-peptide linkage, and the acquisition of one-carbon units.

One-carbon units at various levels of oxidation are generated metabolically and are reactive only as moieties attached to the N5 or N10 positions of the folate molecule. The range of oxidation states for folate one-carbon units extends from methanol to formate as methyl, methylene, methenyl, formyl or formimino moieties (**Table 1**). When one-carbon units are incorporated as folate derivatives, they may also be converted from one oxidation state to another by the gain or loss of electrons.

The source of one-carbon units for folate   One-carbon units at the oxidation level of formate can enter directly into the folate pool as formic acid in a reac-

Table 1   Structure and nomenclature of folate compounds (see Fig. 1)

Compound	R	Oxidation state
5-formyl-THF	–CHO	Formate
10-formyl-THF	–CHO	Formate
5-formimino-THF	–CH=NH	Formate
5,10-methenyl-THF	–CH=	Formate
5,10-methylene-THF	–CH2–	Formaldehyde
5-methyl-THF	–CH3	Methanol

tion catalysed by 10-formyl-THF synthase (**Fig. 2**). Entry at the formate level of oxidation can also take place via a catabolic product of histidine, formiminoglutamic acid. The third mode of entry at the formate level of oxidation involves the formation of 5-formyl-THF from 5,10-methenyl-THF by the enzyme serine hydroxymethyl transferase (SHMT). The 5-formyl-THF may be rapidly converted to other forms of folate. A final mode of entry of formate arises from carbon-1 of the ribose moiety of methylthioribose, a by-product of the conversion of *S*-adenosylmethionine to polyamines.

The enzyme SHMT is involved in the entry of one-carbon units at the formaldehyde level of oxidation by catalysing the transfer of the β-carbon of serine to form glycine and 5,10-methylene-THF. Other sources of one-carbon entry at this level of oxidation include the glycine cleavage system and the choline-dependent pathway, both enzyme systems generating 5,10-methylene-THF in the mitochondria of the cell.

The removal and utilization of one-carbon units from folate   Single carbon units are removed from folate by a number of reactions. The enzyme 10-formyl-THF dehydrogenase provides a mechanism for disposal of excess one-carbon units as carbon dioxide. (Folate administration to animals enhances the conversion of ingested methanol and formate to CO_2, diminishing methanol toxicity.) Alternatively, single-carbon units from 10-formyl-THF are used for the biosynthesis of purines (Fig. 2).

The one-carbon unit of 5,10-methylene-THF is transferred in two ways. Reversal of the SHMT reaction produces serine from glycine but since serine is also produced from glycolysis via phosphoglycerate this reaction is unlikely to be important. However, one-carbon transfer from 5,10-methylene-THF to deoxyuridylate to form thymidylic acid, a precursor of DNA, is of crucial importance to the cell. While the source of one-carbon units – namely 5,10-methylene-THF – is at the formaldehyde level of oxidation, the one-carbon unit transferred to form thymidylic acid appears at the methanol level of oxidation. Electrons for this reduction come from THF itself to generate dihydrofolate (DHF) as a product, which must in turn be reduced back to THF in order to accept further one-carbon units.

A solitary transfer of one-carbon units takes place at the methanol level of oxidation. It involves the transfer of the methyl group from 5-methyl-THF to homocysteine to form methionine and THF. This reaction is catalysed by the enzyme methionine synthase and requires vitamin B_{12} as cofactor. The compound 5-methyl-THF is the dominant folate in the body and remains metabolically inactive until it is

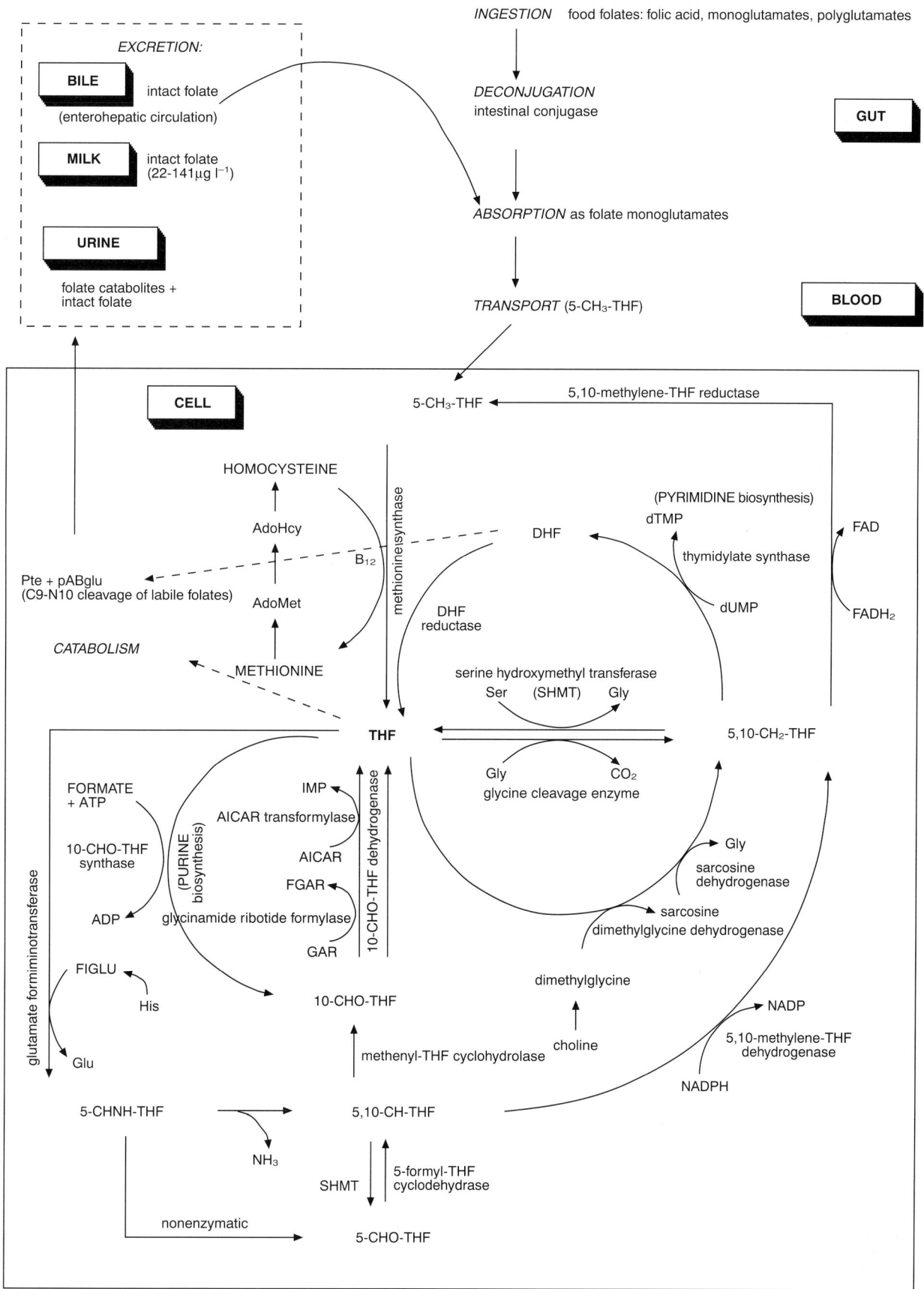

Figure 2 Human folate metabolism. FIGLU: formiminoglutamate, IMP: inosine monophosphate. See text for other abbreviations.

demethylated to THF, whereupon polyglutamylation takes place to allow subsequent folate-dependent reactions to proceed efficiently. The inhibition of methionine synthase due to vitamin B_{12} deficiency induces megaloblastic anaemia that is clinically indistinguishable from folate deficiency. The haematological effect in both cases results in levels of 5,10-methylene-THF inadequate to sustain thymidylate biosynthesis. Clinically, it is essential to ascertain whether the anaemia is the result of folate or vitamin B_{12} deficiency by differential diagnostic techniques. Vitamin B_{12} is essential for the synthesis of myelin in nerve tissue (See: **Cobalamins**: Physiology, Dietary Sources and Requirements), a function probably related to methionine production from the methionine synthase reaction and the subsequent formation of S-adenosylmethionine (ADOMET). Hence, vitamin B_{12} deficiency will lead to nervous disorders in addition to the haematological effects. While the latter respond to folic acid treatment, the neurological effects do not. Thus, inappropriate administration of folic acid in vitamin B_{12} deficiency may treat the anaemia but mask the progression of the neurological defects.

In summary, the biochemical function of folate coenzymes is the transfer and utilization of these one-carbon units in a variety of essential reactions (Fig. 2), including (1) de novo purine biosynthesis (formylation of glycinamide ribonucleotide (GAR) and 5-amino-4-imidazole carboxamide ribonucleotide (AICAR)); (2) pyrimidine nucleotide biosynthesis (methylation of deoxyuridylic acid to thymidylic acid); (3) amino acid interconversions – the interconversion of serine to glycine, catabolism of histidine to glutamic acid, and conversion of homocysteine to methionine (which also requires vitamin B_{12}); and (4) generation and utilization of formate.

Many of the enzymes involved in these reactions are multifunctional, and are capable of channelling substrates and one-carbon units from reaction to reaction within a protein matrix. Another feature of intracellular folate metabolism is the compartmentation of folate coenzymes between the cytosol and the mitochondria: 5-methyl-THF, for instance, is associated with the cytosolic fraction of the cell whereas most of 10-formyl-THF is located in the mitochondria. Similarly, some folate-dependent enzymes are associated with either one compartment on the other, though some are found in both. Metabolic products of folate-dependent reactions such as serine and glycine are readily transported between both locations, but the folate coenzymes are not.

Folate deficiency and hyperhomocysteinaemia An important consequence of folate deficiency is the inability to remethylate homocysteine (Fig. 2). Indeed, there is an inverse correlation between the levels of folate and homocysteine in the blood of humans. Many clinical studies, beginning with the observations of children with homocysteinuria presenting with vascular abnormalities and thromboembolism, have demonstrated an association between hyperhomocysteinaemia and increased risk of premature atherosclerosis in the coronary, carotid and peripheral vasculature. The prevalence of hyperhomocysteinaemia was found to be 30% among patients with cardiovascular disease and the risk of premature occlusive vascular disease was about 30 times greater for people with hyperhomocysteinaemia compared with normal controls. Even mild hyperhomocysteinaemia is recognized to be an independent risk factor for cardiovascular disease. Metabolically, homocysteine may be disposed of by the methionine synthase reaction (dependent on folate as well as vitamin B_{12}), the transsulfuration pathway (dependent on vitamin B_6) and by the choline degradation pathway. Marginal deficiencies of these three vitamins are associated with hyperhomocysteinaemia. Of the three, however, folic acid administration has been shown to be the most effective in lowering homocysteine, blood levels. Convincing evidence of the potential role of folate intake in the prevention of vascular disease, probably by lowering blood levels of homocysteine, has been demonstrated by a significant inverse relationship between serum folate levels and fatal coronary heart disease.

Absorption of folates

Food folates mainly consist of reduced polyglutamates hydrolysed to monoglutamates in the gut prior to absorption across the intestinal mucosa. The conjugase enzyme that hydrolyses dietary folates has been found on the luminal brush border membrane in the human jejunum and has equal affinity for polyglutamates of varying chain length. Transport is facilitated by a saturable, carrier-mediated uptake system, although changes in luminal pH, or the presence of conjugase inhibitors, folate binders or other food components, can adversely affect the rate of hydrolysis and intestinal absorption. Such factors account for the wide variation in bioavailability of the vitamin in foods of plant and animal origin. Some metabolism of the resultant monoglutamate, mainly to 5-methyl-THF, appears to occur during the absorption process, though this may not be necessary for transport across the basolateral membrane of the intestinal mucosa into the portal circulation. The degree of metabolic conversion of dietary folic acid depends on the dose, pharmacological amounts being transported unaltered into the circulation.

Transport in the circulation, cellular uptake and turnover

Folate circulates in the blood predominantly as 5-methyl-THF. A variable proportion circulates freely or bound either to low-affinity protein binders such as albumin (which accounts for about 50% of bound folate) or to a high-affinity folate binder in serum (carrying less than 5% of circulating folate). The physiological importance of serum binders is unclear, but they may function to control folate distribution and excretion during deficiency.

Though most folate is initially taken up by the liver following absorption, it is delivered to a wide variety of tissues for which many types of folate transporters have been described. Because these transporters have affinities for folate in the micromolar range, they would not be saturated by normal ambient concentrations of folate. Therefore, folate uptake into tissues should be responsive to any serum folate levels found after folate supplementation. An important determinant of folate uptake into cells is their mitotic activity, as would be expected given the dependence of DNA biosynthesis on folate coenzyme function. Folate accumulation is more rapid in actively dividing cells than in quiescent cells, a factor probably related to the induction and activity of folylpoly-γ-glutamate synthase. This enzyme catalyses the addition of glutamate by γ-peptide linkage to the initial glutamate moiety of the folate molecule. Although polyglutamate derivatization may be considered a storage strategem, this elongation is the most efficient coenzyme form for normal one-carbon metabolism. The activity of folylpoly-γ-glutamate synthase is highest in the liver, the folate stores of which account for half of the estimated 5–10 mg adult complement. Retention within the cell is also facilitated by the high proportion of folate associated with proteins, and this is likely to be increased in folate deficiency.

The mobilization of liver and other stores in the body is not well understood, particularly in deficiency states, though some accounts describe poor turnover rates in folate-depleted rats. Transport across cell membranes during redistribution requires deconjugation of the large negatively charged polyglutamates. Mammalian γ-glutamyl hydrolases that hydrolyse glutamate moieties residue by residue and transpeptidases that can hydrolyse folylpolyglutamates directly to mono- or diglutamate forms of the vitamin have been described for a number of tissues. Thus mammalian cells possess two types of enzymes that can play a key role in folate homeostasis and regulation of one-carbon metabolism: the folylpolyglutamate synthetase which catalyses the synthesis of retentive and active folate, and a number of deconjugating enzymes that promote release of folate from the cell. Polyglutamate forms released into the circulation either through cell death or by a possible exocytotic mechanism would be hydrolysed rapidly by plasma γ-glutamyl hydrolase to the monoglutamate form.

Excretion

Folate is concentrated in bile, and the enterohepatic recirculation from the intestine accounts for considerable reabsorption and reutilization of folate (about 100 μg per day). Faecal folates mostly arise through gut microflora biosynthesis of the vitamin, with only a small contribution from unabsorbed dietary folate. Urinary excretion of intact folates accounts for only a small fraction of ingested folate under normal physiological conditions. The greater amount of excretion in urine is accounted for by products of an intracellular scission of the folate molecule at the C9–N10 bond, consisting of one or more pteridines and p-acetamidobenzoylglutamate. The rate of scission of the folate molecule is increased during rapid mitotic conditions such as pregnancy and early stages of growth in young animals. Scission of folate perhaps constitutes the major mechanism of folate turnover in the body.

Human Folate Requirements

Folate requirement is the minimum necessary to prevent deficiency. Dietary recommendations for populations, however, must allow for a margin of safety to cover the needs of the vast majority of that population. As with most nutrients this margin of safety corresponds to two standard deviations above the mean requirement for a population, calculated to meet the needs of 97.5% of the population. Thus, dietary recommendations such as the recommended dietary allowances (RDA) in the USA, the reference nutrient index (RNI) in the UK and the World Health Organization/Food and Agriculture Organization (WHO/FAO) safe level of intake contain allowances for individual variability, the bioavailability of folate from different foodstuffs, and periods of low intake and increased utilization (**Table 2**). International recommendation tables are constantly subject to review, taking into account the most recent population surveys relating intake to indicators of folate status as well as experimental laboratory findings. The maintenance of adequate folate status throughout the life span is under scrutiny in view of findings relating folate status with the risk of neural tube defects and specific chronic diseases including coronary artery disease and cancer.

Table 2 Folate reference values and recommendations for various population groups

Population category	US recommended dietary allowance,[a] 1989 (μg per day)	UK reference nutrient intake,[a] 1991 (μg per day)	WHO/FAO safe level, 1988 (μg per day)
Infants (months)			
0–0.5	25	50	16–24
0.5–1.0	35	50	32
Children (years)			
1–3	50	70	50
4–6	75	100	50
7–10	100	150	102
Men (years)			
11–14	150	200	170
15–18	200	200	200
19–24	200	200	200
25–50	200	200	200
51+	200	200	200
Women (years)			
11–14	150	200	170
15–18	180	200	170
19–24	180	200	170
25–50	180	200	170
51+	180	200	170
Pregnancy	400	300	370–470
Lactation			
First 6 months	280	260	270
Second 6 months	260	260	270

[a]Defined as two notional standard deviations above the mean requirement.

The crucial role of folate in at least one of its functions, the biosynthesis of precursors for DNA, suggests that folate requirements may vary with age, though folate utilization is most obviously increased in pregnancy and lactation.

Pregnancy and prepregnancy

Maintaining adequate folate status in women in their child-bearing years is particularly important since a large proportion of pregnancies are unplanned and many women are likely to be unaware of their pregnancy during the first crucial weeks of fetal development. Pregnancy implies considerable mitotic activity related to fetal growth, uterine expansion, placental maturation and expanded blood volume. Therefore, it imposes demands on folate supply large enough to lead to deficiency more often than the nonpregnant state. The highest prevalence of poor folate status in pregnant women occurs among the lowest socioeconomic groups and is often exacerbated by the high parity rate of these women. Indeed, the megaloblastic anaemia commonly found amongst the malnourished poor in pregnancy probably reflects the depletion of maternal stores to the advantage of the fetoplacental unit as indicated by the several-fold higher serum folate levels in the newborn compared with the mother. From the baby's viewpoint considerable evidence indicates that maternal folate deficiency leads to fetal growth retardation and low birthweight. The higher incidence of low-birthweight infants born to teenage mothers compared with their adult counterparts is probably related to the additional burden of adolescent growth on folate resources.

The amount of supplemental folate required to satisfy fetal and maternal needs is still debated. The UK recommended intake for folate during pregnancy is set at 100 μg daily above that recommended for nonpregnant women on the basis that this is the amount required to maintain plasma and erythrocyte levels at or above those of nonpregnant women. Based on these and similar observations, international recommendations for folate in pregnancy since 1989 have been set at a level of 300–470 μg daily, substantially less than the level of 800 μg set in 1980 in the USA. The lack of evidence about the supplemental requirement level in pregnancy prompted the development of a laboratory-based assessment of metabolic turnover which involved the assay of total daily folate catabolites (along with intact folate) in the urine of pregnant women. The rationale of the procedure was that this catabolic product represented an ineluctable daily loss of folate, the replacement of which should constitute the daily requirement. After correction for individual variation in catabolite excretion and bioavailability of dietary folate, the recommended allowances based on this mode of assessment were approximately 50% higher than current international recommendations. The data produced by the catabolite excretion method may represent a more accurate reflection of requirement in the light of the uncertainty in the estimation of food folate content as well as the problem of underreporting of intakes.

Folate and neural tube defects   The debate on folate requirements of normal pregnancy has been overtaken by the finding that periconceptual consumption of folic acid has a significant protective effect against the occurrence and recurrence of neural tube defects (NTD). This malformation in the developing embryo consists of a failure of the neural tube to close properly during the fourth week of embryonic life. Incomplete closure of the spinal cord results in spina bifida, while incomplete closure of the cranium results in anencephaly. It appears that folic acid exerts its protective effect by overcoming a partial block in folate metabolism rather than by correcting a nutritional deficiency. A functional variant of the gene for 5,10-methylene-THF reductase, the 'thermolabile variant' associated with NTD, may express its aberrancy through an inability to bind its flavin cofactor properly, an inability shown to be corrected experimentally (in the bacterial enzyme at least) by increasing the folate concentration. It is likely that other variants of this gene and/or variants of other genes associated with folate metabolism are involved not only in NTD but also in vascular diseases related to hyperhomocysteinaemia (see above).

International agencies have published folic acid recommendations for the prevention of NTD. To prevent recurrence, 5 mg folic acid daily in tablet form is recommended, while 400 μg daily is recommended for the prevention of occurrence, to be commenced prior to conception and continued until the twelfth week of pregnancy. Given the high proportion of unplanned pregnancies, the latter recommendation level is applicable to all fertile women.

The strategies for supplying women with folate in the periconceptual period take three forms: firstly, supplementation in the form of a tablet; secondly, educating women to choose folate-rich foods; thirdly, fortification of staple foods with folic acid either by regulation or in a nondirective way by industry.

By avoiding the widespread introduction of extraneous material into the food supply the first two options have the potential to cause least harm to nontargeted population groups. However, experience with supplementation has shown that women are unlikely to use supplements through unawareness of the benefit, forgetfulness or lack of motivation because of the low risk involved. The varied diet advocated by the second approach is least likely to benefit those most at risk – the poor. The third strategy, food fortification, is considered to be the most practical approach of delivering the recommended amount of folate. This approach requires that sufficiently high levels of fortification are achieved to ensure that almost all women receive the daily recommended amount of folic acid. Meeting this goal, however, gives rise to the potential problem that those for whom it was not primarily intended would be likely to receive excessive amounts of the vitamin. The issue of greatest concern which has prevented the implementation of folic acid fortification programmes has been the possibility that the diagnosis of cobalamin deficiency due to pernicious anaemia in the elderly might be delayed by the administration of folic acid. This is because high oral doses of folic acid pass into the circulation unaltered and are metabolized by tissues independently of cobalamin. Correction of the haematological abnormality of cobalamin thus occurs while the neuropathy may proceed unabated and undiagnosed. The key to the fortification debate lies in the determination of the minimum effective dose required to achieve folate status associated with lowest risk of NTD, a status calculated to correspond to 400 ng ml^{-1} maternal red cell folate.

Lactation

Unlike pregnancy, where the bulk of folate expenditure arises through catabolism, the increased requirement in lactation is chiefly due to milk secretion. Several observations indicate that mammary tissue takes precedence over other maternal tissues for folate resources. For instance, maternal folate status deteriorates both in early and late lactation but milk folate concentration is maintained or increased. Moreover, supplemental folate appears to be taken up by mammary epithelial cells preferentially over haematopoietic cells in lactating women with folate deficiency, indicating that maternal reserves are depleted to maintain milk folate content in lactating women. Recommendations are based on the maintenance requirement of nonpregnant, nonlactating women plus the estimated folate replace the quantity lost in milk 60–100 μg daily is based on a 40–60 μg l^{-1} and an absorpt sources of 50–70%. The off may be underestimates, how a less efficient absorption r diet is more likely, and on estimations of milk folat

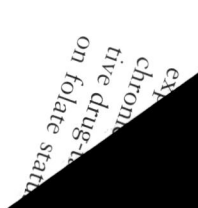

as 100 μg daily. Therefore an additional 200 μg folate daily or a total of 500 μg daily seems a more realistic recommendation for lactating women.

Infants and children

The high concentration of circulating folate in newborn infants coincides with the rapid rate of cell division that takes place in the first few months of life and is reflected in the higher folate requirement for infants on a weight basis compared to adults. Though the recommendation standards (see Table 1) may underestimate the quantities consumed by many breast-fed infants, intake is generally higher than these levels so that folate deficiency is unlikely.

Data on requirements for older children is sparse, so recommendations up to adolescence are based on interpolations between the values for very young children and adults. Daily recommended levels are ensured to be above 3.6 μg kg^{-1} body weight, an amount associated with no overt folate deficiency in children and shown to maintain plasma folate concentrations at a low but acceptable level.

Adolescents and adults

Folate recommendations for adolescents are set at a similar level to those for adults, the smaller weights of the former age group being compensated for by higher rates of growth. The general approach in setting recommendations for adults has been based on intake data. Canadian studies demonstrated that a mean intake of 150–200 μg daily was associated with no overt signs of folate deficiency and suboptimal folate status in less than 10% of subjects. This value is close to the reported median folate intake in Britain of 209 μg daily in women, but lower than the 300 μg daily in men. In contrast to the US recommendations, there is no difference in the UK recommendations for men and women, since it is argued that the lower requirement due to smaller lean body mass in women is offset by their potentially greater need during pregnancy.

Elderly people

Although folate deficiency occurs more frequently in the elderly than in young adults, recommendations are set at the same level for both groups. Reference recommendations apply to healthy subjects. However, a significant proportion of the elderly population are likely to suffer clinical conditions and be exposed to a range of environmental factors such as smoking, alcohol consumption and prescription taking which may have a detrimental effect

Food Sources of Folate

Folate is synthesized by microorganisms and higher plants, but not by mammals for whom it is an essential vitamin. The most concentrated food folate sources include liver, yeast extract, green leafy vegetables, legumes, certain fruits and fortified breakfast cereals. Prolonged exposure to heat, air or ultraviolet light is known to inactivate the vitamin, thus food preparation and cooking can make a difference to the amount of folate ingested; boiling in particular results in substantial food losses. Foods that contain a high concentration of folate are not necessarily those that contribute the most to overall intakes of the vitamin in a population. For example, liver is a particularly concentrated source, providing 320 μg folate per 100 g, but it is not eaten by a sufficient proportion of the population to make any major contribution to total dietary folate intakes. Beer, in contrast, contains at most 9 μg per 100 g but is consumed often enough by the British, for example, to account for about 10% of their daily folate intake. **Table 3** shows the percentage contribution made by the main food groups to average daily intake of folate in British adults.

The contribution of different foodstuffs depends on cultural differences and national eating habits. For instance, orange juice is the main contributor of folate in the US diet. Much of the current international contribution of folate to the diet is skewed towards fortified breakfast cereals and this foodstuff is likely to be joined shortly in this regard by the contribution from fortified flour products. In the main, though, adherence to dietary recommendations to increase consumption of folate-rich foods

Table 3 Contribution made by main food groups to the average daily intake of folate in British adults, from a survey conducted in 1987

Food	Contribution(%)
Cereal products	21
Bread	12
Breakfast cereals[a]	3
Meat, meat products	9
Milk, milk products	8
Vegetables excluding potatoes	16
Beans	3
Green leafy vegetables	3
Potatoes	14
Fruit and fruit juice	5
Beers	10
Soft drinks	3
Tea	3

[a]Many breakfast cereals were not fortified with folic acid at the time of the survey.

is likely to enhance not only folate intake but also other nutrients essential to health.

See also: **Adolescents**: Dietary Habits and Nutrient Requirements. **Anaemia (Anemia)**: Megaloblastic Anaemia. **Children**: Nutritional Requirements of School Children. **Cobalamins**: Physiology, Dietary Sources and Requirements. **Lactation**: Dietary Requirements. **Older People**: Nutritional Requirements. **Pregnancy**: Safe Diet for Pregnancy; Preconception Nutrition and Prevention of Neural Tube Defects.

Further Reading

Bailey LB, ed. (1995) *Folate in Health and Disease.* New York: Marcel Dekker.

Blakley RL and Benkovic SJ, eds (1984, 1985) *Folates and Pterins*, vols 1 and 2. New York: Wiley.

Blakley RL and Whitehead VM eds (1986) *Folates and Pterins* vol. 3. New York: Wiley.

Botez MI and Reynolds EH, eds (1979) *Folic Acid in Neurology, Psychiatry and Internal Medicine.* New York: Raven Press.

Chanarin I (1979) *The Megaloblastic Anaemias*, 2nd edn. Oxford: Blackwell.

Herbert V and Das K (1994) Folic acid and vitamin B_{12}. In: Shils ME, Olson JA and Shike M (eds) *Modern Nutrition in Health and Disease*, 8th edn. Philadelphia: Lea & Febiger.

Institute of Medicine, Food and Nutrition Board (1994) *How Should the Recommended Dietary Allowances be Revised?* Washington, DC: National Academy Press.

Picciano MR, Stokstad ELR and Gregory JF, eds (1990) *Folic Acid Metabolism in Health and Disease.* New York: Wiley-Liss.

Scott JM and Weir DG (1994) Folate/vitamin B_{12} interrelationships. In: Tipton KF (ed.) *Essays in Biochemistry*, vol. 28, pp. 63–72. London: Portland Press.

Scott JM, Kirke PN and Weir DG (1990) The role of nutrition in neural tube defects. *Annual Review of Nutrition* 10:277–295.

Selhub J and Miller JW (1992) The pathogenesis of hyperhomocysteinemia: interruption of the co-ordinate regulation by *S*-adenosylmethionine of the remethylation and transsulfuration of homocysteine. *American Journal of Clinical Nutrition* 55:131–138.

FOOD AID

Overview

D J Shaw, formerly UN World Food Programme, Rome Italy

Copyright © 1998 Academic Press

Food security and adequate nutrition are crucial to the quality of human life and general wellbeing. They also have important economic and social implications for nations. The main cause of hunger and food insecurity is poverty. Adequate dietary intake (including micronutrients) at critical times of life is a major factor determining physical and mental development and resistance to disease. This article focuses on the reasons for the growing need for food aid, the sources of its supply, the different types of food aid distribution programmes, and the kinds of food commodities that are contained in food aid programmes.

The Need for Food Aid

Food aid is a controversial form of development assistance. Detractors point to the political and commercial motives that stimulate donors to provide food aid. They emphasize the possible disincentive effect food aid can have on local food production in countries that receive such aid and its potential disruption to trade, as well as the problem of creating dependence on the part of governments and beneficiary groups in developing countries.

Many of the criticisms levelled at food aid, however, are equally – and in some cases more – applicable to other forms of aid. Its value also deserves equal prominence. Food aid plays a vital role in saving lives in emergencies. Properly applied, it can assist developing countries that are short of food achieve more rapid and more equitable development. Owing to its history, constituency and inherent nature, food aid has special advantages in addressing the major problems of poor people, supporting food security programmes, and reducing the social costs of economic reform and adjustment measures that poor, food-deficient countries are undertaking. It is also an additional form of aid in the sense that donors are unlikely to increase their financial assistance to replace food aid. Food aid has also helped the domestic agricultural policies and programmes of donor countries faced with large surplus stocks of food.

Food aid should also be put in proper perspective. It represents a small fraction of food production in developed and developing countries. In recent years, it has accounted for about 9% of the cereal imports of developing countries and some 7% of cereal stocks in developed countries. However, its importance in the cereal imports of the poorest countries, especially in sub-Saharan Africa, has grown.

Reasons for increasing need

The indications are that food aid will be required, on an increasing scale, well into the twenty-first century. In many poor developing countries, particularly in sub-Saharan Africa, the number of malnourished people is increasing, and food production is not keeping pace with population growth, resulting in higher food imports. These countries are finding it increasingly difficult to pay for commercial food imports owing to their falling foreign exchange earnings and high level of debt repayments. To these difficulties must be added the social cost of economic reform and structural measures, and the considerable increase in the number, scale and duration of disasters that have resulted in a large increase in the need for emergency food aid. This, in turn, has increased the demand for aid, including food aid, for rehabilitation and reconstruction programmes in the aftermath of emergencies. Similarly, assistance is required for disaster prevention, preparedness and mitigation programmes. These programmes could reduce the negative effects of future disasters on economic development and human welfare and the need for further emergency aid.

The world's population in 1997 is estimated to be 5.6 billion people. Although the rate of population growth is declining, additions to the world population have been increasing, and exceed 86 million people a year, mostly in developing countries. United Nations population projections indicate that the world population may reach 11.9 billion by the year 2050.

Despite appreciable worldwide improvements, some 780 million people in developing countries do not have access to enough food to meet their basic daily needs. This includes increasing numbers of malnourished children under 5 years of age: 192 million children suffer from protein–energy malnutrition. More than 2 billion people, mostly women and children, are deficient in one or more micronutrients.

The burden of hunger falls disproportionately on women and children. Over 40% of women in developing countries are underweight and/or anaemic. Growth failure affects one-third of children. An estimated 40 000 children die each day from malnutrition and related diseases: 150 million who live on suffer from illness and poor growth. Clinical vitamin A deficiency, endemic in 40 developing countries, blinds some half a million preschool children a year and leaves 2.8 million with eye damage. Iodine deficiency, which affects some 1.5 billion people worldwide, remains the most common preventable cause of mental retardation. The problem of iron deficiency is increasing in many parts of the developing world.

More than a third of rural people in developing countries have income and consumption levels below nationally defined poverty lines. Urban poverty is also growing rapidly in the developing world as people move into towns and cities in search of work and welfare. In the four decades since 1950, the urban population of developing countries grew, to 1.6 billion people.

Overlying these problems is the rapid increase in disasters, particularly those caused by war. In 1970, there were 2.5 million refugees in the world. A decade later, there were 11 million. In 1993, the number was over 18 million. In addition, an estimated 24 million persons were displaced from their homes in their own countries.

Armed conflict is not the only human disaster affecting the developing countries and their people. A silent 'economic emergency' continues, often accompanied by misplaced economic reform and adjustment programmes, which is resulting in the economic and social isolation of the poorest people in developing countries. Since the 1980s such factors as unemployment, falling commodity prices, rising military expenditure, poor returns on investment, the debt crisis and economic adjustment programmes have drastically reduced the real incomes of some 800 million people in 40 developing countries. In Latin America, the reduction has been as much as 20%; in sub-Saharan Africa, often much more. At the same time, cuts in essential social services have resulted in even fewer programmes in nutrition, health, education and training, especially for the poor.

While the majority of undernourished people (over 500 million) are in Asia, their number has been falling since the 1970s. In contrast, in sub-Saharan Africa poverty and food insecurity are expected to increase by the year 2000 to affect nearly 200 million people. Projections indicate that food imports to that region are likely to at least double during the 1990s. In addition, if the food security of millions of Africans is to be improved through programmes that increase their access to food, even higher food imports will be required. Since overall economic prospects are unfavourable, food aid will continue to play an important part in meeting the region's food deficits.

Food aid targets and supplies

An annual target of at least 10 million tonnes of cereals and adequate quantities of other food commodities was established at the World Food Conference in 1974. Subsequent projections of annual food aid requirements to the year 2000 indicate the need to increase current food aid supplies. These projections range from 20 million tonnes to maintain the existing share of food aid in developing countries' food imports and the current level of nutrition in developing countries, to 55 million tonnes with the aim of improving nutritional standards throughout the developing world.

In contrast, global food aid, as currently defined and statistically recorded, fell sharply to 9.5 million tonnes in 1995 as food prices increased, reducing the amount of food that could be bought from donors' aid budgets, and food stocks in donor countries, from which food aid supplies are drawn, fell to their lowest levels for many years (**Table 1**). Three other negative developments have also occurred. First, an increasing proportion of food aid has gone to meet emergencies rather than support development. Secondly, a significant part of food aid deliveries has gone to the countries in transition, such as the former Yugoslavia and the former Soviet Union, rather than

to the traditional developing countries. Thirdly, a large part of food aid continues to be supplied as programme aid bilaterally, mainly for donor commercial and foreign policy interests, and is sold in urban markets in developing countries where it does little to benefit the poor and malnourished. At the same time, total food aid commitments under the Food Aid Convention of 1995 (see below) have been reduced from 7.5 million tonnes under the previous Convention to 5.36 million tonnes. The USA, the largest food aid donor, has reduced its commitment under the Convention by more than half in response to mounting pressure to reduce the huge US federal budget deficit at a time when US farm exports are expected to reach record levels.

What is Food Aid?

Food aid is distinguished from the commercial food trade by the size of the discount food exporters allow from the commercial price. The *Principles of Surplus Disposal and Consultative Obligations of Member Nations* of the Food and Agriculture Organization (FAO), originally adopted in 1954 as a code of conduct to avoid food aid having any harmful effect on normal food production in recipient countries and on international trade, defined food aid as including: gifts or loans of food commodities by governments, intergovernmental organizations (principally the World Food Programme, the food aid organization of the United Nations), and private, voluntary or

Table 1 Global food aid deliveries 1988–1995 (in tonnes – cereals in grain equivalent)

	1988	1989	1990	1991	1992	1993	1994	1995
By food aid category								
Total	14 848 249	11 733 718	13 641 761	13 195 903	15 219 004	16 846 085	12 644 753	9 524 693
Relief	3 265 289	2 388 289	2 767 652	3 565 372	4 964 029	4 159 654	4 243 151	3 236 072
Project	4 011 745	2 871 992	2 836 174	2 980 796	2 576 152	2 491 018	2 801 074	2 478 241
Programme	7 571 215	6 473 437	8 037 935	6 649 735	7 678 823	10 195 413	5 600 528	3 810 379
By commodity type								
Cereals:	13 152 273	10 727 023	12 458 920	12 014 499	13 393 250	15 033 848	10 786 884	8 416 176
Wheat and wheat flour	10 066 401	7 379 403	7 979 328	7 908 916	7 802 838	7 501 031	6 802 830	4 974 967
Rice	997 332	873 402	732 054	938 738	1 007 284	1 045 430	727 606	1 187 016
Coarse grains	1 765 004	2 062 275	3 322 847	2 829 051	4 163 725	6 038 442	2 724 325	1 823 013
Blended/fortified	323 536	412 143	424 691	337 794	419 403	448 945	532 123	431 180
Noncereals:	1 695 976	1 006 495	1 182 841	1 181 404	1 825 754	1 812 237	1 857 869	1 108 517
Dairy products	340 502	156 624	135 458	226 811	308 631	225 131	133 458	63 190
Vegetable oil and fats	882 439	527 730	551 675	362 780	542 927	484 586	427 618	305 216
Meat and fish	52 954	59 117	70 571	86 965	161 005	69 119	61 294	27 482
Pulses	203 046	155 637	182 112	282 907	356 962	410 767	434 736	323 306
Other noncereals	217 038	107 388	243 026	221 941	456 230	622 637	800 761	389 320

1995 data are provisional. Source: WFP/INTERFAIS

nongovernmental organizations; cash grants tied to food purchases; and sales and loans of food commodities on credit terms with a repayment period of 3 years or more.

The Development Assistance Committee of the Organization for Economic Cooperation and Development, which comprises the major donor countries, has agreed on a level of 25% below the commercial price as an arbitrary definition of the grant element in official development assistance. Some immediate problems arise for defining and recording food aid.

A large part of so-called 'food trade' does not take place as straight market sales at free international prices. It is conducted through a labyrinth of various forms of bilateral agreements between governments that provide discounts from the 'commercial' price (itself depressed by the huge surpluses that have existed in the major food-exporting countries) in many direct and indirect ways. These food transactions, which have come to be called 'grey area' food aid, are perhaps more than quadruple the level of statistically recorded food aid (9.5 million tonnes in 1995), and are carried out largely for donor short-run political and commercial (market protection and penetration) purposes. If this hidden food aid was brought out into the open and focused on the needs of poor, food-insecure people, a major step would be taken in dealing with the world hunger problem and, by extension, the eradication of poverty and food insecurity.

The countries that signed the Final Act of the Uruguay round of multilateral trade negotiations in 1994, including the major aid donors, recognized that during the reform programme leading to greater liberalization of trade in agriculture, the least-developed and net food-importing developing countries may experience negative effects in terms of the availability of adequate supplies of basic foodstuffs from external sources on reasonable terms and conditions, including short-term difficulties in financing normal levels of commercial imports. They therefore agreed to establish mechanisms to ensure the availability of food aid at a level sufficient to meet the food needs of those countries. While the demand for food aid will increase as a result of the higher cost of commercial food imports resulting from the Uruguay round, the supply of food aid is now threatened by both a reduction of surplus stocks and by higher food prices, which will mean a smaller volume of food aid from the donor budgetary allocations that are made in monetary terms. A balance between the two forces will be found by maintaining food aid at an 'adequate' level, presumably in volume terms to offset fluctuations in production and prices.

Sources of Food Aid

Donor countries

Food aid is a highly complex system of food transactions and transfers involving at any one time some 120 countries as donors, recipients and sources of supply. The conventional conception of food aid has been one of grants or concessional sales by food-exporting or surplus-producing countries to developing countries with food deficits and either long-term problems of undernutrition or immediate problems of emergencies and distress. Donors provide different resources, money as well as food commodities, on different terms, and different types of foods, allocate their resources differently and accord different priorities to humanitarian relief, economic and social development, and political and commercial interests. Developing countries are intermittent donors of food aid and have become increasingly the source of food commodities used in food aid programmes.

The bulk of food aid is, however, supplied by a small number of food-exporting developed countries (**Table 2**). The USA is the main source of food aid, although its proportion of world food aid supplies has declined as the volume of its deliveries has declined and the number and supplies of other donors have increased. In 1995, the USA supplied 41% of the volume of global food aid; the second largest source was the Commission of the European Communities (CEC) and member countries of the European Union (39%), followed by Japan (9.2%), Canada (5.1%), Australia (2.4%) and the Republic of Korea (1.6%). Together, these sources provided over 98% of food aid deliveries in 1995.

Food aid conventions

Special arrangements have been established with the aim of providing an adequate and assured supply of food aid both for development purposes and in times of emergency. A series of Food Aid Conventions commenced in 1967, guaranteeing minimum amounts of food aid in cereals irrespective of fluctuations in production, price and stocks. Each signatory to the Conventions undertakes to provide a minimum contribution of cereals converted into the equivalent amount in wheat using standard conversion factors.

The signatories to the Convention of 1995 were Argentina (35 000 tonnes), Australia (300 000 tonnes), Canada (400 000 tonnes), the European Union (1 755 000 tonnes), Japan (300 000 tonnes); Norway (20 000 tonnes); Switzerland (40 000 tonnes) and the USA (2 500 000 tonnes). The figures in brackets are the minimum annual guaranteed

Table 2 Food aid deliveries in 1995 by donor and commodity type (in tonnes – cereals in grain equivalent)

Donor	Cereals					Noncereals					Total noncereals
	Wheat and wheat flour	Rice	Coarse grains	Blended/ fortified	Total cereals	Dairy products	Veg. oil and fats	Meat and fish	Pulses	Other noncereal	
Total	**4 974 968**	**1 187 016**	**1 823 013**	**431 180**	**8 416 176**	**63 190**	**305 216**	**27 482**	**323 306**	**389 320**	**1 108 517**
Argentina	0	0	13 400	0	13 400	0	0	0	0	0	0
Australia	170 467	43 266	14 412	84	228 229	0	931	0	2 225	1 467	4 623
Austria	10 900	0	0	0	10 900	1 173	0	0	0	0	1 173
Belgium	17 011	4 176	18 132	0	39 319	0	40	0	900	2 781	3 721
Canada	404 746	7 240	22 790	0	434 776	30	26 171	3 971	19 543	240	49 955
Cuba	0	0	0	0	0	0	0	0	0	2211	2211
Denmark	57 475	940	17 717	0	76 132	797	1 392	2 530	18 566	231	23 516
CEC	1 749 078	85 549	494 803	11 319	2 340 749	40 672	62 779	5 043	78 007	28 872	215 373
Egypt	0	1 689	0	0	1 689	0	0	0	0	0	0
Finland	2 298	0	300	79	2 677	1 029	2 153	412	40	296	3 930
France	130 645	26 222	49 424	83	206 374	472	1 568	4 249	0	2 025	8 314
Germany	47 038	21 219	108 370	8 336	184 963	0	13 223	1 367	17 149	5 925	37 664
Greece	18 748	0	0	0	18 748	0	0	0	0	50	50
Hungary	0	0	0	0	0	0	0	42	0	0	42
India	6 004	0	0	0	6 004	0	0	196	0	10	206
Ireland	4 775	20	1 643	0	6 438	0	0	0	0	15	15
Italy	44 970	13 302	4 560	0	62 832	424	4 258	393	621	2 664	8 360
Japan	261 750	578 071	29 740	787	870 348	50	1 033	3 756	2 299	541	7 679
Korea, Rep.	0	150 000	0	0	150 000	0	0	0	0	0	0
Luxembourg	1 376	0	0	0	1 376	0	200	0	0	114	314
Netherlands	13 485	16 987	65 313	3 518	99 303	2 736	5 032	1 725	17 497	2 566	29 556
Norway	19 501	3 673	20 689	303	44 166	15	3 318	3 653	0	988	7 974
Pakistan	0	4 715	0	0	4 715	0	0	0	0	0	0
Saudi Arabia	0	0	1 000	0	1 000	40	60	0	0	951	1051
Spain	0	48	685	0	733	9	9	2	0	0	20
Sri Lanka	0	0	0	0	0	0	0	0	0	52	52
Sweden	45 337	28 421	37 013	383	111 154	0	2 104	0	7 811	1 742	11 657
Switzerland	1 362	20 027	21 006	3 716	46 111	2 482	509	96	4 419	1 697	9 203
Turkey	5 596	0	0	0	5 596	0	0	0	0	0	0
UK	76 304	1 200	87 430	4 470	169 404	0	222	0	9 701	2 242	12 165
USA	1 868 774	170 180	803 285	397 148	3 239 387	12 816	178 551	0	142 175	328 231	661 773
Vietnam	0	500	0	0	500	0	0	0	0	0	0
NGOs	17 326	9 571	10 689	952	38 538	444	1 628	51	2 355	3 410	7 888
Others	0	0	609	0	609	0	34	0	0	0	34

1995 data are provisional. CEC, Commission of the European Communities; NGO, nongovernment organization. Source: WFP/INTERFAIS.

contributions of each signatory in wheat equivalent. In most years, members have exceeded their minimum commitments.

International emergency food reserve

An International Emergency Food Reserve was established in 1975 as an international standby facility to respond rapidly to emergencies. This continuing reserve has a target of 500 000 tonnes of cereals made up of voluntary contributions and is administered by the World Food Programme. An Immediate Response Account of US $30 million in cash was established in 1991 as an integral part of the Reserve for the purchase of food as close as possible to where an emergency has occurred and its speedy delivery to the victims of disasters prior to the arrival of further food aid from donor countries. Contributions to the Reserve and its special account have been neither sufficient nor flexible enough in recent years to respond adequately and quickly to emergencies whenever and wherever they have occurred.

Obtaining food aid commodities in developing countries

While the bulk of food aid commodities are provided from the major donor countries, a small but increasing amount has been procured in the developing countries themselves. About 16% of the total volume of global food aid deliveries (1.5 million tonnes, mostly in cereals) were obtained in developing countries in 1995. Food produced in developing countries is used as food aid through a variety of arrangements. In what are called 'triangular transactions', a donor purchases food in one developing country for use as food aid in another developing country. In 'trilateral operations', a donor country may provide a food commodity to one developing country where it is exchanged for another commodity, which is used as food aid in another developing country. Donors may also buy food commodities in a developing country, which are used as food aid in the same country. Finally, under 'exchange arrangements', a food commodity provided by a donor, such as wheat, may be swapped for a locally produced crop such as maize, which is used as food aid. In 1995, two-thirds of the food procured in developing countries was obtained through triangular transactions. Most was obtained in sub-Saharan Africa (mainly maize and sorghum) and south and east Asia (mostly rice).

These arrangements have gained increasing favour among food aid donors and agencies. They are seen as providing an incentive for increasing food production and trade in developing countries, reducing

transport costs, increasing the speed of food aid deliveries, and providing food commodities more in keeping with the food habits and customs of food aid beneficiaries. However, there are many difficulties in the way of increasing the scale of these operations, many of which will require more financial and technical aid to remove.

Distribution Programmes

Over half the volume of food aid supplied in 1995 was provided bilaterally on a government-to-government basis; 30% was supplied multilaterally through the UN system, almost all (98%) through the World Food Programme; and 20% was distributed by nongovernmental organizations (NGOs), mainly on behalf of bilateral aid agencies.

Food aid has traditionally been classified into three distribution programmes, each with its own set of donor legislation, procedures, sources of financing and method of operation (see Table 1).

Programme food aid

Programme food aid is provided exclusively on a bilateral, government-to-government basis, as a grant or as a credit on low repayment terms. It helps to fill the food gap between a country's demand for food and national food production and the current level of commercial food imports, thereby avoiding increases in local food prices and additional food imports. By replacing additional commercial imports, it provides balance of payments support, as the foreign exchange that would have been used to pay for those imports is saved. It also provides budgetary support as the food aid commodities supplied are usually sold in the recipient country, mainly in urban markets, providing local currency for the government. This allows increased development expenditure without causing inflation or balance of payments problems. It also helps to shield development expenditures that would otherwise be cut during times of economic crisis, reform and adjustment.

Project food aid

Project food aid is targeted on poor and food-insecure people through specific types of development projects. It is provided on a grant basis for specific groups of people and identified development purposes. The food aid helps to meet the additional demand for food generated by implementing development projects, provides income in the form of food for project workers, or helps to meet a minimum nutritional need. A wide range of development projects can be supported. These include those designed to improve the nutrition and health of mothers and preschool children by providing supplementary food at mother and child health centres during pregnancy, lactation and weaning; education, especially primary schools, and training programmes by providing meals at schools and training centres; labour-intensive works programmes, including the construction or improvement of irrigation, roads, land improvement and protection, urban renewal and low-cost housing through food-for-work programmes in which food is provided as part-payment of wages; land settlement and new farming systems during which food is provided in the early years of settlement or during the transition period until food self-reliance is achieved; and market reform and price stabilization through the establishment and maintenance of food reserves.

Food aid commodities are provided directly to project beneficiaries, mainly free of charge. However, they may be sold in one of three ways: first, to designated project workers, often at subsidized prices, thereby increasing their wages; second, as part of the purpose of an assisted project (for example, in dairy development schemes where the food aid commodities dried skim milk and butter oil are mixed with locally produced milk and the reconstituted milk is sold, or food reserve schemes where the food aid commodity, such as wheat or rice, is sold at certain times of the year to stabilize prices for poor consumers); and third, a small proportion of the food aid commodities provided may be sold on the local market to generate local currency to help offset the internal transport, storage and handling costs of delivering the food aid commodities or to buy local tools, materials or equipment needed for the food-aided development project, thereby generating more employment and income. Funds saved from governments' budgets through the provision of food aid can also be used to expand or improve development projects or social services.

Emergency food aid

Food aid may be required in response to emergencies. These emergencies may be classified into four types.

Firstly, there are sudden, short-term natural disasters (hurricanes, floods, tidal waves, volcanic eruptions, earthquakes) that may arise without warning in a limited area; for these disasters relief supplies are needed for a short time until normal food supplies can begin again.

Secondly, there are slow-maturing, longer-term natural disasters caused by crop failure due to drought or pest and disease attacks; relief food supplies are needed until the next harvest, normally a period of 6 months to 1 year, unless prolonged drought occurs over more than 1 year continuously. Unlike short-term natural disasters, there is usually some warning before a disaster of this kind occurs. Generally, these disasters cover a larger area, ranging from a region of a country to a number of neighbouring countries.

Thirdly, there are disasters caused by armed conflict, leading to large numbers of refugees and persons displaced from their homes, and the disruption of food production and supplies and normal economic activities. The scale, complexity and duration of these emergencies is increasing. Most conflicts now occur not between countries but within them. Most of the victims are not soldiers but citizens, especially women and children, the most vulnerable group. Most of the conflicts have occurred in poor countries, or newly created states with economies in transition following the collapse of the old political order. Few have the resources, administration or logistics to cope without external assistance. Several of these disasters have been made worse by the lethal combination of war and drought.

Fourthly, there are economic emergencies caused by internal or external factors that can seriously hurt a national economy. The economic reform and adjustment measures to overcome the problem may adversely affect poor people. Food aid can play one of four roles in these situations. It can provide general financial support by saving foreign exchange on food that would otherwise have to be imported commercially, and the food aid commodities provided can be sold in local markets thereby providing extra revenue for the recipient government. It can support reform programmes in different sectors of the national economy, for example market reform and pricing policy in the agricultural sector that would give an incentive price to producers to grow more food without pricing the poor consumer out of the market. It can increase investment in specific development programmes and projects that generate additional employment and income for poor people. And, finally, it can support employment and nutrition schemes as compensatory measures for people who lose their jobs or cannot afford the increased price of basic food commodities as a result of economic adjustment measures.

Regional differences

There have been marked differences among the developing regions of the world in the ways in which food aid has been used (**Fig. 1**). Between 1989 and 1992, most food aid to Latin America and the Caribbean, North Africa, the Middle East, Eastern Europe and the former Soviet Union was provided as

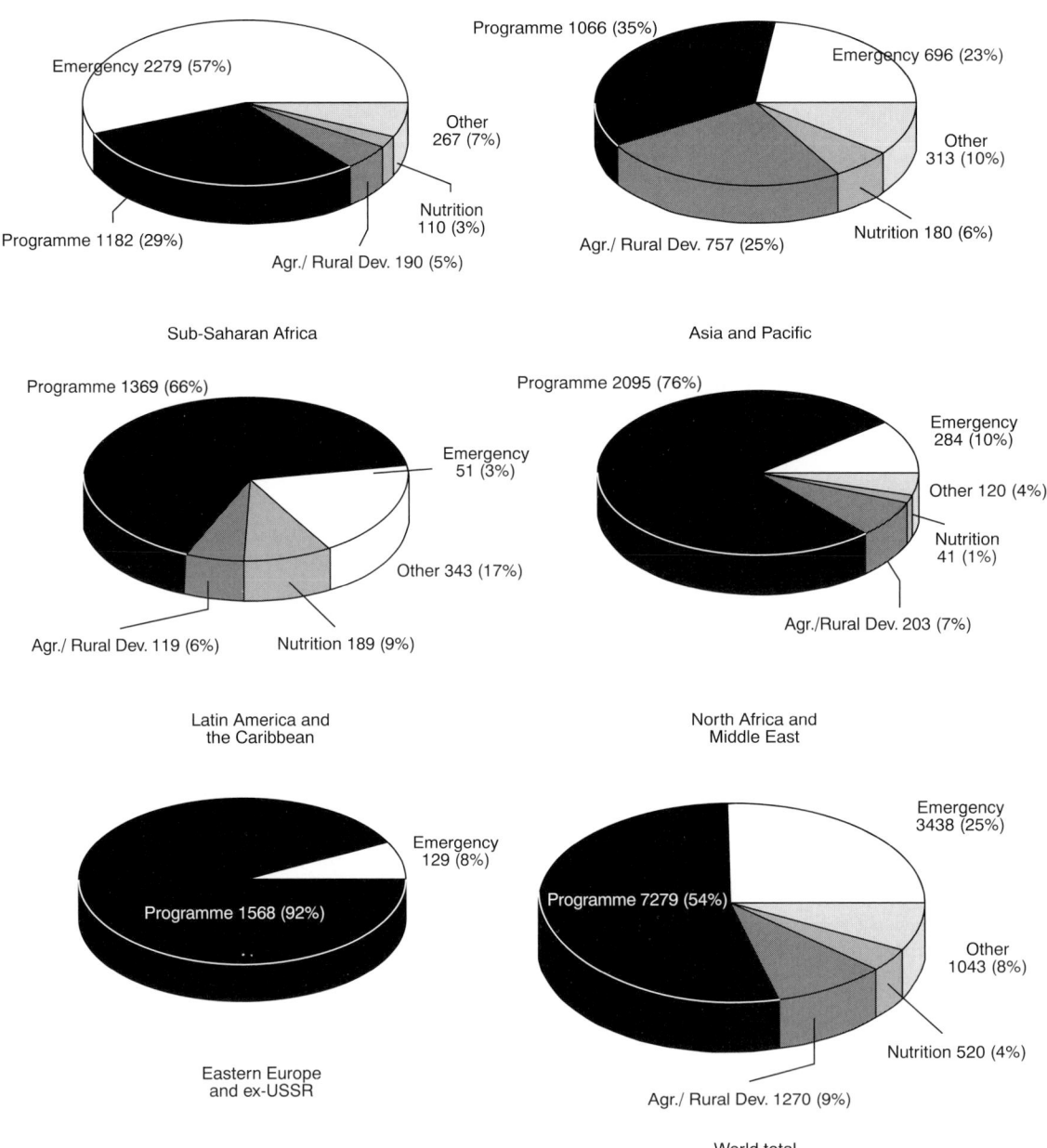

Figure 1 Food aid deliveries by category and regions: 4-year average, 1989–1992. Figures are in thousands of tonnes (rounded); cereals in grain equivalent. Note: 'Agr./Rural Dev.', 'Nutrition' and 'Other' comprise project food aid. Source: WFP INTERFAIS.

programme food aid. In contrast, the largest part of food aid to the Asia and the Pacific region was project food aid, while in sub-Saharan Africa the largest proportion of the food aid supplied was for emergencies. Taking the world as a whole, less than a quarter of the food aid provided was directly targeted on poor and food-insecure people through development projects designed to improve their nutrition, education, training and employment. Over half of global food aid was in the form of programme aid, and a quarter was emergency aid.

Commodities

Most of food aid is supplied in the form of cereals, with much smaller amounts as noncereal commodities (see Table 1). In 1995, of the 9.5 million tonnes of food aid delivered, 8.4 million tonnes (88%) was provided in cereals and the remaining 1.1 million tonnes (12%) in noncereal food commodities.

Wheat and wheat flour are the main cereal commodities in food aid, followed by coarse grains (maize, sorghum, barley, oats), rice and cereal-based blended or fortified foods.

Of the noncereal foodstuffs provided in food aid, vegetable oil and fats and pulses are the most common, followed by dairy products, meat and fish.

See also: **Food Aid Organizations**: History and Role. **Malnutrition**: Definition, Classification and Epidemiology. **Nutrition Policies**: In Developing Countries. **Population, Development and Nutrition**: Overview. **Refugees**: Nutritional Management.

Further Reading

Clay E and Stokke O, eds (1991) *Food Aid Reconsidered: Assessing the Impact on Third World Countries*. London: Frank Cass.

FAO (1985) *Food Aid for Development*. FAO Economic and Social Development Paper no. 34. Rome: Food and Agriculture Organization of the United Nations.

FAO (1992) *FAO Principles of Surplus Disposal and Consultative Obligations of Member Countries*, 3rd edn. Rome: Food and Agriculture Organization of the United Nations.

Relief and Development Institute, London (1987) *A Study of Triangular Transactions and Local Purchases in Food Aid*. WFP Occasional Paper no. 11. Rome: World Food Programme.

Relief and Development Institute, London (1990) *A Study of Commodity Exchanges in WFP and Other Food Aid Operations*. WFP Occasional Paper no. 12. Rome: World Food Programme.

Ruttan VW ed. (1993) *Why Food Aid?* Baltimore: Johns Hopkins University Press.

Shaw J (1995) Future directions for development and relief with food aid. In: von Braun J (ed.) *Employment for Poverty Reduction and Food Security*, pp 252–274. Washington, DC: International Food Policy Research Institute.

Shaw J (1996) *The World Food Programme and Emergency Relief*. Advanced Development Management Programme Series No. 20. Tokyo: Sophia University.

Shaw J and Clay E, eds (1993) *World Food Aid. Experiences of Recipients and Donors*. Rome, London and Portsmouth (NH): World Food Programme Currey/Heinemann.

Shaw J and Singer H, eds (1988) Food policy, food aid and economic adjustment. *Food Policy* (special issue) 13(1).

Shaw J and Singer H (1995) *A Future Food Aid Regime: Implications of the Final Act of the GATT Uruguay Round*. IDS Discussion Paper no. 352, September. Brighton: Institute of Development Studies, University of Sussex.

Singer H, Wood J and Jennings T (1987) *Food Aid: The Challenge and the Opportunity*, Oxford: Clarendon Press.

UN (1975) *Report of the World Food Conference, Rome 5–17 November 1994*. Document E/CONF. 65/20. New York: United Nations.

Wallerstein MB (1980) *Food for War – Food for Peace. United States Food Aid in a Global Context*. Cambridge: MIT Press.

World Bank and World Food Programme (1991) *Food Aid in Africa: An Agenda for the 1990s*. A Joint Study. Washington, DC/Rome: World Bank/World Food Programme.

World Food Programme (1994) *Food Aid for Development*, Beijing: China Agricultural Press.

World Food Programme and Government of The Netherlands (1983) *Seminar on Food Aid*. Rome/The Hague: World Food Programme/Government of The Netherlands.

FOOD AID ORGANIZATIONS

History and Role

D J Shaw, formerly UN World Food Programme, Rome, Italy

Copyright © 1998 Academic Press

This article describes food aid organizations, and gives a brief history of their work, a summary of their direct and indirect nutritional activities, and an account of issues that have arisen in food-aided nutrition programmes (*See:* **Food Aid**: Overview). While food is provided by aid organizations to the poor in developed countries through various forms of food subsidy, food stamps and food distribution programmes, this article focuses on the work of food aid organizations in developing countries.

Definition

Food aid organizations provide aid in the form of food commodities on grant or concessional terms, or provide money to buy food commodities to be used as food aid. They include bilateral government organizations set up in donor countries; multilateral organizations in the United Nations system; and private and nongovernment organizations.

Bilateral government organizations

About half of all food aid is channelled through government agencies in donor countries. These countries have set up organizations, mainly within (or related to) ministries of foreign affairs, to handle their aid programmes. Within these aid organizations, separate food aid units are established to administer food aid separately from the financial and technical assistance that donor countries provide. Food aid has therefore acquired its own institutions, legislation and procedures, often quite different from financial and technical aid, making it difficult to coordinate food with other forms of aid, and impeding the flexibility of transferring food aid to developing countries.

The legal and administrative arrangements for food aid are more elaborate and diverse than for other types of aid. The framework within which food aid is organized is often complex, reflecting distinctive legal and constitutional arrangements, and the particular history of aid, in each donor country. Thus, for example, five ministries and agencies are directly involved in the financing and administration of German food aid, and four in the case of Japan. An added complexity of food aid is its links to ministries and government bodies responsible for national agricultural policy and trade.

The US food aid programme was initiated under legislation for managing its agricultural trade surpluses. It continues to be part of the Farm Bill, which is approved every 5 years, and not part of the foreign assistance legislation governing other types of US aid. Until recently, US food aid was managed by an interdepartmental committee, as is still the case in some other food aid donor countries, such as Canada. The US 1990 Farm Bill legislation divided responsibility between the US Department of Agriculture for bilateral programme food aid, provided on credit terms, and designed mainly to expand US food trade, and the Agency for International Development, which is responsible for food aid provided on a grant basis for development projects and humanitarian purposes.

Agricultural ministries and agencies and the food industry and suppliers have been involved in food aid donor countries in the management, procurement and transportation of food aid commodities from within those countries, and in relation to their national agricultural policies and trade considerations. This close association of food aid with agricultural policies and trade agencies has been increasingly seen as a constraint to organizing food aid to serve developmental and humanitarian objectives in developing countries.

Another layer of complexity has been the separation between food aid for development and food aid for emergencies and disaster relief. Ministries of foreign affairs have tended to be given responsibility for food aid and other forms of assistance in times of emergencies because of their high visibility and political sensitivity. This has led to the division of external aid in donor countries into 'development' and 'emergency' aid, each with its separate agenda, terms, legislation, financing and operating agencies (even separate units within the same aid agency).

Emergency aid has been restricted to an immediate and short-term response to help the victims of disasters. As a result, inadequate assistance has been given for reconstruction and rehabilitation work after disasters have happened, and for programmes that could prevent disasters from occurring, or prepare for them, and reduce their effects in countries where natural disasters (hurricanes, floods, earthquakes, volcanic eruptions) regularly occur. In those countries, disasters are a fact of life and continually interrupt the development process. An attempt is now being made, led by the United Nations, to link emergency and development assistance in a 'continuum' of action, in which emergency assistance supports and protects development programmes and projects, and development activities reduce the effects of disasters.

Multilateral food aid organizations

An increasing proportion of food aid, 30% in 1995, has been channelled multilaterally through organizations of the United Nations (UN). Almost all (98%) is now supplied through the World Food Programme (WFP). Small amounts are also provided by the UN Children's Fund for its child development and relief programmes, the UN High Commissioner for Refugees for refugee feeding, and the UN Relief and Works Agency for Palestinians in the Middle East.

The WFP began operations in 1963 as the food aid organization of the UN on a 3-year experimental basis with a target of US $100 million of resources. It has grown to become the largest source of grant aid for poor people in developing countries in the UN system, and the primary source of international food aid for both development and disaster relief. In 1995, the WFP reached an estimated 50 million of the poorest people in the developing world with 2.8 million tonnes of food at a cost of US $1.6 billion. Over 25 million people were the victims of natural and man-made disasters in 41 developing countries, over two-thirds of whom were women and children. Most (21 million) were the victims of man-made disasters. The remaining 4 million were affected by drought and other natural disasters. In addition, 25 million received WFP aid through 240 development projects in 83 developing countries.

World Food Programme assistance takes three forms: support for economic and social development programmes and projects; meeting emergency food needs and providing associated transport and logistics support; and generally promoting world food security. With its dual role of providing emergency relief and development aid, WFP is well placed to play a major role in linking relief and development. Special attention is given to using its development resources to support disaster prevention, preparedness and mitigation projects, and post-disaster reconstruction and rehabilitation activities, as part of national development programmes. Conversely, its emergency assistance is used, to the extent possible, to serve both relief and development purposes. In both cases, the overall aim is to build self-reliant households and communities.

The two main areas of WFP development assistance have been agricultural and rural development, and the development of human resources. The former include a range of development projects designed to increase agricultural production, protect the environment, improve rural infrastructure (roads, storage, housing, etc.), support agricultural settlement schemes on new land, and help change low-yielding traditional farming to higher-production modern systems, with small amounts allocated for the establishment of food reserves. The main functions of WFP development aid have been to increase employment and incomes in food-for-work programmes in which food forms part of the wage; to provide an incentive for communities to work together in development programmes for their common benefit; and to tide poor people over periods of settlement on new lands, or during changes in the farming systems, until they are able to provide their own food.

The development of human resources through improvements in nutrition, health, education and training has also been a major concern of WFP. The main support has been given to the most vulnerable groups – to pregnant and lactating women and pre-school children through mother and child health programmes, and to primary-school children through school feeding programmes – with smaller amounts given to secondary and higher education institutions and training programmes.

In emergencies, WFP performs a number of vital tasks. It provides emergency relief food from its own regular resources. It administers the International Emergency Food Reserve, an international emergency standby facility. Increasingly, the WFP has been called upon to help coordinate the food aid aspects of large-scale international relief operations. In so doing, WFP makes its unique transportation and logistics services available to the international community. With the cooperation of donor countries, the WFP has helped to improve port, storage and inland transportation systems in developing countries during relief operations, the benefits of which remain after the emergencies have passed. Services have been provided to food aid donors for the purchase, transportation and monitoring of food commodities for their own bilateral food aid programmes, and a WFP International Food Aid Information System has been developed which provides a database for decision-making on food aid operations throughout the world.

The WFP has the largest global operational network with staff in 85 country offices serving 90 developing countries. They can assist in the assessment of food aid needs, help in obtaining food, and organize its distribution from borrowed stocks. The WFP can divert ships carrying its food aid consignments to ports close to where emergencies have occurred and help coordinate airlift and airdrop operations.

A major change in WFP operations has taken place as emergencies and disasters have increased. Whereas in 1992 two-thirds of WFP assistance was given for development project and one-third for emergencies, the reverse is now the case, with increasing focus on the poorest countries, especially in sub-Saharan Africa.

Nongovernmental organizations

Although nongovernmental organizations (NGOs) finance only a small part of total food aid directly from their own resources (less than 1% in 1995), an increasing amount is channelled through them (20% in 1995), mainly on behalf of bilateral government food aid programmes, and particularly for the growing emergency relief supplies. The NGOs are seen to have the special advantages of being in direct contact with poor and vulnerable people in developing countries, aware of their needs, and able to arrange distribution systems to reach them.

A large number of NGOs, both internationally and in the developing countries themselves, have been involved in food aid for many years. Only a small number of international NGOs, however, have the staff and resources to handle and distribute food aid on a large scale. In the USA, for example, the two largest NGOs, Cooperative for American Relief Everywhere (CARE) and Catholic Relief Services (CRS) handle the bulk of US food aid channelled through NGOs. An international network of 11 independent CARE organizations has been established in Australia, Austria, Canada, Denmark, France, Germany, Italy, Japan, Norway, the UK and the USA, which provide food and other forms of aid. Contributions are made by the general public in many of these countries as a repayment for the benefits received in the form of food aid parcels distributed by CARE as part of the large US aid programme to European countries after World War II. In Canada, a group of 10 NGOs have established a Canadian Foodgrains Bank, a common facility from which to provide emergency food aid. In Europe, two international NGOs, the International Committee of the Red Cross and the League of Red Cross and Red Crescent Societies, play prominent roles in providing food aid during emergencies. Other NGOs that handle food aid are Caritas, the NGO of the Roman Catholic church; the Oxford Committee for Famine Relief (Oxfam), which uses food aid in development projects and for emergency operations; Médecins sans Frontières, which combines food aid with its medical assistance; and Save the Children Fund, which uses food aid in its child development and protection programmes. Groups of NGOs have formed associations to coordinate their food aid operations and to provide advocacy on food aid policies to governments and the general public. In the USA, a Coalition for Food Aid, which includes the major NGOs, has played an important part in helping to shape US food aid legislation and programmes. Food Aid Management, a consortium of some of the major NGOs involved in the US food aid programme, has been working to promote the adoption of common policies and management standards, to design training programmes, to provide a forum for discussion on management concerns, and generally to facilitate collaboration among NGOs. A coordinating body for NGOs in member states of the European Union, known as EuronAid, was established in 1980 to provide logistical and financing services to NGOs using food aid provided by the Commission of the European Communities.

History

Early history

Food aid has existed for as long as civil society itself. Communities have provided succour to their members in times of natural disasters, war or other emergencies. In the ancient civilizations, food was stored in good years to be distributed when harvests were poor. In countries such as China and India, a tradition was developed of mobilizing the rural labour force to construct irrigation channels, roads and other infrastructure through large-scale food-for-work programmes, and to provide relief to those affected by frequent disasters caused by drought, floods, hurricanes and earthquakes.

Nineteenth century: international relief assistance

The modern history of international food aid provided by governments may be said to have begun in the early nineteenth century. The first recorded legislative act of this kind was in 1812 when the US congress passed an Act for the Relief of the Citizens of Venezuela, authorizing the president to purchase goods to the value of US \$50 000, a considerable sum at that time. During the Great Irish Famine of 1846–1847, the British government provided £100 000 for the purchase of Indian corn (maize) in the USA for distribution in Ireland. The colonial powers also accepted famine relief for their colonies as a routine duty of colonial administration.

Twentieth century: large-scale food aid

The first major food aid operation occurred after World War I from 1918 to 1926 for reconstruction programmes in the war-torn countries of Europe when the US congress voted to provide special postwar relief credits. A total of 6.23 million tonnes of food was provided under these programmes. With the end of these programmes, the USA was still producing considerable surpluses of cereals that could not be sold on the international market. Other ways of disposing of these burdensome food stocks were sought, which were costing the taxpayer increasingly more to store. In 1933, during the Depression, a way was found of increasing 'food aid', and enabling farmers to earn an income, by allowing surplus food to be exported from the USA at prices below the international market price. The Grain Stabilization Board was set up to finance these exports. The Commodity Credit Corporation was also created to manage releases from the increasing food stocks for food aid and subsidized export, thereby stabilizing, supporting and protecting farm income and prices in the USA.

World War II gave a further boost to US food aid. Under the Lend-Lease Act of 1941, the USA provided some US \$6 billion of agricultural products to the Allied powers. At the end of the war, as at the end of World War I, the USA came to the aid of European countries in a massive reconstruction programme that involved the largest aid programme in world history. Under this European recovery programme, more popularly known as the Marshall Plan (after its originator, Secretary of State George C. Marshall), US \$13.5 billion of aid was provided between 1948 and 1952, almost one-third of which consisted of food, feed and fertilizer.

Formalizing food aid

With the continued growth of US food stocks, further legislation was passed after World War II to use the surplus food commodities as food aid abroad. However, it was the Agricultural Trade Development and Assistance Act of 1954 – which was to become widely known by its number, Public Law (PL) 480 – that was to formalize and provide the legal framework for US food aid basically in the form that has remained to the present time. The passing of PL 480 marked a recognition that world food shortages and US surplus agricultural production could no longer be considered to be isolated or temporary. It established a relationship between US national agricultural and foreign policy interests and external assistance that shaped the country's food aid policies and programmes. The first objective mentioned in the PL 480 legislation was to develop new markets for US agricultural commodities on a mutually beneficial basis.

Under PL 480, US food aid increased rapidly during the 1950s and 1960s. By the mid 1960s, it reached over 18 million tonnes a year at a cost of US $1.6 billion. Since PL 480 was passed in 1954, the USA has provided more than US $45 billion in food aid to every quarter of the developing world. Although its share of total food aid has fallen as other countries have become food aid donors, and increased their food aid supplies, it still provides nearly 40% of all cereal food aid and 60% of all noncereal food aid. At the same time, the value of agricultural commodities exported under credit, guarantee and export enhancement programmes (so-called 'grey area' food aid) has increased considerably since PL 480 was enacted in 1954. The total value of these programmes was almost three times the value of agricultural exports designated as 'food aid' in 1993, and accounted for 18% of the total value of US agricultural exports.

Multilateral food aid

A United Nations Relief and Rehabilitation Administration was set up in 1943 to distribute aid to countries that had been occupied by the enemy forces during World War II. Between 1943 and 1948, this organization distributed US $3.7 billion of aid, about half in the form of food. It was closed when that aid programme came to an end. Various proposals were made to establish a multilateral food aid organization through the UN system following the creation of the Food and Agriculture Organization (FAO) of the UN in 1945. None of these proposals was approved, mainly because the world's leading food exporters (especially the USA) and the main food importers (principally the UK) were reluctant to yield their power and sovereignty in world agricultural trade to a multilateral body whose decisions were arrived at by consensus, not on the basis of economic strength. A multilateral code of conduct for food aid was agreed upon in 1954, however, in the form of the FAO *Principles of Surplus Disposal*, to avoid harmful interference of food surplus programmes with normal patterns of food production in developing countries and international food trade, and a special body was appointed to monitor the application of those principles.

An important milestone in the history of food aid was the setting up of the World Food Programme as the food aid arm of the UN. A number of factors contributed to agreement in the early 1960s to establish the WFP despite the failure of earlier proposals; one of these factors was a major change in the political climate following the election of President John F. Kennedy in the USA. During his presidential campaign in 1960, Kennedy had spoken favourably about the general idea of a multilateral food aid programme, and after his election he showed strong support for the UN. In his first address at the UN General Assembly in 1961 he proposed that the decade of the 1960s be designated the 'United Nations Decade for Development' under which 'the United Nations' existing efforts in promoting economic growth can be expanded and coordinated'.

One of President Kennedy's first acts was to establish an Office for Food for Peace within the executive office of the president, with the aim of expanding US food aid to promote development in the developing countries. A newly accepted principle of international solidarity in the UN had led to greater willingness to give assistance to developing countries. A continuous campaign in the UN and unanimous adoption of a resolution to provide surplus food to poor and hungry people through the UN system led to a report by a group of experts which was to provide a framework for what eventually became the World Food Programme. The USA took the lead in proposing the establishment of the WFP as a small experimental programme by offering to provide 40% of the target of US $100 million of resources for a period of 3 years (1963–1965). The success of the experiment led to the continuation of the WFP after 1965. The earlier experience of providing US PL 480 food aid had an important influence on the size and form of the WFP. All contributions to the WFP's resources were voluntary, supplementary to bilateral food aid, and in addition to other forms of assistance. Most of PL 480 food aid had been provided as programme aid, mainly to further US political and commercial interests. This had attracted considerable criticism and controversy.

The WFP was deliberately kept small so as not to compete with the large bilateral food aid programmes. It was also restricted to supporting emergency operations and development projects (as opposed to providing general programme aid for balance of payments and budget support), to test out the use of food aid in pilot activities such as school feeding and labour-intensive works programmes, and because it was felt that it would be easier to monitor and evaluate results. The USA was also anxious to share with other countries some of the burden of providing food aid to developing countries that it had borne almost alone for many years.

The advantages of channelling food aid through the UN system were recognized from the beginning. Food aid would be provided without any political or commercial strings attached. The WFP could combine food commodities provided by a number of food-exporting countries; a broader choice could then be offered to recipients, and a wider scope could also be provided for nutritional aims. Countries with too small, or intermittent, surpluses to set up their own food aid programmes could make contributions to the WFP. Small contributions of high symbolic importance could be made by developing countries. Richer countries with no food to offer could make contributions in cash or services to buy food or administer and transport the food aid commodities provided. Finally savings could be made in transport and administrative costs by drawing on a 'food basket' located in different parts of the world and by using competing transport and logistics services.

Food aid conventions: guaranteeing food aid

The broadening and consolidation of participation in food aid by donor countries, which was started with the creation of WFP, was taken further with the establishment of a Food Aid Convention as part of the International Grains Agreement in 1967. International agreements on wheat, later expanded to cover all grains, had been entered into since 1949 with the objective of ensuring fair and stable prices for both importing and exporting countries. During the 1960s, the USA had already indicated that it was no longer prepared to assume the major burden of providing food aid without the cooperation of other donors. At the same time, the European Community (now European Union) and its member countries had accumulated large surpluses through their agricultural protection policy that affected the US agricultural trade.

During discussions on a new agreement to succeed the International Wheat Agreement of 1962, the USA proposed that the agreement cover world trade in grains and include a provision for food aid. Other countries were reluctant to agree, but with the prospect of stabilization of the world grain market they eventually accepted. As new aid commitments on a regular basis would be costly for non-traditional food aid donors to undertake, they were offered concessions in industrial trade as part of the bargaining process. As a result, a unique facility was established for food aid in 1967, a Food Aid Convention by which member countries guaranteed to provide a minimum physical amount of food aid in cereals irrespective of fluctuations in production, stocks and prices. Under the Convention of 1967, eighteen member countries agreed to provide a minimum of 4.5 million tonnes of cereal food aid. This was later increased to 7.5 million tonnes under the Convention of 1986, but was reduced to 5.36 million tonnes under the Convention of 1995 as a result of the decision by the USA to cut its commitment by over a half. Members have, however, exceeded their minimum commitments in most years since 1967.

World food crisis of early 1970s: World Food Conference 1974

Another milestone was reached in the history of food aid with the world food crisis of the early 1970s. Food production and stocks fell. World food prices increased steeply. At the same time, world oil prices reached unprecedented levels. Poor, food-importing countries were particularly affected. Food aid fell to its lowest level at a time when it was most needed. Food surpluses were no longer available. A number of food aid donors bought less food with the money they had allocated in their aid budgets for food aid as food prices rose and transport became more costly as oil prices increased.

A World Food Conference was called by the UN in 1974 to address the crisis. Concern was expressed not only about the need to increase food production in the developing countries, but also to have an adequate and dependable level of food aid to protect poor, food-importing countries against future crises, and to establish effective coordination of food aid operations worldwide. Among the Conference's resolutions, it was agreed that all efforts be made to ensure that at least 10 million tonnes of cereals be provided as food aid a year (almost double what was provided at the time). The Conference also recommended an international arrangement on world food security, included the establishment of grain reserves at strategic locations. This led to the creation of the International Emergency Food Reserve (IEFR) in 1975 with a target of not less than 500 000 tonnes of food as an international standby arrangement. Resources in food and money were to be kept readily available in contributing countries. The IEFR was placed at the disposal of the WFP to allow it to respond quickly to emergencies. At the same time, the governing body of the WFP was reconstituted as the Committee on Food Aid Policies and Programmes (CFA) to help coordinate food aid programmes carried out by bilateral, multilateral and nongovernmental organizations, including emergency food aid.

Uruguay round of multilateral trade negotiations: the Final Act 1994

The need for continued food aid was recognized in 1994 at the end of 7 years of multilateral trade negotiations (known as the 'Uruguay round' because it was started in Uruguay in 1986) involving 117 states, almost three-quarters of them developing countries, and the signing of a Final Act that, among other things, began a process of freeing world agricultural trade. The major food-producing and exporting developed countries, particularly the USA and those of the European Union, were paying huge amounts to support their farmers and subsidize their exports; this resulted in large surpluses, unfair trading practices and low agricultural prices, to the disadvantage of food-exporting developing countries.

The Final Act established for the first time a system of multilateral controls over agricultural trade, and a new UN body, the World Trade Organization, was set up. A process was also begun that will change the way in which national agricultural policies operate and will bring about a gradual reduction in subsidies paid to farmers and for exports. It is generally recognized that the Uruguay round will bring substantial benefits and increase opportunities for trade expansion and economic growth. At the same time, it is realized that the poorest and food-importing developing countries may suffer from reduced food stocks and higher food prices that may result from the Uruguay round agreements. It has been agreed, therefore, to establish ways of ensuring that they receive appropriate amounts of food aid.

Activities

Food-aided activities have a built-in element of improving nutrition when they provide food to poor and hungry people. There are certain types of activities, however, where the primary aim is to improve the nutritional status of the beneficiaries through distributing food directly to them. In addition, there are other food-assisted activities where improved nutrition may be obtained indirectly.

Emergency relief

The provision of emergency food aid to victims of natural and man-made disasters, including refugees and persons displaced from their homes (**Fig. 1**), has played a vital, often life-saving, role. Sustaining people at basic nutritional levels has not only helped them to survive but has enabled them to engage in reconstruction, rehabilitation and development activities when emergencies have ended.

No two emergencies are alike. The most appropriate type of feeding programme to prevent malnutrition and death occurring during and after disasters will depend on such factors as the nature of the disaster itself (sudden, short-term natural catastrophes; slow-maturing, longer-term disasters caused by drought; disasters caused by war and civil strife; and economic disasters affecting poor households, communities and nations); where they happen; what time of year they happen; the characteristics of the people affected; and the length of time during which relief food supplies are needed.

Better provision can be made for the nutritional needs of victims of disasters that have been anticipated through early warning than those that occur suddenly. Nutrition and related problems are quite different in short-term and longer-term relief feeding operations. In the longer-term, more attention must be paid to food supplies being adequate and assured in quantity and quality, to adjust diets more closely to the needs of particular groups of the afflicted population, especially mothers and children, and to provide other basic needs.

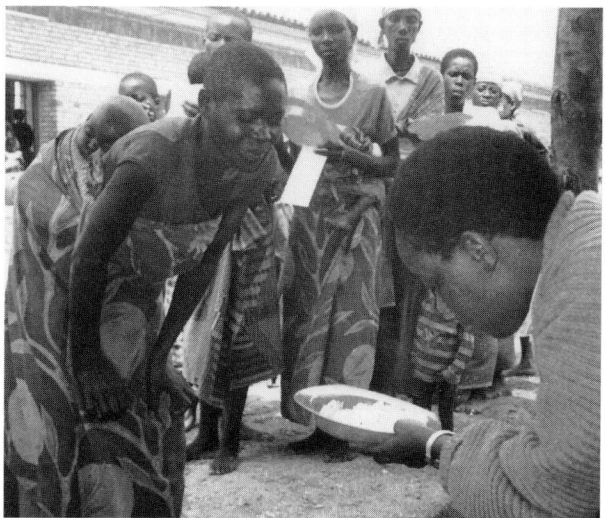

Figure 1 Emergency food assistance to victims of civil conflict in Rwanda. Women and children displaced by civil strife queue to receive a meal prepared using WFP rations in a camp near Gikongoro (WFP/Tom Haskell).

Protracted refugee and displaced people operations

In recent years, a special concern has been the large increase in the number of refugees and displaced persons caught up in emergency situations that have lasted for many months, even years. These people depend almost entirely on help from the host government and international community (**Fig. 2**). Some situations are so protracted that children are born and mature in feeding camps. Given the length of time involved, the afflicted people must be treated not only in terms of their survival and subsistence but also their individual capacities for growth and independence.

Solutions to three basic problems have to be found. First, how to provide an assured and continuous food supply that is not only adequate for good health but sufficiently varied to avoid a monotonous diet, and flexible enough to meet changing needs. Second, how to supply other, non-food, basic needs in the absence of which the dependent population would have to sell or exchange part of the food rations. Third, how to cater for developmental as well as survival needs in terms of nutrition, health, education and training, and, where possible, to provide employment and income-earning opportunities.

Supplementary feeding programmes for mothers and infants

Pregnant and lactating women and pre-school chil-dren in developing countries are particularly vulnerable to nutritional deficiencies. Malnutrition results in high child mortality and widespread disabling diseases, and can inhibit physical growth and mental development. Food supplements have been provided through food aid programmes throughout the developing world to protect the nutrition and health of women and their children, taking up about 4% of all food aid supplied annually in recent years. These supplements are distributed through mother and child health centres, where they exist, or through other channels, such as social welfare organizations, schools, women's clubs and voluntary associations (**Fig. 3**). Supplementary rations are provided for the mother to take home or through cooked meals or snacks at the distribution centres. Mothers and children attracted to health centres by the distribution of food can be checked, screened and immunized, serious cases of malnutrition can be detected and treated, and health and nutrition education and child-care guidance can be provided. Distinctions should be made between generalized supplementary feeding programmes which provide a food supplement for all children of a certain age in order to prevent malnutrition, and therapeutic feeding programmes for life-saving and rehabilitation of the most seriously malnourished children who need specific and intensive nutritional and medical attention. These children are treated at special feeding centres, hospitals or clinics, where they are fed several times a day.

The food aid provided has played a synergistic role. It has acted as a stimulus to encourage governments to invest more to extend health and nutrition

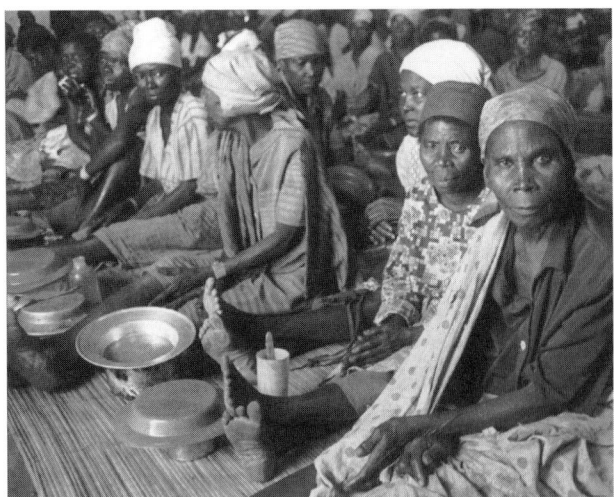

Figure 2 Food assistance to displaced and war-affected people in Angola. Displaced women and children at a feeding centre run by Concern, an Irish NGO, in Malanje, about 500 km east of the Angolan capital of Luanda. The WFP provided food commodities (corn-soy blend, dried fish, maize, pulses, rice, salt, sugar and vegetable oil) to displaced persons, returnees, conflict-affected people and drought victims in this protracted emergency operation (WFP/Chris Sattleberger).

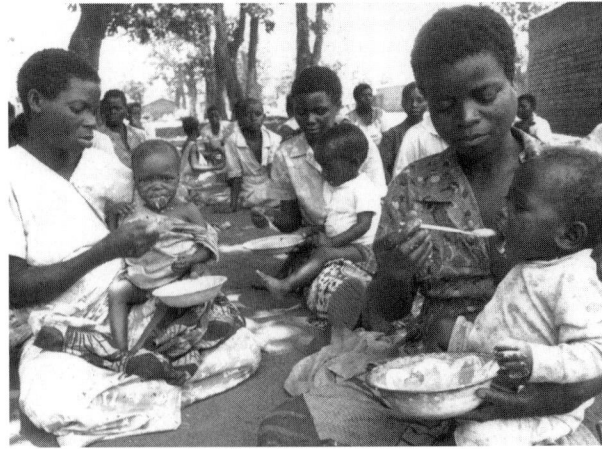

Figure 3 Vulnerable group feeding in Malawi. Mothers feeding their children supplementary rations provided by WFP to improve food security and nutrition among selected vulnerable groups, including children under 5 years old, expectant and nursing mothers, women heading single households, and children suffering malnutrition (WFP/Crispin Hughes).

services to the poor. It has supported and fostered the involvement of local communities and voluntary organizations as well as other aid agencies in such programmes, which have helped in institution-building. Organizational, managerial and logistics systems have been set up, or strengthened, to reach out to the poor and provide them with food and basic health and nutrition services.

School feeding programmes

Provision of meals at primary schools has been a prominent feature of food aid programmes for many years (**Fig. 4**). Such schemes accounted for about 8% of total annual food aid supplied in recent years. Apart from their educational benefits, school meals programmes complement food eaten at home, thereby bringing nutritional and health improvements, and can be used to teach children improved food habits and the hygienic handling of food.

Hunger and malnutrition reduce the physical and mental capacity of children. Large numbers of schoolchildren in developing countries suffer from both wasting and stunting. Many do not have an adequate intake of vitamins and minerals, which may result in illness that reduces school attendance and increases the drop-out rate. When children go without food, their alertness, attention span and learning capacity are significantly reduced. School meals can also act as an incentive for poor parents to send their children to school, thereby increasing the range of enrolment (particularly for girls) and reducing the drop-out rate.

Food-for-work programmes

The provision of food in labour-intensive works programme is another prominent way of improving nutrition, directly and indirectly. About 9% of annual food aid supplies in recent years has been used in these food-for-work (FFW) programmes (**Fig. 5**). The food aid provided for FFW (usually in the form of family rations for a worker and family members) increases the food consumption of participants whose incomes are too low for them to buy sufficient food for a healthy and fully productive life. The additional food increases the capacity to work on projects that increase food production, employment and income, which, in turn, lead to increased food consumption.

Food is provided in one of three ways. In most cases, family rations are distributed to workers at centres close to the work site in return for labour. In some cases, workers are given coupons along with their cash wages to buy food commodities at designated shops or stores, often at prices lower than those in the local markets, thereby increasing their wages and increasing the amount of food that they can buy. In other situations, the food aid commodities are sold on the market in recipient countries and the funds raised used to pay workers' wages in cash.

Food-for-work programmes can therefore provide nutritional benefits in a number of ways. They can help to mobilize poor people's most abundant resource, their own underutilized labour, by generating jobs quickly, increasing the incomes of the very poor and increasing productivity. They are also self-

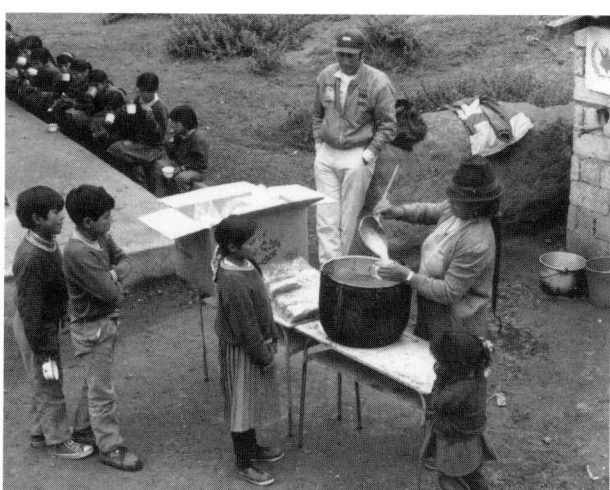

Figure 4 Primary school feeding in Ecuador. Students aged 5–12 years receive meals for attending school. The WFP uses food assistance to encourage attendance, reduce drop-out rates, enhance nutrition and to serve as a small income transfer to increase the household budget in depressed areas (WFP/Rhodri Jones).

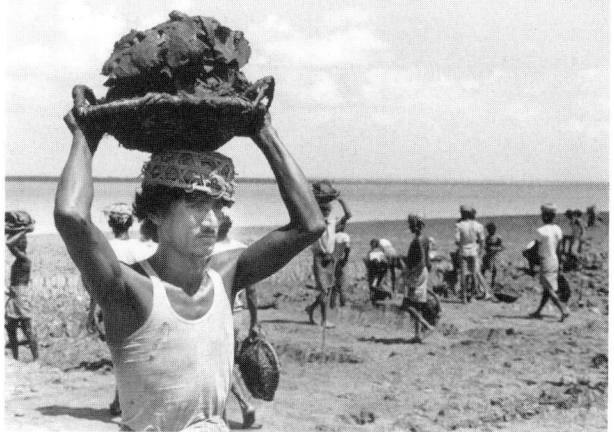

Figure 5 Food-for-work programme for water and land development in Bangladesh. Workers receive food rations in exchange for labour on FFW programmes designed to prevent the loss of life and property from flooding while increasing the availability of arable land by constructing and rehabilitating rural infrastructure. More than 2 million unskilled labourers are employed through such programmes during the agricultural off-season (WFP/WIF).

targeting on the most destitute, as only the poorest will work for food. In Asia, FFW has been used extensively as a relief measure in times of emergencies and disasters. It has been a means of addressing the seasonal dimensions of poverty and hunger in work programmes outside the agricultural season, and it has brought particular benefits to women in poor households or as single heads of households. Women often make up a high proportion of the work force in FFW programmes, frequently because the structure of the regular labour market excludes women. The FFW programmes are flexible and women find their timing compatible with their domestic and other responsibilities. Payment in food is also attractive to women who often have more command over food than cash in the household. Women play a pivotal role in alleviating poverty and food insecurity owing to their strategic position in the household and the productive work they do outside, especially in food production. The FFW approach serves to support and fortify this role.

Public food distribution and subsidy programmes

Food distribution and subsidy programmes have been used in developing countries with the aim of getting basic foods to poor people at low cost, thereby increasing their food consumption and income. These schemes can take the form of general price subsidies or rationing of basic food commodities at prices lower than their market value (or free). Food stamp programmes have been used to increase food consumption among the poor and reduce the administrative burden and costs of handling, transporting and distributing food directly. Food aid has been used to support these programmes. Their effects have depended largely on the nature of the programme, including the degree of targeting, the choice of the food commodities distributed, and the design and implementation of the programmes. Each programme should be designed to suit the particular local situation. There is no ideal single type: a programme that is efficient and effective in one place may be unsuitable in another.

Public food distribution and subsidy programmes can be powerful and cost-effective tools for reaching certain social, economic and political aims, or they can be harmful to economic growth and equity. As with so many other policy tools, the question is not whether they are good or bad, but when and how they are applied. There are other ways of making food available at low prices. Like other measures, they are open to abuse. This raises the question as to which type of programme is most efficient in each situation, in reaching and benefiting a target population at least cost, and within an acceptable level of leakage.

Market reform and food reserves

The price of food has an important effect on the nutritional status of both small food producers and poor consumers. Governments in developing countries face the dilemma of providing incentive prices to producers to increase production without pricing poor consumers out of the market. Food aid can help resolve this problem in several ways. Ensuring that food is physically available in an area throughout the year can help to stabilize food prices. Food aid has been provided to help governments establish food reserves for price stabilization schemes by releasing food from the stocks when prices rise above a certain level and for emergency stocks to make food available in times of disaster. In many developing countries, food produced by small farmers often cannot be increased or taken to market because the road network is inadequate to get production services to them and to get the harvest out. Food has also been lost after production because of inadequate storage facilities. Food aid has helped to improve market infrastructure, such as rural roads and storage facilities, through food-for-work programmes. Warehouse management has also been strengthened through training programmes and the provision of pesticides to prevent food losses during storage. These measures have helped to increase the income of small farmers, who are often net food purchasers, and to increase employment for landless agricultural labourers. They have also helped to reform the marketing system by increasing private trading and by reducing the control of high-cost and inefficient government marketing organizations with a monopoly on grain marketing.

Credit for food security

A number of innovations in the 1980s involved the provision of credit to poor women's groups with the help of food aid to assist them establish private enterprises in the growing and diversifying economies of developing countries, thus improving their food security. An example is WFP-supported programme working exclusively for the poorest women in Bangladesh, the 'ultra-poor', with no land, most of whom are single heads of households with four or five children, and a literacy rate below 10%. A supplementary feeding programme for mothers and their children has been gradually transformed since the mid 1980s to enable the beneficiaries to look after themselves when food aid comes to an end. Each woman participant received a monthly family ration, valued at about US $6, for 2 years, a significant addition to their own resources. While receiving their rations, participants deposited the equivalent of about US $0.70 every month into a savings and credit scheme. After 2 years, each woman had built up a small amount of capital, but not enough to go into business. A credit scheme was, therefore, set up with money from the sale of wheat provided by a group of food aid donors. The money was put into a revolving fund managed by a national NGO. At the same time a package of development services was provided, including training in income-generating activities, group formation and marketing skills, savings and credit, functional literacy, and mother and child health care. A women's centre provided training in the production and marketing of poultry, sericulture, fish farming, tailoring and food processing, for which there are ready markets in Bangladesh. Between 1988 and 1993, over 100 000 women received loans totalling the equivalent of US $3.5 million; the repayment rate has been almost 100%.

Economic reform and adjustment programmes

Many developing countries would benefit from adjusting their economies to the realities of internal and international conditions through economic reform measures. However, these measures often involve drastic reduction in public expenditure, which particularly affect the poor by reducing the subsidies of basic foods, increasing unemployment and cutting support for basic social services in nutrition, health, education and training. Food aid can help to mitigate these adverse effects on the poor. A major contribution has been in providing general financial support. Programme food aid provided bilaterally by donor governments can replace part of commercial food imports, thereby releasing the foreign exchange that would have been spent on buying those imports. As the food aid commodities are sold in the markets of recipient countries, they generate income for the government's budget. Both the savings and income can then be spent on programmes of benefit to poor, food-insecure people.

Food aid can also be used in compensatory measures to rescue and preserve basic social services for the poor, provide employment to those who lose their jobs, and nutrition support to those who cannot afford the increased food prices brought about by the adjustment process. The most appropriate compensatory measure in both cases would be to provide productive, income-earning employment. It may be necessary in the short run, however, to provide food directly through compensatory nutrition programmes.

Issues in Food Aid for Nutrition

A number of issues have arisen where food aid has been used with the aim of improving nutrition, directly or indirectly.

Targeting and registration

Targeting is a key concern in the design and implementation of food intervention programmes. It is a strategic factor in ensuring access and outreach to needy people. Various ways of identifying and reaching the target group have been adopted in order to provide food aid to those in most need. Medical, nutritional and household surveys have been carried out, or rapid appraisal and beneficiary participation techniques, and risk and vulnerability mapping have been used. In supplementary feeding programmes, selection criteria for mothers have included teenage pregnancy, low prepregnancy weight, low birthweight of previous children, and multiple pregnancies. For preschool children, selection criteria have included different degrees of malnutrition, low birthweight, lack of weight gain, and sudden loss of weight due to illness. In armed conflicts, 'corridors of tranquility' have been negotiated with the warring parties to ensure that food and other essential items can get through to the civilian population caught up in the fighting.

Research findings have pointed to the importance of targeting by age. Providing nutrition supplements early in life, preferably before the age of 3 years, can have important benefits in terms of growth, learning capacity and cognitive performance and, later in life, pregnancy and work capacity. However, food supplements distributed as take-home family rations or fed at mother and child centres or schools do not necessarily result in additional consumption for the target groups. The supplements may be shared with other family members or replace foods that otherwise would be eaten. Information is required on how food is shared within the household before food supplements can be effectively distributed. Targeting by type of food might help to overcome some of these problems. Providing 'low-status' but nutritious foods can help in ensuring that they reach the poorest people in both relief operations and development projects. Providing premixed weaning food is more likely to reach young children. The timing of food supplements is also important; They are most valuable, for example, outside the agricultural year when the seasonal dimensions of hunger are most marked, or at times of the year when work output is highest, or at the beginning of the school day for children who would not have had breakfast.

Targeting involves difficult choices in terms of the

costs and benefits in nutritional and other terms. A balance may need to be struck between criteria that focus on the very poor and worst affected, and less exacting criteria that address need on a community or area basis, without spreading resources too thinly to obtain results, or favouring any particular group. Targeted interventions may fail because it is not possible, or too costly, to carry them out on a sustainable basis. Many difficulties can be overcome by involving the beneficiaries themselves in the design, implementation and evaluation of nutrition intervention programmes. Inadequate registration systems have led to donor mistrust of the number of people estimated to require assistance. As a result, too little or too much aid has been provided, leading to either waste and corruption or unnecessary hardship, especially for women and children, the least influential and most vulnerable group.

Food rations

Considerable controversy has surrounded what should be the appropriate size and content of food rations, particularly during emergencies. The food rations provided are determined by many factors, including the food commodities available either from donor countries or through purchase or exchange in recipient countries; the specific nutritional requirements of the beneficiaries; their food habits and preferences; the roles and purposes for which food rations are provided; government policies and priorities; possible market displacement; the cost of provision; logistical considerations, such as the availability of transportation, storage, handling, preparation and processing facilities; the need for special packaging and containers; and the risk of damage, spoilage and waste.

For mothers, the general aim is to supply the additional energy and protein requirements for pregnancy and lactation. Food supplements for young children are generally designed to provide about half their daily energy, and most of their protein, requirements. In school feeding programmes, the aim is to complement food consumed at home in order to make up for deficiencies in protein, fat and certain minerals and vitamins, the absence of which could lead to greater exposure to disease and to undermining the general health of school children. For refugees, the World Food Programme and the UN High Commissioner for Refugees have agreed that when they have no other resources, food rations should meet all nutritional requirements. They should provide no less than 1900 kilocalories of energy per person per day, of which at least 8% should be provided in the form of protein and 10% in the form of fat.

The energy content can be modified depending on the circumstances of the refugees.

Food aid rations are usually calculated on the basis of the nutritional requirements of the beneficiaries. They can also be based on the amount of income they can give to the receivers. In this case, the food commodities provided are those most expensive for the beneficiaries to buy in the local market, thereby creating the greatest saving in the household budget, which can be used to buy other foods, and other essential items, which can bring further nutritional benefit.

Micronutrient deficiencies can be addressed through food aid rations in several ways. Foods rich in certain miconutrients can be included, such as groundnuts for their niacin content, or fortified cereal blended foods, such as corn-soy blend and wheat-soy blend. Certain foods can be fortified with vitamins, such as vitamin A in wheat, vegetable oils and dried skimmed milk. Iodine-fortified salt can be distributed in goitre-prevalent areas. Food aid distribution systems can also be used to provide vitamins and minerals in capsule form, including iron supplements to prevent anaemia, iodine supplements to prevent goitre and cretinism, and vitamin A supplements to prevent blindness, as well as oral rehydration therapy to prevent dehydration in young children by diarrhoea.

Guidelines have been issued for food supplement programmes to promote breast-feeding, the use of weaning foods based on locally prepared mixtures, and the safe use of dried milk powder. Supplements are usually not provided to infants under 6 months so as not to discourage breast-feeding. Food produced in developing countries has been bought and used as food aid in the development of weaning food mixtures. When skim milk powder is provided (which is enriched with vitamin A) in a take-home ration, mothers are encouraged to use it as an additive to a weaning food, and not as a reconstituted drink, in order to avoid problems arising from unsafe drinking water and unclean feeding bottles.

Changing food habits

Food-aided nutrition programmes have been accused of changing food habits and creating a demand for more expensive foods that cannot be produced locally, thereby creating a disincentive for local food production. However, a change in commodities can lead to a more efficient diet. Food habits are not unchangeable. They can be transformed by many factors, such as government import and pricing policies; changes in the relative prices of food commodities; increasing income; transport and logistics improvements; migration to urban areas; fuel costs;

and changes when women take part in income-earning activities outside the home. To the extent that food aid substitutes for food imports that would have occurred in any case, the causes of change in food habits must lie elsewhere. As food supplements are provided as additions to the diet, they are unlikely to cause farmers to produce less food. The use of local foods as food supplements, and in the production of weaning foods based on local foods, can create additional demand for locally grown foods, thereby stimulating increased food production.

Coordination

Integrating food aid with financial and technical assistance in national development programmes that give priority to improving the wellbeing of the poor is the best way of using it to help overcome hunger and malnutrition in sustainable ways. Food-aided nutrition interventions are likely to be more effective if they are part of a package of assistance which includes health care, nutrition education and employment programmes to increase incomes. In addition to adequate food, other essential items may need to be provided, including safe drinking water, basic medicines, improved shelter, fuel and human security. Without these items, nutrition and health may not be protected even though sufficient food is supplied. These items are provided by different government departments and aid agencies. Coordination of their provision is necessary to ensure that they are provided together.

See also: **Food Aid**: Overview. **Malnutrition**: Definition, Classification and Epidemiology. **Nutrition Policies**: In Developing Countries. **Population, Development and Nutrition**: Overview. **Refugees**: Nutritional Management.

Further Reading

Administrative Committee on Coordination/Subcommittee on Nutrition (1993) *Nutritional Issues in Food Aid*. ACC/SCN Symposium Report. Nutrition Policy Discussion Paper no. 12. Geneva: United Nations.

Beaton G and Ghassemi H (1982) Supplementary feeding programmes for young children in developing countries. *American Journal of Clinical Nutrition* 35(4):864–916.

FAO (1992) *Principles of Surplus Disposal and Consultative Obligations of Member Nations*, 3rd edn. Rome: Food and Agriculture Organization of the United Nations.

FAO and WHO (1992) *International Conference on Nutrition. World Declaration and Plan of Action for Nutrition*. Rome: Food and Agriculture Organization of the United Nations and World Health Organization.

Gillespie S and Mason J (1991) *Nutrition-relevant Actions: Some Experiences from the Eighties and Lessons for the Nineties*. ACC/SCN State-of-the-Art Series. Nutrition Policy Discussion Paper no. 10: Geneva: United Nations.

Greaves JP and Shaw DJ, eds (1986) *Food Aid and the Well-being of Children in the Developing World*. New York: United Nations Children's Fund and the World Food Programme.

Jennings J, Gillespie S, Mason J, Lotfi M and Scialfa T, eds (1991) *Managing Successful Nutrition Programmes*. ACC/SCN State-of-the-Art Series. Nutrition Policy Discussion Paper no. 8. Geneva: United Nations.

Pinstrup-Andersen P (1988) *Food Subsidies in Developing Countries: Costs, Benefits and Policy Options*. Baltimore: Johns Hopkins University Press for the International Food Policy Research Institute.

Pollitt E (1979) *Malnutrition and Infection in the Classroom*. Paris: United Nations Educational, Scientific and Cultural Organization.

Quisumbing A, Brown L, Feldstein H, Haddad L and Pena C (1995) *Women: The Key to Food Security*, Washington, DC: International Food Policy Research Institute.

Shaw J and Singer H, eds (1988) Food policy, food aid and economic adjustment. *Food Policy* (special issue) 13(1).

Shoham J (1994) *Emergency Supplementary Feeding Programmes*. London: Overseas Development Institute.

UN (1975) *Report of the World Food Conference, Rome 5–17 November 1974*. Document E/CONF. 65/20. New York: United Nations.

WFP (1978) Modalities of operation of the international emergency food reserve. *Report of the Sixth Session of the United Nations/FAO Committee on Food Aid Policies and Programmes*. Document WFP/CFA 6/21, Annex IV. Rome: World Food Programme.

WFP (1990) *Food Aid and Education: Past Experience and Future Directions*. Rome: World Food Programme.

WFP (1992) *Food Aid Working For Women. The World Food Programme and Women in Development*. Rome: World Food Programme.

FOOD ALLERGIES

Contents
Aetiology
Diagnosis and Management

Aetiology

T J David, L Patel and **C I Ewing**, Booth Hall
Children's Hospital, Manchester, UK

Copyright © 1998 Academic Press

The concept that certain foods can produce adverse reactions in susceptible individuals has a long history. Hippocrates (460–370 BC) reported that cow's milk could cause gastric upset and urticaria. Later, Galen (AD 131–210) described a case of intolerance to goat's milk. It was Lucretius (96–55 BC) who said 'What is food to one man may be fierce poison to others'. In the 1920s and 1930s a fashion developed of blaming food intolerance for a large number of hitherto unexplained disorders. The uncritical and overenthusiastic nature of the claims, plus the anecdotal evidence upon which they were based, generally discredited the whole subject. Indeed, the field of food intolerance has been described as 'a model of obstruction to the advancement of learning'. The whole area has provoked much controversy. The introduction of double-blind provocation tests has placed studies on a more scientific footing, but they are impractical in routine management. The lack of objective and reproducible diagnostic laboratory tests which could eliminate bias has ensured that controversy about food intolerance continues.

Definitions

The word 'allergy' is frequently misused, and applied indiscriminately to any adverse reaction, regardless of the mechanism. An allergic response is a reproducible adverse reaction to a substance mediated by an immunological response. The substance provoking the reaction may have been ingested, injected, inhaled or merely have come into contact with the skin or mucous membranes. 'Food allergy' is a form of adverse reaction to food in which the cause is an immunological response to a food. The much broader term 'food intolerance' does not imply any specific type of mechanism, and is simply defined as a reproducible adverse reaction to a specific food or food ingredient. In North America the terminology used is different: the term 'food sensitivity' is used to cover all adverse reactions to food, which are then subdivided into 'food hypersensitivity' (i.e. immunologically mediated) and 'food intolerance', which implies a non-immunologically mediated event.

The term 'food aversion' comprises food avoidance, where the subject avoids a food for psychological reasons such as distaste or a desire to lose weight, and psychological intolerance. The latter is an unpleasant bodily reaction caused by emotions associated with the food rather than the food itself. Psychological intolerance will normally be observable under open conditions, but will not occur when the food is given in an unrecognizable form. Psychological intolerance may be reproduced by suggesting (falsely) that the food has been administered.

The term 'anaphylaxis' or 'anaphylactic shock' is taken to mean a severe and potentially life-threatening reaction of rapid onset, with circulatory collapse. 'Anaphylaxis' has also been used to describe any allergic reaction, however mild, that results from specific immunoglobulin E (IgE) antibodies, but such usage fails to distinguish between a trivial reaction (e.g. a sneeze) and a dangerous event.

An antigen is a substance that is capable of provoking an immune response. An antibody is an immunoglobulin that is capable of combining specifically with certain antigens. An allergen is a substance that provokes a harmful (allergic) immune response.

Immunological tolerance is a process which results in the immunological system becoming specifically unreactive to an antigen which is capable in other circumstances of provoking antibody production or cell-mediated immunity. The immunological system nevertheless reacts to unrelated antigens given simultaneously and via the same route.

Atopy means the ability to produce a weal and flare response to skin prick testing with a common antigen such as house dust mite or grass pollen. The atopic diseases are asthma (all childhood cases but not all adult cases), atopic eczema, allergic rhinitis, allergic conjunctivitis and some cases of urticaria.

Mechanisms of Food Allergy

Understanding of the mechanisms of food allergy is poor, and in many cases the precise mechanism is obscure.

Sensitization

Possible factors contributing to immunological sensitization leading to food intolerance include:

1. Genetic predisposition: food allergy is commonly familial, suggesting the importance of genetic factors.
2. Immaturity of the immune system or the gastrointestinal mucosal barrier in newborn infants may predispose to sensitization. The numerous studies investigating whether food allergy or atopic disease can be prevented by interventions during pregnancy or lactation are based on the idea that there is a critical period during which sensitization can occur.
3. Dosage of antigen: it may be that high dosage leads to the development of tolerance, and low dosage leads to sensitization. This may help to explain the well-documented phenomenon of infants who become allergic to traces of foods that reach the infant through the mother's breast milk.
4. Certain food antigens are especially likely to lead to sensitization, for example egg, cow's milk and peanut. The reasons why certain foods are more likely to provoke an allergic reaction than others is poorly understood.
5. A triggering event, for example a viral infection: the evidence is anecdotal, but there is a suggestion that food allergy may develop in a previously nonallergic subject after a viral infection such as infectious mononucleosis (glandular fever).
6. Alteration in the permeability of the gastrointestinal tract, permitting abnormal antigen access: the best example of this is the suggestion that acute viral gastroenteritis may damage the small intestinal mucosa, allowing abnormal absorption of food proteins, leading to sensitization. Thus there is some evidence suggesting that in a few cases the onset of cow's milk protein allergy follows shortly after an episode of gastroenteritis.

Immunological and molecular mechanisms

Despite the gastrointestinal barrier, small amounts of immunologically intact proteins enter the circulation and are distributed throughout the body. In normal individuals, the gut-associated lymphoid tissue (GALT), although capable of mounting a rapid and potent response against foreign substances, develop tolerance to ingested food antigens. The means by which tolerance develops is poorly understood, but it is believed that failure to develop tolerance leads to food allergy. The relatively low salivary secretory IgA concentrations together with the large amount of ingested protein contributes to the large amount of food antigens confronting the immature GALT. In genetically predisposed infants, these food antigens may stimulate the excessive production of IgE antibodies or other abnormal immune responses.

Heat treatment

Heat treatment clearly affects certain (but not all) foods, rendering them less likely to provoke an allergic reaction in a subject who is allergic. Occasionally the reverse occurs, as in the celebrated case of Professor Heinz Küstner, who was allergic to cooked but not raw fish.

In cow's milk, whey proteins are easily denatured by heat but casein is highly resistant. This observation led to the suggestion that the heat treatment of whey proteins may be a simple and logical strategy for producing a hypoallergenic infant milk formula. However, double-blind, placebo-controlled oral challenges gave rise to immediate hypersensitivity reactions to heat-treated whey protein in four out of five children with cow's milk protein intolerance. The reason for these reactions is not known, but one possibility is a reaction to residual casein, which is often present in trace amounts in commercial whey preparations. The small proportion of patients with cow's milk protein intolerance likely to tolerate heat-treated cow's milk, such as evaporated milk, means that heat-treated milk is unlikely to be suitable as a substitute for a cow's milk infant formula.

Cooking reduces the allergenicity of eggs by 70%. However, one of the major allergens in eggs, ovomucoid, a heat-resistant glycoprotein which contributes to the gel-like structure of egg white, is resistant to heating. Heat appears to render a large number of fruits and vegetables less likely to provoke adverse reactions in subjects who are intolerant. Thus, for example, it is not uncommon to see children who are allergic to raw potatoes or fresh pineapple, but almost all such children can tolerate cooked potatoes or tinned pineapples. In some situations it appears that heat can accelerate a process of denaturation which can in time occur on its own. For example, there have been studies of patients who reacted to fresh melon, pear, peach, pineapple, grape and banana. In each case, stewed or tinned fruit caused no reaction. Studies of fresh extracts of these fruits showed that when stored in a refrigerator, the extracts lost their ability to provoke a positive skin test after approximately 3 days.

Prevalence

Unreliability of self-reported food allergy

Reports of food allergy from individuals or parents of children are notoriously unreliable. Such reports have to be treated with scepticism. It is common for parents to believe that foods are responsible for a variety of childhood symptoms. Double-blind provocation tests in children with histories of reactions to food confirm the story in only one-third of all cases. In the case of purely behavioural symptoms the proportion that could be reproduced under blind conditions was zero. The same is true of adults' beliefs about their own symptoms. If needless dietary restrictions are to be avoided, one has to be sceptical, and it may be necessary in some cases to seek objective confirmation of food intolerance. The gross overreporting of food allergy has to be borne in mind when looking at data on prevalence that is based on unconfirmed subjective reports.

Population studies

The parents of 866 children from Finland were asked to provide a detailed history of food allergy, and for certain foods the diagnosis was further investigated by elimination and open challenge at home. Food allergy was reported in 19% by the age of 1 year, 22% by 2 years, 27% by 3 years, and 8% by 6 years. In a prospective study of 480 children in the USA up to their third birthday, 16% were reported to have had reactions to fruit or fruit juice and 28% to other food. However, open challenge confirmed reactions in only 12% of the former and 8% of the latter.

Estimates of the prevalence of cow's milk protein allergy are reported to range from 0.3% to 7.5% of subjects. There is little objective data on the prevalence of food allergy in adults.

Natural History

The natural history of food allergy has been little studied. It is well known that a high proportion of children with food intolerance in the first year of life lose their intolerance in time. The proportion of children to which this happens varies with the food and probably with the type of symptoms that are produced. Thus it is common for allergy to cow's milk or egg to spontaneously disappear with time, whereas peanut allergy is usually lifelong. In the North American study referred to above, it was found that the offending food or fruit was back in the diet after only 9 months in half the cases, and virtually all the offending foods were back in the diet by the third birthday. A further study of nine children with severe adverse reactions to food showed

that despite the severity, three were later able to tolerate normal amounts of the offending food and a further four became able to tolerate small amounts.

While it is clear that the majority of children with food intolerance spontaneously improve, it remains to be established to what extent this depends on the age of onset, the nature of the symptoms, the food itself and other factors such as associated atopic disease.

In adults with food allergy, the problem is far more likely to be lifelong. Nevertheless, some adults do become tolerant to foods to which they were allergic. In one adult follow-up study, approximately one-third of adults were found to lose their allergy after maintaining an elimination diet for 1 year.

Cross-Reactions

Cross-reactions may occur between different species, and between different foodstuffs that may or may not belong to the same botanical family.

Animal milk

There is a marked antigenic similarity between the proteins that cause food allergy in the milk of cows, goats, sheep and horses. It is often not appreciated that almost all subjects who are allergic to cow's milk protein are allergic to the milks of these other animals. This is one of the many reasons why goat's milk is not an appropriate milk substitute for an infant with cow's milk allergy.

Eggs

The eggs from turkeys, ducks, geese and seagulls all contain ovalbumin, ovomucoid and ovotransferrin, the major allergens in chicken's eggs. The eggs of chickens and turkeys have a similar relative potency of allergenicity. The immunochemical identity of proteins in the egg white of ducks and geese differs somewhat from that of chickens, and they may have less potency as allergens. Of all the bird's eggs listed above, the eggs of the seagull are the least allergenic, and bear the least immunochemical similarity to chicken eggs.

Legumes

It is not always obvious which plants belong to the same family. Products of the Leguminosae family include beans, peas, soya beans, lentils, peanuts, liquorice, carob and gum arabic. Cross-reactivity is uncommon, and the degree of genetic relationship may be of little relevance. Thus, for example, patients with soya allergy are not uncommonly allergic also to peanuts, although the two legumes are not closely related.

Seafood

The taxonomic diversity of animals classified as 'seafood' (fish, molluscs, crustaceans) suggests that complete cross-reactivity for all seafood is unlikely to be common. In one study, of 20 children with a history of allergy to cod, there was a history of allergy to sole in 11 (55%), to tuna in seven (35%), and to mackerel, anchovy, sardine, red mullet and salmon each in one (5%). Most studies of cross-reactivity are based on skin prick and IgE antibody test results which are of little relevance to clinical sensitivity.

Food and pollen

Cross-reactions can occur between inhaled pollen and ingested food allergens. There is a well-documented association between allergy to birch tree pollen and allergy to apple, carrot, celery, potato, orange and tomato. It is likely that this association might be explained by a structural similarity between birch pollen allergens and one or more antigens that are common to these foods. Similarly, patients with mugwort pollen allergy can have concomitant intolerance to celery.

Special Requirements for the Occurrence of Allergic Reaction to Food

In some individuals, there is a clear one-to-one relationship between the ingestion of a food and a reaction. An example might be an individual with allergy to cod. Every time the subject eats cod, there is an immediate allergic reaction. In other individuals the relationship between the food and an allergic reaction is less precise. There are a number of possible reasons for this, as follows.

Timing of reaction and delayed reactions

Most allergic reactions to foods occur within minutes of ingestion of the food. However, sometimes a reaction may be delayed. This is best documented in cow's milk protein allergy, where three types of reaction are recognized. These are (a) early skin reaction, (b) early gut reaction, and (c) late reaction. An affected individual usually only exhibits one of these types of reaction. In the early skin reaction group, symptoms begin to develop within 45 min of cow's milk challenge. Almost all patients in this group have a positive skin prick test to cow's milk. In the early gut reaction group, symptoms begin to develop between 45 min and 20 h after cow's milk challenge. About a third of patients in this group have a positive skin prick test to cow's milk. In the late reaction group, symptoms begin to develop about 20 h after cow's milk protein challenge. Only about 20% of this late

reaction group have a positive skin prick test to cow's milk, and these are mostly children with atopic eczema. Almost all children in the late reaction group present over the age of 6 months, and as a group their age at presentation is significantly higher than that of the two other groups.

Quantity of food

The quantity of cow's milk, for example, required to produce an allergic reaction varies from patient to patient. Some patients are highly sensitive and develop anaphylaxis after ingestion of less than 1 μg of casein, β-lactoglobulin or α-lactalbumin. In contrast, there are children and adults who do not react to 100 ml of milk but who do react to 200 ml or more. There is a relationship between the quantity of milk required and the time of onset of symptoms. In one study, the median reaction onset time in those who reacted to 100 ml milk challenges was 2 h, but the median reaction onset time in those who required larger amounts of milk to elicit reactions was 24 h.

Food-dependent exercise-induced anaphylaxis

In this unusual condition, attacks only occur when the exercise follows within a couple of hours of the ingestion of specific foods such as celery, shellfish, squid, peaches or wheat. The mechanisms that result in food-dependent exercise-induced anaphylaxis are obscure. This disorder, though rare, is important in the interpretation of dietary challenge studies of food intolerance, because in these patients a simple double-blind food challenge without exercise will fail to validate a history of food intolerance.

Drug-dependent food allergy

Certain individuals only react to specific foods while taking a drug. The best recognized examples of this are individuals who only react to foods while taking salicylate (aspirin).

Effect of disease activity

It is a common but poorly understood observation that children with eczema and food allergy can often tolerate some or all food triggers when the skin disease clears (usually when the child is on holiday in a sunny country).

Other possibilities

It is not known whether food allergy can be confined to occasions when the pollen count is high or when the individual consumes certain other foods. At present there are no objective studies that address the complex issue of the possible additive effect of orally ingested and possibly inhaled antigens. There are people with allergy to foods in whom the severity of adverse reactions clearly varies from time to time, but the reasons for this variability are not known.

See also: **Dairy Products**: Nutritional Value. **Eggs**: Nutritional Value. **Food Allergies**: Diagnosis and Management. **Food Intolerance**: Types and Incidence. **Infants**: Milk-feeding and Weaning. **Legumes**: Types and Nutritional Value.

Further Reading

Bentley SJ, Pearson DJ and Rix KJB (1983) Food hypersensitivity in irritable bowel syndrome. *Lancet* 2:295–297.

Bernhisel-Broadbent J and Sampson HA (1989) Cross-allergenicity in the legume botanical family in children with food hypersensitivity. *Journal of Allergy and Clinical Immunology* 83:435–440.

Bock SA (1987) Prospective appraisal of complaints of adverse reactions to foods in children during the first three years of life. *Pediatrics* 79:683–688.

Bush RK, Taylor SL, Nordlee JA and Busse WW (1985) Soybean oil is not allergenic to soybean-sensitive individuals. *Journal of Allergy and Clinical Immunology* 76:242–245.

David TJ (1987) Reactions to dietary tartrazine. *Archives of Disease in Childhood* 62:119–122.

David TJ (1993) *Food and Food Additive Intolerance in Childhood*. Oxford: Blackwell.

De Martino M, Novembre E, Galli L *et al.* (1990) Allergy to different fish species in cod-allergic children: in vivo and in vitro studies. *Journal of Allergy and Clinical Immunology* 86:909–914.

Dreborg S (1988) Food allergy in pollen-sensitive patients. *Annals of Allergy* 61:41–46.

Eriksson NE (1978) Food sensitivity reported by patients with asthma and hay fever. *Allergy* 33:189–196.

Herian AM, Taylor SL and Bush RK (1990) Identification of soybean allergens by immunoblotting with sera from soy-allergic adults. *International Archives of Allergy and Immunology* 92:193–198.

Kajosaari M (1982) Food allergy in Finnish children aged 1 to 6 years. *Acta Paediatrica Scandinavica* 71:815–819.

May CD (1982) Food allergy: lessons from the past. *Journal of Allergy and Clinical Immunology* 69:255–259.

May CD and Bock SA (1978) A modern clinical approach to food hypersensitivity. *Allergy* 33:166–188.

Pastorello EA, Stocchi L, Pravettoni V *et al.* (1989) Role of the elimination diet in adults with food allergy. *Journal of Allergy and Clinical Immunology* 84:475–483.

Pauli G, Bessot JC, Dietemann-Molard A, Braun PA and Thierry R (1985) Celery sensitivity: clinical and immunological correlations with pollen allergy. *Clinical Allergy* 15:273–279.

Young E, Patel S, Stoneham M, Rona R and Wilkinson JD (1987) The prevalence of reaction to food additives in a survey population. *Journal of the Royal College of Physicians (London)* 21:241–247.

Diagnosis and Management

T J David, L Patel and **C I Ewing**,
Department of Child Health, University of Manchester, UK

Copyright © 1998 Academic Press

The diagnosis of food allergy is made from the history, supported by investigations and by responses to avoidance of specific food triggers.

Documenting Food Allergies

Since the value of investigations is limited, it is especially important to obtain a clear history. There are a number of practical points to be made.

Speed of onset

In general, the quicker the onset of the allergic reaction, the more reliable is the history. If a child develops a violent allergic reaction within a minute or two after ingesting a food, it is much easier to link the reaction to a specific food than if a reaction only occurs 1–2 days after eating a food.

Coincidences need to be excluded

If a child becomes unwell (e.g. starts wheezing) an hour after eating a specific food, the wheezing could be caused by the food, or it could just be a coincidence. The more times that such a sequence has been observed, the more likely it is that there is a cause and effect relationship.

Observations need to be tested for internal consistency

Someone may believe that he or she is allergic to a food if a symptom (e.g. urticaria) occurs on (say) three occasions after eating a specific food. It is important to find out:

1. whether the subject has had the same symptoms on other occasions when the suspect food trigger was not taken.
2. whether the subject has taken the suspect food on one or more other occasions without any adverse effects.

Failure to seek inconsistencies such as these is one factor that is responsible for the overdiagnosis of food allergy.

Documenting a diagnosis of food allergy

If it is reported that someone is allergic to an item, it is important to probe further and find out on what basis the person has been deemed allergic. It is common to find children and adults who are believed to be allergic to a food solely on the basis of skin tests or blood tests, which are in fact almost wholly unreliable (see below). It is also common for people to believe that they are allergic to something because a health professional said so one day, on what further enquiry reveals to be flimsy or nonexistent grounds.

Another common problem is the misinterpretation of a sequence of events. For example, a child with an ear infection is given an antibiotic, and 3 days later develops diarrhoea, so the parents come to believe the child is allergic to the antibiotic. In fact the cause of the diarrhoea is far more likely to be either an underlying viral infection, or a disturbance of the gut flora. Another example is the report of a child who is believed to be allergic to sesame seeds because of reactions occurring after eating buns coated with sesame seeds; most such children are in fact not allergic to sesame seeds but are reacting to the egg glaze that has been used as an adhesive for the seed coating. Another common example is the child with asthma who coughs and wheezes after drinking a diluted orange squash drink, with the result that it is believed that the child is reacting to the colouring agent tartrazine. If fact such reactions are more likely to be due to sulfite preservatives in the squash; sulfites trigger symptoms in 60% or more of children with asthma.

Practical Diagnostic Difficulties

Multiple mechanisms

Reactions to foods are a heterogeneous group of disorders caused by a variety of different immunological and pharmacological mechanisms. In any individual case, the precise mechanism is often not known. No single type of laboratory test could possibly cover all the different possible mechanisms of reactions to foods. Even if one focuses on food allergy, there are a number of different possible immunological mechanisms, including immunoglobulin E (IgE) antibody-mediated and cell-mediated, reactions and circulating immune complexes.

Inability to predict outcome

In many situations (e.g. atopic disease), the subject wants to know whether there will be any benefit from food avoidance (e.g. not drinking cow's milk or not eating apples). Even if there were valid tests for the diagnosis of food intolerance, the outcome of avoidance measures depends on a number of other variables. Allergen avoidance may succeed for the following reasons:

- the patient was intolerant to the item;
- coincidental improvement;
- placebo response.

The reasons why a trial of food avoidance may fail to help can be summarized as follows.

1. The subject is not allergic to the food.
2. The period of elimination was too short. For example, where a child has an enteropathy (damage to the small intestine) due to food allergy, it may take a week or more for improvement in symptoms to occur.
3. The food has been incompletely avoided. This may happen in a subject supposed to be avoiding cow's milk protein who continues to eat food containing cow's milk proteins such as casein or whey.
4. The subject is allergic to other items that have not been avoided, for example a child with cow's milk protein allergy who fails to improve when given a soya-based milk to which there is also an allergy.
5. Coexisting or intercurrent disease, for example gastroenteritis in a child with loose stools who is trying a diet excluding cow's milk.
6. The patient's symptoms are trivial and have been exaggerated, or alternatively do not exist at all and have either been imagined or made up by the parents.

It is unrealistic to expect there to be a test that can overcome all these problems.

Diagnostic Tests

Skin prick tests

The principle of skin prick tests is that the skin weal and flare reaction to an allergen demonstrates the presence of mast-cell-fixed antibody, which is mainly IgE antibody. This antibody is produced in plasma cells, and is distributed in the circulation to all parts of the body, so that sensitization is generalized and therefore can be demonstrated by skin testing. In the presence of specific IgE antibody, mast cells in the skin release histamine, which in turn causes a visible weal and flare reaction in the skin.

The procedure is that a drop of allergen solution is placed on the skin which is then pricked with an hypodermic needle. Two control solutions should also be used. One is the diluent, in order to detect false positive reactions. The other is a positive control (e.g. a histamine solution), to enable comparison with a positive result of an allergen solution. The skin prick test induces a response that reaches a peak in 8–9 min for histamine, and 12–15 min for allergens. The size of the weal reaction (and not the larger red flare) is measured.

There are numerous problems with skin prick tests. These include the following:

- There is no agreed definition about what constitutes a positive reaction.
- The size of the weal depends to some extent on the potency of the extract.
- Antihistamines and tricyclic antidepressants suppress the histamine-induced weal and flare response of a skin test. The suppressive effect of antihistamines may last from a week up to several months for some of the more recently introduced nonsedating antihistamines.
- False positive tests: skin prick test reactivity may be present in subjects with no clinical evidence of allergy or intolerance. This is sometimes described as 'asymptomatic hypersensitivity' or 'subclinical sensitization'. While many with positive skin prick tests will never develop the allergy, some subjects with positive skin prick tests do develop symptoms later. However, since the test cannot identify those who are going to develop symptoms, the skin test information is of no practical value.
- False positive results: skin prick test reactivity may persist after clinical evidence of intolerance has subsided. For example, in a study of children with egg allergy, it was noted that five out of 11 who grew out of egg allergy had persistently positive skin prick tests after egg allergy had disappeared.
- False negative tests: skin prick tests are negative in some subjects with genuine food allergies.
- Skin prick tests mainly detect IgE antibody. However, many adverse reactions to food are not IgE-mediated, in which case skin prick tests can be expected to be negative. Taking cow's milk protein intolerance as an example, patients with quick reactions often have positive skin prick tests to cow's milk protein, but those with delayed reactions usually have negative skin prick tests.
- False negative results are a problem in infants and toddlers, when the weal size is much smaller than later in life.
- There is a poor correlation between the results of provocation tests (e.g. double-blind food challenges) and skin prick tests. For example, in one study of 31 children with a strongly positive (weal > 3 mm in diameter) skin prick test to peanut, only 16 (56%) had symptoms when peanuts were administered.
- Commercial food extracts (sometimes heat-treated) and fresh or frozen raw extracts may give different results (more positives with raw foods), reflecting the fact that some patients are allergic to certain foods only when taken in a raw state. In others the reverse is the case.

The role for skin prick tests is mainly for use in research studies. The results of skin tests cannot be taken alone, and standard textbooks of allergy acknowledge that 'the proper interpretation of results requires a thorough knowledge of the history and physical findings'. The problems in clinical practice are, for example, whether a subject with atopic disease (eczema, asthma or hay fever) or symptoms suggestive of food intolerance will benefit from attempts to avoid certain foods or food additives. However, skin prick test results are unreliable predictors of response to such measures.

Skin test results are known to be misleading in cases of inhalant allergy (e.g. allergy to dust mites or grass pollen), and skin prick tests for food allergy are especially unreliable because of the large number of false positive and false negative reactions.

Intradermal testing

Intradermal testing comprises the intradermal injection of 0.01–0.05 ml of an allergen extract. It can cause fatal generalized allergic reaction (anaphylaxis), and is only performed if a preliminary skin prick test is negative. Intradermal tests are more sensitive than skin prick testing, and hence also produce even more false positive reactions. The number of false positive reactions makes the interpretation of the results of intradermal testing even more difficult than skin prick testing. The difficulty in the interpretation of the results, the pain of intradermal injections and the risk of anaphylaxis mean that intradermal testing has no place in the routine investigation of food allergy.

Skin application of food prior to food challenges

There is one situation where direct application of food to the skin may be of practical value, and that is prior to a food challenge in a child in whom one fears an anaphylactic reaction. An example might be a 6-month-old infant with a history of a severe allergic reaction to egg. If the parents wish to see if the child has outgrown the allergy without directly administering egg and risking a violent reaction, a simple approach is to rub some raw egg white into the skin and observe the skin for a few minutes. If the skin application of egg in this way causes an urticarial reaction, then a gradual diminution and disappearance of this response during the succeeding months and years can probably be taken to indicate the development of tolerance, and a continuing brisk response to skin contact would constitute a deterrent to an oral challenge. This is, however, only an approximate guide, and there are a number of possible reasons why such testing may give a false positive result (e.g. using a raw food when the food is usually eaten cooked, such as egg or potato) or a false negative result (e.g. the child is receiving an antihistamine drug).

Tests for circulating IgE antibodies

The radioallergosorbent test (RAST) is the best known of a number of laboratory procedures for the detection and measurement of circulating IgE antibody. Unfortunately the clinical interpretation of RAST results is subject to most of the same pitfalls as the interpretation of skin prick testing. Additional problems with RAST are the high cost, and the fact that a high level of total circulating IgE (e.g. in children with severe atopic eczema) may cause a false positive result. Depending upon the criteria used for positivity, there is a fair degree of correlation between RAST and skin prick test results.

Provocation tests

A provocation test may be useful to confirm a history of allergy. An example might be a child who developed wheezing and urticaria minutes after eating a rusk. The rusk contained, as its main ingredients, wheat and cow's milk protein. To determine which component, if any, caused the reaction, oral challenges with individual components can be conducted. However, the results of provocation tests cannot prove that improvement in a disease has been *caused* by food avoidance. For example, a child with atopic eczema is put on a diet avoiding many foods, and the eczema improves. The improvement could be a coincidence, it could be a placebo effect, or it could be due to the diet. Just because the child is shown to react to a single food does not prove that avoidance of that food was the cause of the improvement.

Open and blind challenges   Where the subject and the observer know the identity of the administered material at the time of the challenge, the procedure is said to be an *open* challenge. In a *single-blind challenge* the observer but not the patient or family know the identity of the test material. To avoid bias on the part of the observer, a double-blind challenge is required. A *double-blind* challenge comprises exposing the subject to a challenge substance, which is either the item under investigation or an indistinguishable inactive (placebo) substance. Neither the subject nor the observer knows the identity of the administered material at the time of the challenge or during the subsequent period of observation.

The purpose of provocation tests   The aim of a food challenge is to study the consequences of food or food additive ingestion. Provocation tests are helpful:

1. to confirm a history (parents' observations of alleged food allergy are notoriously unreliable, as are adults' beliefs about their own allergies);
2. to confirm the diagnosis, for example of cow's milk protein allergy in infancy, where the diagnostic criteria include improvement on elimination diet and relapse on reintroduction;
3. to see if a subject has grown out of a food intolerance;
4. as a research procedure.

The food challenge should replicate normal food consumption in terms of dose, route and state of food. It should also be performed in such a way that the history can be verified. Thus, for example, it is no use solely looking for an immediate reaction if the parents report a delayed reaction.

Open food challenges are the simplest approach, but open food challenges run the risk of bias influencing the parents' (or doctors') observations. Often this is unimportant, but in some cases belief in food intolerance may be disproportionate, and where this is suspected there is no substitute for a double-blind placebo-controlled challenge. An open challenge may be an open invitation to the overdiagnosis of food intolerance. For example, in the UK parents widely believe that there is an association between food additives and bad behaviour, but in one series, double-blind challenges with tartrazine and benzoic acid were negative in all 24 children with a clear parental description of adverse reaction.

The double-blind placebo-controlled challenge is regarded as the best technique to confirm or refute histories of adverse reactions to foods. The ability to unravel food-related problems is said to be limited only by the imaginations of the physician and dietitian. In fact the technique is subject to a number of potential limitations, not all of which can be overcome.

Effect of dose   In some cases of food intolerance, minute quantities of food (e.g. traces of cow's milk protein) are sufficient to provoke florid and immediate symptoms. In other cases, much larger quantities of food are required to provoke a response. In one study, 8–10 g of cow's milk powder (corresponding to 60–70 ml of milk) was adequate to provoke an adverse reaction in some patients with cow's milk protein allergy, whereas others (with late onset symptoms and particularly with atopic eczema) required up to 10 times this volume of milk daily for more than 48 h before symptoms developed.

Size of dose   Concealing large doses is difficult. Standard capsules containing up to 500 mg of food are suitable for validation of immediate reactions to tiny quantities of food, but concealing much larger quantities of certain foods (especially those with a strong smell, flavour or colour) can be very difficult.

Route of administration   Reactions to food occurring within the mouth are likely to be missed if the challenge bypasses the oral route, for example when foods are given in a capsule or via a nasogastric tube. In practice, patients whose symptoms are exclusively confined to the mouth are unusual, and where there is a history of purely oral reactions an alternative challenge procedure can be employed. In subjects who are intolerant of sulfites, it is recognized that the administration of sulfites in capsules or directly into the stomach via a nasogastric tube usually fails to provoke an adverse reaction, whereas the oral administration of solution will succeed in doing so.

Problems with capsules   Children often cannot swallow large capsules, and this is a major limitation as most cases of suspected food allergy are in infants and toddlers; it is unsatisfactory to allow patients or parents to break open capsules and swallow the contents mixed into food or drink, as the colour (e.g. tartrazine) or smell (e.g. fish) will be difficult or impossible to conceal, and the challenge will no longer be blind.

Anaphylactic shock   There is a danger of producing anaphylactic shock, even if it did not occur on previous exposure to the food. For example, in Goldman's classic study of cow's milk protein intolerance, anaphylactic shock had been noted prior to cow's milk challenge in five children, but another three out of 89 children developed anaphylactic shock as a new symptom after cow's milk challenge. In a study of 80 children with atopic eczema treated with elimination diets, anaphylactic shock occurred in four out of 1862 food challenges. The risk appears to be greatest for those who received elemental diets.

Effect of disease activity   A food challenge performed during a quiescent phase of a disease such as urticaria, eczema or asthma may fail to provoke an adverse reaction.

Additive effect of triggers   Although some patients react repeatedly to challenges with single foods, it is possible (but unproven) that some patients react adversely only when several allergens are given together. There certainly are some subjects who react only in the presence of a nonfood trigger, such as exercise or taking aspirin.

Special types of provocation testing   Other than giving a suspect food by mouth and asking the subject to swallow it, there are some alternative approaches:

Oral mucosal challenge   A small portion of food is applied to the mucosa inside the mouth, and one looks for reactions such as swelling of the lips, and tingling or irritation of the mouth or tongue, possibly followed by other more generalized symptoms such as urticaria, asthma, vomiting, abdominal pain or anaphylactic shock. Patients with food intolerance commonly make use of these oral symptoms, spitting out and avoiding further consumption of a food that provokes the symptom.

Gastric mucosal challenge   An allergen is applied directly to the gastric mucosa via an endoscope, and the mucosa is then observed for signs of a reaction. It is also possible to take biopsies of the gastric mucosa to study the histological changes and measure the tissue concentration of mediators of inflammation such as histamine.

Rectal challenge   The standard test to confirm a diagnosis of coeliac disease is the jejunal biopsy, in which a small portion of jejunal mucosa is obtained with the aid of a special capsule which is swallowed; when it has passed into the small intestine the capsule is triggered and withdrawn, containing a portion of intestinal mucosa which can be examined under the microscope. A suggested alternative test is the instillation of gluten into the rectum, in order to look for a reaction that would signify coeliac disease. The procedure requires several biopsies from the rectum, and it is uncertain whether the results are reliable.

Management

Dietary elimination

The management of food allergy consists largely of elimination from the diet of the trigger food or foods. Elimination diets are used both for diagnosis and treatment of food intolerance. A diet may be associated with an improvement in symptoms because of intolerance to the food or a placebo effect, or the improvement may have been a coincidence. The degree of avoidance that is necessary to prevent symptoms is highly variable. Some patients are intolerant to minute traces of food, but others may be able to tolerate varying amounts. Strict avoidance and prevention of symptoms are the aims in certain instances, but in many cases it is unknown whether allowing small amounts of a food trigger could lead to either enhanced sensitivity or the reverse, increasing tolerance. The duration required for dietary avoidance varies. For example, intolerance to food additives may last only a few years, whereas intolerance to peanuts is usually lifelong. Although food allergy is common in children, most have grown out of the problem by the age of 5 years; an important exception is those with nut allergy.

Malnutrition Malnutrition is a major risk of unsupervised diets.

Calcium Cow's milk is an important source of calcium, and avoidance of cow's milk and its products carries the risk of an inadequate intake of calcium. Unfortunately, it is far from clear what constitutes an adequate intake for various different age groups.

Protein, energy Milk, eggs, fish, meat, wheat and their respective manufactured food products are important sources of protein and energy. Avoidance of these without the provision of alternative sources of protein and energy leads to the risk of an inadequate intake; growth failure, serious malnutrition and weight loss are well-documented sequelae of unsupervised and inappropriate dietary elimination.

Iodine Cow's milk and dairy products are an important source of dietary iodine. Exclusion of cow's milk products and a number of other items from the diet, coupled with the consumption of large amounts of soya milk (which has been reported to cause hypothyroidism by increasing faecal loss of thyroxine), have resulted in hypothyroidism and growth failure due to dietary iodine deficiency.

High risk factors The risk of malnutrition from an elimination diet is particularly high in the following situations:

- The diet is not supervised by a dietitian.
- There is chronic disease prior to diagnosis, or concurrent chronic disease such as severe atopic eczema. The subject's nutrient requirements may be increased.
- Malabsorption or enteropathy increases the risk of malabsorption of nutrients.
- The subject is avoiding sunlight; the risk of vitamin D deficiency compounds the effects of a low calcium intake.
- The subject is already on a diet that excludes numerous foods, e.g. a vegan or macrobiotic diet.

The role of the dietitian The dietitian has three roles in the management of elimination diets. One is to ensure that the resulting diet is nutritionally adequate, and prevent potential deficiency states by recommending (in an infant) appropriate amounts of infant milk formula, and (in older children or adults) supplements of calcium, vitamins and so on. Another role is to advise how to avoid specific foods, particularly those contained in manufactured foods. The third role of the dietitian is to give suggestions as to how to make the diet practical and palatable, and suggest recipes for the use of a limited range of foods (e.g. how to make biscuits with potato flour).

Cow's milk protein avoidance Any form of cow's milk, whether fresh, skimmed, condensed or evaporated, needs to be avoided. Also forbidden are milk products containing casein, whey and nonfat milk solids. Where milk substitutes are required, the choice lies between formulae based on soya protein, casein hydrolysate or whey hydrolysate. Soya formulae are cheaper, but unsuitable for those who are also intolerant to soya.

Butter, margarine, cream, cheese, ice cream and yogurt all need to be avoided. Fats that can be used instead include margarines made from pure vegetable fat (e.g. Tomor) and lard.

Caution is required with baby foods, as a large number of manufactured products (e.g. rusks) contain milk protein.

A common trap is so-called 'vegetarian' cheese, often wrongly believed to be safe for subjects with cow's milk allergy; in fact it differs from ordinary cheese only by the use of nonanimal rennet, and is unsuitable for people with cow's milk allergy.

Meat, game and poultry are all allowed, but sausages and pies should be avoided unless it is known that they are milk-free. Intolerance to cow's milk protein is not a reason to avoid beef.

Eggs are allowed, but not custard or scrambled egg which may contain milk.

Fish is allowed, unless it is cooked in batter (which unless otherwise stated should be assumed to contain milk) or milk.

Lemon curd, chocolate spread, chocolate (unless stated to be milk-free), toffee, fudge, caramels and butterscotch are all unsuitable.

All ordinary cereals (e.g. oats) are allowed, but caution is required with manufactured breakfast cereals, some of which contain milk powder.

It is essential to check the list of ingredients on the label of any manufactured food. There is a special problem with unwrapped foods, because there is no label of ingredients. Examples include bread, sausages and confectionery.

Egg avoidance Eggs (both the white and the yolk), and all products that contain egg or albumen, must be avoided. As well as chicken's eggs, eggs of other birds such as geese, turkeys and quails must be avoided. Eggs are widely used to make cakes, and are sometimes used in the manufacture of bread. Egg wash or glaze is commonly brushed on to the surface of rolls, buns or baps, and also on bread, cakes and pastry used in puddings (e.g. apple pie). Sweets can be a hazard because they are usually sold without information about ingredients, and egg is included in several products.

Mayonnaise should contain egg; custard usually does not, with the exception of egg custard and egg custard tarts. Eggs are an essential ingredient of soufflés and certain sauces, such as béarnaise or hollandaise sauce.

Egg allergy is not a reason to avoid eating chicken.

Soya avoidance   The major difficulty is massproduced bread, because in the UK soya is often included as an ingredient in flour. Soya is also found in manufactured products that contain hydrolysed or textured vegetable protein, and minced beef which unless described as 'pure beef' has been known to include quantities of soya protein.

'Wheat-free' and 'gluten-free'   These terms cause confusion; they are not interchangeable. Subjects who are allergic to wheat cannot tolerate foods that contain any type of wheat. Subjects with coeliac disease can tolerate all wheat proteins other than the gluten fraction.

Peanut avoidance   Peanut is also known as groundnut or arachis, so these three names need to be sought on labels of manufactured foods as well as some pharmaceutical products. The difficulty comes with 'vegetable oil', which may mean peanut oil; only by writing to the manufacturer of individual products can the identity of the vegetable oil be determined. It is not known to what extent subjects with peanut allergy should avoid peanut oil. Most peanut oil used in food manufacture is highly refined, and contains only very minute quantities of peanut protein. In small-scale studies, when subjects with peanut allergy were given highly refined peanut oil there was no reaction. However, it remains possible that such oil contains traces of protein sufficient to result in enhanced reactivity, so that when the subject does ingest peanut accidentally the reaction is worse than previously. On the latter grounds, subjects with peanut allergy are advised to avoid peanut oil.

Drug treatment

Drug treatment has little part to play in the management of food allergy. There are two exceptions. Firstly, in a very small number of cases the reaction to a food is exclusively gastrointestinal, and in these subjects the reaction can be blocked by taking the drug sodium cromoglycate by mouth 20 min before the trigger food is swallowed. Secondly, there are a small number of individuals who develop a lifethreatening reaction, anaphylactic shock, when exposed to a trigger food. If this occurs, urgent medical attention (within minutes) is essential. Subjects who have already had a life-threatening allergic reaction to a food are commonly issued with a preloaded adrenaline syringe to be administered while waiting for medical help. Self-administered adrenaline is not without its hazards, however (e.g. inadvertent intravenous administration causing fatal cardiac arrest), may not be effective in all cases. Nevertheless, it is the best hope for someone who is experiencing a lifethreatening allergic reaction to a food. The need for urgent medical help cannot be overemphasized.

There is little evidence that antihistamine drugs are of any value. It would be reasonable to take a nonsedating, quick-acting antihistamine such as terfenadine if experiencing an allergic reaction to a food, but it is questionable whether it will have much effect.

Desensitization

In theory it ought to be possible to desensitize subjects with food allergy by giving injections of gradually increasing quantities of an appropriate extract of the food trigger. In practice, such treatment is not available. One at present insurmountable difficulty is that desensitization (also known as hyposensitization) treatment carries a small risk of death from the treatment itself. A subject may have a series of injections without any major problem, but develop fatal anaphylactic shock after the next injection. There is some evidence that desensitization performed in this way can work, but such subjects would probably require maintenance injections on a permanent basis, and the very subjects most at risk of fatal anaphylaxis from accidental injection are quite probably also the ones most at risk from fatal anaphylaxis resulting from the desensitization treatment.

See also: **Calcium**: Physiology. **Colonic Diseases and Disorders**: Nutritional Management. **Dairy Products**: Nutritional Value. **Drugs**: Drug-Nutrient Interactions. **Eggs**: Nutritional Value. **Food Allergies**: Aetiology. **Food Intolerance**: Types and Incidence. **Iodine**: Iodine Deficiency Disorders. **Malnutrition**: Definition, Classification and Epidemiology. **Protein**: Requirements and Role in Diet.

Further Reading

Acciai MC, Brusi C, Francalanci S, Gola M and Sertoli A (1991) Skin tests with fresh foods. *Contact Dermatitis* 24:67–68.

Ancona GR and Schumacher IC (1950) The use of raw foods as skin testing material in allergic disorders. *California Medicine* 73:473–475.

Bernstein IL (1988) Proceedings of the task force guidelines for standardizing old and new techniques used for the diagnosis and treatment of allergic diseases. *Journal of Allergy and Clinical Immunology* 82:487–526.

Bock SA, Buckley J, Holst A and May CD (1977) Proper use of skin tests with food extracts in diagnosis of hypersensitivity to food in children. *Clinical Allergy* 7:375–383.

Bock SA, Sampson HA, Atkins FM *et al.* (1988) Double-blind, placebo-controlled food challenge as an office procedure: a manual. *Journal of Allergy and Clinical Immunology* 82:986–997.

Bousquet J (1988) In vivo methods for study of allergy: skin tests, techniques, and interpretation. In: Middleton E, Reed CE, Ellis EF, Adkinson NF and Yunginger JW (eds) *Allergy: Principles and Practice*, pp 419–436. St Louis: Mosby.

Curran WS and Goldman G (1961) The incidence of immediately reacting allergy skin tests in a 'normal' adult population. *Annals of Internal Medicine* 55:777–783.

David TJ (1984) Anaphylactic shock during elimination diets for severe atopic eczema. *Archives of Disease in Childhood* 59:983–986.

David TJ (1987) Reactions to dietary tartrazine. *Archives of Disease in Childhood* 62:119–122.

David TJ (1989) Hazards of challenge tests in atopic dermatitis. *Allergy* 101–107.

David TJ (1993) *Food and Food Additive Intolerance in Childhood*. Oxford: Blackwell Scientific Publications.

Fontana VJ, Wittig H and Holt LM (1963) Observations on the specificity of the skin test. The incidence of positive skin tests in allergic and nonallergic children. *Journal of Allergy* 34:348–353.

Ford RPK and Taylor B (1982) Natural history of egg hypersensitivity. *Archives of Disease in Childhood* 57:649–652.

Fries JH and Glazer I (1950) Studies on the antigenicity of banana, raw and dehydrated. *Journal of Allergy* 21:169–175.

Goldman AS, Anderson DW, Sellers WA, Saperstein S, Kniker WT and Halpern SR (1963) 1. Oral challenge with milk and isolated milk proteins in allergic children. *Pediatrics* 32:425–443.

Hill DJ, Duke AM, Hosking CS and Hudson IL (1988) Clinical manifestations of cows' milk allergy in childhood. II. The diagnostic value of skin tests and RAST. *Clinical Allergy* 18:481–490.

Josephson BM and Glaser J (1963) A comparison of skin-testing with natural foods and commercial extracts. *Annals of Allergy* 21:33–40.

Kagi MK and Wuthrich B (1991) Falafel-burger anaphylaxis due to sesame seed allergy. *Lancet* 338:582–583.

Lessof MH, Buisseret PD, Merrett J, Merrett TG and Wraith DG (1980) Assessing the value of skin tests. *Clinical Allergy* 10:115–120.

Meglio P, Farinella F, Trogolo E and Giampietro PG (1988) Immediate reactions following challenge-tests in children with atopic dermatitis. *Allergie Immunologie* 20:57–62.

Nater JP and Zwartz JA (1967) Atopic allergic reactions due to raw potato. *Journal of Allergy* 40:202–206.

Patterson R (1985) *Allergic Diseases. Diagnosis and Management*, 3rd edn. Philadelphia: Lippincott.

Patel L, Radivan FS and David TJ (1994) Management of anaphylactic reactions to food. *Archives of Disease in Childhood* 71:370–375.

Voorhorst R (1980) Perfection of skin testing technique. *Allergy* 35:247–261.

FOOD CHOICE

Factors Influencing Food Choice

R Shepherd and **D Mela**, Institute of Food Research, Reading, UK

Copyright © 1998 Academic Press

It is commonly recognized that humans raised in a given cultural environment consume and tend to prefer certain customary foods and flavour combinations. However, within a culture or family, different individuals also express varied liking and selection of specific foods. Possible underlying explanations for the emergence of similarities and differences amongst individuals can be drawn from both the social and biological sciences. Factors influencing food choice operate and can be examined at many levels, ranging from very basic, unlearned behaviours, through psychobiologically and socially reinforced preferences, through individual and culturally derived attitudes, beliefs and practices, to external economic and physical constraints on food acquisition, storage and use.

What Influences Food Choice?

From among all the possible foods in the world, why do we choose particular ones to eat? Why are some edible materials not even considered to be foods? Why do people from different cultures eat different foods? Why do two people with the same culture and similar backgrounds have different preferences for foods and hence different diets? The answers to these questions are far from straightforward. Eating provides nutrition and fulfils biological needs but it is also a source of pleasure and comfort, and reflects and conveys information about social status and relationships.

Food choice, like any complex human behaviour, will be influenced by many interrelated influences, and a number of researchers have proposed schemes to describe these. Such models in general do not attempt to explain the likely mechanisms of action of the different factors. They can be useful in pointing to what we need to measure in research, but do not offer a framework within which to design investigations, nor a basis upon which to build theories of the processes of human food choice.

The examples of models shown in **Figs 1–3** illustrate the large number of variables which may be of interest. In general, these variables can be divided into those related to the food, to the person making the choice, and to the external environment. Some of the chemical and physical properties of the food are perceived in terms of flavour, texture or appearance. These sensory attributes do not, of themselves, directly determine whether a person will choose a food but rather the person's liking for an attribute in a particular food will be the determining factor. Sensory perceptions, in turn, develop from and are influenced by both the psychobiological effects of foods and external environmental factors (see below). Within a particular culture there is a great deal of agreement on how appropriate certain sensory attributes are for particular foods, but there are also substantial differences between individuals in their preferences, which will in part lead to different food choices and diets. Understanding these individual differences in preferences and food choice is of major concern in determining the factors influencing patterns of food selection.

In addition to these types of influences there are influences from the wider environment, including social and cultural factors and marketing, advertising and availability of the foods. The influence of many of these marketing and economic variables may be

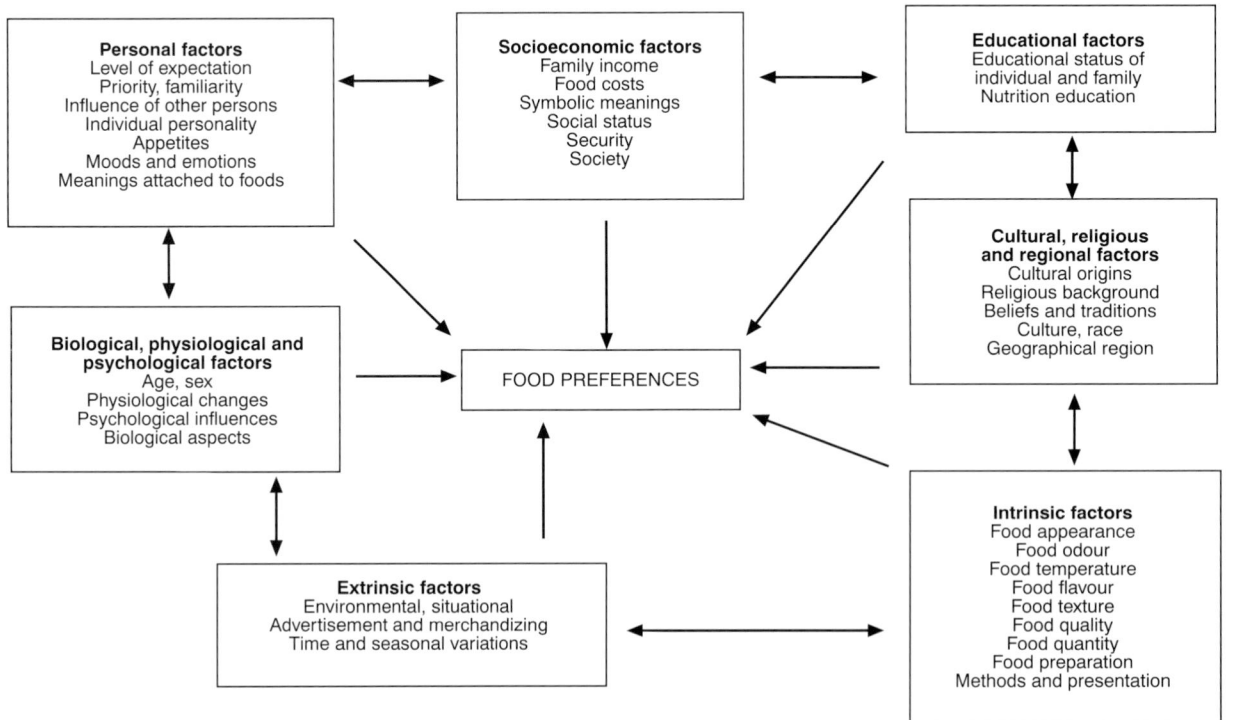

Figure 1 Factors influencing food preferences. Reprinted with permission from Khan (1981) *CRC Critical Reviews in Food Science and Nutrition* 15:129–153. Copyright CRC Press.

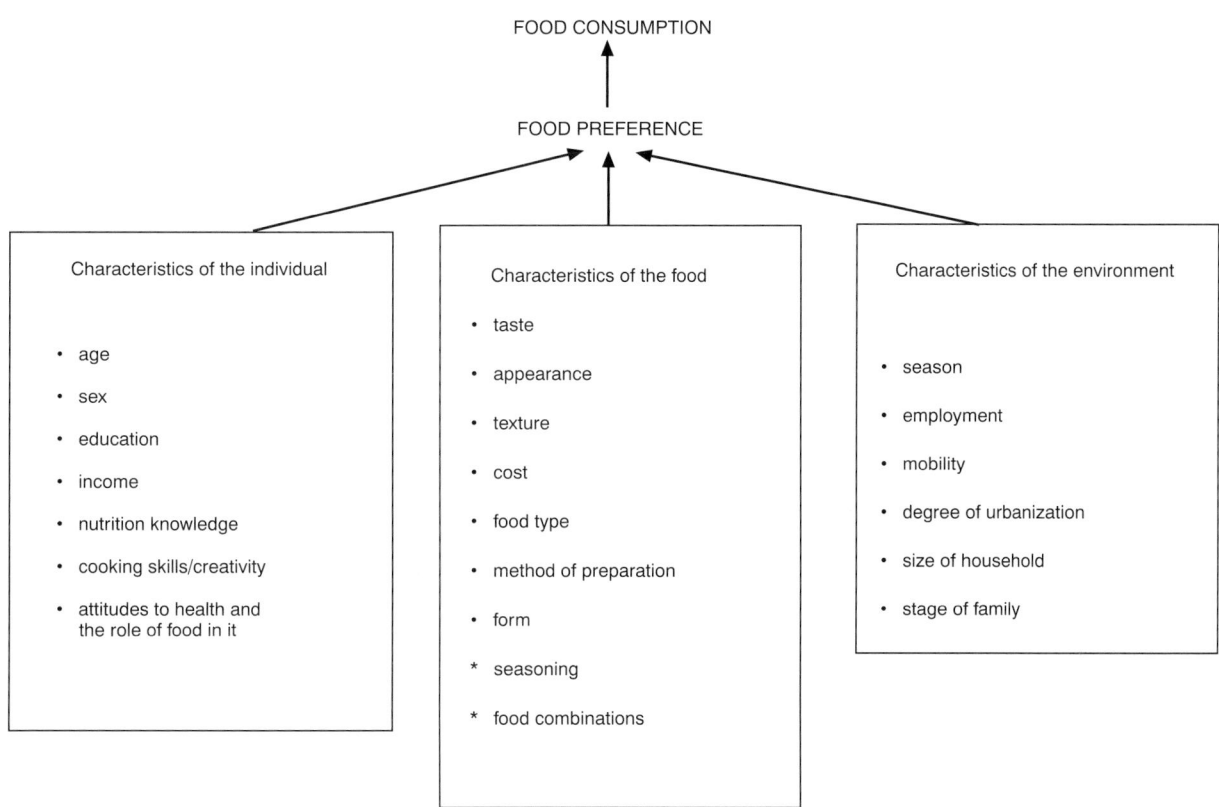

Figure 2 Factors influencing food preferences. From Randall and Sanjur (1981), with permission from Gordon and Breach Science Publishers.

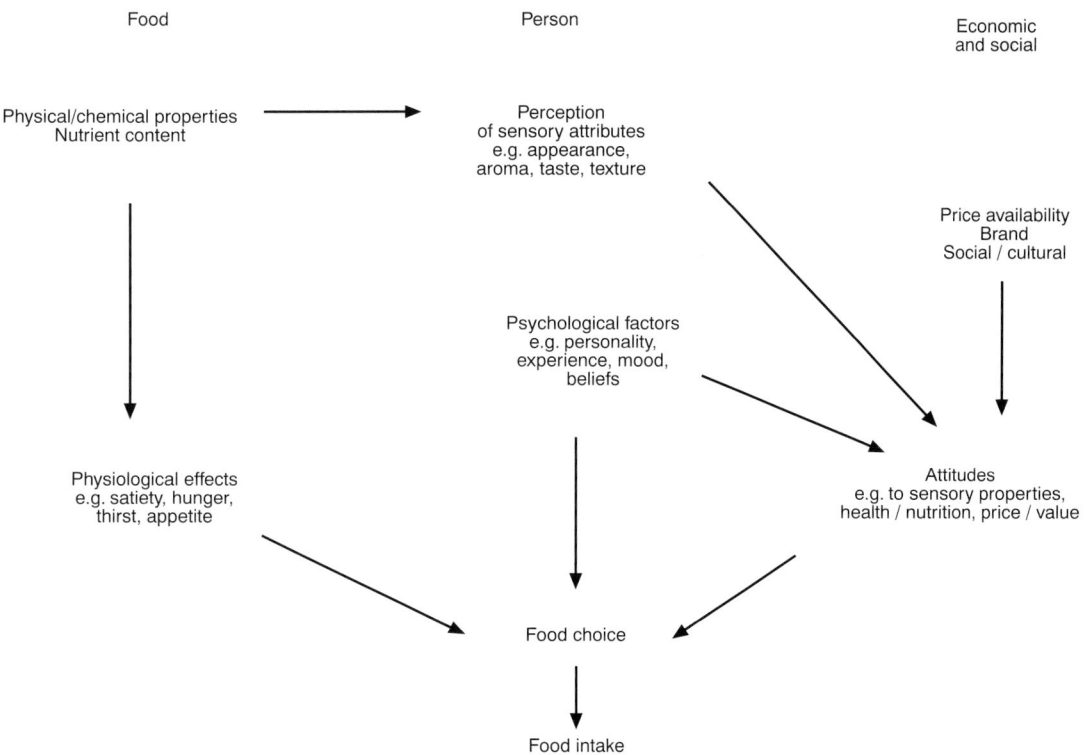

Figure 3 Some of the possible factors affecting food choice and intake.

mediated by people's attitudes and beliefs, as may the influence of social, cultural, religious or demographic factors. So, in addition to sensory qualities, a person's *beliefs* about other less immediately verifiable attributes (such as nutritional quality and health benefits) of a food may be more important than the *actual* attributes in influencing a person's choice.

There has been a good deal of research into how food choice is related to particular people's beliefs, attitudes and intentions. Much of the work has made use of social psychological theories of attitude-behaviour relationships, in particular the theory of reasoned action and its extension in the form of the theory of planned behaviour. Generally, this research has shown a clear prediction of behaviour from intention, which in turn is influenced by attitudes, social pressure and perceptions of control over choices. In turn, attitudes are predicted by beliefs about the outcome of a particular behaviour and the value attached to that outcome by the individual. More recently, emphasis has been placed on the importance of moral, or ethical, considerations in influencing food choices as well as on the issues of image and identity. This line of research tends to characterize people as carefully weighing up all the costs and benefits of their choices in a rational manner, although attempts are made to incorporate the assessment of more impulsive, affective or emotional factors which may also be highly influential in choice decisions.

The Role of Culture

Culture is one of the most obvious influences on food preferences and choice, and often has strong historical antecedents, rooted in the geography, climate and range of native plant and animal species, which are then integrated into 'traditional' rules of cuisine and appropriateness. If we look at people from different cultures they make very different choices from each other, some of which are simply caused by external constraints on food availability, but others of which occur even where the cultural and geographical variations are relatively small (e.g. within northern Europe). This has been explored within the discipline of anthropology following two distinct lines of research, social anthropology and a more 'biocultural' approach.

The approach taken in social anthropology is often one of seeking to understand consumption practices as indicative of wider social structures and relationships: for example, different castes in India are associated with different food consumption practices. Some people would describe food consumption prac-tices as expressing or symbolizing certain social relationships, although such terminology has been criticized as ambiguous. 'Functionalist' theoretical positions would indicate a more 'purposive' element in food choice decisions, emphasizing (for example) how choices might serve to reinforce such social differences and maintain the status quo. Certainly, there is a large body of thinking within the social sciences which would support the notion that food choices may serve to affirm or bolster cultural, social or personal distinctiveness for particular groups and individuals.

The biocultural tradition has argued for an interaction between biological factors and the evolution of cultural traditions. An example of this is the rituals surrounding the preparation of 'blue corn' by the Hopi North Americal native populations. Although maize has been an important crop in North and Central America for a long time, raw maize has serious nutritional shortcomings and if consumed as a staple can lead to pellagra, a disease of niacin deficiency. Treatment with alkali can, however, release significant amounts of otherwise unavailable niacin. Many North and Central American natives use maize to make some form of tortilla or bread, which are traditionally prepared by boiling the maize in alkaline limewater. Thus they have developed an elaborate method of food processing that can have an important nutritional benefit. While people from such societies would not (and do not) describe the reasons for these production methods in terms of any nutritional benefit, and the rituals around them have great symbolic meaning for the people, it can be argued that the benefits conveyed by these forms of production and their establishment into unquestioned rituals give an advantage to that society.

Rituals and traditions surrounding foods occur in every culture. It is, however, far more difficult to strip away the surface of those of our own culture in order to understand any underlying reasons and motivations, because those around us share that culture and hence food practices often remain unquestioned; they 'just seem natural' or they are 'what we have always done'.

Economic and Social Influences on Food Choice

Income can be clearly seen to be related to the foods that people choose. In the UK, for example, there is evidence that unemployed people and those in households where someone is in receipt of state benefits may be at greater nutritional risk. A social gradient in food intakes is particularly apparent for fresh fruits and vegetables. A number of recent reports have pointed to the difficulties encountered by people on low incomes in trying to secure a healthy diet.

However, the relationship between income and food choice is not a simple one and it requires more thorough investigation. While income places constraints on selection, different social groups also develop their own preferences and tastes. Not only are different social groups likely to be associated with particular likes (both in relation to food and otherwise) but knowledge of such classifications may lead to particular food choices because of the value of a particular classification that accompanies that choice. Selection of particular foods is then thought to be influenced not only by, for example, sensory liking and nutritional benefits, but also by the knowledge of the symbolic value associated with a particular food. Thus, for example, consumption of different forms of meat can often be associated with status differences, and a particular type of meat may be consequently consumed (or avoided) in order to attempt to establish or emphasize such associations.

Choices are not made by individuals in isolation and there is a need to consider these choices within the social context. In particular, the family unit appears likely to play a major role in determining the choice of foods, although there has been little work directly on how family decisions are made in this regard. One study found that men had little input into family food selection or food preparation, although they were more involved in older families. In newly married couples husbands changed their eating habits more on marrying than did wives, although there were differences between types of foods in these compromises. On the other hand, there is also some evidence of men's control over the constituents of family diets even though women tend to do most of the shopping and food preparation. The role of gender in food choice and acquisition can vary widely across different cultural and social groups, with some groups having clearly reinforced rules of behaviour. Interactions between family members in decision-making, the influence of family members on the choice of others and the potential changes in the social function of family meals brought about by changes in life style and technology (e.g. microwave ovens, freezers) remain to be more fully researched.

Acquisition of Sensory and Food Preferences

Unlearned preferences

Humans appear to have a limited battery of unlearned and universal sensory preferences. The results of a large number of studies examining responsiveness to simple tastes and smell stimuli by infants suggest that humans are born with positive hedonic responses to sweetness, and probably a dislike for bitter and sour tastes. Ability to sense (and like) salty stimuli probably develops 3–6 months postnatally in humans, and there may also be some postnatal maturation of bitter taste perception. There are a number of lines of evidence that support the view that these responses are truly unlearned (congenital), but this does not exclude the possibility of their subsequent modification by later experience and learning (e.g. the liking for bitterness in coffee or beer). Teleological explanations have often been put forward to account for these apparently universal human chemical sensitivities and preferences. For example, the liking for sweetness is attributed to the fact that naturally occurring sweeteners are associated with safe sources of energy and selected nutrients. Salt taste is suggested to promote ingestion of sufficient sodium and, perhaps, other minerals. Many natural toxicants are bitter-tasting, and it is widely accepted that bitter taste perception provides animals with the capacity to recognize such substances and avoid them.

Compared with studies of simple tastes, far less is established regarding possible unlearned preferences for specific odours (aromas) and foods, and little work has been carried out on volatile odours or more complex systems or food models. Also, there are no discrete, agreed categories of odours from which representative compounds might be easily selected for testing. While likings for a number of food-related and other aromas show many broad general similarities across different human populations, this may better reflect shared experiences with common environmental odours than a specific genetic predisposition. There is good evidence that young infants rapidly learn to recognize and respond to specific environmental and food-related odours. This has been shown with human infants within hours of birth, and animal research demonstrates potentially important learned responses following *in utero* exposure through maternal diets. Recent work also points to an attraction of human newborns to specific maternal odours such as amniotic fluid and lactating breasts, which seems likely to be an expression of associations learned before or during the perinatal period.

Broad similarities in food preferences within ethnic groups or families may result from genetic similarities as well as from social interactions and common environmental exposure. One question which often arises in this area is, within a particular society, how much influence do social and learning factors have when compared with these genetic factors?

While genetic factors are known to markedly influence the ability to sense certain specific taste and odour compounds, less is known about the heritability of taste and smell preferences. As noted, although there are clearly identifiable cultural food preferences, largely conveyed to children by adults, a paradox appears when one moves into a finer analysis, where the food preferences of children are typically found to be no better related to those of their own parents than to another child's parent. They seem to represent cultural norms rather than accounting for differences between families within the same culture.

Studies of twins have had mixed results, but point to significant genetic influences on intakes of nutrients and perhaps some specific foods. The genetic influences tend to be small relative to general environmental effects; however, notably, shared family environment does not appear to be a major contributor to similarities of dietary habits of adult twins. Most of the differences between people in preferences and choices seem to be related to learning, much of which may take place within a social context. While learning within the family is undoubtedly a primary route for the transmission of general cultural norms, the evidence for family background as a determinant of variation in the food preferences and intakes of individuals within a culture is relatively weak.

Learned preferences

What mechanisms might explain the development of preferences with experience? The common notion that increased liking for foods or flavours can occur by 'mere exposure' is supported by experimental studies, although exposure is rarely 'mere'. Usually, foods are not simply presented in a neutral way on repeated occasions, but are instead associated in some way with social situations or postingestive physiological consequences which may prompt the development of likes or dislikes.

Psychobiological influences on development of food preferences Humans and other animals are endowed with the ability to recognize and learn about the consequences – metabolic, physiological, and psychological – associated with the ingestion of specific foods or sensory characteristics. These types of learned responses are highly robust. They can supersede innate preferences and, particulary evident for aversions, may be extremely stable.

Development of prompt and persistent dislike or aversions to specific sensory qualities or foods can occur when they are associated with negative outcomes, particularly nausea and gastrointestinal upset. Such aversions are most readily directed toward novel or less preferred foods. A large proportion (up to 65%) of people report at least one strong food aversion, and it appears that aversions are acquired most frequently during childhood. This is when many foods are tried for the first time and when the frequency of sickness with gastrointestinal symptoms may be particulary high. Some aversions which develop in childhood still persist 50 years later. The dislike of the food typically remains long after the initial incident is forgotten, and often despite knowledge that the item is known to be safe to eat or did not cause the illness. Thus, food aversion learning is a powerful phenomenon which may account for many apparently idiosyncratic and strong dislikes for the 'taste' of particular foods.

In a similar manner, though perhaps less readily, it appears that human sensory preferences can be fostered by pairing specific qualities with positively 'rewarding' physiological or psychological outcomes. It is more difficult to produce convincing examples of conditioned preferences, since the process may occur more gradually than aversions and be less accessible to conscious association. The sensation of a food (i.e. perception of its flavour) is probably unchanged, but the centrally determined affective response is altered. It seems reasonable to ascribe the development or maintenance of liking for such (innately disliked) items such as coffee and alcoholic beverages to their rewarding psychobiological effects. The apparent human preference for the sensory properties of fats in foods also cannot be reliably related to established inborn mechanisms; the available evidence suggests that this is secondary to their association with the metabolic or other aftereffects of ingestion of fat-containing foods.

The significant role of conditioned responses in food preferences is well supported by animal research, though definitive human studies are lacking. Furthermore, the influence of psychological (e.g. mood and performance) effects of foods on subsequent food liking remains to be elucidated. The biological advantage of a capacity to modify preferences based on the benefit derived from consuming a food is obvious, and it is likely that such learning processes play an important role in determining sensory responsiveness, and guiding food choice and intake.

Social transmission of food preferences It is clear that social contacts and settings can have a marked influence on food preference and consumption. This starts early in life, where an important influence motivating initial and repeated experiences with foods is peer pressure. Studies show that the preferences of young children can be readily manipulated by the presence of other children expressing particular preferences. The use of foods as rewards may also have interesting effects on expressed preferences. Food may be used in two different ways: the food itself can be a reward, e.g. a snack given to a child for performing a task, or its consumption can be rewarded, e.g. 'Eat up your greens and you can watch television'. Often eating one food (such as vegetables) will be rewarded with another highly preferred one (such as a sweet dessert item). In experimental trials, when a significant adult such as a teacher used a neutral snack food as a reward this was found to increase liking for the snack. On the other hand, when eating a neutral food was rewarded with being able to play, consumption of the target food initially increased; however, when the reward was subsequently removed, liking for the food fell to *below* its initial level. That is, rewarding consumption of a food has been found to decrease children's liking of it.

One explanation of these results is in terms of a psychological theory of self-perception. If children eat a target food it may well be acceptable and even liked, unless they can see an external reason for eating it. In the rewarded case there is an external reason: 'I'm only doing this so that I can do something I want to'. In the case where the target food acts as a reward, the opposite is true and the child thinks, 'I must like this food because I am eating it without any external force and I am even doing other things in order to earn it'.

Do parents use these techniques to increase children's liking for 'desirable' or 'healthy' foods? In a small survey of American parents the two most popular methods mentioned were helping with preparation of the food and adults displaying how much they liked the food. None spontaneously said they used the food as a reward but a number said they rewarded consumption of the food. Thus, some of the actions of parents are contrary to what the experimental research findings would recommend. One problem with implementing the findings of this research, though, is that it applies to initially neutral foods and not to highly disliked foods. It is unlikely to be effective to offer a highly disliked food as a reward, since children will see this as nonsensical from a very early age.

Although children's food-related learning and attitudinal development progresses towards adult attitudes and preferences, food also offers a means for rebellion and the display of distinctive non-adult behaviours. For example, research on older children has shown a subculture of children's preferred sweets with names, colours and taste sensations differentiating them from ordinary sweets and from other foods, and it is suggested that such sweets represent a rebellion against the adult world. There was also an important element of sharing and trading these items, further emphasizing the social element in this type of food. Other research has shown increased appeal to children of items like walnuts and dates presented in forms differentiated to be more attractive to children, and the appeal of such items can be enhanced by the 'not-for-adults' image.

Use of food to make such social statements is clearly not limited to children, and there are innumerable examples of adult foods and beverages which are heavily marketed using implicit or explicit reference to the social image which would be projected by use of the product. Indeed, there are entire product ranges (e.g. spirits, bottled waters), where objective recognition of the subtle differences between brands would in truth not be possible for most consumers, who make their selection based on a judgment of cost, believed (but not detected) product quality, and the image projected (to others) by the label.

Conclusions

At the broadest level, the geocultural and agroeconomic environment shape food choice by influencing the range of foods available to human populations. These are also incorporated into general cultural rules for cuisine and appropriate eating behaviour, which strongly dictate much of what foods and food combinations will be eaten, when, how, and by whom.

At the individual level, it is possible to identify a number of psychobiological and social forces which act upon the acquisition, maintenance and expression of food choices. Although sensory-affective responses may be an important influence on food choice, it is likely that humans are congenitally endowed with few specific taste preferences. Most of the responses to more complex foods are therefore learned, and some of this learning can begin at a very early point in life. It is clear that humans and other animals are endowed with the ability to recognize and learn from the contexts and consequences associated with ingestion of specific foods or sensory qualities, and many examples of human likes and dislikes for specific foods can be best explained by such processes. Liking for specific sensory qualities can be acquired or modified by their temporal linkage with physiological, psychological, pharmacological or social events and contexts. These various types of experience and learning about foods may form a powerful and lasting force in subsequent food beliefs and acceptance. Indeed, many seemingly idiosyncratic food preferences of individual adults could have their roots in early childhood, suckling or even fetal experiences. However, food preferences are clearly dynamic and responsive to differences and shifts in their associations with particular socio-environmental contexts and psychobiological effects, and therefore liable to change with development and experience.

It is nevertheless important to recognize that food choice may often have little to do with sensory-affective judgments. This is not just because of external (e.g. financial or cultural) influences, but because foods are selected in accordance with individual attitudes toward a wide range of perceived qualities, including nutritional and functional attributes. Food selections also represent a strong medium for expression of personal and cultural values.

See also: **Food Intolerance**: Types and Incidence. **Fruits and Vegetables**: Nutritional Value. **Niacin**: Pellagra. **Religious Customs**: Influence on Diet. **Socioeconomic Status**: Relationship with Diet and Nutritional Status.

Further Reading

Fieldhouse P (1986) *Food and Nutrition: Customs and Culture*. London: Chapman & Hall.

Friedman MI, Tordoff MG and Kare MR, eds (1991) *Chemical Senses*, vol. 4, *Appetite and Nutrition*. New York: Marcel Dekker.

Khan MA (1981) Evaluation of food selection patterns and preferences. *CRC Critical Reviews in Food Science and Nutrition* 15:129–153.

Lyman B (1989) *A Psychology of Food*, New York: AVI.

Meiselman HL and Macfie HJH, eds (1996) *Food Choice, Acceptance and Consumption*. London: Blackie.

Mela DJ and Catt SL (1996) Ontogeny of human taste and smell preferences and their implications for food selection. In: Henry CJK and Ulijaszek SJ (eds) *Long Term Consequences of Early Environment: Growh, Development and the Lifespan Development Perspective*, Society for the Study of Human Biology Symposium Series 37, pp 139–154. Cambridge University Press.

Randall E and Sanjur D (1981) Food preferences – their conceptualization and relationship to consumption. *Ecology of Food and Nutrition* 11:151–161.

Shepherd R, ed. (1989) *Handbook of the Psychophysiology of Human Eating*. Chichester: Wiley.

Solms J, Booth DA, Pangborn RM and Raunhardt O, eds (1987) *Food Acceptance and Nutrition*. London: Academic Press.

FOOD COMPOSITION DATA

Compilation, Uses and Limitations

D A T Southgate, formerly of the Institute of Food Research, Norwich, UK

Copyright © 1998 Academic Press

A knowledge of the composition of foods is essential for the dietary management of patients and for most quantitative research on human nutrition. This information has traditionally been provided by tables of food composition and, since the 1970s, increasingly by computerized nutritional data bases. Data on the composition of foods from these compilations are also widely used in nutritional surveillance and in assessments of the adequacy of food supplies and for nutritional labelling.

Compilation

Assembling compilations on the composition of foods for both food composition tables and nutritional data bases involves the same processes and principles. The process of compilation involves assembling the data in a consistent format which can be used conveniently and accurately by the users of the compilation. Since data bases are essentially 'tools' for the nutritionist and others to use, compilation involves a dialogue with users in order to establish their requirements. In most countries the compilation is carried out centrally either in a government department or agency, or a research institute (usually with government funding). These compilation groups typically have steering committees which include representatives of users to ensure that the data bases develop to meet the users' requirements.

Compilation requires three basic decisions: first, the range of constituents to be included; second, the range of food items to be included; and third, how to obtain the data.

Constituents

Most compilations include a reasonably comprehensive range of nutrients but the growth of nutritional research interests in the role of other biologically active constituents is increasing pressures for extending the number of constituents to include these 'non-nutrients'. The coverage is usually determined by the most demanding of the users, who tend to be nutritional epidemiologists and nutritional researchers. The typical coverage in a nutritional data base is given in **Table 1**.

The inclusion of a constituent is conditional on there being a satisfactory method for analysing the nutrient and the existence of a sufficient body of information on the amounts of the nutrient in a range of foods to assess its inherent variability. This latter factor will determine whether or not it is

Table 1 Coverage of nutrients in nutritional data bases

Constituent	Mode of expression	Notes on extent of coverage
Water		Most
Total nitrogen		Most
Protein	Calculated from total nitrogen	All: some use common 6.25 factor; others use specific factors for different food groups
Amino acids	mg amino acid per g N *or* mg per 100 g food	Usually in subsidiary compilations
Fat (total)		All
Fatty acids	Fatty acid % total fatty acids *or* g per 100 g food	Usually in subsidiary compilations
Carbohydrates (total)	Often by difference *or* by summation of sugars and starches	Summation is the preferred approach
Sugars	May be expressed as the monosaccharides	Many, but individual sugars given in a few data bases
Starches	May be expressed as glucose or as the polymer	Many
Nonstarch polysaccharides (NSP)	Usually expressed as polymer	UK and related data bases
Dietary fibre	NSP in UK; from Total Dietary Fiber method in US and many other compilations	No international agreement on definition or method as yet. Data rather limited
Alcohol	g per 100 g or per 100 ml	Most for relevant foods
Energy value	kcal or kJ, calculated from protein, fat, carbohydrate and alcohol	All, but choice of conversion factors differs between data bases
Inorganic nutrients		
Na, K, Ca, Mg, P, Cl	mg per 100 g food	Most
Cu, Fe, Zn	mg per 100 g food	Many
F, I, Se, etc.	μg per 100 g food	Limited coverage
Vitamins		
Fat-soluble:		Most
vitamin A	As retinol	
vitamin D	As cholecalciferol	
vitamin E	As α-tocopherol	
Carotenes	As β-carotene or as retinol equivalents	Most; a few give values for different carotenoids
vitamin K	Phylloquinone	Very limited
Water-soluble:		
vitamin C	mg per 100 g food	All
thiamin		
riboflavin		
niacin		
vitamin B$_6$		Most
folates	μg per 100 g food	
vitamin B$_{12}$	μg per 100 g food	Most
Pantothenic acid	mg per 100 g food	Many
Biotin		

possible to provide representative data for the amount of the nutrient in a range of foods. In many cases data may only be available for a limited number of foods, or it may only be sensible to give data for a limited number of foods for a variety of reasons, and many compilations include subsidiary or complementary tables giving this more limited coverage.

At this stage the compilers will consider the modes of expression that will be used. These are based on official International Union of Nutritional Sciences (IUNS) nomenclature with the occasional exceptions where national nomenclature rules differ.

Food items

Decisions about which food items to include are the most difficult for the compiler because of the wide range of foods in the human diet. Complete coverage of all the foods on sale in a developed country would require a data base with tens of thousands of food items. However, complete coverage of all the foods consumed, which in the main consist of complex, mixed, cooked dishes, expands this number possibly by two orders of magnitude. All compilers therefore have to consider the priorities for inclusion of food items very critically.

Priorities for inclusion   In a national data base priority will be given to foods that form the major part of the food intake of the population. These are identified using national data on food consumption and a range of other information from market surveys, information on food purchasing patterns, and data from the food industry. In the UK this gives a list of between 200 and 500 food items which provide about 80% of the energy intake. To these must be added the foods consumed by specific groups; thus infant formulae which provide all the dietary intake of young babies must be included. The data base must also include the foods eaten by ethnic groups within the population and those with special dietary restrictions. Finally, most compilers aim to provide food items whose composition can be seen as examples of different types of food. Most national data bases do not provide information on the composition of specific brands of foods, unless the brand name is critical for identifying the food, or more rarely, the brand is an important market leader.

Food descriptions and nomenclature   Accurate use of a data base can only be made if the food item can be properly identified and related to, for example, the foods being consumed by the subjects in an epidemiological survey, and the systems of nomenclature used and deciding on the descriptions of the food items form an important part of the work of compilers. Even within a national data base there are wide differences in the names of foods used in different parts of the country, and most data bases provide a thesaurus of alternative names and the systematic (taxonomic) names of plants and animals to facilitate accurate identification of food items within the data base.

The increase in the number of international nutritional epidemiological studies has resulted in the wider use of national tables. This, in turn, has made the identification of food items and food nomenclature the topics of a number of international studies in attempts to formalize food descriptions. Some national data bases include coding systems developed to facilitate international usage, but this is not widespread at present.

Sourcing the data

It is possible to distinguish two approaches to obtaining the data for use in compilations, direct and indirect. A combination of the two approaches has been used for most compilations in current use. Whichever approach is adopted, careful documentation is required.

Direct approach   This involves the development of sampling and analytical programmes for obtaining the data. This approach has the advantage in that the compilers have control over the sampling protocols to ensure the identity of the food and that the sample is representative. They can also control the choice of analytical methods and the quality assurance schemes in operation in the analytical laboratory. The compilers are thus completely familiar with the provenance and quality of the data. This approach is, however, expensive. It can also be argued that this approach discounts the large amount of information available on the composition of foods in the scientific and other literature.

Indirect approach   In the indirect approach the literature on the composition of foods is searched for suitable data. This involves the compilers in making judgments about the applicability of the samples analysed, their identity and whether or not the sampling protocol ensured that a representative sample was analysed. Judgments also need to be made about the choice of analytical methods and the control of their execution. The modes of expression of data may also need to be converted into the form that will be used in the data base. The assessment process is demanding and time-consuming often because of inadequate documentation in much of the literature. Formal protocols have been developed for assessing the analytical quality of data, but the use of these is limited at present to a few nutrients. Assessing sampling protocols, which are critically important for the compiler, still requires expert judgment.

Combined approach In practice most national compilations are based on a combination of the two approaches, with literature searching typically forming the first stage in the data compilation process, followed by the design of sampling and analytical protocols whenever the reported data are judged to be inappropriate for use, or the search shows that little or no data exist for a food item that is required in the database.

Documentation

Most data bases – especially those available in hard copy versions – give textual introductions which describe the ways in which the data have been obtained, the analytical methods used and the modes of expression used for the nutrients. Many computerized data bases, however, do not contain this documentation, which is vital for the proper use of the data base. All compilers have usually had to adopt compromises when assembling the data, especially when dealing with missing values. They may also have some reservations about the analytical or sampling protocols and the overall quality of the data in the data base of which the users need to be aware. In a printed food composition table the presence of missing data and references to footnotes or the introductory text are easy to accommodate. Such facilities are more difficult, but not impossible, within a computerized system; nevertheless, reading the compilers' textual documentation is essential for proper use of any data base.

Accuracy

The accuracy of a data base can be judged in two senses. Firstly, how accurately does it document the composition of an individual food item? Secondly, how accurately does the data base as a whole perform as it is normally used?

Prediction of the composition of a food item

Prediction of food composition is determined by two factors, first the sampling protocol used to obtain the sample which was analysed (or the samples that were analysed in the literature sources used to provide the data). The compilers of data bases have the task of assembling representative data which apply to the country or region of the country for which the data base is prepared, and possibly also the time of year, for the item in question. This is in contrast to the analyst who is required to provide accurate compositional data on the specific sample presented for analysis.

Natural variability Second, the accuracy of the data given will be limited by the fact that all foods are biological materials and exhibit natural variations in their composition. This variation differs for different classes of foodstuff and for each nutrient. This means that the data base values, assuming that they are representative, will not necessary give the composition of an isolated sample of the same food item.

In general the composition of fresh plant foods, especially those with a high moisture content, shows more variability than drier foods such as cereals. However, with all foods the place of production, the production methods used and the storage conditions are responsible for considerable variability (greater than 10%) in the vitamins and many trace elements. Processed foods tend to show less variation than unprocessed foods, but even processed foods show variability depending on the composition of ingredients, which are controlled but cannot be standardized for all nutrients.

Some nutrients show great variability, either due to natural causes or because they are extremely labile and affected by the conditions under which a food has been stored or heated in cooking; for these nutrients nutritional data bases cannot give an accurate prediction of the amount that may be present in a food. Thus the vitamin C in a plant is profoundly affected by the level of illumination the plant has received and is also very susceptible to oxidation; as a consequence a nutritional data base can only reliably be seen as providing semiquantitative information. The folate vitamins are also heat-labile and readily oxidized, so that folate levels for cooked foods are approximate estimates. Many of the inorganic trace elements in foods are profoundly affected by the soil type and fertilizer treatments, so again it is difficult for compilers to give representative values. The fortification of animal feeds with fat-soluble vitamins can also cause considerable variation in the composition of food such as liver. Ideally a nutritional data base should include a measure of variability (standard deviation, standard error of the mean, or confidence limits) alongside each value in a data base; unfortunately for most nutrients and most foods insufficient analytical data are available to give this information.

Analytical variations Most of the analytical methods for nutrients are well established, and provided that a proper quality assurance system is in operation the methods have reasonable precision.

The precision with which the micronutrients, vitamins and trace inorganic nutrients can be measured is, as one would expect, not as good as that for the macronutrients or inorganic constituents such as sodium, potassium, calcium and phosphorus, which are present at levels exceeding 100 mg per 100 g of food. Compatible methods are available for many nutrients and as a general rule inaccuracies that can be ascribed to analytical causes are not very common. Differences can arise where the values obtained for a nutrient are method-dependent, such as those for fat and carbohydrates, although this is more strictly a question of conceptual definitions. Dietary fibre values are very dependent on the definition adopted and the method selected to translate the chosen definition into values. Folates values measured by microbiological assay depend on the organism used: *Streptococcus faecalis* gives lower values than *Lactobacillus caseii*.

Differences between data bases Differences between data bases are most commonly due to differences in modes of expression or because food items that are nominally the same are actually different foods, whether by formulation, method of preparation, or production under different conditions. Furthermore, the same brand name can be used for different products in different markets and vice versa.

Accuracy in use

Many users of nutritional data bases require a semiquantitative guide in order to give general dietetic advice; however, some dietetic uses require greater precision, for example in formulating diets for diabetic patients and low-sodium diets in hypertension; and even more accuracy is required by those who conduct nutritional analyses using the data base to calculate nutrient intakes from records of food intakes.

Relatively few large formal studies have been undertaken but these show that the calculated values for energy, protein, fat and available carbohydrates are usually within a few percentage points of the analysed values. The calculated values for potassium, calcium, phosphorus and magnesium show similar agreement. Analytical values for sodium are often in excess of calculated estimates because of the addition of salt in cooking, and analytical values for iron are similarly slightly higher, possibly because of iron contamination. The micronutrients are usually predicted with lower accuracy, probably around 10%, except for vitamin C and folates where the calculated values may be substantial overestimates.

It is important when comparing calculated values with analysed values to ensure that the amounts of foods making up the analysed diets are precisely the same amounts as used in the calculations; where collections are not supervised closely, the tendency is to undercollect.

Uses

Data bases can be considered to have three major uses: nutritional analysis, where the data base is used to calculate nutrient intakes from records of food consumption; nutritional synthesis, where the data base is used in calculations to generate diets with specific nutrient contents; and as a source of compositional information.

Nutritional analyses

In nutritional analyses the calculations may be based on food consumption measured at many different levels. These levels have important implications for the compiler of data bases because they set the requirements for compositional information appropriate to the level of measurement (**Table 2**).

Food supplies level Measurements at the food supplies level are widely used by governments and international agencies for assessing the nutritional adequacy of food supplies; the 'food balance sheets' of the Food and Agricultural Organization of the United Nations are one important example of this level of use. National data calculated in this way give information on food disappearance rather than food consumption in the strict sense. In order to meet this type of use the data base must give the composition of raw food at the wholesale level, e.g. the composition of bulk cereals and animal carcasses.

Food purchases level Measurements of food purchases are of two types: household budget studies, usually undertaken primarily for economic reasons where food consumption is derived from records of household purchases in monetary terms, and food surveys where the amounts of food purchased by a household are measured, of which the UK National Food Survey is an example. Both types of study require data for the composition of foods 'as purchased'. Household budgetary surveys also require information on retail prices to convert monetary expenditure into quantities of food.

Individual food intake level For studies of individual food intake, subjects provide records of food consumption either prospectively in a weighed intake study, or retrospectively; the amounts consumed are

Table 2   Requirements for food items and nutrients at different levels of data base usage

Level of use	Food items	Nutrients	General features of data base
Food supplies	Foods measured at raw, bulk or commodity level	Usually restricted to macronutrients and energy	Relatively small data base is required
Food purchases			
Household budget surveys	Foods as purchased, retail raw. Prices	Macronutrients, major inorganic nutrients and vitamins	Information needed on losses of food during preparation
Food consumption surveys	Foods as purchased retail or obtained raw	Macronutrients, major micronutrients	Information needed on losses of food during preparation
Individual food intakes	Foods as consumed, cooked, including mixed dishes	Comprehensive coverage of macro- and micronutrients	Requirements may extend to detailed coverage of constituents

obtained by the dietary recall method or a food frequency questionnaire. These types of study provide the most detailed records of foods consumed and have the most demanding requirements for the inclusion of food items in a data base because the records include specific branded foods and (more importantly) cooked, mixed dishes; that is, foods 'as consumed'.

Nutritional synthesis

Data bases are widely used by dietitians and other health-care professionals to calculate diets that will provide specific amounts of nutrients; for example, low-energy diets for the obese, diets controlling energy, carbohydrate and fats for the diabetic patient, and low-sodium diets in hypertension. This type of calculation requires the data base to contain the range of foods likely to be eaten by the patients in question, but the quantitative requirements may not be very demanding. Where diets with very precise composition are required, for example in metabolic studies, analyses of the foods are necessary.

At present most of these diets are formulated initially by manual calculation from the data base, but nutritional syntheses programs are becoming available to computerize the calculation. Because in principle there are an infinite number of solutions to the problem of planning a diet that will provide a specific nutrient content, these programs require the foods to be selected according to the patients' preferences or meal patterns before the calculations of the diet are executed; such programs can provide a patient with a much more varied diet.

Sources of compositional information

In addition to their use in providing compositional data for guiding food choices for health reasons, nutritional data bases are now widely used in nutritional labelling where this forms part of food regulation. In most countries where nutritional labelling is required (or permitted), the data taken from an authoritative nutritional database are acceptable. Food manufacturers or distributors are thus relieved from carrying out analyses on their own products. The regulations have the requirement that the item in the data base must correspond to the food being labelled; generic labelling of foods such as meats, fruits and vegetables is often permitted.

In the USA the nutritional labelling regulations require manufacturers to carry out their own analyses, using specified methods defined by the Association of Official Analytical Chemists, and also specifies that the sample shall be representative of production within certain limits. This has provided the US national data base with a great deal of manufacturers' data on branded foods. The UK data base also uses some manufacturers' data where the requirements about choice of analytical method and that the sampling was representative can be met.

Limitations

Many of the limitations have been mentioned briefly above. They fall under three headings.

Coverage of foods

No existing data base is truly comprehensive in the sense of covering all the foods likely to form part of the human diet. The analytical resources required to construct such a comprehensive data base are very great indeed and coverage of all cooked mixed dishes is virtually impossible. Additionally, the production of new food products and the reformulation of existing products is a continuous activity of the food industry. This means that complete coverage of all food items is a practically impossible aim. Users of nutritional data bases therefore have to evolve strategies for dealing with missing foods.

In most cases choosing a food that is biologically related or similar to the missing food is satisfactory. In the case of cooked dishes calculation from the recipe using data on the loss of weight on cooking provides an acceptable strategy, but the estimation of vitamin losses in cooking means that the calculated values must be regarded as approximate.

Coverage of nutrients

Most data bases provide coverage of all the macronutrients and most of the vitamins and major inorganic nutrients. The principal gaps at present are the trace elements for which, despite their nutritional desirability, it is difficult for the compilers to provide representative values for the reasons discussed earlier. The coverage of the carotenoids in most data bases is limited, but reliable methods for separating the various forms have now become available and in the future one should expect better coverage. The same applies to the different folate vitamins although the analytical methods are possibly less well developed. Many data bases give limited coverage of the carbohydrates in foods but newer methods will almost certainly remove this limitation in the future. Coverage of the non-nutrient biologically active components represents a greater problem because of the number of candidate constituents coupled with the lack of agreed methods, but nutritional research interest in these components should eventually resolve this limitation.

Data quality

Quality implies fitness for its purpose, so the uses made of data bases need to be considered in any discussion of the limitations on the quality of the data in data bases.

The accuracy of data bases will always be limited by the natural variability in the composition of foods and this places a limit on the predictive accuracy of any data base both for predicting the composition of any one sample of a food and in the calculations made from the data base. These limitations decline as the number of the food records used in the calculations increases, so that, in effect, the foods eaten approach a representative sample size.

The major limitation in producing data bases is the documentation of sampling and the analytical methods used, and particularly the use of quality assurance schemes in analytical laboratories. In many countries the need for such quality assurance schemes in laboratories producing data on food com-

position, particularly for use in data bases, is becoming accepted. Research is needed to develop objective quality assurance schemes for sampling protocols to ensure that this important aspect of data quality is covered. However, the quality of the data in most nutritional data bases at present is considerably superior to the quality of food intake data, and this is the major limitation in using nutritional data bases to assess nutrient intakes.

Presentation

Overall formats

Most compilations of nutritional compositional data take the form of a matrix where one dimension is provided by the nutrients or other constituents and the second is the food items. In food composition tables the dimensions of the matrix have physical constraints set by the physical dimensions of the printed page and the overall size of the printed tables. In some tables the data for a single food are presented on one page but it is more common to have a page with several foods on it. Where the number of nutrients exceeds the page width this format means that several pages are needed to present all the data for the foods. Thus the UK *Composition of Foods* uses four pages to give the proximates, carbohydrate fractions, vitamins and inorganic constituents respectively. These tables also contain a range of subsidiary tables giving more data for nutrients where the information is limited. The German tables adopt the one page per food format and include values for many minor constituents. The Australian tables also use this format. One page per food gives more scope for describing the food item and enables additional food items to be inserted as the data become available.

In computerized data bases there are virtually no physical limits on the size of the food/nutrient matrix, but most compilers prefer to group the foods into foods of related type (**Table 3**). In practice it is often difficult to produce an unequivocal classification of foods, especially mixed dishes, and most data bases rely on a thesaurus or index to enable users to locate foods. The problem is greater with large tables where searching for an item can be frustrating until one understands the logic of the compilers. In a computerized system searching for a food or nutrient is very easy indeed, given the appropriate software.

Documentation

Most tables contain a detailed textual introduction which describes the mode of compilation, the

Table 3 Examples of major food groups in nutritional compilations. The Food and Agriculture Organization (FAO) data base is most widely used for measurements of food purchases and includes mainly raw foods. The groupings are linked to classes of foods used to categorize economic aspects of food production and consumption. The UK data base is widely used for studies of individual food intakes and therefore includes many cooked dishes within the food group which appears most appropriate

Groups used in FAO tables	Groups used in UK tables
Cereals and grain products	Cereals and cereal products
Starchy roots, tubers and fruits	(within vegetables)
Grain legumes and legume products	(within vegetables)
Nuts and seeds	Nuts
Vegetables and vegetable products	Vegetables
Fruits	Fruits
Sugars and syrups	Sugars, preserves and confectionery
Meat, poultry and game	Meat and meat products
Eggs	Eggs
Fish and shellfish	Fish and fish products
Milk and milk products	Milk and milk products
Oils and fats	Oils and fats
Beverages	Beverages
	Alcoholic beverages
Miscellaneous	Miscellaneous

provenance of the data, analytical methods used and the modes of expression adopted. Understanding the introduction is essential for the proper, accurate use of the tables, because in the introduction the compilers can direct the users on the limitations of the data. Ideally all data bases should have comparable documentation readily available to the user, and the more sophisticated data bases do include the documentation accessible on screen. In the absence of computerized documentation the users of computerized data bases need to read the hard copy version if they are to use the data base correctly.

Computerization

In many cases the data base compilers have created the data bases on disk and allowed software providers to write the software for using the data base and market a data base package where the data base itself is licensed to the software company who in turn licence it to the users. Such software packages typically contain search programs and programs for performing nutrient analysis calculations using a range of types of food intake inputs. The software often provides programs for comparing calculated intakes with recommendations or dietary targets defined by the user. Simplified software packages use limited food or nutrient data sets and produce comparisons with recommendations. Most of the more developed

packages contain provision for entering one's own compositional data. It is important to recognize that there are potential disadvantages in being able to write in your own data, because the user may not have the facilities or judgment to assess the data being entered to the same standard as the original compilers.

INFOODS

International Network Food Data Systems (INFOODS) is an international group set up under the auspices of the United Nations University to improve the standard of nutritional data bases worldwide. The group saw the need for making sure that data bases were compatible internationally, because otherwise international epidemiological studies could not be carried out with confidence. Originally the creation of a single world data base was discussed, but abandoned in favour of a network of regional centres linked to the national data bases in their region. INFOODS has addressed the major issues of data quality, especially the choice of compatible analytical method. It also developed a system for the interchange of nutrient data and made a start on the difficult topic of food nomenclature and descriptors. This latter activity is continuing, although INFOODS now acts primarily as a clearing house for communication between the regional centres which provide the main foci of activity.

See also: **Dietary Surveys**: Surveys of National Food Intake; Surveys of Food Intake in Groups and Individuals. **Dietetics**: The Role of Dietetics in Health Care. **Nutritional Status**: Dietary Assessment.

Further Reading

Cashel K, English R and Lewis J (1989) *Composition of Foods*. Canberra: Australian Government Printing Service.

Deutsche Forschungsanstalt für Lebensmittelchemie (1994) *Food Composition and Nutrition Tables*, 5th edn. Stuttgart: Wissenschaftliche Verlagsgesellschaft.

Greenfield H and Southgate DAT (1994) *Food Composition Data; Production, Management and Use*. London: Chapman & Hall.

Holland B, Welch AA, Unwin ID, Buss DH, Paul AA and Southgate DAT (1991) *McCance and Widdowson's The Composition of Foods*, 5th edition. Cambridge: Royal Society of Chemistry.

Klensin JC, Feskanich D, Lin V, Truswell AS and Southgate DAT (1989) *Identification of Food Components for INFOODS Data Interchange*. Tokyo: United Nations University.

Loughridge JM, Walker AD and Towler G (1993) *Inventory of Nutritional Software.* FLAIR Concerted Action Programme no. 12. Wageningen: Department of Human Nutrition.

Rand WM and Young VR (1983) International Network of Food Data Systems (INFOODS) report of a small planning meeting. *Food and Nutrition Bulletin* 5:15–23.

Siminopoulos AP and Butrum RR, eds (1992) *International Food Data Bases and Information Exchange. Concepts, Principles and Designs.* World Review of Nutrition and Dietetics no. 68. Basel: Karger.

Sullivan DM and Carpenter DE (eds) (1993) *Methods of Analysis for Nutrition Labeling.* Arlington: Association of Official Analytical Chemists.

Trichopoulou A, ed. (1992) Methodology and public health aspects of dietary surveillance in Europe: the use of household budget surveys. *European Journal of Clinical Nutrition* 46 (supplement 5).

Truswell AS, Bateson DJ, Madafiglio KC, Pennington JAT, Rand WR and Klensin JC (1991) INFOODS guidelines for describing foods: a systematic approach to facilitate exchange of food composition data. *Journal of Food Composition* 4:18–38.

FOOD CONTAMINANTS

Contents

Mycotoxins – Occurrence and Toxic Effects

F S Chu, University of Wisconsin, Madison, Wisconsin, USA

Copyright © 1998 Academic Press

The term 'Mycotoxin' is a convenient generic name for the toxic substances formed during the growth of fungi or mould ('myco', fungal; 'toxin', poison). In contrast to the bacterial toxins, which are mainly proteins with antigenic properties, the mycotoxins encompass a considerable variety of low molecular weight compounds with diverse chemical structures and biological activities. Like most microbial secondary metabolites, the functions of mycotoxins for the fungi themselves are still not clearly defined.

In considering the effect of mycotoxins on the animal's body, it is important to distinguish between mycotoxicosis and mycosis: 'mycotoxicosis' is used, in general, to describe the action of mycotoxin, which is frequently mediated through a number of organs, notably the liver, kidney and lungs, and the nervous, endocrine and immune systems; 'mycosis' refers to a generalized invasion of living tissues by growing fungi.

Mycotoxins and mycotoxicosis are an especially significant problem for human and animal health, because under certain conditions foodstuffs can provide a favourable medium for fungus growth and toxin production. Because of the relative stability of mycotoxins to heat and other treatments, they may remain in food materials for a long period. Mycotoxins have caused great economic losses because not only is there a loss of crops and animals when a severe outbreak occurs, but there are also a number of unseen losses, such as declines in productivity of milk and eggs, toxin residue problems, effects on animal product quality, increased susceptibility to infection, refusal to eat by animals, manifestation of nutritional status, decline in reproductive success, and the costs of controlling the problems.

The mycotoxin problem is an old one. Ergotism and mushroom poisoning, for example, have been known for centuries. Outbreaks of other types of toxicoses associated with the ingestion of mouldy food by humans and animals have also been recorded in the twentieth century. A well-documented example is the outbreak of a disease called alimentary toxic aleukia (ATA) which resulted in more than 5000 deaths in humans in the Orenberg district of the USSR during World War II. The cause of this outbreak was later determined to be trichothecene mycotoxins produced by fungi growing on grain allowed to stand in the field during winter.

Since the discovery in the early 1960s of aflatoxins, highly potent carcinogens produced by *Aspergillus flavus* and *A. parasiticus*, research has focused new attention on mycotoxins. Many newly identified fungal poisons are attracting attention because of their association with foods and animal feeds and because of their diverse toxic effects.

Growth of Toxicogenic Fungi

Invasion of fungi and production of mycotoxins in commodities can occur under favourable conditions in the field (preharvest), at harvest, and during processing, transportation and storage (**Table 1**).

Most of the mycotoxin-producing fungi belong to one of three genera, namely *Aspergillus*, *Fusarium* and *Penicillium*. However, not all the species are toxicogenic.

Genetic, environmental and nutritional factors as well as time of incubation greatly affect the formation of mycotoxins (**Table 2**). In general, adequate mould growth in the grains or foods is necessary before subsequent production of toxin, and optimal conditions for toxin formation generally have a narrower window than those for mould growth. For example, the optimal temperatures and water activity (A_w) for the growth of *Aspergillus flavus* and *A. parasiticus* are around 35–37°C (range 6–54°C) and 0.95 (range 0.78–1.0), respectively; for aflatoxin production, the values are 28–33°C and 0.90–0.95 (range 0.83–0.97), respectively. The production of fumonisin by *Fusarium moniliforme* on maize is another good example. Fumonisin levels decreased 3-fold when A_w was lowered from 1.0 to 0.95, with no change in fungal growth. However, a 300-fold reduction in fumonisin production was found when

Table 2 Factors affecting the formation of mycotoxins

Genetics
Environmental factors
Nutritional factors
Time of incubation

In the field

Weather conditions
Biological–plant stress
Invertebrate vectors
Species and spore load of infective fungi
Variations within plant and fungal species
Microbial competition

During storage and transportation

Water activity
Temperature
Crop damage
Time
Blending with mouldy components
Chemical factors, e.g. aeration (oxygen and carbon dioxide levels)
Type of grain
pH
Presence or absence of specific nutrients, inhibitors and minerals
Chemical treatment

A_w was lowered from 1.0 to 0.90 with only 20% decrease in fungal growth.

Natural Occurrence and Toxic Effects of Selected Mycotoxins

Some of the most frequent naturally occurring mycotoxins, the toxin-producing fungi, and their major toxic effects in human and animals are shown in **Table 3**. It is apparent that whereas some mycotoxins, e.g. aflatoxin (AF), are produced only by a few species of fungi within a genus, others, e.g. ochratoxin A (OA), are produced by fungi across several genera. A number of commodities can be contaminated with different types of mycotoxins. In general, most mycotoxins affect specific organs, but owing to their diverse structure, the trichothecenes (TCTCs) affect many organs. Among the mycotoxins, AF, OA, fumonisin (Fm), deoxynivalenol (DON) and several other TCTCs are some of the most frequent contaminants in human and animal foodstuffs.

Aflatoxins

General considerations Aflatoxins have chemical structures containing dihydrofuranofuran and tetrahydrofuran fused with a substituted coumarin. At least 16 different structurally related toxins have been found and the structures of the major AFs are

Table 1 Occurrence of toxicogenic fungi

Stage	Fungal species
In the field	*Aspergillus flavus, Alternaria longipes, Alternaria alternata, Claviceps purpura, Fusarium moniliforme, Fusarium graminearum*, other *Fusarium* spp.
Introduced at harvest	*Fusarium sporotrichioides, Stachybotrys atra, Cladosporium* spp., *Myrothecium verrucaria, Trichothecium roseum, Alternaria alternata*
Introduced during storage	*Penicillium* spp. – *P. citrinum, P. cyclopium, P. citreoviride, P. islandicum, P. rubrum, P. viridicatum, P. urticae, P. verruculosum, P. palitans, P. puberulum, P. expansum, P. roqueforti* *Aspergillus* spp. – *A. parasiticus, A. flavus, A. versicolor, A. ochraceus, A. clavatus, A. fumugatus, A. rubrum, A. chevallieri* *Fusarium* spp. – *F. monoliforme, F. tricinctum, F. nivale*, other *Fusarium* spp.

Table 3   Natural occurence of selected mycotoxins

Mycotoxins	Major producing fungi	Typical substrate in nature	Biological effect
Alternaria mycotoxins	Alternaria alternata	Cereal grains, tomato, animal feeds	A, M, IIm
Aflatoxin B$_1$ and other aflatoxins	Aspergillus flavus, A. parasiticus	Peanuts, corn, cottonseed, cereals, figs, most tree nuts, milk, sorghum, walnuts	A, H, C, M, T
Citrinin	Penicillium citrinum	Barley, corn, rice, walnuts	Nh, C, M
Cyclopiazonic acid	A. flavus, P. cyclopium	Peanut, corn, cheese	Nr, Cv
Deoxynivalenol	Fusarium graminearum	Wheat, corn	Nr
Cyclochlorotine	P. islandicum	Rice	A, H, C
Fumonisins	F. monoliforme	Corn, sorghum, rice	A, H, Nr, C(?), R
Luteoskyrin	P. islandicum, P. rugulosum	Rice, sorghum	A, H, C, M
Moniliformin	F. moniliforme	Corn	Nr, Cv
Ochratoxin A	A. ochraceus, P. viridicatum, P. verrucosum, etc.	Barley, beans, cereals, coffee, feeds, maize, oats, rice, rye, wheat	A, Nh, T
Patulin	P. patulum, P. urticae, A. clavatus, etc.	Apple, apple juice, beans, wheat	Nr, C(?), D, T
Penicillin acid	P. puberulum, A. ochraceus, etc.	Barley, corn	Nr, C(?), M
Penitrem A	P. palitans	Feedstuffs, corn	Nr
Roquefortine	P. roqueforti	Cheese	Nr
Rubratoxin B	P. rubrum, P. purpurogenum	Corn, soyabeans	A, H, T
Sterigmatocystin	A. versicolor, A. nidulans, etc.	Corn, grains, cheese	H, C, M
T-2	F. sporotrichioides	Corn, feeds, hay	A, D, ATA, T
12,13-Epoxytrichothecenes other than T-2 and	F. nivale, etc.	Corn, feeds, hay, peanuts, rice	D, Nr
Zearalenone	F. graminearum, etc.	Cereals, corn, feeds, rice	G, M

From CAST (1989). The optimal temperatures for the production of mycotoxin are generally 24–28 °C, except for T-2 toxin which is generally produced maximally at 15 °C.
A, apoptosis; ATA, alimentary toxic aleukia; C, carcinogenic; C(?), carcinogenic effect is still questionable;
Cv, cardiovascular lesion; D, dermatoxin; G, genitotoxin and oestrogenic effects; H, hepatotoxic; Hr, haemorrhagic;
M, mutagenic; Nh, nephrotoxin; Nr, neurotoxins; R, respiratory; T, teratogenic.

shown in **Fig. 1**. The toxins are primarily produced by *Aspergillus flavus* and *A. parasiticus* in a number of important agricultural commodities in the field and during storage. Recent studies have shown that some strains of *A. nominus* and *A. tamarii* are also AF producers. Because the four major toxins were originally isolated from fungal cultures of *A. flavus*, the first few letters of the fungus were used to form the name. These toxins fluoresce either blue or green under ultraviolet light, and this distinguishes the B or G types of toxins. Aflatoxin B$_1$ is most toxic in this group and is one of the most potent naturally occurring carcinogens; other AFs are less toxic (B$_1$ > G$_1$ > B$_2$ > G$_2$). Because AFB$_1$ frequently contaminates several major commodities, extensive studies have been done on its toxicity, biological and biochemical effects. Consumption of AFB$_1$-contaminated feed by dairy cows results in the excretion in milk of a hydroxylated metabolite of AFB$_1$ known as AFM$_1$. This compound is about 10 times less toxic

than AFB$_1$, but its presence in milk is of concern for human health.

The main target of AF is liver. Typical symptoms of aflatoxicoses in animals include proliferation of the bile duct, centrilobular necrosis and fatty infiltration of the liver, and hepatomas, as well as generalized hepatic lesions. In addition to these acute hepatotoxic effects, the carcinogenic effects of AFB$_1$ are of great concern. Because of their presence in foods and strong evidence of their association with human carcinogenesis, aflatoxins are still a serious threat to human health even after more than thirty years of research.

Biosynthesis of aflatoxin   The biosynthetic pathway for AFB was postulated in the 1980s, and the major genes and enzymes involved in the biosynthesis have now been identified and characterized. Starting with polyketide precursors such as acetate, at least 20

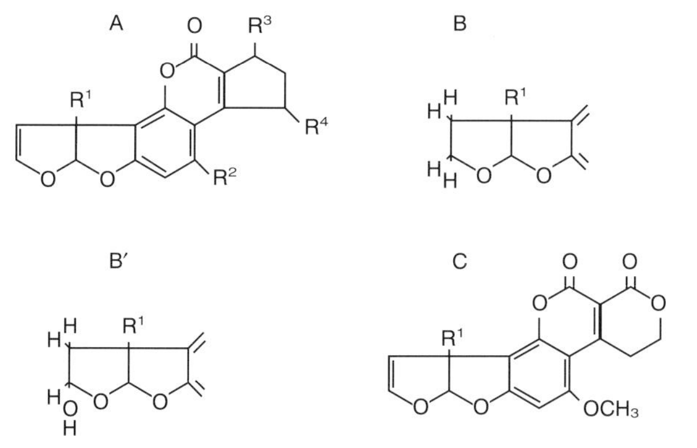

Aflatoxins	Structure	R^1	R^2	R^3	R^4
B_1 (F)	A	H	OCH_3	=O	H
M_1 (F,M)	A	OH	OCH_3	=O	H
P_1 (M)	A	H	OH	=O	H
Q_1 (M)	A	H	OCH_3	=O	OH
R_0 (M)	A	H	OCH_3	OH	H
R_0H_1 (M)	A	H	OCH_3	OH	OH
B_2 (F)	AB	H	OCH_3	=O	H
B_{2a} (F,M)	AB'	H	OCH_3	=O	H
M_2 (F,M)	AB	OH	OCH_3	=O	H
G_1 (F)	C	H	-	-	-
G_2 (F)	BC	H	-	-	-
G_{2a} (F,M)	B'C	H	-	-	-
GM (F,M)	BC	OH	-	-	-

Figure 1 Structures of aflatoxins; (F), aflatoxin produced by fungi; (M), metabolite of aflatoxin. From Chu (1977).

steps involving 17 postulated enzymes have been identified.

Aflatoxins in human foods Aflatoxins have been found in corn, peanuts and peanut products, cotton-seeds, rice, pistachios, tree nuts (brazil nuts, almonds, pecans), pumpkin seeds, sunflower seeds and other oil seeds, copra, spices and dried fruits (figs, raisins). Of most concern is the frequent contamination with high levels of AF in peanuts, corn and cottonseed, mostly due to infestation by mould in the field. Soyabeans, beans, pulses, cassava, grain sorghum, millet, wheat, oats, barley and rice are resistant or only moderately susceptible to AF contamination in the field. It should be reiterated that resistance to aflatoxin contamination in the field does not guarantee that the commodities are free of AF contamination during storage. Inadequate storage conditions, such as high moisture levels and warm temperatures (25–30°C), can create conditions favourable for the growth of fungus and production of AF. High levels of AFB_1 have been reported in rice, cassava, figs, spices, pecans and other nuts.

The potential hazard of AFs to human health has led to worldwide monitoring programmes for the toxin in various commodities as well as regulatory actions by nearly all countries. Levels varying from zero tolerance to 50 parts per billion (ppb) have been set for total AFs. Most countries, including the USA, have a regulatory level around 20 ppb in foods. For AFM_1 in dairy products, a level between zero tolerance to 0.5 ppb has been used. To avoid contamination of milk and other dairy products with AFM, rigorous programmes regulating AFB_1 in feed have also been established. Most governments set a lower tolerance level for AFs in the feed for dairy cows. In the USA, the level of AFs in feed for dairy cows is 20 ppb; for other animals, it is 100 ppb.

Aflatoxin and human carcinogenesis Whereas AFB_1 has been found to be a potent carcinogen in many animal species, the role of AF in carcinogenesis in humans is complicated by hepatitis B virus (HBV) infections. Epidemiological studies have shown a strong positive correlation between AF levels in the diet and primary hepatocellular carcinoma (PHC) incidence in some parts of the world, including certain regions of China, Kenya, Mozambique, Philippines, Swaziland, Thailand and South Africa (Transkei). Aflatoxin – DNA and AF – albumin adducts as well as several AF metabolites (mainly AFM_1) have been detected in serum, milk and urine of humans in these regions. However, the prevalence of HBV infection is also correlated with liver cancer incidence in these regions. Several studies have indicated that AF exposure is the more important factor. Since multiple factors are considered to be important in carcinogenesis, environmental contaminants such as AFs and other mycotoxins may, either in combination with HBV or independently, be important aetiological factors.

Ochratoxins

General considerations Ochratoxins (OT), a group of dihydroisocumarin-containing mycotoxins (**Fig. 2**), are produced by a number of fungi in the genera *Aspergillus* and *Penicillium*, including *A. sulphureus*, *A. sclerotiorum*, *A. melleus*, *A. ochraceus*, *A. awamori*, and *P. viridicatum*, *P. palitans*, *P. commune*, *P. variabile*, *P. purpurescens*, *P. cyclopium* and *P. chrysogenum*. *Aspergillus ochraceus* and *P. viridicatum*, two species that were first reported as OA producers, occur frequently in nature. Because of its distinct chemotype, *P. viridicatum* has been reclassified as *P. verrucosum*. Other fungi, such as *Petromyces alliceus* (isolated from onion), *Aspergillus citricus* and *A. fonsecaeus* (h in *A. niger* group), have also been found to produce OA.

Because most OA producers are storage fungi, pre-harvest fungal infection and OA production are not a serious problem; the toxins are generally produced in grains during storage in temperate regions.

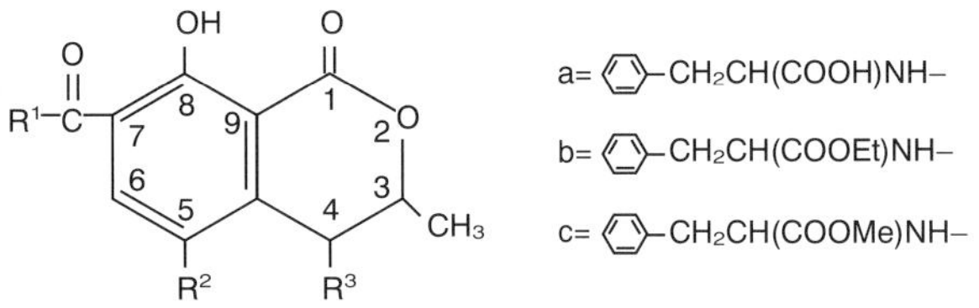

Ochratoxins	R^1	R^2	R^3
A	a	Cl	H
B	a	H	H
C	b	Cl	H
A Methyl ester	c	Cl	H
B Methyl ester	c	H	H
B Ethyl ester	b	H	H
4–OH–OA	a	Cl	OH
α	OH	Cl	H
β	OH	H	H

Figure 2 Structures of ochratoxins. From Chu (1977).

Although most OA producers can grow in a range of temperatures from 4°C to 37°C and at A_w as low as 0.78, optimal conditions for the toxin production are narrower, with temperature at 24–25°C and A_w values greater than 0.97 (minimum A_w for OA production is about 0.85).

Worldwide, OA occurs primarily in cereal grains (barley, oats, rye, corn, wheat) and mixed feeds, and levels higher than 1 ppm have been reported. Ochratoxin A has been found in other commodities, including beans, coffee, nuts, olives, cheese, fish, pork, milk powder, wine, beer and bread. The presence of OA residues in animal products is of concern because it binds tightly to serum albumin and has a long half-life in animal tissues and body fluids. Thus, OA can be carried through the food chain and the natural occurrence of OA in kidneys, blood serum, blood sausage and other sausage made from pork has been reported.

Toxic effects Ochratoxin A, the most toxic member – median lethal dose (LD_{50}) about 20–25 mg kg^{-1} – and also the most commonly found toxin in this group, has been found to be a potent nephrotoxin causing kidney damage, including degeneration of the proximal tubule, in many animal species. Liver necrosis and enteritis were also observed in these animals. Apart from its acute toxic effects, OA also acts as an immunosuppressor and a teratogen in test animals. Although OA has never been shown to be mutagenic, a weak genotoxic effect has been demonstrated in several systems. Ochratoxin A is considered to be a weak nephrocarcinogen because a high level of toxin and an extended period of exposure is necessary to induce the tumours.

Ochratoxin A and human health The role of OA in human pathogenesis is still speculative. Ochratoxin A has long been considered to be associated with the nephropathy of people residing in certain Scandinavian and Balkan regions, and more recently in Tunisia, where exposure may be 'endemic'. The pathological lesions of nephropathy in humans are similar to those observed in endemic porcine nephropathy which is due to the consumption of feeds contaminated with OA. Since a high proportion of the patients suffering from endemic nephropathy in the Balkan region develop tumours of the renal pelvis and ureter, the possible involvement of nephropathy in tumour development was suggested. Ochratoxin A has been found in human serum in Tunisia and a number of European countries including Bulgaria, Poland, Yugoslavia and Germany. In certain areas of the Balkans and Tunisia, OA levels in the food and in human serum in endemic regions are higher than in nonendemic regions. The toxin also has been found in human milk and kidneys in some endemic regions.

Human exposure to OA could occur through consumption of OA-containing cereals or animal foods. In 1996, it was reported that the mean daily intake of OA by humans in European Union member countries was 1.8 ng per kg body weight (range 0.7–4.7 ng kg^{-1} calculated from data on OA levels in foods, and 0.9 ng kg^{-1} (range 0.2–2.4 ng kg^{-1}) when calculated from the levels of OA in human blood. The main dietary sources (55%) were cereals and cereal products (0.2–1.6 μg of OA per kg). Coffee (mean level 0.8 μg kg^{-1}), beer, pig meat, blood products and pulses also contribute to OA intake in humans. These findings emphasize the possible involvement of OA in human carcinogenesis and the health hazard of exposure to OA in humans. Among 77 countries that have regulations for different mycotoxins, eight have specific regulations for OA, with limits ranging from 1 μg kg^{-1} to 20 μg kg^{-1} in different foods.

Fumonisin

General considerations Fumonisins (Fm) are a group of toxic metabolites produced primarily by *Fusarium moniliforme*, one of the most common fungi colonizing corn throughout the world. More than nine structurally related Fms (**Fig. 3**) have been found since the discovery of fumonisin B_1 (FmB_1, diester of propane-1,2,3-tricarboxylic acid of 2-amino-12,16-dimethyl-3,5,10,14,15-pentahydroxy-icosane) in 1987. Several hydrolysed derivatives of Fms, resulting from removal of the tricarballylic acid and other ester groups, have also been found in nature. *Fusarium proliferatum*, another common

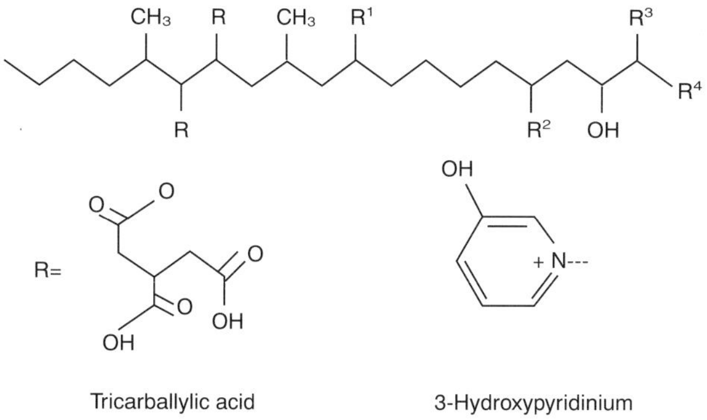

Figure 3 Structures of fumonisins; 3HP, 3-hydroxypyridinium; TCA, tricarballylic acid.

Fumonisins	R¹	R²	R³	R⁴
FmB₁	OH	OH	NH₂	CH₃
FmB₂	H	OH	NH₂	CH₃
FmB₃	OH	H	NH₂	CH₃
FmB₄	H	H	NH₂	CH₃
FmA₁	OH	OH	NHCOCH₃	CH₃
FmA₂	H	OH	NHCOCH₃	CH₃
FmC₁	OH	OH	H	H
FmC₄	H	H	H	H
FmP₁	OH	OH	3HP	CH₃
FmP₂	H	OH	3HP	CH₃
FmP₃	OH	H	3HP	CH₃

naturally occurring species, also produces Fms. Although *F. anthophilum*, *F. napiforme* and *F. nygamai* are capable of producing Fms, they are not commonly isolated from human or animal food. Other related fusaria, including *F. subglutinans*, *F. annulatum*, *F. succisae* and *F. beomiforme*, are not Fm producers. In addition to fusaria, *Alternaria alternata* f. sp. *lycopersici* produces a group of host-specific toxins named AAL toxins, which have a chemical structure similar to the Fms and induce similar toxic effects. Production of FmB by *Alternaria alternata* f. sp. *lycopersici* has been found in some cultures. Likewise, some Fm-producing isolates also produce small amounts of AAL toxins.

Fumonisins are most frequently found in corn, corn-based foods and other grains (such as sorghum and rice). The level of contamination varies considerably in different regions and different years (range from zero to more than 100 ppm, generally below 1 ppm). Fumonisin B₁ is most commonly found in the naturally contaminated samples; FmB₂ generally accounts for a third or less of the total. Although production of the toxin generally occurs in the field, continued production of toxin during storage after harvesting also contributes to the overall levels. In the laboratory, the highest yield was achieved in corn culture and less in rice culture; peanut and soya bean were found to be poor substrates for toxin production. The toxin is very stable to heat as well as resistant to other treatments. Acid hydrolysis causes the loss of tricarballylic acid, but the hydrolysed products may still have toxic effects. Transmission of FmB to the edible portion of meat or egg is unlikely to occur because of the rapid excretion of the toxin in animals. No significant amount of FmB₁ is transmitted to milk.

Toxicologic effects of FmB₁ Fumonisin B₁ is primarily a hepatotoxin and carcinogen in rats. Earlier studies showed that feeding culture material from *F. moniliforme* to rats resulted in cirrhosis and hepatic nodules, adenofibrosis, hepatocellular or ductular carcinoma, and cholangiocarcinoma. Later studies indicated that the kidney is also a target organ.

Results from these earlier observations were confirmed with the studies of purified Fms. Although FmB₁ was originally found to be a potent cancer promoter, subsequent studies showed that it is also a carcinogen. The effective dose of FmB₁ for cancer initiation in rat liver depended both on the levels and the duration of exposure. For tumour formation, there appears to be a balance between the compensatory cell proliferation due to the hepatotoxicity of FmB₁ and the inhibitory effect on the subsequent hepatocyte cell proliferation. All of the three major Fms, – FmB₁, FmB₂ and FmB₃ – show cancer initiation and promoting activities in rats. In cell culture systems, FmB₁ was found to be a mitogen and cytotoxic to the cells but had no genotoxic effect.

Impact on human and animal health While Fms are commonly detected in corn-based foodstuff, the impact of low levels of Fms in human foods is not known. Current data suggest that they may have more impact on the health of farm animals than on humans. Thus, the Mycotoxin Committee of the American Association of Veterinary Laboratory Diagnostics recommended that the FmB₁ levels be limited to 5 ppm, 10 ppm, 50 ppm and 50 ppm for feeds to be used for horses, swine, beef cattle and poultry, respectively. Several reports indicated that significantly higher levels of Fms, sometimes together with AFs and TCTC mycotoxins, were present in corn samples collected from areas with high rates of human oesophageal cancer. The ability of *F. moniliforme* to produce nitrosamines (carcinogens) suggests that a combination of several aetiological agents in the mouldy corn, including FmB₁, may play an important role in carcinogenesis in humans. Currently, only Switzerland regulates the Fm level (1.0 ppm) in human food.

Trichothecene mycotoxins

General considerations Trichothecenes are a group of naturally occurring toxic tetracyclic sesquiterpenoids produced by many species of fungi in the genera *Fusarium* (most frequently), *Myrothecium*, *Trichoderma*, *Trichothecium*, *Cephalosporium*, *Verticimonosporium* and *Stachybotrys*. The term 'trichothecene' is derived from the first compound, trichothecin, to be isolated in this group. All the mycotoxins in this group contain a common 12,13-epoxytrichothecene (six-membered oxygen-containing ring) skeleton and an olefinic bond with different side chain substitutions.

The chemical structures for some of the most common naturally occurring TCTC are shown in **Fig. 4**. Based on the presence of a macrocyclic ester or ester-ether bridge between C4 and C15, TCTCs are generally classified as macrocyclic (type C) or nonmacrocyclic. The nonmacrocyclic TCTCs are further divided into two types: type A TCTCs, including T-2 toxin, HT-2 toxin, neosolaniol (NESO), diacetoxy-scirpenol (DAS) and T-2 tetraol (T-4ol), which contain a hydrogen- or ester-type side chain at the C8 position; and type B TCTCs, including DON, nivalenol (NIV), and fusarenon-x (FSx, or 4-acetyl-NIV), which contain a ketone. Type C group TCTCs, including roridins and verrucarins, contain a macrocyclic ring. In addition to fungi, extracts from a Brazilian shrub, *Baccharis megapotamica*, also contain macrocyclic TCTCs.

The structural diversity of TCTC mycotoxins results in different toxic effects in animals and humans. Unlike AFB_1 and OA toxicoses, where primary effects and clinical manifestations are well defined in the liver and kidney, TCTC mycotoxicoses are difficult to distinguish because they affect many organs, including the gastrointestinal tract and the haematopoietic, nervous, immune, hepatobiliary and cardiovascular systems. Ingestion of food containing TCTC mycotoxins causes many types of mycotoxicoses in humans and animals, including mouldy corn toxicosis, scabby wheat toxicosis (red mould, akakabi-byo disease or scabby barley poisoning), feed refusal and emetic syndrome (in swine), fusaritoxicoses, haemorrhagic syndrome and alimentary toxic aleukia. More than a hundred TCTC have been identified in the laboratory; only a few selected toxins that have been found in foods are described here.

Type A TCTCs The T-2 toxin, a highly toxic type A TCTC, was isolated in the middle 1960s. It was originally found to be produced by a strain of *Fusarium tricinctum* isolated from mouldy corn, and later to be produced by *F. sporotrichioides* (major), *F. poae*, *F. sulphureum*, *F. acuminatum* and *F. sambucinum*. Unlike most mycotoxins, which are usually synthesized at around 25°C, the optimal temperature for T-2 toxin production is around 15°C. Higher temperatures (20–25°C) are needed for the production of related metabolites, such as HT-2 toxin. Although T-2 toxin occurs naturally in cereal grains, including barley, corn, corn stalk, oats, wheat and mixed feeds, contamination with T-2 toxin is less frequent than with deoxynivalenol. However, T-2 toxin (LD_{50} in mice 2–4 mg kg^{-1}) is much more toxic to animals, perhaps also to humans, than DON (LD_{50} in mice 50–70 mg kg^{-1}).

Most of the type A TCTCs, including T-2 toxin, are cytotoxic and cause haemorrhage, oedema, and necrosis of skin tissues. Inflammatory reactions near the nose and mouth of animals are similar to some lesions found in humans suffering from ATA disease. The severity of lesions is also related to chemical structure. Macrocyclic toxins such as verrucarin A are most active, followed by group A toxins (T-2 toxin); least active are type B toxins such as NIV.

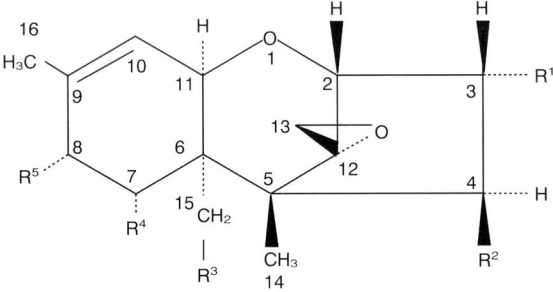

Trichothecenes	R^1	R^2	R^3	R^4	R^5
DAS	OH	OAc	OAc	H	H
4-MAS	OH	OAc	OH	H	H
15-MAS[a]	OH	OH	OAc	H	H
Scirpentriol	OH	OH	OH	H	H
DON	OH	H	OH	OH	=O
NIV	OH	OH	OH	OH	=O
FSx	OH	OAc	OH	OH	=O
T-2	OH	OAc	OAc	H	ISV
HT-2	OH	OH	OAc	H	ISV
T-2 triol	OH	OH	OH	H	ISV
3′-OH-T-2	OH	OAc	OAc	H	OH-ISV
T-2 tetraol	OH	OH	OH	H	OH
NESO	OH	OAc	OAc	H	OH
Roridin A, B, E, H, J	H	MC[a]	MC	H	H
Roridin K	H	MC	MC	H	OH
Verrucarin A, B, J, K	H	MC	MC	H	H
Verrucarin L	H	MC	MC	H	OH
Satratoxin F, G, H	H	MC	MC	H	H
Verrucarol	H	OH	OH	H	H

[a] Macrocyclic

Figure 4 Structures of selected trichothecenes. The abbreviations Oac, ISV and OH-ISV represent $OCOCH_3$, $OCOCH_2CH(CH_3)_2$ and $OCOCH_2C(OH)(CH_3)_2$ respectively, and MC represents a macrocyclic structure with a chain of atoms joining the C4 and C15 positions where R^2 and R^3 become OCOCROCO with different macrocyclic (R) structures. DAS, diacetoxyscirpenol; DON, deoxynivalenol; FSx, fusarenon-x; MAS, monoacetoxyscirpenol; NESO, neosolaniol; NIV, nivalenol. From Chu (1997).

Neurologic dysfunctions, including emesis, tachycardia, diarrhoea, refusal of feed/anorexia and depression, were also observed. Some TCTCs including, T-2 toxin also induce major gastrointestinal lesions such as perioral dermatitis, stomatitis, oesophagitis, gastritis, radiomimetic lesions and sometimes haemorrhage in the intestines. However, the major lesion of T-2 toxin is its devastating effect on the haematopoietic system in many mammals, including humans. Typically, there is a marked initial increase in the number of circulating white blood cells, especially lymphocytes, followed by a rapid decrease to 10–75% of normal values. Platelet counts are also reduced. There is also extensive cellular damage in the bone marrow, intestines, spleen and lymph nodes, and in severe cases complete atrophy of bone marrow and marked alteration of plasma coagulation factors. Of the known mycotoxins, T-2 toxin and related TCTCs are the most potent immunosuppressants and cause significant lesions in lymph nodes, spleen, thymus and the bursa of Fabricius. The heart and pancreas are other target organs for T-2 toxin. Although urinary and hepatobiliary lesions have been observed for T-2 toxin and DAS, these effects are considered to be secondary.

Deoxynivalenol Deoxynivalenol is a major type B TCTC mycotoxin produced primarily by *Fusarium graminearum* and other related fungi fungi such *F. culmorum* and *F. crookwellense*. Because DON causes feed refusal and emesis in swine, the name 'vomitoxin' is also used. Although DON is considerably less toxic than most other TCTC mycotoxins, the level of contamination of this toxin in corn and wheat is generally high, usually above 1 ppm, sometime greater than 20 ppm. Contamination of DON in other commodities, including barley, oats, sorghum, rye, safflower seeds and mixed feeds have also been reported. Deoxynivalenol has been found in cereal grains in many countries, such as Australia, Finland, France, Germany, Hungary, Italy, South Africa, the UK, China, Japan, India and many others including the USA and Canada.

With wet and cold weather during maturation, grains are especially susceptible to *F. graminearum* infection, which causes 'scabby wheat' and simultaneously produces the toxin. The optimal temperature for DON production is about 24°C. Outbreaks of DON in winter wheat in the USA, Finland and Canada usually occur when continental chilly and humid weather favouring the fungal infection is followed by a humid summer favourable for toxin production. For other crops such as corn and rice, a continental humid, warm summer is more favourable. Depending on the weather conditions, the infestation

of *F. graminearum* in wheat and corn and subsequent production of toxins in the field varies considerably from year to year as well as in different regions. Thus, the levels of DON in these commodities are difficult to predict.

Toxicologically, DON induces anorexia and emesis both in humans and animals. Because of the frequent occurrence of high levels of DON in wheat and corn, its stability, and reported food poisoning outbreaks in humans, contamination of cereals with DON is a major concern of both the government and the food and animal feed industries. Contamination of DON in wheat and corn may be associated with other toxic effects because other *Fusarium* toxins, including zearalenone and other TCTCs, may also present. Other type B TCTCs such as nivalenol and acetylated DON, which are more toxic than DON to test animals, occur naturally in some parts of the world.

The impact of TCTC on human and animal health Because of their diverse toxic effects and also because of frequent contamination by toxins or toxicogenic fungi in foods and feeds, TCTCs are potentially hazardous to human and animal health. However, among the many types of TCTC mycotoxicoses mentioned earlier, only ATA and scabby wheat toxicosis have been demonstrated in human populations. The former, ATA, was attributed to the human consumption of overwintered cereal grains colonized by *Fusarium sporotrichioides* and *F. poae*; it caused the deaths of hundreds of people in the USSR between 1942 and 1947. Later studies indicated that T-2 toxin and related TCTCs were the primary cause. The signs and symptoms of ATA disease, which include skin inflammation, vomiting, damage to haematopoietic tissues, leucocytosis and leucopenia, are common in humans and animals.

Deoxynivalenol has been found to be primarily responsible for outbreaks of scabby wheat toxicosis in humans that occur quite commonly in several countries, but these toxicoses rarely cause death. Between 1961 and 1985, for example, 35 outbreaks involving 7818 cases were found to be caused by consumption of foods made from either scabby wheat or mouldy corn in China. In one well-documented study, 362 persons in a commune were involved. The symptoms, which occurred within 15 min to 1 h after eating foods made out of flour from mouldy corn, included nausea (90%), emesis (61%) and headache and drowsiness (78%), and 5–6% had abdominal pain, diarrhoea and a low fever. People generally recovered 2–4 days after ingestion of the foods. Analysis of the leftover mouldy corn revealed that the samples had 0.34–93.8 ppm of

DON; no T-2 toxin or nivalenol were found. Similar cases have been reported for people consuming scabby wheat flour.

The widespread natural occurrence of DON in wheat in Canada and the USA in the late 1970s and early 1980s alerted the general public to the potential hazard of this mycotoxin. Although DON is not as toxic as other TCTCs, the level of contamination in wheat and corn in high and intoxication of humans by DON occurs more often. The tolerable daily intakes of DON for adults and infants were estimated to be 3 μg kg^{-1} and 1.5 μg kg^{-1} body weight, respectively. Consequently, a tolerance level of 1 ppm for DON in grains for human consumption has been set by a number of countries, including USA. In Canada, the guideline for DON in the uncleaned soft wheat used for nonstaple foods is 2 ppm, but 1 ppm for infant foods. Although inadequate storage may lead to the production of some other TCTC mycotoxins, fusarial infestation in wheat and corn in the field is of most concern because of the DON problem.

Trichothecenes may also be involved in the 'sick building' syndrome in humans. *Stachybotrys atra* was isolated from a badly water-damaged home in a Chicago suburb whose occupants complained about headaches, sore throats, hair loss, flu symptoms, diarrhoea, fatigue, dermatitis, and general malaise.

Other selected mycotoxins

In addition to the mycotoxins discussed above, a number of other mycotoxins also occur naturally. The impact of some of these mycotoxins on human and animal health is discussed below.

Other mycotoxins produced by *Aspergillus* Sterigmatocystin (ST) is a naturally occurring hepatotoxic and carcinogenic mycotoxin produced by fungi in the *Aspergillus*, *Bipolaris*, and *Chaetomium* genera and by *Penicillium luteum*. Structurally related to AFB$_1$ ST is known to be a precursor of AFB$_1$. Although the carcinogenicity of ST is less than that of AFB$_1$ in test animals (10 to 100 times less), this mycotoxin has been found to be mutagenic and genotoxic. Sterigmatocystin occurs naturally in cereal grains such as barely, rice and corn, coffee beans and foods such as cheese. It has also been found in pickled foodstuffs in Linxian, a region of China with a high incidence of oesophageal cancer, and in foods from Mozambique where high PHC incidence was reported. Toxicogenic fungi have been isolated from patients with oesophageal cancer, and these strains are capable of producing ST in many commodities. The role of ST in human carcinogenesis appears to be indirect and inclusive.

Aspergillus terreus and several other fungi (*A. flavus* and *A. fumigatus*) have been found to produce tremorgenic toxins territrem A, B and C, aflatrem and fumitremorgin.

Aspergillus terreus, *A. fumigatus* and *Trichoderma viride* also produce gliotoxin, which is an epipolythiopiperazine-3,6-diones sulfur-containing piperazine antibiotic, that may have immunosuppressive effects in animals. In addition, *A. flavus*, *A. wentii*, *A. oryzae* and *Penicillium atraovenetum* are capable of producing nitropropionic acid (NPA), a mycotoxin causing apnoea, convulsions, congestion in lungs and subcutaneous vessels, and liver damage in test animals. This toxin was also identified as an aetiological agent for deteriorated sugar cane poisoning, a fatal food poisoning that occurred in China. However, the fungi involved in the contamination in the sugar cane and NPA production were *Arthrinium sacchari*, *A. saccharicola* and *A. phaeospermum*.

Other mycotoxins produced by *Penicillium* Other than OA, *Penicillium spp.* produce many mycotoxins with diversified toxic effects. Cyclocholortine, luteoskyrin and regulosin have long been considered to be possibly involved in yellow rice disease during World War II. They are hepatotoxins and also produce hepatomas in test animals. However, incidences of food contamination with these toxins have not been well documented. Several other mycotoxins, including patulin, penicillic acid (PA), citrinin, cyclopiazonic acid (CPA), citreoviridin and xanthomegnin, which are produced primarily by several species of *Penicillium*, have attracted some attention because of their frequent occurrence in foods.

Patulin and PA are produced by many species in the *Aspergillus* and *Penicillium* genera, and a heat-resistant fungus *Byssochlamys nivea* frequently found in foods also produces patulin. Both toxins are hepatotoxic. Patulin is frequently found in damaged apples, apple juice, apple cider and sometimes in other fruit juices and feed. Penicillic acid has been detected in 'blue eye' corn and meat. Owing to its highly reactive double bonds which readily react with sulfhydryl groups in foods, patulin is not very stable in foods containing these groups. Nevertheless, patulin is considered a health hazard to humans. At least 10 countries have regulatory limits, most commonly at a level of 50 μg kg^{-1} for patulin in various foods and juices. Frequently associated with the natural occurrence of OA is citrinin, also a nephrotoxin, produced by *P. citrinum* and several other species of *Penicillium* and *Aspergillus*. One of the mycotoxins closely associated with the natural occurrence of AF in peanuts is cyclopiazonic acid, which causes hyperaesthesia and convulsions as well as liver, spleen, pancreas, kidney, salivary gland and myocardial damage. The toxin was originally found to be produced by *P. cyclopium*; but a number of other species of *Penicillium* (*P. crustosum, P. griseofulvin, P. puberulum, P. camemberti*) and *Aspergillus* (*A. versicolor, A. flavus* but not *A. parasiticus*, and *A. tamarii*) produce CPA. Natural occurrence of CPA in corn, peanuts and cheese has been reported. *Penicillium rubrum* and *P. purpurogenum* produce two highly toxic hepatotoxins (LD$_{50}$ in mice 3.0 mg kg^{-1} i.p.) called rubratoxins A (minor) and B (major), which are complex nonadrides fused with anhydrides and lactone rings. Rubratoxin B has shown to have synergistic effects with AFB$_1$.

In addition to the above hepatotoxins and nephrotoxins, *Penicillium* species produce many mycotoxins with strong pharmacological effects on neurosystems. For example, *P. crustosum* and *P. cyclopium* produce tremorgenic indoloditerpenes called penitrem A–F. Penitrem A, the major toxin in this group, causes tremorgenic effects in mice. Roquefortines A–C (C is most toxic), which are produced by *P. roqueforti* and several other *Penicillium* species, have neurotoxic effects in animals and have been found in cheese. Tremorgens in the paspalitrem group (paspalicine, paspalinine, paspalitrem A and B, paspaline and paxilline) are produced by *Claviceps paspali* and some *Penicillium* species.

Other mycotoxins produced by *Fusarium*

Some *Fusarium* species can also produce mycotoxins other than TCTCs and Fm. Zearalenone (ZE), 6-(10-hydroxy-6-oxo-*trans*-1-undecenyl)-β-resorcyclic acid-lactone, is a mycotoxin produced by the scabby wheat fungus, *F. graminearum* (*roseum*), which also produces DON. Also called F-2, it is a phytooestrogen causing hyperoestrogenic effects and reproductive problems in animals, especially swine. Natural contamination with ZE primarily occurs in cereal grains such as corn and wheat. Contamination with this mycotoxin, sometimes together with DON, in feed may result in a large economic loss in the swine industry. *Fusarium moniliforme* also produces several other mycotoxins including fusarins A–F, moniliformin, fusarioic C, fusaric acid, fusaproliferin and beauvericin in addition to Fms. Although the impact of these mycotoxins on human health is still not known, fusarin C (FC) has been identified as a potent mutagen. In addition to *F. moniliforme* and *F. subglutinans*, several other *Fusarium* species including *F. graminearum* have also been identified as FC producers. *Fusarium moniliforme* was also found most effective, among a group of several fungi tested in reducing nitrates to form potent carcinogenic nitrosamines. These observations further suggest that

the contamination of foods with this fungus could be one of the aetiological factors involved in human carcinogenesis in certain regions of the world.

Mycotoxins produced by other species

Other than the fungi in the *Aspergillus*, *Penicillium* and *Fusarium* genera, mycotoxins are also produced by *Alternaria*, a plant pathogen and another genus of fungi commonly found in our environment. The toxins can be produced in both preharvest and postharvest commodities by these fungi. *Alternaria alternata* and other *Alternaria* species are capable of producing dibenzopyrone types of mycotoxins: alternariol, alternariol monomethyl ether (AME), altenuene, isoaltenuene and altenuisol, tetramic acid metabolites tenuazonic acid (TzA) and related compounds, and perylene derivatives altertoxins (ATX) I, II (also called stemphyltoxin II), III and stemphyltoxin. Although most of those compounds are relatively nontoxic, AME has been shown to be positive in Ames test at relatively high concentrations. Tenuazonic acid is a protein synthesis inhibitor and is capable of chelating metal ions and forming nitrosamines. This mycotoxin is also produced by *Phoma sorghina* and *Pyricularia oryzae*, and may be related to *onyalai*, a haematological disorder of humans in sub-Saharan Africa. Although no extensive survey has been conducted to determine the occurrence of these mycotoxins in human foods, limited studies indicate that some of them (such as AME and TA) could occur frequently in apple and tomato products. The structural and functional similarity between fumonisins and AAL toxins further shows the importance of mycotoxins produced by fungi in the *Alternaria* family.

Classical examples of intoxication by fungal metabolites

Two classical examples related to the mycotoxins are ergotism and mushroom poisoning. Because these intoxications result from ingestion of a fungal body containing toxic metabolites, these two types of poisons sometimes are excluded from the modern discussion of mycotoxins. Ergots and poisonous mushrooms still can be unintentionally introduced into the food chains. Some phytoalexins elaborated by plants as a result of alteration of their metabolism by either fungal infection or other damage have also been found to be toxic to human and animals.

Ergotism   Ergotism is a human disease that results from consumption of the ergot body (the sclerotium of the fungus) in rye or other grains infected by a parasitic fungus in the *Claviceps* genus (*C. purpurea*; *C. paspali* may also be involved). Pharmacologically active alkaloids produced by the fungus in the ergot body are the major cause of human intoxication. Two types of ergotism have been documented. In the convulsive type, affected persons have general convulsions, tingling sensation of muscles ('pins and needles') and sometimes the entire body is racked by spasms. Epidemics occurred between 1581 and 1928 in European and other countries. Although it has been suggested that the consumption of ergots that cause convulsive ergotism may have played a role in the Salem 'witchcraft' incidents, this is still controversial. In the gangrenous type of ergotism, the affected parts become swollen and inflamed, with violent, burning pains, hence its name, 'fire of St Anthony'. In general, the affected area became numb first, turned black, then shrank, and finally became mummified and dry. Outbreaks occurred from the Middle Ages to the nineteenth century. In some areas of France, grain contained as much as 25% ergots and people died after consuming about 100 g ergot over a few days. Between 1770 and 1771, about 8000 people died in one district alone in France. In general, 2% ergots in the grain is sufficient to cause an epidemic. European and most other countries have a regulatory limit of 0.1–0.2% ergots in flour. Biochemically, ergotisms are due to the intoxication of ergoline alkaloids that are produced by the fungus present in the sclerotia of *C. purpurea*. The most active components are amides of D-lysergic acid, including both cyclic peptide and nonpeptide amides of ergot alkaloids. These alkaloids causing smooth muscle contraction and blocking neurohormones have both vasoconstriction and vasodilation effects and also affect the central nervous system. Thus, they have some therapeutic uses.

Toxic metabolites of fungal-damaged plants   Phytoalexins are a group of compounds produced in plants as a result of physical or biological damage, which alters the metabolism of the host plant. Some of these compounds are toxic to humans and animals. One example is the fungal-infected sweet potato. Prior to World War II, Japanese investigators found that sweet potatoes infected by black rot mould *Ceratocystis fimbrita* (*Ceratostomella fimbriata*) were toxic to animals. A number of compounds, including ipomeamarone, ipomeanine, β-furoic acid and batatic acid, which contained a furan moiety with side chain attached at 3 or β-position, were isolated. Ipomeamarone (IPMone) gives a bitter taste to the sweet potato and is most abundant. It is considered as a hepatotoxin but may also be toxic to the lungs. Ipomeanol and IPMone are produced by *Fusarium solani javanicum* (in the USA). Although these metabolites are considered to have diverse toxic effects in farm animals, their impact on humans is not known. Another group of compounds that may have a role in human carcinogenesis are nitroso compounds produced by some common fungi. A number of nitrosamines have been identified in foods, and their presence in food regions of China with high rates of oesophageal cancer suggests that they may play a part in human carcinogenesis.

Conclusions

Mycotoxins are a group of naturally occurring, low molecular weight, fungal secondary metabolites, frequently contaminating agricultural commodities, foods and animal feeds. Numerous moulds can produce mycotoxins both before and after harvest, but not all are toxicogenic. The mycotoxins causing most concern are aflatoxins, ochratoxins, fumonisins and some tricothecene mycotoxins such as DON. Whereas natural occurrence of toxic fungi and mycotoxins in human and animal foods has been reported and outbreaks of mycotoxicoses have been documented, there are still some mycotoxicoses that have not been well characterized. Production of mycotoxins is controlled by such environmental conditions as kind of mould, substrate, water activity or moisture and relative humidity, temperature, time, atmosphere and microbial interaction. Although some mycotoxins are related to the cause of certain mycotoxicoses, others are not. Many mycotoxins are highly toxic to animals and probably to humans, although the toxicities vary considerably. Owing to their diversified toxic effects and high stability to heat treatment, the presence of mycotoxins in foods stuff is a potential hazard to human and animal health, and many measures have been established to control this problem.

See also: **Cancer**: Epidemiology and Associations Between Diet and Cancer. **Cereal Grains**: Dietary Significance and Nutritional Value.

Further Reading

Bhatnagar D, Lillehoj EB and Arora DK, eds (1991) *Handbook of Applied Mycology*, vol. 5, *Mycotoxins in Ecological Systems*. New York: Marcel Dekker.

Busby WF Jr and Wogan GN (1979) Food-borne mycotoxins and alimentary mycotoxicoses. In: Riemann H and Byran FL (eds) *Food-borne Infections and Intoxications*. New York: Academic Press.

CAST (1989) *Mycotoxins, Economic and Health Risks*. Task force report no. 116. Ames: Council of Agricultural Science and Technology.

Chu FS (1977) Mode of action of mycotoxins and related compounds. In: Perlman D (ed.) *Advances in Applied Microbiology* 22:33–43. New York: Academic Press.

Chu FS (1991) Mycotoxins: food contamination, prevention, mechanisms and carcinogenic potential. *Mutation Research* **259**:291–306.

Chu FS (1997) Trichothecene mycotoxicoses. In: *Encyclopedia of Human Biology* 8:511–522. New York: Academic Press.

Cole RJ and Cox RH (1981) *Handbook of Toxic Fungal Metabolites*, New York: Academic Press.

Dutton MF (1996) Fumonisins, mycotoxins of increasing importance: their nature and their effects. *Pharmacology and Therapeutics* **70**:137–161.

Hui YH, Gorham JR, Murrell KD and Cliver DO (1994) *Foodborne Disease Handbook*, vol. 2, *Fungal Diseases*. New York: Marcel Dekker.

Jackson L, DeVries JW and Bullerman LB, eds (1996) *Fumonisins in Food*. New York: Plenum.

Marasas WFO, Nelson PE and Toussoun TA (1986) *Toxigenic Fusarium Species: Identity and Mycotoxicology*. University Park, Pa: Penn. State Univ. Press.

Miller JD and Treholm HL (1994) *Mycotoxins in Grain: Compounds Other Than Aflatoxin*. St Paul: Eagan Press.

Riley RT, Norred WP and Bacon CW (1993) Fungal toxins in foods. *Annual Review of Nutrition* **13**:167–189.

Sharma RP and Salunkhe DK (1991) *Mycotoxin and Phytoalexins in Human and Animal Health*. Boca Raton: CRC Press.

Pesticides

M Saltmarsh, Alton, Hampshire, UK

Copyright © 1998 Academic Press

What are Pesticides?

Pesticide is a generic term that covers a wide range of natural and synthetic chemicals (over 700 in total) that are used to protect crops from attack from pests, both before and after harvest. There are many different sorts of pests. The term includes insects, slugs and snails, nematode worms, mites, rodents, weeds, moulds, bacteria and viruses. The chemicals can be applied before and during growth of the plant or on to the stored crop as, for example, fumigants which are used to kill pests which have infested stored cocoa or grain. Chemicals used to treat pests on animals are not included; they are considered as veterinary medicines.

The pesticide formulation used by the farmer will include the pesticide chemical itself and a number of other chemicals that enable it to be applied and to work as effectively as possible. These will include solvents, adhesives and surface-active agents such as emulsifiers. In some cases other chemicals, known as 'safeners' are applied to minimize the damage done to the crop while maintaining the effectiveness of the spray on the target.

It is estimated that worldwide usage of pesticides is around 2.5 million tonnes with a cost in 1997 of $21 billion.

Why Do We Need Pesticides?

Food crops are subject to attack by a multitude of pests and diseases and pesticides are applied to minimize the damage to the crop. It has been estimated that without protection world cereal crop yields would fall by between 46 and 83%. History is littered with records of crop failures and famine caused primarily by rodent, insect or fungus. Some of these events have had a wide-ranging and long-lasting effect, like the 1845–1846 Irish potato famine and the 1917–1918 German 'turnip winter', the latter so called because the potatoes rotted and turnips were the only stored root crop that was available to feed the population through the winter. Both these events, in which 1.5 million and 700 000 people died, respectively, were caused by potato blight, infection by the fungus *Phytophthora infestans*. Famine caused by massive swarms of locust is still all too common in Northern Africa and Arabia. Less spectacular but as disastrous is the loss of an estimated 30% of harvested crops in India to rodents.

In addition to the loss of the crop, pesticides are used to control agents which make the crop toxic rather than healthy. Two examples are the toxins caused by fungi. When an insect bores into a peanut it allows spores of the fungus *Aspergillus flavus* to enter and grow, producing the aflatoxins, a series of carcinogens. When rye (*Secale cereale*) grows in damp conditions a fungus, *Claviceps purpurea*, can grow on the seed. If this seed is subsequently ground into flour and made into bread it can cause consumers to suffer hallucinations, gangrene and death. Outbreaks amounting to epidemics were common in the Middle Ages in Europe and one occurred as recently as 1951 in France.

A second reason relates not so much to quantity as to quality. Supermarkets in the developed nations offer a wide range of fresh produce at competitive prices. Consumers do not like holes made by slugs and snails in their fresh lettuce. They do not expect scab marks on their apples, nor holes made by small maggots in their carrots. Flour millers do not expect to have to clean the grain from weed seeds before milling. Even small defects can dramatically reduce the value of the crop, or indeed make it unsaleable, and the need for a competitive price requires minimal labour input so that application of pesticide is essential.

Types of Pesticides

There are currently around 600 pesticides, both natural and synthetic. Natural pesticides include both chemicals derived from plant sources and biological agents such as parasitic wasps, mites, bacteria and chemicals contained within or exuded by plants or bacteria. While there is no inherent reason why natural products should be any safer than synthetic ones (after all, insect venoms and toxins and poisonous plants are natural), it appears that the risks do lie in their potential impact on the environment rather than on their effect in food. There are also increasing numbers of cases where plants have been given a gene which expresses a natural pesticide (see *Bacillus thuringiensis*, below).

At the time of writing, naturally derived pesticides make up less than 5% of the world pesticide market, but a great deal of work is being devoted to the screening of natural sources and this proportion will certainly increase. The most successful natural product development so far has been that of the pyrethrin insecticides, of which 33 are currently available.

The largest classes of pesticides are pyrethrins, organochlorines, organophosphates and carbamates, although there are many smaller classes with only one or two members. The chemical structures of the key members of the major groups are given in **Table 1**.

Important Pesticide Groups

This list covers the important pesticide groups and some individual pesticides but does not attempt to be comprehensive.

Pyrethrins

Pyrethrins are chemically related to pyrethrin, which is a secondary metabolite found in the flowers of the pyrethrum plant (*Chrysanthemum cinerariaefolium*). Dried pyrethrum flowers were used as an insecticide in ancient China and in the middle ages in Persia. The dried flowers are still used. Current production is around 20 000 tonnes per annum centred in Kenya and Tanzania. The pyrethrins are effective insecticides, having very low dose rates and rapid knockdown of insects but being harmless to mammals under all normal conditions. Natural pyrethrins break down rapidly under the influence of oxygen and UV light. This limits their use in agriculture, but recently synthetic analogues have been developed to overcome these problems. Starting from the structure of the natural product a large number of synthetic compounds have been made. It is worth noting how they differ in effectiveness: deltamethrin is a broad range insecticide; allethrin is particularly toxic to house flies (*Musca domestica*) but much less effective with other insects; flumethrin is active against cattle ticks; while others are acaricides or miticides with little or no insecticidal activity.

Bacillus thuringiensis

Bacillus thuringiensis is a widely distributed bacterium that during sporulation produces a crystal inclusion which is insecticidal when ingested by the larvae of a number of insect orders. Susceptible orders include Lepidoptera, Diptera and Coleoptera. The action of *B. thuringiensis* was first observed in 1901 as the cause of a disease of silkworms. Several strains of the bacterium have been identified with activity against a range of insects including cabbage looper, tobacco budworm, mosquito, black fly and more recently nematodes, ants and fruit flies. While the bacterium appears an ideal insecticide (having a toxicity 300 times greater than synthetic pyrethroids), it requires careful use. It is most effective against neonates and early larval instars so that spraying must be timed for egg hatch. It also has no contact activity and must be ingested so the plant must be well covered to ensure the insect receives a lethal dose. Furthermore it has a half-life in the field as short as 4 h, so careful timing is essential for it to be effective. Despite these limitations, it has been shown to be an important component of crop management programmes.

One way of overcoming the problems of application of *B. thuringiensis* is to incorporate the gene responsible for expression of the protein into the crop plant. This has been achieved with maize (*Zea mays*) to protect against the European corn borer, with cotton (*Gossypium hirsutum*) to protect against a range of budworms and bollworms, and with potato (*Solanum tuberosum*) against Colorado beetle. (Cotton may seem irrelevant in a text on food but cottonseed oil is used extensively in cooking oils, margarines and industrial fats.) This genetic modification has great benefits but care has to be taken that the food product has not changed in some unpredicted way. All genetically modified foods have to be extensively tested and cleared by regulatory agencies before release.

Neem oil

This is an oil obtained from the neem tree, *Azadirachta indica* A. Juss. It has been used as an insecticide in India and Africa but is increasingly being being developed as a significant commercial product. It contains a number of compounds, one of the most

Table 1 Chemical structure and Acceptable Daily Intake (ADI) of some pesticides

Compound	Class	Structure	ADI (mg per kg body weight)
Deltamethrin	Pyrethrin		0.01
DDT	Organochlorine		0.02
Lindane (HCH)	Organochlorine		0.008
Chlorfenvinphos	Organophosphate (mixture of two isomers)		0.002
Malathion	Organophosphate		0.02
Propoxur	Carbamate		0.02
Simazine	Triazine		0.005
Glufosinate			0.02
Glyphosate			0.3

active being azardirachtin, which is an insect anti-feedant but also shows growth inhibitory and endocrine disrupting effects. This product and its individual components is at the beginning of its commercial development which is likely to result in a series of products as significant as those from pyrethrum.

Microbial phytotoxins

These are herbicides and include the highly commercially successful glufosinate, a synthetic form of phosphinothricin, first isolated from *Streptomyces hygroscopicus*, a soil-borne microbe. This compound is a potent, irreversible inhibitor of glutamine synthetase which is used in plants for photorespiration. Many attempts have been made to make synthetic variants of phosphinothricin without success. Other members of this group include anisomycin and herboxidiene, derived from other *Streptomyces* strains. The veterinary insecticide, avermectin is derived from *Streptomyces avermitilis*.

Organochlorines

The organochlorines were the first group of synthetic insecticides and without them the dramatic decrease in malaria observed in the 1950s would have been impossible. The best known of this class is DDT (dichlorodiphenyltrichloroethane) but others include 2,4 DD, hexachlorbenzene and lindane. Of these only lindane (γ-hexachlorocyclohexane, see Table 1) is still in use in the developed world.

These compounds are very slow to break down in the environment and one result of this persistance was the decline in bird numbers graphically described by Rachel Carson in the book *Silent Spring*. The problem was that DDT was concentrated through the food chain and predator birds in particular were failing to raise chicks. Since the organochlorine pesticides and other sources of organochlorines in the environment have been largely phased out, numbers of many species of birds are rising again. It is recognized that pesticides are still having an adverse influence on numbers of some birds that inhabit farmland. However, this is not a straightforward effect. In the case of the Grey Partridge, for example, it is because herbicides have reduced the number of weeds, which in turn has reduced the number of insects which feed on the weeds, resulting in fewer insects for the chicks to eat.

The mechanism of action of the organochlorines is not known in detail although they appear to act on the central nervous system. In humans the organochlorine compounds tend to accumulate in the body fat and in mothers' milk. While there is no direct evidence that they cause mutations or cancers, there is concern that lindane may be a carcinogen and its role in breast cancer is still under review. However, in contrast, DDT and γ-HCH have both been shown to inhibit tumours in mice initiated by aflatoxin B_1.

Although organochlorine pesticides have largely been phased out in Europe, analysis for them continues and low levels of lindane are still being detected in milk in the UK (typically at 0.005 mg kg^{-1} compared with the Maximum Residue Limit (see below) of 0.008 mg kg^{-1} and an Acceptable Daily Intake (see below) of 0.05 mg per kg body weight)

Organophosphorus compounds

Organophosphorus compounds generally contain both sulfur and phosphorus linked to carbon atoms. Their discovery was a by-product of the development of nerve gases. The group includes parathion, malathion, dimethoate, diazinon and chlorfenvinphos. They are used as herbicides, insecticides and fungicides. They break down quickly in the environment and do not concentrate in body fats, although they may be stored for some time. However, their mode of action – inhibition of acetylcholine esterase – means that they affect both insects and mammals and their use depends on the effective dose in the target species being below the sensitivity of other species.

Acute effects of sublethal doses of organophosphates in man include sweating, salivation, abdominal cramps, vomiting, muscular weakness and breathing difficulties. Concern has also been expressed about long-term effects following acute exposure. Research suggests that some victims may show reductions in in some neurobehavioural tests when tested some months after exposure. There are also concerns that people who do not appear to have suffered acute poisoning, have subsequently developed debilitating illnesses. Symptoms include extreme exhaustion, mood changes, memory loss, depression and severe muscle weakness.

Carbamates

Carbamates are derived from carbamic acid and are used against both insects and weeds. They are also acetylcholine esterase inhibitors. They are very reactive and are used up rapidly after application.

Methyl bromide

Methyl bromide was for many years the fumigant of choice for destroying insects in stored crops, but it is now being withdrawn as part of the general restriction on volatile organohalogen compounds because of their damaging effect on the ozone layer. It is being replaced by a number of less environmentally damaging compounds, including phosphine, although none currently available is as effective or as cheap as methyl bromide.

Phosphine

Phosphine has been used as a fumigant for many years. It is highly reactive and leaves no residues but great care has to be taken in its application because it is very toxic to humans.

Control of Pesticides

The control over pesticides is exercised in two ways: stringent testing on new pesticides before they are permitted and measurement of the residue in the crop.

Testing pesticides

There are a number of national and international bodies that approve new pesticides within their areas of responsibility. These include Codex Alimentarius, the European Union and the US Food and Drug Administration (USFDA). Currently, within the European Union, registration of pesticides is being harmonized under Directive 91/414 EEC. Annexe 1 of this Directive will identify all active ingredients permitted in pesticides. As yet this Annexe is incomplete and member states are still acting under their National laws.

Within the UK pesticide registration is carried out under the Control of Pesticide Regulations 1986 and is the responsibility of the Ministry of Agriculture, Fisheries and Food who are advised by the Advisory Committee on Pesticides.

In the USA a new Food Quality Protection Act of 1996 replaced both the Food, Drug and Cosmetic Act and the Insecticide, Fungicide and Rodenticide Act to provide a comprehensive regulatory scheme for pesticides.

In order to gain approval for use, pesticides are subjected to an extensive testing programme including toxicity tests on mammals, plants, insects, fungi, birds, bees, fish, earthworms and other soil organisms. The toxicity studies include effects of pesticides on fetuses and infant animals. There are also environmental tests which include laboratory tests on the breakdown and movement of the chemical in plants, soil, water, air, mammals, birds and fish. These latter tests determine the rate of decay in the various species. Laboratory tests are followed by prolonged field trials to determine the fate of the chemical and its breakdown products in the environment and to estimate how the pesticide is concentrated up the food chain. On average it takes about 10 years to develop a new pesticide at a cost of about £50 million. The complete dossier of results has to be submitted to the approval body who determine whether the tests have been sufficiently rigorous to allow an Acceptable Daily Intake (ADI) of the pesticide to be set. The ADI is defined as the amount of a pesticide which can be taken in each day throughout a person's life with the practical certainty, on the basis of all known facts, that no harm will result. This is determined on the basis of the highest level at which the pesticide has no observable effect in animal tests. This is then reduced by a factor of 10 in case humans are more sensitive than the animals used in the tests, and by a further factor of 10 to allow for cases where some humans may be more sensitive than others. In some cases, where the data show unusual effects, the safety factor can be increased from 100 to 500 or 1000. In practice the amount of pesticides to which the population is exposed is far below this level. Table 1 includes the ADI for a number of the more common pesticides. There is no evidence that there are any cases where the combined effects of two pesticides are greater than the sum of their individual effects, in other words there is no evidence of synergy in toxicology between the different pesticides. Once Maximum Residue Limits (MRL see below) for foodstuffs have been set on the basis of good agricultural practice, a total dietary intake is determined by considering all commodities in which the pesticide is likely to be used, and assuming the upper range of consumption, all foodstuffs at the MRL and no losses during transport, storage or food preparation. This figure is then compared with the ADI. For all permitted pesticides in the UK the figure is below the ADI.

Maximum residue limits

Maximum Residue Limits (MRLs) are statutory limits set on individual active ingredient and foodstuff combinations. They are based on residue levels which result when the pesticide is used according to the instructions on the label and in accordance with good agricultural practice (GAP). MRLs may be used to ensure that the pesticides are only being used in accordance with GAP. Many countries have codes of good operating practice with training for farmers and operators to ensure that pesticides are used at optimal levels. Some countries rely on the Codex Alimentarius Committee on Pesticide Residues to establish MRLs, while others set their own. (Codex Alimentarius is an international body which has over 120 countries as members and their standards are increasingly being accepted as the basis of world trade in foodstuffs.)

In the USA the FDA used to set tolerances for pesticide/foodstuff combinations but under the 1996 Act it sets a level for each pesticide in all foods based on the principle of a reasonable certainty of no harm. This is defined as a lifetime cancer risk of less than 1 in a million. There is also a requirement that residue tolerances must be specifically determined as being safe for children.

Within the EU, individual Member States have historically set their own MRLs which differ from state to state. Directive 76/895 established a common MRL setting regime and a series of subsequent Directives has fixed the levels for a series of pesticides in fruit, vegetables, cereal products and products of animal origin. There is an ongoing programme to harmonize the levels throughout the Union.

Most industrialized countries have pesticide surveillance programmes which cover both home-produced and imported commodities and these report annually. The EU has an annual specific coordinated programme to check compliance in nominated combinations of pesticide and foodstuff. MRLs require sophisticated equipment for their determination because the levels are so low and the minimum detectable limit depends on the foodstuff. For example the tolerance for aldrin and dieldrin (two organochlorines) in the USA is between 0.05 and 0.1 mg kg^{-1} (parts per million), depending on the foodstuff. There are over 600 different active ingredients available commercially. Because there are so many, laboratories around the world have developed sophisticated rapid analytical techniques to allow them to screen pesticides by class so that retailers, food manufacturers and governments can carry out analyses as a matter of routine.

The MAFF 7th Report of the UK Working Party on Pesticide Residues in 1996 showed 68% of samples had no detectable residue, 31% had residues below the MRL and <1% were over the MRL. Similar results were obtained by the FDA who report results with relation to the tolerance to the pesticide/commodity combination. In 1995, of over 9000 samples analysed, 64% had no detectable residues, 34% had residues below the tolerance, <1% had residues over the tolerance and <1% had residues for which there is no tolerance in that particular pesticide/commodity combination.

In all cases where MRLs or tolerances are exceeded follow-up action is taken. For home-produced materials, this involves investigation of the grower and prosecution if necessary. For imports, exceeding the level causes the consignment to be refused entry.

Maximum levels of pesticides are also set for drinking water. Pesticides get into water from spraying, runoff, percolation or from treatment of fish in aquaculture. Good practice is increasingly being developed to minimize the levels in raw water and treatment works are developing systems to reduce incoming levels to levels acceptable for drinking water.

Endocrine Disruption

The possibility that a number of chemicals discharged into the environment as a result of human activity may disrupt the endocrine system of a wide range of mammals has recently been given considerable prominence. Among the chemicals cited are the organochlorine pesticides, most of which have now been withdrawn for other reasons. While there is no doubt that there are a significant number of cases of endocrine disruption, the evidence to point to any particular chemical as a cause is lacking. It is also worth noting that deliberate endocrine disruption is

a mechanism of a number of natural insecticides which act so as to inhibit development of juvenile larvae to adults. Fortunately these pesticides are reactive and usually have a short life in the field.

It is also true that there are very many naturally occurring endocrine disruptors, including the phyto-oestrogens present in vegetables, notably soya beans, peas, beans, cabbage and hops. However, since this issue is very serious a considerable amount of work has now been initiated and its results will have implications for future testing of pesticides.

Future Prospects

In many parts of the world it is recognized that there has been too great a reliance on pesticide use and not enough on improving agricultural practices. There is increasing pressure to move towards minimizing pesticide usage in order both to improve the environment and to reduce cost. This is being done by using newer, more specific pesticides and by adopting improved agricultural practices and integrated pest management (a combination of biological and chemical control).

Biological control is not new. It the 1930s *Macrocentrus homonae* was introduced into Sri Lanka from Indonesia to control the Tea Small Leaf Roller (*Adoxophyes*) with such success that no chemical control measures are needed for this pest even today. More recently there have been some impressive results from using predator insects, for example in the control of cassava green mite (*Mononchellus tanajoa*) in West Africa and white fly in European greenhouses.

In terms of agricultural practice, improved crop hygiene, crop rotation, better understanding of optimal timing of application and varying sowing dates, together with the development of more powerful and more discriminating pesticides has brought about a decrease in pesticide inputs. This is seen dramatically in the case of oil seed rape (canola). Less than 1% of the weight of herbicide applied to this crop in 1983 was applied in 1993.

Unfortunately pests develop resistance to individual pesticides over time and research is continually needed to develop both new pesticides and resistant varieties of crops to keep the pests in check. There has been some success with new pesticides having new modes of action such as the antifeedants and antimoulting agents, but this will be a continuing battle for the foreseeable future.

See Colour Plate 6.

See also: **Phytochemicals**: Classification and Occurrence; Epidemiological Factors.

FOOD FOLKLORE

Overview

A R P Walker, South African Institute for Medical Research, Johannesburg, South Africa

Copyright © 1998 Academic Press

Introduction

In all countries there are folklore beliefs in the use of a variety of foodstuffs to remedy illness and to promote long life. Some of the views and practices of the ancients and of later populations are discussed here in relation to current dietary guidelines. It appears that much that was taught and applied in the past has basic soundness, and is in harmony with present-day advice on the attainment of a 'prudent' diet and lifestyle.

Ancient Beliefs

Beliefs in the value of eating particular foods date back for thousands of years. It was believed that certain foods could prevent or heal various diseases, and prolong life, could fan sexual desire and overcome impotence, produce euphoria and enhance general wellbeing.

The knowledge that certain plants, mineral and animal substances have healing properties is as old as humanity. In most cultures, drug lore developed as a key part of folk medicine, and the rural habitat of most societies up to recent times meant that the vast majority of the population knew something of the healing properties of plants and other natural resources at least of those found in their own region. Such knowledge was handed down by word of mouth from one generation to the next, a procedure that worked well for the needs of small, scattered communities. In time, a flourishing trade in *materia medica* developed, with a ready market in the towns, to which growing numbers of people migrated. Many early writers, such as Pliny in Roman times, admonished the public for its gullibility over the often extravagant claims of doctors, druggists and healers. Inevitably, however, greed, ignorance and credulity sustained the drug markets; indeed, even some of the better educated were prey to the claims of quack doctors, so anxious and hopeful were patients for a cure.

In classical Greek and later in Roman times, there was considerable interest in the nature of foods and their sequelae. There was a detailed classification of food and drink according to their perceived properties – strong, weak, drying, moistening, cooling, heating, binding, laxative, and so forth. Thus, beef was strong and binding, beans were astringent and laxative, seafood was dry and light, and cheese strong and nourishing. The type and the quantity of food consumed would be adjusted for each individual to maintain a balance between the elemental fire and water of which all living creatures were thought to be composed.

The importance and significance of food in the everyday lives of people was well recognized. Thus, the English language has numerous allusions to food. We eat our words and swallow our wrath, we sink our teeth into a problem, drink in a message, find an explanation indigestible, and reject it with biting comments. Additionally, we speak of 'taste' in many areas of flavours to describe people and situations – spicy, flat, sour, sweet, delectable, and so on. We also speak of sensations associated with food – of coolness, bland, tart, smooth as cream, an oily personality, and so forth.

In early times, numerous individual foods and their benefits became important. As examples, in the time of the biblical patriarchs, Rachel quarrelled with Leah over who should partake of the mandrakes gathered by Reuben; for each wife wanted to eat them in order to kindle desire in Jacob. At the siege of Masada, the Roman general, Flavius Silva, described the foods and the concoctions that he ate and of the rigours he underwent in seeking to overcome his impotence. Included in his treatment was the drinking 'of a daily potion of egg whites, cinnamon and hot mead until I retched at the thought of another . . .'. Pliny reported that the Emperor Nero ate leeks seven days each month to clear his voice. At much the same period, there was Cato's medicine, which was a mixture of magical incantations and animal and vegetable remedies. Cabbage administered both internally and externally was his favourite 'cure-all'.

It is interesting that some foods were given much more attention than others. Thus, honey, when used externally, has been known to have wound healing properties for four thousand years. Egyptian art depicts the collecting and processing of honey as worthy of being offered to the gods. For the children of Israel, the 'promised land' of Canaan was 'flowing with milk and honey'. In the time of Hippocrates, honey was given as oxymel (vinegar and honey) for pain, hydromel (honey and water) for thirst, and as a mixture of honey, water and various medicinal substances for acute fevers.

Garlic was used by all early civilizations. The Egyptians fed large doses to their labourers to keep them healthy and invigorated as they built the pyramids and other buildings. Garlic was one of the items that the children of Israel cried out for in the wilderness. Its position as a leading food with numerous beneficial properties was often mentioned. Thus, Dioscorides, about AD 65, wrote five books on *De Materia Medica*, the product of a lifetime study. Therein it was claimed, *inter alia*, that garlic was an excellent food, both to clean out the blood vessels and to remedy obstructions. However, a warning was made that when taken in excess, garlic would stir up bodily lusts and become a source of lechery. The Romans thought that garlic gave physical strength.

As to bread, it has been pointed out that, 'If it is possible to condense three thousand years of history into a few lines of print, the best way to do so perhaps is to consider the various groups of people who have pressed for bread to be white or brown'. The difference in food value between the two was well recognized by Hippocrates, who maintained, 'Thy food shall be thine remedy', and, more to the point, 'And this I know, moreover, that to the human body it makes a great difference whether the bread be fine or coarse, of wheat with or without the hull . . .'. In some countries, bread has more importance than in others. In modern Italy, where bread is eaten every day and at every meal, an emotional tone surrounds it. The people consider it wrong to waste any food, but sinful to waste bread; the *thrifty* housewife is so described because she uses much more of bread than of other accompanying foods.

Salt and its symbolism is one of the fascinating stories in folklore. It was the earliest condiment, and it has been almost universally used. Homer referred to salt as 'divine', and he separated those nations that knew of salt from those that did not. Faithfully living Christians were called 'the salt of the earth'. Salt was eagerly sought and even used as money. The Roman saltcellar was a symbol of hospitality and friendship. In ancient days, salt was used as a form of purification, as a medicine, and in embalming after death. Wars have even been fought for salt rights. One of the causes of the French Revolution was reported to be the tax on salt. In Africa, a salt mixture was sometimes obtained from wood ashes. In ancient times,

pepper also reached fame, and reparations after wars often were made partially in payments of pepper.

Historical Beliefs

In medieval times, many believed that both animals and plants reflect, in their outward characteristics, the nature of their curative potential. Thus, the lungs of the longwinded fox were recommended for asthma, the juice of the red beet for anaemia, and the root of the mandrake for male impotence.

The pain of love was healed with Horace's prescription of pigeons and turtledoves. The mood of love was wooed with pistachio nuts, radishes, celery, dates, mint, parsley, quinces and walnuts. Italians thought that tomatoes had an amorous effect, and Italian sauces became popular. Lettuce was initially thought to be a sexual stimulant, but later, it was looked upon as a repressor.

In the late 1600s the potato was brought from South America to many Western countries. Spanish peasants marvelled at its lush growth, but somehow came to think that it poisoned the soil, spread the plague and could cause diarrhoea and leprosy. This poor reputation may have arisen from the views of the strict clergy in that country, who held that there was no authority in the Bible for the potato's existence. Some governments, however, regarded the potato as an answer to periodic famines. Its real popularity in Europe did not develop for another two centuries. In Ireland, even although it became a staple, the potato was thought by some to be immoral, since it was so easy to grow and left the hands of the farmers idle.

In the sixteenth century, native Americans used an infusion of spruce and pine needles to cure what was later described as scurvy. In Europe, it was reported that parsley, chervil, lettuce and strawberries were good to heal spongy gums. Walnut juice was lauded as the key to perfect nutrition; it was thought to be a source of good health and long life. A shortage of iron, as manifested by 'pale ears', was treated by drinking the liquid resulting from rusty iron shavings steeped in vinegar overnight. Another early treatment was to stick rusty nails into a sour apple and allow them to stand overnight, and then to remove the nails and eat the apple. An English surgeon claimed that sugar alone could provide the basis for good nutrition, good disposition and a cure for all wounds.

In the early 1800s, a London physician, Dr Cadogan, wrote, 'It is a custom of some to give a little roast pig to an infant which, it seems, cures it of all of its mother's longings'. It was believed in this period that 'walking barefoot on the dewy grass provided contact with basic life force that is being evoked from the living soil . . . put your hands in the soil as much as you can . . . handle living plants and drain their health giving electrical charges into your body. Man should live where he can take his shoes off occasionally and walk barefeet'. For the very overweight, the instruction was, 'You will take sitz baths, live on fruits and green vegetables alone. Soon you will become indeed a much healthier man'. Saffron was regarded as a specific for jaundice, and was also prescribed in cases of measles to hasten the eruptive state.

In the USA in the 1830s, when cholera broke out on the eastern seaboard, several cities banned the sale of fruits, thinking they were the cause, along with salads and uncooked vegetables. Sylvester Graham in the USA wrote, 'Tea can produce delirium tremens. Condiments, like sexual excess, cause insanity'. John Harvey Kellogg wrote, 'Coffee cripples the liver'. As to tea, he also quoted an early opinion that tea was the main cause of insanity.

Good old-fashioned sea water was often recommended in April or May as part of the general spring cleaning. In the eighteenth century in the UK it was held that sea water could cure many ills. The well-circumstanced flocked to Brighton to drink the sea water and to bathe in it. The Prince of Wales (later King George IV) took sea water to cure swollen glands. It was also considered to be a cure for haemorrhoids.

Other Beliefs

In Australia, aborigines believed that to eat the flesh of the parrot or cockatoo is to risk developing, like the birds, a hollow in the top of one's head and a hole under one's chin. Believing the liver to be the seat of mercy, others forcibly fed the organ to the sly or the mean in their communities.

In East Africa, young girls and women were often not permitted to eat eggs lest they become infertile or acquire extra lovers. Eating eggs could result in baldness. During pregnancy, drinking cow's milk could later spoil the mothers' breast milk.

In the eighteenth-century Madagascar, soldiers were forbidden to eat hedgehog, . . . as it is feared that this animal, from its propensity of coiling up into a ball when alarmed, will impart a timid, shrinking disposition to those who partake of it'.

In Jamaica, it was believed that drinking sorrel may initiate premature contractions during pregnancy, and the eating of pepper may cause the baby to become blind.

Twentieth Century Beliefs

The twentieth century saw a further emphasis on the use of garlic, which was regarded as a means of curing low blood pressure, of inhibiting germs, and of cleansing blood and the intestines. It was even urged to put a piece of garlic in the rectum at night. Patients could expect to taste it in their mouths the next morning, and would then be assured that the full cleansing task had been accomplished while they slept.

A theory was advanced by Rodale and others that healthy living required natural foods to be eaten with no cooking: 'No animal eats cooked foods'. There should be avoidance of sugar and of fluoridated water. A chemical-free diet, a supplement of rose hips, and natural vitamins and minerals should be eaten daily. It was predicted that this diet if faithfully followed could prolong life to a hundred years.

In *Folk Medicine: A Vermont Doctor's Guide to Good Health*, the author revived interest in vinegar. He maintained that the principal American health problem is an excess of alkalinity. Hence, patients were advised to avoid meat, wheat foods, citrus fruits, white sugar and maple syrup, and to precede each meal with two tablespoons of apple cider vinegar. By such means the acidity of the body would be increased. Others held vinegar to be of value in weight reduction.

Organic foods were and are strongly held by some to be the more nutritious. However, the criticism was made that organic foods tend to become the most contaminated of all. Organic fertilizers of animal or of human origin are more likely to contain gastrointestinal parasites. Among other beliefs, royal jelly from the queen bee was believed to be of great healing importance. Postmenopausal women after eating royal jelly were said to regain their fertility. Yogurt was and still is credited with the capacity to lessen infections in the bowel.

How Sound Are Present Convictions?

When we were young we were told to eat crusts to make our hair curl, beetroot to give colour to our cheeks, carrots to make our eyes sparkle, parsley and onions to promote breast development, fish to nourish brains, and an apple a day to keep the doctor away. It may be wondered, whether our beliefs are any sounder than the convictions of the past, when we imbibe 'tonics' to whet jaded appetites, consume various proprietary foods or prescriptions to put 'beef' into us, seek to combat undernutrition during the night hours, to keep the memory alert at examination times, and to provide athletes with extra energy and *élan*.

As to the specific efficacy of remedies, in the past there was the drinking of lemon juice and like preparations to prevent or treat scurvy, of cod liver oil to avoid rickets, and the eating of 250–500 g liver a day to control pernicious anaemia – these certainly are valid remedies today. The scientific reasons for the effectiveness of these and other earlier practices are now well understood, and if need be, the appropriate remedies can be taken in pill form.

What of present advice and belief in the benefits of some of our everyday foodstuffs? There is good reason to believe that a lettuce or a cupful of spinach a day will help to protect against megaloblastic anaemia and neural tube defects; legumes (beans, peas, lentils and peanuts) will help to reduce blood glucose level; oatmeal, or almonds or walnuts, will promote a reduction of serum cholesterol level; garlic (yet a further use) has a pronounced enhancing effect on blood fibrinolytic activity; grapefruit reduces elevated haematocrit, cabbage and brussels sprouts are potentially cancer preventatives, and, conceivably, a quarter of a cupful of olive oil taken daily may have a significantly protective effect against cancers of the breast and colon, and against coronary heart disease, as exemplified by the experience of some Mediterranean populations. The old adage of 'an apple a day . . .' has actually given rise to a health philosophy. Not least, the antibacterial and antifungal properties of honey have now been well documented.

Folklore beliefs: are they 'in' or 'out'?

With the substantiation of some old folklore beliefs, and with newly advanced guidelines for a 'prudent' diet, what kind of message regarding what to eat, or what to avoid, is being received through the popular media? Rather mixed, alas, with much overclaiming and overblaming. The authoritative nutritional guidelines to all Western populations and to most urban developing populations are: eat less, eat less fat especially animal fat, and double the intakes of bread and vegetables, with fruit up by a half. So what message is being actually received? An assistant editor of the *British Medical Journal* wrote rather sarcastically, 'When the message does contain explicit nutritional comment, often the comment is false or nonsensical . . . It is often antimedical, antichemical, or antiindustrial . . . "Eat (or drink) this and you will enjoy it, or be happy, or be seen to be successful, or beautiful, or sexually attractive".' In despair at the numerous contradictions in advice, a London housewife was led to cry, 'First they say bread's good for you, then they say it's bad; butter used to be good for you, now they say it's bad; I don't listen to any of them anymore!'. In the USA, in a recent study of food advertisements on Saturday morning television, most were considered to be the antithesis of what is recommended for healthful eating.

It could be asked – are doctors themselves persuaded? In this regard it is interesting to note that in a recent review on the physician's role in health promotion in the USA, it was concluded that physicians are actually *less* attentive to their patient's diet than in the past. Only half of the large series of doctors questioned considered diet to be 'very important' in health regulation. Their scepticism was attributed in part to their opinion of the lack of valid and consistent data to support many official dietary recommendations.

How do medical journals regard old and more recent folklore advice? In some reviews, there have been endorsements, albeit lightheartedly, of beliefs of the past. In an editorial in *Annals of Internal Medicine*, the author reminded us of 'our mother's health behavioral prescriptions regarding the injunctions "Don't smoke, drink, or let yourself get fat. Drive safely. Eat your fish and vegetables," and so on'. It was concluded, ironically, that 'these prescriptions are supported by extensive and costly investigations. Perhaps our most sensible public health recommendation should be moderation in all things, and moderation in *that*'. A like message was echoed in an article in *Nature* entitled, 'Eat your broccoli (and brussels sprouts) . . .' 'Every month or so another "broccoli" story makes news, reflecting an understandable desire for a silver bullet, a single answer. But given the present level of knowledge, there is only one right answer about diet and health. Do what your mother told you to do – eat a balanced diet and get some exercise. And hope you inherited good genes'. Intriguingly, 'a single answer' is but an echo of the age-old quest in centuries past for the 'elixir of life'.

For the enthusiasts, the strict vegetarians, the fruitarians and others, it is well to allow that the foods that they consume, and in whose value they have great faith, can confer a feeling of wellbeing and of associated good health beyond that measured by chemical analysis or by biological evaluation. In this connection, one of the modern founders of social medicine was Professor John Ryle of Cambridge. One of his tenets was that the study of the unfit should be balanced in endeavour by the study of the fit. Little research is directed into this field. With the hugely increasing interest in alternative medicine, greater attempts should be made to learn why the consistently well keep well, no matter how bizarre may be their beliefs and their dietary and nondietary practices.

In brief, while many of the beliefs of old were fanciful, others, regarding the beneficial properties of certain foodstuffs and of not overeating, have a sound physiological basis.

Food Information, Misinformation and Danger

In Western populations nutrition is now a very popular subject, but even with all of the current knowledge, it seems to be no easier to educate the public today than it was in the past. Indeed, in the USA it has been stated that more food notions – correct and incorrect – flourish there than in any other Western country. Nutrition is one of the biggest drawing cards on the newsstands. While the public is increasingly food conscious, nutritional understanding has shown limited improvement. One result is continuing, perhaps increasing, food faddism. This term includes many aspects of nutritional misinformation. It is characterized by exaggerated beliefs about the value of nutrition in health and disease. While food fads are popular they are usually followed enthusiastically only for short periods. Most fads may be physically harmless, but they may be costly for poor people. Some fads may lead to nutritional inadequacies, and could lead to serious deficiencies. Furthermore, a fad may be harmful because a person adopts this therapy rather than seeking the advice of a physician, and hence may delay appropriate medical treatment. Children tend to accept their parent's beliefs, which develop into relatively fixed patterns which are difficult to change in later years. Teenagers are particularly susceptible to food fads because of pressure from their associates.

Two common advertising claims that require comment are that foods are 'natural' or 'organic'. The use of the word 'natural' and similar terms in food labelling and advertising has been a source of concern for some years. In the UK in July 1989 the Ministry of Agriculture, Fisheries and Food issued guidelines on such claims. These advanced some principles on which such labelling should be based. It was stated that the term 'natural' without qualification should be used to describe single foods of a traditional nature to which nothing has been added. Claims such as 'natural goodness', 'naturally better' or 'nature's way' have very limited meaning and should not be used. Moreover, 'natural', meaning no more than plain or unflavoured, should not be used.

Regarding 'organic' claims, in the UK in June 1991 a regulation on 'organic' indications in relation to agricultural products and foodstuffs was adopted. Claims that a food has been produced organically may be made only where prescribed principles of organic production at farm level have been satisfied. The principles are that the fertility and biological activity of the soil must be maintained or increased, where appropriate, by procedures such as the cultivation of legumes, green manures or deep-rooting plants, in an appropriate multiannual rotation programme. Other organic or mineral fertilizers (listed in the regulation) can be applied only when secured by adequate crop rotation or soil conditioning. For compost activation, appropriate microorganism or plant-based preparations (biodynamic preparations) may be used. Pests, diseases and weeds shall be controlled by a combination of the measures including appropriate rotation programmes, protection of natural enemies of pests through provisions favourable to them (e.g. hedges, nesting sites, release of predators), and natural and mineral materials listed in the regulation.

In the USA, the Food and Drug Administration (FDA) has made the criticism that 'the use of the word "health" in connection with food implies that these products have health giving or curative properties, when in general, they possess simply the nutritive qualities to be experienced in any wholesome food product'. At present, if a food product makes false or misleading claims on the label, the FDA can take action because of mislabelling. Until recently, manufacturers were only allowed to make nutritional claims on labels, such as 'good source of vitamin C'. Claims that the product might prevent, treat or cure a disease were prohibited on the grounds that it was being marketed as an 'unapproved drug', not as a food. However, within the past few years, there have been changes, due to the results of experimental studies on animals and humans, epidemiological observations, and so forth. As an example, a cereal manufacturer has advertised bran products with the claim that they can help to decrease the risk of certain life-threatening diseases, particularly colon cancer.

At present, with certain limits, products can be legally promoted in books, magazine articles and on radio or television talk shows. The unknowns of medicine, and disagreement among reputable scientists regarding interpretation of research findings, tend to foster nutritional misinformation. Magical solutions appeal to those who distrust the medical profession. Given the right circumstances, potentially everyone is capable of exchanging sound judgment and common sense for miraculous cures. In the USA, France and certain other countries, it has been reported that patients now turn for help to the various alternative healers, rather than to their own physician. This indicates that beliefs in food folklore are far from being discarded.

See also: **Food Choice**: Factors Influencing Food

Choice. **Health Foods**: Dietary Supplements - Micronutrients. **Religious Customs**: Influence on Diet.

Further Reading

Adams F (1939) *The Genuine Works of Hippocrates*, p 9. Baltimore: Williams & Wilkins.

Bingham S (1991) Dietary aspects of a health strategy for England. *British Medical Journal* 303: 353–355.

Cameron AG (1971) *Food Facts and Fallacies*. London: Faber.

Coetzee R (1982) *FUNA Food from Africa: Roots of Traditional African Food Culture*. Durban: Butterworths.

Davis A (1970) *Let's Eat Right to Keep Fit*. New York: Harcourt Brace.

Deutch RM (1977) *The New Nuts Among the Berries*. Palo Alto: Bull Publishing.

Jackson R (1988) Physicians and their medicine. In: *Doctors and Diseases in the Roman Empire*, chap. 3, pp 75–76, 78. London: British Museum Press.

Lowenberg ME, Todhunter EN, Wilson ED, Savage JR and Lubawski JL (1979) *Food and People*, 3rd edn. New York: John Wiley.

Majno G (1975) *The Healing Hand: Man and Wound in the Ancient World*. Cambridge: Harvard University Press.

Melville B and Francis V (1992) Dietary habits and superstitions of rural Jamaican women during pregnancy. *European Journal of Clinical Nutrition* 46:373–374.

Rinzler CA (1991) *Feed A Cold, Starve A Fever*. New York: Ballantine.

Trant H (1954) Food taboos in East Africa. *Lancet* 267:703–705.

Walker ARP (1995) Dietary advice: from folklore to present beliefs. *Nutrition Reviews* 53:8–10.

Whelan EM and Stare FJ (1976) *Panic in the Pantry*. New York: Atheneum.

Wynder EL, Stellman SD and Zang EA (1996) High fiber intake: indicator of a healthy lifestyle. *Journal of the American Medical Association* 275:486–487.

Zumla A and Lulat A (1989) Honey – a remedy rediscovered. *Journal of the Royal Society of Medicine* 82:384–385.

FOOD FORTIFICATION

Importance in the Diet

U Arens, British Nutrition Foundation, London, UK

Copyright © 1998 Academic Press

Food fortification is a long-standing practice, and is even a legal requirement for some products in some countries. The addition of nutrients to foods can substantially reduce the risk of nutrient deficiency diseases in population groups. The basis for the fortification of foods should ideally be the assessment of nutrient intakes in population groups in relation to scientific recommendations about requirements for health. However, fortification practices are influenced by many other considerations including legislative requirements and marketing benefits. Some scientists are concerned that unregulated food fortification may lead to the risk of excessive intakes of particular nutrients, and may also confuse nutrition education messages. However, many consider nutrient enrichment of foods to be the most effective way to improve the intakes of particular nutrients, and thus some health indices, within populations.

Definitions

Restoration

The term 'restoration' describes the replacement, either fully or partially, of nutrients lost during some stage of food production or distribution. Restoration should be considered in situations where the original food was an important source of one or more nutrients prior to processing, especially where there is also evidence of inadequate intakes of such nutrients in population groups. A report issued by the Food and Agriculture Organization/World Health Organization (FAO/WHO) *Codex Alimentarius* Food Standards Programme suggested that the criteria for restoration should be 'where the edible portion of the food, prior to processing, storage or handling, contains an essential nutrient in an amount equal to, or greater than, 10% of the Recommended Daily Amount (RDA) in a reasonable daily intake'.

Fortification or enrichment

The term 'fortification' describes the addition of nutrients to a food above levels that would normally occur. In some cases nutrients added to a food would not normally be present at all. The latter practice is sometimes described more specifically as 'supplementation', although the term may be confused with the practice of the consumption of nutrient concentrates in tablet form. In most cases the terms 'fortification' and 'enrichment' can be used interchangeably, but some caution is needed with the American legislative description of certain products as 'enriched', as such products have a standard of identity that requires nutrients to be added in accordance with regulations issued by the US Food and Drug Administration (FDA). The term 'nutrification' is sometimes used.

Rationale

The public health rationale for fortification is that additional intakes of nutrients will be beneficial to a population group. Nutrient intakes from unfortified food sources should be assessed and population groups identified. From this information, decisions can be made on the most suitable foods to be used as 'carriers', and the appropriate types and amounts of nutrients to be added to the foods.

When a population group at risk of deficiency selects foods not typically consumed by other sections of a population, targeted fortification using these particular foods will be the most effective strategy. However, in many cases risk groups do not consume foods that are different. The targeted supply of higher intakes of particular nutrients to small numbers of an easily identifiable population group may be more effectively achieved by giving supplements, e.g. iron tablets to pregnant women.

Where the benefits of higher intakes of a nutrient extend to wider groups within a population, fortification of staple foods is an appropriate strategy. The variation in intakes of staple foods often broadly relates to energy requirements. The use of staple foods should ensure that while nearly all the population obtains additional amounts of the nutrient, individuals consuming higher amounts of a staple food are not put at risk of excessive intakes of the nutrient being fortified (the fortificant).

If the intakes of a micronutrient in a population are assumed to follow a normal distribution (**Fig. 1**), the effect of fortification of a staple food can be predicted to shift the distribution curve to the right, as a result of increased intakes of the micronutrient in (nearly) all sections of the population. The percentage of the population with low and possibly inadequate intakes of the micronutrient becomes smaller, thus reducing the risk of nutrient deficiency associated with poor health. Conversely, the percentage of the population with higher intakes of the micronutrient becomes larger, and consideration must be given in formulation decisions, to ensure that adverse

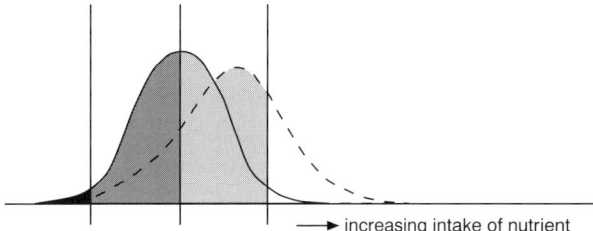

Figure 1 Predicted effects of fortification of a staple food on the distribution of intakes of a micronutrient in a population. Solid line, 'normal' distribution of a micronutrient; dashed line, distribution of the micronutrient after fortification. The density of the shading of the area under the curve reflects the degree of risk of inadequate intake: solid, high risk; medium, moderate risk; light, low risk.

effects of higher intakes of the micronutrient are unlikely to occur.

The decision to fortify foods includes consideration of many aspects including the following.

Legislative requirements

The addition of nutrients to particular foods may be mandatory in some countries. In the UK, for example, legislation requires the addition of vitamins A and D to margarine, and thiamin, niacin, calcium and iron to all flour except wholemeal. In the USA, the term 'enriched' carries defined legal specifications in relation to the nutrient content of certain foods, e.g. milk, flour, cornmeal, pasta and margarine.

Expert recommendations

For some product sectors, expert committees establish recommendations for nutrient parameters. For example, infant formula manufacturers consider the views of recognized panels with expertise on the nutritional requirements of infants – in Europe such recommendations are set by the European Society for Paediatric Gastroenterology and Nutrition (ESPGAN). Some trade and professional organizations also provide general guidelines to manufacturers on fortification practice.

Research data

Scientific studies may indicate the benefits of higher intakes of particular nutrients in subgroups of the population. Where expert committee or policy guidance is not available, the fortification of certain products may be based on such research data. In the absence of formal guidance, considerable care needs to be taken with the application of scientific research data into food fortification decisions, to ensure public safety and responsible practice.

Dietary survey data

In many countries dietary survey data are available indicating amounts and distributions of nutrient intakes in sections of the population. Such data are a useful basis for decisions on the nutritional rationale for the addition of nutrients to foods, the quantities of nutrients to be added, and the most suitable food vehicles.

Labelling requirements

Legislative criteria for nutrient declarations or claims may have an effect on fortification practice. Where a 'minimum' nutrient content is required to allow claims to be made on food labels, nutrients will often be added to products to achieve levels sufficient to enable such claims to be made.

Marketing aspects

The addition of nutrients to a food may provide a positive feature to communicate to consumers. The marketing advantage is likely to be strongest where competitor products are not fortified, and where consumers have some awareness of the 'benefits' of the nutrient being added. Conversely, public perception may consider the fortification of some products to be 'unnatural', or indicative of the poor nutritional quality of the original ingredients in a food product.

Technical benefits or complications

Some vitamins function effectively as antioxidants or colouring agents – vitamin C, for example, is particularly valued for its ability to reduce oxidative spoilage in certain foods. When the prime purpose for the addition of a vitamin to a food becomes its functional rather than its nutritional properties, it should be considered a food additive. In some cases, the addition of nutrients to particular products may not be possible for technical reasons. The stability of individual nutrients varies widely, and the formulation of nutrient mixtures needs to consider factors affecting deterioration. Vitamin B_{12}, for example, is sensitive to light, is unstable in both acid and alkaline conditions. Added nutrients may also affect food quality: iron salts in particular may accelerate oxidative rancidity, resulting in adverse taste and colour changes in some foods. Differences in the biological availability of different nutrient forms will need to be considered in relation to respective technical aspects of suitability.

Costs

The addition of a vitamin or mineral to a food increases costs to the food manufacturer (including additional costs for the mixing process and quality control procedures). Costs will also vary depending on the particular fortificant selected and the level of addition. Such costs, however, are often minimal in relation to other manufacturing costs, and may not affect pricing of the final product. In some instances, the addition of nutrients to a product may allow it to be sold at a higher price.

Fortified Foods in the UK Diet

A wide range of food products sold in the UK are fortified. The most significant foods are described by product sector.

Margarine

Margarine has been fortified in the UK since 1925 on a voluntary basis, but in 1940, the government made the addition of vitamins A and D to all margarine sold for domestic use compulsory, so that levels are comparable with, or higher than, those found in butter (**Table 1**). Policies requiring the mandatory fortification of margarine also exist in many other countries, e.g. Belgium, Denmark, Australia, Sweden and Portugal. Margarine makes a particularly important contribution to the dietary intake of vitamin D. Data from the UK National Food Survey in 1988 indicated that margarine alone provided 40% of average household intakes of vitamin D and 10% of vitamin A (butter provided 2% and 5% respectively).

In 1991 a UK government report reviewing the fortification of yellow fats recommended that the addition of vitamins A and D to margarine should continue to be mandatory, and that manufacturers should be encouraged to extend the practice of fortification to low-fat spreads. The report emphasized that although most people in the UK obtained vitamin D principally from the action of sunlight on skin, in housebound or elderly people, vitamin D from fortified margarines may be vital in preventing osteomalacia in an already vulnerable group. Other groups in the UK at risk of poor vitamin D status include Asian children and women.

Table 1 Content of vitamins A and D in butter and margarine sold in the UK

Vitamin	Margarine, fortified (μg per 100 g)	Butter (μg per 100 g)
Vitamin A	780	815
Vitamin D	7.94	0.76

From Holland et al. (1991).

Bread and flour

All wheat flours, except wholemeal, are required by UK legislation to contain certain levels of thiamin, niacin, calcium and iron (**Table 2**). The addition of these nutrients to flour was introduced partly to replace nutrients lost during processing. In 1981, a UK government committee reviewed the need for this legislation, and recommended that such restoration should no longer be mandatory. For example, concerning calcium, it was suggested that 'the original reasons, and all the subsequent reasons for the addition of calcium to flour that have been put forward over the years, are not longer valid ... there is no longer any nutritional justification for the compulsory addition of calcium to flour'. However, revised regulations were opposed during public consultation, and fortification remains a legal requirement in the UK.

The nutrients added to flour provide about 14% of average household intakes of thiamin and 11% of calcium intakes, whereas the contribution to iron and niacin intakes are much smaller (6% and 2% average intakes). The withdrawal of thiamin fortification from bread and flour, was predicted to double the number of those whose thiamin intake was below an arbitrary 1 mg a day, from 21% to 43% of a sample of UK adults. An assessment of dietary intakes of UK adolescents predicted that withdrawal of calcium fortification from bread and flour would result in a 13% reduction in average calcium intakes in a population group whose intakes should be increased.

As a result of scientific data describing the protective effects of higher intakes of folic acid in the maternal diet in relation to the incidence of neural tube defects in babies, recommendations have been made that additional folate/folic acid should be consumed by all women prior to conception and during early pregnancy. Most women are not able to achieve the intakes recommended (600 μg per day) by increased consumption of folate-rich foods, so routine fortification of bread and breakfast cereals with folic acid has been proposed in the UK.

Table 2 Micronutrient composition of different flours in the UK

Micronutrient	Unfortified white flour (mg per 100 g)	Fortified white flour (mg per 100 g)	Wholemeal flour (mg per 100 g)
Calcium	15	140	38
Iron	1.5	2.0	3.9
Thiamin	0.1	0.3	0.5
Niacin	0.7	1.7	5.7

From Holland et al. (1988).

Breakfast cereals

Most ready-to-eat breakfast cereals have been fortified on a voluntary basis for many years with a range of vitamins and iron. Breakfast cereals make a useful contribution to intakes of micronutrients in the typical UK diet, especially of thiamin, riboflavin, vitamin B_6, folic acid, vitamin D and iron. The levels of micronutrients added to breakfast cereals are usually between 17% and 50% of the labelling recommended daily allowance (RDA) per serving, and are well below levels identified as being potentially adverse.

A UK government expert advisory group recommended that more breakfast cereals should be fortified with folic acid. Although about 70% of breakfast cereals sold in the UK are fortified with folic acid, levels of intake achieved are still well below the 600 μg per day recommended for women prior to and during early pregnancy, and debate continues in support of mandatory fortification and greater emphasis on the use of supplements.

Drinks

Most soft drinks are not fortified, although products based on fruit juice often contain additional vitamin C to compensate for losses during processing, and to function as an antioxidant. Several soft drinks are marked specifically as 'sports drinks' and these products typically contain a greater variety and higher levels of added vitamins and minerals.

Vegetable protein foods

A variety of food products attempt to simulate the taste qualities of meat for people choosing not to consume meat products. Because meat is an important source of several nutrients not readily available from other foods, there has been some concern that the substitution of meat by vegetable protein foods may result in lower intakes of these nutrients. A UK government committee examining meat substitute foods recommended that such foods contain specified levels of thiamin, riboflavin, vitamin B_{12}, iron and zinc. Levels advised were higher than those typically present in meat because consideration was given to the predicted lower bioavailability of nutrients from these foods, e.g. the lower absorption of nonhaem iron compared with the haem iron present in meat. In practice, the levels suggested for products that resemble meat are only achievable through fortification.

Meal replacements

Meal replacement products are intended to replace one or several meals normally consumed, e.g. milk-based drinks intended for consumption during periods of poor appetite or illness, or food products to support attempts at weight loss. The assumption is made that people will depend on such products as a principal or complete source of nutrition, so meal replacements are typically fortified. A UK government committee specifically considered the composition of very low-calorie diet (VLCD) products used during weight loss programmes, and stated that such products should provide 100% RDA levels of specified micronutrients. In practice this means that such products have to be fortified to achieve these levels of micronutrients.

Milks

Low-fat liquid milks are sometimes fortified with vitamins A and D, and occasionally also with additional calcium. Vitamins A and D are usually added to low-fat dried milk powders.

Infant formulae are modified milks developed for infants. It is recognized that breast milk is uniquely suited to the requirements of young infants, and substitute products should be formulated to mimic as closely as possible the nutrient features of breast milk. As a result of closely defined nutrient ideals agreed for infant formulae, legal specifications prescribe minimum and maximum levels for nutrient components than any other food products. To ensure compliance with legislation and also, where appropriate, with expert committee recommendations, all products in this sector are fortified with vitamins and minerals, in many cases with particular amino acids, and in some cases with long-chain fatty acids.

Weaning foods

Weaning foods are progressively introduced into the diets of infants from the age of 4–6 months. Many manufactured weaning foods are available, and these are often fortified in the line with the particular nutritional requirements of older infants.

Other foods

Other individual food items may contain added nutrients, and such fortification is most commonly observed where foods are marketed to particular groups with nutritional concerns. Vitamin B_{12} is sometimes added to foods aimed at vegetarians and more especially vegans, and various vitamins and minerals are typically added to foods promoted as 'sports' or 'slimming' products.

Labelling

A major consideration in the fortification of foods is the legislative control over the provision of information on labelling. Usually minimum levels of nutrient are required before labelling claims can be made, to protect consumers being misled by emphasis on insignificant quantities of nutrients in a food. The reference points used within legislation or guidelines for the declaration of nutrients include:

- per unit weight (e.g. per 100 g);
- per unit energy (e.g. per 100 kJ);
- per food serving;
- per quantity of food that can reasonably be consumed in a day.

Nutrient declarations

The presentation of nutrition information on food labelling is often defined by legislation. The European Union directive on nutrition labelling sets out the following general provisions for nutrient declarations:

- Declarations are voluntary, unless a nutrient claim is made.
- The format for labelling can be the 'big four' nutrients (energy, protein, carbohydrate and fat) or the 'big four' plus the 'little four' (saturates, sugars, fibre and sodium).
- Vitamins and minerals can only be listed when present in significant amounts: this means at least 15% of the recommended daily allowance of the labelling values per 100 g or 100 ml of a food, or per single-portion package of a food (**Table 3**).

In the USA, numeric criteria for nutrient declarations are defined within legislation under the Nutrition Labelling and Education Act (NLEA).

Nutrient claims

Information about the presence or modification of a nutrient in a food described on labelling is referred to as a 'claim'. Such nutrient claims are usually accompanied by a descriptor, e.g. 'high', 'reduced', 'low' or 'no added' in relation to the nutrient being described. Nutrient declarations are not considered to be nutrient claims.

In the UK, the food labelling regulations of 1996 prescribe minimum levels of vitamins or mineral in a food to allow a claim to be made on a food label. Thus a claim that a food or drink is a source of a scheduled vitamin or mineral (see Table 3) requires the product to contain at least 17% of the RDA in the quantity of that food that can reasonably be consumed in one day. A product claiming to be a 'rich' or 'excellent' source of a micronutrient should contain at least 50% of the RDA. A typical daily serving of drink, for example, would require a vitamin C

Table 3 Criteria for vitamin or mineral declarations in the European Community

Micronutrient	Labelling RDA	Nutrient declaration (minimum amount per 100 g, 100 ml or package)
Vitamin A (μg)	800	120
Vitamin D (μg)	5	0.75
Vitamin A (mg)	10	1.5
Vitamin C (mg)	60	9
Vitamin B$_1$ (mg)	1.4	0.21
Vitamin B$_2$ (mg)	1.6	0.24
Niacin (mg)	18	2.7
Vitamin B$_6$ (mg)	2	0.3
Folate (μg)	200	30
Vitamin B$_{12}$ (μg)	1	0.15
Biotin (mg)	0.15	0.023
Pantothenic acid (mg)	6	0.9
Calcium (mg)	800	120
Phosphorus (mg)	800	120
Iron (mg)	14	2.1
Magnesium (mg)	300	45
Zinc (mg)	15	2.25
Iodine (μg)	150	22.5

From EC (1990).

content of about 10 mg to allow the claim 'contains vitamin C', and 30 mg to allow the claim 'high in vitamin C'.

In decisions on the voluntary fortification of foods, the cut-off values for claims defined within legislation or guidelines are evidently an important consideration in formulation decisions. Regulatory scrutiny and enforcement require analytical values of nutrient content to be within reasonable parameters of levels declared on labelling; predictions in the changes in nutrient content of a food over expected shelf life must be made, so that initial formulation 'overages' ensure that levels declared on labelling are met (or exceeded) throughout the period in which the food can be assumed to be suitable for consumption. Some micronutrients are particularly labile to factors such as heat or light, and so proportionately greater overages may be calculated into the initial formulation to be added to a carrier food.

Potential Overdosage

Nutrients can have adverse effects when consumed in excess, especially when high levels of intake occur over a long time. There are particular concerns about the potentially toxic effects of the fat-soluble vitamins. Some nutritionists are concerned that marketing-led pressures to add nutrients to food may lead to greater levels of some nutrients in more and more

food products. In addition, the proportion of the population regularly consuming vitamin and mineral supplements has increased in many countries, so some individuals could be consuming very high levels of some nutrients.

Evidence of the adverse effects of fortification in the UK was observed with vitamin D in the mid 1950s. Symptoms occasionally observed in infants and young children (failure to thrive and hypercalcaemia) were a result of high intakes of this vitamin, as infant milks and cereals and even cod liver oil compounds were fortified with vitamin D. As a result of a report published in 1957, fortification levels were much reduced, so that average vitamin D intakes in young infants had been halved by the end of 1958.

Potential overdosage problems due to the potency of nutrient concentrates must be avoided by precision in formulation and mixing, and regular assessment by analysis to monitor the outcomes of fortification practice. Extreme variation in analytical data indicate inadequate manufacturing procedures, or unsuitability of the carrier food.

Reports from the USA on the vitamin D content of fortified milks indicated considerable variation, and consequently major inaccuracy in the labelling declarations. Only about one quarter of milk samples analysed contained between 80% and 120% of the amount of vitamin D declared on the label. Excessive vitamin D in milk (500 times the amount stated on the label) was demonstrated to have been the reason for several cases of hypervitaminosis D, and recommendations were made in the USA for more frequent monitoring of vitamin D levels in fortified foods.

For most micronutrients there is a wide margin between RDA levels and amounts that would be considered undesirable in relation to adverse health effects. Nutrient quantities typically added to foods are nearly always below RDA levels. Where fortification practice receives government support, recommendations are often made for specific carrier foods to restrict the range of products being fortified. Some fortification recommendations relate nutrient levels to the energy content of a food (e.g. x mg of a vitamin per 100 kJ), thus ensuring some relationship between energy intakes (and possibly energy requirements) and micronutrient intakes.

See also: **Bioavailability**: Definition and General Aspects. **Community Nutrition**: Definition and Approaches. **Food Processing**: Nutritional Influences. **Vitamin Supplementation**: Role.

Further Reading

Anderson S, Vickery C and Nicol A (1986) Adult thiamin requirements and the continuing need to fortify processed cereals. *Lancet* **ii**:85–89.

Codex Alimentarius Commission (1985) *Report of the 14th Session of the Codex Committee on Foods for Special Dietary Use.* Joint FAO/WHO Food Standards Programme. Geneva: WHO.

Crawley H (1993) The role of breakfast cereals in the diets of 16–17 year old teenagers in Britain. *Journal of Human Nutrition and Dietetics* **63**:205–215.

Department of Health (1991) *The Fortification of Yellow Fats with Vitamins A and D.* Committee on Medical Aspects of Food Policy: Report on Health and Social Subjects no. 40. London: HMSO.

Department of Health and Social Security (1980) *Foods Which Simulate Meat.* Committee on Medical Aspects of Food Policy: Report on Health and Social Subjects no. 17. London: HMSO.

DHSS (1981) *Nutritional Aspects of Bread and Flour.* Committee on Medical Aspects of Food Policy: Report on Health and Social Subjects no. 23. London: HMSO.

European Commission (1990) EC Directive of 24 September 1990 on nutrition labelling for foodstuffs (90/496/EEC) O.J. 33 L276 40–44, Brussels.

Holland B, Welch PA, Unwin ID, Buss DH, Paul AA and Southgate DAT (1991) *McCance & Widdowson's The Composition of Foods*, 5th edn. Cambridge: Royal Society of Chemistry.

Hurrell RF and Cook JD (1990) Strategies for iron fortification of foods. *Trends in Food Science and Technology.* Sept: 56–61.

Moynihan P, Adamson A, Rugg-Gunn A, Appleton D and Butler T (1996) Dietary sources of calcium and the contribution of flour fortification to total calcium intake in the diets of Northumbrian adolescents. *British Journal of Nutrition* **75**:495–505.

Schorah C and Buss DH (1995) Should flour fortification with folic acid be mandatory to reduce the incidence of neural tube defects? *Nutrition Bulletin* **76(20)**:292–301.

Food intake *see* **Dietary Intake Measurement**: Methodology; Validation. **Dietary Surveys**: Surveys of National Food Intake; Surveys of Food Intake in Groups and Individuals. **Nutritional Status**: Dietary Assessment.

FOOD INTOLERANCE

Types and Incidence

T J David, L Patel and **C I Ewing**, Booth Children's Hospital, Manchester, UK

Copyright © 1998 Academic Press

Definition of Food Intolerance

Food intolerance can be defined as a reproducible adverse reaction to a specific food or food ingredient, which is not psychologically based. Although this appears straightforward, there are a number of difficulties with this definition, and these are discussed below.

Lack of definition of 'adverse reaction'

One problem with our definition of food intolerance is the lack of definition of what constitutes an adverse reaction. All eating causes reactions, which include satiety, feeling warm, the urge to defecate (due to the gastrocolic reflex) and weight gain.

Variation in tolerance

People vary in their tolerance of events. For some, flatus is an unacceptable and embarrassing problem, whereas for others it is the normal effect of eating baked beans.

Any food in excess may be harmful

The definition above does not take into account dosage. Large quantities of certain foods may result in disease in certain individuals, although such disorders are not usually included in the category of food intolerance. Any food, however harmless, can be harmful if taken in excess. Notable examples of this include the following:

- Apples, pears and honey are rich sources of fructose, a sugar which in early childhood is not well absorbed if taken in large quantities. Thus if a child takes a quantity of fructose in excess of what can be absorbed in the gastrointestinal tract, the result will be loose stools (diarrhoea) due to the osmotic effect of unabsorbed fructose. It should be noted that whereas this applies to normal children, there are in addition a small number of children who are especially poor at handling ingested fructose, and in these children even small quantities of fructose-containing foods will cause florid diarrhoea.

- Chicken liver is a rich source of vitamin A. There are reported cases of infants who were fed large quantities of chicken liver, and who as a result developed raised intracranial pressure as a consequence of vitamin A toxicity.
- In those who are genetically predisposed, ingestion of an excess of purine-rich foods contributes to hyperuricaemia, leading to gout, a disorder which is not usually regarded as a form of food intolerance.

Principal Mechanisms and Pathophysiology

The principal mechanisms resulting in food intolerance and the pathophysiology (where this is understood) are discussed below.

Food allergy

The term 'allergy' implies a definite immunological mechanism. This could be antibody-mediated, cell-mediated, or due to circulating immune complexes. The clinical features of an allergic reaction include urticaria (nettle rash), angioedema, rhinitis (sneezing, nasal discharge, blocked nose), worsening of pre-existing atopic eczema, asthma (wheezing, coughing, tightness of the chest, shortness of breath), vomiting, abdominal pain, diarrhoea and anaphylactic shock (*See:* **Food Allergies**: Aetiology; Diagnosis and Management).

Enzyme defects

Inborn errors of metabolism may affect the digestion and absorption of carbohydrate, fat or protein. In some subjects the enzyme defect is primarily gastrointestinal, causing defects in digestion or absorption. An example is lactase deficiency, described below. In other subjects, the enzyme defect is systemic. An example is the rare disorders of hereditary fructose intolerance, described below.

Lactase deficiency   An example of an enzyme defect causing food intolerance is lactase deficiency. In this condition, which is a disorder primarily affecting infants and young children, there is a reduced or absent concentration of the enzyme lactase in the small intestinal mucosa. Affected subjects are unable to break down ingested lactose, the main sugar found in milk. If lactose is not absorbed it passes into the large intestine, where there are two consequences: one is an osmotic diarrhoea; the other is that some of the unabsorbed lactose is broken down by intestinal bacteria, accompanied by the production of gas (hydrogen) leading to abdominal distension and flatus and the production of organic acids which cause perianal soreness or excoriation. The production of hydrogen, its absorption into the bloodstream and its excretion in the breath, are the basis for a simple and elegant test for sugar intolerance, the breath hydrogen test. In this test, the subject suspected of lactase deficiency swallows a portion of sugar; breath is collected every half an hour, and the hydrogen content is measured. In the normal individual, the sugar is absorbed and hydrogen is not produced. In the intolerant individual, the sugar is not absorbed, hydrogen is produced, and a steep rise in hydrogen concentration is found in the exhaled air.

The management of lactose intolerance is the avoidance of foods that contain lactose (mainly cow's milk and its products). For infants it is worth noting that the soya-based infant formulae are lactose-free. In theory, an alternative is to add to cow's milk microbial β-galactosidase, which can produce a lactose-free milk, with the inconvenience that it has a sweeter flavour and requires a 24 h incubation period at 4°C.

In infants and young children, lactase deficiency is usually a transient problem occurring after an episode of gastroenteritis, but it is commonly a feature of any disease that causes damage to the intestinal mucosa (e.g. coeliac disease). Levels of lactase tend to fall during mid to later childhood, and in a number of populations (e.g. in Africa, Mexico and Greenland) a high proportion of adults have very little lactase activity. This adult deficiency is believed to have a genetic basis. Humans are the only animal apart from the domestic cat that drinks milk after weaning, and deficiency of lactase in adults could in certain populations be considered the normal state.

Hereditary fructose intolerance   In this condition, which is inherited as an autosomal recessive, there is deficiency of the liver enzyme fructose 1,6-bisphosphate aldolase. As a result, fructose 1-phosphate accumulates in liver cells, and acts as a competitive inhibitor for phosphorylase. The resulting transient inhibition of the conversion of glycogen to glucose leads to severe hypoglycaemia (low blood glucose concentration). Affected infants are symptom-free as long as their diet is limited to human milk. If they receive milk formulae or any food that contains fructose they develop attacks of hypoglycaemia, shock, coma and convulsions. There may be jaundice, an enlarged liver and sometimes progressive liver disease. The treatment requires the complete elimination of fructose from the diet, which may be difficult as fructose is a widely used food additive and sweetener. A trivial but interesting feature of the condition, in survivors, is a notable reduction in dental caries, a beneficial result from the need to avoid many types of confectionery.

Pharmacological mechanisms

Caffeine A good example of a pharmacological agent with the ability to cause adverse reactions and to be found in food is caffeine. The stimulant effects, which may be welcome at times but unwelcome at others, of 60 mg caffeine in a cup of tea or 100 mg caffeine in a cup of coffee are well recognized. What is less well recognized is that heavy coffee or tea drinkers can suffer a number of other side effects of caffeine, which stimulates gastric secretion and can cause heartburn, nausea, vomiting, diarrhoea and intestinal colic. Also common are irregular heartbeats, episodes of rapid pulse, sweating, tremor, anxiety and sleeplessness. Caffeine also has a diuretic effect.

Sodium nitrite Another pharmacological effect occurs when unusually large quantities of sodium nitrite are ingested. Sodium nitrite is an antioxidant used as an antibacterial agent, and in quantities of 20 mg or more it can cause dilatation of blood vessels resulting in flushing and headache, and urticaria.

Tyramine, histamine and other vasoactive amines A further example of a pharmacological mechanism is the adverse effect of various vasoactive amines such as tyramine, serotonin, tryptamine, phenylethylamine and histamine, which are found in a range of foods such as tuna, pickled herring, sardines, anchovy fillets, bananas, cheese, yeast extracts (such as Marmite), chocolate, wine, spinach, tomato and sausages. There appear to be three main mechanisms in operation:

- An abnormally high intake of vasoactive amines, such as histamine or tyramine, either because of a high content in food or because of synthesis of these chemicals in the gut by bacteria.
- An abnormal effect whereby drugs or chemicals in food interfere with the enzymes which break down vasoactive amines.
- An abnormal release from mast cells of histamine

and other mediators of inflammation, triggered by eating certain foods such as strawberries, shellfish and alcohol.

Vasoactive amines are the normal constituents of many foods. They arise mainly from the decarboxylation of amino acids, but they may also develop during normal food cooking and during the storage of food. An example is histamine, found at different levels in various types of sausage (**Table 1**). The term 'semidry' when applied to sausages means sausages that are fermented for varying periods. During this sausage ripening process, the histamine concentration increases, depending upon the length of the process. It is estimated that 70 mg to 1000 mg of histamine ingested in a single meal is necessary for the onset of toxicity, depending on individual sensitivity. Thus 130 g of the pepperoni sample that contained 55.0 mg histamine per 100 g would be necessary to cause symptoms in the most sensitive individuals.

The largest amount of histamine and tyramine are found in fermented foods such as cheese, alcoholic drinks, sausage, sauerkraut and tinned fish. Badly stored food (see below) such as mackerel and tuna can contain large amounts of histamine.

The effects of large doses of tyramine, histamine and other vasoactive amines are extremely variable. Histamine causes flushing (by dilation of blood vessels), constriction of smooth muscle in the intestine and the bronchi, increased heart rate, headache, fall in blood pressure and asthma. Tyramine causes

Table 1 Histamine levels in sausages obtained from retail markets in the San Francisco Bay area

	Histamine level (mg per 100 g)	
	Mean	*Range*
Cooked sausages[a]		
Bologna	0.55	0.19–0.84
Cooked salami	0.83	0.47–5.86
Kosher salami	0.50	0.33–0.97
Semidry sausages		
Thuringer cervelat	2.35	1.03–3.63
Thuringer	1.19	0.31–2.56
Dry sausages		
Italian dry salami	2.14–24.5[a]	0.42–36.4[a]
Pepperoni	1.03–38.1[a]	0.72–55.0[a]
Chorizo	2.29	0.60–8.08

From Taylor SL, Leatherwood M and Lieber ER (1978) A survey of histamine levels in sausages. *Journal of Food Protection* 41:634–637. With permission. Copyright held by the International Association of Milk, Food and Environmental Sanitarians, Inc.
[a]Depending upon the brand tested.

constriction of blood vessels, and it stimulates the release of noradrenaline from nerve endings. It can also cause the release of histamine and prostaglandins from mast cells. Dietary tyramine is known to induce hypertension and headache in patients who are taking monoamine oxidase inhibitor drugs. This effect has been shown to be due to inhibition, by these drugs, of intestinal and hepatic metabolism of tyramine, so that the amine accumulates.

The variable effect of histamine taken by mouth is in part due to the varying degree of inactivation in the gastrointestinal tract. Histamine is inactivated by mucoproteins which are produced in the gastrointestinal tract mucosa, but this inactivation can be blocked by other amines such as cadaverine and putresceine, which also bind strongly to mucoproteins. Thus, when food is taken which contains cadaverine and putresceine, more histamine can therefore be absorbed. In fact most of the histamine that is absorbed is degraded, as it is transported across the mucosa, by the intestinal enzyme diamine oxidase. Cadaverine and putresceine also have a high affinity for diamine oxidase, and so they can also interfere with the inactivation of histamine by this enzyme. Another barrier to the absorption of histamine is provided by the liver enzyme methyltransferase.

Thus the effect of histamine and other vasoactive amines on an individual will depend on a number of factors, which include:

1. the amount of vasoactive amine that is present in food;
2. the amount of histamine released (as a result of an allergic process);
3. the permeability of the gastrointestinal tract, including inactivation by mucus and by mechanisms in the gut mucosa;
4. interference with the synthesis or release of enzymes involved in amine breakdown (e.g. liver damage, causing reduced activity of methyltransferase).

Tyramine and migraine   There has been interest in a possible relationship between dietary tyramine and migraine. One hypothesis is that some patients with migraine have defective metabolism of ingested tyramine in the intestinal wall, which leads to increased absorption, apparently explaining why foods containing tyramine can provoke attacks in susceptible individuals. However, there is no evidence that the activity of monoamine oxidase, the main tyramine metabolizing enzyme, is lower in patients with food-induced migraine than in other individuals prone to migraine, although levels of monoamine oxidase in platelets are generally lower in patients with migraine.

Set against these theoretical arguments, most attempts to induce migraine by tyramine challenge in children and adults have been unsuccessful. Furthermore, a controlled study of exclusion of dietary vasoactive amines in children with migraine failed to demonstrate benefit. In the latter study, patients were randomly allocated to either a high-fibre diet low in dietary amines or a high-fibre diet alone. Although there was no significant difference in the results for the two groups, both groups showed a highly significant decrease in the number of headaches, emphasizing the need for a control diet in studies designed to show that dietary manipulation improves disease.

Of the foods reported to be common triggers of attacks of migraine, only cheese is rich in tyramine. Chocolate is low in this and other vasoactive amines, and red wine usually contains no more tyramine than white wine. Alcoholic drinks, particularly red wine, are commonly reported to provoke attacks of migraine. Whether these attacks are due to alcohol itself or some other compound has been disputed. The major chemical difference between red and white wines is the former's high concentration of phenolic flavonoids such as anthocyanins and catechins, which as well as having direct effects on blood vessels may also inhibit the enzyme phenol sulfotransferase. Patients with food-induced migraine were shown to have significantly lower levels of platelet phenol sulfotransferase activity, and it has been hypothesized (but not proved) that low activity of this enzyme could lead to an accumulation of phenolic or monoamine substrates which in turn might directly or indirectly provoke attacks of migraine.

Regardless of the possible mechanism, a number of people with migraine are made worse by specific dietary triggers such as cheese or wine, for whatever reason, and avoidance of specific food triggers in susceptible subjects may prove helpful in reducing the frequency of attacks.

11β-Hydroxysteroid dehydrogenase and liquorice   Liquorice contains an enzyme that inhibits 11β-hydroxysteroid dehydrogenase, resulting in sodium and water retention, hypertension, hypokalaemia and suppression of the renin–aldosterone system.

Irritant mechanisms

Certain foods have a direct irritant effect on the mucous membranes of the mouth or gut, e.g. coffee and curry. In certain individuals, food intolerance only occurs in the presence of a coexisting medical disorder. For example, the ingestion of spicy food, coffee or orange juice provokes oesophageal pain in some patients with reflux oesophagitis. This effect is unconnected to the temperature or acidity of the food, or to any effect on the lower oesophageal sphincter. The treatment, in susceptible individuals, is to avoid the trigger food item.

Specific drug–food combinations

One example of drug-induced food intolerance is potentiation of the pressor effects of tyramine-containing foods (e.g. cheese, yeast extracts and fermented soya bean products) by monoamine oxidase inhibitor drugs. Another is the effect of taking alcohol in patients with alcohol dependence during treatment with disulfiram (Antabuse). The reaction, which can occur within 10 min of alcohol ingestion and may last several hours, consists of flushing and nausea.

Toxic mechanisms

Nature has endowed plants with the capacity to synthesize substances that are toxic, and thus serve to protect them from predators whether they be fungi, insects, animals or humans. Thus many plant foods contain naturally occurring toxins. On a worldwide scale, reactions to naturally occurring toxins may outnumber allergic reactions, although it is currently fashionable to pay more attention to the latter.

Protease inhibitors   Soya beans were originally introduced into the USA as a source of oil, the extracted meal being used as a by-product that could provide animals with a source of protein. However, it was recognized that it was necessary to subject soya beans to heat treatment if they were to support the growth of animals. It was later found that the substance responsible for growth inhibition in raw soya beans was a protease inhibitor, trypsin inhibitor, and it is now known that protease inhibitors are widely distributed throughout the plant kingdom, particularly in legumes, but to a lesser extent in cereal grains and tubers. In addition to inhibition of growth, one of the most characteristic responses of most animals to trypsin inhibitor is enlargement of the pancreas. The depression of growth is believed to result from endogenous loss of protein (i.e. loss into the gastrointestinal tract) due to hypersecretion of the pancreas. Soya bean products that have been adequately heat-treated to inactivate trypsin inhibitor are safe for consumption.

Lectins   Most legumes and cereals contain a group of proteins that have the property of being able to agglutinate the red blood cells of various species of animals – the phytohaemagglutinins or lectins. Some of these lectins, such as ricin from the castor bean, are extremely toxic. Others, such as those in the soya bean, are nontoxic. Lectins appear to be responsible for the fact that many other legumes, unless properly cooked, not only fail to support the growth of animals but lead to death. Lectins are found in many food items commonly consumed in the human diet including tomatoes, bean sprouts, raw vegetables, fruits, spices, dry cereals and nuts, and it is not known whether these are harmful in any way. However, it is well recognized that inadequate cooking of red kidney beans can cause severe gastrointestinal upset, with vomiting and diarrhoea. It is for this reason that it is recommended that uncooked red kidney beans should be cooked by boiling hard for 10 min.

Lathyrogens   Lathyrism is a paralytic disease that is associated with the consumption of chickling pea or vetch, *Lathyrus sativus*. The causative factor is believed to be an amino acid derivative, β-N-oxalyl-α,β-diaminopropionic acid, a metabolic antagonist of glutamic acid, a substance which is involved in the transmission of nerve impulses in the brain.

Mimosine   Mimosine is an amino acid that comprises 1–4% of the dry weight of the legume *Leucaena leucocephala*, and consumption of the leaves, pods and seeds leads to hair loss. In animals, as well as producing hair loss, mimosine is also a goitrogen.

Djenkolic acid   In parts of Sumatra the djenkol bean is a popular item of consumption. The bean is a seed of the leguminous tree, *Pithecolobium lobatum*, and resembles the horse chestnut in size and colour. Consumption of this seed leads to kidney failure, which is accompanied by blood and needle-like clusters in the urine, and the latter have been identified as containing the amino acid djenkolic acid.

Goitrogens   Substances capable of producing goitre are present in plants belonging to the cabbage family, including cabbage, turnip, broccoli, cauliflower, Brussels sprouts, kale, rapeseed and mustard seed. Cow's milk is a vector for the transmission of goitrogens from animals fed kale and turnips, and may have been responsible for endemic goitre in countries such as Australia and Finland.

Cyanogens   A number of plants are potentially toxic because they contain glycosides from which hydrogen cyanide may be released by enzymatic hydrolysis. The most common plants eaten by humans, in order of their potential cyanide content, are lima beans (*Phaseolus lunatus*), sorghum, cas-

Table 2 Examples of toxic constituents of plant foodstuffs and their role in plant physiology

Toxic constituent	Type of food containing toxic constituent	Physiological role of toxic constituent	Role in plant defence: mechanism of toxic constituent
Protease inhibitors	Legumes, cereals, potatoes, pineapple	?Prevents degradation of storage protein during seed maturation	Part of defence against invading microbes following mechanical damage to leaves
Haemagglutinins	Legumes, cereals, potatoes	(a) Attach glycoprotein enzymes (b) Role in embryonic (c) development/differentiation Protect against seed predators (c) Role in sugar transport or store (d) ?Involved in root nodule nitrogen-fixing bacteria symbiosis	(a) Counteract soil bacteria (b) Antifungal (c) Protect against seed predators
Glucosinolates	Radish, horseradish, turnip, cabbage, rapeseed	?Disease and insect resistance	
Cyanogens	Almonds, cassava, corn, peas, butter beans, bamboo shoots		
Saponins	Alfalfa, French beans, soya beans		

From Leiner (1980).

sava, linseed meal, black-eyed pea (*Vigna sinensis*), garden pea (*Pisum sativum*), kidney bean (*Phaseolus vulgaris*), Bengal gram (*Cicer arietinum*) and red gram (*Cajanus cajans*).

Vicine and convicine Vicine and convicine are β-glucosides that are present in broad beans (*Vicia faba*). When consumed by individuals with deficiency of the enzyme glucose-6-phosphate dehydrogenase, these substances precipitate the condition of favism, which is characterized by anaemia caused by haemolysis of red blood cells. The enzyme deficiency is a genetic disorder that is confined largely to inhabitants of countries surrounding the Mediterranean basin (Italy, Sicily, Lebanon, Israel and north Africa), although individuals of the same ethnic background residing in other countries may also suffer from favism.

Cycasin Cycad seeds or nuts are obtained from *Cycad circinalis*, a palm-like tree that grows throughout the tropics and subtropics. The seeds, unless thoroughly washed, are extremely toxic, causing poisoning in humans and tumours in experimental animals. The toxic ingredient methylazoxymethanol, the aglycone of cycasin, is released on hydrolysis of cycasin by intestinal bacteria.

Pyrrolizidine derivatives Pyrrolizidine alkaloids are found in a wide variety of plant species. The toxic ingredient belongs to a class of compounds that are derivatives of pyrrolizidine. Large numbers of people have been poisoned through consumption of cereal and grain crops contaminated with pyrrolizidine-containing plants. It is also possible that milk from cows grazing on pastures that contain such plants could act as a vector for the transmission of pyrrolizidine to humans. In one part of the western USA one such plant, the tansy ragwort (*Senecio jacobea*) is readily consumed by cows and goats, and the milk from such animals has been shown to contain significant amounts of a pyrrolizidine derivative jacoline.

Lupin alkaloid Milk from animals that have eaten plants from the lupin family, notably *Lupinus latifolius*, may contain quinolizidine alkaloids such as anagyrine. There is strong evidence that these alkaloids are teratogenic in animals, causing severe bony deformities, and there is some evidence that similar defects may occur in the offspring of human mothers who drink alkaloid-containing milk in pregnancy.

Other examples There are numerous other examples of toxic substances present in foodstuffs.

Table 3 Examples of foodborne toxins or toxin-producing organisms, excluding plant foodstuffs

Pathogen or toxin	Principal symptoms	Common food source
Bacillus cereus	(a) Diarrhoea	Proteinaceous food, vegetables, sauces, puddings
	(b) Vomiting	Fried rice
Bacillus subtilis	Vomiting, diarrhoea, flushing, sweating	Meat and pastry, meat or seafood with rice
Bacillus licheniformis	Diarrhoea	Cooked meat and vegetables
Clostridium botulinum	Neuroparalytic disease (botulism)	Meat, fish, vegetables, hazelnut conserve
Clostridium perfringens	Diarrhoea, abdominal pain	Meat, poultry
Salmonella enteridis	Diarrhoea, abdominal pain, fever, vomiting	Poultry, eggs
Staphylococcus aureus	Vomiting, abdominal pain, diarrhoea	Numerous, especially cooked high-protein foods
Verotoxin-producing Escherichia coli	Haemorrhagic colitis	Ground beef
Listeria monocytogenes	Listeriosis	Unpasteurized cheese, undercooked meat
Dioxins and dibenzofurans	Adverse effects uncertain when consumed in quantities found in food	Fish
Cantharidin	Sensitivity to urethra and genitalia; priapism	Frogs which have Meloidae (blister beetles)
Methylmercury	Brain damage	Fish, bread
Toxic alkaloid (saxitoxin) in dinoflagellates and plankton	Diverse gastrointestinal and neurological disorders (paralytic shellfish poisoning)	Clams, oysters, scallops and mussels
Brevetoxins	Paraesthesia, abdominal pain, diarrhoea, transient blindness, paralysis, death (neurotoxic shellfish poisoning)	Clams, oysters, scallops and mussels
Ciguatera toxin	Diverse gastrointestinal and neurological disorders	Fish (especially reef predators)
Tetrodotoxin	Diverse gastrointestinal and neurological disorders	Puffer fish, certain newts
Domoic acid	Vomiting, diarrhoea, hyperexcitation, seizures, memory loss (amnesic shellfish poisoning)	Mussels
Okadaic acid, dinophysis toxins, yessotoxin, pectenotoxins	Diarrhoea, vomiting, abdominal pain (diarrhetic shellfish poisoning)	Mussels, scallops
Scombrotoxin (usually histamine)	Headache, palpitations, gastrointestinal disturbance	Mackerel, tuna and related species
Tetramine (red whelk poisoning)	Diplopia, dizziness, leg pains	Whelks
Grayanotoxins (in honey from areas of Turkey where rhododendrons are grown)	Hypotension, bradycardia, vomiting, sweating	Honey
Unknown (? in algae) (turtle flesh poisoning)	Cardiorespiratory failure, death	Turtles

These include solanidine in potatoes, cyanide in tapioca, mycotoxins in mushrooms and cereal grains, and phototoxic furocoumarins in angelica, parsley, dill and celeriac, which in sufficient quantities can give rise to a wide variety of toxic reactions (**Table 2** and **Table 3**).

Food storage

Chemical changes in food during storage can produce substances that cause food intolerance. An example is intolerance to ripe or stored tomatoes in subjects who can safely eat green tomatoes, where ripening of the fruit produces a new active glycoprotein. Some adverse reactions resulting from food storage come into the category of toxic reactions, such as the rise in levels of histamine and tyramine in certain foods during storage as a result of bacterial decarboxylation. An example of this is the production of histamine in badly stored mackerel and other fish, scombroid fish poisoning. Contamination of food by antigens such as storage mites or microbial spores may give rise to adverse effects, particularly asthma and eczema. Contamination of food by microorganisms may result in adverse effects. For example, celery, parsnip and parsley may become infected with the fungus *Sclerotinia scleriotiorum* (pink rot), resulting in the production of the photosensitizing chemicals psoralen, 5-methoxypsoralen and 8-methoxypsoralen.

Practical Applications

Food arouses not only the appetite but also the emotions. The passion for food that is natural (i.e. free from extraneous ingredients) is not new; in 1857, a survey of adulterants in food showed that childrens' sweets were commonly coloured by red lead (lead oxide), lead chromate, mercuric sulfide and copper arsenite. By the late 1850s, 'pure and unadulterated' had become the stock advertising slogan of those anxious to cash in on the then newly awakened fears of the public. The current scale of the use of additives in food comes as a surprise to most people, and it is understandable that many should find these substances vaguely menacing. Nonetheless, the current phobia of food additives and food processing, and the obsession with so-called 'natural' or 'health' food arises largely out of misinformation and ignorance. Obsession with natural food ignores the wide range of naturally occurring toxins in foods. The concept of 'health food' is wholly misleading. For example, a survey of 'crunchy' peanut butter showed that 11 out of 59 samples from health-food producers contained over 100 μg kg^{-1} of aflatoxins, over 10 times the proposed maximum permitted level for total aflatoxins. Only 1 of the 26 samples from other producers contained aflatoxins in excess of 10 μg kg^{-1}, and none contained more than 50 μg kg^{-1}.

See also: **Antioxidants**: Diet and Antioxidant Defence. **Caffeine**: Chemistry and Physiological Effects. **Drugs**: Drug-Nutrient Interactions. **Food Allergies**: Aetiology. **Fructose**: Absorption and Metabolism. **Hypoglycaemia (Hypoglycemia)**: Dietary and Metabolic Aspects. **Legumes**: Types and Nutritional Value.

Further Reading

Ashwood-Smith MJ, Ceska O and Chaudhary SK (1985) Mechanism of photosensitivity reactions to diseased celery. *British Medical Journal* 1249.

Bjarnason I, Levi S, Smethurst P, Menzies IS and Levi AJ (1988) Vindaloo and you. *British Medical Journal* 297: 1629–1631.

Bleumink E, Berrens L and Young E (1967) Studies on the atopic allergen in ripe tomato fruits. *International Archives of Allergy* 31:25–37.

Ciegler A (1975) Mycotoxins: occurrence, chemistry, biological activity. *Lloydia* 38:21–35.

Conning DM and Lansdown ABG, eds (1983) *Toxic Hazards in Food*. London: Croom Helm.

Edwards CRW (1991) Lessons from licorice. *New England Journal of Medicine*, 325:1242–1243.

Farese RV, Bigieri EG, Shackleton CHL, Irony I and Gomez-Fontes R (1991) Licorice induced hypermineralocorticoidism. *New England Journal of Medicine* 325:1223–1227.

Forsythe WI and Redmond A (1974) Two controlled trials of tyramine in children with migraine. *Developmental Medicine and Child Neurology* 16:794–799.

Gibson GG and Walker R, eds (1985) *Food Toxicology – Real or Imaginary Problems?* London: Taylor & Francis.

Gumbmann MR, Spangler WL, Dugan GM and Rackis JJ (1986) Safety of trypsin inhibitors in the diet: effects on the rat pancreas of long-term feeding of soy flour and soy protein isolate. In: Friedman M (ed.) *Nutritional and Toxicological Significance of Enzyme Inhibitors in Foods*, pp 33–79. New York: Plenum Press.

Hall MJ (1987) The dangers of cassava (tapioca) consumption. *Bristol Medico-Chirurgical Journal* 102:37–39.

Harris JB, ed. (1986) *Natural Toxins. Animal, Plant, and Microbial*. Oxford: Clarendon Press.

Horwitz D, Lovenberg W, Engelman K and Sjoerdsma A (1964) Monoamine oxidase inhibitors, tyramine, and cheese. *Journal of the American Medical Association* 188:90–92.

Kaufman HS (1986) The red wine headache: a pilot study of a specific syndrome. *Immunology and Allergy Practice* 8:279–284.

Knudson EA and Kroon S (1988) In vitro and in vivo phototoxicity of furocoumarin-containing plants. *Clinical and Experimental Dermatology* 13:92–96.

Leiner IE, ed. (1980) *Toxic Constituents of Plant Foodstuffs*, 2nd edn. New York: Academic Press.

Lessof MH (1992) *Food Intolerance*. London: Chapman & Hall.

Littlewood JT, Glover V, Davies PTG, Gibb C, Sandler M and Rose FC (1988) Red wine as a cause of migraine. *Lancet* i:558–559.

Mahoney CP, Margolis MT, Knauss TA and Labbe RF (1980) Chronic vitamin A intoxication in infants fed chicken liver. *Pediatrics* 65:893–896.

Masyczek R and Ough CS (1983) The 'Red Wine Reaction' syndrome. *American Journal of Enology and Viticulture* 34:260–264.

Moffett A, Swash M and Scott DF (1972) Effect of tyramine in migraine: a double-blind study. *Journal of Neurology, Neurosurgery and Psychiatry* 35:496–499.

Moffett AM, Swash M and Scott DF (1974) Effect of chocolate in migraine: a double-blind study. *Journal of Neurology, Neurosurgery and Psychiatry* 37:445–448.

Morgan RGH, Crass RA and Oates PS (1986) Dose effects of raw soyabean flour on pancreatic growth. In: Friedman M (ed.) *Nutritional and Toxicological Significance of Enzyme Inhibitors in Foods*, pp 81–89. New York: Plenum Press.

Noah ND, Bender AE, Reaidi GB and Gilbert RJ (1980)

Food poisoning from raw red kidney beans. *British Medical Journal* **281**:236–237.

Price SF, Smithson KW and Castell D (1978) Food sensitivity in reflux esophagitis. *Gastroenterology* **75**:240–243.

Rackis JJ, Wolf WJ and Baker EC (1986) Protease inhibitors in plant foods: content and inactivation. In: Friedman M (ed.) *Nutritional and Toxicological Significance of Enzyme Inhibitors in Foods*, pp 299–347. New York: Plenum Press.

Salfield SAW, Wardley BL, Houlsby WT *et al.* (1987) Controlled study of exclusion of dietary vasoactive amines in migraine. *Archives of Disease in Childhood* **62**:458–460.

Sandler M, Youdim MBH and Hanington E (1974) A phenylethylamine oxidising defect in migraine. *Nature* **250**:335–337.

Taylor SL (1986) Histamine food poisoning: toxicology and clinical aspects. *CRC Critical Reviews in Toxicology* **17**:90–128.

Wuthrich B and Ortolani C, eds (1996) *Highlights in Food Allergy*. Basel: Karger.

FOOD PROCESSING

Nutritional Influences

A E Bender, Leatherhead, Surrey, UK

Copyright © 1998 Academic Press

Food processing is defined as any and all processes to which food is subjected after harvesting for the purposes of optimizing its appearance, texture, palatability, nutritive value, keeping properties and ease of preparation, and for eliminating microorganisms, toxins and other undesirable constituents including contaminants. It thus includes domestic cooking and preparation.

Processes can be divided into physical methods – such as heating, concentration, grinding and freezing – and chemical or more severe methods. There is no sharp division between the two, but a distinction has arisen from attempts to define 'natural' foods: a term that scientifically has no meaning since all foods come from natural sources, but which some authorities have allowed for single foods that have been subjected only to mild (physical) processing. The difficulty is illustrated by the 'simple' physical process of baking bread, and the domestic process of toasting bread, which damages the lysine and the thiamin. Similarly, the simple physical process of grinding grain and sieving flour to remove bran also leads to loss of the germ with considerable loss of nutrients.

Nutritional Losses

High temperatures damage heat-sensitive nutrients and wet processes cause some loss of water-soluble nutrients. Vitamins, in particular thiamin, folate and ascorbic acid, are sensitive to heat, while others are relatively stable to heat. Some are water-soluble, others are sensitive to light, acidity, alkalinity and oxidation (**Table 1**). In addition, mild heat in the presence of moisture and reducing substances (e.g. glucose) reduces the availability of the amino acid lysine by combining it in a form that is resistant to digestion.

Water-soluble nutrients partially lost in wet processes include vitamins of the B complex and ascorbic acid, and there is a relatively insignificant loss of water-soluble carbohydrates, proteins and mineral salts.

A number of principles should be borne in mind when considering losses of nutrients in food processing.

Some losses are inevitable

Processes that are intended to remove inedible or unwanted parts of the raw foodstuffs, such as intestinal contents of fish and meat, inedible husks such as paddy rice (40% of the grain) to form brown rice, the less palatable outer layers of some vegetables, and (to suit some palates) skin and peel, inevitably result in some nutrient losses. Preparation of white flour from wheat results in some loss of dietary fibre, vitamins B_1, B_2 and B_6, niacin, pantothenate, biotin and folate – some of which are partially replaced – and a small amount of protein. In addition, any wet processes, even simple washing and certainly cooking in water, will result in some loss of water-soluble nurients. When foods are preserved by canning, water-soluble nutrients are divided between the solid and liquid phases; the extent of loss will depend on whether the water phase is consumed as is usually the case with canned fruits, or discarded as with

Table 1 Stability of vitamins

	Air	Light	Heat	Acidity	Neutrality	Alkalinity
Fat-soluble						
A	−	−	+	−	+	+
Carotene	−	−	−	−	+	+
D	+	−	−	−	+	−
E	−	−	−	+	+	+
Water-soluble						
B_1	−	+	−	+	−	−
B_2	+	−	−	+	+	−
Niacin	+	+	+	+	+	+
B_6	+	−	−	+	+	+
Folate	−	−	−	−	−	+
C	−	−	−	+	−	−
Pantothenate	+	+	−	−	+	−

Key: +, stable; −, sensitive.

many canned vegetables. In this context 'drip-thaw', the liquid exuded from some frozen foods, represents a (small) loss of nutrients, whereas the juices exuded when meat is cooked are usually consumed and so are recovered.

The domestic pressure cooker in general results in fewer losses than conventional boiling since the time needed is shorter and less water is used; although reported results are not always consistent, it appears that microwave cooking causes less damage than conventional heating. Commercial drying or concentration under vacuum causes much less damage than drying at atmospheric pressure, and the slow process of sun-drying can result in complete loss of some vitamins because of the long time required – a matter of considerable importance in developing regions.

Destruction of microorganisms (a biological process) increases 10-fold for every 10°C increase in temperature, while destruction of vitamins (a chemical process) only doubles for every 10°C rise in temperature. For this reason high-temperature, short time (HTST) pasteurization and ultra-high-temperature (UHT) sterilization cause less damage than older methods of pasteurization and sterilization con-tinued for longer times, although at lower temperatures.

Major losses

Most discussion of nutrient losses is limited to the most sensitive of the nutrients, namely ascorbic acid, thiamin, folate and available lysine. At one time losses of ascorbic acid were incorrectly taken as an index of overall nutritional losses, but it can serve as an index of staleness.

Factory and domestic losses Manufacturing and processing losses, where they do occur, are often in place of rather than in addition to losses that inevitably accompany domestic cooking. For example, canned foods are cooked during the process and require only heating (or may be consumed, as in the instance of fruits, without further preparation); and dried and frozen foods that have been initially blanched need less domestic cooking than the corresponding fresh food. **Table 2** shows that a food purchased in the fresh, unprocessed state and subjected to the full cooking process in the home, differs little in content of the most sensitive nutrient, vitamin C,

Table 2 Vitamin content of garden peas after processing and cooking

	Fresh		Processed			
	Variety 1	Variety 2	Frozen	Freeze-dried	Air-dried	Canned
Time boiled (min)	10	10	3.5	2	15	Brought to boil
Volume of water[a]	1.2	1.2	1	12.3	23.6	−
Vitamin C content (mg per 100 g)	16.4	18.5	14.0	15.8	11.3	9.2

From Robertson and Sissons (1966).
[a]As a multiple of the volume of food.

Table 3 Peas: cumulative percentage loss of vitamin C at each stage of processing

Fresh		Frozen		Canned		Air-dried		Freeze-dried	
Stage	Loss (%)	Stage	Loss (%)	Stage	Loss (%)	Stage	Loss (%)	Stage	Loss (%)
		Blanching	25	Blanching	30	Blanching	25	Blanching	25
		Freezing	25	Canning	37	Drying	55	Drying	30
		Thawing	29						
Cooking	56	Cooking	61	Heating	64	Cooking	75	Cooking	65

Data from Mapson (1956).

from food processed in the factory and reheated at home. **Table 3** indicates the losses of vitamin C at various stages of processing. Since factory processing is usually in the hands of trained food technologists it is likely that the average, controlled factory process involves less damage than the average domestic procedure.

Relative importance of the food in the whole diet

Where losses of nutrients do take place the relative importance of the food in question to the diet as a whole must be taken into account. For example, an investigation of the comparison of nutritive values of free-range and intensively farmed chickens showed that the meat of broiler chickens contains less thiamin than that of free-range chickens, but since chicken meat supplies less than 1% of the thiamin in the average British diet such differences are of no importance (Vipond, Robertson and Tapsfield, 1964).

The vitamin C content of pasteurized milk is lower than that of fresh milk, but milk is in general an insignificant source of vitamin C in the average diet. On the other hand, while potatoes are not rich in vitamin C they provide a significant part of the average Western intake so damage may be important to some consumers.

Table 4 illustrates this principle in whole meals

canned and stored for long periods. Half the vitamin C was lost in the process and all was lost after 1.5 years of storage, but the amount present in the raw food was only some 2% of the recommended daily allowance (RDA) and so the loss is trivial. On the other hand, there is so much thiamin in the meal that even after the loss of 75% after 5 years' storage there is still sufficient left to provide a full day's recommended intake.

Correct comparisons

When discussing nutritional changes it is necessary to compare the foods 'as eaten', that is to say, not simply before and after processing. 'Fresh' foods may have become available several days after harvesting and then been cooked; frozen foods may have been harvested and frozen within a few hours of harvesting, and then stored in the frozen state before being heated. Similarly, 'fresh' fish may have been stored in ice for days or weeks before being cooked, while frozen fish may have been frozen within a few hours of catching and then stored frozen for some time.

The term 'fresh' is usually qualified as 'garden fresh' for fruits and vegetables that are eaten within a few hours after harvest, while 'market fresh' foods may be several days old, kept at room temperature or cooled.

Table 4 Vitamin losses after canning and storage of whole meals (22 ± 2°C)

	Initial value	Loss after canning (%)	Loss after storage (%)		
			1.5 years	3 years	5 years
Vitamin A (μg)	16.5	50	100	–	–
Vitamin E (mg)	80	0	0	50	50
Thiamin (mg)	9	50	75	75	75
Riboflavin (mg)	6	0	0	0	0
Pyridoxine (mg)	5	0	0	0	0
Vitamin B_{12} (μg)	18	0	0	0	0
Niacin (mg)	110	10	20	20	20
Pantothenate (mg)	21	25	50	50	50
Folic acid (μg)	14	0	0	0	0
Inositol (mg)	26	0	0	0	0
Choline (mg)	27	0	0	0	0

From Hellendoorn et al. (1969).

Losses should be balanced against advantages

There may be loss of nutrients even when the processing is carried out under carefully controlled conditions and such losses are the price that is paid for the advantages of the process. For example, pasteurization of milk causes losses of vitamins C, B$_1$ and B$_2$, but is considered a price worth paying for safety. Another example of the balance between loss and benefit is the use (in Great Britain) of sulfur dioxide to preserve comminuted meat; this rapidly destroys thiamin but this loss is considered to be outweighed by the safety benefits. A third example is the use of sulfur dioxide to prevent browning in ready-peeled, ready-chipped potatoes, which destroys some of the thiamin. Since potatoes are an important source of thiamin in many diets the price of convenience may be considered too high. There is also a small loss of available lysine and thiamin from the outer part of roasted meat and from the crust of bread and from biscuits. The processes involved improve the flavour but the losses are unimportant since only the outer surface of the food reaches a high temperature.

Beneficial Effects

Processing can have beneficial effects such as destruction of antienzymes, antivitamins and various toxins. Methods of preservation such as canning and heat treatment destroy microorganisms and greatly extend the shelf-life of food.

Among the nutritional benefits of processing is the liberation of bound niacin from cereal products. Niacin is present in many cereals in a form, niacytin, from which it is not liberated by the digestive enzymes. Indeed, when calculating the niacin equivalent of cereals (niacin plus that derived from the amino acid, tryptophan) the niacin determined chemically is ignored (apart from any added in enrichment programmes). Baking, especially under alkaline conditions, liberates the niacin. The classical example is the traditional method of making tortillas in Mexico in which the maize is first soaked in lime water which liberates the niacin – a process that helped the population to avoid pellagra which was common in maize-eating communities.

Another example of benefit is the conversion of trigonelline to niacin during the roasting of coffee beans.

Stability of Nutrients

Damage to nutrients, particularly vitamins, is caused by leaching, heat, oxidation, acidity or alkalinity, and exposure to light (Table 1). While the relative stability of pure, isolated nutrients can be assessed, the kinetics of their destruction in a food or a mixture of foods may differ from that determined on isolated nutrients, so Table 1 serves only as a general guide.

Assessment of overall losses requires investigation of the specific product including the particular process and equipment. There are many contradictions in reported values, as exemplified by Tables 2 and 3, owing to different samples and conditions of processing and to differences in sampling and analytical techniques. Clearly, damage to nutrients depends on the intensity and length of time of exposure to the various processes, and since comparisons are usually made between 'fresh' foods (cooked at home) and processed foods, much depends on the conditions of home cooking. Such comparisons are invidious since home cooking obviously covers an enormous range; however, figures from standard food tables (**Table 5**) indicate that vegetables lose 20–40% of their water-soluble vitamins on boiling, and fruits lose 25% of all vitamins except for an 80% loss of folate.

Nutrient Additions

A wide variety of nutrients are added to foods during processing; over the years every nutrient and source of energy has been added to foods. Some are added by law as a public health measure, and others are added to proprietary foods either as a public health measure or as a marketing attraction. In many countries vitamins B$_1$, B$_2$, niacin, iron and calcium – or some of these – are added to white bread (or to the flour). In some instances other cereals are fortified. This is intended to partially replace milling losses in the preparation of white flour and white rice, and in a few instances nutrients are added to maize and pastas. Replacement is partial because in the instance of white bread, fortification brings the level of nutrients up to that of 85% extraction flour, not the level in whole grain.

The other widely practised enrichment is the addition of vitamins A and D to margarines to raise levels to the equivalent in butter which the margarine replaces, or, in the instance of vitamin D, to higher levels.

Apart from fortification, some nutrients are used for functional purposes: for example, ascorbic acid is added to some processed foods to prevent oxidation such as browning of cut fruits and vegetables and fruit juices. Vitamin E is also used as an antioxidant in some infant foods as being a 'natural' and therefore presumably a harmless preservative.

The use of ascorbic acid in dough-making (the Chorleywood process) has no nutritional effect since

Table 5 Typical losses of vitamins in cooking

Vitamin	Percentage vitamin loss			
	Boiling	Baking	Roasting[a]	Stewing[b]
Cereals and cereal dishes				
Thiamin	40	25		
Riboflavin	40	15		
Niacin	40	5		
Vitamin B$_6$	40	25		
Folate	50	50		
Pantothenate	40	25		
Biotin	40	0		
Vitamin C	50	10–70		
Meat dishes (excluding losses recovered in gravy)				
Thiamin			0–40	40–70
Riboflavin			0–30	0–40
Niacin			10–30	30–70
Vitamin B$_6$			0–40	30–60
Folate[c]			–	30
Pantothenate			20	30–50
Vegetables				
Carotene	0			
Vitamin E	0			
Vitamin B$_1$	35			
Vitamin B$_2$	20			
Niacin	30			
Vitamin B$_6$	40			
Folate	40			
Vitamin C	45			

From Holland *et al.* (1991).
[a]Roasting, frying and grilling.
[b]Stewing and boiling.
[c]Applies only to liver and kidney (content too low in other meats).

it is destroyed in the overall process, but the use of ascorbic acid in the curing of meat, e.g. ham, can leave residues in amounts sufficient to make a significant contribution to intake.

Soya bean and other protein sources are added to some foods for functional reasons but incidentally make a contribution to protein intake.

Production of nutritionally favourable products

In the preparation of convenience foods and dishes it is possible to increase amounts and range of nutrients:

1. It is possible to prepare complete meals so as to provide a 'balanced' meal, i.e. one supplying a range of nutrients in adequate amounts.
2. While selecting the components of a ready-made dish there is an opportunity to include specific varieties with high content of vitamins, and to a lesser extent other nutrients. This has led to the development of so-called 'functional' foods which, because of the relatively high content of a particular ingredient, are claimed to confer special

health benefits beyond that of providing the RDA of nutrients, and include other postulated beneficial substances.

3. It is possible to provide foods that satisfy recommended nutritional guidelines such as foods with reduced amounts of saturated fatty acids, increased dietary fibre or reduced energy content.

Conclusion

Developments in food processing, including modifications of traditional techniques, tend to result in milder treatment in attempts to retain flavour, texture and general palatability as far as possible. Such treatments tend to retain more of the sensitive nutrients, even if that was not the original intention. These developments, together with interests in public health as well as for marketing reasons tend towards greater retention of nutrients.

See Colour Plates 7 and 8.

See also: **Catering**: Nutritional Aspects. **Dairy Products**:

Nutritional Value. **Food Fortification**: Importance in the Diet.

Further Reading

Bender AE (1978) *Food Processing and Nutrition*. London: Academic Press.

Bender DA and Bender AE (1997) *Nutrition – A Reference Handbook*, pp 437–466. Oxford University Press.

Harris RS and Karmas E (1975) *Nutritional Evaluation of Food Processing*, 2nd edn. Westport: Avi Publishing.

Hellendoorn EW, Groot AP de, Mijlldekker LP van der *et al.* (1971) *Journal of the American Dietetics Association* 58:434–441.

Holland B, Welch AA, Unwin ID *et al.* (1991) *McCance and Widdowson's The Composition of Foods*, 5th edn. London: Royal Society of Chemistry.

Mapson LW (1956) *British Medical Bulletin* 12:73–77.

Ministry of Agriculture, Fisheries and Food (1976) *Food Quality and Safety; A Century of Progress*. London: HMSO.

Robertson J and Sissons DJ (1966) *Nutrition* 20(1):21–27.

Vipond MS, Robertson J and Tapsfield D (1964) *Proceedings of the Nutrition Society* 23:38.

Food Service *see* **Catering**: Nutritional Aspects.

Fortification *see* **Food Fortification**: Importance in the Diet.

FRUCTOSE

Absorption and Metabolism

J M Johnson, Virginia Polytechnic Institute and State University, Blacksburg, Virginia, USA

Copyright © 1998 Academic Press

Fructose, a monosaccharide, is widely used in food products as a sweetener. This article discusses the development of the production of fructose in both the syrup and crystalline form and its application in food products. The physical, chemical and sensory properties are also discussed.

Sources

Fructose, commonly referred to as 'fruit sugar', occurs both as a free sugar and in combination with other sugars in plants and animals. Fructose and glucose are the component monosaccharides of sucrose, the most common sugar constituent of plants and animals; it is a constituent of blood and other body fluids. In plants, fructose is found in abundance in fruits and honey and in lesser amounts in tuberous vegetables such as potatoes and onions (**Table 1**). However, the major source of fructose as an ingredient in foods is from starch which has been hydrolysed to form glucose followed by conversion to fructose (*See*: **Carbohydrates**: Chemistry and Classification (Including Dietary Fibre).

In the late nineteenth century, starch was hydrolysed with dilute acid to yield glucose and dextrins for commercial purposes. The source of the starch was corn or potato. In the 1940s, cornstarch was the primary choice for the production of glucose, and the introduction of enzyme technology for hydrolysis reactions contributed to the development of glucose syrups of specific glucose content. The conversion of glucose syrups to fructose syrups by immobilized enzyme technology was introduced in the 1960s.

The major source now of fructose as a food ingredient is high-fructose corn syrup (HFCS) produced from cornstarch that has been hydrolysed by enzyme treatment to yield glucose followed by isomerization of the glucose and fructose. The process has been refined over the years with better control of the hydrolysis stage, new bacterial sources of the isomerizing enzyme, and new techniques for immobilization of the isomerizing enzyme.

Crystalline fructose is relatively unstable in that moisture is readily absorbed from the atmosphere by the anhydrous form, causing quick reversion to syrup. A high concentration and purity are necessary to achieve nucleation and crystallization of the sugar from the syrup. Crystallization of fructose has also been accomplished by the use of organic solvents, generally methanol, and by the formation of a salt complex.

Table 1 Free fructose in selected fruits and vegetables (% fresh weight basis)

Food	D-Fructose
Fruits	
Apple	6.04
Grape	7.84
Peach	1.18
Pear	6.77
Cherry	7.83
Strawberry	2.40
Vegetables	
Beet	0.16
Broccoli	0.67
Carrot	0.85
Cucumber	0.86
Endive	0.16
Onion	1.09
Spinach	0.04
Sweet corn	0.31
Sweet potato	0.30
Tomato	1.34

Adapted from Whistler RL and Daniel JR (1985) In: Fennema O (ed.) *Carbohydrates in Food Chemistry*, 2nd edn. New York: Marcel Dekker. With permission.

Isolation and Purification

The isolation of fructose begins with a starch slurry (commonly corn) that has been heated and gelatinized. A thermostable α-amylase is added for liquefaction. The temperature of the slurry is elevated to 105°C or 148°C, depending on whether a low- or high-temperature liquefaction process is selected. The enzyme randomly cleaves the starch molecules to glucose and dextrins. The pH of the slurry is adjusted for the optimum action of the enzyme. Low-pH α-amylase is available which requires a pH adjustment of approximately 4–5 but is more tolerant of variation in pH. Glucoamylase is added for saccharification and allowed to react until the mixture is approximately 95% glucose. Filters remove impurities such as proteins and oils and carbon columns remove colour, flavours and odour. An ion-exchange unit removes minerals and anions from the stream, leaving primarily pure glucose. Some water from the slurry may be evaporated to concentrate the syrup. Spray drying of the slurry produces solids used as a corn syrup solid ingredient.

The glucose slurry is then passed through an immobilized enzyme reactor of glucose isomerase to convert the glucose to fructose. The initial treatment by the immobilized enzyme converts 40–45% of the glucose to fructose. The syrup is evaporated to 71% solids and sold as HFCS-42 or a syrup containing 42% fructose, 50% glucose and 8% other saccharides (dry weight). This syrup may also be fractionated to yield two syrups; one that is 90% fructose (HFCS-90) and one primarily glucose. HFCS-90 is blended with HFCS-42 to produce a syrup that is 55% fructose, 41% glucose and 4% other sugars, and is the syrup of choice by the soft drink industry (**Fig. 1**).

Physical and Chemical Properties

Fructose is a levorotatary ketose generally found as a five-member furanose cyclic unit. The less common isomer from is β-D-fructopyranose, which makes up

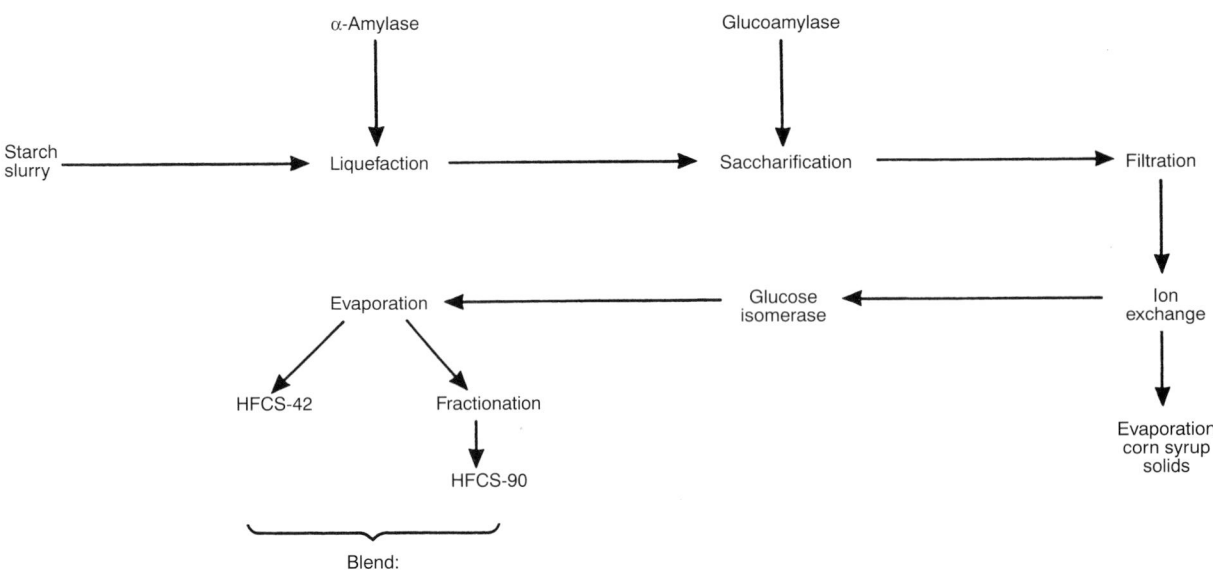

Figure 1 A flow diagram for the manufacture of HFCS from starch.

the mutarotational equilibrium of β-D-fructofuranose. Fructose is hygroscopic and does not crystallize easily from solution. At 20°C, approximately 78 g of fructose is soluble in 100 ml of water compared with 65 g for sucrose and 20 g for lactose. The crystalline hydrate form is less soluble than the anhydrous crystalline form and has very low solubility in nonpolar solvents. Fructose is a reducing sugar and is a reactive component of nonenzymatic browning or the Maillard reaction.

Sensory Properties

Fructose is perceived to be sweeter relative to sucrose. β-D-Fructose in solution has been rated with values from 100 to 175 compared to a sucrose sweetness value of 100. In the crystalline form, β-D-fructose was rated 180 relative to crystalline sucrose at 100. The most common theories of why some molecules vary in perceived sweetness is based on hydrogen bonding and geometrical shape of the molecule. Intramolecular hydrogen bonding enhances sweetness, as well as intermolecular bonding with a receptor site that has a complementary configuration to the molecule to allow for efficient bonding. Typically, a proton donor site, designated as AH, is located approximately 0.3 nm from an electronegative site, designated as B. The fructose molecule meets these requirements to elicit the sweet taste. The AH is designated to be the anomeric hydroxyl group and B is designated as the oxygen atom of the primary alcohol group. A third site capable of hydrophobic bonding, designated as γ, is the methylene carbon atom.

The sweetness of fructose has been reported to decrease with time or age of the solution and is accounted for by mutarotational equilibrium with other forms which are not perceived as sweet. Increased temperature of solution also depresses the sweetness value of a fructose solution; at the same time the specific rotation is increased and there is a shift in the equilibrium. The age and temperature of the solution may account for the reported differences of the sweetness of fructose when compared with sucrose ranging from twice to one-third as sweet. The specific rotation of fructose increases with increasing concentration, although not as rapidly as with increased temperature. The relative sweetness of different concentrations is temperature–concentration dependent. At lower temperatures, the relative sweetness of fructose decreases with increasing concentration, but at higher temperatures (37°C) the relative sweetness increases. This reflects a complex dependence on the shift in equilibria, shifts of forms, and other phenomena.

Food Applications

The most widely used form of fructose as a sweetener ingredient in foods is HFCS. HFCS is theoretically equal in sweetness to sucrose. The presence of a proportion of glucose diminishes the greater sweetness of fructose, making it approximately equal to sucrose, which is sweeter than glucose but less so than fructose. The consumption of HFCS dramatically increased in the 1980s with the incorporation of HFCS as the only sweetener in soft drinks. However, the popularity of soft drinks sweetened with non-nutritive sweeteners in recent years has reduced the use of HFCS for this purpose. HFCS is also widely used in confectionery, breads, biscuits, sweet doughs, cakes, beverages, soups and canned fruit.

The use of HFCS in baked products was limited for a time owing to excessive browning. Recent research resolved the problems of incorporating HFCS in baked products by adjusting the pH of the batter or dough. However, the increased acidity necessary to control browning increases the sharpness or tartness of flavour, which was resolved with added flavourings. Baked products containing HFCS generally have a lower volume than those made with sucrose. The presence of fructose lowers the gelatinization temperature of the starch in the batter and, thus, the structure is set earlier in the baking process than the sucrose counterpart. The use of HFCS in soft, chewy biscuits extends the shelf life because of the ability of HFCS to retain moisture. The use of HFCS in biscuits is limited to about a 50% replacement because of a limited biscuit spread and undesirable surface texture of large cracks. HFCS in breads provides a readily fermentable sugar source for the action of the yeast in addition to providing a residual sweet taste. Frozen desserts and ice cream containing HFCS have a softer texture at low temperatures since fructose depresses the freezing point below that when sucrose is used. The resistance of fructose to crystallization results in a frozen dessert that is smooth and less grainy. HFCS is also used in other dairy products such as yoghurt, chocolate milk and cheese spreads. The sweetener selected for fruit-flavoured drinks and pie fillings is often HFCS because of the nonmasking property of HFCS, allowing for more fruit flavour. The use of HFCS in salad dressings enhances the spice flavours. HFCS is used in combination with sucrose and dextrose syrups in canned fruit packs with the proportions largely determined by the most economical pack. HFCS is used as the partial or complete sweetening agent in tomato products such as ketchup and sweet pickles. The limited tendency of fructose to crystallize makes HFCS a good choice of sweetener for table syrups and dessert toppings.

Utilization of HFCS in foods with health claims has been controversial. The perceived sweetness of fructose may allow less to be used as a replacement for sucrose with the loss in volume compensated for by the addition of a bulking agent such as polydextrose, which results in a product of lower energy than the sucrose-sweetened counterpart. However, some research has shown that when HFCS-42 is combined in food products the sweetness may be less than that of sucrose because of the presence of glucose and other sugars in the food product that have a lower perceived sweetness than sucrose. HFCS-90 is successfully used to obtain an equisweet product when compared with sucrose with an approximately one-third reduction in energy. HFCS used with saccharin also appears to have a synergistic effect on sweetness and reduces the bitter aftertaste. HFCS is also used in rehydrating sports drinks since fructose is efficiently absorbed through the lumen of the intestine and passes through the portal vein for further metabolism in the liver. Orally administered fructose does not significantly increase the release of enteroglucagon and insulin, making a limited amount a possibility as a sweetener for diabetics. However, the long-term effect on plasma glucose levels in diabetics is not known. Similarly, any correlation between severity of diabetes and tolerance for fructose is not known.

Fructose has also been found to reduce the fat and consequent energy intake significantly when taken as a preload dose before a meal. Therefore, the consumption of fructose may serve to control the appetite.

Only two rare inborn metabolic problems with the ingestion of fructose have been reported; essential fructosuria and fructose intolerance. In essential fructosuria, fructokinase is deficient and, with fructose intolerance, fructose-1-phosphate aldolase is deficient. In both cases, individuals should avoid foods containing sucrose and fructose. Other digestive problems have been reported in individuals who have an allergy to corn products since the primary source of fructose added to foods is HFCS from corn.

The use of fructose as a food ingredient, especially in the form of HFCS, has wide acceptance in many food products. The advantages of availability, syrup form, crystalline control and sweetness make it a desirable ingredient for food systems. The use of crystalline fructose is largely limited to speciality foods because of the hygroscopic properties and economics of producing the crystalline product.

See also: **Carbohydrates**: Chemistry and Classification (Including Dietary Fibre).

Further Reading

Johnson JM and Harris CH (1989) Effects of acidulants in controlling browning in cakes prepared with 100% high fructose corn syrup or sucrose. *Cereal Chemistry* **66**:158–161.

Johnson JM, Harris CH and Barbeau WE (1989) Effects of high fructose corn syrup replacement for sucrose on browning, starch gelatinization, and sensory characteristics of cakes. *Cereal Chemistry* **66**:155–157.

Lee CK (1987) The chemistry and biochemistry of the sweetness of sugars. *Advances in Carbohydrate Chemistry and Biochemistry* **45**:199–351.

Lineback DR and Inglett GE, eds (1982) *Food Carbohydrates*. Chicago: Institute of Food Technologists.

Shallenberger RS (1982) *Advanced Sugar Chemistry*. West-port: AVI.

FRUITS AND VEGETABLES

Nutritional Value

A E Bender, Leatherhead, Surrey, UK

Copyright © 1998 Academic Press

Fruits and vegetables have considerable potential as a source of nutrients but the amounts eaten vary enormously both within and between countries. Some 3000 species are known to be edible and there are said to be more than 1500 species of wild tropical plants. In the foreword to *Traditional Plant Foods*, published by the Food and Agriculture Organization of the United Nations, it is stated that 'rural Africa is rich in nutritious plant foods but in recent decades social and economic changes have militated against their propagation and use'. This is because the promotion of major cereals has led to the eclipse of traditional plants. Furthermore, in developing regions many plant foods are regarded as being 'merely' children's food or poor man's food. Indeed, more fruits and vegetables are eaten in industrialized countries where there is an abundance of foods of all kinds than in developing countries, where any addition to the food supply is valuable.

For example, the average daily intake of fruit and vegetables in some underdeveloped regions is only 10–12 g per day compared with the recommendation in Western countries of five (and even up to nine) helpings (at least 375 g per day).

Definition

Plant foods are usually divided into seeds (including cereals), nuts and a third combined group of fruits and vegetables.

Fruits are the fleshy seed-bearing parts of plants while stems, roots, shoots, leaves, some seeds (including peas, beans and lentils), tubers (underground storage organs such as potato, Jerusalem artichoke, sweet potato, yam), underground stems (taro, onion) and flower buds and flowers (cauliflower, broccoli) are all classed as vegetables.

However, through popular usage some fruits such as tomato and cucumber are classed as vegetables, and rhubarb, a stem, as fruit. So the group includes a large number of very diverse foods which differ considerably in nutritional value.

Macronutrients

Fruits and vegetables contain a very high proportion of water (e.g. up to 96% in cucumber) and so, with some exceptions, supply only small amounts of macronutrients. The exceptions are those few eaten in sufficiently large amounts as to constitute a staple food, such as potato, plantain, cassava, taro (colocasia, also known as eddo, dasheen and old cocoyam). These are also lower in water content than many other members of the group and make a significant contribution to the carbohydrate and so the energy intake, and a small contribution of protein. For example, a 1000 kcal (4200 kJ) portion of plantain (*Musa* spp.) supplies 10 g protein. Cassava (manioc, *Manihot utilissima*) is extremely hardy and prolific and is a valuable staple in some communities, although a poor source of protein (1%).

Even in Western countries the potato (*Solanum tuberosum*) makes a contribution to the carbohydrate and protein of the diet, as well as supplying significant amounts of thiamin and ascorbic acid, because several hundred grams are often eaten per day.

One fruit, avocado (*Persea americana*), is a source of fat – 17–27% – two-thirds of which is monounsaturated. Olives (*Olea europea*) contain 10–12% fat, two-thirds of which is monounsaturated and which, of course, are a commercial source of oil. Leafy vegetables are very watery (80–90%) and make an insignificant contribution to the intake of macronutrients. However, such proteins that are supplied are relatively rich in the amino acid lysine, and to some extent, depending, of course on the amount eaten, complement the relative deficiency of lysine in cereals (see Leaf Protein below).

The legumes – peas, beans and lentils – play a special role in the diet since, as eaten, they contain more dry matter than most fruits and vegetables, around 30%. Unlike fresh fruits and vegetables they are usually stored for long periods in the dry state. After rehydration and cooking most of them including 'baked beans' (mature haricot beans, *Phaseolus vulgaris*) supply 5–8 g protein, 10–15 g carbohydrate, 300–400 kJ (80–100 kcal) and 4–5 g dietary fibre per 100 g. Legumes are sometimes described as rich sources of protein, but this is based on the dried product, not as eaten. When rehydrated and cooked their protein content is less than that of cereal products.

Garden peas (*Pisum sativum*) are commonly cooked from the fresh or frozen state, i.e. wet, but the macronutrient content is similar to that quoted above.

Green beans/French beans (pods and seeds of *Phaseolus vulgaris*) contain only 10% dry matter and 2 g protein, 100 kJ (25 kcal) and 2 g dietary fibre per 100 g.

Sprouted beans, commonly mung beans (*Vigna radiata*) but also alfalfa (lucerne, *Medicago sativa*) and adzuki beans (*Vigna angularis*), are also low in dry matter content and supply macronutrients in amounts similar to those in French beans.

Micronutrients

The major contribution of fruits and vegetables to the diet lies in their content of vitamins and minerals, but there are enormous variations between different types and between varieties of the same type.

Vitamins

The vitamin C content of different types of fruits ranges between some thousands of milligrams per 100 g in the instance of the West Indian cherry (acerola/Barbados cherry, *Malpighia punificolia*) to a few milligrams in apples (species of *Malus sylvestris*) and pears (varieties of *Pyrus communis*). The yellow–orange coloured fruits (e.g. apricots, *Prunus armeniaca*, pawpaw, *Carica papaya*) supply carotene, as also do all green vegetables, while it is absent from white types. Leafy vegetables are rich sources of vitamin K and many fruits and vegetables are significant sources of folate.

Growing conditions including soil, fertilizer (type, amount and time of application) and the state of maturity influence the vitamin content, particularly of vitamin C. In some foods, such as citrus fruits and tomato, the vitamin C is influenced by exposure to sunshine. One further cause of variation in vitamin content, again applying particularly to vitamin C and to a lesser extent to folate, is the loss after cropping, particularly from leaves that are bruised or wilted. Consequently it is not possible, apart from very broad generalizations, to state the vitamin content of a particular fruit or vegetable. Furthermore, new varieties have been and are being developed that are particularly rich in some vitamins.

Comparisons between food composition tables from various national authorities are unrealistic. Thus among six such tables (Australia, Germany, Great Britain, Spain, Italy and the USA) the range of carotene in pumpkins is quoted from 0.24 to 19 mg per 100 g; for thiamin between 0.15 and 0.5 mg per 100 g; and for vitamin C between 10 and 50 mg per 100 g. For tomato the carotene ranges between 0.8 and 4 mg per 100 g. Even within one set of tables, in which the same sampling and analytical techniques are presumably used, there is a range of carotene in sweet potatoes (*Ipomea batatas*) from 0.3 to 4.6 mg per 100 g; and for lettuce (*Lactuca sativa*) from 0.16 to 1.6 mg per 100 g.

Mineral salts

These are stable compared with some of the vitamins but the amounts can vary with different growing conditions, though to a lesser extent than described above for vitamins. Chemical analysis can be misleading since part of the mineral may be present in the food in a bound, unavailable form which is not liberated during digestion. In addition there may be other substances present in the same food or eaten at the same meal that interfere with absorption. Substances such as oxalates, phytates, tannins and dietary fibre reduce the amount absorbed.

Generally, vegetables are good sources of potassium with a very high potassium/sodium ratio, but rather poor sources of iron of low availability, although the amount absorbed is a balance between enhancement by the vitamin C present and various factors that reduce absorption. Vegetables are also a minor source of iodine depending on the content in the soil water.

Both fruits and vegetables are often described as sources of calcium but they are minor sources, i.e. many supply around 50 mg per 100 g compared with milk at 120 mg (which is consumed in much larger quantities) and cheese at several hundred mg per 100 g. Some common fruits and vegetables do not contain any calcium and the richer sources such as parsley at 330 mg and watercress at 220 mg per 10 g are eaten in relatively small amounts. Spinach stands out with 600 mg calcium per 100 g, but this is partly unavailable.

Dietary Fibre

All fruits and vegetables are sources of dietary fibre – more precisely nonstarch polysaccharides – but in different amounts. Thus, taken from the same food composition tables, they vary in fruits from around 0.5 g per 100 g in grapes, lychees, melons, cherries, through 1.5 g per 100 g in oranges, peaches, pineapple, plums, rhubarb, apples, 2.5 g per 100 g in mangoes, olives, pears, to nearly 4 g per 100 g guava, blackberries and blackcurrants (Englyst method of analyis). Similarly vegetables vary from 1–1.5 g (potatoes, cauliflower, celery, lettuce), 2 g (aubergine, French beans, cabbage), 4 g (baked beans, lentils, Brussels sprouts), to 6–7 g per 100 g (broad beans, kidney beans)

Leaf Protein

Leafy vegetables contain so little protein that excessive amounts would have to be consumed to make a significant contribution to the diet: such amounts would include unacceptable intakes of dietary fibre (chiefly cellulose). This problem has been overcome by extracting the protein from leaves, including grass; the soluble proteins are separated from the fibrous parts and concentrated by heat coagulation. This product can be added on the domestic scale without further purification to foods such as stews, or can be further refined to remove colour, and dried for storage, which adds to the cost and the technology required. Since grass and many leaves provide a continuing crop leaf protein offers considerable possibilities in developing countries, but has been little exploited.

Developing Regions

As quoted in the Introduction, there are numerous species of wild plants that could make useful contributions to the diet. The Food and Agriculture Organization has frequently drawn attention to the possibility of collecting wild plant foods, of growing them under protection or of cultivating them. It has been calculated, for example, that adding 100 g of leafy vegetables to the diet of a 6-year-old child whose staple is cereal or cassava could supply three times the daily need for vitamins A and C, all the folate, calcium and iron, 15% of the B vitamins and 15% of the protein. Regular consumption of amaranth leaves and leaves of the drumstick tree (*Moringa olifera*) is recommended for children as a public health measure in many areas of the world, particularly to overcome the widespread problem of vitamin A deficiency.

Vegetarians

Although there is little evidence that the avoidance of animal products results in malnutrition, indeed, in some instances the reverse may be true, the intake of some nutrients may be at risk if all animal foods (including fish, eggs and milk products) are shunned. Vitamin B$_{12}$ is present only, with very few exceptions (e.g. some yeasts), in animal foods, so supplementation of the diet is virtually essential.

The average intake of carnitine by strict vegetarians is only one-tenth of that of people eating a mixed diet but plasma levels are within 'normal' limits. However, dietary carnitine may be required by premature infants and possibly by full-term infants and may be required by adults taking certain drugs.

There are very few plant sources of taurine and it is not known to what extent this may be a dietary essential. However, plasma levels in strict vegetarians are close to the 'normal' range.

Toxins and Contaminants

Fruits and vegetables contain large numbers of non-nutrients, some of which are toxic, but they are rarely harmful under ordinary conditions. Anti-nutritional substances in plant foods include anti-enzymes that interfere with digestion, antivitamins, and substances such as oxalates, phytates, tannins and dietary fibre that can interfere with the absorption of some minerals. Glucosinolates, which are responsible for the characteristic flavour of vegetables of the families Cruciferae and Brassicaceae, are goitrogenic but appear to be an insignificant hazard to human health in the amounts usually eaten. In addition some legumes contain lectins in amounts sufficient to have been the cause of occasional cases of food poisoning when incompletely destroyed by cooking.

Most of these substances are destroyed by heat and have been found harmful to animals when included in feed in the raw state. Some are present in salad vegetables that are eaten raw, but in amounts too small to be harmful.

Cassava, especially the bitter variety, contains cyanide. This is usually removed in traditional food processing but not infrequently is a source of harm when the food is not properly treated.

Plantains eaten as a staple provide sufficient 5-hydroxytryptamine to affect central and peripheral nervous systems. Unripe ackee fruit (*Blighia sapida*) contains a toxin (hypoglycin) which causes vomiting sickness and hypoglycaemia. Rhubarb contains oxalate, and although the amounts in stems are harmless, poisoning has resulted from eating the leaves which contain a much higher concentration.

Potatoes contain small, usually harmless, amounts of solanine, but this is increased to toxic levels by exposure to light and subsequent 'greening'.

Some plant foods have been the cause of occasional outbreaks of poisoning in special circumstances. For example Jimson weed, *Datura stramonium*, contains alkaloids including scopolamine which produce hallucination; and the hemp plant, *Cannabis indica*, and the peyote, containing mescaline, have been consumed deliberately for their psychic effects.

Contamination

Some vegetables accumulate environmental toxins such as lead and radioactive fallout but the main cause for concern is from residues of agricultural chemicals, pesticides and weedkillers. The danger of these chemicals is mainly to those handling them in production and manufacture, but there is concern over the small amounts remaining in the crops since these may be consumed over a long period, and the toxins may possibly be cumulative. Among these are the organochlorine insecticides including DDT and dieldrin. Both the substances and their degradation products persist in crops and so find their way into the human food chain. The fact that they are fat-soluble and accumulate in the adipose tissue has given rise to concern but there is no evidence that these quantities merit alarm. Nevertheless, they are restricted in use and are under continuous observation.

Table 1 Sources of vitamin C in the average British diet

Food	% Average intake
Potatoes	16
Other vegetables	19
Fruit juices	18
Fruit	17
Salad vegetables	8
Milk products	5
Meat	4
Soft drinks	4
Enriched cereal products	3

From Gregory et al. (1990).

Role in Diet

There is considerable epidemiological evidence that a high intake of fruits and vegetables is protective against certain forms of cancer. Vitamins C, E and β-carotene, when individually subjected to trials by dietary supplementation, have not been shown to be protective and it has been suggested either that there may be a synergistic effect between the various antioxidants found in plant foods or that some of the numerous other substances in the food may be the protective agent(s). These include lycopene, lutein, indoles and phenols. Overall there are many hundreds of nonnutrients in plant foods whose functions in the diet, if any, have been little investigated.

See Colour Plate 9.

See also: **Antioxidants**: Observational Epidemiology; Intervention Studies. **Bioavailability**: Definition and General Aspects. **Dietary Fibre (Fiber)**: Physiological Effects and Effects on Absorption. **Food Contaminants**: Pesticides. **Legumes**: Types and Nutritional Value. **Nutrition Policies**: In Developing Countries. **Nuts and Seeds**: Nutritional Value. **Phytochemicals**: Epidemiological Factors. **Quasi-Vitamins**: Definition and Examples. **Vegetarian Diets**: Nutritional Adequacy.

Further Reading

FAO (1988) *Traditional food plants*. Food and Nutrition, Paper 42, Rome.

Gregory J, Foster K, Tyler H and Wiseman M (1990) *The Dietary and Nutritional Survey of British Adults*. London: HMSO.

Holland B, Welch AA, Unwin ID, Bass DH, Paul AA and Southgate DAT (1991) *The Composition of Foods*, 5th edn. Cambridge: Royal Society of Chemistry.

Liener IE (1980) *Toxic Constituents of Plant Foodstuffs*, 2nd edn. New York: Academic Press.

Oomen HAPC and Grubben GJH (1978) *Tropical leaf vegetables in human nutrition*. Communication 69, Department of Agriculture Research, Amsterdam.

Souci SW, Fachmann W and Kraut H (1989) *Food Composition and Nutrition Tables*. Stuttgart: Wissenschaftliche Verlagsgesellschaft mbH.

Watson DH (ed.) (1987) *Natural Toxicants in Food*. Chichester: Ellis Horwood.

FUNCTIONAL FOODS

Definition and Potential for Nutritional Role[a]

D P Richardson, Nestlé UK Ltd, Croydon, UK

Copyright © 1998 Academic Press

Nutrition Science and Product Development

The incorporation of nutrition research efforts and thinking into product design has a long and respectable history. Products conceived with micronutrients in mind are well established in the range of everyday shopping items, for example breakfast cereals containing B vitamins and minerals; margarines and spreads with vitamins A, D and E; soft drinks with vitamin C; and iodized salt. These fortified foods and drinks, and indeed nutrient supplements, originate from research on individual nutrients going back to the beginning of the twentieth century. The principle of adding very small quantities of active ingredients to a component of the food supply to achieve a health benefit is well demonstrated by the addition of fluoride to drinking water to delay the onset of dental caries. Several nutrients are added to food and drink products around the world as public health measures and as cost-effective ways of ensuring the nutritional quality of the food supply. Additions of nutrients have also formed the basis of several marketing strategies in new product development. More recently, products with lower fat and saturated fatty acid contents and higher contents of different fibres have had success in the marketplace, and have their origins in the disease risk-management phase of nutrition research, e.g. diets low in fat and saturated fatty acids to reduce risk of heart disease and some cancers. The current national and international scientific investigations linking the role of diet to disease prevention and optimization of human performance will no doubt create further opportunities for

---

[a] This article is adapted from a paper by the same author which was published in 1996 in *Nutrition Reviews* **54**(11): S174–S185.

product development, especially as there is likely to be an upswing in public interest in physical fitness and overall physical and mental wellbeing.

Functional foods, designer foods, pharmafoods, nutraceuticals

Poor food choices and restricted diets can affect the nutritional status of individuals at any stage of life, and potentially their long-term health. Hence, there are many opportunities for the food and pharmaceutical industries to manufacture added-value products to meet the special nutritional requirements of young children, adolescents, women of childbearing age, athletes, the middle-aged and the elderly. Although confusion still exists about how best to define these evolving areas of food and ingredient technology, the common thread is that the foods or components found within them have a potential beneficial role in the reduction of risk of disease. Pharmaceutical companies are motivated to isolate components in foods into tablets or supplement forms, whereas food manufacturers want to develop products containing beneficial components as part of a varied diet, based on the principles of good nutrition, e.g. a wide variety of foods eaten in moderation. The advantage of improved dietary intakes of functional foods and/or food fortification over supplements is that the latter provide only selected components in a concentrated form, not the diversity of nutrients and phytochemicals that occur naturally in foods.

There is a widespread perception that the food and drink industries are growing closer by vertical integration, strategic alliances, mergers and acquisitions, involvement in product developments and collaborative research. Whatever happens in the commercial environment, the use of specific nutrients and ingredients or combinations thereof which are claimed or perceived to be beneficial to health will stimulate the reformulation and repositioning of existing 'on-the-shelf' (OTS) and over-the-counter (OTC) products as well as product and process innovation. Key areas of interest include antioxidant substances including β-carotene, vitamins C and E (the 'ACE' nutrients), mineral nutrients such as calcium, magnesium, zinc and selenium, disease-preventive phytochemicals such as the flavonoids, probiotics such as Bifidus and *Lactobacillus*, fatty acids and lipids including fish oils, and a range of macromolecules including dietary fibres and oligosaccharides.

Potential Legislative Limitations to Market Development

It costs money to research, develop and add health-enhancing ingredients and nutrients to foods, and the commercial benefits of doing so would soon be lost if regulatory controls were too prohibitive. Regulators will need to satisfy the needs of industry for innovation and marketing but protect consumers from false and misleading claims about products.

Whereas current regulatory provisions may well accommodate the topic of functional foods and health claims, even at these early stages of their development, there is a need for researchers, industry and regulators to collaborate on a regular basis so that the principles and criteria for substantiating claims can be assessed properly. It is also extremely important to involve consumer representatives with the aim of establishing more clearly their points of concern and any ideas for action. Internationally, there are enormous variations in regulatory approach (**Table 1**). In the USA, health claims are permitted by the Food and Drug Administration in a total diet context, in several areas where there is 'significant agreement among qualified experts supported by the totality of publicly available evidence'. However, the functional foods industry in the USA dislikes the lack of owner-specific health claims and the lack of data protection. In Japan, the decision process focuses more on the active constituents in particular foods, but there the licensing procedure

Table 1 International comparison of regulatory approaches to functional foods

	Standard for functional foods	Position on health claims
European Community	No regulation	Not permitted
USA	No regulation	As addressed in NLEA
Codex	No regulation	Not permitted
Japan	FOSHU	Permitted only in FOSHU context
Australia	Under review	Not permitted (under review)
Canada	No regulation	Not permitted
New Zealand	No regulation	Not permitted
Sweden	No regulation	Specified health claims permitted

FOSHU, Food for Specified Health Use; NLEA, Nutrition Labelling and Education Act.

and the conditions for approval are believed to be too stringent and costly. Most countries are maintaining a responsible and cautious approach to the issue of health claims and they will learn from the experiences of others. The implications for international harmonization are unclear if individual countries were to proceed to regulate with completely different approaches. However, efficient, innovative and profitable investment by the food industry requires international markets and free movement of goods.

Regulatory control in the UK and Europe

As in many other countries, the regulation of functional foods and beverages in the UK and Europe falls into the grey area between food and drugs. As shown in Table 1, a legal definition for a functional food is not in place in Europe, and neither is there any specific regulatory control on health claims. However, in August 1995, the Ministry of Agriculture, Fisheries and Food (MAFF) in the UK developed a working definition, which is 'a food that has had a component incorporated into it to give a specific medical or physiological benefit, other than a purely nutritional effect'. This distinguishes functional foods from foods that are fortified with vitamins and minerals to enhance their nutritional benefits, such as breakfast cereals, and from food supplements that are marketed primarily as aids to ensure an increased intake of beneficial nutrients. The Ministry accepts that the concept of functional food encompasses a special health benefit, and the presentation of a functional food requires making a claim that relates to its special benefit, otherwise there is little point in developing and marketing the product.

Currently, MAFF has the power under the Food Safety Act 1990 to introduce regulations on the labelling, marking, presentation or advertising of food. All foods must be safe and wholesome, and a claim is any presentation that states, suggests or implies a food has certain characteristics relating to its origin, nutritional properties, nature, production, processing, composition or any other quality. For functional foods, health claims could relate to the prevention of a certain disease or a positive health benefit. Discussions are taking place in the UK and the European Union (EU) to find a formula for allowing certain types of health claims. The authorities appear not to be against claims establishing a link between nutrition and health and wellbeing, but they have not reached a consensus on what to do, if anything. However, some recent health claims in the UK have been the subject of complaints from consumer associations and MAFF have announced that

they are reviewing the situation. The Committee on Medical Aspects of Food Policy (COMA), an independent group of experts appointed by the UK Department of Health, has also taken initial steps to clarify the situation with MAFF. All health claims require careful interpretation of existing national and international rules. Any unscrupulous attempts to by-pass existing regulatory constraints would be unwise and would incur the wrath of industry, government and consumer organizations.

Label information   In the UK, the legal position is as follows and it has several interesting points and general principles for compliance. The main statutory controls are the Food Labelling Regulations 1984 (as amended) (FLR 1984), the Food Safety Act 1990 (FSA 1990) and the Trade Descriptions Act 1968 (TDA 1968). In addition, the Food Advisory Committee (FAC), a committee of independent experts which advises MAFF and the Department of Health, published a report in 1991 in which it defined health claims as 'any statement, suggestion or implication in food labelling and advertising (including brand names and pictures) that a food is in some way beneficial to health, and lying in the spectrum between, but not including, nutrient claims (i.e. high/low/reduced components in foods) and medicinal claims'. The FAC recommended that health claims should only be permitted if they can be justified according to any recommendations that have been made or supported by the Chief Medical Officer. The FAC also laid down some general principles:

- The claim must relate to the food as eaten rather than to the generic properties of any of the ingredients.
- A food, when consumed in normal dietary quantities, must be able to fulfil the claim being made for it, and adequate labelling information must be given to show consumers that the claim is justified.
- The labels should give a full description of the food to ensure that selective claims, even if true, do not mislead.
- Any claim must trigger full nutrition labelling, namely Group 2 of the EC 'Nutrition Labelling' Directive 90/496/EC including energy; protein; carbohydrate, of which sugars; fat, of which saturates; fibre and sodium, expressed per 100 g or per 100 ml. In addition, information may be given voluntarily as consumed per serving size as quantified on the label.
- The role of the specific food should be explained in relation to the overall diet and other factors.

Although the FAC approach was systematic, the UK

government decided not to adopt its report while there was a prospect of further European controls on claims. Nevertheless, the FAC confirmed that health claims relate to common or normal foods with the same appearance as conventional foods, but with amended composition, which are still eaten as part of the usual diet. If this is the case, it may be that the provisions of existing legislation are perfectly adequate. The FLR 1984 prohibits the presentation of food in such a way that a purchaser is likely to be misled to a material degree as to the nature, substance or quality of the food. The FSA 1990 makes it an offence to render and sell food that is injurious to health and to present food so as to mislead as to the nature, substance or quality of the food; interestingly, there is no reference to misleading 'to a material degree' and 'presentation', which in this context includes shape, appearance, packaging or the setting of food when it is on sale. The TDA 1968 makes it an offence to apply a false description to goods in the course of a trade or business. One area this law covers is fitness for purpose, strength, performance, behaviour or accuracy, and it is the headings 'fitness for purpose' or 'performance' that could be used in dealing with inaccurate and unsubstantiated health claims. Although there is no case law yet relating to health claims, it is likely that any offence could in part be avoided by the provision of accurate and detailed labelling. For a claim to be covered at all under the FLR 1984 and FSA 1990, it must be expressed positively, i.e. a food *is* capable of something, whereas a number of products on the market state that a food *may* have certain properties. Hence, with regard to enforcement of existing laws, the wording of a health claim if not positively expressed, together with the detailed and accurate information on pack and the availability of data to support the claim, could help prevent an offence being committed.

The point has been made that functional foods are no different from any other foodstuffs on the market about which the manufacturer wishes to make a claim, and that it is unnecessary to have particular rules covering functional foods. The claims currently being made in the UK relate generally to maintenance of good health, which the FAC accepted should be permitted. In the future, food manufacturers will seek to justify their claims by linking them to scientific research which has been endorsed by COMA and current advice on healthy eating. This is what the FAC recommended should be required of manufacturers, and to date, it has become their practice without the use of additional statutory controls.

Along with many other EU member states, the UK makes a clear distinction between foods and medi-cines. The FLR 1984 stated that if a claim is made either expressly or by implication that a food is capable of preventing, treating or curing human disease, it is a medical claim requiring a human medicinal licence issued under the Medicines Act 1968. Disease includes any injury, ailment or adverse condition of body or mind. In some cases, the distinction between a nutritional health claim and a medical claim may be unclear. However, the purpose of a drug is to prevent or cure a disease. This is not the main function of food, and a direct link between food and disease prevention is not permitted. Functional foods are not pills or capsules.

Industry initiatives on health claims in the marketing of food products There is no doubt that the responsibility for a health claim lies with the company involved and it is important for manufacturers and their trade associations to take the necessary initiatives to comply with the legislation and activities of the relevant authorities and also to take measures aimed at eliminating consumer problems and flaws in the market which could undermine credibility. For example, in Sweden the Federation of Swedish Food Industries, in consultation with the National Food Administration and the National Board for Consumer Policies, prepared a set of food industry rules for the use of health claims in the marketing of food products. Industry took the lead by demonstrating a commitment to the promotion of responsible marketing and advertising (including labels, leaflets, recipes, brochures, videos, films, etc.), and a willingness to accept the main burden of responsibility regarding the use of health claims. The rules are based on up-to-date research findings and it is intended that they are updated to keep pace with new developments. The rules will also be amended, where necessary, to conform to current and future international standards.

The Swedish industry rules are:

- Marketing and information material containing health claims should promote consumer awareness of the connection between food and health. The claims should be presented in such a way as to enhance public confidence in food products and the food industry. Therefore, the use of health claims must not result in a loss of confidence in food products, whether in individual cases or in general.
- The claims are to be consistent with official Swedish recommendations on diet and nutrition and should be based on scientific facts generally accepted in Sweden today. They should give a balanced overall picture of the causes and effects described in the marketing material, with

particular reference to the food product in question. They must therefore be formulated to take into account the need for a balanced diet providing all the essential nutrients. Such claims should only be made when marketing products whose normal consumption has a substantial effect on the diet as a whole.

- The claims are to be sufficiently detailed to enable the consumers themselves to form an opinion of the claims made. Packages should be supplied with a complete declaration of the nutrient content.

Table 2 shows the Swedish rules which list eight connections between physiological conditions and diet which they consider well established.

Scientific consensus and the substantiation of health claims

A major challenge for those involved in the research and development of functional foods is the scientific validation and substantiation of a claim in the eyes of the law. It is already clear that in some areas manufacturers will need better clinical evidence of the overall relationship between diet and disease, and they may need to carry out specific clinical trials on their products. The issue of substantiation of claims covers not only the safety and efficacy of the food components themselves, but also the finished food as it would be used by people. For parts of the food industry, this is a move towards the greater use of the biomedical sciences more akin to the pharmaceutical industries.

Like dietary recommendations, guidelines and quantified targets for intakes of micro- and macronutrients, the substantiation of health claims must be based on sound science – a synthesis of epidemiological, metabolic and animal studies, human clinical evaluations and mechanistic data. The diet and health relationship is complex, data are often difficult to interpret, and hence there is a need for caution in evaluating the results of nutrition research. In some areas of nutrition, scientific consensus does not exist, and some of the confusing nutritional advice in the public domain reflects the conflicting beliefs of medical, scientific and nutritional experts, the effects of media advertising and even political expediency.

Safety evaluations   If a functional food is a novel food or contains a novel ingredient (i.e. one that has not hitherto been used for human consumption to a significant degree or that has been produced by an extensively modified or entirely new food production process), a manufacturer in the UK would typically request a safety clearance by submitting a dossier of evidence to the Advisory Committee on Novel Foods and Processes (ACNFP). This process is voluntary in the UK, although a similar approval procedure will

Table 2   Swedish industry approach to health claims in the marketing of food products

Physiological condition	Link with diet
Obesity	A diet with low or reduced energy content is a significant factor in the prevention and treatment of obesity
Blood cholesterol level	Reduced intake of saturated fats, either by reducing the total fat content or replacing them by monounsaturated or polyunsaturated fats, can help to lower blood cholesterol levels
Blood pressure	Reduced intake of salt (sodium chloride) can counteract high blood pressure
Atherosclerosis	High blood cholesterol level and high blood pressure are diet-related risk factors for atherosclerosis
Constipation	Dietary fibre speeds up the passage of food through the intestinal tract and counteracts constipation caused by low intake of dietary fibre or lack of exercise
Osteoporosis	A calcium intake corresponding to official recommendations, together with physical activity and abstention from smoking, provides the best protection against osteoporosis
Caries	The absence of sucrose and other easily fermentable carbohydrates in products that are eaten between meals reduces risk of caries
Iron deficiency	Foods that are rich in iron provide protection against iron deficiency. Another significant factor is whether food constituents stimulate or inhibit absorption

become mandatory once the European draft Council Regulation on Novel Foods and Novel Food Ingredients is adopted.

Up to now, considerations of food safety have been limited to the potential for producing acute and chronic toxic effects or nutrient deficiency. However, in future, nutritional assessments of novel foods will need to be carried out against a background of rapidly advancing knowledge about the role of diet in the causation and prevention of many diseases, from classical nutrient deficiencies to coronary heart disease and some cancers which are major determinants of human mortality and morbidity. Functional foods, whether novel or not, could have the potential to influence dietary habits in ways that can decrease risks for chronic or other diseases, or adversely, lead to increased risks for the populations consuming them. The increasing recognition that dietary bioactive molecules have a multiplicity of actions which, although physiological, may entrain sustained changes in metabolism of pathological significance, also blurs the boundary between nutrition and toxicology.

Table 3 summarizes the main areas for the substantiation for nutritional safety and efficacy of functional foods and ingredients which may or may not be defined as novel. It can serve as a useful guide to

Table 3 Basis for the scientific dossier to substantiate nutritional safety

Nutritional composition

Dietary significance; intake; extent of use

Interactions with other components of diet; bioavailability

Presence of antinutritional factors

Implications for possible changes in gut microflora

Quantitative effects; dose responses

Impact on metabolic pathways and physiological function in humans

Overall toxicological assessments including allergy/intolerance factors

Potential effects on vulnerable groups, young, elderly, etc.

History of safe use; previous human exposure

Storage, preparation and instructions for use

Direct effects on pathophysiological processes

Relation to current dietary recommendations/targets

Technical details of processing and product specification

If probiotic, history of organism, consistency and stability of organism, survivability, colonization, replication, amplification in human gut

manufacturers on how to prepare a comprehensive scientific dossier to support health claims.

The food industry recognizes that the greater use of health messages must be consistent with substantiated medical fact and best practice around the world. However, what could be extremely frustrating to reputable manufacturers is that functional foods backed by considerable research efforts and investment could be undermined by, and appear to be the same as, those that are crude, carelessly made, have no real substantiating evidence and, at worse, are fraudulent. If the consumer does not believe or trust the ability of a product to provide the stated benefits, the long-term credibility of the industry would soon be damaged. The process for the establishment, verification and use of claims and messages must, therefore, be scientifically sound and credible. At the same time, the process needs to be flexible and pragmatic. It must evolve responsibly with a consensus of regulatory, academic, industry and consumer bodies rather than being a system of rigid product registration, closed lists of authorized claims, predefined wording and regulatory constraints.

Research and Development

The number of major research programmes designed to investigate and clarify the therapeutic value of foods and food components is forecast to continue to grow, particularly where serious debilitating diseases are concerned, such as heart disease, cancers and osteoporosis. This growth is happening in both the private and public sectors and we are seeing converging technologies and scientific disciplines throughout the food supply chain as well as in basic and applied research. There are also increasing opportunities for partnerships and collaborative efforts between researchers, government and industry. For example, in Europe, the objectives of the European Commission's Science Research Development Work Programme 1994–1998 include the promotion and harmonization of research in the major European primary food production sectors of agriculture and its links with the processing industries and the consumer. The programme is diverse, covering all aspects of the production and utilization of biological raw materials with the aim of developing new markets, products and processes for raw material derived from agriculture. One of the key areas is 'Generic Science and Advanced Technologies for Nutritious Foods' and the major objective is to improve the competitive position of the food industry, which is composed of leading multinationals and a wide range of specialist small and medium enterprises (SMEs) throughout Europe. The research efforts are aimed to improve the competitiveness and growth position of European industries in the agro-industrial sector.

There is a recognition that European research expertise must be at the forefront in understanding the role of food in the maintenance and improvement of human health and wellbeing and in the prevention of major diseases. The work programme of research is expected to lead to the design of special or tailored foodstuffs and ingredients for specific population groups and for special health benefits. The European Commission has stated categorically that this will be an expanding area for the food industry in the future and will involve multidisciplinary research projects combining the expertise of scientific partners in academia, government and industry. Specific research areas are to improve knowledge of the role of nutrient intake and nutritive properties of products, interactions and metabolism, especially trace elements and minerals (e.g. zinc, selenium, calcium, iron), vitamins (e.g. tocopherols, folic acid, vitamin C), other biologically active non-nutrients (e.g. antioxidants, polyphenols, carotenoids, flavonoids), n-3 and n-6 fatty acids and phytoprotective substances.

Similarly, in the UK, government departments, research councils and industry have participated fully in the development of national strategies for establishing a healthy diet in humans leading to an improved quality of life. In addition to fundamental issues relating to the quality of life, it is emphasized that there is the potential for wealth creation through the exploitation of such research by the food industry. The findings of the UK Technology Foresight Programme (Food and Drink and the Health and Life Sciences Panels) have also identified the relationship between food and health as a significant factor in the quality of life and future competitiveness of the UK. The main objectives of these new research initiatives include:

- increasing understanding of the mechanisms underlying the physiological, metabolic and behavioural effects of specific components of the diet from molecular to the whole organism level;
- linking food and plant science with nutrition research;
- taking advantage of the opportunities of the European nutrition research programme and supporting complementary research in the UK;
- encouraging technology interaction through LINK schemes (jointly funded research projects between science and industry in the priority areas identified by the Technology Foresight Programme), and by

promoting dissemination of research findings to industry and the consumer.

An 'Agro Food Quality Link Programme Functional Foods Initiative' has been sponsored by MAFF in which over a hundred companies from all sectors of the food industry have taken part. A series of focus groups are concentrating on specific topics and LINK projects have already been approved, including one on methodologies for measuring antioxidant status and indices of oxidative stress in humans.

This current emphasis on research is considered important to underpin the development of safe, efficacious dietary advice and products.

Consumer education: changing people's eating habits

An equally important research objective of the UK government and the European Commission is to improve the understanding of the role of food and other life-style factors, such as physical exercise, in the general health and wellbeing of the consumer. Undoubtedly, education is the key to the development of the market for functional foods and positive eating. Although the food industry is serving consumers whose overall standard of living is increasing, market research continues to show that it is the relatively older, wealthy and better educated consumers (social groups A and B) who are aware of and understand diet and health issues. Questions have already been raised about the possibility of social division between those able to afford foods for 'positive eating' and those who cannot.

Research efforts in the UK are now being focused on ways to underpin the provision of advice and information to enable consumers to make informed choices as well as on the factors determining food choice, including the development of taste preferences and hedonic, social, emotional and cognitive influences in food choice. Similarly, the Council of the European Parliament has adopted a programme of 'Community Action on Health Promotion, Information and Training'. This initiative is supported by the European food industry, and the Confédération des Industries Agro-alimentaires de la CEE (CIAA) together with representatives of the UK Food and Drink Federation (FDF) have submitted a policy document and scientific data with a view to becoming a full partner in the development of a sound framework for the health promotion policy in Europe. The food industry's representative bodies have also offered expertise and the technical and scientific resources of its member companies to facilitate future developments. The opportunities for industry to meet the challenge of science communications are highlighted in **Table 4**.

Table 4   Meeting the challenge of science communications

Consider identification of new industry food science communicators

Prepare updated position papers for timely responses to current and emerging issues

Identify a greater number of opportunities to comment on food policy issues at the early stages of development

Increase collaborative activities with other professional and trade associations

Ensure that the voice of food science is enhanced by presenting expert testimony and written commentaries

Establish collaborative alliances among government, industry and academia for strategic investment of public and private resources

Focus on the importance of the food sector to the economy and benefits of safe and quality food to a healthy population

Promote targeted basic and applied research into food science, technology and nutrition

Capitalize on the current and long-term emphasis on health

Seize the opportunity to be part of the health-care industry

Conclusions

The food industry has created efficient and safe food processing and delivery systems around the world, and it is willing and able to capitalize on new technologies and research with the development of tasty, pleasurable and healthy products. The development of functional foods requires careful attention to safety, labelling and claims, as well as to the nutritional and physiological rationale, cost and sensory qualities, all of which are keys to food choice and acceptability. **Table 5** and **Table 6** summarize the main areas for further action in an area of rapid change from the scientific, technical, legislative and consumer points of view. Developments in the area of functional foods will be heavily dependent on scientific substantiation of which safety and efficacy will be the principal components.

Table 5   Research areas requiring further action

Investigation of health-enhancing diets, foods, ingredients, nutrients – safety, dose response, efficacy over time, public health

Substantiation of potential health benefit claims

Communication of health benefits/appropriate labelling/marketing

Pioneering and innovative technological advances in the food industry

Appropriate and secure regulatory framework to commit resources

Table 6   How health claims and statements may create confusion, questions and problems

Scientific proof	'I'd want to know ...'
Dosage	'How often?' 'How much?'
Effect on natural balance	'What if the balance is upset?'
Overdosage	'What happens if I eat too much?'
What's the difference?	'Is yours really better for me?'
More precise information	'How does it help you?'
Exact effects on body	'I need more information'

Functional foods represent one of the most challenging areas of food technology and nutrition science. The pace of innovation, however, is dependent on the economic state of the organizations and institutions paying the bills, and the level of imaginative research funding to match an area rich in ideas. Another major influence affecting the expansion of the functional food business is the attitude and involvement of the retail trade. The creation of a regulatory climate which encourages fair trade, free movement of goods, the harmonization of controls to ensure validity of claims, and consumer protection is fundamental to the future role of functional foods for consumers and food markets. Ultimately, however, we should always remember that enjoyable eating and drinking involves balance, variety and moderation within the framework of a healthy, active life style.

Acknowledgment

A version of this paper appeared in *Nutrition Reviews*, vol. 54, no. 11, pt. II (November 1996) published by the International Life Sciences Institute.

See Colour Plate 10.

See also: **Food Fortification**: Importance in the Diet. **Food Processing**: Nutritional Influences. **Nutritional Labelling**: European Perspectives. **Probiotics and Prebiotics**: Definition and Role.

Further Reading

American Dietetic Association (1995) Position paper on phytochemicals and functional foods. *Journal of the American Dietetic Association* 95(4):493–496.
Australian National Foods Authority (1994) *Functional Foods Policy Discussion Paper*. Canberra; NFA.
Australian National Food Authority (1994) *Proceedings of*

the International Workshop: Functional Foods – The Present and the Future. Canberra: NGA.

BIBRA Toxicology International (1995) *BIBRA Research on Functional Foods*. Woodmansterne Road, Carshalton, Surrey SM5 4DS.

Biotechnology and Biological Science Research Council (1995) *Food Directorate Strategy*. Polaris House, North Star Avenue, Swindon SN2 1UH.

Cabinet Office/Office of Public Service and Science/Office of Science and Technology (1995) *Forward Look of Government-funded Science, Engineering and Technology*. London: HMSO.

Campden & Chorleywood Research Association, Chipping Campden GL55 6LD. 1995

Cockbill C (1994) Food law and functional foods. *British Food Journal* 96(3):3–4.

Confédération des Industries Agro-Alimentaires de la CEE (1994) Submission to the European Commission. NUT/031/94E. CIAA, Rue de la Loi 74, B-1040 Brussels.

Department of Health (1991) *Guidelines on the Assessment of Novel Foods and Processes*. Advisory Committee on Novel Foods and Processes. Report on Health and Social Subjects 38. London: HMSO.

Department of Health (1993) *The Nutritional Assessment of Novel Foods and Processes*. Report of the Panel on Novel Foods of the Committee on Medical Aspects of Food Policy. Report on Health and Social Subjects 44. London: HMSO.

European Commission (1992) Proposal for a Council Regulation (EEC) on novel foods and novel food ingredients. Off. J. Euro. Comm C190/3.

European Commission. A programme of community action on health promotion, education, information and training COM(94)202 Final. Adopted 2nd June 1995.

European Commission Science Research Development (1994) *Agriculture and Fisheries 1994–1998*. Brussels: EC.

Federal Register (1993) *Nutrition Labelling*. Final Rules 58(3).

Federation of Swedish Food Industries (1990) Health claims in the marketing of food products. The Food Industry's Rules. Sveriges Livsmedelsindustri förbund August.

Food Advisory Committee (1991) *Report on its Review of Food Labelling and Advertising 1990*. Report Fd AC/REP/10. London: HMSO.

Food and Drink Federation (1995) Research Strategy Group, 6 Catherine Street, London WC2B 5JJ.

Furukawa T (1993) The nutraceutical rules: health and medical claims: 'Foods for specified health use' (FOSHU) in Japan. *Regulatory Affairs* 5:189–202.

Goldberg I, ed. (1994) *Functional Foods Designer Foods, Pharmafoods, Neutraceuticals*. London: Chapman & Hall.

Labuza TP (1994) Shifting food research paradigms for the 21st Century. *Food Technology* 48:50–56.

Leatherhead Food Research Association (1993) *Market Intelligence Section Multiclient Study on Future Opportunities for Functional and Healthy Foods in Europe*. Leatherhead Food Research Association, Randalls Road, Leatherhead, Surrey KT22 7RY.

Leatherhead Food Research Association (1995) *Future Opportunities for Functional Foods. An In-depth Analysis of Consumer Attitudes*. Randalls Road, Leatherhead, Surrey KT22 7RY.

Ministry of Agriculture, Fisheries and Food (1994) Food Safety Directorate. *MAFF Food Research Requirements Document 1995–96*. London: MAFF Publications.

Ministry of Agriculture, Fisheries and Food (1995) *Annual Report of the Advisory Committee on Novel Foods and Processes (ACNFP) 1994*. London: MAFF Publications.

Ministry of Agriculture, Fisheries and Food (1995) *Food Standards and Labelling Division Discussion Paper on Functional Foods and Health Claims*. London: HMSO.

PA Cambridge Technology Centre (1995) *Nutritional Healthcare – A Continuing Global Trend*. Melbourn, Royston, Herts SG8 6DP.

PA Consulting Group (1990) *Functional Foods: A New Global Added Value Market*. London.

Potter D (1990) Functional foods – a major opportunity for the dairy industry. *Dairy Industry International* 556:16–17.

Potter D (1995) *Functional Foods – Challenges and Opportunities*. Royston: PA Cambridge Technology Centre.

Richardson DP (1993) The role of the food industry in developing and communicating better nutrition. In: Leathwood P, Horisberger M, and James WPT (eds) *For a Better Nutrition in the 21st Century*. Nestlé Nutrition Workshop Series 27, pp 179–196. Vevey: Nestec Ltd. New York: Raven Press.

Riemersma RA (1995) *LINK Agro Food Quality Programme. Dietary Antioxidant Vitamins and Oxidative Stress*. Cardiovascular Research Unit, University of Edinburgh in collaboration with Nestlé UK Ltd, Van den Bergh & Jurgens Ltd and Roche Products Ltd.

Seymour Cooke Food Research International (1995) *Positive Eating. An International Report on the Interface between Food, Health and Nutrition*. 42 Colebrooke Row, London N1 8AF.

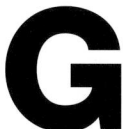

GALACTOSE

Absorption and Metabolism

Adel Abi-Hanna and **Jose M Saavedra**, Johns
Hopkins University School of Medicine, Baltimore,
Maryland, USA

Copyright © 1998 Academic Press

Lactose, a disaccharide composed of glucose and galactose, is the principal sugar of mammalian milk and the principal carbohydrate energy source for infants and children; thus galactose plays a central metabolic role in human nutrition. Lactose is hydrolysed in the intestine into glucose and galactose, which together with other sources of these monosaccharides are absorbed and metabolized and used as energy. Galactose additionally is an important constituent of complex polysaccharides, galactolipids and other glycoconjugates of structural and functional importance. Both absorptive as well as metabolic defects affecting galactose have been described.

Dietary Sources of Galactose

Lactose is by far the most abundant source of galactose in the diet of most humans. However, lactose can also be found in a considerable number of sources. These include drugs and medications, which use lactose as an excipient, in part because of its excellent tablet-forming capacity. Additionally, small amounts of galactose can be present in many fruits and vegetables, and considerable amounts can also be found in legumes (beans and peas) and in other food plants. Galactose polysaccharides with various glycolytic linkages such as $\alpha(1-6)$, $\beta(1-3)$ and $\beta(1-4)$ are ubiquitous in animals and plants. The bioavailability of galactose in these linkages found in foods is not well known. Some galactosidasis in plants can liberate galactose, and foods fermented by microorganisms for preparation or preservation may also contain free galactose. The role of free and bound galactose in cereals, fruits, legumes, nuts and other vegetables may contribute to sources of galactose that are not readily obvious. Bound galactose is also present in raffinose oligosaccharides and other sugars.

Galactose Absorption

Lactose is hydrolysed in the intestine by the enzyme lactase-phlorizin hydrolase to glucose and galactose. In humans, D-glucose and D-galactose are the only nutritionally significant monosaccharides that are actively absorbed. Although glucose and galactose can cross the intestinal mucosa down a diffusion gradient, the slowness of this method is such that water would diffuse in the opposite direction leading to a lessening in the concentration gradient. Thus, a rapid transport mechanism exists for glucose and galactose, particularly in infants. The 'coupled carrier' hypothesis is generally accepted as the main mechanism. In the small intestine and proximal tubule of the kidney, D-glucose is absorbed by epithelial cells via a sodium-dependent cotransport system existing at the luminal membrane level and a sodium-independent transport system at the basolateral membrane level. It is suggested that the potential difference across the brush border membrane of the cell also plays an important role in the mechanism which concentrates sugar in the cell.

The genetic functional defects of this cotransport system are expressed in two main clinical entities; selective congenital glucose and galactose malabsorption by the intestine discussed below, and familial renal glycosuria. Once galactose is absorbed, it must be converted to glucose for utilization. This occurs primarily by the pathways explained below. Three distinct enzymatic defects are responsible for the conditions generally described as galactosaemia.

Glucose–Galactose Malabsorption

Pathophysiology and clinical manifestation

Glucose and galactose malabsorption is a rare congenital disease resulting from a selective defect in the intestinal transport of glucose and galactose. It is characterized by the neonatal onset of severe, watery, acidic diarrhoea. The diarrhoea is profuse and contains sugar. In children given lactose, faecal sugar mainly consists of glucose and galactose with only small amounts of lactose, since lactase activity is usually adequate. Hyperosmotic dehydration and metabolic acidosis are the rule. Related gastrointestinal signs and symptoms include increase of abdominal gas, distension and vomiting. Intermittent or permanent glycosuria after fasting or after a glucose load is frequent. Thus the combination of reducing sugar in the stool and slight glycosuria despite low blood glucose levels is highly suggestive of glucose–galactose malabsorption.

The major characteristic in glucose–galactose malabsorption is the lack of intracellular glucose or galactose accumulation against a concentration gradient. The transport of other molecules such as alanine or leucine via a sodium cotransporter is typically intact.

The abnormality of carbohydrate metabolism is confined to glucose transport in the small intestine and the proximal renal tube. The main defect appears to be the absence of a functional sodium-dependent glucose contransporter. Electrolytes can be secreted in the jejunal mucosa together with fluids, suggesting that the combined glucose-sodium water absorption process is effective. Sucrose can undergo normal hydrolysis and fructose can be absorbed typically without problems. Glucose entry into the erythrocytes is normal and so are fasting blood glucose levels. Oral glucose tolerance tests usually yield a flat glucose curve while breath hydrogen tests done separately for glucose and galactose are consistent with malabsorption.

The functionality of the cotransporter at the brush border membrane is either absent or reduced. Additionally, the participation of a mutarotase in sugar transport has recently been suggested in the absence of this enzyme, and has been demonstrated in glucose-galactose malabsorption. However, full understanding of this condition requires additional information on the liquid composition of the membrane and on other characteristics and genetic control of this transport system.

Diagnosis

Children affected with glucose-galactose malabsorption are of diverse origin. There is high consanguinity rate and no clear-cut vertical transmission, suggesting an autosomal recessive mode of inheritance.

The diagnosis can be established by a clinical history of watery diarrhoea with glucose-water solution or milk and rapid cessation of the problem when these are discontinued. Oral glucose or galactose tolerance tests and breath hydrogen analysis can aid in the diagnosis. The differential diagnosis includes congenital lactase deficiency, sucrose-isomaltose deficiency and congenital chloride-secreting diarrhoea. Most other monosaccharide malabsorption and intolerance is secondary to mucosal injury and responds to adequate nutritional management with complete resolution.

Management

Treatment consists of immediate rehydration, adequate maintenance of hydration and initiation of a glucose- and galactose-free diet. Since fructose is tolerated, most of the carbohydrate initially can be given as fructose, using other dietary modular products of protein and fat as well as micronutrients.

Biochemistry and Physiology of Galactose

The main pathway of galactose metabolism in humans is the conversion of galactose to glucose, without disruption of the carbon skeleton. The name 'galactosaemia' has been associated with a syndrome of toxicity associated with the administration of galactose to patients with an inherited disorder of galactose utilization, leading to multiple clinical manifestations, including malnutrition, mental retardation, liver disease and cataracts. The clinical manifestations are linked to specific enzymatic defects. Thus the term 'galactosaemia' should be qualified by the specific defect. Three enzymatic steps are required to metabolize galactose to UDP-glucose. Two alternate pathways, oxidation and reduction, are used in the absence of enzymes of the main route (**Fig. 1**).

Step 1: galactokinase

Galactose is phosphorylated by galactokinase with ATP to form galactose 1-phosphate. The equilibrium is far in the direction of sugar phosphorylation, but the reaction is reversible. Galactokinase has been studied in detail in human red cells, leucocytes, fibroblasts, placenta, liver and various human fetal tissues. It is detectable in fetal liver from 10 weeks of gestation onwards and the activity of the enzyme in liver and red cells is higher in the second and third trimester. Its activity is higher in red blood cells from human infants than in cells from adults, and in reticulocytes than with aged red cells. Cultured human fibroblasts show enhanced galactokinase activity when grown in the presence of galactose, whereas in the liver the activity does not appear to be regulated by dietary galactose. The red cell enzyme, like that of the liver, undergoes substrate and product inhibition.

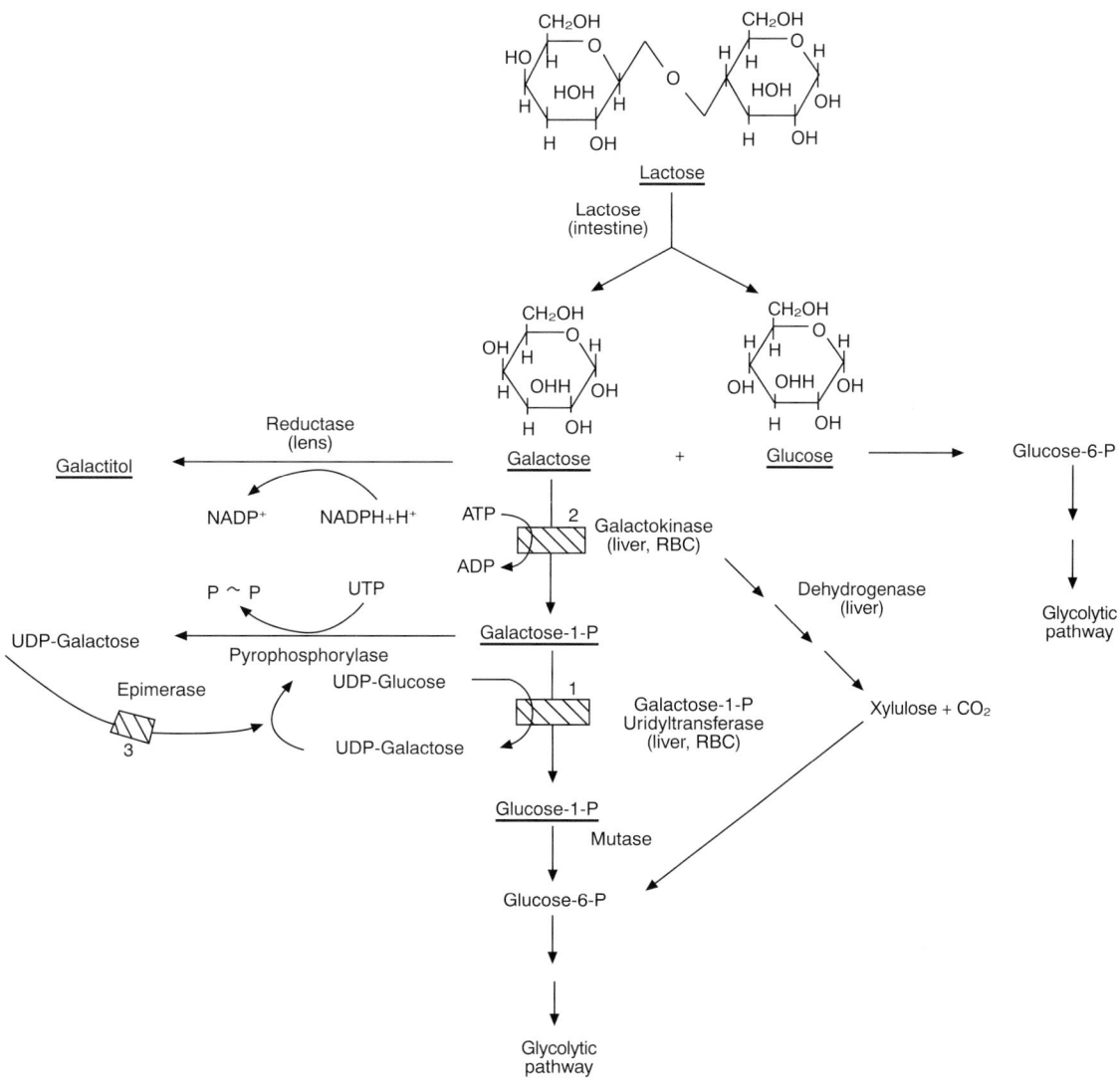

Figure 1 Metabolic pathways of galactose metabolism. The hatched areas indicate metabolic blocks due to the specific enzyme deficiencies: 1, galactose-1-phosphate uridyltransferase; 2, galactokinase; 3, UDP-galactose; 4'-epimerase. P, phosphate; RBC, red blood cell. Adapted from Elsas LJ and Acosta PB (1994) Nutrition Support of Inherited Metabolic Disease, in Shils, Olson and Shike, *Modern Nutrition in Health and Disease*, Lea and Febiger, Philadelphia, 8th edn, vol. 2, p 1198.

The assignment of the gene for galactokinase has been made to human chromosome 17, and its regional localization of the chromosome has been assigned to band q21–22.

Step 2: transferase

Galactose 1-phosphate reacts with UDP-glucose to produce UDP-galactose and glucose 1-phosphate. This step is catalysed by galactose-1-phosphate uridyltransferase, an enzyme present in bacteria and most mammalian tissues. Like galactokinase, galactose-1-phosphate uridyltransferase is detectable in fetal liver from 10 weeks of gestation, with the liver enzyme-specific activity being highest at 28 weeks of gestation. The rate of reaction may be regulated by substrate concentration and limited by UDP-glucose substrate inhibition of transferase. Glucose 1-phosphate is a potent inhibitor of the enzyme. Uridine nucleotides such as uridine di- and triphosphate are powerful competitive inhibitors of substrate UDP-glucose.

Galactose-1-phosphate uridyltransferase deficiency is the most commonly reported defect in galactosaemic patients. In the young infant galactose is a major energy source and its metabolism to glucose 1-phosphate is essential, but this is not the case in the fetus in whom glucose is the main energy source. However, the metabolism of galactose in the fetus is important to prevent accumulation of toxic galactose metabolites. Thus in galactose-1-phosphate uridyltransferase deficiency the fetus could be at a disadvantage as early as the 10th week of gestation. Dietary and hormonal influences on the liver enzyme have not been reported. In the rat a galactose-rich diet increases transferase activity.

Galactose-1-phosphate uridyltransferase is localized on chromosome 9p13. At least 32 variants in the nucleotide sequence of the galactose-1-phosphate uridyltransferase gene have been identified, with the most frequent being change in amino acid codon position 188 in which an arginine is substituted for a glutamine, the Q188R mutation. This Q188R mutation is associated with 'classical' galactosaemia with virtually no galactose-1-phosphate uridyltransferase activity detectable. However, there are other variant forms of the enzyme which have diminished but detectable activity, known as Duarte, Indiana, Rennes, Los Angeles, Münster and Chicago. Heterozygotes for normal and Duarte alleles are presumed to have 75% of normal galactose-1-phosphate uridyltransferase activity. Homozygotes for the Duarte allele could have 50% activity, and compound heterozygotes for the Duarte allele and the classical galactosaemia allele have 25% activity in peripheral erythrocytes.

Step 3: epimerase

The UDP-galactose is converted to UDP-glucose by UDP-galactose 4′-epimerase. The UDP-glucose thus formed can then enter the reaction again in a cyclical fashion until all the free galactose coming into the pathway is converted to glucose 1-phosphate. This enzyme is responsible for the inversion of the hydroxyl group at the C-4 carbon of the hexose chain to form glucose from galactose; it is also important for the conversion of UDP-glucose to UDP-galactose when only glucose is available and galactose is required as a constituent of complex polysaccharides. The epimerase maintains a cellular equilibrium of UDP-glucose to UDP-galactose in a ratio of about 3 : 1.

The purified enzyme is a dimer of identical subunits that consists of a mixture of catalytically active subunits (epimerase-NAD$^+$) and inactive subunits (epimerase-NADH-uridine nucleotide). The NAD binds to the enzyme and induces a conformational change resulting in enzymatic activity. For liver enzyme activity, exogenous NAD is required and NADH is a potent inhibitor of the enzyme. Any process disturbing the NAD/NADH ratio, such as ethanol metabolism which generates NADH, will impair galactose utilization. Cellular levels of UDP-glucose and other uridine nucleotides may also exert rate-regulating effects. Cells not exposed to free galactose form the sugar from glucose in adequate amounts to satisfy normal growth and development. Epimerase activity of the intestinal mucosa increases with age, whereas human red cells have a higher activity in newborns than adults. The intestinal enzyme activity can be enhanced by feeding diets high in glucose or galactose content. Less information is available on fetal levels of UDP-galactose 4′-epimerase, but one fetus of 16 weeks' gestation had liver enzyme activity comparable with that of children and adults. In epimerase deficiency, when the amount of entering galactose is low, an elevated level of galactose 1-phosphate in red blood cells may be reduced to normal but the UDP-galactose level stays elevated. The gene for epimerase has been assigned to human chromosome 1.

Alternative pathway: reduction

The polyol pathway was first identified in placenta and seminal vesicles, and is responsible for the fructose content of seminal fluid. Two enzymatic reactions involving aldose reductase and sorbitol dehydrogenase catalyse the conversion of glucose to fructose with sorbitol as the intermediate. In certain cells, such as renal collecting duct cells, retinal pigment epithelial cells and renal glomerular endothelium, and under certain conditions, aldose reductase functions to produce sorbitol which acts as an intracellular osmolyte. The acyclic polyols such as sorbitol, galactitol and mannitol are the end product of metabolism and have osmotic properties. The presence of galactitol in the urine and plasma of patients with transferase-, galactokinase- and epimerase-deficiency galactosaemia is suggestive of the importance of the reduction of galactose as an alternative pathway. However, the high K_m of this enzyme indicates that reduction will occur only when galactose levels in tissues are very high.

Patients with classical galactosaemia have markedly elevated levels of galactitol in plasma and urine, which remain above age-matched control levels after treatment with galactose-free diet, whereas high urinary galactose levels return to normal in all patients. Aldose reductase has been localized to the Schwann cells of peripheral nerves and to renal paptillae cells. Kinetic studies suggest that neither glucose nor galactose are preferred substrates. Only when tissue levels of galactose are much elevated would reduction be important. Aldose reductase activity of lens and other tissue is stimulated by sulfate ions and ATP and is inhibited by various keto acids, fatty acids and ADP. Increased production of galactitol is felt to play an important role in the pathogenesis of cataracts in the infant with galactose-1-phosphate uridyltransferase, galactokinase and UDP-galactose epimerase deficiency. The toxicity of polyols in the ocular lens is probably related to their ability to act as osmotically active particles within the lens cells, which leads to accumulation of water and eventually cell dysfunction.

Cataracts are the primary manifestation of disease in untreated patients with galactokinase deficiency, who manifest accumulation of galactitol but not galactose 1-phosphate in tissues. Thus the galactose 1-phosphate and not galactitol toxicity is probably a necessary mediator in both transferase and epimerase deficiencies for expression of hepatic disease, renal tubular dysfunction and increased red blood cell turnover.

Alternative pathway: oxidation

In the absence of galactose-1-phosphate uridyltransferase activity, galactose 1-phosphate and galactose accumulate behind the block. The second alternate pathway, besides reduction of galactose to sugar alcohol, galactitol, is the oxidation of galactose to sugar acid, galactonate. Galactonate, for example, appears in the urine of transferase-deficient individuals. Galactonate can be further metabolized to xylulose, a sugar capable of further metabolism. This pathway accounts for about 50% of oxidation of galactose by galactosaemic patients. Patients with transferase-deficient galactosaemia excrete galactonate in urine after galactose is administered, and galactonate has been found in the liver of a transferase-deficient subject.

Disorders of Galactose Metabolism

Clinical manifestations

Galactose is an important constituent of the complex polysaccharides which are part of cell glycoconjugates, key elements of immunologic determinants, hormones, cell membranes structures, endogenous animal lectins and numerous other glycoproteins. In addition galactose is incorporated in galactolipids, important structure elements of the central nervous system. It is not difficult to assume that the abnormal galactose metabolism in galactosaemic patients could have profound and widespread effects on glycoconjugate structures and their biological function.

Classically, the term 'galactosaemia' was associated with an inherited disorder of galactose utilization characterized by malnutrition, liver disease, cataracts and mental retardation, resulting from the specific deficiency of galactose-1-phosphate uridyltransferase. However, other enzymatic defects with variations of clinical presentation can also lead to galactosaemia (**Table 1**). Thus it is preferably better to refer to these abnormalities of metabolism by the specific enzymatic deficiencies which are described below.

Transferase deficiency   Failure to thrive is the most common initial clinical sign of galactose-1-phosphate uridyltransferase deficiency, and it is present in all cases. Vomiting or diarrhoea is present in almost all patients, usually starting within a few days of milk ingestion. Jaundice, hepatomegaly or both are present almost as frequently after the first week of life. The jaundice of intrinsic liver disease may be accentuated by severe haemolysis in some patients. Abnormal liver function tests and ascites may develop. The reason for liver toxicity remains obscure. The liver of affected patients has a characteristic acinar formation, and liver biopsy on occasion has been helpful in establishing the diagnosis. There is high frequency of neonatal death due

Table 1   Disorders of galactose metabolism

Enzyme deficiency	Primary clinical manifestations
Galactose-1-phosphate uridyltransferase	Failure to thrive
	Emesis/diarrhoea
	Jaundice, hepatomegaly
	Cataracts
	Galactosuria
	Gonadal dysfunction
	Developmental delay, neurologic symptoms
	Cataracts
Galactokinase	Similar manifestations as transferase deficiency, but with no liver, kidney or gonadal dysfunction
UDP-galactose 4′-epimerase	Mostly asymptomatic
	Rarely same manifestations as transferase deficiency but with no gonadal dysfunction

to *Escherichia coli* sepsis, possibly caused by the inhibition of leucocyte bactericidal activity.

Galactose 1-phosphate and galactitol have been detected in the kidneys of patients with galactosaemia. Renal toxicity may manifest as renal tubular dysfunction and a defect in urine acidification mechanisms. Galactosuria, hyperchloraemic acidosis, albuminuria and aminoaciduria may also occur. Hyperchloraemic acidosis could be also secondary to the gastrointestinal disturbance and poor food intake. Galactosuria may be intermittent, depending on oral intake, and can disappear within 3–4 days with the use of intravenous glucose. The finding of urinary reducing substances which do not react in a glucose oxidase test should raise the suspicion of galactosaemia. This finding, however, does not establish the diagnosis, since galactosuria can also occur in intestinal lactase deficiency and in severe liver disease due to other causes.

Ovarian atrophy appears to be an important manifestation of galactose toxicity, with clinical and biochemical evidence of ovarian dysfunction present in nearly all affected females. The basis of the toxicity has not been defined. The consequences of the gonadal dysfunction range from failure of pubertal development, through primary amenorrhoea to secondary amenorrhoea or premature menopause (75–76% of affected females). Although gonadal function has been described as early as infancy based on elevations of follicle stimulating hormones (FSH) and abnormal stimulation testing, no predisposing factor for gonadal dysfunction can be found. Previous recommendations that dietary lactose restriction from birth may be beneficial have in fact not prevented gonadal dysfunction. In the galactosaemic male, a complete understanding of gonadal dysfunction has not yet been described. The majority – but not all – of male galactosaemic patients had normal pubertal development, and a few individuals have been found to have normal semen.

Cataracts have been observed within a few days of birth. These may be found only on slit-lamp examination and can be missed with an ophthalmoscope, since they consist of punctate lesions in the fetal lens nucleus. Several hypotheses have been postulated to account for their formation and are mentioned above. It seems conclusive that the initiator of the process in rats is galactitol and not galactose 1-phosphate. Galactose 1-phosphate accumulates only late in the process and is absent in patients with galactokinase deficiency who present with cataracts.

Development of mental retardation may be apparent after the first months of life. Signs of increased intracranial pressure and cerebral oedema have been observed as a presenting feature.

Many of the toxicity symptoms can rapidly resolve with institution of dietary lactose restriction. However, a substantial percentage of children have subnormal IQs and speech and language deficits, but rarely devastating neurological sequelae. Most galactosaemic patients with lactose restriction are deficient of cognitive functioning in one or more areas. The deficits are variable, and do not appear to be related to the age, diagnosis or the severity of illness at presentation. The pathophysiology of these impairments in galactosaemia remains unknown. Several hypotheses are suggested, including toxic oedema due to increased brain galactitol concentrations, changes in the second messenger pathway, and changes of the energy status of the brain.

Galactokinase deficiency   Galactokinase deficiency is characterized by the occurrence of cataracts without liver, kidney or ovarian dysfunction and no increased risk of infections. A number of infants are reported to have pseudotumour cerebri, with very rare neurological involvement, suggesting that retardation is not a feature. The absence of liver and kidney damage in galactokinase deficiency and the presence of damage to these organs in transferase deficiency make it likely that toxicity in the later condition is in some way associated with galactose 1-phosphate formation.

Epimerase deficiency   Elevated red cell levels of galactose 1-phosphate with absence of UDP-galactose 4′-epimerase have been described in a patient with normal growth, development and normal ability to metabolize ingested galactose. Several cases of biochemical deficiency have been described but symptomatic cases are extremely rare. A few had cataracts, sepsis, liver, kidney and brain abnormalities, including a few with neurosensory deafness. There appears to be no ovarian dysfunction. The absence of ovarian dysfunction suggests that elevated UDP-galactose levels may protect the ovary from damage observed in transferase deficiency. Screening programmes have been established in Japan, where the incidence is reported to be 1 in 23 000. In epimerase deficiency, when dietary galactose is low, galactose 1-phosphate concentrations in red blood cells may be reduced to normal, but UDP-galactose concentrations remain elevated. Despite the many phenotypic similarities between transferase and epimerase deficiency, the latter is characterized by elevated red cell levels of UDP-galactose even with modest galactose intake.

Diagnosis

The presence of reducing substance in urine which does not react with glucose oxidase reagents is consistent with galactosuria; however, occasionally some infants (particularly premature babies) also develop galactosuria. It is important to note that the presence of lactose, fructose and pentose in the urine may give the same results. The presence of cataracts in infants without other systemic symptoms suggests the possibility of galactokinase deficiency. The presence of cataracts in older patients with the absence of gastrointestinal dysfunction or failure to thrive in galactosaemic patients helps to differentiate between galactokinase deficiency and transferase deficiency.

The diagnosis of transferase deficiency is suggested by abnormally high amounts of red cell galactose 1-phosphate and confirmed by direct assay of red cell transferase activity. The red cell UDP-glucose consumption test may help to differentiate homozygous patients with a complete absence of transferase in red cells from heterozygous patients who have intermediate levels. Normal red cell values are of 6 mmol UDP-glucose consumed per hour per millilitre of red blood cells. In galactokinase deficiency the diagnosis can be made by the presence of normal amounts of galactose-1-phosphate uridyltransferase and the absence of galactokinase in the red blood cells.

Galactose-1-phosphate uridyltransferase deficiency can be diagnosed prenatally, by assay of galactose-1-phosphate uridyltransferase activity in cultured amniotic fluid cells or chorionic villi, and by galactitol measurement in amniotic fluid supernatant. The perinatal diagnosis is undertaken rarely, because the transferase deficiency is seen as a treatable condition.

Methods for mass screening of newborns for galactosaemia are available, although galactosaemia is rare. The incidence in Norway is 1 in 96 000, in Sweden 1 in 81 000, in the USA 1 in 62 000, in Switzerland 1 in 58 000, in Germany 1 in 40 000, and the worldwide incidence is about 1 in 70 000. Newborn screening has not been introduced in Great Britain, the Netherlands or in some states of the USA. Most newborn screening programmes designed for the detection of anomalies of galactose metabolism use tests to measure either blood galactose or the activity of galactose-1-phosphate uridyltransferase. Beutler and Baluda developed a fluorescence test in which the activity of uridyltransferase in the dried blood spot is required for the reduction of NADP, yielding fluorescence under long-wave ultraviolet light; the intensity of the fluorescence corresponds to the activity of uridyltransferase. The main advantage of this test is that it can be completed in short time, although false positive results do occur. The disadvantage of this test is that patients with galactokinase deficiency are not detected by this method. Guthrie and Paigen described a more efficient test using the principle of metabolite inhibition; galactose inhibited the growth of an E. coli mutant strain lacking uridyltransferase. Later, Paigen used an E. coli mutant strain which lacks UDP-galactose 4'-epimerase activity. Using the Paigen test it is possible to detect galactokinase and uridyltransferase deficiencies. Epimerase deficiency can also be detected by the Paigen test if alkaline phosphatase is added to hydrolyse galactose phosphatase. In many screening laboratories the Beutler test is combined with the microbiological Paigen test.

Management

A galactose-free diet is the current treatment for galactosaemia. It is important to know that galactose is present not only in milk but in other sources of food. A strict galactose-free diet in galactosaemic patients with transferase deficiency is not harmful. The quality of the galactose-free diet and patient compliance are usually monitored by measuring free galactose in plasma and galactose 1-phosphate in erythrocytes.

Growth retardation, cognitive impairment, speech impediment, tremor, ataxia and ovarian failure are frequent complications in spite of a strict galactose-free diet. Elevated galactose phosphate levels may occur in erythrocytes of even well-treated galactosaemic patients. This elevation is attributed to endogenous production of the metabolite. A galactose-free diet is recommended from birth. It is recommended to restrict galactose in the diet of pregnant mothers diagnosed perinatally with transferase deficiency; a galactose-free diet should be started as soon as the diagnosis is made in the infant regardless of any preexisting manifestation of toxicity. The strict galactose-free diet will cause regression of symptoms and findings. It is important for the families to be aware of the high incidence of verbal dyspraxia even on a very strict diet. The speech intervention programme and language stimulation are recommended as early as the first year of life. Many patients with normal IQ values who were treated from birth have learning disabilities, speech and language deficit, and psychological problems. Neurological sequelae have been described also in patients on strict galactose-free diets. These sequelae include cerebellar ataxia, tremor, choreoathetosis and encephalopathy. Gonadal dysfunction in female galactosaemic patients is an almost universal finding, even with a strict galactose-free diet. There is no current therapy for ovarian dysfunction except palliative replacement of oestrogen and progesterone. This is suggested in galactosaemic females to develop secondary sexual characters and establish regular menses. There is no universal recommendation for the management of newborns screened positive nor for galactosaemic heterozygotic patients.

In patients with epimerase deficiency, UDP-glucose cannot be converted to UDP-galactose. Thus a complete absence of galactose from the diet and the lack of formation of UDP-galactose via transferase would have serious consequences. There would be an inability to form complex polysaccharides and an inability to provide an adequate galactose component for brain cerebrosides. The treatment of epimerase deficiency relies on providing a small amount of dietary galactose.

See also: **Fetal Origins of Disease**: Fetal Development and Later Disease. **Glucose**: Chemistry, Dietary Sources and Glycaemic Index; Metabolism and Maintenance of Blood Glucose Level; Glucose Tolerance. **Inborn Errors of Metabolism**: Classification and Biochemical Aspects. **Liver Disorders**: Nutritional Management. **Renal Function and Disorders**: Nutritional Management of Renal Disorders.

Further Reading

Acosta PB and Gross KC (1995) Hidden sources of galactose in the environment. *European Journal of Paediatrics* **154**(supplement 2):S87–92.

Berry GT (1995) The role of polyols in the pathophysiology of hypergalactosemia. *European Journal of Paediatrics* **154** (supplement 2):S53–64.

Beutler E and Baluda M (1996) Biochemical properties of the human red cell galactose-1-phosphate uridyl transferase (UDP Glucose: alpha-D Galactose-phosphate uridyl transferase) from normal and mutant subjects. *Laboratory and Clinical Medicine* **67**:947.

Gitzelmann R and Boshard NU (1995) Partial deficiency of galactose-1-phosphate uridyltransferase. *European Journal of Paediatrics* **154**(supplement 2):S40–44.

Jakobs C, Vleijer W, Allen Y and Holton JB (1995) Prenatal diagnosis of galactosemia. *European Journal of Paediatrics* **154** (supplement 2):S33–36.

Jakobs C, Schweitzer S and Dorland B (1995) Galactitol in galactosemia. *European Journal of Paediatrics* **154** (supplement 2):S50–52.

Kaufman FR, McBride-Chang C, Morris F, Wolf J and Nelson M (1995) Cognitive functioning, neurologic starters and the brain imaging in galactosemia. *European Journal of Paediatrics* **154**(supplement 2):2–5.

Liu Y, Vanhooke JL and Perry PA (1996) UDP-galactose 4-epimerase: NAD⁺ content and a charge-transfer band associated with the substrate-induced conformational transition. *Biochemistry* **35** (23):7615–7620.

Ng WG, Xu YK, Kauffman DR and Donnell GN (1989) Deficit of uridine diphosphate galactose in galactosemia. *Journal of Inherited and Metabolic Disease* **12**:257–266.

Sagal S (1995) Defective galactosylation in galactosemia; low cell UDP galactose an explanation? *European Journal of Paediatrics* **154**(supplement 2):S65–71.

Segal S (1989) Disorders of galactose metabolism. In: Scriver CR, Beaudet AL, Sly WS and Vale D (eds) *The Metabolic Basis of Inherited Disease*, 6th edn, pp 453–480. New York: McGraw-Hill.

Segal S (1995) Galactosemia unsolved. *European Journal of Paediatrics* **154** (supplement 2):S97–102.

Schweitzer S (1995) Newborn mass screening of galactosemia. *European Journal of Paediatrics* **154** (supplement 2):S37–39.

GALL BLADDER DISEASE

Nutritional Therapy

A B Williams and **Josef E Fischer**, University of Cincinnati, Ohio, USA

Copyright © 1998 Academic Press

Parenteral nutrition has allowed long-term survival of patients with intestinal compromise. The realization of the importance of enteral stimulation and its interaction among multiple systems of the host, especially hepatic protein synthesis and systemic immunity, has influenced the routine use of parenteral nutrition. Enteral nutrition is preferred, with parenteral nutrition if enteral nutrition is insufficient. Nonetheless, advances in parenteral formulations, catheter technology and a greater understanding of essential micronutrients have decreased the septic and metabolic complications associated with this mode of therapy and improved survival of those patients with crippling intestinal disorders. Complications remain, however, for those patients who require total parenteral nutrition (TPN), apart from the immediate consequences of catheter placement and the ateleologic administration of foodstuffs. Hepatobiliary dysfunction due to cholestasis remains an important sequela of long-term TPN. Though the prime pathophysiologic mechanism for an increase in gall bladder disorders is thought to be a lack of muscular contraction and bile stasis, the presence of comorbid conditions in these patients make identification of a single pathologic entity difficult. Often these patients have disordered enterohepatic biliary circulation from ileitis or ileal resection, clinical malnutrition before beginning TPN, global liver dysfunction, or other septic or metabolic derangements which predispose to lithogenesis or sludge formation. Lack of enteral stimulation with the addition of TPN only compounds the biliary dysfunction.

Normal Biliary Physiology

Bile is secreted by the hepatocyte into the biliary canaliculi and stored during periods of fasting in the gall bladder, when the sphincter of Oddi is contracted, permitting reflux of bile into the gall bladder. Bile is composed of water, electrolytes, cholesterol, phospholipids (primarily lecithin) and bile salts. Bile salts are derivatives of cholesterol, conjugated by the hepatocyte with hydrophilic amino acids, glycine or taurine. The epithelial cells of the bile ducts secrete a fluid rich in bicarbonate through an active transport mechanism influenced by secretin, vasoactive intestinal peptide and cholecystokinin (CCK). Cholesterol and phospholipids are insoluble in water but are solubilized into micelles by the bipolar moieties of the primary bile salts, cholate and chenodeoxycholate (**Fig. 2**). Upon stimulation by fat or amino acids in the duodenum, CCK is released, relaxing the sphincter of Oddi and allowing gall bladder contraction. Bile then flows from the gall bladder and admixes with ingested fats to aid in solubilization, enzymatic degradation and absorption. Ninety-five per cent of the bile acids are then reclaimed at the terminal ileum and returned to the hepatocyte via the portal vein and resecreted into the bile. Colonic bacteria can convert the primary bile salts to the secondary bile salts, lithocholate and deoxycholate, through hydrolytic enzymatic processes. Deoxycholate is reutilized as a bile salt; however, lithocholate is insoluble and is eliminated in the faeces. Approximately 6 g of bile acids per day are efficiently circulated: the 500 mg per day lost in the faeces are restored through *de novo* synthesis (**Fig. 1**).

Pathogenesis of Cholelithiasis

The pathogenesis of predominantly cholesterol gallstones is related to three important factors: supersaturation of bile with cholesterol, gall bladder stasis and the presence of nucleating factors.

The relationship between the three components of

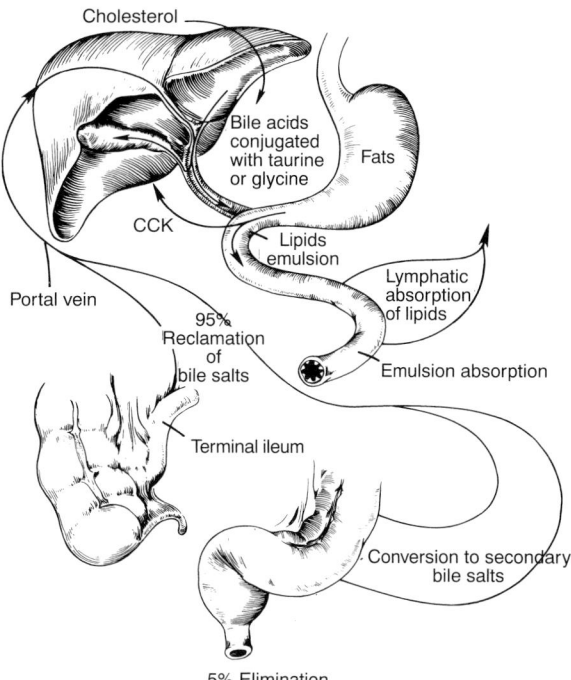

Figure 1 The enterohepatic circulation of bile salts. Cholesterol-derived bile salts are conjugated with taurine or glycine by the hepatocyte and secreted into the bile canaliculi. During fasting, bile is stored in the gall bladder and released under the regulation of cholecystokinin (CCK) upon the presence of fat or amino acids in the stomach and duodenum. The bile acids emulsify the ingested lipids and aid in absorption. At the terminal ileum, 95% of the bile salts are reclaimed and returned to the liver via the portal vein. The 5% not reclaimed is either excreted or reabsorbed after deconjugation by colonic bacteria. From Lamonte *et al.* (1981) with permission.

bile (cholesterol, lecithin and bile salts) was first described by Admirand and Small in 1968. Using a triangular diagram with the three compounds on each arm of the triangle, they described a curve determined from the relative concentrations of each substance which demarcated the limits of cholesterol's solubility (**Fig. 3**). The saturation point of cholesterol can be attained by increasing the concentration of cholesterol itself, or by decreasing the concentration of bile acids. Increased ingestion or increased hepatocellular synthesis increases cholesterol secretion. Increased synthesis and hypersecretion is influenced by certain hormones, e.g. oestrogens, and perhaps through genetic influences, as seen in certain Native American populations. Malabsorption of bile salts at the terminal ileum or resection of the ileum can decrease the circulating pool of bile salts and tip the balance of interactions toward cholesterol lithogenesis. Patients without a functional ileum are dependent upon *de novo* synthesis of bile salts to keep cholesterol in solution.

Supersaturation of cholesterol alone, however, is

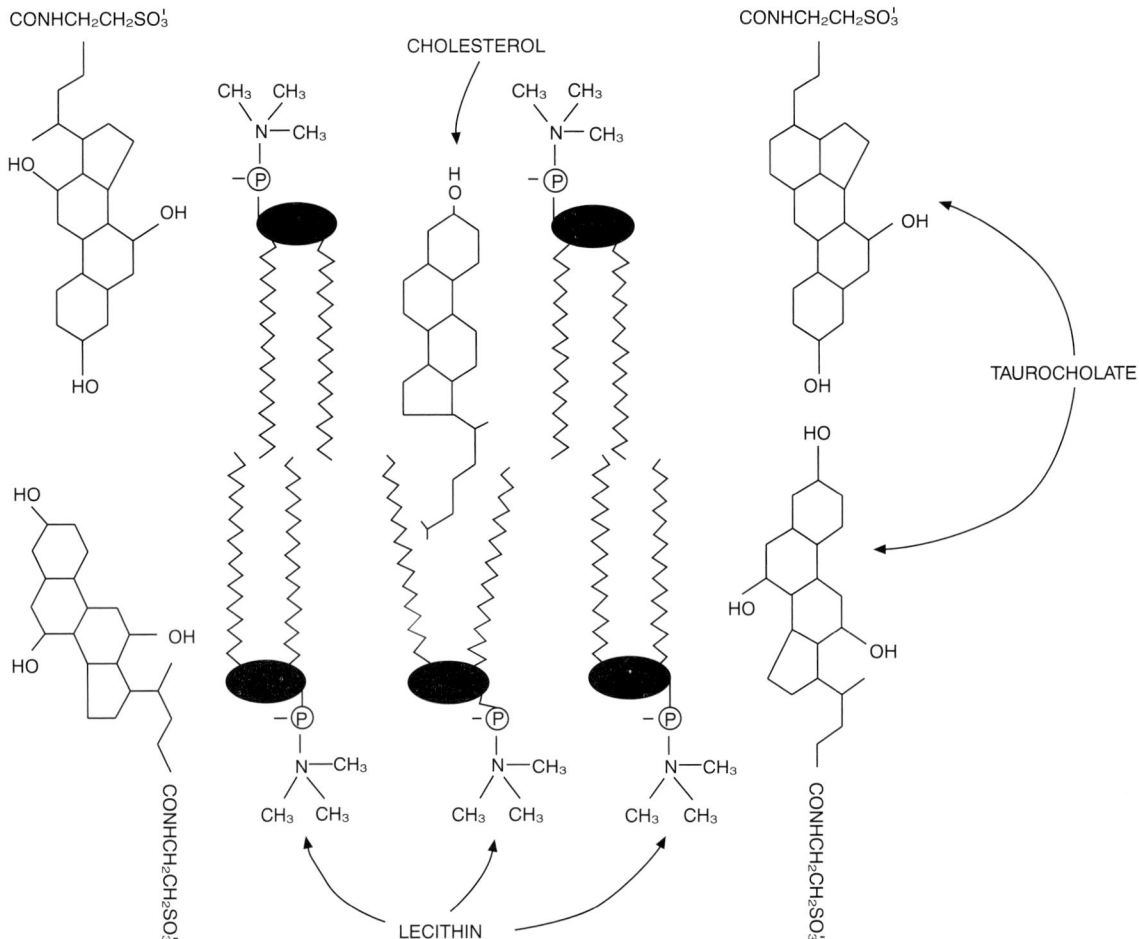

Figure 2 The formation of micelles. The bipolar moieties of the bile salt taurocholate and lecithin emulsify and keep cholesterol in solution. From Lamonte *et al.* (1981).

not enough to induce lithogenesis. Patients with supersaturated bile do not always develop gallstones. A nucleating factor is needed to initiate stone formation. Bacteria, calcium salts, cellular debris, mucus and pigmented salts have all been implicated as nidi for stone formation. Spontaneous nucleation requires a marked degree of supersaturation to develop clinically significant stones, owing to the continuous counterbalancing processes of aggregation and disaggregation. However, a heterogeneous nucleating factor can sequester the cholesterol crystals and impede the disaggregating influence of the bile salts.

Finally, stasis of the gall bladder allows reabsorption of water and precipitation of the supersaturated solution. With intermittent, complete gall bladder emptying, even supersaturated bile cannot coalesce into stones. Prolonged fasting, diabetes, truncal vagotomy and pregnancy all decrease gall bladder emptying and predispose to cholelithiasis.

In contrast to predominantly cholesterol stones, pigmented gallstones are of two varieties. Black pig-

mented stones are found in patients with haemolysis or cirrhosis, and are composed of polymers of bilirubin and calcium bilirubinate. Earthy calcium bilirubinate stones are found in patients whose bile ducts are probably colonized with pathogenic organisms; these stones are found predominantly within the bile ducts and are seen in patients with recurrent cholangitis, biliary enteric anastomoses, biliary strictures or parasitic infestation. The mechanism of formation of these stones is not entirely certain; however, it is thought that conjugated bilirubin is deconjugated by bacterial glucuronidases and may precipitate as calcium bilirubinate stones. The presence of bacteria and bacterial glycocalix found in 90% of these stones supports this theory. In the absence of bacteria, a supersaturation of bile with unconjugated bilirubin (as seen in haemolytic anaemias or multiple transfusions) may lead to formation of black pigmented stones in much the same way as cholesterol stones are formed. There is some evidence that suggests biliary sludge seen in patients with gall bladder dysmotility is composed of calcium bilirubinate and

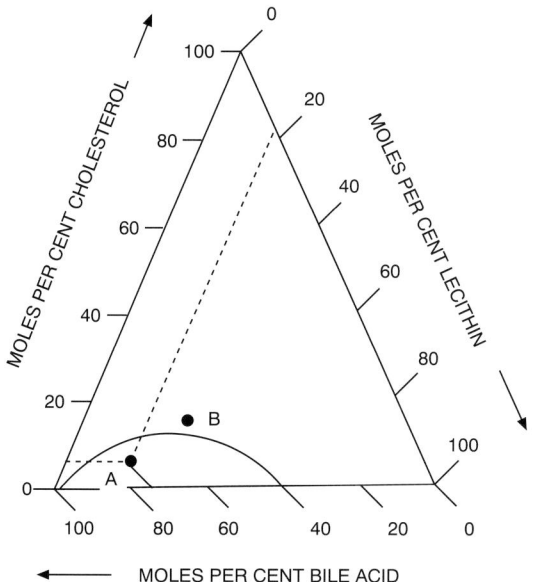

Figure 3 Amerind diagram. The curved solid line describes the limit of solubility of various concentrations of the components of bile. Bile with the concentrations of cholesterol, lecithin and bile acid marked at point A would not be supersaturated with cholesterol. However, the composition of bile seen at point B would be supersaturated with cholesterol and would predispose to lithogenesis. From Amerind and Small (1968).

not predominantly cholesterol; nonetheless the pathogenesis of both may be tied to bile salt-induced solubility, stasis and the presence of nucleating material.

Route of nutrition and its effects on the gall bladder and extrahepatic biliary tree

Total parenteral nutrition has been implicated in the formation of gallstones, biliary sludge, acalculous cholecystitis, hepatic steatosis and hepatic cholestasis. It is by no means certain that all forms of hepatic damage are the same. Gallstones are probably a manifestation of stasis arising from other causes (see below). Hepatic steatosis seems to be related to excess carbohydrate, lack of a clearance cycle and perhaps the hormonal milieu of the portal system. Studies in the rat have shown that infusion of solutions containing 20% dextrose is associated with an elevated portal insulin/glucagon molar ratio as well as hepatic steatosis. Addition of glucagon to TPN formulations both prevents and reverses the TPN-associated hepatic steatosis. However, hepatic steatosis in adults and the cholestatic syndrome in infants and children may not be the same disease. The former rarely goes on to cirrhosis, while the cholestatic syndrome in children not uncommonly leads to cirrhosis and death from liver failure.

In one convincing study of the effects of TPN on the biliary tree, there was a 6% incidence of biliary sludge after 3 weeks of TPN, 50% at 4–6 weeks, and 100% after 6 weeks. The biliary sludge resolved 4–6 weeks after discontinuation of the TPN and resumption of enteral feeding. Furthermore gallstones develop in 30–40% of adult patients after 24 months of TPN. One trial comparing enteral with parenteral nutrition in patients with inflammatory bowel disease found 61% of patients on TPN had elevated levels of hepatic and biliary tract enzymes, compared with 6% on enteral nutrition. Infants receiving TPN for short bowel syndrome commonly have elevated bilirubin levels within 2 weeks of starting TPN, hepatic enzymes elevated by 4–6 weeks and liver biopsies consistent with hepatic cholestasis at the same time. Upon discontinuation of the TPN, enzyme and bilirubin concentrations normalize in 4–6 weeks.

What, then, is the mechanism of TPN-induced changes in the hepatobiliary system? Are the intrahepatic and extrahepatic processes aetiologically similar? Several theories have been proposed; these fall into two schools of thought. The apparent sludging of bile throughout the biliary tree seen with TPN has been ascribed either to a manifestation or intrinsic toxicity of the TPN itself, or to the absence of enterocyte-induced stimulation of bile flow and its effects on bile composition. Evidence for both theories is equivocal, and both are likely to play a role in the pathogenesis of hepatobiliary dysfunction. Probably the intrahepatic and extrahepatic biliary processes represent slightly different manifestations of the same pathologic process. (As mentioned above, the process of steatosis may be aetiologically different.) Because the gall bladder is able to effectively concentrate bile, stone formation predominates in the extrahepatic system, while cholestasis and hepatocellular damage predominate in the intrahepatic biliary system owing to the continuous interaction of toxic bile salts and the canalicular cell membranes.

The addition of lipids to TPN regimens in the early 1970s, with the concomitant reduction in the percentage of energy from carbohydrate, led to a reduction in hepatic steatosis. This led investigators to examine the effects of other components of parenteral nutrition and their possible role in hepatobiliary complications.

Both animal and clinical studies have implicated amino acids in biliary stasis. Intrahepatic cholestasis in the neonate seems to be related to the volume of amino acids infused. Infants develop cholestasis faster when larger concentrations of amino acids are infused and only after prolonged administration. Additionally, studies performed whereby lipids and carbohydrate were administered by the intravenous route and proteins and amino acids by the naso-gastric route showed a dramatic decrease in cholestasis, implicating the parenterally administered amino acid as toxic to the canalicular membrane. Specifically, methionine in large concentrations, is a known hepatotoxin. Intravenous alanine, arginine and tryptophan have all been implicated in animal studies to reduce bile flow. It is thought that perhaps the enterocyte serves a gatekeeper's role in preventing the influx of large concentrations of toxic amino acids. It is difficult to distinguish, however, whether the improvement in cholestasis seen in these comparative studies is a function of parenterally supplied amino acid toxicity or the beneficial effects of enteral stimulation.

Conversely, other studies have shown a beneficial effect of large volume amino acid administration. Rapid infusion of amino acids (2.1 g min^{-1}) resulted in improved gall bladder contractility by inducing the release of CCK, whereas a more typical rate of amino acid infusion did not result in CCK release and did not enhance gall bladder contractility. Whether this translates into improved hepatobiliary outcomes is only conjectural at this point.

Further evidence exists to implicate a lack of certain amino acids in parenteral formulations as the cause of cholestasis. The addition of serine, a methyl donor, in one study reversed the cholestatic effects of TPN. Taurine, a major conjugate of bile acids, is not an essential amino acid in adults; however, a relative deficiency in neonates has been implicated as a cause for cholestasis. Taurine has been shown to promote bile flow, but clinical improvement with the addition of taurine to TPN has not been conclusively proved. Animal studies have not shown any correlation between serum taurine levels and changes in bile composition during TPN, suggesting that decreased serum taurine levels would not predispose to cholelithiasis.

Glutamine may protect against TPN-related hepatobiliary dysfunction through enhancing gut mucosal immunity, or more probably by changing the insulin/glucagon ratio in the portal blood. Glutamine is the primary energy source for enterocytes and can enhance mucosal immunologic function in rats. However, the evidence in other species is less compelling. Nonetheless, studies have noted a similarity between TPN-induced hepatocellular damage and sepsis-related hepatic parenchymal injury, implying that increased translocation and portal endotoxaemia are the culprits for TPN-associated hepatotoxicity. By improving mucosal immunity and decreasing mucosal atrophy, glutamine may reduce portal endotoxaemia and attenuate hepatobiliary complications.

Because bacteria serve as a nidus for stone formation and employ glucuronidases to deconjugate bilirubin (which is the major component of pigmented stones and the sludge of acalculous cholecystitis), they seem essential to the pathophysiology of stone or sludge formation. On the other hand, a small amount of translocation may be beneficial to the host as an immunologic surveillance mechanism. Paradoxically, by furnishing glutamine in TPN solutions, investigators have noted an increase in bacterial translocation. Increased hepatobiliary complications during TPN may be the price paid for an enhanced enterohepatic immune system.

Advances in lipid emulsion therapy have shed light on the effects of TPN on bile composition and flow. Studies in the acholecystic rat have shown that TPN formulations with 1% lipid vessel suspension (Intralipid) decrease bile flow, increase biliary cholesterol concentration and increase the lithogenic index independent of the route of administration (enteral or parenteral). Other reports in both rats and prairie dogs (whose hepatobiliary system is similar to humans) have also found a decrease in bile flow but no changes in biliary composition or lithogenicity. A definitive clinical answer remains to be obtained concerning the intrinsic role of lipids on biliary stone formation; however, a study of preoperative patients on TPN for 48 h comparing the effects of medium-chain and long-chain triacylglycerols on bile composition and lithogenicity found that the medium-chain group had a significantly larger biliary cholesterol concentration, a higher biliary total lipid concentration and a faster nucleation time than the long-chain group, despite lower serum levels of cholesterol ester, triacylglycerol and phospholipids in the medium-chain group. It is thought that perhaps the difference is due to the more rapid hydrolysis of the medium-chain triacylglycerols and oxidation of free fatty acids to acetyl-CoA in the mitochondria which upregulate *de novo* cholesterol and phospholipid synthesis and secretion by the hepatocyte. While the impact of medium-chain triacylglycerol on biliary complications is unclear, this work may point to a role for certain intravenous lipids in the lithogenesis of predominantly cholesterol stones.

Noting the high incidence of pigmented stones and sludge in patients on TPN has led others to investigate the role of TPN on biliary bilirubin metabolism. Investigators noted a 4-fold increase in conjugated bilirubin and a 7-fold increase in unconjugated bilirubin in the bile of animals on TPN compared with those on enteral feedings. Biliary calcium levels were also significantly higher in the TPN group. Interestingly, these animals had no biochemical evidence of haemolysis. Biliary stasis and increased bilirubin deconjugation seem the most likely explanation for the increase in bilirubin insolubility.

In summary, in both human and animal studies, TPN slows the flow of bile but has equivocal effects on cholesterol solubility. There may be some intrinsic effects of TPN on the liver's ability to secrete bilirubin and calcium, the two major components of pigmented stones and sludge, but bile stasis seems to be the prime pathophysiologic event in initiating stone and sludge formation.

Another compound implicated in TPN-induced hepatic cholestasis and/or cholelithiasis is phytosterol. Found in lipid emulsions derived from vegetable sources (parenteral lipid is derived primarily from soya bean oil), phytosterol is poorly metabolized to bile salts and may be less soluble than cholesterol in solution. It is thought that enterocytes poorly absorb phytosterol, accounting for the low serum levels found in enterally fed patients. The higher levels found in patients on TPN may predispose to sludging and stone formation, especially in those patients who have an altered enterohepatic circulation of bile salts and are dependent upon *de novo* synthesis to keep cholesterol in solution. Though the evidence implicating phytosterol is plausible, it is somewhat circumstantial and awaits further investigation.

Effects of Stagnation

Though parenterally administered nutrition has some intrinsic effects on bile composition and flow, its primary effect on cholelithiasis stems from the lack of enterocyte-mediated gall bladder contraction and the resultant extrahepatic biliary stasis. The want of biliary stimulation by gut hormones, notably cholecystokinin, is the *sine qua non* of cholelithiasis. Prevention of this stasis by sphincterotomy, exogenous CCK administration, or periodic small-volume enteral feedings, all ameliorate the hepatobiliary complications associated with TPN. This biliary stasis is the common denominator for patients with an increased risk of cholelithiasis during pregnancy, after truncal vagotomy, after major trauma or surgery, and patients on prolonged parenteral nutrition. The frequent comorbid conditions (malnutrition, sepsis, hepatic failure) and dysfunctional enterohepatic circulation associated with the latter group often exacerbate the lithogenic effects of biliary stasis.

Further evidence suggests the absence of gut stimulation in patients receiving total parenteral nutrition can lead to bacterial overgrowth in the intestine with an increase in the production of lithocholate. Increased levels of lithocholate have been associated with TPN-related cholestasis, and lithocholate is a known hepatotoxin. Patients on TPN treated with oral metronidazole or gentamicin have shown some improvement in the incidence of hepatobiliary disorders. However, animal studies with oral antibiotics have shown equivocal effects.

Diagnosis

The diagnosis of gall bladder disorders relies firstly on a thorough history and physical examination. The history should specifically elicit frequency of right upper quadrant pain, any postprandial symptoms, fever, jaundice, acholic stools, and any medications that might affect gall bladder emptying time (e.g. opiates, oestrogen replacement therapy, oral contraceptives). On examination, a distended gall bladder is sometimes palpable in asthenic individuals and may elicit a Murphy's sign if significant inflammation is present.

Laboratory examination may reveal an elevation in concentrations of the enzymes found in the cells lining the biliary tract. Alkaline phosphatase and γ-glutamyltransferase levels may be elevated; however, alkaline phosphatase may be nonspecifically elevated in patients with bony abnormalities. Leucine aminopeptidase or 5'-nucleotidase, both specific for the biliary tract, can distinguish biliary abnormalities in patients with suspected bone pathology. Other liver enzymes, as well as bilirubin, may be elevated depending on the degree of cholestasis, presence of common bile duct obstruction, and/or consequent liver damage. Though nonspecific for gall bladder pathology, the white blood cell count may also be elevated depending on the degree of inflammation.

Plain radiographs are generally not useful in the diagnosis of gall bladder disorders, as only 10–15% of stones are radioopaque. Real-time grey-scale ultrasonography is purportedly 98% sensitive and specific for identifying gallstones. Additionally, ultrasound can identify gall bladder wall thickening, pericholecystic fluid, sludge or ductal enlargement suggesting pathology of the biliary system. Cholescintigraphy, using [^{99m}Tc] iminodiacetic acid, can identify acute cholecystitis with a reported 100% sensitivity and 95% specificity. With a normal biliary system, this nuclear medicine scan outlines the liver and biliary system and reveals flow into the small intestine. Failure of visualization of the gall bladder or failure of flow of the nuclide into the intestine suggests an obstruction presumably due to stones. However, investigators have noted an increased false positivity with the hepatobiliary scans for acute cholecystitis when examining patients on TPN. The administration of morphine during the performance of the test may increase the diagnostic specificity of this test by allowing prolonged biliary exposure of the nuclide. Oral cholestography has generally been replaced by radionuclide scanning in the diagnosis of acute biliary disease. The oral agents are sometimes poorly absorbed in patients with ileus, emesis or diarrhoea, and poorly excreted in patients whose bilirubin concentration is greater than 50 μmol l^{-1} (3 mg dl^{-1}).

Management

The mainstay of therapy for patients with acute or chronic, calculous or acalculous cholecystitis is cholecystectomy. The advent of laparoscopic cholecystectomy has allowed a safe, minimally invasive alternative to conventional coeliotomy. However, most patients dependent upon TPN have had multiple abdominal operations with resultant dense adhesions, making even traditional, open cholecystectomy technically challenging. Investigators have therefore sought alternatives ways to prevent the formation of these troublemaking stones.

One measure proposed for patients with short bowel syndrome who are likely to require long-term TPN is removal of the gall bladder during the initial operation or during subsequent explorations before the onset of any biliary disease. In one retrospective series, 31% of patients on TPN with less than 180 cm of remaining bowel developed biliary complications requiring operation with an associated mortality rate of 18%. The authors of this study advocated prophylactic cholecystectomy when the gall bladder can be easily approached, when the anatomy is straightforward, and the patient is haemodynamically stable and can tolerate the added procedure. Cholecystectomy not only removes the potentially static reservoir of bile, but also promotes rapid turnover of bile acids. Because the bile acids can no longer can be sequestered in the gall bladder, there is an improvement in the physical characteristics favouring biliary solubility. Elective prophylactic cholecystectomy as a separate procedure should not be undertaken, however.

Cholecystostomy is another form of treatment for patients too unstable to undergo formal cholecystectomy under local anesthesia, the gall bladder can be drained through a biliary-cutaneous fistula and the pericholecystic inflammation can be relieved. Unless the stone impacted in the cystic duct is removed, however, cholecystostomy does not resolve the inciting inflammatory object, and therefore the procedure should be a bridge to, not a replacement for, formal cholecystectomy when feasible. Additionally, patients on TPN with acalculous cholecystitis often have delays in diagnosis secondary to concomitant liver enzyme elevations, frequent catheter-related septic episodes, and multiple operations requiring intensive care unit stays with an inability to report symptoms. This delay in diagnosis results in an increased frequency of ischaemic, necrotic and gangrenous complications of the gall bladder for which treatment with cholecystostomy would not suffice and would probably lead to further septic complications. Nonetheless, a very high success rate for percutaneous cholecystostomy in the critically ill patient has been reported, with a comparable morbidity and mortality to traditional open cholecystostomy. Careful judgment must be employed when deciding which procedure to undertake.

Because cholecystectomy is often fraught with difficulty in these patients, other investigators have sought medical alternatives to reduce or avoid gall bladder disorders. The most rational and cost-effective mode of therapy is enteral stimulation. Indeed, if tolerated, some form of enteral feeding should be an adjunct to any parenteral alimentation therapy. As little as 20–25% of total energy delivered enterally is beneficial. By stimulation of the stomach and duodenum with amino acids or lipid, cholecystokinin is released, relaxing the sphincter of Oddi and stimulating muscular wall contraction. However, not all patients tolerate enteral feedings, owing to obstruction, large-output fistulas or malabsorption. For these patients, exogenous CCK has been shown to be effective in preventing sludging, by stimulating gall bladder contraction and preventing biliary stasis. In fact, some reports have indicated that CCK can relieve the intrahepatic cholestasis associated with TPN, provided the associated liver damage is not too severe. Some patients did notice side effects with this therapy, though not particularly disabling. Abdominal cramping and increased ostomy outputs were the most commonly reported side effects. A further issue, cost, may make this mode of therapy impractical.

To recruit endogenous CCK, rapid administration of amino acids has been proposed and has been shown to affect gall bladder emptying time. Pulsed intravenous amino acid administration, through its effects on release of CCK, can increase gall bladder ejection fractions and decrease residual gall bladder volumes. Though effective, this therapy may be limited by the large osmotic load needed to induce a response and has not been shown in a clinical trial to improve outcome.

Other helpful measures include avoidance of narcotic analgesics and cholinergic antagonists, which contribute to biliary stasis through contraction of the sphincter of Oddi. Ursodeoxycholic acid has been widely used for gallstone dissolution and for patients with cholestasis due to intrinsic liver disease. It is thought to be a choleretic agent, which may explain its benefit in patients with disordered bile secretion. It may also augment the bile acid pool in patients dependent upon *de novo* synthesis. Its efficacy in TPN-related cholestasis is currently being evaluated, and preliminary investigations have shown efficacy in both children and adults in reducing the cholestatic picture associated with home TPN.

Conclusions

Nutritional therapy for patients with gall bladder disorders should strive to decrease the lithogenicity of bile. For patients who can tolerate nutrition via the enteral route, its beneficial effects on the hepatobiliary system cannot be overemphasized. For patients who are reliant upon intravenous delivery of foodstuffs, a careful balance of amino acids, carbohydrates and lipids along with adequate essential micronutrients are necessary to avoid global malnutrition and to ensure proper hepatobiliary function. A high index of suspicion for biliary complications must be maintained with these patients, and prompt recognition and treatment should follow the onset of symptoms. Methods of avoidance of biliary disease for patients on TPN range from intermittent gall bladder stimulation to prophylactic cholecystectomy. Sound clinical judgment is needed to weigh the benefits of life-propagating parenteral nutrition and its potentially life-threatening biliary complications.

See also: **Gastrointestinal Tract**: Structure and Function of the Small Intestine. **Liver Disorders**: Nutritional Management. **Nutritional Support**: Enteral Feeding; Parenteral Nutrition.

Further Reading

Amerind WH and Small DM (1968) Physical-chemical basis of cholesterol formation in man. *Journal of Clinical Investigation* 47:1043–1052.

Fischer JE (1996) *Nutrition and Metabolism in the Surgical Patient*. New York: Little, Brown.

Fisher RL (1989) Hepatobiliary abnormalities associated with total parenteral nutrition. *Gastroenterology Clinics of North America* 18(3):645–663.

Holzbach RT (1983) Gallbladder stasis: consequence of long term parenteral hyperalimentation and risk factor for cholelithiasis. *Gastroenterology* 84(5):1055–1058.

Lamonte WW, Matolo NM, Birkett DH and Williams LF (1981) Pathogenesis of cholesterol gallstones. *Surgical Clinics of North America* 61(4):765–774.

Roslyn JJ, Pitt HA, Mann LL, Ament ME and DenBesten L (1983) Gallbladder disease in patients on long-term parenteral nutrition. *Gastroenterology* 84:148–154.

Zoli G, Ballinger A, Healy J, O'Donnell LJD, Clark M and Farthing MJG (1993) Promotion of gallbladder emptying by intravenous aminoacids. *Lancet* 341:1240–1241.

GASTROINTESTINAL TRACT

Contents

Structure and Function of the Stomach

J P Pearson, University of Newcastle, Newcastle upon Tyne, UK

D Hutton, Bioprocessing Ltd, Consett, UK

Copyright © 1998 Academic Press

The stomach is an organ of the upper digestive tract. Its major function is to store and liquefy food to allow its further digestion and absorption by the small intestine. Liquefaction is achieved by the action of acid, pepsin and strong rhythmic muscle contractions. The stomach is well suited to carry out its digestive functions: it is expandable to accommodate a meal, muscular to allow strong contractions to mix and break up the food, and the acid and pepsin needed for digestion are released on demand from specific gland structures.

Structure

The stomach is an expandable chamber between the oesophagus and the duodenum. Its volume is only about 50 cm³ when empty, yet it can expand up to 1000 cm³ when full with food. The stomach can be divided anatomically into four regions (**Fig. 1**). The oesophageal squamous epithelium ends at the gastro-oesophageal opening, where the columnar epithelium of the stomach begins. The first region of the stomach is the *fundus*, which lies above the opening of the oesophagus. The next region is the *body*, or *corpus*, which together with the fundus forms a food storage reservoir. This allows control of the rate of food delivery to the small intestine, so as to synchronize it with maximal digestion and absorption. The distal part of the stomach, the *antrum*, has a thicker muscle layer and its major function is to generate vigorous mixing of food with the gastric secretions to produce a slurry known as chyme. The stomach ends in the *pylorus*, a muscular sphincter which controls the release of chyme into the duodenum.

Histology of the stomach

The wall of the stomach consists of four types of tissue: connective, smooth muscle, neural and epithelial (**Table 1**). Within these layers is a vascular system with arterioles supplying the external muscle layers and gastric arteries supplying a plexus of arterioles in the gastric submucosa, which in turn provide nutrients for the mucosal secretory cells. The cells producing the gastric secretions are located in the mucosa of the stomach arranged in structures called gastric pits (**Fig. 2**). Pits are made up of several gastric glands and are distributed throughout the mucosa. Glands in the body and fundus of the stomach contain chief (peptic) cells deep within them which synthesize, store and secrete the inactive enzyme precursor, pepsinogen. Parietal (oxyntic) cells are found more widely distributed within the gland extending towards the top. These cells secrete hydrochloric acid (HCl) and intrinsic factor into the gland lumen. Also present near the base of the glands

Table 1　Layers of the stomach wall

Outside	Serosa	Connective tissue
	Muscularis arterioles distributed throughout this layer	Longitudinal muscle Myenteric autonomic nerve plexus Circular muscle Submucosal autonomic nerve plexus
	Submucosa	Plexus of arterioles
	Mucosa	Muscularis mucosa – smooth muscle Gastric glands – endocrine cells, chief (peptic) cells, parietal cells and mucus neck cells Lamina propria – connective tissue and lymph nodes
Inside (lumen)		Epithelium – surface mucus cells

in this region of the stomach are endocrine ECL (enterochromaffin-like) cells, which secrete histamine. The antral glands lack parietal cells so no acid is secreted from this region; however they do contain peptic cells, and therefore secrete pepsinogen. In addition they contain endocrine G cells. These secrete the polypeptide hormone gastrin, which together with histamine is involved in the control of acid secretion. G cells also contain intrinsic factor.

Throughout the gastric mucosa the mucus neck cells are continually dividing and either migrating out of the pits to replace shed surface epithelial cells or down into the pits where they can differentiate into acid or pepsin secreting cells. In this way the whole mucosa is replaced every 72 h. The major secretion of the surface epithelial cells is mucus. Mucus forms a continuous surface layer and is the first line of defence against gastric juice; however, it does not extend up into the oesophagus. The gastric mucus layer stops at the gastro-oesophageal junction, so the oesophagus must have a different protection mechanism (**Fig. 3**). In the human stomach the thickness of this mucus layer varies from 50 to 450 μm (median thickness of 180 μm). Without this layer gastric juice acid and pepsin would destroy the mucosa. Bicarbonate secreted into this layer by the epithelial cells neutralizes the acid diffusing from the lumen in an unstirred aqueous environment.

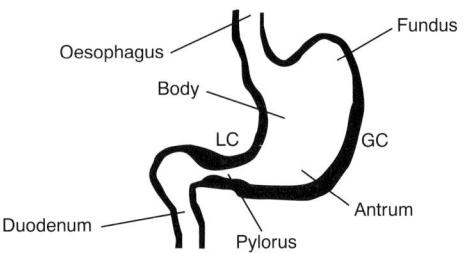

Figure 1　Stomach anatomy. The extent of the smooth muscle is shown by the darkened areas. LC, lesser curvature; GC, greater curvature.

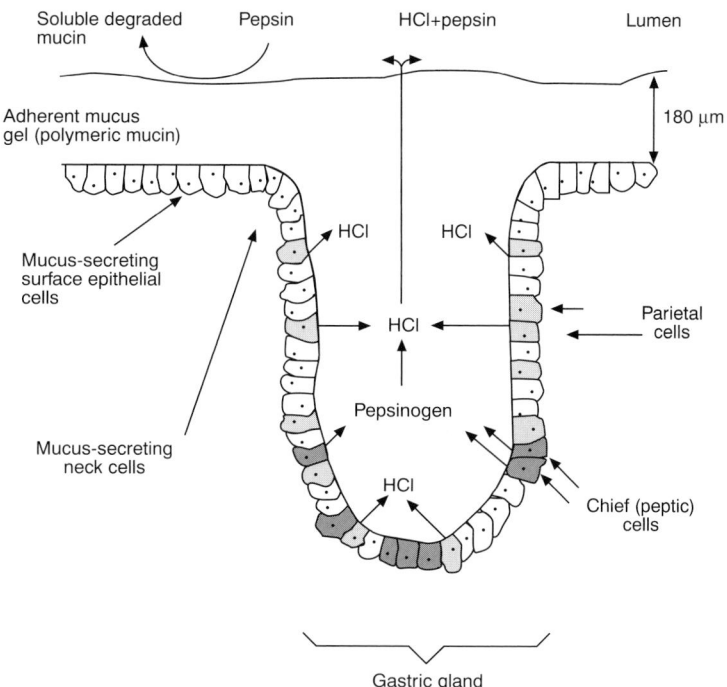

Figure 2 Structure of the human gastric mucosa.

Consequently a pH close to 7 is maintained at the epithelial cell surface. The thickness of the layer is maintained by secretion of new mucus balancing that lost by pepsin digestion and mechanical shear. Along with mucus the epithelial cells also secrete trefoil peptides, which have growth factor-like activities (see below).

Composition of Gastric Juice and Regulation of Production

Table 2 lists the components of gastric juice. The main enzymes involved are the lipases and pepsins; acid secretion also play an important role in gastic digestion with mucus having a protective role. Intrinsic factor and haptocorrins are discussed in a later section.

Lipases

Lipases are a minor but significant enzyme secretion. Partial digestion of fat occurs in the adult stomach and preliminary digestion of triacylglycerols aids the action of pancreatic lipases. These enzymes are particularly important in infants with respect to breakdown of milk fat, 30–60% of which is lipolysed in the gastric lumen. Gastric lipases are glycoproteins with molecular weights of about 45 000. Lipase secretion is highest in the body and fundus of the stomach and very low in the antrum. Secretory granules containing lipases are located in peptic cells, particularly in the fundic mucosa. Gastric lipases

have a broad pH optimum (2.5–7.0) and are stable down to pH 1.5. They are therefore able to survive in the stomach's acidic environment and will be active during feeding when the gastric pH rises to around 5.0. Secretion of gastric lipase is coupled with pepsin secretion by peptic cells in response to pentagastrin (a functional analogue of gastrin).

Lipase secretion from isolated human gastric glands is stimulated by cholecystokinin (CCK) and carbachol, but histamine has no effect. In the dog secretin and prostaglandin E_2 stimulate lipase secretion. There is also a positive feedback loop in gastric lipase secretion: release of long-chain fatty acids from triacylglycerols by lipases stimulates CCK secretion, which in turn stimulates the secretion of pancreatic and gastric lipases.

Pepsins

Pepsins are the major enzyme secretions of the stomach, digesting protein in the diet to yield peptide fragments. Pepsins are members of the aspartate proteinase family with two asparate residues at the active site. They are broad-specificity endopeptidases with a preference for peptide bonds between hydrophobic amino acids. Human gastric juice contains two groups of pepsins, namely pepsin A, which contains six isoenzymes, and pepsin C, which contains two isoenzymes (**Table 3**). Once secreted into the lumen, the acidic conditions convert pepsinogens to pepsin. Unlike the activation of other proteinases,

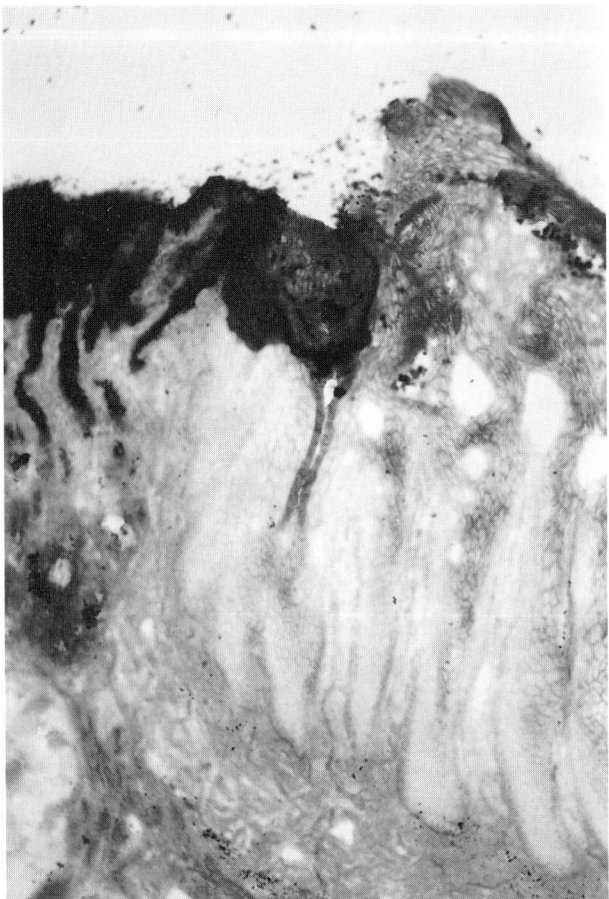

Figure 3 The mucus gel at the gastro-oesophageal junction. This section of pig gastric/oesophageal mucosa is stained with alcian blue/periodic acid–Schiff. To the left of the picture is the gastric mucosa showing a darkly staining mucus layer; to the right is the oesophageal mucosa showing no stained mucus layer. The human gastro-oesophageal junction shows an identical picture. Magnification 100×. (This slide was prepared by Dr Jane Dixon.)

Table 2 Composition of gastric juice

Mucus (salivary and gastric)
Lipases (EC 3.1.1.3)
Pepsins 1–6 (EC 3.4.23.1)
Urea
[a]Intrinsic factor and haptocorrin
H_2O
$Na^+, Mg^{2+}, H^+, K^+, Cl^-, HPO_4^{2-}$
[b]HCO_3^-
Salivary amylase

[a]Dealt with in their own section of text.
[b]Only present secreted into the mucus layer. Once out in the lumen HCO_3^- will react with H^+ to form H_2CO_3, which can decompose to $H_2O + CO_2$.

Table 3 Pepsins of human gastric juice

Pepsin group	Chromosome location	Individual pepsins
A	11q13	1, 2, 3a, 3b, 3c, 4.
C (gastricsin)	6	5 and 6

These isoenzymes can be separated by agar gel electrophoresis at pH 5.0 or anion exchange HPLC.

e.g. trypsinogen to trypsin via a proteolytic cleavage by another enzyme (enterokinase), pepsinogen activation is autocatalytic. The process is understood in detail for porcine pepsinogen. Secreted pepsinogen has an N-terminal peptide of 44 amino acids blocking the active site. On exposure to pH values below 5 carboxyl groups become protonated, abolishing charge–charge interactions. This allows part of the N-terminal protein into the active site where it is cleaved, releasing a 16 amino acid peptide. The enzyme is now partially activated; full activation occurs with cleavage of a further 28 amino acids from the N-terminal by either another partially activated pepsin or a fully activated enzyme.

The majority of proteinase activity in human gastric juice is pepsin 3 (70.3 ± 2.6%), although variable amounts of pepsin 5 are also present (16.9 ± 2.0%). The only other isoenzyme found in significant amounts is pepsin 1. This differs from other pepsins in that it is an ionic complex of a 14 500 molecular weight protein and proteoglycan. Also, unlike the other pepsins, pepsin 1 is secreted only in the fundic and not the pyloric glands, and is only present in significant amounts in stimulated juice. Pepsin 1 has the largest molecular weight (44 500), while the others have molecular weights around 35 000. The pH optimum against protein substrates for all pepsins is in the acidic range 1.9–3.6. Pepsin 1 secretion is elevated in peptic ulcer disease (PUD) and is therefore the ulcer-associated pepsin. Also associated with peptic ulcer disease is the bacteria *Helicobacter pylori* (HP), which colonizes the stomach at the epithelial surface under the mucus layer. HP is believed to protect itself from the acid environment of the stomach by the action of a membrane-bound urease, which generates ammonia from the urea present in gastric juice. Interestingly, approximately 50% of all people in the UK over 50 years old are HP positive, yet only a small proportion of these will develop peptic ulcer disease. The increased secretion of pepsin 1 in PUD may be explained by HP infection.

Pepsinogen secretion   The initial stimulus for pepsinogen secretion is feeding; there is a basal level of secretion which is 20% of the stimulated secretion. Maximal secretion produces gastric juice with a pepsin concentration approaching 1 mg ml^{-1}. There is a biphasic response with initial release of stored pepsinogen in a rapid phase (20–40 min) followed by a less rapid steady state of secretion. Pepsinogen secretion is stimulated by CCK, forskolin and by insulin-induced hypoglycaemia mediated by the vagus nerve. Gastrin stimulates pepsinogen secretion but it is much less effective than CCK. Secretion is also stimulated by the peptide hormones secretin and VIP (vasoactive intestinal peptide), by adrenaline acting through β_2-adrenergic receptors, and by prostaglandins; all these agents alter intracellular cAMP levels. Pepsinogen secretion is stimulated by cholinergic agents acting on muscarinic M3 subtype receptors; these agents also stimulate acid secretion. Acetylcholine and the CCK/gastrin family act through altering intracellular Ca^{2+} and inositol triphosphate (IP_3) levels. Pepsinogen is secreted by compound exocytosis with granules fusing together and with the plasma membrane. The enzyme is condensed within the vesicle in association with a divalent cation, e.g. Ca^{2+}. Initial fusing with the plasma membrane produces a small pore releasing the Ca^{2+}, causing the vesicle contents to swell. This produces a larger pore through which the pepsinogen is released.

Acid

Acid is secreted by the gastric gland parietal cells via the action of the gastric H^+, K^+ ATPase, a transmembrane pump. In non-stimulated parietal cells the pump is present in cytoplasmic vesicles. On stimulation the pumps are transported to the apical membrane along the actin cytoskeleton. For activity the pump requires to be associated with K^+ and Cl^- conductive pathways. Because there is a huge H^+ concentration gradient across the parietal cells (the lumen has 2–4×10^6 greater H^+ concentration than the blood), the cells require a great deal of energy and 34% of the cell volume is mitochondria. The processes of HCl secretion are shown in **Fig. 4**. The H^+, K^+ pump is a dimer of an α- (catalytic subunit) and a β-glycosylated subunit, with between 8 and 10 membrane-spanning segments. Most of the α-subunit is on the intracellular side and contains the ATP binding site, while the β-subunit extends out into the extracellular milieu. Hydrophilic amino acids in the membrane-spanning portions form the ion pathway. The mechanism of action of the pump is shown in **Fig. 5**.

Control of acid secretion   Four cells are involved in the control of acid secretion: the parietal, the entero-

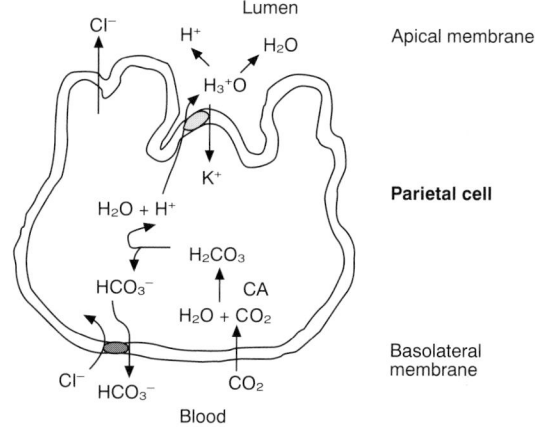

Figure 4 Ion movements in HCl secretion. Na^+ can be transported instead of H_3^+O. HCO_3^- transport back into the blood during acid secretion is the so-called alkaline tide. Cl^- entry via the basolateral membrane may be linked to Na^+ entry. Cl^- exiting across the apical membrane into the lumen may be linked to K^+ efflux. Light grey area indicates cation exchanger; dark grey area indicates anion exchanger; CA, carbonic anhydrase.

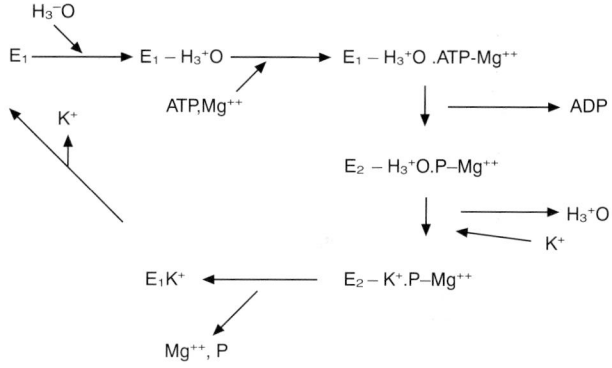

Figure 5 The mechanism of action of the H^+, K^+, ATPase in acid secretion from the parietal cells. E_1 is the transporter with its ion binding site exposed on the cytoplasmic side of the cell membrane. E_2 has the the site exposed on the outside (extracellular surface).

chromaffin-like (ECL), the G and the D cells. The three major stimulatory compounds are gastrin, histamine and acetylcholine, and the major inhibitory compound is somatostatin. The interaction between the four cell types, the four controlling agents and other factors is shown in **Fig. 6**.

Acid secretion can be divided into four phases: basal, cephalic, gastric and intestinal. In the basal phase, secretion is only 10% of maximum. In the cephalic phase secretion is 45% of maximum. In response to smell, taste, sight, chewing and swallowing, the fundic and oxyntic mucosa are stimulated by the vagus (parasympathetic) nerve. Acid is secreted by the parietal cells following direct stimulation, with acetylcholine binding to M3 muscarinic

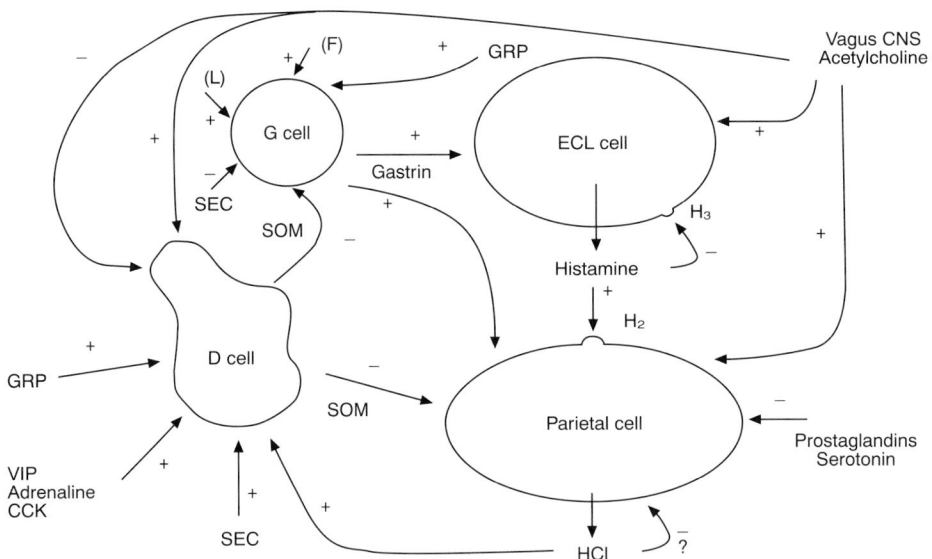

Figure 6 Control of gastric acid secretion. Key: + shows a stimulatory effect on cell secretion; − shows an inhibitory effect on cell secretion; [F], food and aromatic amino acids; [L], local and long reflex loops; SEC, secretin; SOM, somatostatin; GRP, gastrin-releasing peptide from parasympathetic nerve fibres; VIP, vasoactive intestinal peptide; CCK, cholecystokinin; ?, suggested effect.

receptors. Acetylcholine also stimulates histamine release from the ECL cells which binds to H_2 receptors on the parietal cells, causing an increase in cAMP stimulating acid secretion. The vagus also stimulates G cells of the antrum to release gastrin into the blood. This further stimulates the parietal cells via binding to CCK-B receptors and increasing intracellular Ca^{2+}, leading to an increase in HCl secretion.

During the gastric phase acid secretion is 45% of maximum. Food entering the stomach causes distension, and gastrin is released from the antrum. This release occurs via two mechanisms: (a) local enteric and long loop parasympathetic-mediated reflexes; and (b) stimulation of G cells to release gastrin directly by the products of protein digestion, i.e. peptides and amino acids, particularly hydrophobic amino acids. This second effect is interesting considering that the G cells must be covered with a mucus gel layer and the amino acids must diffuse through it before eliciting a response. The gastrin produced by both mechanisms stimulates the parietal cells to produce HCl directly and via histamine release from ECL cells.

The intestinal phase is mainly an inhibitory phase; however, there is a small stimulatory phase in which amino acids and peptides in the jejunum promote release of gastrin from the intestine. Two groups of factors lead to the inhibitory phase. First, fat, acid, hypertonicity and distension of the duodenum cause release of secretin from duodenal S cells, which inhibits gastrin release and thereby acid secretion. This works partly through the release of somatosta-

tin from D cells in the stomach. In addition, a smaller effect on acid secretion results from gastric inhibitory peptide, released from intestinal K cells, VIP released from nerve endings and CCK released by intestinal cells, again probably via a somatostatin-mediated pathway. Second, stimulation of G cells is reduced as food leaves the stomach and pH falls as buffering from food is lost. This high H^+ concentration will stimulate the D cells to release somatostatin, further inhibiting gastrin release. As well as inhibition of gastrin secretion, gastrin is also destroyed by a neutral endopeptidase present in stomach cells. With removal of stomach distension the vagal and intrinsic nerve stimuli for acid secretion are lost.

Mucus

The mucus covering the surface of the stomach consists of a mixture of many secretions and exfoliated cells. The major viscous and gel-forming component of the mucus gel is mucin, present at approximately 50 mg ml^{-1}. Mucin is also present in gastric juice as a result of pepsin erosion of the surface of the gel. It is secreted by the surface epithelial cells and mucus neck cells and is a glycoprotein, about 80% carbohydrate. The core protein of mucin has large regions of amino acid tandem repeats (TR) which are different for different mucins. The TR regions are the sites of heavy glycosylation. The N- and C-terminal regions of the protein core are globular and rich in cysteine and contain domains like those in von Willebrand factor, a glycoprotein involved in blood clotting which polymerizes via disulfide bridges. Mucin units are therefore polymerized via disulfide bridges into polymers with molecular weights of about 10×10^6 (**Fig. 7**). Polymerization is essential for gel formation, which results from noncovalent interactions between polymers. Also present in the gel and the juice, secreted by mucin secretory cells, are IgA, which combats bacterial invasion, and trefoil peptides (mol. wt 5000–10 000), which may interact with mucin to stabilize and strengthen the gel. They also inhibit acid secretion and gastric motility, however their major function is as growth factors, promoters of gastric healing and suppressors of tumour growth.

Mucin secretion   Mucin secretion is by compound exocytosis and may be linked to Cl^- secretion, with the mucin polyanion stored inside granules condensed with Ca^{2+}-mediated charge shielding. The exocytosis mechanism is similar to that for pepsinogen. There are two routes: (1) constitutive, with a steady release from the cells; and (2) regulated, with release from storage granules. Muscarinic receptors mediate mucin secretion. Cholinergic agonists stimulate secretion via protein kinase C and IP_3, leading to an increase in intracellular Ca^{2+}. Beta-adrenergic agents, secretin and prostaglandins E_2 and $F_2\beta$ stimulate secretion via a cAMP-mediated mechanism and NO acts via cGMP. Inflammation and infection as well as epithelial damaging agents, e.g. free radicals and mustard oil, stimulate mucin secretion.

Intrinsic Factor

Gastric intrinsic factor (IF) is defined as a substance required for the absorption of vitamin B_{12} (cobalamin, Cbl), which is essential for the formation of red blood cells. In the absence of IF, Cbl fails to be absorbed, erythrocyte production is defective and pernicious anaemia results. The most detrimental effect of gastric mucosal atrophy is the loss of IF. Two other Cbl binders exist in the body that are distinct from IF – these are haptocorrin (Hc) and transcobalamin II (TCII), the plasma binder then transports Cbl from the terminal ileum.

Dietary Cbl is always bound to proteins and is released by cooking and pepsin digestion. In gastric juice free Cbl is faced with both gastric IF and Hc mainly derived from saliva. At pH 2.0 Cbl affinity for Hc is 50 times higher than for IF, therefore free Cbl binds to Hc in the stomach. However, in the small intestine trypsin degrades Hc and Cbl is bound by IF. The Cbl–IF complex is absorbed in the terminal ileum after interaction with a receptor (IFRC) specific to IF–Cbl.

The gene for IF is found on chromosome 11. Purified IF is a glycoprotein of approximately 57 kDa. Its protein component varies between 341 and 351 residues and the carbohydrate moiety, consisting of 30–37 residues, 49–68% hexoses, 27–37% hexosamines and 13–18% sialic acid, constitutes 9.2–15%

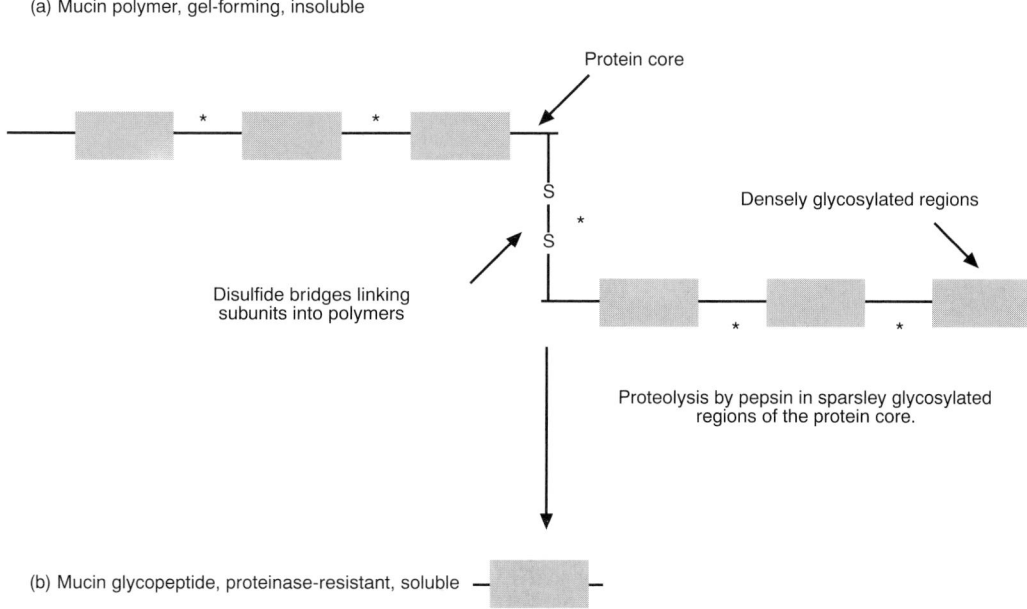

(a) Mucin polymer, gel-forming, insoluble

Protein core

Densely glycosylated regions

Disulfide bridges linking subunits into polymers

Proteolysis by pepsin in sparsley glycosylated regions of the protein core.

(b) Mucin glycopeptide, proteinase-resistant, soluble

Figure 7   Model for the structure of gastric mucin. Mucin genes expressed and secreted in the stomach are MUC 5 AC and MUC 6; both are coded for on chromosome 11 on the p arm at position 15 (11p15.5). The * indicates regions susceptible to proteolysis.

of the molecule (6.1–6.6 kDa). The sugar chains are either *O*-glycosidically or *N*-lactosaminically linked. *In vitro* transcription/translation studies have shown that removing 12% of the *C* terminus of the molecule results in all Cbl binding activity being lost, and the receptor binding region is at residues 25–44.

Intrinsic factor is classically described as being secreted by stomach fundus and body parietal cells. However, the use of immunocytochemistry and *in situ* hybridization has shown it is also found randomly in chief cells, G cells and in secretory ducts of the salivary glands. This may explain the fact that control of IF secretion is apparently multifactorial, in common with that of other gastric juice components, and can be activated by gastrin, histamine, acetylcholine and cholecystokinin. IF secretion in man varies between 50 and 100 nmol l^{-1}, considerably greater than daily requirements.

Absorption

Alcohol, drugs and fatty acids are absorbed in the stomach whereas the products of carbohydrate and protein digestion are not. Partially digested carbohydrate and protein products are not lipid-soluble and are too large to cross cell membranes. Unlike in the intestine, no specialized nutrient transporters are present in the stomach mucosa. The continuous mucus gel layer also provides a physical barrier to diffusion of anything other than low molecular weight solutes ($M_r \sim 1300$). There are also no specialized transport systems for ingested non-lipid-soluble electrolytes such as Ca^{2+}.

Gastric lipase activity is largely overlooked. Initial digestion of dietary fat in the stomach is a prerequisite for efficient intestinal lipolysis. In infants gastric lipolysis of milk is extensive and the medium-chain fatty acids released in the stomach are absorbed through gastric mucosa.

Ethanol and a number of drugs readily pass across the gastric mucosa. Ethanol is partially lipid-soluble and can therefore diffuse through the epithelial cell membranes and into the submucosal capillaries.

Nonsteroidal anti-inflammatory drugs, e.g. acetylsalicylic acid (aspirin), oral anticoagulants (e.g. dicoumarol) and sulfonylurea oral antidiabetic agents can all be absorbed through the gastric mucosa. These weakly acidic drugs are nonionized at gastric pH. In this form they are lipid-soluble and can therefore be absorbed quickly by crossing the plasma membrane of the epithelial cells.

Alcohol and nonsteroidal anti-inflammatory drugs can cause gastric mucosal damage and have been used in models of gastroduodenal ulceration. They rapidly diffuse through the protective adherent mucus gel layer (in the case of ethanol causing its dehydration) and in these models cause epithelial damage, cell exfoliation and, in more severe cases, vascular damage, haemorrhage and visible lesions. Following acute damage rapid repair occurs by a process of re-epithelialization. The repairing epithelium is protected from the endogenous damaging agents of acid and pepsin by a thick gelatinous coat mainly composed of a fibrin gel formed on the mucus gel template.

Gastric Motility and Emptying: The Role of the Stomach as a Reservoir and a Churn

Motility of the stomach allows it to serve as a reservoir, to act as a churn to fragment food and mix it with gastric secretions to aid digestion, and to empty gastric contents into the duodenum at a controlled rate.

Gastric motility and storage are complex and subject to multiple regulatory mechanisms. The first aspect of gastric motility is gastric filling. Accommodation of large changes in volume when a meal is eaten is achieved by the plasticity of the stomach smooth musculature and by receptive relaxation. Plasticity means that smooth muscle can maintain constant tension over a wide range of lengths without changing tension. Mechanoreceptors in the proximal stomach signal the degree of distension and, beyond a certain level, a stretch-activated contraction is initiated and pacesetter cells are depolarized. These properties are augmented by receptive relaxation of the deep folds of the stomach (known as rugae) which is mediated by the vagus nerve and associated with eating, possibly via stimulation of the taste buds.

A group of pacesetter cells is located high on the greater curvature of the stomach, generating slow wave potentials sweeping down the length of the stomach three times per minute. These spontaneous depolarizations are known as the basic electrical rhythm (BER) of the stomach. The stomach's circular smooth muscle layer may be stimulated to contract in peristaltic waves synchronized with the BER. The contractions in the thinly muscled fundus and body are weak but become stronger in the thickly muscled antrum. Food emptied into the stomach from the oesophagus is therefore stored in the body of the stomach and gradually fed into the antrum where mixing takes place. The antrum can contain 30 ml of chyme but only a few ml of chyme are forced through the pyloric sphincter into the duodenum with each peristaltic wave. Each wave causes the sphincter to contract more forcefully, blocking passage into the duodenum. This process is called retropulsion and achieves thorough mixing of chyme in the antrum. These events are known as the gastric phase of digestion, which is initiated as soon as food enters the stomach. The dominant hormone of the gastric phase is gastrin (**Table 4**). When gastrin levels are high the fundus and body of the stomach are relaxed and serve mainly to store chyme. Gastrin stimulates pyloric contraction and increases cardiac sphincter tone, preventing reflux. Gastrin also stimulates acid and pepsinogen secretion and antral motility, thus facilitating gastric digestion. These antral peristaltic contractions also provide the driving force for gastric emptying, which is regulated by multiple gastric and duodenal factors.

The main gastric factor influencing gastric emptying is the amount of chyme in the stomach. Simplistically, emptying rate is proportional to the volume of chyme. Distension triggers an increase in motility via stretching of smooth muscle as well as involvement of the intrinsic plexuses, the vagus nerve and gastrin. The rate of emptying also depends on the degree of liquefaction of the contents.

Duodenal factors are of prime importance in contolling gastric emptying rate. As soon as food begins to enter the duodenum the intestinal phase of digestion begins. Distension and the presence of acid, hypertonicity and fat in the duodenum stimulates receptors triggering neural or hormonal factors to suppress gastric motility and emptying by reducing gastric smooth muscle excitability. Neural responses are mediated by intrinsic nerve plexuses (short reflex) and autonomic nerves (long reflex), collectively known as the enterogastric reflex. The hormonal response is mediated by several hormones released from duodenal mucosa; these are known as enterogastrones and include secretin, CCK and GIP.

The volume of chyme in the duodenum is detected by mechanoreceptors and results in reflex inhibition of gastric motility and increase in pyloric tone by the vagally mediated enterogastric reflex.

The pH of duodenal contents affects gastric emptying. A pH less than 4.5 inhibits further emptying by stimulating the release of secretin. This inhibits gastric motility and gastrin release while stimulating pancreatic bicarbonate secretion. Conversely, when the duodenal chyme is above pH 5.0, motilin is released which increases the strength of the gastric contractions and the tone of the pyloric sphincter (Table 4).

Hypertonicity can result because digestion releases large amounts of amino acid and glucose molecules. If absorption of these substances does not keep pace, then the osmolarity of the duodenal contents increases. This results in large volumes of water entering the intestine from plasma, causing circulatory disturbances and resulting in reflex inhibition of gastric emptying. Duodenal osmoreceptors trigger the release of GIP which decreases gastric motility and secretion of both pepsin and acid.

The ingestion of fat is the most potent stimulus for inhibition of gastric motility, fat being digested more slowly than carbohydrates and proteins. Fats and fatty acids are detected by duodenal chemoreceptors

Table 4   Gastrointestinal peptide hormones affecting gastric motility and emptying

Hormone	Amino acid No. (chromosome)	Cell source	Stimuli	Effects on stomach
Gastrin	34 (17) 17 14	G cells	Amino acids Distension pH > 3.0 Parasympathetic activity	↑ Antral motility
Gastric inhibitory peptide	43	K cells of intestinal mucosa	Glucose Distension Hypertonicity	↓ Gastric motility and secretion
Motilin	22	Enterochromaffin cells of small intestine	pH > 5.0	↑ Gastric motility
Secretin	27	Duodenal S cells	Hypertonicity pH < 4.5	↓ Gastric motility and secretion
Cholecystokinin	58 (3) 39 12 8	Upper small intestinal mucosa	Fats Amino acids	↓ Gastric motility and secretion

stimulating the release of cholecystokinin. This hormone has multiple effects including inhibition of gastric emptying.

After a meal is completely emptied from the stomach there are no more gastric factors to enhance gastric excitability.

See also: **Alcohol**: Absorption, Metabolism and Physiological Effects. **Cobalamins**: Physiology, Dietary Sources and Requirements. **Drugs**: Drug-Nutrient Interactions. **Fatty Acids**: Metabolism.

Further Reading

Allen A, Hutton DA, Leonard AJ, Pearson JP and Sellars LA (1989) Pepsins. In: Wallace JL (ed.) *Endogenous Mediators of Gastrointestinal Disease*, chap. 3, pp 54–69. Boca Raton: CRC Press.

Forstner G (1995) Signal transduction, packaging and secretion of mucins. *Annual Review of Physiology* 57:585–605.

Hamash M (1994) Gastric and lingual lipases. In: Johnson LR (ed.) *Physiology of the Gastrointestinal Tract*, 3rd edn, chap. 32. New York: Raven Press.

Kent-Lloyd KC and Debas HT (1994) Peripheral regulation of gastric acid secretion. In: Johnson LR (ed.) *Physiology of the Gastrointestinal Tract*, 3rd edn, chap. 39, pp 1185–1225. New York: Raven Press.

Lefebure O *et al.* (1996) Gastric mucosa abnormalities and tumourigenesis in mice lacking the pS2 trefoil protein. *Science* 274:259–262.

Moffett, D, Moffett S and Schauf C (1993) The gastrointestinal tract In: *Human Physiology*, 2nd edn, section VI, chaps 21 and 22, pp 591–651. St Louis: CV Mosby.

Newvonen PJ and Kivisto KT (1994) Enhancement of drug absorption by antacids. *Clinical Pharmacokinetics* 27(2):120–128.

Nicolas JP and Guéant JL (1995) Gastric intrinsic factor and its receptor. In: *Baillière's Clinical Haematology*, Vol. 8, no. 3, chap. 5, pp 515–531. London: Baillière Tindall.

Quigley EMM (1996) Gastric and small intestinal motility in health and disease. *Gastroenterology Clinics of North America* 25(i):113–145.

Sachs G (1994) The gastric H, K ATPase In: Johnson LR (ed.) *Physiology of the Gastrointestinal Tract*, 3rd edn, chap. 27, pp 1119–1138. New York: Raven Press.

Sands BE and Padolsky DK (1996) The trefoil peptide family. *Annual Review of Physiology* 58:253–273.

Wank SA (1995) Cholecystokinin receptors. *American Journal of Physiology* 269:G628–G646.

Structure and Function of the Small Intestine

R D E Rumsey, University of Sheffield, UK

Copyright © 1998 Academic Press

The small intestine is the barrier between the external environment and the human interior, through which all nutrients must pass. Transport is only possible following the complex processes of digestion, which take place largely within the small intestine. Complete digestion and absorption take place if the optimal motility patterns of the small intestine are employed. Each facet of small intestinal function, absorption, digestion and motility is dependent on the other to produce human nutrition.

Within the regulatory capacity of the small intestine exist mechanisms to alter the rate of nutrient absorption, to signal the passage of nutrients and to change the phases of metabolism. The complexity of function in the small intestine is also related to the structure, architecture and cellular kinetics of the system and this is a logical point at which to begin.

Structure

The small intestine is the main site of digestion and absorption within the gastrointestinal tract. It is a hollow tube more than 6 m in length with a luminal diameter of about 4 cm. The first 20 cm distal from the pylorus is the duodenum, the next 2.5 m is the jejunum and the final half is the ileum. There are no anatomically distinguishing characteristics along the small intestine; any alterations in architecture are gradual.

All segments of the small intestine possess a mucosa with the same sophisticated structural pattern along its length. The mucosal lining is surrounded by two muscle layers; the innermost layer consists of circular, smooth muscle sheets oriented radially around the lumen. The second, thinner layer is of longitudinal sheets, surrounded by a thin serosal layer. The regulation of muscular movement (motility) is achieved by the enteric nervous system which consists of two matrices of interconnecting neurons. The outermost matrix is the myenteric plexus situated between the two muscle layers. Situated between the mucosa and the circular muscle layer is the submucosal plexus from which sensory neurons extend into the mucosa. Interneurons connect the two plexuses, which in turn receive postganglionic parasympathetic nerve fibres.

The enteric nervous system is a complex system exhibiting a high degree of autonomy over gut function. It is recognized that the enteric neurons use as many as 20 neurotransmitters and neuromodulators, as well as the classical neurotransmitter mechanisms of the autonomic nervous system. The enteric nervous system is only surpassed by the brain and spinal cord in its capacity for information processing.

Mucosal structure

The lining of the small intestine is remarkably adapted for the function of absorption by increasing the surface area for transmucosal transport at three levels of magnitude (**Fig. 1**).

- The inner surface has circular folds which increases the area by a factor of about 3.
- The mucosa projects from the folds into the lumen with fingerlike structures (villi) about 1 mm in length. Villi increase the surface area a further 10 times. The surface of each villus is covered with epithelial cells known as enterocytes. Absorption takes place across the enterocyte barrier.
- Small, hairlike filaments known as microvilli project from the luminal surface of each enterocyte into the lumen. Microvilli increase the surface area for absorption by a further 20 times.

The three structures combine to increase the surface area by some 600 times. Each villus is supplied with its own connective tissue support known as the lamina propria, its own arteriolar and venous microcir-culation with capillaries draining the basolateral regions of all the enterocytes, and its own lymphatic system.

Cell kinetics of the enterocyte

The life span and kinetics of small intestinal enterocytes are particularly important in understanding the process of absorption. Enterocytes have a short life of 2–3 days in humans. New cells are born in a proliferative zone below the villus in the crypts of Lieberkühn. After birth, new cells begin to move in the direction of the lumen and mitosis continues for two or three more divisions while each cell remains within the crypt. As the enterocyte emerges from the crypt, proliferation ceases and the process of differentiation proceeds so that the cell, by now passing up the outer surface of the villus, reaches functional maturity with a full capacity of enzymes towards the villus tip. On reaching the tip, enterocytes are sloughed off into the intestinal lumen and digested.

The short life span of the enterocyte bestows massive adaptive potential within the tissue since the process of differentiation may be influenced by changes in any nutrient or other luminal factor to induce a rapid functional response.

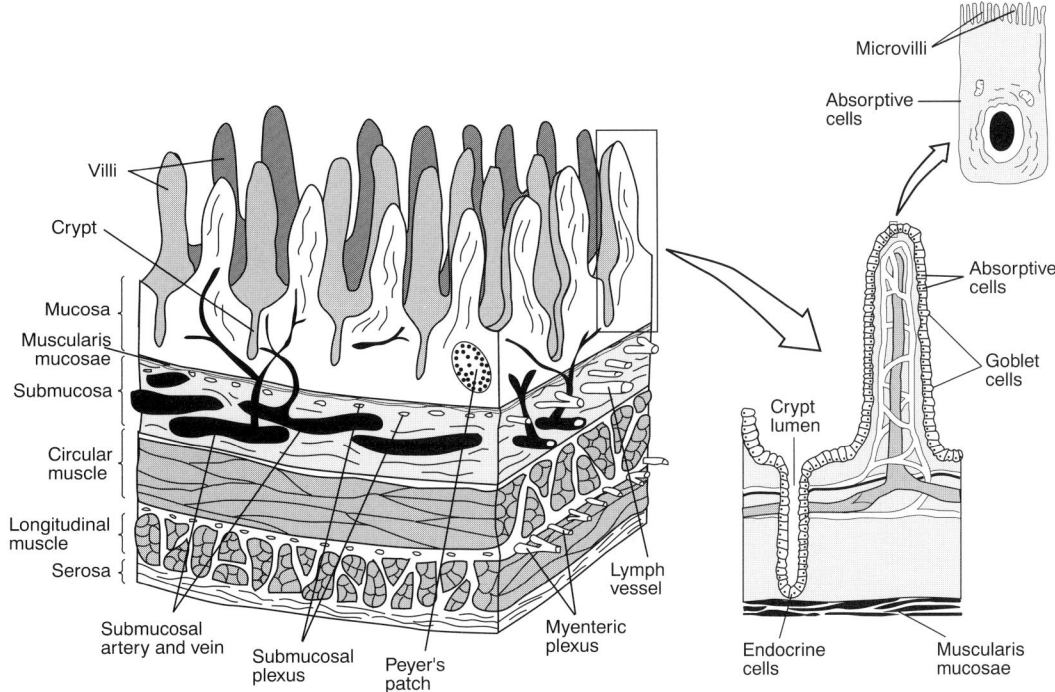

Figure 1 Wall of the small intestine. The intestinal surface area is enhanced by finger-like villi.

Motility

Vigorous controlled movement of the intestinal wall is essential for the two basic properties of segmentation or mixing and peristalsis or aboral propulsion (**Fig. 2**). The two properties are interdependent since neither segmentation nor peristalsis alone would result in optimal digestion and absorption. The peristaltic export of chyme from the duodenal segment in an aboral direction is only effective following considerable segmentation to optimize the homogeneous distribution of digestive juices.

While the neural basis of peristalsis has been acceptably modelled, the answers to basic questions concerning the receptors involved and the occurrence of reverse or retroperistalsis in particular circumstances remain elusive. The precise sensory messages that are needed to switch motility from segmentation to peristalsis and vice versa are also unclear, except that the signals must be both chemical and physical, being related to the passage and characteristics of the nutrients along the gastrointestinal tract.

The migrating motor complex

When the small intestine is emptied after the passage of a meal, segmentation contractions stop and are replaced by a pattern of motility called the migrating motor complex (MMC). The MMC is a series of weak peristaltic rushes in the aboral direction, each rush only occurring along a short distance of the total length. The series begins at the level of the stomach and takes about 2 h to reach the ileocaecal valve at the distal ileum. It is considered that the MMC performs a 'housekeeping' function by sweeping debris such as sloughed cells, residual chyme and bacteria aborally in the interval between meals. These patterns continue in the absence of eating. When food is introduced into the stomach, MMC patterns are replaced by segmentation contractions.

The passage of chyme along the small intestine

Chyme is expelled from the stomach into the duodenum in 'packets' in response to the hormonal (cholecystokinin and secretin) influence on gastric emptying. The aqueous component of the meal is emptied first as larger solid particles are reduced by the activity of the gastric musculature. The lipid component of the meal is liable to separate within the stomach lumen and remain as one of the last fractions of the meal to be emptied.

Chyme appears to mix rapidly within the duodenum, presumably by segmentation action, and the early parts of the meal pass rapidly along the duodenum and jejunum, possibly because the nutrient content of this initial 'packet' is aqueous and therefore lower. Some observations suggest that certain meals produce retroperistaltic movements within the proximal small intestine. The transit rate of chyme is reduced gradually through the second half of the small intestine, the ileum. The remnants of the meal are released across the ileocaecal valve as the pressure of contents within the ileum rises.

Nutrient regulation of motility and transit

Traditional experimental techniques in which simple nutrient substrates were introduced by tube into the 'starved' human duodenum found that, under these conditions, most nutrients were absorbed immediately within the proximal tenth of the small intestine. Real food offers a more complex problem for the small intestine since the processes of digestion only begin within the lumen of the stomach. It is now apparent that digestion takes place along a significant fraction of the whole small intestine, with the processes of absorption occurring, as a consequence, along the majority of segments. Certainly enterocyte functional capacity on ileal villi is comparable with those on the jejunal villi.

These observations have been supported by findings that meals of a high nutrient density are more slowly emptied from the stomach and pass along the small intestine at a reduced rate. Evidence exists for a regulatory mechanism situated within the mucosa of the terminal ileum capable of sensing the presence of nutrients such as lipid, and providing feedback

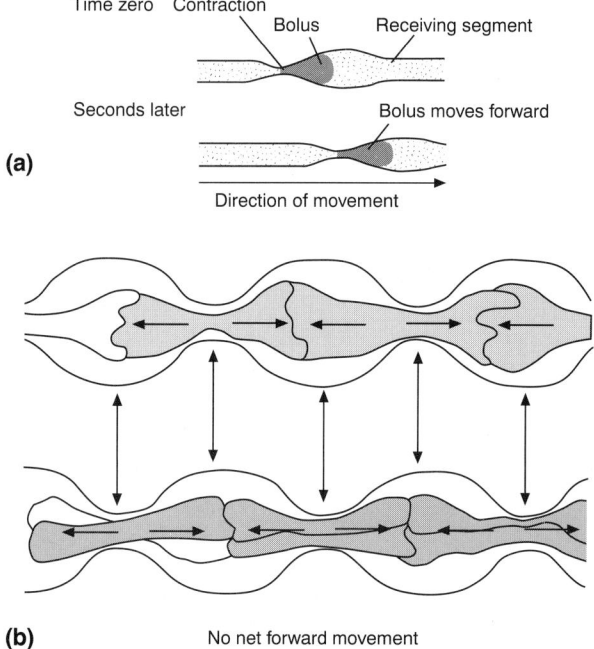

Figure 2 Contractions in the gastrointestinal tract. (a) Peristaltic contractions are responsible for forward movement; (b) segmental contractions are responsible for mixing.

restraint on motility patterns in the stomach, duodenum and jejunum to slow the passage of meals in proportion to their nutrient density. This mechanism, the 'ileal brake', taken with the hormonal control of gastric emptying, explains the almost complete absorption of meals of the highest nutrient density.

Digestion

The chyme from the stomach is mixed in the duodenum with digestive juices from three sources: the pancreas, the liver and the intestinal mucosa itself.

The pancreas

The pancreas is an elongated gland situated beneath the stomach (**Fig. 3**); it has two separate roles, both essential for human nutrition. Exocrine pancreatic function is the production of pancreatic juice for secretion into the duodenal lumen. Pancreatic juice is a potent mixture of enzymes and solutes which are essential for the process of digestion of protein, lipid and carbohydrate, and for producing the optimal pH environment within the duodenal lumen. The juice is secreted as an ultrafiltrate of plasma from acini, composed of clusters of secretory cells connected to

Table 1 Volumes absorbed by the small intestine per day

	Volume (ml)
Volume entering the small intestine	
Ingestion:	
Food	1300
Drinks	1300
Saliva	1500
Gastric juice	2000
Pancreatic juice	1500
Plasma secretions:	
Bile	500
Intestinal secretion	1500
Total:	9600
Volume absorbed by the small intestine	9000
Volume passing through the ileocaecal valve	600

ducts. The composition of these secretions is listed in **Table 1**.

The second function is the endocrine secretion of the hormones of intermediary metabolism, insulin and glucagon, into the hepatic portal vein supplying blood to the liver.

Pancreatic juice The bulk of pancreatic secretion (**Table 2**) is a dilute solution of sodium bicarbonate ($NaHCO_3$) which neutralizes the acid effluent from the stomach and provides an alkaline environment for the enzymes present in the secretion.

Enzymes Pancreatic proteolytic enzymes are secreted in inactive form to avoid digestion of pancreatic tissue itself. Once within the duodenal lumen the main enzymes – trypsin, chymotrypsin and carboxypeptidase – are liberated and each attacks different peptide linkages in the protein molecule. Pancreatic amylase converts polysaccharides into smaller saccharide molecules, particularly disaccharide. Pancreatic lipase is the only source for the enzymatic

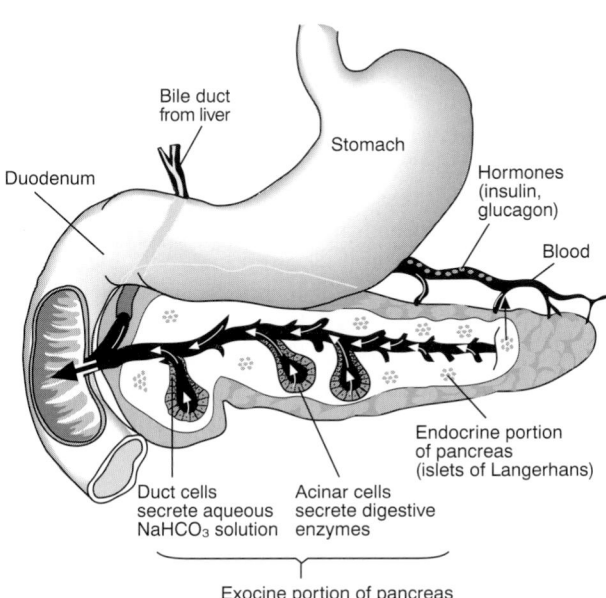

Figure 3 Exocrine and endocrine portions of the pancreas (glandular portions of the pancreas are grossly exaggerated). The exocrine pancreas secretes into the duodenal lumen a digestive juice composed of digestive enzymes secreted by the acinar cells and an aqueous $NaHCO_3$ solution secreted by the duct cells. The endocrine pancreas secretes the hormones insulin and glucagon into the blood.

Table 2 Constitutents of pancreatic juice

Secretion	Function
$NaHCO_3$	Establishes pH environment (pH 7–8)
Amylase	Digests complex carbohydrate
Carboxypeptidase	Digests proteins and polypeptides
Chymotrypsin	Digests proteins and polypeptides
Elastase	Digests elastin
Trypsin	Digests proteins and polypeptides
Lipase	Digests triacylglycerol
Nuclease	Digests nucleic acids

digestion of fat. Lipase hydrolyses dietary triacylglycerols to monoacylglycerols and free fatty acids. Deficiency of pancreatic lipase results in serious fat malabsorption. Pancreatic amylase or peptidase deficiency is less serious since small intestinal enzymes would significantly minimize any loss of activity.

Regulation of pancreatic secretion   Pancreatic juice is stimulated to flow in response to rises in the blood concentrations of two gastrointestinal hormones, secretin and cholecystokinin. Both hormones are liberated from the duodenal mucosa in response to different components of the luminal environment. Secretin is produced in response to acid and stimulates the pancreatic acini to secrete $NaHCO_3$, so that the acid contents emerging through the pylorus are neutralized. Cholecystokinin (CCK) secretion is prompted by the presence of both lipid and protein in the duodenal lumen, and the effect of CCK on pancreatic acini is to promote the secretion of enzymes. All three types of pancreatic enzymes are stored in zymogen granules within the acinar cells and released into the ducts on stimulation. As the final components of the meal finally leave the stomach, acid and nutrient levels fall in the lumen and pancreatic secretion ceases.

Parasympathetic nerve stimulation is also recognized to produce a small stimulation of pancreatic juice flow probably as part of the cephalic and gastric phases, preparing the duodenal environment for a meal.

The liver

The second main source of secretion is the liver. Bile is formed in the liver canaliculi and passes down the bile duct into the duodenum. The opening of the bile duct into the duodenum, the sphincter of Oddi, is controlled by cholecystokinin levels. When the sphincter of Oddi is closed, bile is diverted and stored in the gall bladder.

The role of bile   Bile is a solution of $NaHCO_3$, similar to pancreatic juice but without enzymes and including a number of organic solutes of which the bile salts are essential for the digestion of fat. Bile salts have a detergent action which emulsifies the large droplets of dietary fat into a water-soluble form, a micelle, rendering the fat molecules available for hydrolysis by pancreatic lipase.

The intestinal mucosa

In contact with chyme the intestinal mucosa secretes a mucus-containing watery fluid into the lumen. The mucus protects and lubricates, and water is necessary in excess for the multiple hydrolytic processes of digestion. However, the fluid is devoid of enzymes; pancreatic juice is the sole source of digestive enzymes within the lumen of the small intestine. Enzymes are present within the intestinal mucosa but fixed in the enterocyte cell membrane.

Nutrient Absorption

Absorption is the transfer of the products of digestion together with minerals, micronutrients and water from the gut lumen into the blood. The mucosa of the small intestine is adapted structurally to optimize nutrient absorption and enterocytes posses specific transport mechanisms to facilitate transport. The mechanisms responsible for the absorption of lipid are significantly different from those governing the absorption of other nutrients.

Sodium absorption

Sodium absorption is central to the absorption of the majority of nutrients. Indeed, the interdependence of sodium, water and nutrients (particularly sugars) is an important element in nourishment under pathological conditions, for instance in considering the rationale for rehydration therapy. The enterocyte membrane possesses carrier proteins for the transport of specific substrates. A specific sodium transporter exists on the enterocyte basolateral membrane, exporting sodium from the cell by an energy-dependent process. The effect of the sodium transporter is to maintain a low intracellular sodium concentration.

Different processes permit the passage of the sodium ion from the lumen into the enterocyte across the mucosal membrane. Sodium may pass by passive diffusion down its concentration gradient or be transported by a (second) luminal transporter in association with nutrients such as glucose and amino acids. Thirdly, some sodium may diffuse between the cells directly into the interstitial spaces. Water molecules follow sodium ions across the membranes.

Carbohydrate absorption

The absorption of carbohydrate molecules (**Fig. 4**) is directly linked to the final stage of digestion. Luminal carbohydrate digestion produces largely the disaccharide molecules sucrose, lactose and maltose. The enterocyte luminal membranes are richly endowed with disaccharidases which hydrolyse the disaccharides to the monosaccharides glucose, fructose and galactose. These membrane-bound enzymes are now considered to be associated with the protein transporter

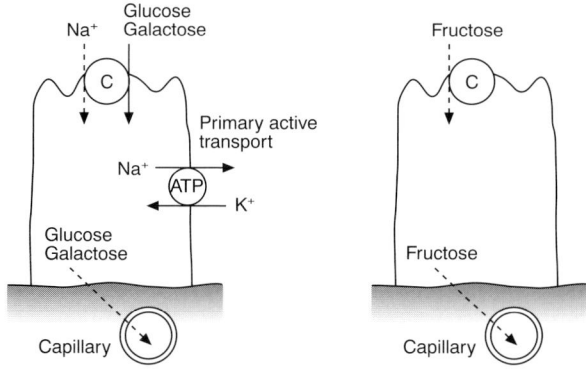

Figure 4 Carbohydrate absorption mechanisms. (a) Secondary active transport: glucose and galactose are absorbed using Na$^+$ cotransport systems. Sodium ions are removed using the (Na$^+$-K$^+$)-ATPase pump (primary active transport). (b) Facilitated diffusion: fructose absorption is passive but relies on a carrier molecule. Solid arrow, movement against concentration gradient; broken arrow, diffusion down concentration gradient; ATP, ATP-dependent pump; C, carrier molecule.

molecules described above which facilitate the transport of sodium across the enterocyte luminal membrane. Sugars are cotransported with sodium ions against their own concentration gradients, a process of great nutritional value. Once concentrated within the enterocyte, the sugars pass by facilitated diffusion across the basolateral membrane into the interstitial spaces and from there diffuse into the capillaries of the intestinal villus.

Protein absorption

Similar to carbohydrate, protein digestion is incomplete within the lumen of the small intestine. However, considerably more amino acid has been produced through protein digestion and amino acids are absorbed by secondary cotransport with sodium ion in the same fashion as sugars (**Fig. 5**). Some simpler

dipeptides remain within the lumen and these final peptide bonds are hydrolysed by aminopeptidase enzymes within the enterocyte luminal membrane.

Lipid absorption

The absorption of fat (**Fig. 6**) is a different process from that of carbohydrate and protein by virtue of the insolubility of the molecules of lipid in water. The products of lipase digestion, fatty acids and monoacylglycerols, are insoluble and so cannot diffuse through the chyme to reach the enterocyte membrane. The role of micelles produced by the action of bile salts is carriage of the lipid molecules to the enterocyte luminal membrane where the fatty acids and monoacylglycerols diffuse from the micelle through the lipid component of the membrane to enter the enterocyte cytoplasm.

Luminal micelles that have donated their fat burden across the mucosa are then free to take up more lipid from the droplet pool. Once within the enterocyte fatty acids and monoacylglycerols are reesterified to reform triacylglycerols under the action of enzymes within the endoplasmic reticulum. The intracellular triacylglycerol droplets are coated with a protein coat called apolipoprotein which renders the lipid soluble once more. The coated droplets are called chylomicrons. Chylomicrons pass across the basolateral membrane of the enterocyte by exocytosis into the interstitial spaces where they are inhibited from passing into villus capillaries by the basement membrane. Instead chylomicrons pass into the lacteals of the villus and, from there, into the lymphatic system draining into the circulation at the

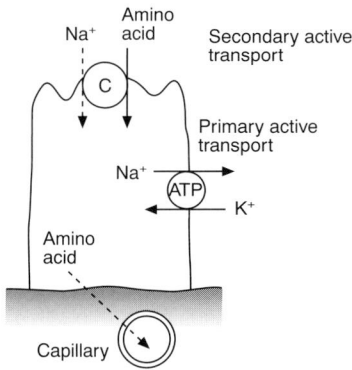

Figure 5 Amino acids (and some short peptides) are absorbed by secondary active transport using Na$^+$ cotransport. Solid arrow, movement against concentration gradient; broken arrow, diffusion down concentration gradient; ATP, ATP-dependent pump; C, carrier molecule.

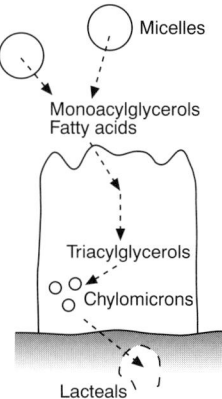

Figure 6 Lipids are absorbed by diffusion after digestion to monoacylglycerols and fatty acids. These are reconstituted into triacylglycerols and packaged as chylomicrons within the cell before entering intravillous lymphatic vessels (lacteals); these have an open endothelium (broken outline) and are therefore more permeable to larger particles than are the blood capillaries.

great lymphatic duct behind the right atrium of the heart.

It is important to realize that lipid absorption is a passive process and the kinetics are, therefore, largely dictated by the luminal concentration of lipid. To this extent lipid absorption might be expected to be more dependent on intestinal mixing and motility than other luminal components.

Absorption of minerals

Mineral absorption is normally proportional to dietary intake, with two important exceptions: iron and calcium, the absorption of which can be regulated according to the needs of the body. Calcium absorption is related to the amount of specific binding protein within the enterocyte. The concentration of the calcium-binding protein that regulates calcium uptake from the gut is itself secondary to vitamin D levels.

Iron absorption occurs more rapidly if the ion is in the ferrous state. Dietary iron binds to the protein transferrin in the lumen which passes into the enterocyte by endocytosis following binding to a receptor in the membrane. The transferrin-bound iron passes across the basolateral membrane into the bloodstream when required for haem synthesis. Short-term storage of iron takes place within the enterocyte in the form of the granular protein ferritin.

Absorption of vitamins

Water-soluble vitamins are absorbed with water and fat-soluble vitamins are absorbed dissolved within the fat droplets in micelles. Vitamin B_{12} is unique in that it may only be absorbed combined with the gastric intrinsic factor by a specific mechanism in the distal ileum.

Gastrointestinal Hormones

The gastrointestinal hormones are a group of peptide molecules of which more are identified every year. Most are extremely potent biological agents exerting their action at some distance from the site of secretion (endocrine) or close to the site of release (paracrine). The hormones are secreted in granules from enteroendocrine cells within the gastrointestinal mucosa in response to nutrient signals from the lumen. The precise physiology of most of these molecules has yet to be clarified and the following review is restricted to those peptides on which there is broad agreement (**Table 3**).

Table 3 Functions of the major gastrointestinal hormones

Hormone	Stimulus	Function
Gastrin	Protein in the stomach	Stimulates gastric secretion Promotes gastric motility Promotes ileal motility Promotes colonic motility Relaxes ileocaecal valve Trophic action on gastric and intesintal mucosae
Secretin	Acid in the duodenum	Inhibits gastric secretion Inhibits gastric motility Stimulates pancreatic juice flow Stimulates bile flow (HCO_3) Trophic action on pancreatic exocrine tissue
Cholecystokinin	Fat/protein in duodenum	Inhibits gastric secretion Inhibits gastric motility and gastric emptying Stimulates pancreatic enzymes Gall bladder contraction Sphincter of Oddi relaxation Trophic action on pancreatic exocrine tissue Satiety signals
GIP	Duodenal chyme	Inhibits gastric emptying Inhibits gastric secretion Stimulates insulin secretion from pancreatic islets

GIP, glucose-dependent insulinotrophic peptide.

Gastrin

Gastrin is secreted from the antral mucosa in response to food in the stomach, particularly a meal high in protein. Gastrin passes into the blood and stimulates a large range of responses along the whole gastrointestinal tract involving both secretions and motility. The general physiology of gastrin is that of a promoter of gut function as food begins to pass along the gut, and as a remover of the remnants of the previous meal. Gastrin secretion ceases as acidity rises within the stomach and duodenum.

Secretin

Secretin is produced by cells in the duodenal mucosa in response to the appearance of acidity and chyme. It performs at least four major functions associated with the passage of the meal through the duodenum. It stimulates the pancreatic duct and acinar cells to produce copious quantities of aqueous $NaHCO_3$ solution; it also promotes a bicarbonate-rich bile flow; it inhibits gastric emptying; and, finally, it inhibits gastric secretion. Secretin secretion rate falls as acidity production from the stomach falls.

Cholecystokinin

Cholecystokinin is secreted from the same general duodenal mucosa as secretin but is produced in response to the lipid and protein components of the meal. It has a multiple role which is not yet completely clear. The CCK molecule exists in a number of peptide chain lengths, each with differing properties but all with extreme potency. Cholecystokinin is the main inhibitor of gastric emptying, slowing the release of nutrient-dense chyme from the stomach at a rate proportional to duodenal and pancreatic digestive function. It stimulates enzyme secretion from the pancreatic acinar cells and causes contraction of gallbladder wall muscle and relaxation of the sphincter of Oddi, allowing bile to flow into the duodenum.

Cholecystokinin levels are now recognized to directly influence feelings of satiety and the perception of fullness in association with meals. The signalling of fullness to the brain by means of CCK release is potentially, therefore, one possible pathway for the peripheral control of food intake and is of particular importance not least by virtue of the presence of CCK receptors known to be present within brain tissue. Secretion of CCK is inhibited by the absence of nutrients in the duodenal lumen.

Glucose-dependent insulinotrophic peptide

Glucose-dependent insulinotrophic peptide (GIP) is also known as gastric inhibitory peptide (both having the same initials). It is the third duodenal peptide hormone and is now recognized to be the 'incretin' peptide important for the mobilization and attenuation of the insulin response to glucose as it is absorbed from the small intestine. It initiates the meal stimulus of the pancreatic islets heralding the absorptive phase of metabolism. Lipid, carbohydrate, acid and duodenal distension all serve to promote the secretion of GIP from the duodenal mucosa.

Trophic action of gastrointestinal hormones

The gastrointestinal hormones, gastrin, cholecystokinin and secretin are recognized to possess trophic properties in that they are responsible for maintaining the cell populations of their target tissues. In the case of gastrin the tissue in question is particularly the gastric mucosa but also the intestinal mucosa; cholecystokinin and secretin are trophic for pancreatic acinar tissue.

See also: **Glucose**: Metabolism and Maintenance of Blood Glucose Level. **Lipids**: Chemistry and Classification. **Protein**: Digestion and Bioavailability. **Sodium**: Physiology. **Sucrose**: Nutritional Role, Absorption and Metabolism.

Structure and Function of the Colon

M A Eastwood, University of Edinburgh, UK

Copyright © 1998 Academic Press

Structure

Embryology

The primitive gut consists of a foregut, midgut and hindgut. The foregut ends and the midgut begins where the bile duct enters the second part of the duodenum. The midgut ends and the hindgut begins at the junction of the right third with the middle third of the transverse colon.

Anatomy

The large intestine is approximately 150 cm in length with six anatomical subdivisions (**Fig. 1**):

- The *caecum*, in the right iliac fossa, is a blind end below the ileocaecal valve, from which the vermiform appendix arises.
- The *ascending colon* extends from the ileocaecal valve to the hepatic flexure.

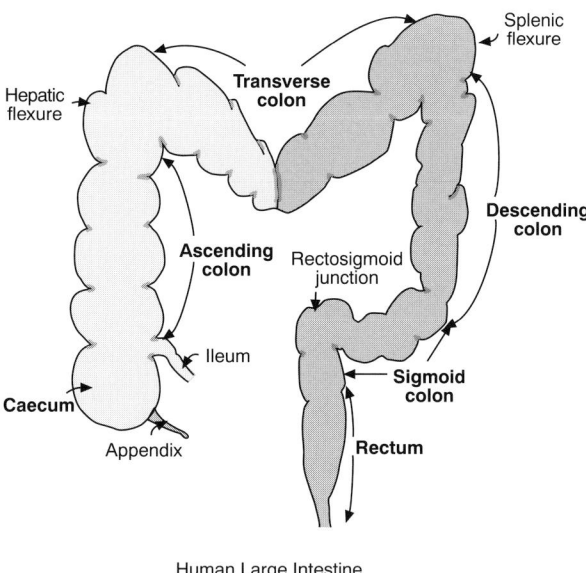

Human Large Intestine
and constituent parts

Figure 1 The anatomical different portions of the colon. The shading indicates their embryonic origins, from the mid and hind gut.

- The *transverse colon* crosses from the hepatic flexure to the splenic flexure.
- The *descending colon* extends down to the sigmoid colon in the left iliac fossa.
- The *sigmoid colon* becomes the *rectum* at the rectosigmoid junction.

Histology

From the lumen to the outside, the walls of the large bowel consist of mucosa, submucosa, muscularis propria and serosa (**Fig. 2**).

Mucosa   The mucosal surface is smooth and without villi. The glands or crypts of Lieberkuhn line the colonic epithelium and extend from the surface to the muscularis mucosae. The crypts secrete mucin which covers the mucosa and lubricates the luminal contents.

Epithelium   The colonic epithelium consists of several types of cells:

1. undifferentiated stem cells, giving rise to epithelial cells;
2. mature columnar cells, which absorb water and electrolytes;
3. mature goblet cells, which are involved in mucus production;
4. endocrine cells, primarily located on the left side of the colon and rectum, which consist of a heterogeneous population of cells producing a variety of hormones including somatostatin,

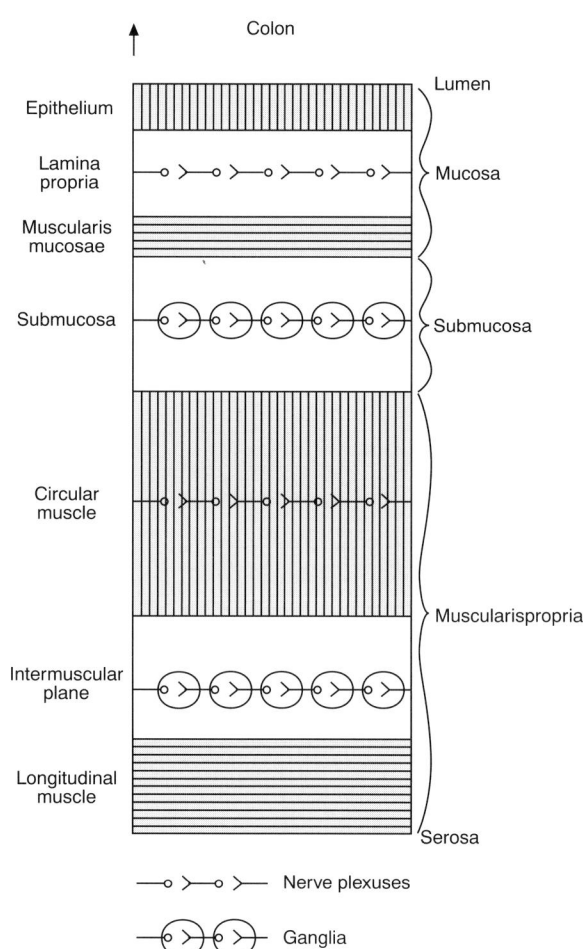

Figure 2   Cross-sections across the walls of the colon.

serotonin, glucagon, pancreatic polypeptide and other peptides of unknown chemistry and function.

Lamina propria   The lamina propria, separating the colonic crypts, lies between the epithelium and the muscularis mucosae. It consists of lymphoid nodules, a stroma of collagen fibres and lymphocytes, plasma cells, eosinophils and macrophages. The viscoelastic properties of the collagen through inter- and intra-molecular crosslinks give the colon elasticity and strength, and help to maintain the colon's shape. These properties deteriorate with advancing age. As the collagen develops increasing crosslinks with age, it becomes more rigid and less strong, which facilitates the development of colonic diverticulosis, pockets in the bowel wall.

Muscularis mucosae   The muscularis mucosae is a continuous sheet of collagen and elastic fibres surrounding smooth muscle cells that lies at the base of the lamina propria.

Submucosa The submucosa is filled with collagen and elastic tissue fibres.

Muscularis propria The main smooth muscle of the large intestine is in two layers, separated by an intermuscular space containing Auerbach's plexus of myenteric nerves. The long axis of the outer layer (the longitudinal muscle) runs along the length of the colon and is thickened to form the three taeniae coli. The thicker inner layer (circular muscle) surrounds the colon, and is thickened in the anal canal to form the internal anal sphincter which is separated from but surrounded by the external anal sphincter. The rectum and the appendix are completely surrounded by muscle.

Serosa The serosal layer is a continuous sheet of squamous epithelial cells. There are localized accumulations of fat cells, protuberances called the appendices epiploicae.

Blood supply and lymphatics

The superior mesenteric artery supplies the midgut (caecum, appendix, ascending colon and most of the transverse colon). The inferior mesenteric artery supplies the hindgut (distal transverse colon to anus). The two colonic arterial blood supplies are linked by the marginal artery, a vascular supply which has the potential to be inadequate at the splenic flexure and the rectum, with resulting ischaemia.

The venous system drains most of the large intestinal blood supply into the portal vein, while blood from the rectum passes to the inferior vena caval system. The portal vein receives blood from the right side of the large intestine through its direct branch, the superior mesenteric vein, and from the left side through the inferior mesenteric vein, a branch of the splenic vein.

The lymphatic plexuses are abundant throughout the gut, especially in the caecum. The lymphatic trunks join in the cisterna chyli, a dilated sac which collects lymph from all of the gastrointestinal tract below the diaphragm and then drains lymph into the thoracic duct and the left subclavian vein.

Nerves of the large intestine

The large intestine receives its extrinsic nerve supply from three sources – the vagus nerve, the mesenteric nerve and the pelvic nerve (**Fig. 3**). The vagal distribution, a parasympathetic innervation, extends to the mid transverse colon, the end of the embryonically derived midgut, and to some extent the limit of the digestive process. The mesenteric (sympathetic) nerves are part of the thoracolumbar

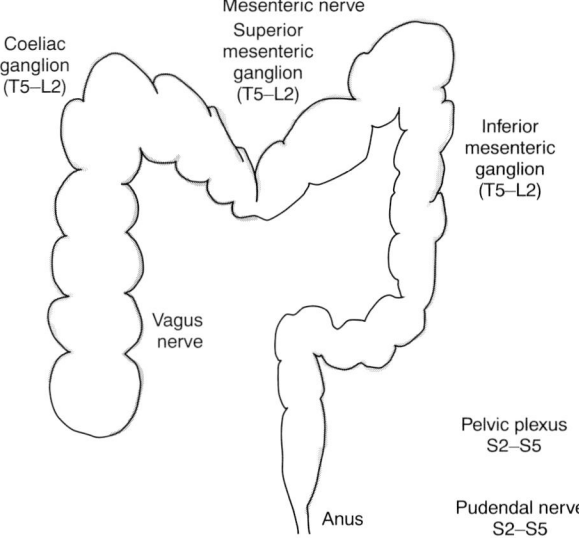

Figure 3 Nerve supply to the colon, showing the vagus nerve (parasympathetic) and the mesenteric nerve and coeliac, superior and inferior mesenteric nerve ganglia (sympathetic).

component of the autonomic nervous system and arise from prevertebral ganglia – the coeliac, superior mesenteric and inferior mesenteric ganglia. The pelvic innervation is parasympathetic and arises from the pelvic plexus.

Motility of the Colon

Chyme is moved through the large bowel from the caecum to the rectum and in that process is converted to solid stool. Contractions of the smooth muscle move or store colonic contents, a process called 'motility'. Most segments of the large bowel have the capacity both to store and to propel contents. Colonic contents arrive in the rectum ready for brief storage prior to evacuation. The mechanism that controls propulsion in the colon is not understood. The right colon contracts at regular intervals, suggesting a critical volume must be reached before the fluids are moved onwards. Various substances have been shown to increase contractility, e.g. bile acids and fatty acids including short-chain fatty acids.

Basis of motility

Colonic muscles have periodic fluctuations of membrane potential ('slow waves' or 'pace-setter potentials'). These start in the longitudinal muscle and pass rapidly and concentrically to circular muscle layers. When excitatory neurotransmitters act on the muscle, spiking and contractions occur. Spikes develop when the membrane potential is maximally depolarized, possibly initiated by the pace-setter potentials. Slow waves are inconsistently present in the human colonic circular muscle, but are recorded more regularly from the longitudinal muscle. The amplitude and frequency of slow waves are sensitive to stretch and to potential stimulatory or inhibitory transmitters.

When electrical oscillations of either muscle layer exceed a frequency of $12–14\ min^{-1}$, individual contractions often fuse as relaxation is incomplete. 'Long spike bursts' of electrical activity in the colon are probably due to this phenomenon. Short spike bursts do not propagate, whereas long spike bursts propagate over long distances.

Colonic muscular contractions may be recorded as changes in intraluminal pressure measured by perfused open-tipped catheters or by small balloons. Movements can be monitored by strain gauges on the serosal surface of the bowel, or by the transit of contents using markers passing through a segment of bowel or the mean transit time of radioopaque solids or radionucleotides.

Disordered motility patterns have been described in both irritable bowel disease and symptomatic colonic diverticulosis. The introduction of coarse wheat bran to the diet of sufferers from the latter is very effective in reducing symptoms. The former is a more complex problem wherein life styles and coping mechanisms are more important, though an increase in wheat bran intake may help some sufferers.

The ileocaecal valve provides a barrier to the reflux of colonic contents into the ileum. Entry of contents into the caecum and reflux of colonic contents are controlled by the integrated actions of the ileocolonic junction and the ileocaecal sphincter. Ileal emptying in humans is intermittent. The distal ileum and the proximal colon act in concert to regulate ileocolonic transit.

The movement of chyme along the colon can be regarded as flow in a disperse system, but does not take account of turbulent flow conditions. During flow through the colon, there can be intense agitation of the contents of the colon, with resultant effects on boundary or surface layers during the flow. The different layers have a physical effect on each other, with substances diffusing from one layer to another. The rate of movement in the centre of the tube is different from that at the boundary layer; the further from the wall, the greater the decrease in fluid velocity. This means that different fractions of intestinal contents will move along the gastrointestinal tract at different rates. This has profound consequences for both the aerobic and anaerobic colonic bacterial population.

Transit through the large intestine takes some 36–48 h, the transit times being comparable in the right colon, the left colon and the rectosigmoid. Faeces move backwards and forwards and stools may be retained for long periods in the right half of the colon. The more viscous polysaccharides extend the mouth to caecum and caecum to rectum transit time; guar, tragacanth and pectin being slower than wheat bran. Total time within the large intestine may well influence contact time between chyme and the mucosa and also the time available for bacterial enzymes to interact with the faecal contents.

Mass movements

Migrating bursts of contractions associated with defaecation consist of contractions at higher force and increased migration velocity. Bursts of electrical spiking activity occasionally seem to propagate over the entire length of the bowel with a 30 s duration and superimposed on high-frequency control oscillations. The propagation velocity of these ranges from $1\ cm\ s^{-1}$ to $16\ cm\ s^{-1}$ with an average of $9\ cm\ s^{-1}$. This activity is associated with propulsive contractile activity over a large part of the colon. Mass movements result in defaecation.

Diurnal patterns

A stimulus is needed to elicit peristaltic activity. Increased colonic output has been related to propagating bursts of spiking activity associated with propulsive contractions. These bursts of spiking activity are observed 1 h after a meal. Propagation can occur over a short section of the colon at about $4\ cm\ s^{-1}$ or from the right colon to the rectosigmoid junction at about $9\ cm\ s^{-1}$. The burst of activity recurs repetitively with a duration of 15–20 s.

In the 2 h period following a meal, the total duration of long spike bursts increases by 16–130%. Short spike burst occurrence does not change with meals. A minimum colonic load of 1.25 MJ (300 kcal) is needed to induce a colonic motor response. Motor responses depend on the type of food ingested. Ingestion of 2.5 MJ (600 kcal), of fat induces a response but isoenergetic amounts of protein or carbohydrate do not. During sleep, migrating long spike bursts are absent. Propulsive contractions over the whole length of the colon with a mean frequency of four per 24 h at a propagation velocity of approximately $1\ cm\ s^{-1}$ are associated with an urge to defaecate.

Anorectal functions

The main function of the ascending colon is faecal storage. Most contractile activity is segmental, promoting both absorption and mixing of gut contents. Electrical oscillatory activity at frequencies of 6–12 cycles per minute or short spike bursts of less than

5 s duration occur within the same frequency. These electrical activities occur in the circular muscle layer and do not propel intestinal contents onwards. The effect is to generate segmental circular muscle contractions, and for a time to retain the contents in one place in the colon.

The holding action of the anal sphincter retains stool, resulting in faecal storage in the rectum. The rectal wall accommodates to distension by faecal residue, having a viscoelastic property that allows reservoir continence. The rate of distension and the degree to which the rectum expands determine the urge to defecate.

Colonic Fermentation and Absorption

The colon can be regarded as two organs. The right side of the colon is a fermenter, with considerable absorptive capacity and more electrolyte absorption than the left side, which is a conserver and regulator of faecal output (**Fig. 4**). The colon is involved in salvage and excretion of:

1. nutrients;
2. chemicals excreted in the bile.

The salvage is primarily that of nutrients, particularly resistant starch, proteins, fats, water and secreted mucoproteins. Bacteria modify these compounds before their absorption. Biliary excreted or digested chemicals may be bacterially modified and conserved in the enterohepatic circulation, or may be excreted in the faeces intact or bacterially altered.

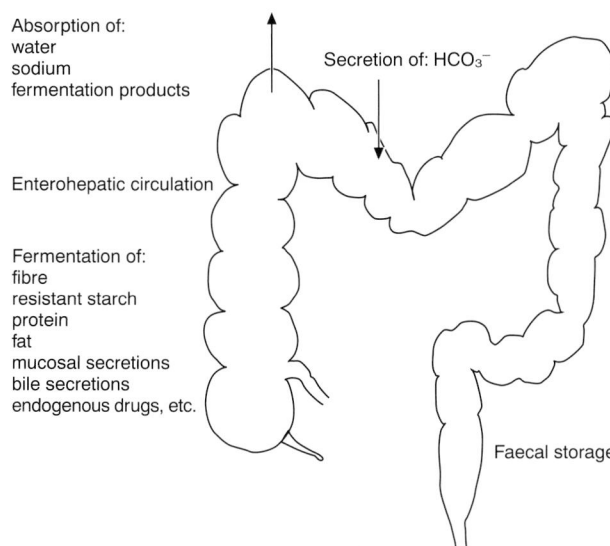

Figure 4 Colonic function: fermentation, absorption, faecal formation and faecal storage.

Absorption

The multiple physical phases in the colon are important in affecting colonic metabolism, absorption and evacuation of faeces.

Two mechanisms bring nutrients into contact with the epithelium. The first is the intestinal contractions, creating turbulence. Secondly, convection currents direct luminal contents from the centre of the lumen to the epithelial surface. The physical interactions include filtration as different components pass through to the colonic epithelium at individual rates, largely determined by component size. Increased luminal content viscosity alters both convection and diffusion of the nutrients.

Colonic bacteria

The colonic flora is a complex ecosystem of more than 400 bacterial species. Anaerobic bacteria outnumber the facultative organisms 100-fold. The total bacterial count in faeces is 10^{10}–10^{12} colony-forming units per ml. The colonic flora of a single individual is remarkably constant over prolonged periods, although there are wide variations in the microflora between individuals. The colonic bacteria should be viewed not as single contributors, but as a total caecal bacterial complex, an organ of intense metabolic activity, complementary to the liver in the enterohepatic circulation. The colonic bacterial flora receive nutrition from the ileum, from dietary and endogenous sources. The dietary sources have neither been digested nor absorbed in the upper intestine. The physical status of the bacteria, whether surface or luminal, adsorbed to solid nutrient material (e.g. fibre) or mucus, influences their growth and metabolic activity.

Colonic bacterial activity is mainly reductive, in contrast to the liver which is oxidative. The wide range of colonic bacterial metabolic transformations include such major enzymes as azoreductase, nitrate reductase, nitroreductase, β-glucosidase and β-glucuronidase. The processes of anaerobic caecal bacterial metabolism are complex and varied, leading to partial or complete breakdown with the end products being absorbed and reexcreted in the enterohepatic circulation, absorbed from the colon to be utilized as nutrients, or excreted in stool.

Bile acids, a degradation product of cholesterol, are conserved in an enterohepatic circulation. The amount and type of bile acids returning to the liver in the portal vein or lost in faeces are important in the control of cholesterol degradation to bile acids. Some gums and pectins reduce ileal bile acid reabsorption thereby increasing the amount of bile acids reaching the colon. In the caecum, bile acids are adsorbed to dietary fibre, increasing faecal loss and thereby reducing body cholesterol. Other fibres, e.g. gum arabic, decrease serum cholesterol without increasing faecal bile acid excretion. The most effective dietary fibres in influencing sterol metabolism (e.g. pectin) are fermented in the colon. Such fibres probably alter colonic bile acid metabolism through altering bacterial metabolism. The mechanism is either by influencing the type of bile acid which is absorbed and returns to the liver in the portal vein, or (more certainly) by the increased numbers of bacteria sequestrating bile acids and increasing faecal loss.

Dietary fibre: nonstarch polysaccharide

An important influence on colonic function is dietary fibre or nonstarch polysaccharide (NSP). Dietary fibre is best regarded as the unabsorbed remnant of plant foods resistant to hydrolysis by human alimentary digestive enzymes. A series of analytical methods have been developed by Southgate, Van Soest and Asp, all improved upon by Englyst and Cummings. However, measuring dietary fibre quantitatively is an incomplete measurement because of the varied actions of the many sources, types and preparations of dietary fibre. Fibre may to varying degrees modulate gastric emptying time, nutrient absorption, caecal metabolism, sterol metabolism and stool weight and constitution.

The fermentation of fibre yields hydrogen, methane and short-chain fatty acids (SCFA) and other polysaccharide degradation products. When pectin in which the methyl, acetyl and C6 are labelled with ^{14}C is fed to rats, the majority of the pectin metabolized in the colon is excreted as carbon dioxide; however, ^{14}C is found in hepatic glycerol phospholipids, protein amino acids and cholesterol esters. The fermentation products of fibre pass into a wide but specific range of metabolites. Similar results have been found with gelatinized bean starch and resistant starch uniformly labelled with ^{14}C.

Hydrogen can be measured in the breath and has a diurnal variation, with its nadir at midday and at maximum some 2 h after meals. The amount exhaled differs with the polysaccharide source. Disaccharides generate hydrogen more rapidly than trisaccharides, and oligosaccharides are the slowest. More complex carbohydrates are fermented more slowly, a process that requires the induction of specific enzymes.

There are wide differences in the proportion of breath methane exhalers between different healthy adult populations, ranging from 33% to 80%. The breath methane status of an individual remains stable throughout the day and over prolonged periods. Yet fermentation of faeces from all healthy individuals will always produce methane. This suggests that everyone produces methane in their caecum, but a critical amount must be produced to spill over into the breath. Methane-producing organisms are strict anaerobes. Significant bacterial methane production only occurs if sulfate-reducing bacteria are not active. The metabolic end product of sulfate reduction could be toxic to methanogenic bacteria. When sulfate is present, sulfate-reducing bacteria have a higher substrate affinity for hydrogen than methanogenic bacteria.

Carbohydrates such as pectin, gum arabic, oligosaccharides and resistant starch are fermented in the colon to short-chain fatty acids (SCFA) (acetic, propionic and n-butyric, molar ratio 60:20:15), carbon dioxide, hydrogen and methane. Small amounts of isobutyrate, valerate and isovalerate, particularly branched-chain fatty acids, originate from protein degradation. Its has been estimated that 40–50 g of carbohydrate will yield 400–500 mmol total SCFA, 240–300 mmol acetate and 80–100 mmol each of propionate and butyrate.

The SCFA are readily absorbed by the colon. Human colonic SCFA absorption is concentration-dependent and involves bicarbonate secretion, a process independent of the chloride-bicarbonate exchange. It is possible that there is also mucosal acetate-bicarbonate exchange. SCFA stimulate sodium absorption from the colonic lumen, involving the recycling of hydrogen ions. Un-ionized SCFA cross into the colonic mucosal cell and dissociate, and hydrogen ions return to the lumen in exchange for sodium. Colonic water absorption is also dependent upon SCFA absorption.

Of the SCFA, only acetic acid is measurable in the systemic circulation. Propionic acid is metabolized in the liver. Butyric acid is used as a fuel by the colonic mucosa. SCFA and butyric acid in particular may be the preferred energy sources and potent stimulants of cellular proliferation in the colon.

SCFA are the predominant anions in human faeces. On the usual intake of fermentable carbohydrate, faecal SCFA concentrations and molar ratios remain relatively constant. Faecal SCFA estimations do not reflect caecal and colonic fermentation.

The different ways in which dietary fibre or NSP affects colonic function can be grouped into three functional types:

1. *Guar gum and pectin:* increased caecal fermentation and increased SCFA production, but no effect on stool output.
2. *Tragacanth, karaya, xanthan:* a reduced effect on

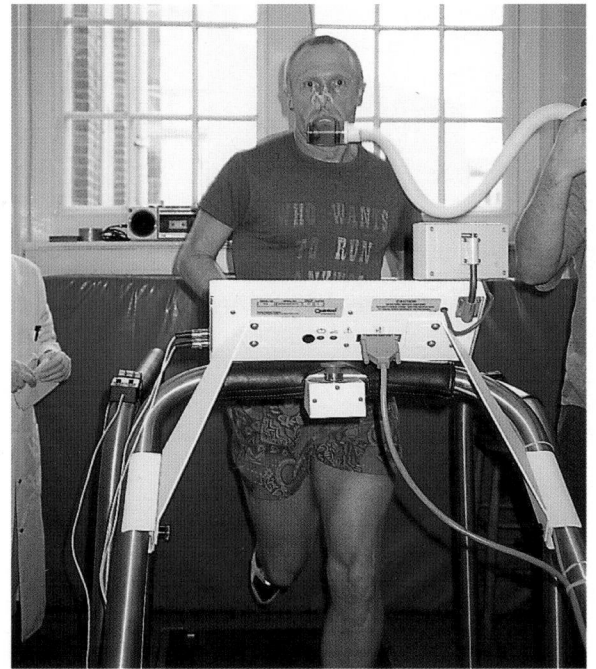

Plate 1 Energy. Indirect calorimetry instrument to measure energy expenditure by gas exchange. (With permission from W. Walker/ Chichester Institute of Higher Education).

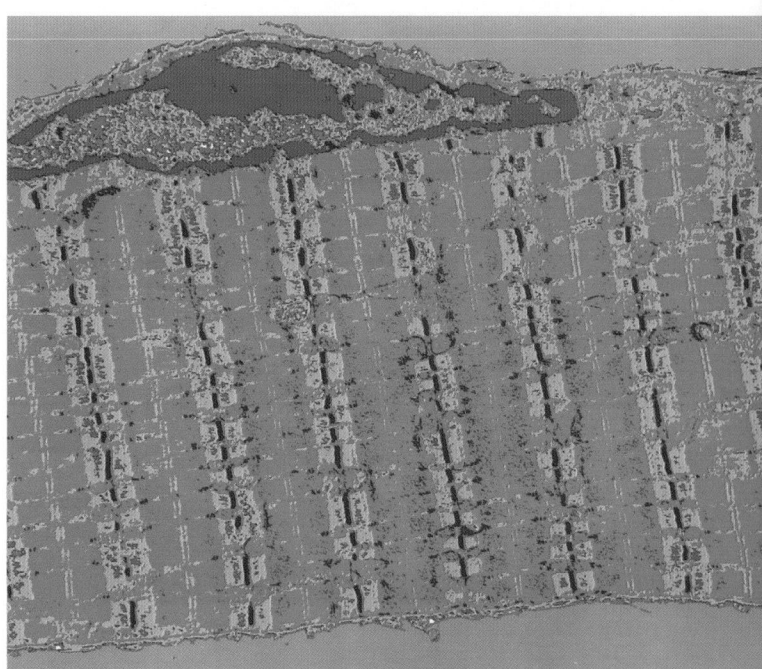

Plate 2 Striated muscle. Coloured transmission electron micrograph (TEM) of a longitudinal section through striated skeletal muscle. The striated banding pattern of the muscle fibrils is seen. The fibrils run in parallel (from left to right) and between them runs sarcoplasmic reticulum that transmits nerve impulses to the fibrils. At the top is a cell nucleus (purple). Within each fibril are contactile units called sarcomers, separated by black lines. A sarcomere has protein filaments of myosin (red) and actin (green) that slide over each other, thereby causing the whole muscle to contract. (With permission from Quest/ Science Photo Library).

Plate 3 Oils and fats. Assortment of dietary oils and fats. In the front row are butter, lard and soya margarine. The back row has oil made from (left to right): corn (maize), sunflowers, groundnuts (peanuts) and olives. (With permission from Cordelia Molloy/ Science Photo Library).

Plate 4 Fetal development and later disease. Babies of different weights and sizes at birth. (With permission from MRC Southampton).

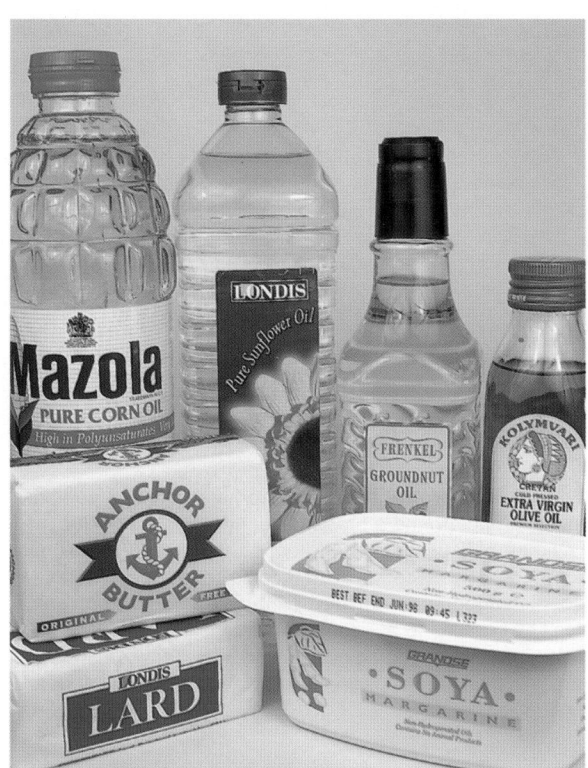

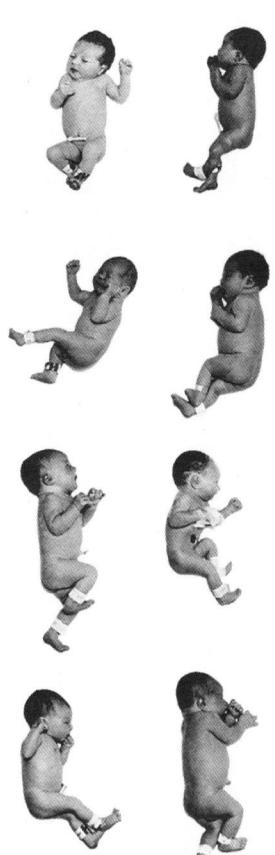

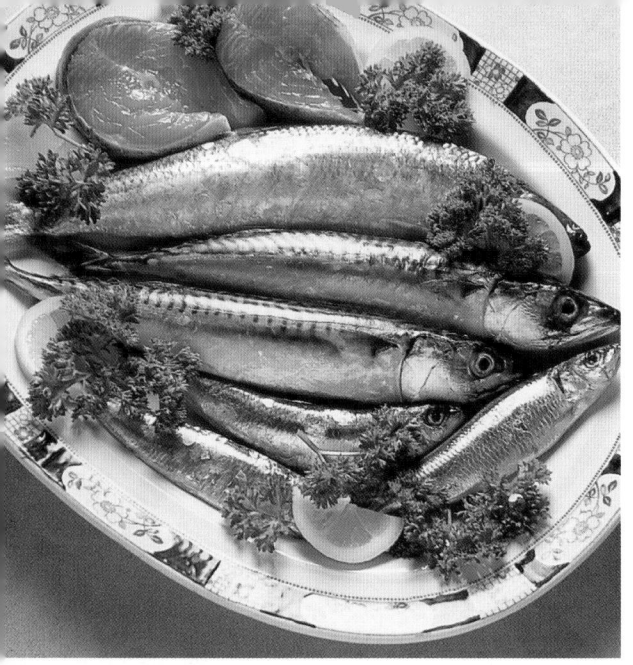

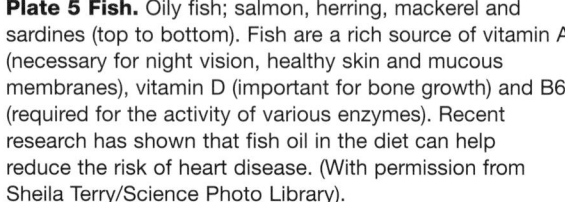

Plate 6 Pesticides. Late spraying barley with fungicide. (With permission from CTC/Zeneca).

Plate 5 Fish. Oily fish; salmon, herring, mackerel and sardines (top to bottom). Fish are a rich source of vitamin A (necessary for night vision, healthy skin and mucous membranes), vitamin D (important for bone growth) and B6 (required for the activity of various enzymes). Recent research has shown that fish oil in the diet can help reduce the risk of heart disease. (With permission from Sheila Terry/Science Photo Library).

Plate 7 (below) **Confectionery production.** Workers by a conveyer belt on a production line at a chocolate factory. They are removing defective bars of chocolate as part of quality control. Chocolate is made from cocoa beans which are the seeds of the cacao tree, *Theobroma cacao*. Chocolate is a source of carbohydrates, fats, protein, vitamins and minerals. (With permission from Rosenfeld Images Ltd/Science Photo Library).

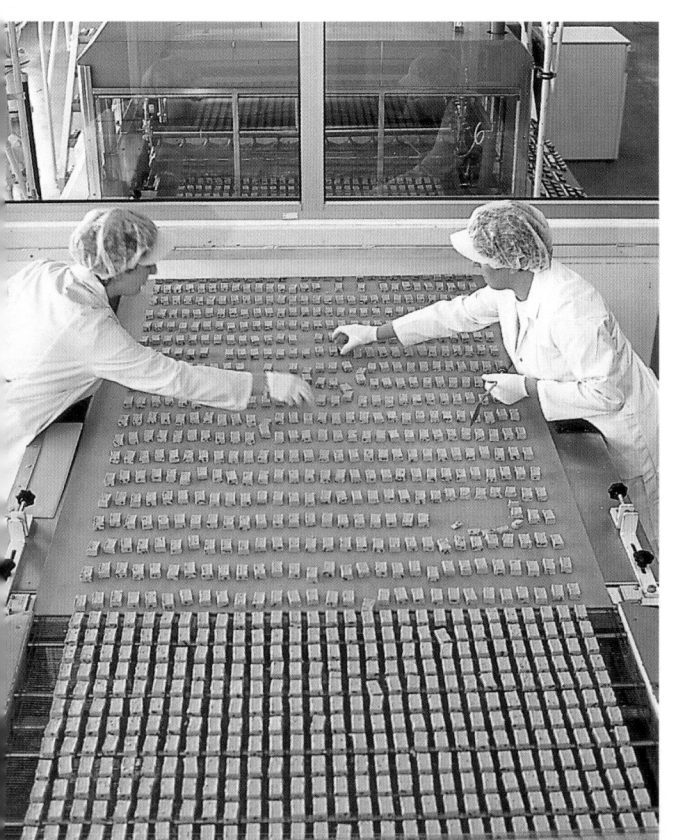

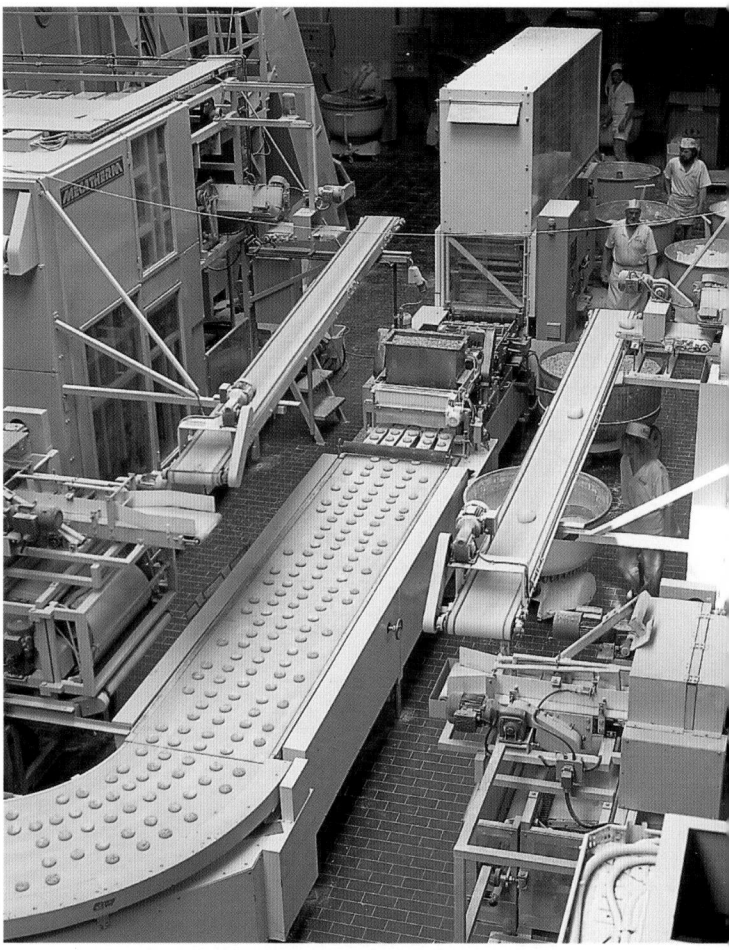

Plate 8 (above) **Bread production line.** Workers watching portions of dough being carried around a bread bakery on conveyer belts. Dough is a mixture of flour, water or milk and usually some sugar, salt and fat. If light, porous, leavened bread is to be made, the yeast of baking powder is added as well. These produce carbon dioxide gas, which causes tiny bubbles to appear in the dough mixture. The dough is baked into bread, inspected, packaged and then distributed to customers. (With permission from Rosenfeld Images Ltd/Science Photo Library).

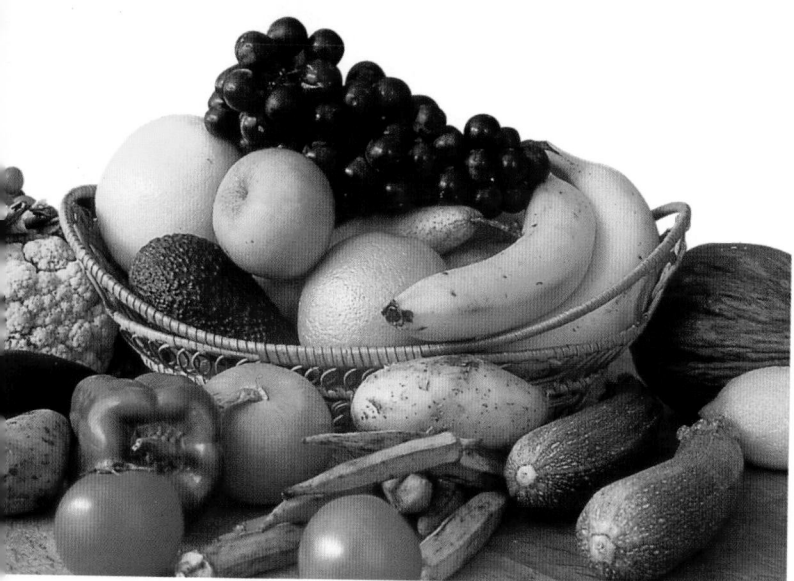

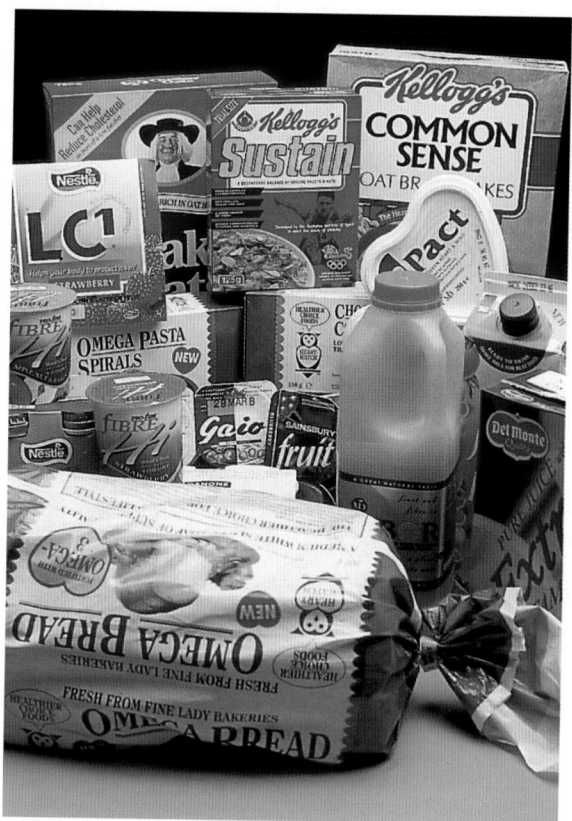

Plate 9 *(above)* **Fruits and vegetables.** A selection of fruits and vegetables. (With permission from CTC/Zeneca).

Plate 10 *(right)* **Functional foods.** A selection of pre-packaged foods. (With permission from John Young/Leatherhead Food RA).

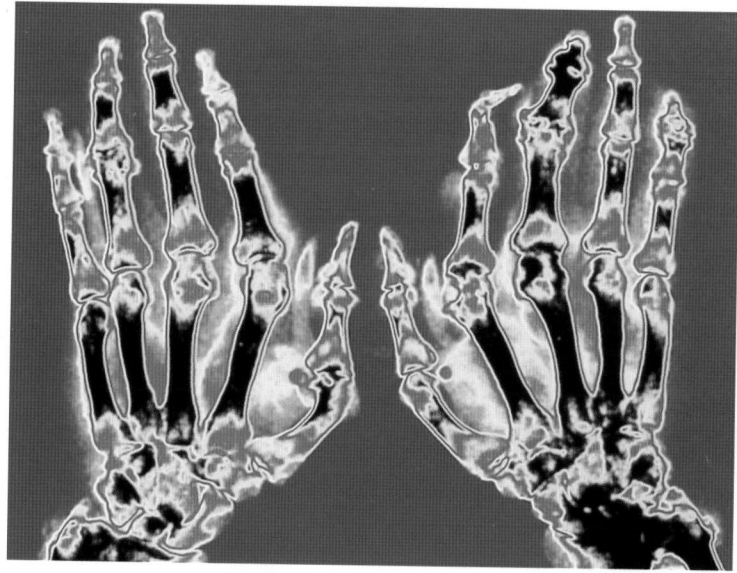

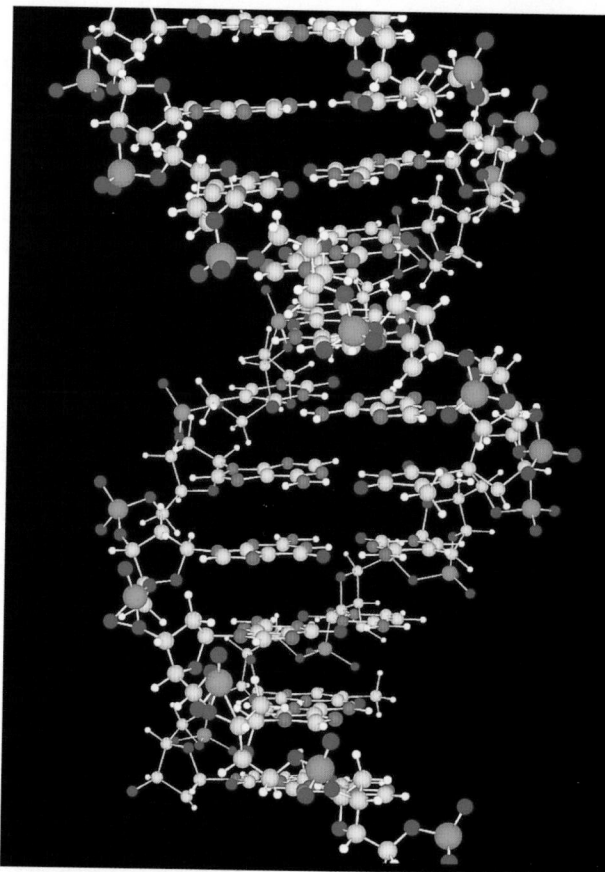

Plate 11 *(above)* **Gouty hand.** Coloured X-ray image of the hands of a patient suffering from gout. The joints between the individual bones are clearly swollen and arthritis has caused bone erosion in several finger joints. Gout is caused by a defect in uric acid metabolism. This causes an excess of uric acid and its salts (sodium urate) to accumulate in the bloodstream and the joints. These collect in the joint capsules causing an acute inflammation, with accompanying swelling, redness and pain. Gout has traditionally been associated with overeating and overdrinking. Treatment involves the use of anti-inflammatory drugs and abstention from rich foods and excessive alcohol. (With permission from Alfred Pasieka/Science Photo Library).

Plate 12 *(above right)* **DNA molecule.** Computer graphic and stick model representing a segment of the molecule *Deoxyribonucleic Acid* (DNA). This is the alpha form of the DNA in that the spiral winds anti-clockwise when viewed from above. DNA contains the inherited instructions that produce a living organism. Atoms are depicted as colour-coded balls with stick bonds: phosphorus (orange), oxygen (red), carbon (grey), nitrogen (blue), and hydrogen (white). The DNA molecule is made of two strands of atoms twisted into a helical shape. Each strand consists of an outer sugar-phosphate backbone (orange-red), from which nucleotide bases project (grey-blue). The bases are paired forming the genetic code. (With permission from Alfred Pasieka/Science Photo Library).

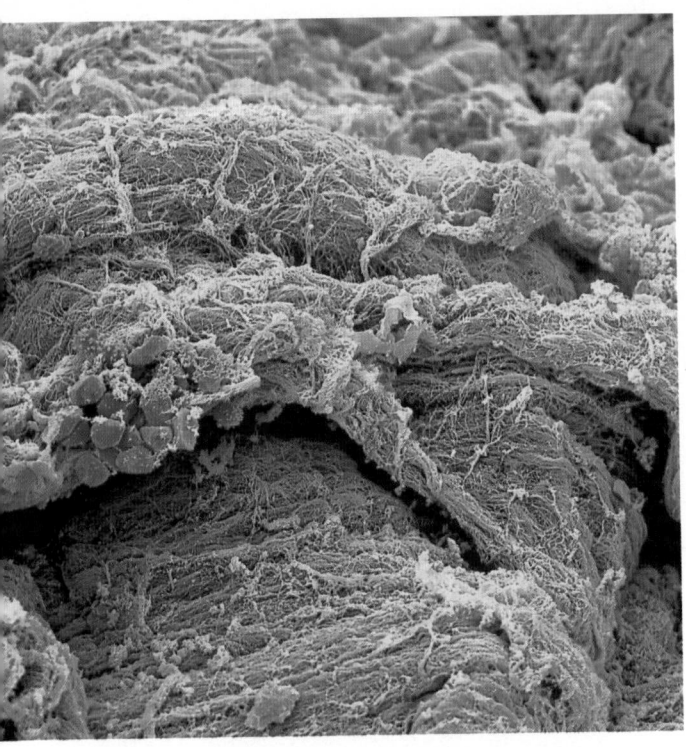

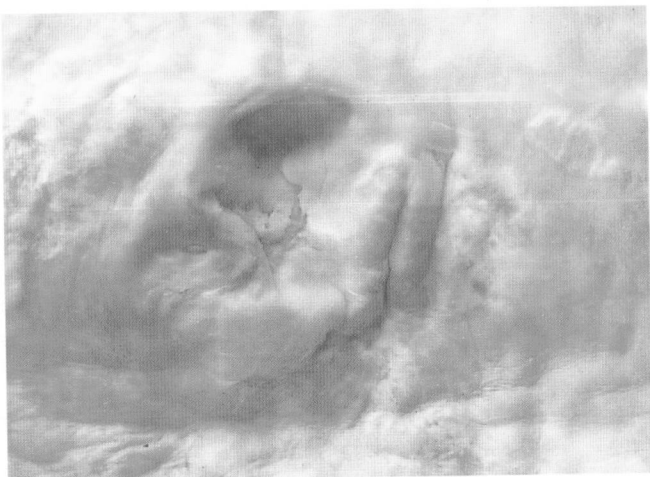

Plate 13 *(above)* **Atheroma.** View of the lining of a human aorta showing fatty plaques of atheroma. Atheroma is a mixture of low-density lipoproteins, decaying muscle cells, fibrous tissue, clumps of blood, platelets and cholesterol. The plaques narrow the arteries causing the disease atherosclerosis. The deposits interfere with blood flow and can trigger the formation of abnormal clots that block arteries. (With permission from Science Pictures Ltd/Science Photo Library).

Plate 15 *(above)* **Atherosclerosis.** Coloured Scanning Electron Micrograph of the surface of a plaque (atheroma) which is partially blocking an artery to cause atherosclerosis. The plaque consists of a deposit containing a mixture of fats (such as cholesterol) and proteins (such as fibrin) which appears yellow/green. A number of dead blood cells (*erythrocytes*, red) lie of the atheromaís surface. (With permission from Eye of Science/Science Photo Library).

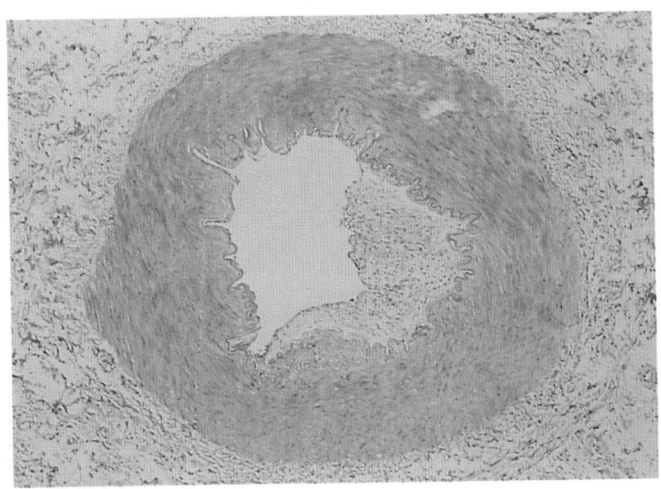

Plate 14 *(right)* **Atherosclerosis.** Light Micrograph of a cross section through an artery with mild atheroma. The artery wall is pink. The formation of a fatty plaque or atheroma (grey, centre) has greatly narrowed the side of the artery lumen (white, centre). This causes a considerable reduction in blood flow. In severe cases heart attacks or stroke may occur. The condition occurs naturally with aging but is accelerated by high fat diets, cigarette smoking, obesity and inactivity. (With permission from Biophoto Associates/Science Photo Library).

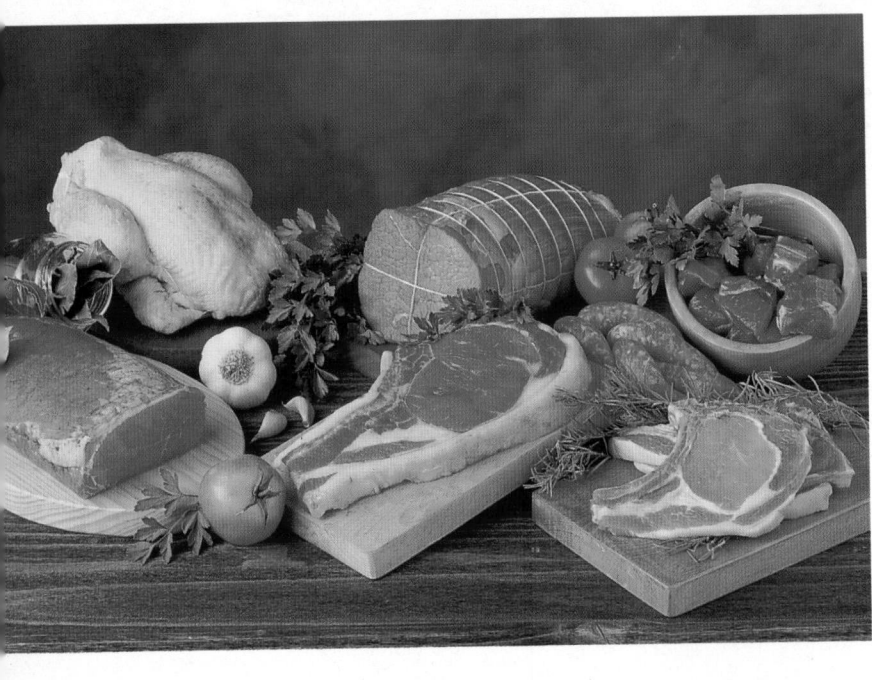

Plate 16 Assorted meats. A selection of fresh meats–chicken, ham, lamb and pork chops, and beef pieces. (With permission from Ricardo Arias, Latin Stock/Science Photo Library).

caecal colonic activity, increased caecal SCFA and increased faecal water and weight.

3. *Gellan, ispaghula, wheat bran:* no increase in caecal SCFA concentration, but an increase in faecal SCFA output (wet and dry weights).

Other examples of colonic metabolism

Salicylazosulfapyridine Salicylazosulfapyridine (5-aminosalicylic acid moiety joined through an azo link to sulfapyridine) is used in the treatment of ulcerative colitis. Less than 10% is absorbed from the small intestine. The remainder passes to the colon where bacteria split the 5-aminosalicylic acid from the sulfapyridine, which is absorbed. The majority of the 5-aminosalicylic acid passes through the colon and is excreted in stool.

Beetroot Beetroot pigment is a red pigment which is excreted in the urine (beeturia) and faeces by approximately 14% of the population. The beetroot vegetable is rich in oxalic acid, a reducing agent and antioxidant. The beetroot pigment itself is a redox indicator and sensitive to oxidation, which is readily decolorized by gastric acid and colonic bacteria, a decolorization that does not happen in the presence of oxalic acid. Thus beeturia occurs in individuals in whom a critical amount of oxalic acid passes down into the colon, protecting the red pigment from bacterial decolorization before colonic absorption and urinary excretion. Individuals not having beeturia may have insufficient colonic oxalic acid to protect the colour, and excrete the pigment as a brown metabolite in urine.

Faeces

Studies of stool weight

Many population studies of faecal weight and bowel habit have resulted from the Burkitt and Trowell hypothesis that colon cancer, faecal weight and dietary fibre intake are closely related. Painter proposed that colonic diverticulosis and dietary fibre intake are related. The hypothesis is that the high dietary fibre intake of Africans is protective against colonic disease, mediated through a faecal weight of 200–500 g per day. It has been suggested that for individuals living in Western societies a dietary fibre intake of 25 g per day (fibre source not defined) and a stool weight of 150 g per day are protective against colonic cancer. In one Scottish study in individuals aged 18–80 years the faecal weight in men was 100 ± 50 g and in women 75 ± 34 g on a daily dietary fibre intake of 16 g (men) and 13 g (women). The range of mean daily stool weights was 15 g to 280 g.

The individual variation over 7 days was 25 g to 250 g per day. Bowel frequency in Britain is one bowel movement per day (range three times a day to every third day). All these wide variations make a simple method of defining normal colon function difficult. The fit and active elderly show no difference in stool weight from the young, in contrast to the frail elderly where stool output may fall to less than 50 g per 24 h.

Effect of fibre on stool weight

There have been few studies of how the colon adjusts to the addition of fibre to the diet over time and the effect on stool weight; 3 weeks is the usual trial period, a convenient rather than a physiological time period. Different fibres have different effects on stool weight.

Stool consists of a mixture of water (75%), bacteria (12%) and residual fibre (12%). Wheat bran increases stool weight in a linear manner and decreases intestinal transit time, independent of the initial stool weight. Wholemeal bread has little or no effect on stool weight. The particle size and water-holding capacity of the wheat bran is all-important. Coarse wheat bran is more effective than fine wheat bran. The greater the water-holding capacity of the bran, the greater the effect on stool weight. The water bound by the bran also dilutes but does not increase the output of faecal constituents, e.g. bile acids, and hence their concentration decreases. The increment in stool weight per gram of wheat bran varies in different populations. For control subjects the increase in stool weight, depending on bran particle size, is 3–5 g wet stool weight per gram of fibre. In patients with irritable bowel syndrome and symptomatic diverticulosis the increment is 1–2 g wet stool weight per gram of fibre. **Table 1** summarizes some experiments with fibre supplementation in human subjects and the effects on faecal weight.

Colonic microbial growth may be stimulated by fermentable fibre sources as apple, guar or pectin, which have little or no effect on stool weight. There may also be an added osmotic effect of products of bacterial fermentation on stool mass. Pectin is fermented very rapidly, ispaghula slowly and wheat bran hardly at all. Colonic SCFA concentration relates to faecal water. Continued fermentation in the distal colon of some complex carbohydrates, e.g. ispaghula, results in increased faecal SCFA; faecal water, osmolality and stool weight.

The formation of faeces

The ileal contents change across the colon from a viscid material to a malleable, plasticine material. During this change, the nature of the physical state

Table 1 The efficacy of a fibre may be expressed as wet stool increment per gram of ingested fibre. This varies from fibre to fibre. The higher the g wet stool weight increase per g ingested fibre, the more effective is the fibre in increasing stool weight and hence improving laxation. The table summarizes the results of three separate studies

Fibre supplement	g wet stool increment per gram fibre
Citrus pectin	0.3
Gum arabic	0.6
Potato fibre	1.5
Gum karaya	0.4
Fruit, vegetables and bread	3.4
Fruit and vegetables	4.9
Raw carrot	5.8
Gum tragacanth	6·3
Wheat bran[a]	7.9
	10.5

[a]Results from two separate studies.

dictates events in the colon. The phases in the colon include solid, liquid, colloidal and gas bubble phases, as well as hydrophobic and hydrophilic and possibly micellar phases. Plasticization is an increase in workability, flexibility and extensibility. Water is the most important plasticizer in biological systems, changing mobility and rheologic viscoelastic and mechanical properties.

Water is all-important in the gastrointestinal tract. It is present largely as free fluid but is also held within bacterial cells and residual nutrients (fibre, resistant starch and protein). The traditional concept of 'bound water' suggested discrete free and bound physical states of water (free, loosely bound and tightly bound states) in a complex system. The terms 'bound' and 'free' imply that there are two types of water, which can be distinguished chemically or physically. The terms 'plasticizing' and 'nonplasticizing' describe two different operational conditions for different amounts of water, but not different types of water. The solute specific value is the maximum amount of water that can act as a plasticizer or a particular solute, rather than the amount of water that is bound. The less mobile water molecules are freely exchangeable with all of the water in the solution, i.e. the water is not bound. In the development of the plasticine form, the initial sorbed water fraction is most strongly plasticizing and unfreezable or bound. The later sorbed water fraction is nonplasticizing, freezable, and is free, mobile or loosely bound.

Polymers

Polymers in the colon may be in several and changing forms, secondary to the constituents and their con-

centration in the luminal contents and bacterial degradation of these polysaccharides. The mechanism whereby polymers contribute to the translation of a viscous ileal fluid to a Plasticine-like faecal material is uncertain. This process may well include concentration of the colonic contents, colloids, gels, sols and lipid-containing micelles and bacteria. In the gastrointestinal tract there are complex lipid–micellar–aqueous–hydrocolloid phases. Colloids can be lyophilic (solvent-attracting) or lyophobic (solvent-repelling), and hydrophilic or hydrophobic in water. Sols are dispersions of solids in liquids, which consist of water, free monomers and small aggregates coexisting within and intimately dispersed throughout the liquid-solid phase network. Gels contain two dispersed components or phases: one gives a solid character to the gel and the other is a liquid. A conversion from sol to gel involves aggregation and growth of particles or macromolecules with periods of very rapid growth in aggregate size. At a critical point of aggregation, the gel point, viscosity changes rapidly and a gel network or gel phase results. Gel point is dependent upon pH, ionic strength, presence of small particles and specific ions and the aqueous and lipid environment.

Micelles are stable, colloid-sized clusters of lipids held in a detergent, at concentrations above the critical micelle concentration. An important small intestinal micelle consists of bile acids, triacylglycerols, cholesterol and di- and monoacylglycerols. It is not known if micelles exist in the colonic contents, but if they do they could contribute to the formation of a stool readily moving along the colon.

In the colon water is distributed in three ways:

1. free water which can be absorbed from the colon;
2. water that is incorporated into bacterial mass;
3. water that is held by fibre.

The effect of fibre in the colon may be summarized as:

Stool weight =
$$W_f (1 + H_f) + W_b(1 + H_b) + W_m(1 + H_m)$$

where W_f, W_b and W_m are, respectively, the dry weights of: fibre remaining after fermentation in the colon, bacteria present in the faeces, and osmotically active metabolites and other substances in the colonic contents which could reduce the amount of free water absorbed; and H_f, H_b and H_m denote their respective water-holding capacities (i.e. the weight of water resistant to absorption from the colon, per unit dry weight of each faecal constituent).

See also: **Colonic Diseases and Disorders**: Nutritional

Management. **Dietary Fibre (Fiber)**: Physiological Effects and Effects on Absorption. **Fatty Acids**: Metabolism. **Gastrointestinal Tract**: Structure and Function of the Small Intestine. **Microflora of the Intestine**: Role and Effects.

Further Reading

Eastwood MA (1992) The physiological effect of dietary fibre: an update. *Annual Review of Nutrition* **12**:19–36.

Kirsner JB and Shorter RG (1988) *Diseases of the Colon, Rectum and Anal Canal.* Baltimore: Williams & Wilkins.

Kritchevsky D and Bonfield C (1995) *Dietary Fiber in Health and Disease.* St Paul: Eagan Press.

Molerus O (1993) *Principles of Flow in Disperse Systems.* London: Chapman & Hall.

Phillips SF, Pemberton JH and Shorter RG (1991) *The Large Intestine: Physiology, Pathophysiology and Disease.* New York: Raven Press.

Geriatric nutrition *see* **Older People**: Nutritional Requirements; Physiological Changes; Nutritionally Related Problems; Nutritional Management of Geriatric Patients.

GLUCOSE

Contents

Chemistry, Dietary Sources and Glycaemic Index

David J A Jenkins, St Michael's Hospital, Ontario, Canada

Copyright © 1998 Academic Press

Glucose and its polymers are important energy sources for living organisms and structural components of plants. Because of the diversity of compounds in which glucose occurs it may be helpful first to discuss nomenclature.

Nomenclature and Chemical Structure

Glucose

The compound D-glucose (Greek *gleucos*, 'sweet wine') or dextrose is 2,3,4,5,6-pentahydroxyhexaldehyde, more conventionally expressed as $C_6H_{12}O_6$, with a molecular weight of 180.16. Glucose is readily soluble in water, in powder form. Below 50°C, α-D-glucose hydrate is the stable form, at 50°C the anhydrous form is obtained, and at higher temperatures, β-D-glucose is obtained. Glucose is also present in the diet as part of the disaccharides sucrose (glucose and fructose) and lactose (glucose and galactose).

Glucose oligosaccharides

Oligosaccharides (Greek *oligo*, 'few') are sugar polymers; the term usually refers to compounds containing 2 to 9 units, but may include polymers containing up to 19 units. The dimer, trimer and tetramer forms in which glucose molecules are joined by (1–4) linkages are referred to as maltose, maltotriose and maltotetrose, since these substances are the products of starch digestion in the malting process.

Starches

Starches are large molecular weight, α-linked polymers of glucose $(C_6H_{10}O_5)_n$. Most starches show a mixture of α(1–4) and α(1–6) linkages. The α(1–4)-linked polymer forms a linear structure which allows for hydrogen bonding between polymer chains and a more compact starch structure. Introduction of (1–6) linkages introduces branch points and a more open structure which allows the (1–4) linked backbone with the hemiacetal bond in the alpha configuration to coil like a spring into a helical form. Branched starches with the (1–6) linked are more readily hydrated and digested in contrast to the (1–4)-linked linear starch. The (1–4)-linked starches are referred to as *amylose starch* and (1–6)-linked starches are *amylopectin starches*.

Resistant starch

Resistant starches are defined by their resistance to digestion in the human upper gastrointestinal tract. As with the term 'dietary fibre', the definition is largely physiological. One proposed classification divides resistant starches into three classes: RS_1, RS_2 and RS_3. The first class, RS_1, is starch that escapes small intestinal digestion owing to the food form and incomplete enzymatic attack (e.g. large particle size or compact nature of food, or starch entrapment by dietary fibre). The second, RS_2, includes the more crystalline starches which resist digestion (e.g. high-amylose starches which resist gelatinization). The RS_3 starches are retrograded starches (e.g. high-amylose starches which on cooling after cooking form a compact, hydrogen-bonded crystalline structure which excludes water).

Cellulose

Like starch, cellulose is a (1–4)-linked glucose polymer $(C_6H_{10}O_5)_n$, but in this instance the glucose molecules are β-linked allowing the development of a linear polymer with strong intrachain hydrogen bonding. Cellulose polymers may consist of as many as 10 000 glucose monomer units. Cellulose is both resistant to small intestinal digestion and insoluble in cold or hot water and most dilute acids and alkali. It is partially degraded by colonic bacteria; the proportion degraded is dependent on the source, with cellulose from vegetables broken down to a greater extent than cellulose from cereals, such as wheat.

Beta-glucans

In many ways, these predominantly β(1–4)-linked glucose polymers are the cellulose equivalent of the starch amylopectin. Here, it is the β(1–3) linkages interspersed throughout the polymer that prevent the compact structure achieved with the cellulose polymer where only the β(1–4) linkages exist. As a result of the more open molecular structure of the β-glucan, unlike cellulose, it is readily hydrated and soluble in water, forming a solution of high viscosity. The viscosity in turn is dependent on the molecular weight and the presence of the (1–3) linkages. The greater the molecular weight, the greater the viscosity. Thus reduction of molecular weight by acid or enzymatic hydrolysis, which may also occur during food processing, may greatly reduce viscosity. The common feature shared by both cellulose and the β-glucans is that both are resistant to digestion by small intestinal enzymes. However, whereas cellulose is only partially fermented by the colonic bacteria, β-glucans are completely fermented.

Hemicellulose

The term 'hemicellulose' should not be taken to imply a class of β(1–4)-linked glucose polymers. The similarity with cellulose lies not in the chemical structure but in the fact that hemicellulose is also insoluble in hot or cold water or hot dilute acid. It is, however, soluble in dilute alkali. The polymeric structure is heterosaccharitic with two or more sugars, e.g. arabinoxylans found in cereals, with a relatively small molecular size (50–200 saccharide units).

Occurrence

Glucose is the primary carbohydrate energy source of vertebrates. In healthy humans, fasting blood glucose levels lie in the approximate range 3.5–5.5 mmol^{-1} (depending on the laboratory) and rise postprandially to values considerably less than 10 mmol/l^{-1} (the renal threshold for complete reabsorption, above which glucose 'spills' over into the urine). Blood levels over 7.8 mmol l^{-1} 2 h after a 75 g glucose load are one of the diagnostic criteria for diabetes. Glucose is stored as glycogen, an α-linked polymer, predominantly in the liver and muscles ('animal starch'). On average, a 70 kg man may store 500 g of glycogen. Glucose can also be synthesized *de novo* by gluconeogenesis from the gluconeogenic amino acids.

Glucose is present in fruit and vegetables and, although less sweet on a per gram basis than fructose or sucrose, it is responsible together with fructose and sucrose for the sweet taste of vegetables and fruit. With the exception of fruit such as green banana, seeds (grain and dried legumes) and tubers, where starch is the major carbohydrate form, foods containing glucose, fructose and sucrose in various ratios form the major available (i.e. absorbable in the small intestine) carbohydrate sources. The relative proportions of the sugars have not been generally determined and figures are not yet available for most foods.

The chief sources of dietary starch are cereal grains, dried legumes and tubers. The major part of the available carbohydrate in these foods is starch. Starches contain both α(1–4) and α(1–6) linkages, i.e. amylose and amylopectin (**Fig. 1**). In most studies amylose predominates, with a ratio of amylose to amylopectin of 2–3 : 1. In general, legumes contain higher amylose levels than do cereals. Cultivars of corn have been bred with high amylose levels.

Resistant starches form a small proportion of most industrialized Western diets. Increased starch malabsorption may be induced by coarse milling or large particle size of cereal grains (e.g. whole-grain

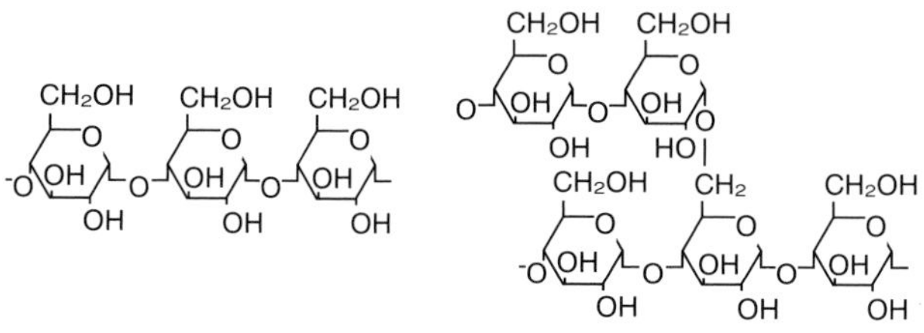

Figure 1 Partial structures of amylose (linear) and amylopectin (branched) starches.

pumpernickel or bulgur wheat). Such foods may be said to contain resistant starch (RS_1). Resistant starches that are crystalline in nature and resist hydration (RS_2) are found in green banana, high-amylose corn and relatively high-amylose legumes (peas, beans and lentils). Starches, especially high-amylose starches that are cooked and then allowed to cool, undergo retrogradation with more crystalline realignment. These starches (RS_3) are produced in common foods such as potato, rice and bread. Resistant starches in this category are produced commercially from high-amylose cornstarch by enzymatically debranching the remaining (1–6) linkages and allowing the resulting (1–4)-linked starch to 'retrograde' into a highly crystalline, digestion-resistant starch.

Cellulose is an important structural component of plant cell walls. In human nutrition, it forms an important part of the 'insoluble' dietary fibre component reported in food composition tables. However, values for the actual proportion of the total dietary fibre that is composed of cellulose are only available in special food composition tables for a relatively small number of foods.

From the standpoint of human nutrition, β-glucans are found predominantly in cereals, notably oats and barley, with trace amounts in wheat. In oats, the β-glucan is concentrated in the outer bran layer and may comprise 50% of the dietary fibre value and possibly 8–9% of the so-called oat bran derived from standard milling practices. In barley, the β-glucan is more dispersed through the endosperm and thus a bran concentrate is less easy to achieve. In both cases, high β-glucan cultivars may greatly increase the yield of β-glucan. In addition, 'wet' processing techniques may yield a high-concentration β-glucan bran and purified β-glucan oat gum.

Analysis

Analysis of glucose may involve chemical, enzymatic, electrochemical and high-performance liquid chromatography (HPLC) systems. Prior to the introduction of enzyme-based analyses, chemical techniques were

based on the reducing ability of glucose, and techniques employing copper sulfate were popular. Such techniques were influenced by other reducing sugars and reducing substances including uric acid and vitamin C. With the introduction of the more specific glucose oxidase-based tests the chemical tests were abandoned, although there was debate over the potential carcinogenicity of the early chromogens, o-dianizadine and o-toluidine. Later, more specific, hexokinase-based enyzme assays were introduced. Current methods for rapid determination of blood glucose, which no longer require prior precipation of plasma proteins, involve electrochemical detection. These methods rely on silver electrodes to detect electrons generated by the oxidation of glucose by glucose oxidase contained in membranes on the surface of the electrodes. For determination of glucose and α-limit dextrins resulting from starch digestion, HPLC techniques have proved useful.

Much attention has been given to the analysis of the glucose polymers – starches, resistant starches, cellulose and β-glucans – in the context of dietary fibre. The ultimate assessment depends on the use of specific enzymes or enzyme systems to break the macromolecules down to their component glucose and other sugars where mixtures containing other polymers (dietary fibres) are being analysed. These are then assessed by gas chromatography or HPLC and the ratios of the sugars determined. More routine assessment may involve a variety of chemical techniques combined with enzymatic digestion and, in the case of a popular Association of Official Analytical Chemists (AOAC) approved technique for dietary fibre analysis, with a gravimetric determination. There is, however, debate as to whether the resistant starch, which in the gravimetric AOAC technique is analysed as dietary fibre, should be included as fibre or whether it is physiologically distinct. It is also debated whether a determination of β-glucan is sufficient without knowledge of its viscosity and molecular weight, factors that determine its physiological effect.

Physiology

The physiology of the gastrointestinal absorption of (and the energy retrieved from) the glucose molecule along the length of the gastrointestinal tract in its various forms are discussed below, together with the influence of other dietary factors (**Fig. 2**).

Absorption

In its simplest form, glucose ingested by mouth is rendered isotonic in the stomach by the gastric juices and expelled through the pylorus into the duodenum

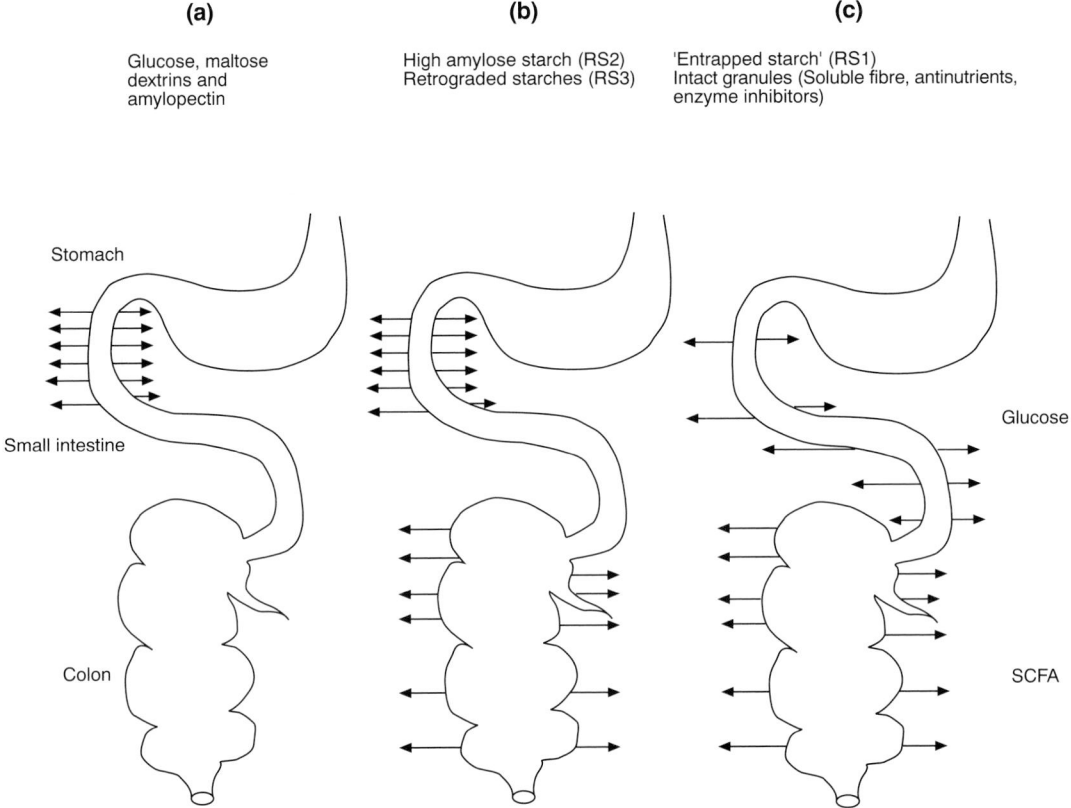

Figure 2 Effect of different forms of glucose on glucose absorption and short-chain fatty acid (SCFA) production and uptake from the gut: (a) glucose, maltose, dextrins and amylopectin; (b) high-amylose starch and retrograded starches; (c) entrapped starch and intact granules.

where active transport takes place at the brush border by way of a sodium-linked glucose transporter. The absorbed glucose which is taken up by way of the portal vein suppresses hepatic glucose output but does not markedly alter the glucose balance across the liver. The major part of the absorbed glucose is taken up by muscle and also adipose tissue under the action of insulin. Similarly, sucrose and lactose are both split and absorbed at the brush border by the brush border enzymes sucrase-isomaltase and lactase. Although sucrose deficiency is exceedingly rare, hypolactasia is common in adult life in most of the world's populations with the exception of those of northern European origin. Thus, unlike sucrose malabsorption, small-intestinal lactose malabsorption is common, with significant amounts of lactose entering the colon, resulting in gas production, short-chain fatty acid (SCFA) synthesis and, in some instances, diarrhoea.

Purified, fully hydrated, cooked amylopectin starch, on the other hand, commences digestion in the mouth under the action of salivary amylase. Enzyme activity ceases under the acidic conditions of the stomach and resumes in the duodenum under the action of pancreatic amylase. Amylolytic digestion in

both mouth and stomach results predominantly in the production of free glucose, maltose, maltotriose and the α-limit dextrins of greater polymeric length. The free glucose is taken up by the brush border glucose transporter and the uptake of maltose and maltotriose are effected by brush border enzymes, notably the sucrase–isomaltase complex. In both these situations, absorption in the small intestine is considered to be complete.

However, foods as eaten do not usually comprise pure glucose and pure amylopectin starch as their carbohydrate components. Many factors influence small-intestinal absorption both in terms of rate and amount (**Table 1**). Some of these factors have already been discussed in connection with amylose and resistant starch.

Food components

Insoluble fibre may form a coat around starchy foods limiting the penetration of enzymes and so reducing the rate and amount digested. Viscous soluble fibres may also reduce the rate of absorption through prolonging gastric emptying and acting as a barrier to diffusion in the small intestine. Starch–protein interaction (as seen with gluten in wheat products) and

Table 1 Factors influencing glycaemia and gastrointestinal events

Factors influencing the availability of carbohydrate	Glycaemia	Stomach	Small intestine		Colon	
		Gastric emptying	Absorption rate	Motility	Bacterial fermentation	Faecal bulk
Food components						
Fibre soluble (viscous)	−	− − −	− −	−?	+ + +	+
Insoluble	0?	+	+	+	+	+ + +
Macronutrients						
Protein–starch interaction	−	−?	− −	?	+	?
Fat–starch interaction	−	−	− −	?	+	?
Starches						
Amylopectin	+	?	+ +	?	0	0
Amylose	−	−	− − −	?	+ +	+
Sugars and glucose polymers						
Glucose	+ +	−?	+	0	0	0
Maltose	+ +	−?	+	0	0	0
Maltodextrins	+ +	0	+	0	0	0
Antinutrients						
Phytates	−	?	−	?	+	?
Tanins	−	?	−	?	+	?
Saponins	?	?	−	?	+	?
Lectins	−	−	−	?	+	?
Amylase inhibitors	−	0	−	?	+	?
Alpha-glucosidase inhibitors	−	0	−	?	+	?
Food processing						
(a) Cooking						
Starch gelatinization	+	0	+ +	?	0	0
Starch retrogradation	−	?	− −	?	+	+
Parboiling (e.g. rice)	−	?	−	?	?	0
(b) Particle size						
Milling	+	+	+	?	0	0
Crushing	+	?	+	?	0	0
Flaking	+	?	+	?	0	0
Extruding	−	?	−	?	0	0

Key: +, increase, promote; −, inhibit, reduce; 0, no effect; ?, uncertain.

starch–fat interactions have been shown to reduce the rate of digestion, and fat is known to slow gastric emptying. A number of the so-called 'antinutrients' present in foods, notably lectins, phytates and tannins, have been shown to reduce the digestibility of foods. For example, it is considered that phytate, by binding calcium ions which catalyse starch digestion by amylase, reduces the rate of small-intestinal starch digestion.

Food processing may influence the rate of digestion by removing or reducing the level and activity of inhibitory food components. It may also modify the structure of the food or its components to make the food more available to digestive enzyme attack. Examples of these are cooking, resulting in starch gelatinization, and reducing the particle size (and hence increasing the surface area) by milling, crushing or flaking. On the other hand, processing may also reduce digestibility by parboiling, cooking with retrogradation of the starch, and extrusion, as in the production of pasta, producing a more compact physical structure.

Increasing the frequency of meals and reducing their size spreads the nutrient load over time and hence prolongs the time spent in the absorptive state. It is perhaps the 'clearest' model of slowing the rate of absorption and is referred to again to explain the metabolic consequences of reducing the absorption rate.

Finally, enzyme inhibitors of carbohydrate absorption have been developed for pharmacological use in the treatment of diabetes which reduce the rate of carbohydrate uptake from the small intestine. One example of this class of substance is acarbose, an α-glycoside hydrolase inhibitor, which has antiamylase and antisucrase-isomaltase activity and so inhibits both intraluminal and brush border carbohydrate digestion and absorption of starch, sucrose and maltose.

Possible effects of prolonging absorption time of carbohydrate

The question remains as to what physiological effects are produced when carbohydrate is absorbed more slowly (**Table 2**). A broad spectrum of effects are seen which appear beneficial when glucose is sipped slowly rather than drunk as a bolus or when starchy meals are eaten more frequently but in smaller amounts. Studies by Ellis in the 1930s first demonstrated a reduction in insulin requirements in patients with diabetes when glucose and insulin were administered in small, frequent doses. Since then, a range of metabolic benefits have been ascribed to increased meal frequency (the 'nibbling versus gorging' phenomenon). Early studies reported lower total cholesterol levels with increased meal frequency. Subsequent studies showed low-density lipoprotein (LDL) cholesterol reduction in subjects eating three meals a day, compared with those eating from six to as many as 17 meals daily for periods of 2–8 weeks. An extreme model of slowing absorption, where 17 meals daily were fed, demonstrated lower levels of apolipoprotein B in addition to total and LDL cholesterol. Population studies also indicated that total cholesterol levels were lower in those who ate more meals daily. Studies using stable isotopes showed

Table 2 Possible effects of prolonging absorption time of carbohydrate

---

Flatter postprandial glucose profile
Lower mean insulin levels postprandially and over the day
Reduced gastric inhibitory polypeptide response
Reduced 24 h urinary C peptide output
Prolonged suppression of plasma free fatty acids
Reduced urinary catecholamine output
Lower fasting and postprandial serum total and LDL
  cholesterol levels
Reduced hepatic cholesterol synthesis
Lower serum apolipoprotein B levels
Lower serum uric acid levels
Increased urinary uric acid excretion

---

that cholesterol synthesis was reduced at greater meal frequencies. Furthermore, mevalonic acid excretion (a water-soluble marker of cholesterol synthesis) suggested that the change in cholesterol levels was also related to the change in urinary mevalonic acid output. Since insulin is known to stimulate HMGCoA reductase activity, a rate-limiting enzyme in cholesterol synthesis, the depressed cholesterol synthesis was attributed to the lower insulin levels observed. In addition, the reduction in serum cholesterol levels on 'nibbling' may have resulted from increased bile acid losses due to more frequent bile acid cycling through the gut following increased meal frequency.

Studies of non-insulin-dependent diabetes have shown depressed glucose and insulin levels during the day with increased meal frequency. In nondiabetic subjects, the major effect of reducing the absorption rate (by sipping glucose over 3 h instead of taking the same amount of glucose as a bolus within 5 min) was to reduce insulin secretion. In addition, insulin suppression of free fatty acids and branched-chain amino acid levels was prolonged, and following glucose challenge no counter regulatory response was observed.

Finally, serum uric acid, an independent risk factor for coronary heart disease, was reduced and increased urinary uric acid excretion were seen with increased food frequency. As with the reduction in serum cholesterol levels, the effects of lower insulin levels were used to explain these differences. It was suggested that insulin promoted renal reabsorption of uric acid as demonstrated in the context of sodium reabsorption and hypertension in hyperinsulinaemic states.

Further effects of food frequency on diabetes have been assessed. It has been suggested that increased food frequency may limit obesity by reducing adipose tissue enzyme levels. Acute studies in humans failed to show an increased thermogenic response with increased meal frequency. Nevertheless, when satiety was assessed in acute studies, fluctuations in satiety were less over the whole day; long-term studies have yet to be undertaken. Concern still remains that 'snacking' may increase body weight in susceptible individuals. Despite these concerns, the demonstration that increased meal frequency can improve certain aspects of lipid and carbohydrate metabolism makes it a valuable model for other methods of 'spreading the nutrient load', e.g. reducing the rate of glucose absorption.

Colonic function

A portion of the starch, together with dietary fibre including cellulose and β-glucan, enters the colon and is fermented by the colonic microflora with the growth of the faecal biomass and the production of SCFA, hydrogen and methane. The extent to which this occurs varies from individual to individual, the nature of the resistant starch and the source of the cellulose, e.g. vegetable cellulose is more readily fermented than cereal cellulose. Although some individuals will be found to have starch in their faeces, the majority of subjects show little or no faecal starch. Furthermore, all the β-glucan is broken down by bacterial action in the colon. Only a proportion of the cellulose escapes colonic bacterial fermentation and contributes directly to faecal bulk. Thus a significant proportion of glucose molecules are not absorbed in the small intestine but enter the colon and are salvaged after conversion to SCFA. The SCFA are rapidly absorbed and contribute to the host's energy metabolism. They are usually produced in the ratio of 60% acetate, 20% propionate and 20% butyrate, but the relative ratios of these three fatty acids vary depending on the substrate and the rate of fermentation. Of the three SCFA, only acetate appears in the peripheral circulation to any significant extent. Propionate is of interest since it is gluconeogenic and has been suggested to inhibit hepatic cholesterol synthesis. It is largely extracted by the liver at first pass. Butyrate, on the other hand, is taken up and used by colonocytes. The slower the fermentation the higher the butyrate levels. Starches have been claimed to increase colonic butyrate and in some instances propionate production, and butyrate is said to have antineoplastic properties.

The Glycaemic Index

The differing effects of different carbohydrate foods in raising the blood glucose concentration postprandially have long been recognized. The glycaemic index classification was proposed to indicate the rates at which different starchy foods were digested. It was hoped that selection of foods with lower glycaemic indices would contribute to prolonging the absorption of nutrients, and so improve the glycaemic profile and reduce levels of fasting blood lipids.

However, a number of acute (up to 1 day) mixed meal studies during the mid to late 1980s suggested that a glycaemic index classification of foods had no clinical utility. Nevertheless, a number of subsequent reports have documented improved glycaemic control in both type I and II diabetes as judged by serum fructosamine and glycosylated haemoglobin levels in studies of 2 weeks' to 2 months' duration. Furthermore, some studies also noted reductions in serum lipids. Many high-fibre foods which lower LDL cholesterol levels also have low glycaemic indices (barley, beans, etc.). Extensive glycaemic index tables have now been published which will help in food selection for therapeutic and study purposes.

Many of the traditional starchy foods from different cultures have a low glycaemic index (**Table 3**). Finally, results of cohort studies suggest that consumption of foods with a low glycaemic index, especially in the context of a high-fibre diet, protects from the development of type II diabetes. One is therefore left to wonder whether the rapid increase in diabetes in cultures in transition from traditional to Western life-style patterns is in part due to the high glycaemic index of the diets eaten, in addition to the excess consumption of energy and reduced physical activity.

Calculation of the glycemic index

The glycaemic index (GI) has been defined as (area under the blood glucose response curve for 50 g carbohydrate from the test food) divided by (area under the blood glucose response curve for 50 g carbohydrate from the standard source) × 100. The standard carbohydrate source for modern assessments is white bread. In the early studies, however, 50 g glucose was used rather than bread. On the 'bread scale' the glucose GI is approximately 130%. Other food GI values can be adjusted accordingly to allow direct comparison of the two scales.

The area under the blood glucose curve includes the area above the fasting level only. Any area

Table 3 Glycaemic index of staple foods from different cultures

Food	Average GI	Culture
White bread rolls	100	North American, European
Pumpernickel	70–90	North European
Pasta	50–70	Mediterranean
Cracked wheat (tabouli)	60–70	Mediterranean, Middle Eastern
Beans, lentils, dried peas	40–70	Southern USA, Latin American, Middle Eastern, Indian, Oriental
Parboiled long-grain rice	70	Asian, North African

Glycaemic index (GI) is rounded to the nearest 10%.

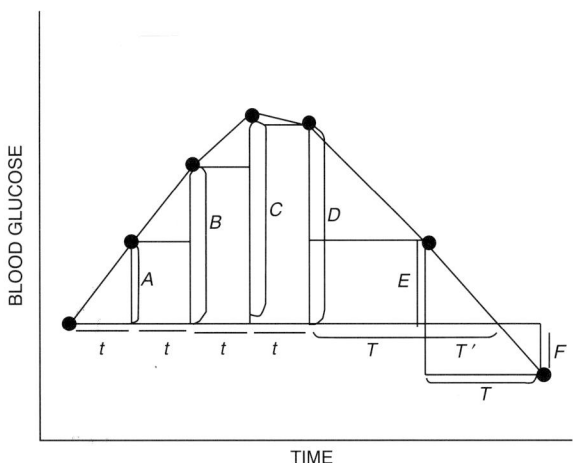

Figure 3 Schematic representation of postprandial blood glucose response (Wolever and Jenkins, 1986).

beneath the fasting level is ignored. The incremental area under the blood glucose response curve is the sum of the areas of the triangles and rectangles. In Fig 3, A, B, C, D, E and F represent the blood glucose increments above the baseline value (fasting level) at sequential time points and t and T represent different time intervals between blood samples.

When the blood glucose concentration at F falls below the fasting concentration (**Fig. 3**), only the area above the fasting level is included in the total area represented by the triangle ET, where T' represents the portion of the time interval T when the blood glucose level between E and F is above the fasting level.

The overall equation simplifies to:

$$\text{Area} = \left(A + B + C + \frac{D}{2}\right)t + \frac{(D+E)\,T}{2} + \frac{E^2 T}{2(E+F)}$$

If the last blood glucose concentration F is above the fasting level, then the term $(E + F)T/2$ is substituted for the last term in the equation, namely $E^2T/2(E + F)$. An example of the incremental area calculation is shown in **Table 4**.

Calculation of mixed meal or total day's GI Each carbohydrate component is expressed as a percentage of the total carbohydrate in the meal or day and multiplied by the relevant glycaemic index. The sum of these values represents the meal's or the day's glycaemic index.

Calculation of glycemic load

Glycaemic load = diet glycaemic index
× daily dietary carbohydrate intake in grams per day

See also: **Carbohydrates**: Resistant Starch and Oligosaccharides. **Diabetes Mellitus**: Classification and Chemical Pathology. **Glucose**: Metabolism and Maintenance of Blood Glucose Level; Glucose Tolerance.

Further Reading

Bertelsen J, Christiansen C, Thomsen C *et al.* (1993) Effect of meal frequency on blood glucose, insulin, and free fatty acids in NIDDM subjects. *Diabetes Care* **16**:3–7.

Brand JC, Calagiuri S, Crossman S *et al.* (1991) Low-glycemic index foods improve long-term glycemic control in NIDDM. *Diabetes Care* **14**:95–101.

Crapo PA, Reaven G and Olefsky J (1976) Glucose and insulin response to orally administered simple and complex carbohydrates. *Diabetes* **25**:741–747.

Englyst HN, Wiggins HS and Cummings JH (1982) Determination of the non-starch polysaccharides in plant

Table 4 Example of calculation of incremental area under the blood glucose response curve for glycaemic response where the last glucose value falls below baseline

Time (min)	Corresponding letter on Fig. 3	Blood glucose (mg dl⁻¹)	Blood glucose increment (mg dl⁻¹)
0	–	100	–
15	A	120	20
30	B	140	40
45	C	160	60
60	D	150	50
90	E	120	20
120	F	90	−10

Calculation:

$$\text{Area} = (20 + 40 + 60 + 25) \times 15 + (25 + 10) \times 30 + \frac{20^2 \times 30}{2 \times (20 + 10)} = 3425 \text{ mg min dl}^{-1}$$

From Wolever and Jenkins (1986).

foods by gas-liquid chromatography of constituent sugars as alditol acetates. *Analyst* **107**:307–318.

Fontvieille AM, Acosta M, Rizkalla SW *et al.* (1988) A moderate switch from high to low glycemic index foods for 3 weeks improves the metabolic control of type 1 (IDDM) diabetic subjects. *Diabetes Nutrition and Metabolism* **1**:139–143.

Foster-Powell K and Brand Miller J (1995) International tables of glycemic index. *American Journal of Clinical Nutrition* **62**:871S–893S.

Jenkins DJA, Wolever TMS, Taylor RH *et al.* (1980) Rate of digestion of foods and post-prandial glycaemia in normal and diabetic subjects. *British Medical Journal* **2**:14–17.

Jenkins DJA, Wolever TMS, Taylor RH *et al.* (1981) Glycemic index of foods: a physiological basis for carbohydrate exchange. *American Journal of Clinical Nutrition* **34**:362–366.

Jenkins DJA, Wolever TMS, Ocana AM, Vuksan V, Cunanne SC and Jenkins MJA (1990) Metabolic effects of reducing rate of glucose ingestion by single bolus versus continuous sipping. *Diabetes* **39**:775–781.

Jones PJH, Leitch CA and Pederson RA (1993) Meal frequency effects of plasma hormone concentrations and cholesterol synthesis in humans. *American Journal of Clinical Nutrition* **57**:868–874.

Salmeron J, Manson JA, Stampfer M, Colditz GA, Wing AL and Willett WC (1997) Dietary fiber, glycemic load, and risk of non-insulin-dependent diabetes mellitus in women. *Journal of the American Medical Association* **277**:472–477.

Schauberger G, Brinck UC, Sulder G, Spaethe R, Niklas L and Otto H (1977) Exchange of carbohydrates according to their effect on blood glucose. *Diabetes* **26**:415.

Wolever TMS and Jenkins DJA (1986) The use of the glycemic index in predicting the blood glucose response to mixed meals. *American Journal of Clinical Nutrition* **43**:167–172.

Metabolism and Maintenance of Blood Glucose Level

T Wolever, University of Toronto, Ontario, Canada

Copyright © 1998 Academic Press

This article describes the role of glucose in the body as a fuel and as a precursor of other compounds, some of which are essential and some of which are potentially toxic. The metabolic pathways of glucose metabolism (glycolysis, glycogen and lipid synthesis, the pentose phosphate shunt and the glycosylation of proteins) are described together with a discussion of some of the factors that control them and the relative proportions which they contribute to total glucose use in the body. Finally, the roles of the liver, muscle and pancreas in the regulation of blood glucose are described, with particular reference to the pathogenesis of diabetes mellitus.

Significance of Glucose in the Body

Glucose has many functions and is essential for the metabolism of all plants and animals. In most human diets, it is the most abundant nutrient absorbed by the intestine; about 85% of dietary carbohydrate is absorbed as glucose, and this single compound contributes 35–50%, or more, of total energy intake. Nevertheless, glucose is not an essential dietary component and it can be synthesized in the body from many precursors. Thus, some populations, such as the Greenland Eskimo, can survive on diets containing virtually no carbohydrate.

Glucose as fuel

For most tissues, glucose is a preferred fuel and for some, such as red blood cells, it is essential. Of particular importance is the fact that, under normal circumstances, the brain requires glucose as a fuel; loss of consciousness occurs if the concentration of glucose in the blood becomes too low. Thus, a finely tuned and rapidly responding system has evolved which controls the blood glucose concentration within a narrow range despite large changes in the rate at which glucose enters the body from the diet. During periods of fasting when the rate of entry of glucose from the intestine is zero, to prevent the blood glucose concentration from falling, the nonessential use of glucose as a fuel has to be reduced and the rate of glucose output from the liver (release from stores and synthesis from other substrates) has to be increased. During periods of feeding when the rate of entry of glucose into the body from the intestine is high, the rate of use of glucose as a fuel has to be increased because only a limited amount can be stored. As will be discussed below, this is accomplished primarily by a switch of the fuel used by muscle from fat to glucose.

After an overnight fast, the blood glucose concentration is maintained by glucose release from the liver, the rate of glucose use by muscle is low, the concentration of free fatty acids in blood is high and the use of fat as fuel is high. After a carbohydrate-containing breakfast is consumed, the rate of entry of glucose into the blood from the intestine increases, the rate of entry of glucose into the blood from the liver falls, the glycogen content of liver increases, the use of glucose as a fuel (glucose oxidation) increases and the use of fat as a fuel falls; the time course of these events is shown in **Fig. 1**.

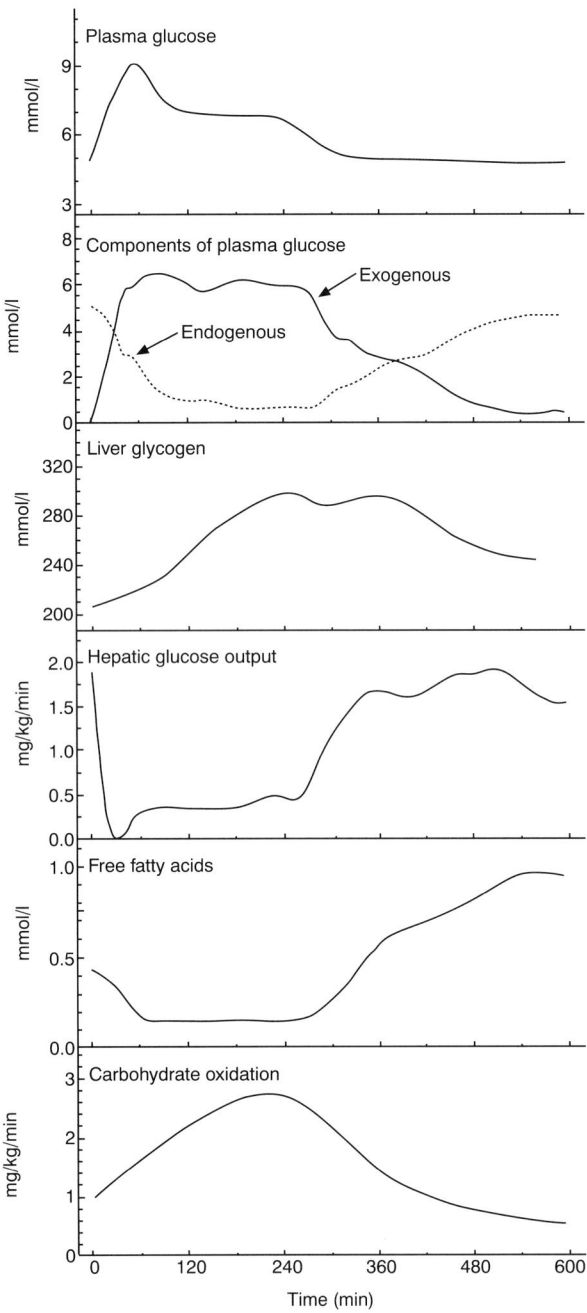

Figure 1 Time courses of the changes in (from top to bottom) plasma glucose, the exogenous (solid line) and endogenous (dotted line) components of plasma glucose, hepatic glucose output, liver glycogen, plasma free fatty acids and carbohydrate oxidation in normal subjects for 10 h after a liquid meal containing (824 kcal) 67.3% of energy from carbohydrate as glucose, 18.5% fat and 14.2% protein. Redrawn from Taylor *et al*. (1996).

up by peripheral tissues, about 80% is taken up by muscle and 15% by brain. Of the glucose taken up, about 30–40% is oxidized and the rest is stored as glycogen. The amount and rate of carbohydrate oxidation after a meal depends upon the amount of carbohydrate in the diet and rate at which it is absorbed. The dependency of glucose oxidation on glucose absorption is illustrated in Fig. 1. In this study, glucose absorption (shown by the concentration of exogenous glucose in the plasma) rapidly reached a peak and remained relatively constant for 4–5 h after the meal. During this time the rate of glucose oxidation continued to increase until the exogenous glucose availability began to fall. Once glucose absorption began to fall, the rate of glucose oxidation fell and the rate of fat oxidation increased, as indicated by the rise in plasma free fatty acids (FFA). High-carbohydrate meals promote greater carbohydrate oxidation and suppress plasma FFA for longer than lower-carbohydrate meals. In addition, carbohydrates which are more slowly digested delay the postprandial rise in plasma FFA and result in a somewhat lower peak, but prolonged increase in the rate of glucose oxidation.

Glucose storage and release

Glucose can be stored as glycogen in liver and muscle. About two-thirds of total body glycogen is in muscle, but muscle glycogen is used by the muscle and is not available for other tissues. The maximum amount of glycogen that can be stored in the body is about 500 g, but this amount is not usually achieved unless a diet very high in carbohydrate is consumed. The normal pattern of glycogen storage in liver after a single meal is shown in Fig. 1. Typically, during a day when three carbohydrate-containing meals are consumed, liver glycogen content continues to increase at a constant rate until approximately midnight. Glycogen is formed directly from glucose in a series of reactions via glucose-6-phosphate, glucose-1-phosphate and UDP glucose (**Fig. 2**). Glycogen in the liver can also be formed indirectly from glucose synthesized from precursors such as glycerol, lactate and alanine (gluconeogenesis). Surprisingly, even 3–5 h after a carbohydrate-rich meal when liver glycogen content is increasing at a rapid rate, the formation of glycogen directly from glucose makes up only about 70% of total glycogen synthesis, with gluconeogenesis contributing 30% of total glycogen accumulation.

There is some evidence that the exact proportions of glucose taken up by the various tissues and the proportion stored and oxidized varies with the type and amount of carbohydrate consumed. The amount of glycogen stored increases with the amount and

Ultimately, during weight stability the fuels used by the body for energy are the same as those consumed in the diet. In normal subjects, after an oral glucose load of 1 g kg^{-1} body weight, about 70% of the ingested glucose load is taken up by peripheral tissues and 30% by the liver. Of the glucose taken

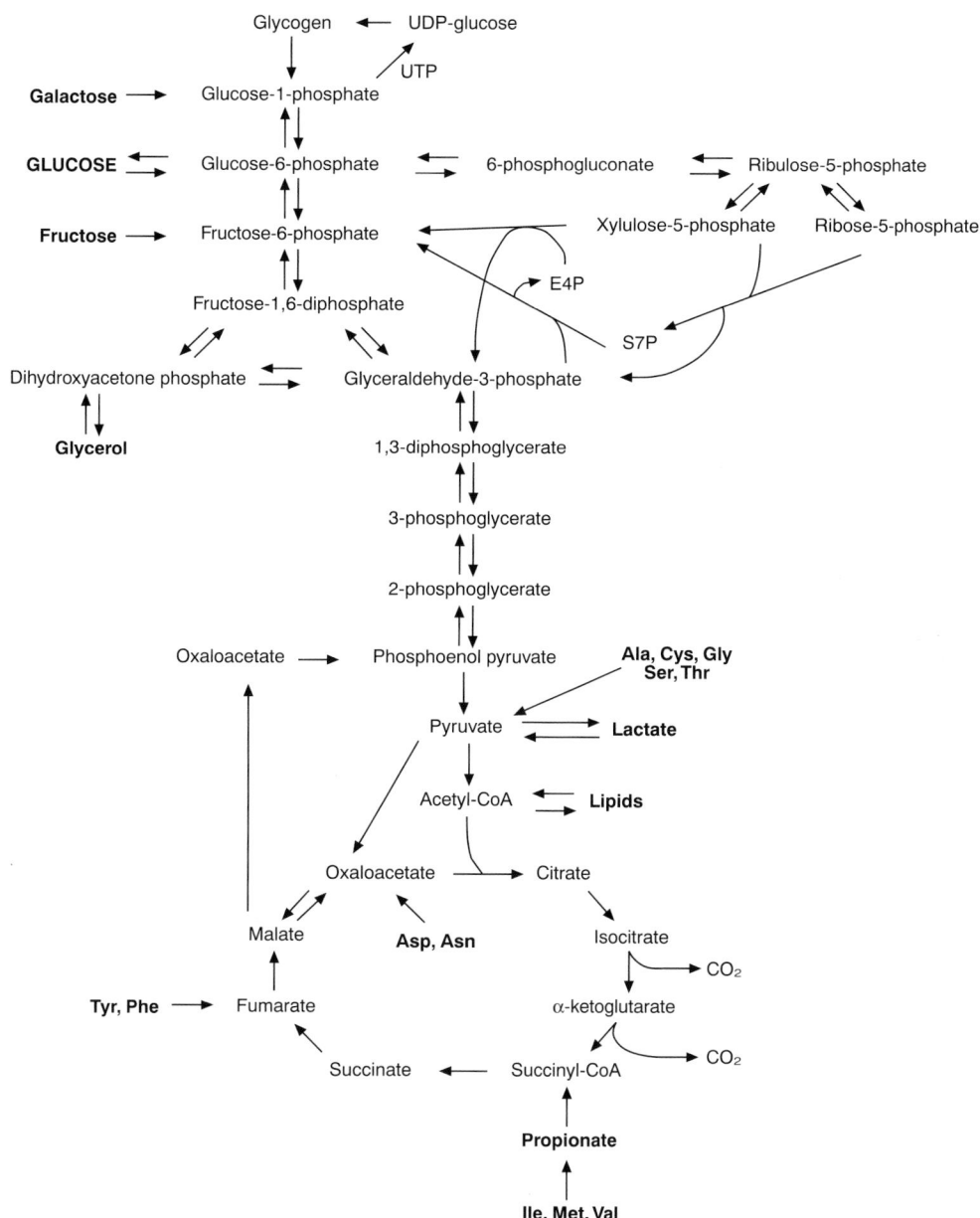

Figure 2 Pathways of glucose metabolism. Compounds in bold represent precursors or end products. E4P, erythrose-4-phosphate; S7P, sedoheptulose-7-phosphate; Ala, alanine; Cys, cysteine; Gly, glycine; Ser, serine; Thr, threonine; Asp, aspartate; Asn, asparagine; Ile, isoleucine; Met, methionine; Val, valine; Tyr, tyrosine; Phe, phenylalanine. Reactions involving xylulose-5-phosphate, ribose-5-phosphate, E4P and S7P are reversible but are shown with single arrows for clarity.

frequency of feeding and the amount of glycogen stored is greater if the carbohydrate is rapidly digested and absorbed, producing higher blood glucose and insulin responses. Muscle glycogen is of importance to endurance athletes because exhaustion begins to occur when muscle glycogen runs out. Muscle glycogen can be maximized before the start of an endurance event by a carbohydrate loading diet. Starting about a week before the event, muscle glycogen is depleted by hard training on a relatively low-carbohydrate diet for about 3 days. This is fol-

lowed by a very high-carbohydrate diet (500–700 g per day) for the 3–4 days immediately before the event. Muscle glycogen, and hence performance, can also be maintained during ultralong events, such as the Tour de France, by regular consumption of carbohydrate (usually in sports drinks) during the event.

During fasting, the liver releases glucose into the bloodstream. Traditionally it has been considered that hepatic glucose output is derived from the breakdown of liver glycogen during the first 12–24 h of fasting, by which time hepatic glycogen has been exhausted. In fasts of longer than 24 h, hepatic glucose output is maintained by gluconeogenesis. However, the results of recent studies using nuclear magnetic resonance spectroscopy to measure hepatic glycogen in humans *in vivo*, suggest that the traditional view of hepatic glycogen metabolism needs revising. In normal human subjects who had been consuming a diet containing 60% of energy from carbohydrate for 3 days, the liver contained about 110 g glycogen 4 h after their last meal. During a prolonged fast, liver glycogen content declined linearly by about 3.3 g h^{-1} for the first 22 h, by which time the liver contained about 35 g glycogen. After this, the rate of loss of glycogen slowed so that by the end of the fast at 64 h, the liver still contained 8.5 g glycogen. The results suggest that during the first 22 h of fasting, nearly two-thirds of total glucose output by the liver came from gluconeogenesis and only one-third from glycogen breakdown (**Fig. 3**).

The substrates for gluconeogenesis are shown in Fig. 2. In prolonged fasting, the major gluconeogenic substrates are amino acids derived from muscle protein. Alanine, cysteine, glycine, serine and threonine enter the gluconeogenic pathway via pyruvate, which is carboxylated to oxaloacetate in the mitochondrion. Oxaloacetate itself cannot be transported out of the mitochondrion, so it reaches the cytoplasm via malate, which is converted back to oxaloacetate, and then to phosphoenol pyruvate and 'up' the glycolytic pathway to glucose-6-phosphate (Fig. 2). Aspartate and asparagine enter the pathway at oxaloacetate and tyrosine and phenylalanine at fumarate.

Methionine and the branched-chain amino acids isoleucine and valine are converted to glucose via propionate and succinyl-CoA. Propionate is of interest as a gluconeogenic substrate because it is a product of the fermentation of unabsorbed carbohydrate in the colon. It has been shown that infusion of propionate into the human rectum raises blood glucose.

Lactate and glycerol are the other major gluconeogenic substrates. One source of lactate is that produced during anaerobic metabolism of glucose in muscle. The cycle whereby lactate is released from muscle, converted to glucose in the liver, and the glucose returns to muscle to be converted back to lactate is called the Cori cycle.

Glycerol is released from adipose tissue when triglyceride is hydrolysed to glycerol and free fatty acids, and glycerol is the only portion of fat which can be converted to glucose. Fatty acids are oxidized to acetyl-CoA, but no net glucose synthesis can occur from fatty acids because, for each turn of the tricarboxylic acid (TCA) cycle, two carbon atoms in acetyl-CoA are added, and two are lost as carbon dioxide (Fig. 2). The two carbon atoms of acetyl-CoA (C1 and C2) enter the TCA cycle by condensing with oxaloacetate to form carbons C4 and C5 of citrate (**Fig. 4**). Citrate carbon atoms C6 and C1 are lost as carbon dixoide and, with the randomization at fumarate, carbon C1 from acetyl-CoA becomes C1 or C4 of oxaloacetate and carbon C2 from acetyl-CoA becomes C2 or C3 of oxaloacetate. If the oxaloacetate is converted to glucose, its C1 carbon, derived from C1 of acetate, becomes C3 or C4 of glucose and its C2 and C3 carbons, derived from C2 of acetate, become C1, C2, C5 or C6 of glucose (Fig. 4(b)). If the oxaloacetate remains in the TCA cycle, its carbon atom derived from C1 of acetate is lost as carbon dioxide during its second turn through the cycle, and the carbon atom from acetate C2 has a 50% chance of being lost as carbon dioxide on its third turn of the cycle (Fig. 4(a)).

Role of the pentose phosphate pathway

The majority of glucose is metabolized via the glycolytic pathway, which goes from glucose-6-phosphate to pyruvate (Fig. 2). However, some tissues possess another pathway, the pentose phosphate pathway (also known as the phosphogluconate pathway, the Embden–Meyerhof pathway or the hexose monophosphate shunt), whose main purpose is to generate reducing power in the cytoplasmic compartment in the form of NADPH. These reducing units are required for the synthesis of fatty acids and sterols (such as cholesterol) from small precursors (e.g. acetate). Thus, tissues such as liver, mammary gland, adipose tissue and adrenal cortex, which synthesize lipids, possess the pentose phosphate pathway, but it is virtually absent from muscle which does not make fatty acids. Another important function of the pentose phosphate pathway is to generate pentoses, and particularly ribose used in the synthesis of nucleic acids for the formation of DNA and RNA. In Fig. 2 the pentose phosphate pathway is to the

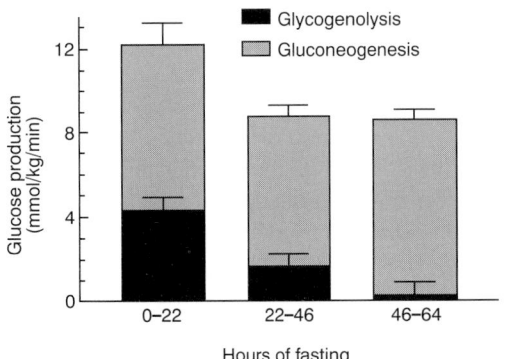

Figure 3 Contributions of gluconeogenesis and glycogen breakdown (glycogenolysis) to total hepatic glucose output during a 68 h fast in humans. Data from Rothman *et al.* (1991).

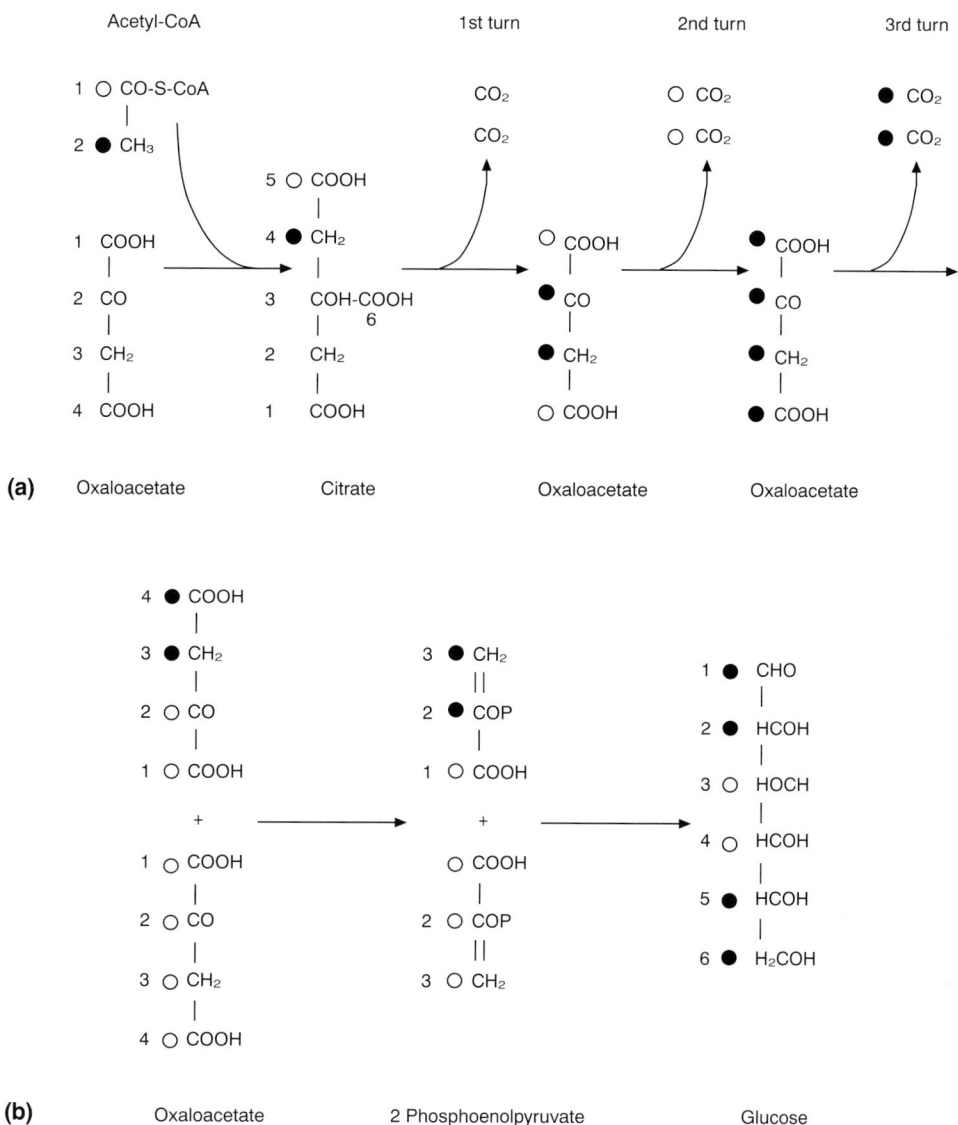

Figure 4 (a) Fate of carbon atoms in acetyl-CoA which enter the tricarboxylic acid cycle and remain in it for at least three turns. (b) Fate of carbon atoms in the conversion of oxaloacetate to glucose. The carbon atoms represented by open and filled circles can be derived from carbon atoms 1 and 2, respectively, of acetate.

right of glucose-6-phosphate, via 6-phosphoglu-conate, ribulose-5-phosphate, xylulose-5-phosphate, ribose-5-phosphate, sedoheptulose-7-phosphate (S7P) and erythrose-4-phosphate (E4P).

Lipid synthesis from glucose

Theoretically, glucose can be converted into fatty acids and sterols via acetyl-CoA. Obviously, if carbohydrate intake is so high that it exceeds both the body's need for energy and the capacity of glycogen stores, then carbohydrate will be converted into lipids for disposal. However, the quantitative importance of this pathway in humans is not clear. In favour of a major role for *de novo* synthesis of fatty acids from carbohydrate is evidence that, on a high-carbohydrate diet, fasting serum triglycerides tend to increase. However, this is not a universal finding. In addition, recent studies using mass isotopomer dilution analysis suggest that *de novo* fatty acid synthesis from carbohydrate is very small (less than 1 g per day) unless carbohydrate intake is extremely high, the illness is severe (burns and AIDS), or with total parenteral nutrition. An alternative explanation for the triglyceride-raising potential of a high-carbohydrate diet is that such a diet raises plasma insulin which, in turn, promotes triglyceride synthesis from fatty acids. In favour of this hypothesis is evidence showing that reducing the blood glucose and insulin-raising potential of the diet by using low-glycaemic index foods reduces serum triglycerides in subjects with raised triglycerides. The low-glycaemic index diets used in these studies had the same carbohydrate fat and protein content as the control, high-glycaemic index diets. The reduction in diet glycaemic index was achieved by exchanging starchy carbohydrate foods, and this was shown in other studies to reduce 24 h urinary C peptide excretion as an index of insulin secretion.

Some studies suggest that fructose (or sucrose) feeding is especially likely to raise serum triglycerides. Again, this is not a universal finding, and in some studies even very high levels of sucrose (over 200 g per day) tended to reduce serum triglycerides rather than raise them. The lack of consistency in the literature has prompted the suggestion that only some individuals are sensitive to a serum triglyceride-raising effect of fructose. Fructose has been suggested to raise serum triglycerides by the following mechanism: in liver, fructose can enter the glycolytic pathway by a different route from that shown in Fig. 2; namely, by the action of the enzyme fructokinase which converts fructose to fructose-1-phosphate, which, in turn, is cleaved to glyceraldehyde and dihydroxyacetone phosphate. In this way fructose bypasses the enzyme phosphofructokinase which converts fructose-6-phosphate to fructose diphosphate, one of the major steps controlling flux through glycolysis. Thus, excess fructose is converted to acetyl-CoA in an uncontrolled fashion; if this occurs at a faster rate than the TCA cycle can use the acetyl-CoA, the excess acetate is converted to fatty acids. However, there are other possible fates of fructose-1-phosphate entering the glycolytic pathway, such as glycogen synthesis. In addition, some fructose is converted into glucose and released into the bloodstream, which accounts for the rise in blood glucose after the ingestion of fructose.

Glycosylation of proteins

Glucose irreversibly combines with long-lived protein-containing macromolecules to form advanced glycation end products (AGE) by a process illustrated in **Fig. 5**. The AGEs so formed cause changes in extracellular components such as collagen, which can affect cell adhesion, growth and matrix accumulation and modify the function of cells such as macrophages and endothelial cells lining blood vessels. These changes can lead to extracellular matrix overproduction, focal thrombosis and vasoconstriction and may, in part, be responsible for the long-term complications which occur in diabetes mellitus, and some of the changes which occur with ageing.

The complex series of dehydrations, rearrangements and reactions which form irreversible AGEs are poorly understood. The process begins with the formation of reversible early glycation products. These are formed from the condensation of a sugar aldehyde or ketone with a free amino group via nucleophilic addition, resulting first in the rapid formation of a Schiff base. Equilibrium is reached in a matter of hours at a steady-state level proportional to the ambient glucose concentration. These Schiff base adducts then undergo rearrangement to form the more stable 1-amino-1-deoxyketose (Amadori) product. Equilibrium of this reaction is reached over several weeks, so that, even on very long-lived proteins, the amount of Amadori product is only proportional to the integrated glucose concentration over the previous 4 weeks. The Amadori product is degraded into various highly reactive carbonyl compounds, such as 3-deoxyglucosone and sugar fragmentation products that react again with free amino groups to form various intermediate and advanced glycation products. The formation of AGE *in vivo*

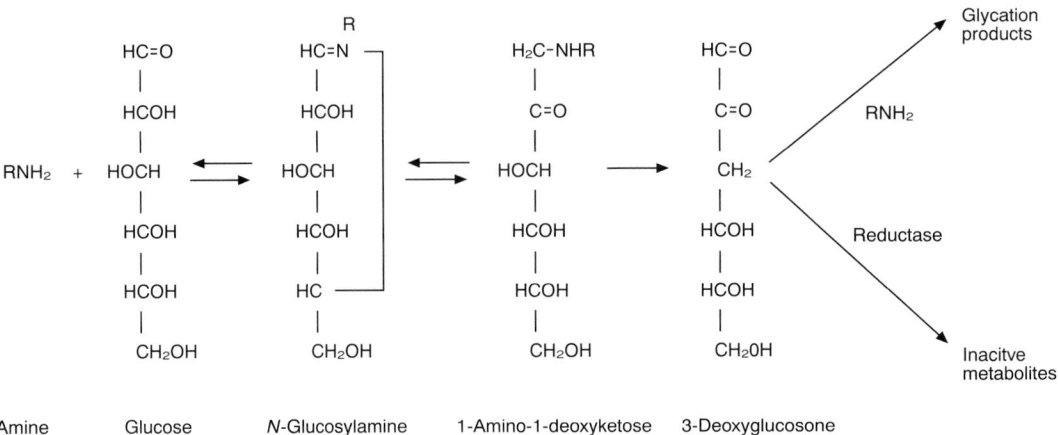

Figure 5 Formation of advanced glycation end products from glucose. Redrawn from Brownlee (1992).

may be slowed by the action of reductase enzymes that reduce compounds such as 3-deoxyglucosone to less reactive ones such as 3-deoxyfructose (Fig. 5).

The rate of AGE formation does not have a linear relationship with the concentration of sugar, and even modest elevations of glucose significantly increases AGE accumulation. Since AGEs are irreversibly attached to macromolecules, the levels of AGE do not decline when hyperglycaemia is corrected, but continue to accumulate at varying rates over the lifetime of the diabetic tissue component. There is evidence that the rate of AGE formation is increased markedly by various oxidative processes. This, perhaps, explains recent observations that vitamin E reduces blood glycosylated haemoglobin (HbA1c) concentrations in diabetes. Haemoglobin, the oxygen-carrying protein found in red blood cells, has a half-life in the blood of about 3 months. Since the extent of glycosylation of haemoglobin depends upon the concentration of blood glucose over the life of the protein, HbA1c is used as an indication of the overall blood glucose control of patients with diabetes over the previous 3 months. Changes in HbA1c are used as a measure of the efficacy of treatments designed to reduce blood glucose. However, it is difficult to see how vitamin E could reduce blood glucose, and it is more likely that vitamin E reduces blood HbA1c by reducing the rate of glycosylation of haemoglobin.

Regulation of Blood Glucose

The regulation of blood glucose is complex and a matter of much debate and continued research interest. At the simplest level, the concentration of glucose in the blood depends upon the balance between the rate at which glucose is entering the blood and the rate at which glucose is leaving the blood. There are three major organs involved in regulating blood glucose: liver, muscle and pancreas.

Fasting blood glucose

Muscle After a 12 h overnight fast, the plasma insulin concentration is low, the blood free fatty acid (FFA) concentration high, and muscle is utilizing primarily fat as fuel. The FFAs originate from the hydrolysis of triglyceride stored in adipose tissue which produces FFA and glycerol by the action of hormone-sensitive lipoprotein lipase. The glycerol produced in this way cannot be used to be re-esterify FFA but is released into the circulation and reaches the liver where it can be used as a gluconeogenic substrate. The FFAs formed by the hydrolysis of triglyceride are released into the circulation. The rate at which muscle uses FFA as fuel is directly proportional to the concentration of FFA in blood. The oxidation of FFA by muscle inhibits the utilization of glucose, thus preserving blood glucose for essential tissues such as brain (**Fig. 6**). A reduction of the insulin-stimulated ability of muscle to take up glucose, termed insulin sensitivity, has little effect on the fasting blood glucose concentration, because in the fasting state, the muscle is not taking up glucose.

Liver In the fasting state, the liver releases glucose into the circulation. The rate of glucose output from the liver can be determined by intravenous infusion of a small amount of glucose labelled with deuterium or tritium and measuring the rate at which the tracer is diluted by glucose being released from the liver. Across the range of nondiabetic fasting plasma glucose concentrations ($3.5-7.8$ mmol l^{-1}) hepatic

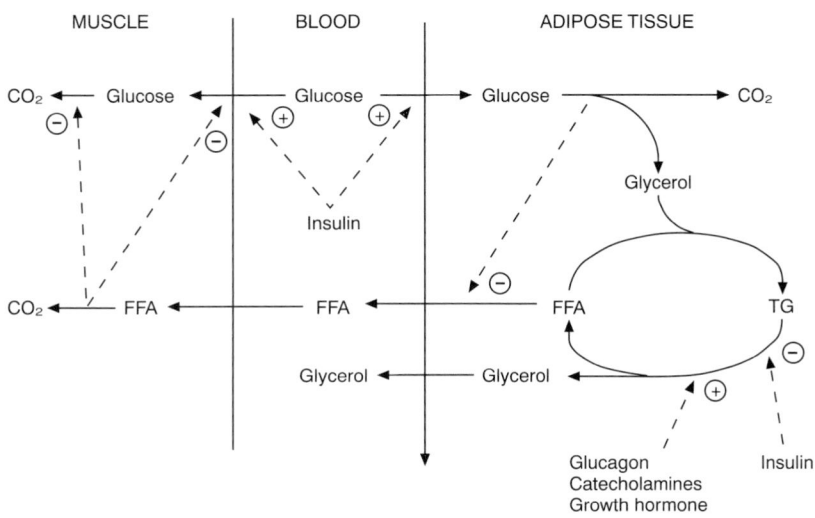

Figure 6 The glucose–fatty acid cycle.

glucose output is low and is not related to the plasma glucose. However, at fasting plasma glucose concentrations above normal, hepatic glucose output is directly related to the plasma glucose concentration. Thus, the fasting plasma glucose concentration is elevated in diabetes because of increased hepatic glucose output.

The exact mechanisms which regulate hepatic glucose output are not known. Insulin induces a reduction in hepatic glucose output in the presence of hyperglycaemia, and suppression of glucose production is much more sensitive to insulin than peripheral glucose utilization. However, insulin also reduces the mobilization of gluconeogenic substrates from the periphery which contributes to the reduction of hepatic glucose output. Insulin also reduces FFA release in the periphery, which also may contribute to the reduction in hepatic glucose output, since a rise in plasma FFA increases hepatic glucose output. Finally, other factors such as glucagon, or even glucose itself, have a role in regulating hepatic glucose output. In the NMR studies illustrated in Fig. 1, the changes in hepatic glucose output were closely mirrored by changes in the ratio of glucagon to insulin. The exact role of these various factors in the regulation of hepatic glucose output is unknown and is still a matter of debate and research.

In the normal situation, the pancreas secretes insulin into the portal system which reaches the liver via the portal vein; the insulin concentration in the portal vein is higher than that in the general circulation, and thus the liver is exposed to higher insulin concentrations than other tissues. However, portal delivery of insulin does not appear to be important in determining the effect of insulin on the liver. Experiments in dogs in which portal insulin concentrations are reduced to peripheral levels show that peripheral insulin levels suppress hepatic glucose output just as effectively as portal insulin.

Pancreas   The pancreas secretes a number of hormones which regulate plasma glucose, including insulin and glucagon. The main role of the low level of insulin in blood in the fasting state is to maintain a brake on the rate of FFA release from adipose tissue and a brake on ketone body production in the liver. In type II, noninsulin-dependent diabetes (NIDDM), the ability of the pancreas to secrete insulin in response to a rise in blood glucose is reduced, and fasting plasma insulin may even be lower than normal despite very high plasma glucose. In type II diabetes, plasma FFAs are raised, but there is enough insulin to prevent unchecked ketone body production in the liver. A complete lack of insulin, as in type I, insulin-dependent diabetes (IDDM), leads to

a marked increase in ketone body production in the liver which, if untreated, this results in ketoacidosis and death. Plasma glucose is also markedly raised, but this is more because of a marked increase in hepatic glucose output than because of a reduction in glucose uptake by muscle. In states of insulin resistance, which may occur with obesity and impaired glucose tolerance, fasting plasma glucose is normal or only slightly elevated, but plasma insulin is markedly raised.

Postprandial blood glucose

Muscle   After a meal, under the influence of insulin, the muscle switches from taking up fat for fuel to taking up glucose. There are two components to glucose uptake: insulin-mediated and non-insulin-mediated. Insulin stimulates glucose uptake directly by upregulating glucose transporters from intracellular storage sites to the cell membrane. It has been estimated that, in normal individuals, about 60% of total glucose uptake is insulin-mediated. However, in states of insulin resistance, insulin-mediated glucose uptake is reduced and noninsulin-mediated glucose uptake (NIMGU) accounts for a larger proportion of total glucose disposal. NIMGU accounts for 60% of glucose uptake in states of mild insulin resistance, such as pregnancy, and in severe diabetes may account for nearly 100% of total glucose uptake. However, the mechanism of noninsulin-mediated glucose uptake is not clear.

According to the glucose–fatty acid cycle (Fig. 6), muscle uptake of glucose is facilitated by the reduction in the blood FFA concentration. The reduction in plasma FFA occurs because the rise in insulin after eating inhibits hormone-sensitive lipase in adipose tissue, and thus, reduces FFA release. The inhibition of FFA release is one of the earliest effects of insulin, and the concentration of insulin required for this is one-tenth that needed to stimulate glucose uptake directly by muscle. FFA release from adipose tissue is also reduced because the glucose taken up by adipocytes produces glycerol which can be used to re-esterify intracellular FFAs rather than releasing them.

Mild impairment of insulin-stimulated glucose uptake, i.e. insulin resistance, is manifested first as a rise in postprandial plasma insulin and, when more marked, as an increase in postprandial blood glucose responses. The inset of **Fig. 7** shows that young, normal subjects were more sensitive to insulin than obese, middle-aged subjects who, in turn, were more insulin sensitive than subjects with impaired glucose tolerance. The main part of Fig. 7 shows that the middle-aged obese subjects were able to overcome their insulin resistance and have a normal post-

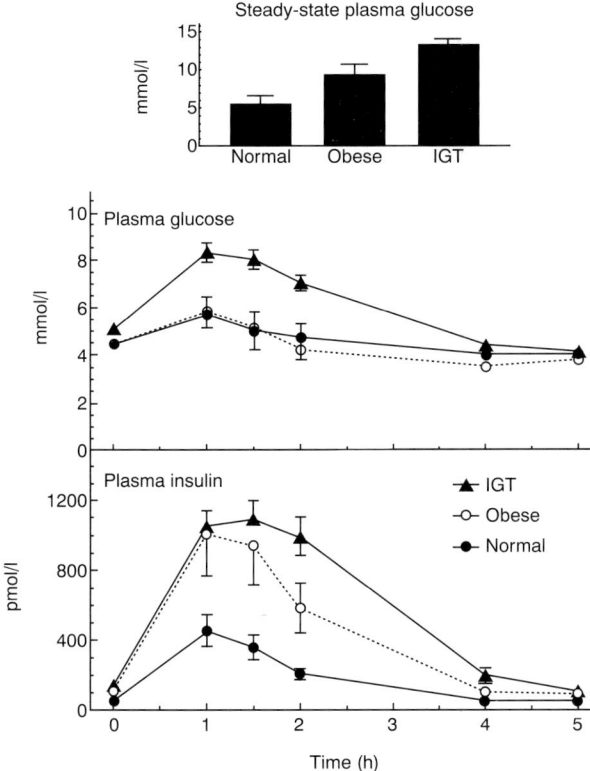

Figure 7 Mean ± SEM plasma glucose (top) and insulin (bottom) concentrations of 10 young lean and eight middle-aged obese subjects with normal glucose tolerance, and 21 subjects with impaired glucose tolerance after a liquid breakfast test meal. The inset (top) shows their steady-state plasma glucose concentrations (SSPG) during intravenous infusion of somatostatin, glucose and insulin on a separate day. SSPG is inversely related to insulin sensitivity, i.e. the higher the SSPG, the lower the insulin sensitivity.

prandial plasma glucose response by secreting much more insulin. Subjects with impaired glucose tolerance were unable to secrete enough insulin to overcome their insulin resistance, as shown by their raised postprandial plasma glucose. In the normal subjects, about 35% of whole body glucose disposal during a euglycaemic insulin clamp is accounted for by glucose oxidation, and the rest is glucose storage. In states of insulin resistance, the reduction in glucose uptake is due mostly to a reduction in glucose storage; glucose oxidation is reduced by 20–30%, but glucose storage is reduced by 40–60%.

Liver   As shown in Fig. 1, endogenous glucose, i.e. hepatic glucose output, accounts for part of the glucose in blood in the postprandial state. In normal subjects, hepatic glucose output is reduced to zero quite rapidly after a meal. However, as noted above, in diabetes hepatic glucose output is increased, and after eating it is not suppressed as effectively as in normal subjects. In addition, the liver contributes to

the control of postprandial blood glucose by taking up glucose and storing it. In diabetes, hepatic glycogen content is low, and in type I diabetes, the rise in hepatic glycogen concentration during the day is only 30% that of normal subjects. Thus, part of the postprandial elevation in blood glucose in diabetes is due to increased hepatic glucose output and reduced hepatic glucose storage.

The liver extracts about 50% of the insulin entering it from the portal vein, and thus has an important role in regulating peripheral insulin concentrations, which in turn influence peripheral insulin sensitivity. There is evidence that plasma FFAs compete for insulin binding sites on the liver. Thus, in states of insulin resistance such as abdominal obesity and diabetes, where portal FFA concentrations are increased, the fraction of insulin the liver extracts is reduced. Another cause of reduced hepatic insulin extraction is cirrhosis of the liver. The reason for this is that cirrhosis causes fibrosis, which disrupts the architecture of the liver, resulting in direct shunting of portal blood to the peripheral circulation. Reduced hepatic insulin extraction increases the peripheral insulin concentration which, in turn, results in a downregulation of insulin receptors in the periphery leading to insulin resistance and a further exacerbation of postprandial hyperglycaemia and hyperinsulinaemia.

Pancreas   The β cells of the pancreas secrete insulin in response to several factors including neurological signals stimulated by the sight, smell and taste of food (the cephalic phase of insulin secretion), blood glucose and amino acids, and the gut hormones GIP and GLP-1. Plasma insulin concentrations vary on a minute-by-minute basis, suggesting that insulin is secreted in discrete pulses every few minutes. This presumably allows for the most efficient control of blood glucose because less insulin is required to produce a given reduction of plasma glucose if it is infused in a pulsatile fashion than if continuously infused. There are two phases of insulin secretion after a meal: the first phase is a large, rapid burst which occurs within a few minutes of starting to eat and is only detected if plasma insulin is measured very frequently after eating; the second phase is a slower but more prolonged secretion of insulin which lasts for as long as plasma glucose is elevated over the fasting level.

As noted above, about 60% of glucose disappearance is mediated by insulin; in particular the first phase of insulin secretion appears to be critical in controlling postprandial plasma glucose. The evidence for this is that a defect in first-phase insulin secretion appears early in the pathogenesis of type

II diabetes, despite markedly elevated second-phase insulin secretion. If insulin resistance is present, normal postprandial glucose can be maintained by markedly increased plasma insulin (Fig. 7). However, a protein called amyloid is secreted with insulin, and it is thought that this protein accumulates around the β cells in the pancreas and impairs their ability to secrete insulin. In addition, there is evidence that even small increases of blood glucose, if sustained, reduce β cell responsiveness, a process called glucose toxicity. Thus, sustained hyperinsulinaemia and sustained elevations of postprandial plasma glucose may lead to a reduced ability of the pancreas to respond rapidly to a rise in plasma glucose because of amyloid accumulation and/or glucose toxicity. The progressive loss of the early rise in plasm insulin after an oral glucose load with the progression from obese normal to impaired glucose (IGT) to diabetes (NIDDM) is shown in **Fig. 8**. Obese subjects have a much higher rise in plasma insulin between 0 and 15 min than normal subjects and manage to maintain a nearly normal plasma glucose response. However, IGT subjects have a lower insulin response at 15 min than obese subjects despite higher plasma insulin during the 60–120 min period, and the subjects with NIDDM have no rise in plasma insulin at all until after 30 min, despite a markedly increased plasma glucose.

Nevertheless, a relative reduction in insulin secretion is not the only reason why an individual

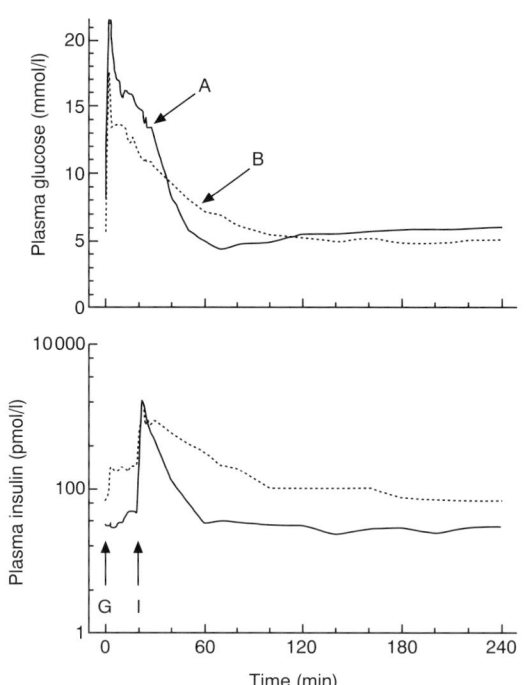

Figure 9 Plasma glucose (top) and log plasma insulin (bottom) concentrations after intravenous glucose injection at time 0 min (G) and insulin injection at time 20 min (I) of two subjects with glucose intolerance. Subject A has reduced insulin secretion and subject B has impaired insulin sensitivity.

may develop impaired glucose tolerance. **Fig. 9** shows the results of a frequently sampled intravenous glucose tolerance test in which glucose is injected intravenously at 0 min followed by a bolus of insulin at 20 min. The results illustrated are from two subjects with glucose intolerance; subject A has almost no insulin secretion in response to the glucose injection, but a relatively rapid rate of disappearance of plasma glucose after the insulin injection; subject B has a prompt insulin response, but a slow rate of glucose disappearance. Thus, insulin resistance, reduced first-phase insulin secretion, or a combination of both may be responsible for glucose intolerance.

See also: **Amino Acids**: Metabolism. **Diabetes Mellitus**: Classification and Chemical Pathology. **Fructose**: Absorption and Metabolism. **Insulin Resistance**: Aetiology and Association with Disease. **Lipids**: Chemistry and Classification; Composition and Role of Phospholipids in the Body. **Liver Disorders**: Nutritional Management.

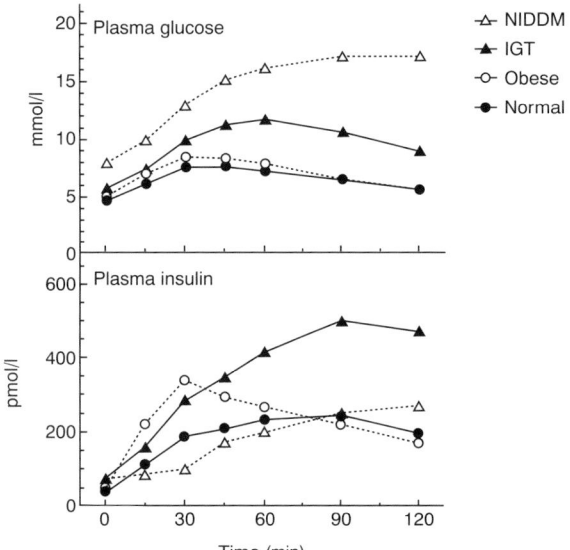

Figure 8 Mean plasma glucose (top) and insulin (bottom) of eight lean normal subjects, seven obese normal subjects, seven subjects with impaired glucose tolerance and three subjects with mild diabetes mellitus for 2 h after a 75 g oral glucose tolerance test. Each subject repeated the test four times.

Further Reading

Bergman RN (1989) Lilly Lecture 1989: Toward physiological understanding of glucose tolerance: Minimal-model approach. *Diabetes* 38:1512–1527.

Brownlee M (1992) Glycation products and the patho-genesis of diabetic complications. *Diabetes Care* **15**:1835–1843.

DeFronzo RA (1988) Lilly Lecture 1987: The triumvirate: β-cell, muscle, liver: a collusion responsible for NIDDM. *Diabetes* **37**:667–687.

Flatt JP (1995) McCollum Award Lecture, 1995: Diet, life-style, and weight maintenance. *American Journal of Clinical Nutrition* **62**:820–836.

Frayn KN and Kingman SM (1995) Dietary sugars and lipid metabolism in humans. *American Journal of Clinical Nutrition* **62**(supplement):250S–263S.

Hawley JA and Burke LM (1997) Effect of meal frequency and timing on physical performance. *British Journal of Nutrition* (supplement) in press.

Matthews DR (1993) Insulin secretion: pulsatility and sig-nalling attributes. In: Marshall SM, Home PD, Alberti KGMM and Krall LP (eds) *The Diabetes Annual*, no. 7, pp. 18–29. Amsterdam: Elsevier Science.

Pedersen O (1993) Glucose transporters and diabetes mel-litus. In: Marshall SM, Home PD, Alberti KGMM and Krall LP (eds) *The Diabetes Annual*, no. 7, pp. 30–54. Amsterdam: Elsevier Science.

Porte D, Jr (1991) β-cells in type II diabetes mellitus. *Diabetes* **40**:166–180.

Radziuk J and Barron P (1995) Does pancreatic portal venous drainage matter? In: Marshall SM, Home PD and Rizza RA (eds) *The Diabetes Annual*, no. 9, pp. 141–158. Amsterdam: Elsevier Science.

Rothman DL, Magnusson I, Katz LD, Shulman RG and Shulman GI (1991) Quantitation of hepatic glyco-genolysis and gluconeogenesis in fasting humans with ^{13}C NMR. *Science* **254**:573–576.

Rossetti L, Giaccari A and DeFronzo RA (1990) Glucose toxicity. *Diabetes Care* **13**: 610–630.

Taylor R, Magnusson I, Rothman DL, Cline GW, Caumo A, Cobelli C and Shulman GI (1996) Direct assessment of liver glycogenstorage by ^{13}C nuclear magnetic reson-ance spectroscopy and regulation of glucose homeo-stasis after a mixed meal in normal subjects. *Journal of Clinical Investigation* **97**:126–132.

Wolfe RR (1992) *Radioactive and Stable Isotope Tracers in Biomedicine: Principles and Practice of Kinetic Analysis*. New York: Wiley-Liss, Inc.

Glucose Tolerance

T Wolever,
University of Toronto, Ontario,
Canada

Copyright © 1998 Academic Press

Glucose tolerance is the response of the blood glu-cose concentration in an individual after consuming an oral load of glucose. Abnormal glucose tolerance covers a spectrum from so-called impaired glucose tolerance to frank diabetes mellitus. Diabetes is a major health problem, not only for those who have it, but it is also very costly for society as a whole because of the direct costs of treatment and the indirect costs due to loss of productivity. Currently in Western countries, although only 2–5% of the population have diabetes, the cost of the treatment of diabetes and its complications may account for up to 20% of total expenditure for health care. Unless effective preventative measures can be developed, over the next 25 years the problem of treating dia-betes is likely to increase to epidemic proportions globally. In Western countries diabetes will become more common because its prevalence is higher in eld-erly individuals, and the proportion of the popu-lation over the age of 65 years, currently about 15%, will increase to 25% early in the next century. In developing countries, increased affluence is accompanied by an increased incidence of chronic diseases; amongst the earliest of these to appear is diabetes, sometimes at astoundingly high rates. In some Pacific island populations, the incidence of dia-betes is 5–10 times that in Europe or North America.

Any attempt to reduce the public health burden of diabetes by earlier detection and treatment or by delaying or preventing the onset of the disorder will involve one or more diagnostic tests to assess the degree of elevation of blood glucose. It is believed by many that the most accurate test for this purpose is the glucose tolerance test. This article will describe the glucose tolerance test and its potential role in the early detection and prevention of diabetes, discuss some of the advantages and disadvantages of the glu-cose tolerance test and other types of tests which have been proposed to replace it, and show the prevalence of abnormal glucose tolerance in different populations around the world.

Definition

Principle of the glucose tolerance test (GTT)

The principle of the GTT is to determine an individ-ual's blood glucose response to an oral load of glu-cose under standardized conditions. The dose of glu-cose used has varied over the years, in different parts of the world and in different situations, from 50 g to 100 g; surprisingly, in normal subjects this makes little difference to the blood glucose response (**Fig. 1**). It is generally agreed that the test should be car-ried out after a 12 h overnight fast and after having consumed a diet containing at least 250 g carbo-hydrate per day for at least 3 days. The subject should remain at rest without smoking for the dur-ation of the test. The glucose response is most com-monly measured in plasma obtained from forearm venous blood taken into tubes containing an additive

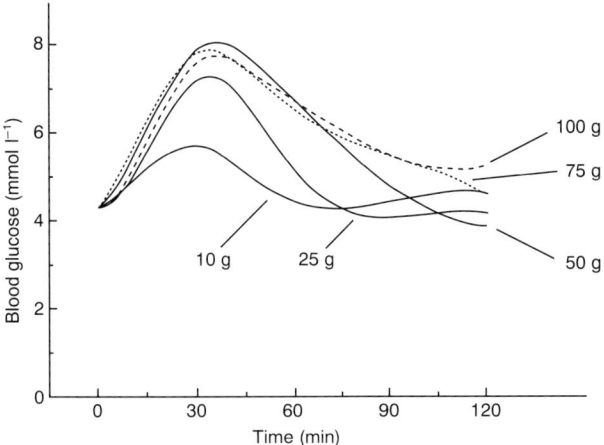

Figure 1 Blood glucose responses in normal subjects following 10, 25, 50, 75 or 100 g oral glucose. From Wolever TMS (1993) Glucose tolerance and the glycaemic index. In: *Encyclopaedia of Food Science, Food Technology and Nutrition.* Macrae R, Robinson R, Sadler M (eds), Vol. 4, pp. 2214–2220. London: Academic Press.

to prevent blood clotting and inhibit red cell glucose metabolism (e.g. sodium fluoride or potassium oxalate). Valid results can be obtained using other types of blood sample but the diagnostic criteria may differ from those in venous plasma. The blood glucose level must be measured fasting and 2 h after the oral glucose load which is dissolved, commonly 250–300 ml of fruit-flavoured water. Additional blood samples may be taken at more frequent intervals, and the test is sometimes prolonged to 3–5 h.

Measurement of blood glucose

The measurement of blood glucose is deceptively complex. Blood can be obtained from the venous, capillary or, uncommonly, the arterial circulation. The glucose concentration in arterial blood is usually higher than that in venous blood, with capillary blood being intermediate, because body tissues remove some of the glucose from arterial blood before it reaches the veins; however the difference varies depending upon the rate of blood flow, the metabolic activity of the tissues, whether the individual is in the fasting or postprandial state and whether the subject has normal or impaired glucose tolerance or diabetes. In addition, glucose can be measured in plasma or whole blood. Since the concentration of glucose in red blood cells is less than that in plasma, the concentration of glucose in whole blood is less than that in plasma. **Fig. 2** shows that the difference between glucose measured in venous plasma and simultaneously obtained whole capillary blood depends upon glucose tolerance status. The concentration of glucose in fasting capillary blood was 0.5–1.0 mmol l⁻¹ less than that in venous plasma in nor-

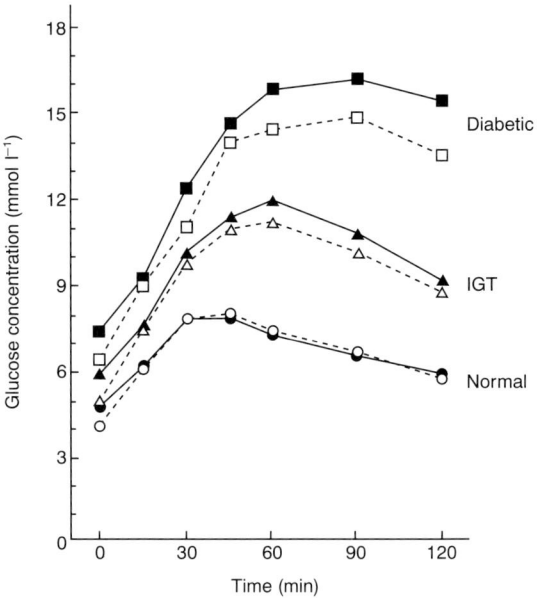

Figure 2 Mean glucose concentration in simultaneously obtained venous plasma and whole capillary blood in normal subjects and subjects with impaired glucose tolerance (IGT) and diabetes after consumption of 75 g oral glucose. Solid symbols, venous plasma; hollow symbols, capillary blood. (Wolever TMS, Chiasson JL, Ross SA, Ryan EA and Hunt JA. Unpublished observations.)

mal, impaired glucose tolerance (IGT) and diabetic subjects. However, after 75 g oral glucose, capillary blood glucose was similar to venous plasma glucose in normal subjects, was about 0.5 mmol l⁻¹ less than venous plasma in IGT subjects, and was 1–2 mmol l⁻¹ less than venous plasma in diabetic subjects. To make matters even more complex, in some methods of measuring glucose whole blood is used but the plasma concentration is measured; for example in some glucose meters a drop of whole blood is applied to a multilayered strip, the outer layer of which allows only the plasma to come into contact with the reagents.

The GTT as a diagnostic tool

The most common use of the GTT is as a test for diabetes mellitus, but it is also used to diagnose hypoglycaemia. Until recently the 75 g oral GTT was accepted as the standard diagnostic test for diabetes by both the World Health Organization (WHO) and the National Diabetes Data Group (NDDG) from the USA. Both groups had similar diagnostic criteria with diabetes defined as a fasting venous plasma glucose (FPG) concentration ≥7.8 mmol l⁻¹ (140 mg dl⁻¹) or ≥11.1 mmol l⁻¹ (≥200 mg dl⁻¹) 2 h after 75 g GTT. It is not necessary to do a GTT in the presence of classic symptoms of diabetes and if random plasma glucose is ≥11.1 mmol l⁻¹ on more than one occasion. Impaired glucose tolerance is the term used to describe a borderline glucose response, i.e. a normal FPG and a plasma glucose concentration of 7.8–11.0 mmol l^{-1} (140–198 mg dl^{-1}) 2 h after a 75 g GTT. In 1997 an expert committee of the American Diabetes Association (ADA) published new diagnostic criteria (**Table 1**) with a reduced FPG cut-off; diabetes is now defined as FPG ≥7.0 mmol l^{-1} (126 mg dl^{-1}). Plasma glucose ≥11.1 mmol l^{-1} 2 h after a 75 g GTT is still considered diagnostic for diabetes. However, the GTT was not recommended for routine screening because of the drawbacks described below. The ADA recommended that measurement of FPG be used to screen for diabetes. In addition, a new diagnostic category of impaired fasting glucose was introduced, defined as FPG of 6.0 to 6.9 mmol l^{-1} (110–125 mg dl^{-1}). It is anticipated that the WHO will recommend the same FPG cut-off as the ADA, but will not use the term 'impaired fasting glucose'. The WHO may continue to recommend the GTT as the preferred method of screening for diabetes because 30–40% of asymptotic people with a plasma glucose ≥11.1 mmol l^{-1} 2 h after a 75 g GTT have a FPG <7.0 mmol l^{-1} and would thus be missed using a screening test based only on FPG.

For the diagnosis of abnormalities of glucose tolerance during pregnancy two sets of criteria are currently recommended by national or international organizations. The WHO recommends the same procedure as used for nonpregnant adults, i.e. a single 75 g oral glucose tolerance test. The NDDG recommends a 3 h test following a 100 g oral glucose load. Since it is recommended that all pregnant women be screened, and since 100 g glucose is quite unpalatable for many people, a two-stage procedure is often used in which the 100 g glucose load is only administered to women with plasma glucose ≥7.8 mmol l^{-1} 1 h after a 50 g glucose load. Both the American and Canadian Diabetes Associations endorse a two-stage procedure. In most other parts of the world the WHO criteria are used.

The diagnostic cutoff points for the GTT are based on prospective studies in which large goups of subjects were given an oral glucose load and followed for periods of 5–10 years or more to determine the relative risk of the later development of vascular and neurological disease.

Assessment

The need for a diagnostic tool

A strategy which may reduce the burden of diabetes is to achieve earlier detection and treatment, and, if possible, prevention of the disorder. Detection of diabetes requires a diagnostic tool. At present glucose tolerance screening is not done widely, partly because of difficulties with the diagnostic test which will be discussed below, and partly because the benefits of earlier diagnosis of diabetes have not been demonstrated. It has been estimated that the average interval between the development of type II diabetes and its diagnosis is 6–10 years, and some individuals have major complications at the time of diagnosis. There is now firm evidence from the Diabetes Complications and Control Trial (DCCT), and other trials, that improving glucose control will prevent diabetes complications in type I, insulin-dependent diabetes. However, 85–90% of people with diabetes have type II diabetes. It is generally assumed, but not yet proven, that the DCCT results can be extrapolated to type II diabetes. The results of the UK Prospective Diabetes Study are expected in 1998; if they show that improved glucose control reduces diabetes complications in type II diabetes, there will be added incentive for diabetes screening.

People with IGT have an increased risk of developing diabetes, and it would be logical to try to identify such individuals and treat them to prevent diabetes. IGT has no symptoms, and the only way to detect it is to do a glucose tolerance test. Screening for IGT is not widely done because, until recently, there was no evidence that treating IGT will prevent or delay the onset of diabetes. A recent economic analysis has suggested that even a modest ability to prevent or delay the onset of diabetes by treatment of IGT may actually save money. In addition, a number of new drugs have been developed which may prevent diabetes. Thus, at the time of writing this article, at least three large prospective trials are underway to see if treatment of IGT will prevent

Table 1 Diagnostic criteria for diabetes mellitus according to the Expert Committee on the Diagnosis and Classification of Diabetes Mellitus of the American Diabetes Association (1997)

Diagnostic category	Fasting plasma glucose	Plasma glucose 2 h after 75 g GTT
Normal	<6.0 mmol l^{-1} (<110 mg dl^{-1})	<7.8 mmol l^{-1} (140 mg dl^{-1})
Impaired fasting glucose	6.0–6.9 mmol l^{-1} (110–125 mg dl^{-1})	
Impaired glucose tolerance*	<7.0 mmol l^{-1} (<140 mg dl^{-1})	7.8–11.0 mmol l^{-1} (140–199 mg dl^{-1})
Diabetes	≥7.0 mmol l^{-1} (≥126 mg dl^{-1})	≥11.1 mmol l^{-1} (≥ 200 mg dl^{-1})

*A diagnostic concentration of fasting plasma glucose for impaired glucose tolerance is not indicated in the expert committee report. It is presumed that fasting plasma glucose must be <7.0 mmol l^{-1}, since a higher level would be diagnostic for diabetes.

diabetes. If these trials show that diabetes can be prevented, then this will provide a strong incentive to screen for the detection of IGT.

Evaluating a diagnostic test

A diagnostic test is used to determine if an individual has a disease or disorder. The test result is either positive or negative. A true positive occurs if the test result is positive and the individual really has the disease, while a false positive occurs if the test result is positive but the individual does not have the disease. Similarly a true negative occurs if the test result is negative in a normal individual, and a false negative when the test result is negative in a person who really has the disease (**Table 2**). The sensitivity of the test is the proportion of individuals who really have the disease with a positive test result. Specificity is the proportion of normal individuals with a negative test result. Predictive value positive is the proportion of positive tests which are true positives and predictive value negative is the proportion of negative tests which are true negatives. Ideally a test will produce no false negatives and no false positives, resulting in 100% specificity and 100% sensitivity. In practice, however, there is always a trade-off between specificity and sensitivity, as illustrated in **Fig. 3**. Increasing sensitivity of a test (i.e. reducing the number of false negatives) results in reduced specificity (i.e. an increased number of false positives), and vice versa.

Problems with the GTT

Although the GTT is considered to be the gold standard test for determining whether an individual has diabetes, it is not widely used because the GTT is perceived as difficult, complicated and time-consuming. The result of the GTT are highly variable and can be abnormal because of physical inactivity or low carbohydrate intake for several days before the test. A false positive result may expose a normal individual to inappropriate treatment. On the other hand, a false negative result could lead to a delay in seeking medical care. Glucose solutions are unpalat-

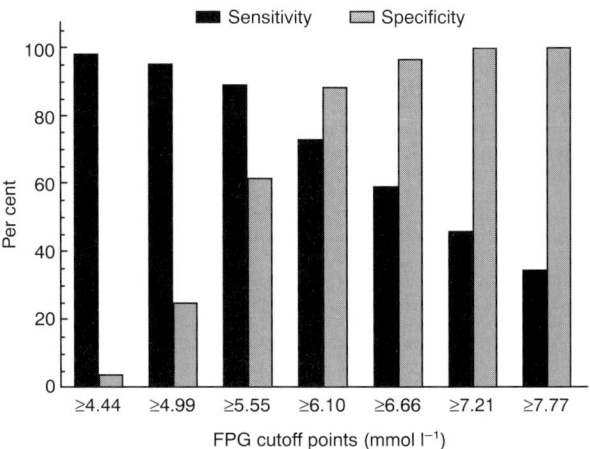

Figure 3 Mean sensitivity and specificity in US and Israel populations aged 40–69 years (total n = 4351) by different fasting plasma glucose (FPG) cutoff points. Diabetes status was determined by 75 g oral glucose tolerance test. Data from Modan M and Harris MI (1994) Fasting plasma glucose in screening for NIDDM in the US and Israel. *Diabetes Care* **17**: 437.

able to many people and nauseating to some. There is also a concern with any screening test that the new diagnosis of diabetes in a person with no symptoms is very alarming and may affect an individual's ability to obtain insurance and employment; from a medical standpoint the diagnosis of diabetes exposes an individual to addional testing, follow-up and treatment which may be bothersome, unpleasant or even hazardous.

Variability of GTT

If an individual is tested with a GTT on repeated occasions, the results on each occasion are quite variable. The degree of variation can be expressed as the coefficient of variation (CV), which is defined as the standard deviation (SD) expressed as a percentage of the mean. Typically, the mean CV of repeated GTTs in the same individuals is about 15%. This degree of variability of the GTT is particularly important in the borderline area and this can be illustrated if one considers a hypothetical individual with a true plasma glucose concentration 2 h after 75 g glucose (2 h pc glucose) of 9.4 mmol l^{-1}, i.e. the midpoint of the IGT range. If the result of repeated GTTs are assumed to be normally distributed with a CV of 15%, the SD = 9.4 × 0.15 = 1.4; thus, only about 75%, or three out of four of this individual's GTT test results will be within the IGT range of 7.8 to 11.0 mmol l^{-1} (i.e. ± 1.13 SD from the mean), and 25% of the tests will incorrectly classify this individual's glucose tolerance. This is borne out in practice. Figure 4 shows the plasma glucose concentrations 2 h after 75 g oral glucose of eight subjects who were given a GTT on four separate occasions over a two-

Table 2 Evaluating a diagnostic test: sensitivity = A/(A + B); specificity = C/(C + D); predictive value positive = A/(A + C); predictive value negative = D/(B + D)

Test result	Presence of disorder	
	Yes	*No*
Positive	True positive (A)	False positive (C)
Negative	False negative (B)	True negative (D)

month period. Each subject's mean 2 h pc glucose was within the range for IGT, however, of the 32 GTTs done by these subjects, 11 (34%) gave incorrect results (**Fig. 4**).

It is not known why the variability of 2 h pc plasma glucose is so high. Error in the measurement of glucose cannot account for it because analytical error typically has a CV in the range of 2–5%. Presumably, therefore, the variation is biological, and may have to do with day-to-day variation in factors such as diet, exercise, emotions, stress, etc. However, there is preliminary evidence that, in nondiabetic subjects, 2 h pc plasma glucose concentrations are less variable after consuming 50 g carbohydrate from a starchy test meal than after consuming 75 g glucose (**Fig. 5**). Theoretically, if the variability of the GTT can be reduced, this would result in increased sensitivity and specificity which would allow more reliable detection of minor degrees of carbohydrate intolerance. Whether this is worth doing or not will depend upon the outcome of currently ongoing studies to see if type II diabetes can be prevented by treating IGT.

Use of other tests for diagnosing diabetes

Measurement of fasting plasma glucose (FPG) is a common way of screening for diabetes in clinical practice, and is a much simpler test than the GTT. FPG lacks sensitivity and specificity: using a low value of FPG as a cutoff point results in high sensitivity (few false negatives) but low specificity (many

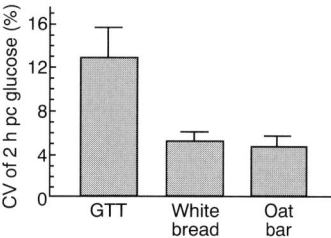

Figure 5 Mean ± SEM within-individual coefficient of variation (CV) of capillary blood glucose 2 h after consumption of 75 g oral glucose (GTT) or 50 g carbohydrate from white bread or a prototype diagnostic oat bar. The results are based on tests in 10 nondiabetic subjects who tested each test meal on three occasions over a six-week period. The differences between GTT and white bread and between GTT and oat bar are significant ($p<0.01$). Data from Wolever TMS et al. (1996) Nutrition Research **16**: 901. (With permission from Elsevier Science.)

false positives). Raising the level of FPG for the diagnostic cutoff improves specificity but reduces sensitivity (many false negatives) (Fig. 3). Since most people do not have diabetes, a reduction in specificity will result in a much larger number of incorrect tests as the same reduction in sensitivity. For example, if the prevalence of diabetes is 10%, for every 100 people screened, 90 will be normal and 10 will have diabetes. If the diagnostic test has a specificity of 90%, nine normal subjects will have a false positive test, whereas with a sensitivity of 90% only one person with diabetes will have a false negative. Thus, when screening for diabetes, the diagnostic test must have high specificity. When using FPG for screening, therefore, a high cutoff value is used and the test is relatively insensitive (Fig. 3). What this means is that the GTT will detect less severe abnormalities of glucose intolerance more reliably than will measurement of FPG. Therefore, the question of whether to use GTT or FPG depends upon the level of abnormality of glucose tolerance that one is willing to accept. If it is not considered important to detect mild abnormalities of glucose tolerance, then FPG is an acceptable test; however, if one wants to detect mild abnormalities of glucose tolerance, then the GTT is preferable to FPG.

Glycosylated hemoglobin (HbA1c), which gives an indication of average blood glucose concentrations over the last 3 months, can also be measured in fasting, or even nonfasting blood, and may also be a useful diagnostic or screening test, alone or when combined with FBG. However, the measurement of HbA1c is not very precise and has not been standardized. In addition, a mildly elevated HbA1c does not reliably distinguish between a normal, IGT or diabetic GTT result.

Studies show that FPG and HbA1c results do not compare well with those of the GTT; but, this may

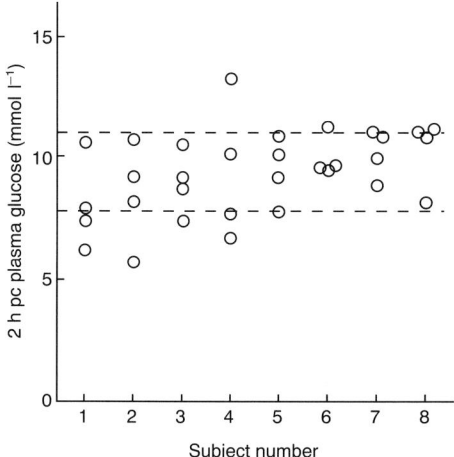

Figure 4 Concentrations of plasma glucose 2 h after 75 g oral glucose (2 h pc plasma glucose) in eight subjects who repeated the test four times over a 2-month period. Mean 2 h pc glucose for each subject was within the range for impaired glucose tolerance (IGT). According to WHO criteria, glucose values below the lower dotted line are normal; values above the upper dotted line are diagnostic for diabetes; values on or between the lines indicate IGT. (Wolever TMS, Chiasson JL, Ross SA, Ryan EA and Hunt JA. Unpublished observations.)

be because of the inaccuracy of the GTT. When 2 h pc glucose, FPG and HbA1c were compared in their ability to predict the presence of diabetes complications, the specificity and sensitivity of the three different tests were similar. Thus, it has been argued that none of the three tests is clearly superior to the others. However, this conclusion only applies to identifying individuals who already have the microvascular complications of diabetes. If diabetes complications are to be prevented, individuals at risk must be identified and treated before the complications have occurred. We do not know yet if diabetes and its complications can be prevented by treating individuals with mild abnormalities of glucose tolerance; but the GTT is more reliable than FPG or HbA1c for detecting mild abnormalities of glucose tolerance.

Incidence and Prevalence

The incidence of a disease is the number of new cases arising within a certain period; prevalence is the total number of cases which exist at a certain point in time. The prevalence of abnormal glucose tolerance (diabetes and IGT) varies over a 30-fold range in different populations around the world (**Fig. 6**). Unfortunately, the populations at greatest risk are those which can least afford to deal with the problem; developing countries, minority groups and disadvantaged communities in industrialized countries. Figure 6 shows the prevalence of all diabetes. Type II, or noninsulin-dependent diabetes (NIDDM), accounts for 80–90% or more of all diabetes in most countries. Type I, or insulin-dependent diabetes (IDDM), accounts for only a small proportion of all diabetes;

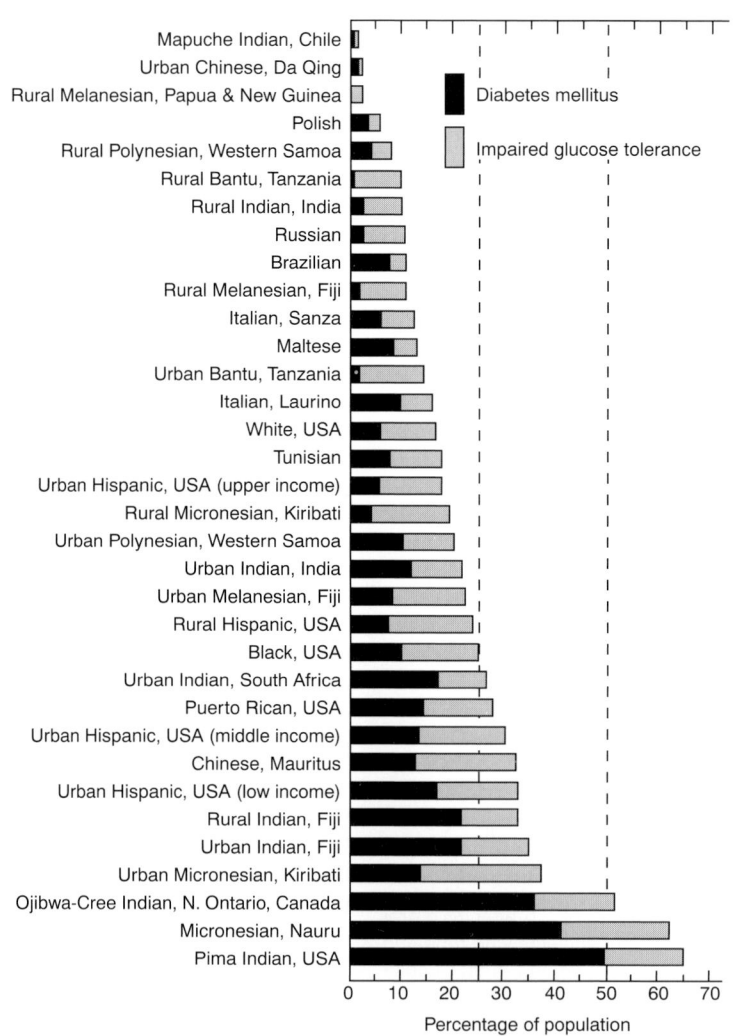

Figure 6 Age-adjusted prevalence of diabetes mellitus and impaired glucose tolerance for individuals 30–64 years of age in different populations. Redrawn from King *et al.* (1993) with data for Ojibwa-Cree Indians added (Harris SB, Gittelsohn J, Hanley A, Barnie A, Wolever TMS, Gao J, Logan A and Zinman B (1997) *Diabetes Care*, **20**: 185–187.

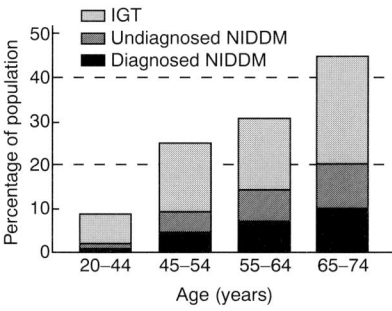

Figure 7 Prevalence of diagnosed and undiagnosed diabetes and impaired glucose tolerance in different age groups of the US population. Redrawn from Kenny *et al.* (1995).

nevertheless, the incidence of IDDM varies widely around the world from 0.7 new cases per 100 000 per year in Shanghai, China, to 10–15 per 100 000 per year in the USA and UK, to as much as 35 per 100 000 per year in Finland.

The prevalence of diabetes varies by age (**Fig. 7**); thus, when comparing rates in different countries where the mean age of the populations differ, the data need to be adjusted for age. In different populations the ratio of prevalence of diabetes in males and females varies markedly, but, overall, diabetes occurs roughly equally in men and women. However, IGT tends to be more common in women, possibly because pregnancy causes insulin resistance, and if glucose intolerance develops during pregnancy it may persist or reappear after delivery.

In the USA, the prevalence of diabetes has been increasing in a linear fashion over the past 35 years (**Fig. 8**). This is partly due to the ageing population, but even when age-adjusted, the prevalence of diabetes has doubled over that period of time.

Conclusions

Diabetes is a major global public health problem, the severity of which is increasing. To reduce the burden of this problem, earlier diagnosis and treatment are necessary. The role of the glucose tolerance test, the meaning of the term glucose tolerance and the diagnostic criteria for diabetes are matters of controversy and debate. Measurement of plasma or blood glucose after an oral carbohydrate load may be the best simple way to identify those with early diabetes or those at risk of developing diabetes. However, there may be revisions in the way tests are conducted and the diagnostic cutoffs which are applied. The resolution of the debate will, not doubt, be influenced by the results of current studies which, in the near future, will provide evidence as to whether earlier detection and treatment of diabetes and IGT is useful.

See also: **Diabetes Mellitus**: Classification and Chemical Pathology; Aetiology and Epidemiology; Dietary Management; Secondary Complications and Their Prevention. **Glucose**: Chemistry, Dietary Sources and Glycaemic Index.

Further Reading

Davidson MB, Peters AL and Schriger DL (1995) An alternative approach to the diagnosis of diabetes with a review of the literature. *Diabetes Care* 18:1065–1071.

Engelgau MM, Aubert RE, Thompson TJ and Herman WH (1996) Screeing for NIDDM in nonpregnant adults: A review of principles, screening tests and recommendations. *Diabetes Care* 18:1606–1618.

Kenny SJ, Aubert RE and Geiss LS (1995) Prevalence and incidence of non-insulin-dependent diabetes. In: National Diabetes Data Group, *Diabetes in America*, 2nd edn, NIH Publication No. 95–1468, pp. 47–67. Bethesda, MD: National Institutes of Health.

King H, Rewers M, WHO Ad Hoc Diabetes Reporting Group (1993) Global estimates for prevalence of diabetes mellitus and impaired glucose tolerance in adults. *Diabetes Care* **16**:157–177.

McCance DR, Hanson RL, Charles MA, Jacobsson LTH, Pettit DJ, Bennett PH and Knowler WC (1995) Which test for diagnosing diabetes? *Diabetes Care* 18:1042–1044.

Knowler WC (1994) Screeing for NIDDM: Opportunities for detection, treatment, and prevention. *Diabetes Care* 17:445–450.

Modan M and Harris MI (1994) Fasting plasma glucose in screening for NIDDM in the US and Israel. *Diabetes Care* 17:436–439.

National Diabetes Data Group (1979) Classification and diagnosis of diabetes mellitus and other categories of glucose intolerance. *Diabetes* 28:1039–1057.

National Diabetes Data Group (1995) *Diabetes in*

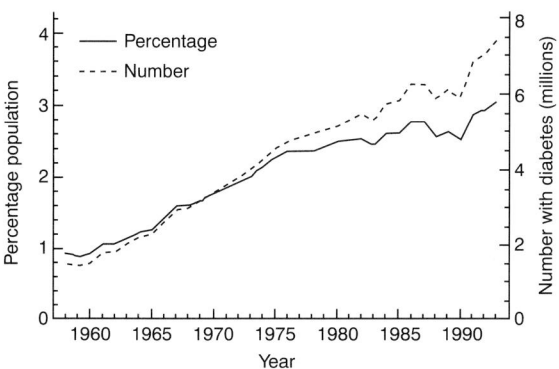

Figure 8 Prevalence of diabetes in the US population from 1958 to 1993. Redrawn from Kenny *et al.* (1995).

America, 2nd edn, NIH Publication No. 95–1468. Bethesda, MD: National Institutes of Health.

Pan X, Li G, Hu Y-H, Wang Ji-x, Yang W, An Z, Hu Z, Lin J, Xiao J-Z, Cao H, Liu P-A, Jiang X, Jiang Y, Wang Jin, Zheng H, Zhang H, Bennett PH and Howard BV (1997) Effects of diet and exercise in preventing NIDDM in people with impaired glucose tolerance. *Diabetes Care* 20:537–544.

Stolk RP, Orchard TJ and Grobbee DE (1995) Why use the oral glucose tolerance test? *Diabetes Care* 18:1045–1049.

The Expert Committee on the Diagnosis and Classification of Diabetes Mellitus (1997) Report of the Expert Committee on the Diagnosis and Classification of Diabetes Mellitus. *Diabetes Care* 20:1183–1197.

WHO (1985) *Diabetes mellitus: report of a WHO study group*. WHO Technical Report Series 727. Geneva: World Health Organization.

Wiener K (1995) Whole blood glucose: what are we actually measuring? *Annals of Clinical Biochemistry* 32:1–8.

Wolever TMS, Vuksan V and Palmason C (1996) Less variation of postprandial blood glucose after starchy test meals than oral glucose. *Nutrition Research* 16:899–905.

Goitre *see* **Iodine**: Iodine Deficiency Disorders.

GOUT

Aetiology and Nutritional Management

Laura C Rall, University of Wisconsin, Stevens Point, USA

R Roubenoff, Tufts University, Boston, Massachusetts, USA

Copyright © 1998 Academic Press

Definition and Aetiology

Gout, from the Latin *gutta* or drop (of evil humour), is an ancient disease that was included in Hippocrates' Aphorisms. In the first edition of his textbook, *Principles and Practice of Medicine* (1892) Osler defined gout as 'a nutritional disorder associated with an excess formation of uric acid'. Today we recognize that this definition is partly true, but that most cases of gout are not due to excess formation of uric acid, but rather to insufficient clearance of the substance. *Hyperuricaemia* occurs when there is too much uric acid in the blood, a condition that is generally agreed to exist when the serum or plasma uric acid exceeds the saturation point at 37°C, which is approximately 7.0 mg dl^{-1}. Hyperuricaemia is a requirement for gout, but it is not always present when a patient presents with a first episode of gout, presumably because the acute deposition of uric acid in a joint reduces blood levels transiently. However, hyperuricaemia is present at some point in virtually all gout patients. It is important to distinguish hyperuricaemia, an asymptomatic condition, from gout, a painful disease which afflicts only a minority of people with elevated uric acid levels. Hyperuricaemia can result from overproduction of uric acid in 10–15% of cases (generally because of enzyme deficiency or overactivity) or from underexcretion of uric acid, which accounts for 85–90% of cases of gout (due to decreased renal clearance of uric acid, even in the setting of a normal glomerular filtration rate).

Chemical Pathology

Uric acid is a by-product of purine metabolism in humans and certain apes, who lack uricase, the enzyme that breaks down uric acid (**Fig. 1**). When uric acid production is normal, and its clearance by the kidneys is normal, this metabolic quirk has no ill effects. However, this minor metabolic inconvenience becomes of pathological importance because uric acid is so poorly soluble in aqueous solutions that it can crystallize and cause the various conditions we recognize as gout. Uric acid can be ingested directly in the diet (especially in organ meats such as liver, kidney and sweetbreads), or it can be produced in the body by two pathways involved in purine metabolism (Fig. 1). The *de novo* synthesis of uric acid proceeds directly from ribose-5-phosphate, while the *salvage* pathway consists of production of

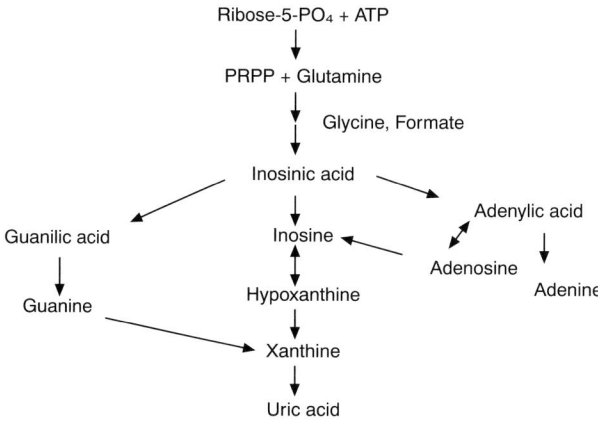

Ribose-5-PO$_4$ + ATP
↓
PRPP + Glutamine
↓ Glycine, Formate
Inosinic acid
Guanilic acid ← Inosinic acid → Adenylic acid
↓ ↓ ↓
Guanine Inosine ← Adenosine ⇄ Adenine
↓ ↓
Hypoxanthine Adenine
↓
Xanthine
↓
Uric acid

Figure 1 Simplified pathway of uric acid metabolism. PRPP, 5-phosphoribosyl-1-pyrophosphate. Modified from Seegmiller, Rosenblum and Kelley (1967) Enzyme-defect associated with a sex-linked human neurological disorder and excessive purine synthesis. *Science* **155**:1682–1684.

the uric acid precursors inosine from adenosine and xanthine from guanine. The medication allopurinol, which blocks the conversion of xanthine to uric acid by xanthine oxidase, is effective because xanthine is far more soluble in aqueous solutions than is uric acid.

The precise mechanism by which uric acid leads to gouty arthritis remains somewhat unclear. However, uric acid is known to be pro-inflammatory, in that it can initiate an immune response with recruitment of white blood cells after uric acid crystals are phagocytosed by polymorphonuclear leucocytes or macrophages. These white blood cells also release tumour necrosis factor and interleukin-1, recruiting more white cells, which release lysosomal enzymes that lead to cartilage destruction and joint erosions with repeated attacks. In addition, ingestion of uric acid leads to death of the phagocytosing cells, leading to release of the uric acid and of additional proteolytic enzymes, thus reinforcing the inflammatory condition. However, the crystals become progressively less phlogistic after several cycles of ingestion and release, and the inflammation relents over a period of 10 to 14 days. The natural history of untreated gout progresses through four stages, from (1) asymptomatic hyperuricaemia to (2) acute gouty arthritis to (3) intercritical gout to (4) chronic tophaceous gout. In addition, renal manifestations of gout develop in up to 50% of patients, depending on the amount of uric acid they excrete.

Prevalence and Risk Factors

Gout is the most common inflammatory arthritis in men, and its prevalence in the USA tripled between 1969 and 1981. This increase is thought to be due to a combination of factors, including ageing of the US population, increased prevalence of diuretic treatment of hypertension, better access to health care, and better diagnosis and reporting of gout. The incidence of gout (i.e. development of new cases) is linked to serum uric acid levels, rising from 0.9 cases per 1000 person-years with uric acid levels under 7.0 mg dl^{-1} to 70 cases per 1000 person-years for those with levels over 10.0 mg dl^{-1}. However, even in this highest category, only 30% of men developed gout over the five years after their uric acid level was determined, confirming that only a minority of hyperuriaemic men develop acute gout.

Risk factors for acute gout other than hyperuricaemia have been identified. All risk factors act either by increasing serum uric acid levels or by reducing the solubility of uric acid in the joints. For example, male sex, alcohol ingestion, obesity and weight gain are associated with increased uric acid production, while diuretics (thiazides and loop diuretics), low-dose salicylates and renal insufficiency lead to reduced clearance of uric acid. Hypertension has been associated with increased risk of gout, but this effect probably operates through renal insufficiency which occurs as a result of hypertension and diuretic therapy. Lead, on the other hand, has been shown to reduce directly the solubility of uric acid in synovial fluid, while lead nephropathy also leads to reduced clearance of uric acid; the gout associated with lead toxicity is known as saturnine gout. Finally, joint trauma and cooling of distal joints reduce solubility of uric acid and increase the risk of an acute attack. Gout was known in the eighteenth century as 'pheasant hunter's toe' when aristocratic gentlemen developed podagra after a day of hunting in the cold marshes and a night of drinking alcohol, especially sherry shipped in lead-lined casks. In more recent times, saturnine gout has been associated with drinking illegal 'moonshine' whiskey distilled through lead-lined stills.

Clinical Features

Gout is typically an episodic monoarthritis, although polyarticular gout (involving three or more joints) occurs in about 10% of cases. The description of the pain of acute gout by Thomas Sydenham in the seventeenth century remains among the best:

> The victim goes to bed and sleeps in good health. About two o'clock in the morning he is awakened by a severe pain in the great toe; more rarely in the heel, ankle, or instep. This pain is like that of a dislocation ... then follow chills and a little fever. The pain ... becomes more intense ... Now it is a violent stretching and

tearing of the ligaments – now it is a gnawing pain and now a pressure and tightening. So exquisite and lively meanwhile is the feeling of the part affected, that it cannot bear the weight of the bed-clothes nor the jar of a person walking in the room. The night passes in torture . . .

Over half of patients present with *podagra*, acute inflammation of the first metatarsophalangeal (MTP) joint, and 75–90% of patients eventually develop podagra. This joint is thought to be most susceptible to gout because it is very prone to trauma and cooling, both of which reduce the solubility of uric acid. After the first MTP, acute gout most commonly involves the ankles, knees, instep, but can also involve the wrists, elbows and small joints of the hands and feet. Large axial joints such as hips, shoulders and vertebral joints are rarely affected. Acute gout often involves a component of tenosynovitis (inflammation of tendon sheaths), and gouty cellulitis (sterile inflammation with urate crystals in the skin) and bursitis have also been described. As Sydenham stated, the onset is generally explosive, but many patients also describe a series of minor attacks leading up to the full-blown episode. Untreated gouty arthritis lasts from days to weeks, but minor bouts may resolve spontaneously in a few hours. At this stage, joint radiographs are normal except for soft tissue swelling. If untreated, acute gout can segue into a deforming, chronic polyarthritis that may be difficult to distinguish from rheumatoid arthritis.

Because a significant proportion of people, perhaps as many as one-third, who have a single acute gouty attack never have another, no further therapy is indicated after the first attack has subsided. Once a patient has demonstrated recurrent attacks of acute gout, or if they have had a uric acid stone (or another type of stone in the setting of hyperuricosuria), treatment aimed at reducing serum uric acid below the point of solubility is indicated. In general, patients who develop a second attack and have a serum creatinine concentration under 2.0 mg dl^{-1} should be evaluated further with a 24 h-urine for creatinine clearance and uric acid output while consuming their regular diet. If the 24-h urinary uric acid totals more than 1000 mg, the patient is classified as an overproducer of uric acid and should be treated with allopurinol if he or she is not allergic. If the 24-h uric acid production is under 700 mg, then the patient is an underexcreter, and may first be treated with a uricosuric agent, which is safer and less expensive than allopurinol. Renal insufficiency will reduce both creatinine clearance and urinary uric acid output, and allopurinol is the drug of choice in this situation, so the utility of a 24-h urine collection is reduced.

Patients who produce between 700 and 1000 mg of uric acid are in a 'grey zone', and clinical judgement regarding optimal therapy is necessary, balancing issues of safety, cost and convenience in the management of a chronic disease.

Chronic tophaceous gout occurs with an average of 10 years of untreated or inadequately treated gout. Over time, the acute attacks become less noticeable, and the patient develops a chronic, often deforming arthritis. This arthritis may mimic rheumatoid arthritis, although it should be less symmetric. At this time, the radiological hallmark of gout, which includes large, well-demarcated erosions in the absence of joint space narrowing ('rat-bite erosions'), are often visible. Tophi, which are subcutaneous deposits of uric acid, may be found in and around joints, bursae (especially the olecranon), tendons (Achilles and infrapatellar), and the extensor surfaces of the forearms. Less commonly, they may arise in the pinna of the ear, cardiac valves, cornea and sclera, and nasal cartilage. Needle aspiration or spontaneous rupture of tophi elicits a white, chalky material that is full of urate crystals under microscopy, and is diagnostic of tophaceous gout. The presence of tophi is always an indication for allopurinol in nonallergic patients.

Dietary Management

The dietary management of gout is focused on two goals: (1) reducing the amount of uric acid which may be deposited as crystals in joints or soft tissues, leading to the clinical syndrome of gout, and (2) managing the disorders that occur with increased frequency among patients with gout, including diabetes mellitus, obesity, hyperlipidemia, hypertension, and atherosclerosis. The focus of the following discussion will be on dietary modifications that may help to achieve these goals.

Low-purine diet

The primary dietary modification that has traditionally been recommended to reduce uric acid production is a low purine diet (less than 75 mg per 24 h, see **Table 1**). Uric acid is the end product of

Table 1 Foods to avoid on a purine-restricted diet

Meats, organ meats (sweetbreads, liver, kidney), fish, eggs, sausages, meat extracts and gravies
Beans, peas, spinach, asparagus, cauliflower, mushrooms
Oatmeal
Legumes
Chocolate
Yeast and yeast extracts
Tea, coffee, cola beverages, alcoholic beverages

purine metabolism in humans, formed by oxidation of its precursors, the oxypurines, hypoxanthine and xanthine. Other diet-related factors that also contribute to increased uric acid levels include obesity and even mild weight gain, starvation and ketosis, and high protein and fat intakes. However, the mechanism by which these factors contribute to increased uric acid levels appears to be different from that which occurs after a high dietary purine intake. In the former case, reduced excretion or an imbalance between the size of the urate pool and the renal clearance of urate seem most important, while high dietary purine intake causes increased production of uric acid.

Current opinion is that although dietary factors may not be the sole cause of hyperuricaemia, they may exacerbate it in patients with other causative factors, including reduced urinary excretion of uric acid. Therefore, although the purine content of the diet typically does not contribute more than 1.0 mg dl^{-1} to the serum urate concentration, a diet moderate in purine content, but not necessarily a severe restriction, is indicated among patients who consume large amounts of purine-containing foods.

The purine content of a food reflects both its nucleoprotein content and turnover. Therefore, foods containing many nuclei, such as organ meats, have a high purine content, as do rapidly growing foods, such as asparagus. It has been suggested that the consumption of large amounts of foods containing a small concentration of purines may provide a greater purine load than the consumption of a small amount of food containing a large concentration of purines. Therefore, the quantity of a particular food that is ingested must be considered in addition to the purine content of that food.

Moreover, data from both human and rat studies have suggested that purine metabolism can be altered by dietary purines, but that not all purines have the same effect. A low-purine diet is devised based on the total purine content of a food, however, some foods that are considered high in purines, such as sardiness and anchovies, actually contain only small amounts of uricogenic bases, adenine and hypoxanthine. In addition, liver, also a high-purine food, contains similar amounts of uricogenic bases as other meats, despite a difference in total purine content.

A recent study was performed to examine this question by measuring changes in serum and urinary uric acid levels among healthy subjects fed beef liver, haddock and soya beans, which supply equal amounts of total purines, but different amounts of the uricogenic purine bases adenine and hypoxanthine. Results indicated that haddock, a hypoxan-

thine-rich food, led to a greater increase in serum uric acid concentration than liver and soya beans, which are adenine-rich foods, despite these items all having the same total purine content. This may be related to a slower breakdown of adenine-rich foods, compared with hypoxanthine-rich foods, into uric acid. Alternatively, the proximity of hypoxanthine to uric acid in the metabolic pathway may increase the proportion of this base that is converted to uric acid, while adenine has more metabolic options that can lead to metabolic end points other than urate. These findings suggest that perhaps levels of uricogenic purine bases, rather than the total purine or nucleic acid content of a food, should be used in making diet recommendations.

Associated disorders

It is crucial to recognize that while gout is not itself fatal, it is often a marker for the presence of risk factors for coronary heart disease, stroke and kidney damage. In several longitudinal studies, gout has been associated with coronary heart disease and with diabetes, and uric acid levels correlate directly with serum triglycerides and cholesterol and inversely with high-density lipoprotein cholesterol. There is also an association between abnormal uric acid excretion by the kidney and increased tubular reabsorption of sodium, hyperinsulinaemia and hypertension. Thus, even though a causal connection between gout and ischaemic heart disease remains elusive, seeing a patient with gout should prompt the clinician to check for the presence of modifiable risk factors for heart disease. Indeed, one study demonstrated that 76% of patients with primary gout had some associated disorder: 43% obesity, 38% hypercholesterolaemia or hypertriglyceridaemia, 36% arterial hypertension, and 6% diabetes. Ten per cent of subjects had the triad of obesity–hypertension–hyperlipidaemia. Thus, managing disorders that are commonly associated with gout may require additional, individualized dietary therapy.

In order to address the above conditions, individualized dietary management is required, although often a diet consistent with recommendations for all people to promote good health can be advised. The most prudent approach would be a diet low in fat, particularly saturated fat, with an emphasis on whole grains, fresh fruits and vegetables, and lean meats, fish and poultry. Such a regimen would not only promote modest weight loss, but would also be of benefit in managing hyperlipidaemia, hypertension and diabetes.

Prognosis

Gout is unusual among the rheumatic diseases in that its aetiology, treatment, and prevention are well understood. Thus, the long-term sequelae of gout should be completely avoidable with adequate treatment, making the overall prognosis excellent. Noncompliance with medication, lack of access to adequate medical care, and inability to tolerate one or more of the medications used to treat gout can lead to a worse outcome. A number of dietary and lifestyle factors may contribute to increased uric acid production among patients with gout. If these factors can be identified and appropriate changes made, the serum uric acid concentration may fall substantially. However, many patients require medication to control the hyperuricaemia. Therefore, while a purine-restricted diet may not be required in most patients with gout, moderation in dietary purine intake, particularly among individuals who habitually consume large amounts of dietary purines, still does seem to be warranted. Additional research efforts directed at differences in the extent to which foods with the same purine content, but different purine base contents, can influence serum uric acid levels, may further redefine the dietary management of gout in the future.

Acknowledgements

Supported by NIH Grant DK02120 (RR), an Arthritis Foundation Clinical Science Grant (RR), USDA Contract 53-K06-01, General Clinical Research Center Grant DRR M01 RR00054, and Boston Obesity Nutrition Research Center Grant PO1DK46200.

The contents of this publication do not necessarily reflect the views or policies of the US, Department of Agriculture, nor does mention of trade names, commercial products, or organizations imply endorsement by the US. Government.

See Colour plate 11.

See also: **Amino Acids**: Metabolism. **Arthritis**: Dietary Aspects of Aetiology and Nutritional Management. **Heavy Metals**: Toxicology. **Hypertension**: Nutritional Management. **Obesity**: Complications of Obesity.

Further Reading

Brand FN, McGee DL, Kannel WB, Stokes J and Castelli WP (1985) Hyperuricemia as a risk factor of coronary heart disease: the Framingham study. *American Journal of Epidemiology* **121**:11–18.

Brule D, Sarwar G and Savoie L (1988) Purine content of selected Canadian food products. *Journal of Food Composition Analysis* **1**:130–138.

Brule D, Sarwar G and Savoie L (1992) Changes in serum and urinary uric acid levels in normal human subjects fed purine-rich foods containing different amounts of adenine and hypoxanthine. *Journal of the American College of Nutrition* **11**:353–358.

Cappuccio FP, Strazzullo P, Farinaro E and Trevisan M (1993) Uric acid metabolism and tubular sodium handling. *Journal of the American Medical Association* **270**:354–359.

Clifford AJ and Story DL (1976) Levels of purines in foods and their metabolic effects in rats. *Journal of Nutrition* **106**:435–442.

Darlington LG, Slack J and Scott JT (1982) Family study of lipid and purine levels in gout patients. *Annals of Rheumatic Disease* **41**:253–256.

Diamond HS, Carter AC and Feldman EB (1974) Abnormal regulation of carbohydrate metabolism in primary gout. *Annals of the Rheumatic Diseases* **34**:554–562.

di Giovine FS, Malawista SE, Thornton E and Duff GW (1991) Urate crystals stimulate production of tumor necrosis factor alpha from human blood monocytes and synovial cells. *Journal of Clinical Investigation* **87**:1375–1381.

Emmerson BT (1996) The management of gout. *New England Journal of Medicine* **334**:445–451.

Garrel DR, Verdy M, Petitclerc C, Martin C, Brule D and Hamet P (1991) Milk- and soy-protein ingestion: acute effect on serum uric acid concentration. *American Journal of Clinical Nutrition* **53**:665–669.

Gonzalez AA, Puig JG, Mateos FA, Jimenez ML, Casas E and Capitan MC (1989) Should dietary restrictions always be prescribed in the treatment of gout? *Advances in Experimental Medicine and Biology* **253A**:243–246.

Kelley WN, Fox IH and Palella TD (1989) Gout and related disorders of purine metabolism. In: Kelley WN, Harris ED, Ruddy S and Sledge CB (eds) *Textbook of Rheumatology*, 4th edn. Philadelphia: WB Saunders.

Levinson DJ and Becker MA (1993) Clinical gout and the pathogenesis of hyperuricemia. In: McCarty DJ and Koopman WJ (eds) *Arthritis and Allied Conditions*, 12th edn. Philadelphia: Lea & Febiger.

Roubenoff R (1990) The epidemiology of gout and hyperuricemia. *Rheumatic Disease Clinics of North America* **16**:539–550.

Roubenoff R (1996) Gout and other crystal diseases. In Stobe JD, Ledenson PW, Traill TA, Petty BG and Helliman DB, eds. *Principles and Practice of Medicine*, 23rd edition. Hartford, CT: Appleton, pp 233–239.

Roubenoff R, Klag MJ, Mead LA, Liang K-Y, Seidler AJ and Hochberg MC (1991) Incidence and risk factors for gout in white men. *Journal of the American Medical Association* **266**:3004–3007.

Scott JT (1980) Long-term management of gout and hyperuricaemia. *British Medical Journal* **281**:1164–1166.

Sydenham T (1850) *The Works of Thomas Sydenham*, translated from Latin by RG Lathan, vol. II, p. 124. London: New Sydenham Society.

Grains *see* **Cereal Grains**: Dietary Significance and Nutritional Value.

GROWTH AND DEVELOPMENT

Physiological Aspects

Marta L Fiorotto, Baylor College of Medicine, Houston, Texas, USA

Copyright © 1998 Academic Press

The term 'growth' is usually taken to mean the gain in weight or height with time. However, in using this term to describe, for example, an infant, it has a broader connotation. Does the infant's body contain the right amount of water, bone, fat and lean tissues? Are its organs the appropriate size? Is the infant functioning appropriately for its age? In this sense 'growth' has a more complex definition, and in order to describe it, it is necessary to consider all of its various aspects. At its most basic, growth is the product of the increase in the number and size of its constituent cells. The mass increment is integrated with the differentiation of the cells into organs and tissues and the consequent development of their specific functions. Various approaches can be used to evaluate the growth process. These include the assessment of the dimensional, compositional and physiologic changes from conception to the end of adolescence.

The growth pattern that an individual ultimately realizes reflects an interaction between the genotype and the environment. An important component of the environment is the individual's nutritional experiences, particularly those in early life. These external influences are signalled to the cellular metabolic pathways via the body's neuroendocrine system. Spontaneous physical activity is important for normal growth during childhood and adolescence, as is evident from the consequences of reduced activity. The effects of exercise on the anabolic processes are mediated by generalized central factors, which are primarily the function of growth hormone and overall energy expenditure, and local factors produced by the cells that are being worked. Catch-up growth describes the rapid growth that follows a period of growth restriction. For the growing organism to realize its genetic potential, nutrients that provide energy, substrates and cofactors must be provided in the right amounts and the correct proportions appro-priate for each stage of development. The specific needs of the fetus, the preterm baby, the young infant, the child and the adolescent, and those required for catch-up growth are influenced by the stage of maturity and growth rate of the organism.

Growth Throughout the Life Span

The growth process

The process of cell growth is broadly similar across all nonregenerating tissues. Initial cell mass increments are achieved by hyperplasia, and in embryonic and fetal life cellular proliferation is the major factor in mass increase. During this phase, cell division is sustained by the actions of mitogens and locally acting growth factors (e.g. the fibroblast growth factor family, the transforming growth factor superfamily, the Hedgehog family) which have a broad specificity. Although at this stage cells are largely undifferentiated and have little cytoplasm, they become committed to specific fates according to the combination of growth factors to which they are exposed. Individual populations of cells enter specific lineages that ultimately result in the formation of discrete organs or systems with common physiological functions (such as the central nervous, the musculo-skeletal, the cardiovascular, the immune and the gastrointestinal systems). The migration and aggregation of cells to form organs and tissues in appropriate locations also are regulated by the extracellular matrix environment and the composition of cell-adhesion molecules on the cells.

The rate of cell division eventually slows and cytoplasm begins to accumulate. Proliferative responsiveness becomes restricted progressively. Continued proliferation is maintained by cell-specific factors (such as epidermal growth factor, nerve growth factors and platelet-derived growth factors) to which the cells become competent to respond. The induction of genes for tissue-specific transcription factors activates and sustains pathways of differentiation by dictating the genes and, ultimately, the proteins that are expressed. Thus, cellular components (i.e. enzymes or subcellular structures) are tissue-specific;

they impart to the cell its functional properties and morphogenic characteristics. In nonaltricial mammals, including humans, birth occurs at the stage when morphogenesis is largely complete, and the functionality of most of the body's physiological systems is such that the organism can sustain itself apart from its mother.

Eventually, the nuclei exit permanently from the cell cycle, and the cells hypertrophy; that is, they expand owing to the accumulation of proteins or fat. Even so, there is continued compositional maturation in which the intrinsic regulation of proteins expressed by the cells is modulated further by hormonal and/or neuronal stimuli derived from the maturing endocrine and central nervous system. These factors effect their changes both at the level of gene transcription and, importantly, at the level of protein turnover. Both the anabolic and catabolic processes required for such turnover are coregulated by an intricate interplay between the actions of hormones and nerve activity in response to changes in the organism's environment, such as changes in nutrient supply, stress, temperature and activity. The mass increase and compositional and functional maturation of each tissue and organ effect profound changes in the body's chemical composition, whether this is viewed from an elemental or macromolecular perspective. Assessment of the chemical composition of the body, therefore, can provide a measure of the state and stage of the organism's growth processes.

This overall pattern of cell growth, i.e. division followed by differentiation and hypertrophy, is seen not only in the long-lived stable tissues of the body, such as nerve tissue, skeletal or cardiac muscle and bone, but also in tissues of the body from which cells are continuously removed and need to be replaced; for example, the skin, blood and intestinal mucosa. These tissues possess nondifferentiated germinative cells that continuously divide to produce new cells which then differentiate, hypertrophy and mature.

The age and rate at which each of these developmental processes occurs vary according to the organ and tissue. There appears to be a broad relationship between the functional importance of an organ at a given postconceptional age and its contribution to body mass. Organs of functional importance to the fetus, such as the central nervous system, the heart and the liver, contribute maximally to body protein mass at birth. Indeed, the brain attains most of its adult size within the first few years of life. After birth, however, as food is ingested, the gastrointestinal tract grows rapidly. Later, as locomotor function and weight-bearing develop, the skeletal musculature grows, and bone ossification progresses. The reproductive tissues are relatively undeveloped until

the onset of puberty; they then attain mature size within a few years. Although the principal growth-related changes are completed with puberty, the relationship between organ mass and functional demand is maintained throughout life. Thus, work load stimulates muscle growth and phenotype change; increased energy expenditure stimulates heart mass; and the intake of food stimulates gastrointestinal, liver and kidney growth according to the composition and amount of food ingested.

Growth assessment

The integrated response of all the individual components of the body is responsible for its changes in shape, mass, composition and function. Thus, a comprehensive growth assessment will include an evaluation of all these components.

Dimensional assessment The specific parameters that best indicate the adequacy of growth vary with age to reflect the dimensions that are undergoing the most active growth. Mass, size and shape are usually assessed from dimensional measures such as weight, lengths, diameters and circumferences. Dimensional assessment after birth is usually based on anthropometric measurements of body weight, skeletal dimensions and limb circumferences. Skeletal growth is assessed from supine crown-heel and crown-rump length (in early infancy) or standing and sitting height, and from body shape measurements (e.g. head circumference and shoulder span). Limb and abdominal circumference measurements, often in conjunction with skinfold measurements, are used as indirect indices of adipose and skeletal muscle masses.

Developments in ultrasonography have made it possible to assess fetal growth; skeletal growth can be determined from measurements of crown-rump length and femur diaphysis length, brain growth from biparietal diameter and head circumference, and liver size from abdominal circumference. The combination of these measurements is highly predictive of fetal weight, and equations based on these measurements give relatively accurate estimates (within 3%) of fetal weight.

Anthropometric data can be analysed in terms of distance and velocities (**Fig. 1**), rate constants and as ratios of dimensions. Distance measurements provide information on how a particular dimension in an individual compares with the same dimension in a similar population. Velocity measurements concern the rate of change of a given dimension over time. Velocities are more informative than distance values because they provide information on how the individual has changed over time. In rate constants, the velocity is expressed as a proportion of the mean absolute value of the growth parameter. Rate constants are useful for purposes of comparison, for example where there are large differences in absolute size across species, or among organs and tissues within an individual, or when comparing growth rates at different developmental ages. Ratios of one parameter to another, such as weight per unit height, or arm-to-head circumference provide a measure of whether growth in linear and mass dimensions are proportional. The denominator often involves skeletal parameters that do not respond to acute aberrations in growth, whereas the numerator is influenced by changes in the soft tissue mass, which is sensitive to environmental factors. Such ratios are used frequently, therefore, in lieu of velocity measurements to identify the presence of a relatively acute change in growth.

The characteristic shape of the human growth curve is shared by other primates and distinguishes itself from that of other mammals by virtue of the slow rate constant of all growth parameters. At 10 weeks of gestation (the time of peak fractional rates of growth), weight and length are increasing by approximately 10% and 5% per day, respectively; immediately before birth, the corresponding values are 0.8% and 0.5% per day, respectively. Growth velocity, however, accelerates during gestation, with maximal rates of gain attained at different ages for individual parameters (**Fig. 2**). Maximal cranial growth velocity occurs at about 20 weeks of gestation and then slows down, whereas the long bones and spine, and hence linear growth velocity in general, attain maximum growth velocity earlier. Weight velocity increases over most of gestation, reaches a maximum at about 34 weeks of gestation and then slows until parturition. All three parameters then accelerate temporarily in the immediate postpartum period, attaining maximum velocities by approximately 2 months postnatal age. For both height and weight, velocity then decreases, reaching a minimum rate between 3 years and 5 years of age (Fig. 1b) which is maintained until puberty. The prolongation of the time between birth and puberty (and hence the attainment of maturity) is characteristic of primates, and represents approximately 25% of the human life span. Puberty is marked by changes in body mass, shape and a temporary acceleration in height and weight velocities. The age of onset, magnitude and duration of the pubertal growth spurt varies considerably among individuals (Fig. 1b), and these variations are largely responsible for gender differences in mature size. In addition to the strong genetic influence, puberty is modified by environmental factors, primarily those of nutritional status and frequency of illness. The end of puberty is marked by fusion of the long-bone growth plates, which causes the cessation of linear growth.

Compositional assessment The concept of chemical maturation is central to the accurate assessment of the adequacy of growth, from the compositional viewpoint. As cells and organs increase in mass, their chemical constituents change, although not necessarily in parallel. For example, as cells hypertrophy, they expand into and displace the extracellular fluid, resulting in a reduction in the tissue's water content (**Fig. 3**). However, once the water content of the tissues reaches a minimum (approximately 73% of the body's lean tissue) by mid-childhood, protein accretion is associated with no further changes in water concentration. Skeletal maturation is associated with mineralization, which proceeds most rapidly during the second and third trimesters of gestation, after the bone collagen matrix has been deposited. Bone mineralization proceeds more slowly postnatally, especially during the first year of life, and attains a maximum level in early adulthood (Fig. 3). Body fat begins to accumulate at the start of the third trimester of gestation after the adipocyte has differentiated, and achieves its maximum contribution to body weight at 6–9 months of postnatal age (Fig. 3). Fat then accumulates at a slower and extremely variable rate determined by the interaction between environment and genetics.

The amounts of the major organic constituents of the body, that is, protein, extracellular fluid, bone and fat, determine the composition and content of both the organic and inorganic elements in the body. Thus, not only is protein the major contributor to body nitrogen, but it is also a determinant of body potassium, the main cation of the cells. The major anion in the extracellular fluid is chloride, and its proportion in the body decreases until it reaches a constant at approximately 3 years of age in parallel to total body water. The amounts of calcium and phosphorus in the body largely reflect skeletal growth and ossification. Similarly, because much of the body's magnesium is found in the bones, its pattern of deposition parallels that of calcium. Adipose tissue, being relatively anhydrous, contains little inorganic material and therefore acts as a diluent.

Body composition assessment can take various approaches. It can be defined in terms of its elemental composition, which can be estimated using nuclear-based techniques. No single elemental measurement, however, defines the various body components exactly. A combination of measurements, e.g. those of potassium and nitrogen, or of nitrogen and carbon, significantly improves the

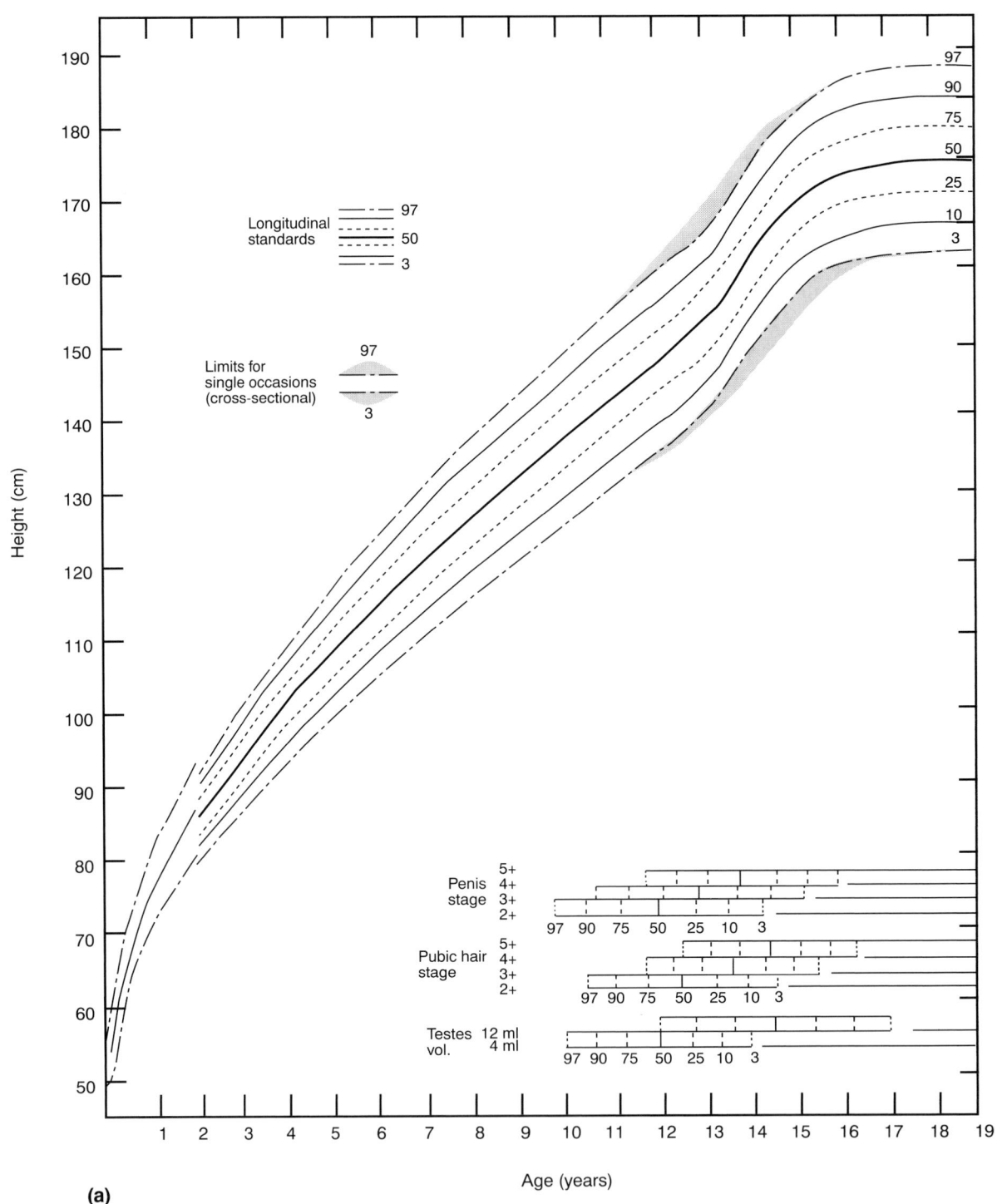

(a)

Figure 1   (a) Individual height attained (or distance) curve for British boys followed longitudinally from birth to 19 years of age. The central line is the 50th centile; it represents the height curve of an average boy, who has his adolescent growth spurt at the average age. Other percentiles are also included; these show the percentage of boys whose height curves fall on or below the labelled line and have their adolescent growth spurt at the average time. The shaded areas above the 97th and below the 3rd centile represent these limits for a cross-sectionally derived measurement. The stages of pubertal development also are shown, together with centile ranges for each stage as they relate to age. The 50th centile represents the age at which the average boy attains the various pubertal stages. Similar charts are available for girls. (b) Individual yearly height velocity curves for British boys followed longitudinally from birth to 19 years of age. The centiles apply to boys who have their adolescent growth spurt at the average age. The shaded areas encompass the range of values from the 3rd to the 97th centile for early-maturing boys whose growth spurt occurs at a younger age, to late-maturing boys whose growth spurt occurs at an older age. Similar charts are available for girls. From Tanner and Whitehouse (1976) *Archives of Disease in Childhood* **51**: 170–179, with permission from BMJ Publishing Group.

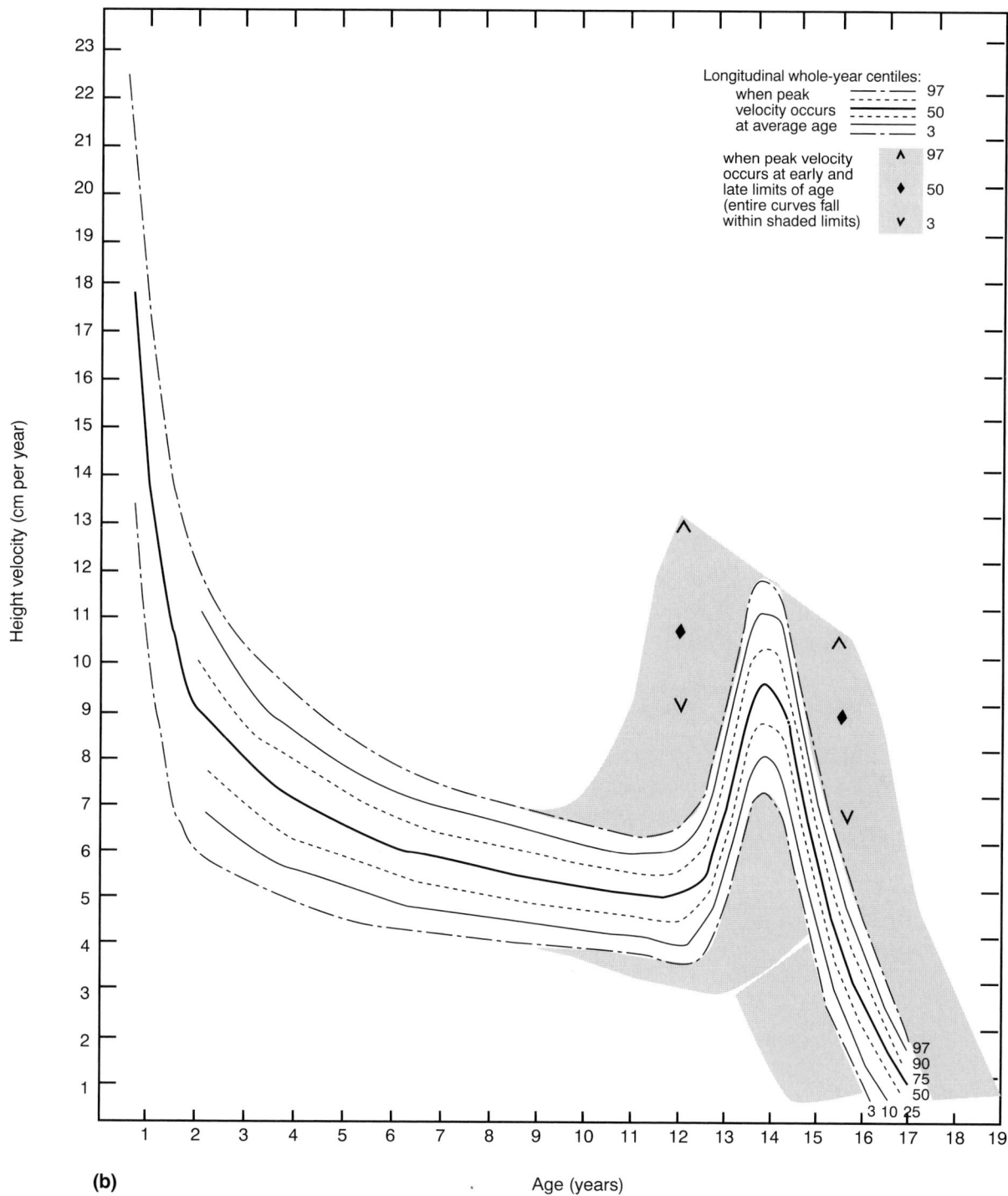

Longitudinal whole-year centiles:
when peak ---·--- 97
velocity occurs ------- 50
at average age ---·--- 3

when peak velocity ∧ 97
occurs at early and
late limits of age ◆ 50
(entire curves fall
within shaded limits) ∨ 3

(b)

Age (years)

Figure 1 Continued.

discriminatory power of this approach to the study of body composition.

The body can also be defined in terms of its physical compartments, and at least five models with varying degrees of complexity have been defined. The most commonly used of these divides the body into two compartments: a fat-free or lean compartment, and a fat one. Various methods can be used to measure either compartment; the other is then obtained by difference from body weight.

Maturational assessment In postnatal life, it is important to assess how far an individual has progressed towards functional maturation. Chronological

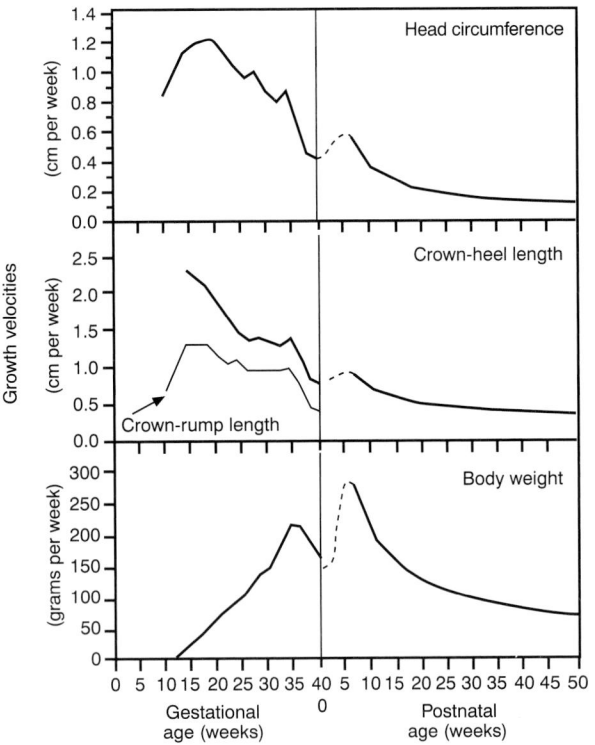

Figure 2 The average values for prenatal and postnatal growth velocities for head circumference, crown-heel and crown-rump (prenatal only) lengths, and weight. Values for velocities between birth and 4 weeks of age have been interpolated.

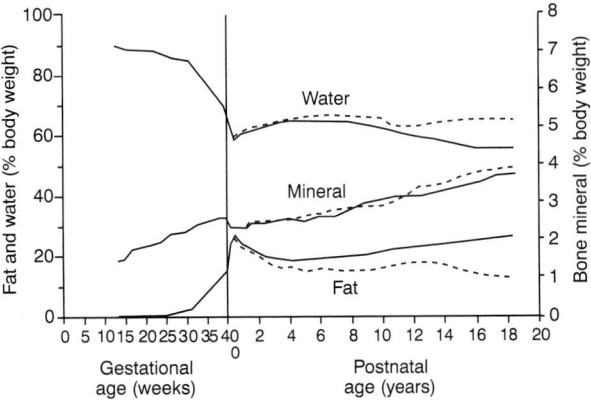

Figure 3 The developmental changes in the water, fat and mineral composition of the body from early gestation to maturity in girls (solid line) and boys (broken line). The difference between 100% and the values for fat represents the body's fat-free mass. The scale for bone mineral is shown to the right of the graph, whereas the scale for water and fat are shown on the left. Note also that the scales for gestational and postnatal ages differ.

age is not reliable because children mature at different rates, and girls on average mature faster than boys. Although certain maturational changes are directly related to size, others are due to physiological maturation itself. Various indices are available

and used depending on the age and process to be assessed.

Bone age Bone age is the most frequently used scale to assess physiologic maturity. The stage of ossification of the bones, their shape and relative position to one another are evaluated radiographically, and their progress towards maturity is determined. The bone age of the individual is the chronological age of a 'normal' child at the same stage of skeletal development. Until 18 months of age the bones of the legs and feet are assessed; thereafter, the hands and wrists are examined. Bone age is closely linked to the age of puberty and is a better predictor of its onset than chronological age.

Dental age The age of primary (4 months to 2 years) and permanent (6 years to 13 years) tooth eruption may also be used to assess maturity. The difference between dental and bone age reflects the difference in the maturation of the head versus that of the rest of the skeleton.

Sexual age Bone and dental ages are not helpful in determining maturational status associated with puberty. However, hormonal changes trigger the onset of growth in the tissues associated with reproductive function. Standards have been developed for assessing the stage of sexual maturity, or sexual age, on the basis of breast and pubic hair development in girls, and genital and pubic hair development in boys (puberty standards for boys are shown in Fig. 1a). The onset of these changes begins earlier in girls and, in both genders, precedes the acceleration in height velocity.

Developmental age The development of the central nervous system is not only key to the regulation and integration of function of most of the body's physiological systems, but is also central to mental and behavioural growth. Unlike other mammals, human babies must develop the skills to stand upright, walk and use their hands for manipulation and purposeful activity, and they must learn behavioural patterns rather than rely on inherited ones. How an infant or child performs various standardized activities is used to assess its developmental age. These activities are categorized to assess gross and fine motor development, speech, vision and hearing, perception or understanding, and social behaviour (**Table 1**). From childhood onward, mental development, or mental age, is often evaluated in terms of 'intelligence' which can be assessed by a variety of tests. Mental age increases at a rate that depends on many intrinsic and environmental variables, although there is a

Table 1 Key developmental milestones during the first 18 months of life

Age (Months)	Gross motor	Visual perceptual/ Fine motor	Language	Adaptive
2	Lifts chest off a table when prone	Visually tracks horizontally and vertically	Social smile	
4	Supports weight with arms extended when prone; rolls over from prone to supine	Moves hands to the midline; manipulates fingers; bilateral reach; mouths objects	Orients to a voice; laughs aloud	Can begin to be spoon-fed
6	Sits with anterior propping; rolls supine to prone	Intentionally grasps objects; transfers an object from hand to hand; rakes at small objects; lifts a cup	Orients to sound in one plane; babbles	Munches; can begin to drink from a cup; demonstrates stranger anxiety
8	Sits erect 10+ min; stands at furniture if put there	Reaches to the side when sitting; holds an object in each hand simultaneously; inspects a bell	Nonspecific 'mama', 'dada'	Chews with tongue lateralization
10	Crawls; pulls to a stand; cruises; walks with hands held at shoulder height for balance	Picks up a small object with finger and thumb; hits a cube against a cup; looks over edge for a fallen toy	Imitates games (peek-a-boo, pat-a-cake); understands 'no'; says 'dada' and 'mama' appropriately	Finger feeds; holds own bottle; demonstrates separation anxiety
12	Walks independently; picks up a toy from the floor without support	Intentionally releases a toy in and out of a container; marks with a crayon; dangles a ring by a string	Two words other than 'mama' and 'dada'; follows one-step gestured commands	Can eat coarsely chopped table foods; drinks mainly from a cup; helps with dressing
18	Runs well; walks down stairs with hand held; walks into a large ball when shown how to kick	Stacks four cubes; scribbles; puts pegs in a pegboard spontaneously	Vocabulary of 7–10 words; points to one body part; points to a picture	Spoon-feeds self

From Gesell (1974).

tendency for physical and mental maturation to be correlated.

Regulation of growth

Genetics The potential form, size and functional capacity of the organism are closely related to its genotype. There are several lines of evidence for this. The mature heights of monozygotic twins reared apart are highly correlated. Similarly, significant correlations are found between the adult stature of parents and their offspring, and between siblings of the same gender. The correlations for indices of soft tissues and fat deposition in these same comparisons, however, are poor. These findings suggest a strong genetic influence on skeletal growth and shape, whereas soft tissue and fat, and hence body weight gain, are primarily influenced by environmental factors. Genetics also exert a strong influence on physiological maturation. Thus, age at menarche and rate of skeletal maturation are correlated within families, especially among monozygotic twins. Differences in

dimensional, compositional and physiological characteristics of various races also are indicative of a strong genetic component in the regulation of growth.

The degree to which the dimensional growth of parents and offspring is similar varies with the age of the offspring. Within an individual, birth dimensions are poor predictors of ultimate stature but improve through infancy, reaching a maximum correlation by about 3 years, provided the individual's environment and health have not been disadvantageous. These observations reveal two further characteristics of the growth process. First, not all genes that regulate stature are expressed at birth. Some are expressed only when the other aspects of maturation have provided an appropriate physiological environment. Second, birth size is markedly influenced by the uteroplacental environment, which in turn depends on maternal stature, nutritional status and the presence of conditions that compromise placental function.

Environment and nutrition In the absence of endocrine disorders, the most important influence on growth is an individual's environment. In this respect, morbidity and poor nutritional status are important because they act synergistically to suppress growth. Illness not only reduces voluntary food intake, but also increases nutrient needs, while poor nutritional status lowers immune competence and hence increases susceptibility to infection. A nutrient intake that is insufficient to meet a child's need will impair normal growth. If episodes of illness are repeated frequently, complete recovery cannot occur between bouts, especially in younger infants, in whom growth rate is high. Thus, frequent episodes of infections and poor nutrient intake are the major factors underlying the delayed growth and maturation and, ultimately, the higher incidence of short stature of individuals among populations of low socioeconomic status, those who live in rural areas, those who are younger siblings in large families, and children who live in stressful conditions. Many geographical differences can also be explained on this basis.

Physiologic The regulation of growth at the physiological level varies according to stage of development. Three phases have been identified. The first of these, which extends from conception to approximately the second year of life, is least understood. As mentioned previously, a multitude of growth factors appears to regulate the growth of individual tissues and organs, and to coordinate their growth with one another. The requirement for a central regulatory system is unclear, as the growth of the bodies of fetuses with no brain is relatively normal. The supply of nutrients and oxygen, in conjunction with thyroid hormone, insulin and the insulin-like growth factors, are believed to be the prime modulators of growth during the latter half of gestation and early infancy. These hormones are extremely sensitive to nutrient supply, and probably mediate the effects of nutrition on cellular anabolic processes. Uterine size and growth factors produced by the placenta also may play a role in regulating the overall growth of the fetus, and presumably ensure that fetal growth is appropriate for maternal size.

The second phase begins toward the end of the first year of life and continues throughout childhood. During this phase, the brain assumes a central role in regulating growth, primarily through the production of growth hormone. Growth hormone either acts directly at the tissue level in synergy with other hormones, such as thyroid hormone and insulin, or indirectly through the production of insulin-like growth factor I (IGF-I), to promote anabolic processes in the body.

The third growth phase is puberty, characterized by the development of secondary sexual characteristics and the pubertal growth spurt. The former result from the production of androgens by the adrenal glands in both boys and girls, testosterone from the testes in boys, and oestrogens from the ovaries in girls. Testosterone is more effective than oestrogens in enhancing muscle and red blood cell growth, which explains their relative increase in boys at puberty. Oestrogens, on the other hand, promote fat deposition, which explains the greater body fat of women relative to men. The secretion of gonadal hormones also underlies the acceleration of linear growth at puberty because they enhance the secretion of growth hormone. A further effect of the gonadal hormones, oestrogens in particular, is to accelerate the maturation and fusion of the epiphyses in the long bones. Thus, the pubertal growth spurt inevitably terminates in the cessation of linear growth.

Physical Activity and Growth

Spontaneous physical activity is important for normal growth and development. Activity influences muscle mass, its vascularization and mitochondrial capacity, the cardiorespiratory system, bone mineralization, and the amount of fat and its distribution in the body. The importance of activity is evident not so much from the effects of training and sports on these anabolic processes but from the compromised growth that accompanies reduced physical activity, whether this is due to injury, illness, a sedentary life style or (more recently) space flight. There is no evidence that in normal, healthy individuals, physical activity influences linear growth. Excessive activity engenders a stress-like response which is detrimental to overall growth. In a broader context, the necessity of activity for normal growth seems to increase with age (with the possible exception of bone), as evidenced by the fact that activity levels are relatively low during periods of most active growth, i.e. in late gestation and infancy.

The mechanisms that link exercise with growth processes are not well understood, although 'central' and 'local' components are believed to be involved. The central components are those through which exercise affects cellular growth throughout the body, for example the cardiorespiratory effects and the increase in the ratio of lean mass to fat. Growth hormone release into the circulation is stimulated by activity, and probably is involved in this pathway. Growth hormone increases tissue and serum levels of IGF-I, which can then enhance the anabolic processes in most tissues. The magnitude of the growth hormone response is moderated by the consumption of high-fat meals. The local effects of exercise are those whereby changes incurred by the activity itself are transformed into signals that stimulate cell growth. These local effects include the production of growth factors; for example, isometric stretch stimulates muscles to produce IGF-I and fibroblast growth factor, both of which stimulate cell growth processes not only in the muscle cells, but also in the tissue's vasculature. The low oxygen tension and pH of exercising muscle have been shown also to stimulate local anabolism.

Normal bone ossification and linear growth, both intra- and extrauterine, require that the bone be subjected to intermittent variations in compression, tension and torsion. These forces are exerted on the bone by muscle contractions and weight bearing; hence, fetal movements are important for normal limb development *in utero*. During a period of rapid growth, prolonged bone compression because of recumbency, muscle paralysis or the presence of a plaster cast, together with the accompanying muscle wasting, can lead to vascular degeneration in the growth plate and eventual closure of the epiphyses and cessation of growth. Differences in activity levels also may contribute to the observed seasonal variation in linear growth.

Activity level is an important determinant of body fatness because it affects energy expenditure. Low levels of physical activity without a compensatory decrease in energy consumption must lead to increased fat deposition and the eventual development of obesity. In industrialized societies, the effects of inactivity on body fat are often exacerbated by coexisting behaviours, such as increased fat intake and alcohol consumption. These not only increase energy intake, but have independent, deleterious effects on the overall health of the individual. Low activity levels also are encountered in children who are severely malnourished and wasted. In this circumstance, reduced activity levels represent an adaptation to minimize the negative energy balance.

Catch-up Growth

Each individual appears to follow a genetically programmed growth curve irrespective of how this growth is expressed. Illness, malnutrition or a lack of appropriate anabolic hormones will cause a child's growth to deviate from the predetermined growth trajectory. However, after the insult has been removed, the growth processes have the capacity to accelerate their velocity to levels above normal for chronological age or maturity (**Fig. 4**). This rapid

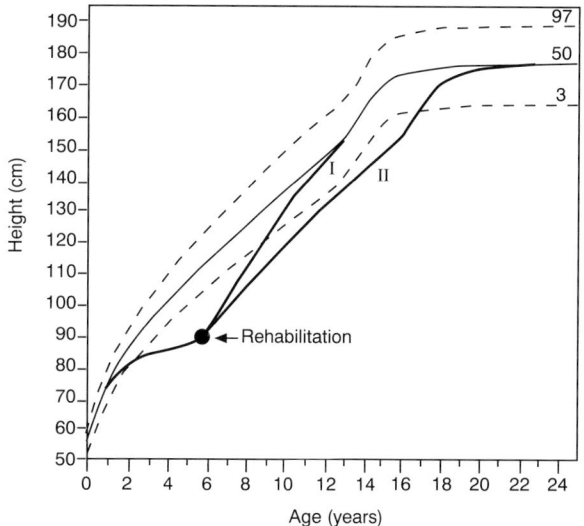

Figure 4 Hypothetical catch-up growth responses in boys following chronic growth restriction. With rehabilitation growth velocity may accelerate to values that are higher than the average for that age until the child returns to the normal growth trajectory along the 50th centile, as in curve I. Alternatively, growth velocity may return to the normal value for age, as in curve II, but growth may proceed for longer because puberty is delayed. Frequently the growth patterns are intermediate to I and II.

growth following the end of a period of growth restriction is called 'catch-up growth'. Complete catch-up growth restores the child to their normal growth trajectory and, thereafter, growth is normal. Complete catch-up growth can occur by appropriate acceleration of velocity so that the original growth curve is attained (curve I in Fig. 4), or growth may be slower but accompanied by delayed maturation (curve II in Fig. 4) that can last as long as 5–6 years. Thus, growth can proceed for longer and permits the child to attain his or her predetermined size. Frequently both a temporary acceleration in velocity and delayed maturation occur.

There are circumstances in which complete catch-up growth does not occur. Disease or undernutrition early in gestation will prevent children from attaining their genetic potential. This may relate to a reduction in the rate of cell multiplication and number which cannot be restored once cells have progressed to the phase of differentiation. The tendency of very premature babies to become small children may be caused by this phenomenon. Studies from developing countries suggest that catch-up growth is incomplete if growth retardation occurs throughout the first 2 years of life, but this is not a universal finding.

Infants whose growth is restricted *in utero* because of extrinsic factors frequently show a period of rapid catch-up growth for the first few months. This continues until they attain a growth trajectory which presumably reflects their genetic programme. The opposite phenomenon, 'catch-down' growth, has also been observed when maternal factors promote enhanced fetal growth. After the infant is born and the maternal influence is removed, the growth rate of these infants decelerates until they return to their genetically determined growth trajectory.

Nutritional Implications

In order for the growing organism to realize its genetic potential, nutrients that provide energy, substrates and cofactors must be available in the right amounts and the correct proportions for each stage of development. During development, the relative requirements of individual nutrients are the amounts needed for their net accretion in the body, to replace inevitable losses, for the maintenance of physiological processes and for physical activity.

The fetus and premature infant

A large component of the nutrient requirement of the fetus is the need for the deposition of protein, fat and minerals in the growing tissues. At a given size, the amounts of nitrogen and minerals retained by the fetus are proportional to its growth rate. The supply of these nutrients occurs exclusively via the placenta which, therefore, determines the amount and form in which they are presented to the fetus. As a consequence, there is a close correlation between placental size and body weight at birth. Moreover, the temporary deceleration of weight gain toward the end of gestation has been attributed to placental insufficiency. The fetus obtains its energy primarily from glucose, lactate and amino acids. The energy is required primarily to sustain anabolic processes and the maintenance of transcellular ionic gradients. The energy requirements vary for different tissues and are highest for the visceral organs and the brain, which have high rates of protein turnover and ion transport. *In utero*, these higher energy needs are countered by the lower energy demands for thermogenesis and muscle contraction. During the last trimester, a significant proportion of energy goes toward fat deposition.

The fetus born prematurely presents a complex challenge in terms of the provision of adequate nutrients to support growth. An overriding concern is that the premature neonate is entirely dependent on its care-givers to provide all the nutrients required for growth, as many of these needs are not known precisely. The energy needs of the preterm infant are greater than those of a fetus of the same postconceptional age owing to the increased demands for thermogenesis and the increased work of breathing. Moreover, the immaturity of the lungs increases the risk of developing lung disease, which will further increase the infant's energy needs. Depending on the degree of prematurity, the normal endogenous energy stores in the form of fat may be very limited. Thus, the premature infant's increased nutrient needs must be met despite the immaturity of the physiological systems in general, and the gastrointestinal system in particular. The ability of the preterm baby to coordinate breathing, sucking and swallowing is not attained until 35 weeks postconceptional age. Although nutrients can be provided by nasogastric tube, their assimilation requires mature peristaltic function, digestive enzymes and transport mechanisms. These functions normally would mature during the third trimester of gestation.

When these immaturities limit the amount of nutrients that can be administered orally, intravenous alimentation is implemented. This method of feeding must take into account the solubilities of various nutrients such as the amino acids tyrosine and cysteine, as well as calcium, which often limit the amount that can be administered. Further considerations include the volume of fluid that the infant can tolerate, given its immature renal function, and the form of the substrates provided to meet the infant's energy needs. Currently, preterm infants are given both fat and glucose. The provision of fat reduces the volume of fluid that must be administered; it decreases the amount of glucose that must be metabolized, thereby reducing the incidence of hyperglycaemia; and it reduces the amount of carbon dioxide that the lungs have to clear. Intravenous feeding has a number of drawbacks inasmuch as the absence of nutrients in the gut is associated with intestinal atrophy, and prolonged use inevitably results in liver dysfunction by mechanisms that are not well understood.

In preterm infants who are mature enough to tolerate oral feedings, neither mature human milk nor standard formulae support optimum growth. Appropriately modified artificial formulae, or human milk fortifiers, have therefore been developed which increase the nutrient density of the feedings to meet the preterm infant's increased needs for energy, protein and minerals, particularly calcium and phosphorus. The provision of increased amounts of calcium and phosphorus salts to support bone mineralization must account for the differences in their solubilities and digestibilities. A consideration in developing these feedings also was the limited capacity of the premature infant to handle excess protein, as the immaturity of key enzymatic pathways and renal immaturity could lead to a hazardous accumulation of amino acids, urea and ammonia. The premature gut cannot completely digest and absorb triacylglycerols, particularly if the fatty acid moieties are saturated. Fat malabsorption not only compromises energy intake but also impairs the absorption of calcium, essential fatty acids and fat-soluble vitamins. These difficulties have been circumvented by providing triacylglycerols that contain a significant proportion of unsaturated fatty acids and also medium-chain triacylglycerols, both of which can be digested more completely.

The young infant

Many aspects of physiological maturation are fairly advanced in the term infant. Its nutrient needs for the first 4–6 months of age are believed to be those consumed by thriving infants breast-fed by healthy, well-nourished mothers. These nutrients are available in forms that are optimally digested and metabolized. The relative functional immaturity of the intestinal tract and metabolic processes necessitates feeds that are relatively small but frequent. Such feeding patterns maximize the efficiency with which dietary nutrients, protein in particular, are used for growth. A significant amount of the nutrient need of newborn infants is for the synthesis of new tissues. However, as the infant's growth rate decreases, this component of the nutrient requirement rapidly falls off, and the nutrient intake per unit body weight decreases accordingly. In a reciprocal manner, a greater proportion of the nutrients is used to replace inevitable losses, and the energy required for normal cell function (i.e. maintenance functions). During the first few years of life the changes in the relative proportions of tissues in the body have an obvious impact on maintenance energy requirements. Skeletal muscle, which has a lower metabolic rate than the visceral organs and the brain, constitutes an increasing proportion of the lean body mass, and this change in body composition contributes to a decrease in the maintenance energy requirement. The concurrent maturation of neuromuscular function has two important implications for the growing infant. First, as chewing and swallowing become coordinated (a process that requires 32 pairs of skeletal muscles), beginning at 6–8 months of age, the child can begin to eat solid foods. This occurs in conjunction with the development of the infant's capacity to sit and, consequently, the ability to feed him- or herself (Table 1). Second, as the child becomes more mobile towards the end of the first year of life, more energy is consumed to support the greater level of physical activity and energy expenditure. Presumably for the same reason, the amount of body fat also begins to decrease at this time.

The child

Beyond infancy, the nutrient requirements for growth are small compared with maintenance needs. However, normal growth is considered the best criterion of whether needs are being met, and, at least for this purpose, the correct measurement of the growth performance of an individual child is crucial. The interpretation of data requires appropriate standards for comparison; this presents a dilemma because it is questionable whether growth standards of children in privileged societies are appropriate for children living in less optimal circumstances. Nevertheless, the nutrient requirements of children of 1–10 years of age are based on the habitual intake of healthy children living in optimal conditions and are the same for both genders. No specific allowance is made for high levels of physical activity. The provision of increased energy for such active children must take into account that children require more energy than adults to do the same amount of work.

The adolescent

The pubertal growth spurt and the changes in body composition that occur during adolescence have several consequences for nutrient intake which differ between boys and girls. Although the requirement for protein increases in both sexes owing to the increased deposition of lean tissues, the timing of this increase varies according to the age at puberty, and therefore tends to occur later in boys than girls. Energy needs are primarily influenced by the changes in the ratio of lean mass to fat and in activity patterns. On average, activity levels decrease with maturation, and more so in girls than in boys. The increased deposition of muscle in boys and adipose tissue in girls also changes the proportion of metabolically active tissues in the body, so that for similar body weights the energy needs of girls are lower. When energy consumption is not adequate because of reduced intake and/or increased expenditure, body fat stores become depleted and the onset and progression of puberty can be disrupted. This phenomenon is observed in young female athletes, such as gymnasts or ballet dancers, who strive for thin bodies, yet need to expend large amounts of energy to train. The higher rate of lean tissue deposition also increases the relative needs for iron and magnesium. In boys, the increase in muscle mass and blood haemoglobin content associated with puberty increases iron needs, while girls need more iron to replace menstrual losses starting at menarche. The accelerated bone growth increases the need for calcium and phosphorus; unlike protein and magnesium, this higher intake is recommended beyond the end of puberty until approximately 25 years of age, when peak bone mineralization is attained. Unfortunately, the eating habits of adolescents frequently are such that their intake does not meet their mineral requirements. This may have long-term repercussions for girls, in that inadequate bone mineralization may predispose them to osteoporosis later in life.

Catch-up growth

The acceleration in the growth rate of all body components necessarily increases the requirement of all nutrients. The actual amount and composition of food that must be provided to meet these needs are influenced by numerous factors including the age and stage of maturity of the child, the desired composition of weight gain and growth rate, the aetiology and the severity of the antecedent growth retardation, and the presence of disease. From estimates of the desired rate of protein and fat gain, the additional amounts of nutrients that must be provided can be estimated. Minerals and vitamins are supplemented, with particular emphasis on those suspected of body store depletion. Because of the rapid deposition of lean tissue, recovering children run the risk of developing hypophosphataemia and hypokalaemia if phosphorus and potassium (the major intracellular anion and cation) are not provided in adequate quantities.

The refeeding of children who are growth-retarded owing to malnutrition presents additional difficulties which must be accounted for in designing appropriate feeding regimens. These difficulties are exacerbated by the presence of gastrointestinal disease, which is common among children in developing countries. Moreover, adaptations in cardiovascular and renal function to chronic malnutrition can limit the initial capacity of these children to handle the increased functional demands incurred by catch-up growth. Thus, the aggressive feeding regimens that support maximum catch-up growth can only be instituted after a short adaptation period of more moderate feeding.

Studies in experimental animals and children have demonstrated a beneficial effect of exercise, as well as nutrients, on linear catch-up growth. Mild to moderate exercise has been shown to enhance linear growth and muscle deposition, independent of nutrient intake. The underlying mechanism has not been determined, but the findings are consistent with those concerning the effects of exercise on growth hormone secretion.

See also: **Bone**: Composition, Metabolism and Bone Growth. **Children**: Nutritional Requirements of School Children. **Exercise**: Physiology of Skeletal Muscle; Diet and Exercise; Beneficial Effects. **Infants**: Nutritional Requirements; Low-birthweight and Preterm Infants.

Further Reading

Cheek DB (1968) *Human Growth: Body Composition, Cell Growth, Energy and Intelligence.* Philadelphia: Lea & Febiger.
Cooper DM (1994) Evidence for mechanisms of exercise modulation of growth – an overview. *Medicine and Science in Sports and Exercise* 26:733–740.
Dietz WH (1996) The role of lifestyle in health: the epidemiology and consequences of inactivity. *Proceedings of the Nutrition Society* 55:829–840.
Falkner F and Tanner JM (1986) *Human Growth: A Comprehensive Treatise*, vols 1–3. New York: Plenum.
Fomon SJ (1993) *Nutrition of Normal Infants.* St Louis: Mosby.
Forbes GB (1987) *Human Body Composition: Growth, Aging, Nutrition, and Activity.* New York: Springer.
Frisancho AR (1990) *Anthropometric Standards for the Assessment of Growth and Nutritional Status.* Ann Arbor: University of Michigan Press.
Gesell A (1974) *Infant and Child in the Culture of Today.* New York: Harper & Row.
Gilbert SF (1997) *Developmental Biology*, 5th edn. Sunderland: Sinauer.
Gluckman PD and Heymann MA (1996) *Pediatrics and Perinatology: The Scientific Basis.* London: Arnold.
National Research Council (1989) *Recommended Dietary Allowances*, 10th edn. Washington: National Academy Press.
Reeds PJ and Fiorotto ML (1990) Growth in perspective. *Proceedings of the Nutrition Society* 49:411–420.
Sinclair D (1989) *Human Growth after Birth.* Oxford: Oxford Medical.
Wang ZM, Pierson RN and Heymsfield SB (1992) The five-level model: a new approach to organizing body-composition research. *American Journal of Clinical Nutrition* 56:19–28.
Widdowson EM and Dickerson JWT (1964) Chemical composition of the body. In: Comar CL and Bronner F (eds) *Mineral Metabolism*, vol. 2. New York: Academic Press.

Growth factors *see* **Cytokines**: Nutritional Aspects.

Gut flora *see* **Microflora of the Intestine**: Role and Effects.

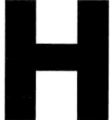

HEALTH FOODS

Dietary Supplements – Micronutrients

D Shrimpton, Cambridge, UK

Copyright © 1998 Academic Press

The widely used expression 'health foods' has the unfortunate implication that foods outside of this category are not healthy. It is preferable to use the term 'dietary supplements', to denote a category of foods that can contribute to the improvement of health and to the maintenance of good health as part of a total pattern of food consumption from all sources that collectively provide a healthy diet.

The dietary supplements discussed below are to be considered as components of a healthy diet. The areas of debate lie chiefly in the identity of a healthy diet, its interaction with both the genetic constitution of the individual consumer and of the consumer's environment, and with the quantification of the dietary constituents necessary to achieve and sustain optimal health.

Because of the interaction between diet and an individual's genetic inheritance and environmental experience, the ideal diet will vary between individuals. Further, through the nearly infinite number of possible nutrient combinations, there may be no single ideal diet but instead a range of diets from which a unique solution can be obtained for each individual.

In the current state of nutritional knowledge it is not possible to match perfectly the characteristics of the individual, including environmental exposure, to a quantified intake of specific nutrients. This is in spite of spectacular advances in understanding the implications for nutrition of the rapidly growing body of knowledge and understanding of molecular biology. The approach, therefore, has been to identify ranges of consumption within which amounts of nutrients can be selected to optimize health. The range for optimization of intake for each nutrient lies at or above the 'recommended daily allowance' (RDA) and below 'an upper safe level'. Currently, the quantification of upper safe levels for micronutrients is a subject of debate.

There is, in addition, the further complication of interaction between nutrients. At many levels of intake the interactions are desirable; but circumstances can arise of imbalance, for example between zinc and copper, which can have consequences that are deleterious for health. Neither are the desirable intakes of micronutrients independent of the intake of macronutrients. For example, it is desirable for the intake of thiamin, vitamin B_1, to be in constant proportion to the total intake of metabolizable energy, the conventional ratio being $72\ \mu g\ MJ^{-1}$. The reader should keep in mind that these supplementary micronutrients not only interact and complement each other, but also interact and complement macronutrients and the micronutrients already present in the diet.

Fat-soluble Vitamins

Vitamin A

Vitamin A has a fundamental role in vision and its deficiency is probably the most important cause of preventable blindness in the world. Its function in the visual process is that of the prosthetic group of the opsins, which act between the light receptors and the initiation of nervous impulses. Vitamin A also has other metabolic functions. It is the carrier for units of mannose when they are required for the synthesis of glycoproteins. It is also involved in the control of cell proliferation and differentiation, although the detail of its mode of action here is not yet completely established.

Vitamin A readily accumulates in the liver. Thus, both the amount and the duration of consumption are important factors in determining an 'upper safe level' for daily intake. Apart from the differing sensitivities to vitamin A between individuals and the effects of age, sex and pregnancy on increasing sensitivity, there is the further confounding factor of wide variations in the content of vitamin A and its precursors in foods. Because of the serious consequences of excessive intakes, particularly in pregnancy where there is a risk of birth defects, regulatory authorities consider that the 'upper safe level' should not exceed 3000 μg retinol equivalents (RE).

Beta-carotene   Beta-carotene is one of many hundreds of carotenoids, relatively few of which have been studied in relation to their impact on human physiology. Metabolically β-carotene is a precursor of vitamin A. It also acts as an antioxidant, quenching singlet oxygen and intercepting peroxyl radicals. There is, in addition, an apparent antiproliferative effect, which may result from its action on cell–cell communication through gap junctions – a property possibly possessed by other carotenoids.

Beta-carotene is nontoxic and, apart from the reversible and harmless yellowing of the skin when large amounts are consumed, has no side effects. Nevertheless, the results of two carefully controlled clinical trials lead to the conclusion that β-carotene could increase the risk for smokers of developing cancer. At present it would be cautious to assume that β-carotene is contraindicated for habitual smokers and, possibly too, for those at risk from passive smoking.

Vitamin D

The major function of vitamin D is to regulate calcium uptake and its deposition and resorption in bone. Vitamin D occurs in two forms: vitamin D_2 (ergocalciferol), associated with plant origins, and vitamin D_3 (cholecalciferol), present in fish liver oils and eggs, with smaller amounts in milk fat and animal liver.

For most humans, the major source of vitamin D is from the action of sunlight on the skin. This action of the ultraviolet (UV) component of sunlight is to convert internally produced 7-dehydrocholesterol to cholecalciferol. Without exposure of the skin to UV light, the individual is completely dependent on ingested vitamin D. Thus the vitamin has been described as a 'sunshine-dependent' hormone. Through the action of calcitriol, vitamin D is fundamentally involved in the formation of bone; when it is deficient, rickets can develop or osteoporotic changes can occur. The formation of vitamin D in the skin is inhibited when the dietary intake is adequate and when the concentrations of the hydroxylated forms of the vitamin in the blood are high. Consequently there is no risk from the formation of large toxic amounts of vitamin D when individuals are excessively exposed to sunlight; although they may be harmed from sunburn.

Excessive and prolonged intakes of dietary vitamin D can result in hypercalcaemia and supplementary vitamin D is contraindicated in cases of renal failure which are also being treated with supplements of calcium. However, the vitamin has only been shown to be toxic in relatively large amounts: in excess of 40 μg per day over long periods in children, and in excess of 50 μg per day for adults.

Vitamin E

Unlike other vitamins, vitamin E has not yet been shown to be directly associated with any enzyme system. Its role is that of an antioxidant and as a scavenger of free radicals. For these reasons it is effective as a protector of the integrity of lipids and of phospholipid membranes and is associated with the reduction of risks associated with the development of cancer and heart disease.

The amounts required by individuals to optimize metabolism in relation to the activity of free radicals are substantially greater, possibly by an order of magnitude, than those required to prevent tissue degeneration. Overall, evidence suggests that 70 mg α-tocopherol equivalents (α-TE) (100 IU) or more vitamin E per day may decrease the risk of coronary heart disease. The lack of toxicity of vitamin E has been consistently reported upon for 20 years, with the exception of individuals whose ability to clot blood is impaired; for these people it is contraindicated.

Water-soluble Vitamins

Thiamin (vitamin B_1)

Thiamin (vitamin B_1) is involved in energy-yielding metabolic systems, especially those involved in carbohydrate metabolism. As thiamin diphosphate it is the coenzyme in three multienzyme complexes involved in oxidative decarboxylation in the mitochondria. In nervous tissue, 2–3% of the thiamin is present as the triphosphate and it is the absence of this form of thiamin which is associated with the rare genetic encephalomyelopathy termed Leigh disease and the similar Wernicke's encephalopathy.

Vitamin B_1 is nontoxic with a long history of safe use as an oral supplement without adverse effects.

Riboflavin (vitamin B_2)

Riboflavin is primarily involved in energy-yielding metabolism. Its function is that of an electron carrier in the oxidation and reduction reactions of the flavin coenzymes. These enzymes have a fundamental role in the mitochondrial electron transport chain. The activities of many of the flavin enzymes are depressed in hypothyroidism and can be stimulated by the administration of thyroxine.

Riboflavin, consumed orally, has no measurable toxicity.

Nicotinamide (vitamin B₃)

Nicotinamide is the active form in two coenzymes (NAD and NADP) that are involved in many oxidation–reduction reactions. It is sometimes incorrectly called niacin and is then confused with nicotinic acid, which has no vitamin activity, although it is useful as an agent for lowering blood cholesterol and is a precursor of nicotinamide.

The biological requirements for this vitamin can be met from dietary protein by conversion of the amino acid tryptophan to nicotinic acid and then to the amide; that is, the dietary requirements depend on the amount and quality of the intake of dietary protein.

There is little published data on the consumption of physiological amounts. It is generally assumed from experience that nicotinamide supplements do not produce any serious side effects. Nicotinamide does not cause flushing and it does not have hypocholesterolaemic effects – in contrast to nicotinic acid.

Pyridoxine (vitamin B₆)

Pyridoxine or vitamin B_6 is involved in the metabolism of amino acids and lipids and in the action of steroid hormones. The metabolically active form is pyridoxal phosphate. However, there are five other forms that are metabolically interconvertible and, apparently, of equal biological activity.

A deficiency of pyridoxine as well as an excess is associated with the occurrence of peripheral neuropathy. The vitamin is commonly consumed as a supplement in the UK and in the USA at daily amounts of 50–200 mg to overcome stressful conditions, particularly premenstrual syndrome (PMS). However, there is considerable debate about the occurrence of PMS, the efficacy of pyridoxine in overcoming it, and on the occurrence or absence at these levels of consumption of a reversible peripheral neuropathy.

The current regulatory position in some European countries who are seeking to restrict the consumption of vitamin B_6 as a dietary supplement to levels of 10 mg daily or less is at variance with the experience of users who claim not to experience side effects at the effective levels of use for PMS (50–200 mg daily).

Folic acid

Folic acid is involved in a wide range of metabolic reactions, promoting normal red blood cell formation and maintaining the nervous system, intestinal tract and normal patterns of growth. The metabolically active form is a conjugate with glutamic acid from which it is released by the zinc-dependent enzyme pteroyl-polyglutamate hydrolase.

A clinical deficiency of folic acid results in a megaloblastic anaemia. The similar anaemia resulting from a deficiency of vitamin B_{12} is accompanied by neurological damage and is termed 'pernicious anaemia'.

It is well established that additional folic acid is essential before conception and in very early pregnancy, at a daily intake of 400 μg, to prevent the occurrence of neural tube defects such as spina bifida. More recently there have been strong indications that comparable daily intakes may reduce the risk of coronary heart disease, through a decrease in one of the risk factors, a high plasma concentration of homocysteine.

Nutritionally the most significant interaction with other metabolites is that of the apparent depression of the absorption of zinc when daily supplementary intakes are 1 mg or more.

Vitamin B₁₂

Vitamin B_{12}, the antipernicious anaemia factor, contains cobalt. No biological role for cobalt independent of vitamin B_{12} has so far been discovered. The various forms of vitamin B_{12} are known collectively as 'cobalamins'.

In humans, vitamin B_{12} is a cofactor in two enzymes that are fundamental in facilitating growth. As methylcobalamin, vitamin B_{12} is the cofactor for methionine synthase, and as adenosylcobalamin, it is the cofactor in methylmalonyl-CoA mutase. Both reactions are involved in promoting the rapid growth and proliferation of the cells of the bone marrow. Vitamin B_{12} is essential for function and maintenance of the central nervous system, and the severe deficiency in pernicious anaemia produces a neurological disease, posterolateral spinal cord degeneration.

No toxic effects have been encountered in humans and the vitamin has no observable adverse effects at any level of recorded use.

Biotin

Clinical deficiency of biotin is rare, but when present it is serious because of the resulting impairment of the enzyme systems associated with cell respiration. These are concerned with the transfer of carbon dioxide in carboxylation, decarboxylation and transcarboxylation reactions through a carboxybiotin intermediate. This is bound to a lysine residue of the carboxylase enzymes as biocytin. The availability of biotin in foods is not well documented and neither is the availability of biotin from microbiological synthesis in the intestine.

There are few reports of the use of biotin as a supplement. The highest daily intake reported for a period of months is 2500 μg. No adverse or toxic effects have been encountered in humans.

Pantothenic acid

The name of this vitamin is derived from the Greek *pantothen*, 'everywhere'. In spite of its widespread occurrence in most foods, no reports of toxicity have been made. Pantothenic acid has a central role in metabolism because it is the functional moiety of coenzyme A. Through this coenzyme it is involved in energy-yielding metabolism, in the elongation of fatty acids, the biosynthesis of steroids and of porphyrins.

Clinically, pantothenic acid can be shown to be associated with neuromotor disorders, mental depression and immune responses.

Vitamin C

Historically, vitamin C (ascorbic acid) is associated with the prevention of scurvy. The behavioural effects of the condition are probably a result of impaired synthesis of catecholamines, some of the hydroxylases being ascorbate-dependent. Most of the other clinical symptoms are probably associated with failures in the synthesis of collagen because of the dependence on ascorbate of some of the hydroxylase enzymes required for its synthesis.

Vitamin C facilitates the absorption of iron, and because of the involvement of copper in some of the hydroxylase enzymes, is also associated with their metabolism.

Vitamin C is a reducing 'sugar' and consequently has the function of a relatively nonspecific reducing agent; however, it has two specific roles. First, it is the cofactor for a variety of hydroxylase enzymes that are involved in redox reactions. Secondly, it acts as an antioxidant and is thought, from *in vitro* studies, to be a major factor in the antioxidant protection system of the plasma, together with vitamin E, β-carotene, selenium and probably other factors.

A major part of the current interest in vitamin C is focused on its ability, as a reducing agent, to act as a quenching agent in free radical reactions. In this context the association is with the promotion of optimal health through support for the immune system and through the defence of tissues against the challenges associated with chronic disease, including cardiovascular disease and carcinogenesis.

There have been concerns expressed in respect of the influence of high intakes of vitamin C on the formation of oxalate stones, but these have been shown to be poorly founded. There has also been doubt expressed concerning its potential to become a prooxidant and through interaction with iron, promote iron-driven generation of hydroxyl radicals. However, the potential for this activity has only been demonstrated in experiments *in vitro* and it seems unlikely to be a significant possibility *in vivo* because there is little free iron, the bulk of it being sequestered by protein.

Mild, transient adverse effects (gastrointestinal symptoms) occur with some regularity at daily intakes of 2000 mg. These effects have little impact on health and perhaps should be termed 'undesirable' rather than 'adverse'. An intake of 2000 mg per day may be identified in some individuals with mild effects, but these do not amount to adverse effects in the sense of an upper limit.

Minerals

Calcium

Bone cannot be formed in the absence of calcium, which is present metabolically in ionic form as simple calcium ions or as orthophosphate or hydroxyl ions. The cellular structure, formation and resorption of bone is complex and involves four types of cell: bone-forming osteoblasts, bone-resorbing osteoblasts, osteocytes (variants of osteoblasts) and bone lining cells. Communication between the cells is mediated by several hormones, including gonadal hormones and the cholecalciferols.

Conceptually there is a potential hazard from a substantial excess of dietary calcium, in that under the influence of excess vitamin D, a small fraction may enter soft tissues. There is, however, consistent evidence in favour of the safety of supplementary amounts up to 1000 mg daily and for as much as 2000 mg daily. Typical consumption in Europe from diets without supplements is 500–1000 mg daily.

Phosphorus

Most of the phosphorus in the body (80–85%) is present within the skeleton as phosphate in the calcium salt hydroxyapatite. The remainder is a component of proteins, phospholipids and nucleic acids. Phosphorus has a fundamental role in energy transfer within the compounds adenosine triphosphate (ATP) and creatine phosphate.

Because of the efficiency of renal excretion, operating in part to maintain homeostasis, excess phosphorus in the tissues is rare. However, it can occur in some disease conditions and, in extreme cases, can precipitate tetany. Toxicity is rare because of the regulatory system based on excretion through the kidneys.

Because phosphorus and calcium are present in the body in approximately equimolar amounts, it is usually assumed that dietary intake should mirror this. Hence the total intake of phosphorus (atomic weight 31) should be 75% of the total intake of calcium (atomic weight 40). This ratio is not critical in adults, although it is considered to be desirable.

Magnesium

Magnesium is present in nearly all cells of the human body. It is a cofactor in more than 300 enzymes and is essential for the structural integrity of mitochondria and of DNA and RNA. Magnesium is also involved in neural and myocardial function. In healthy individuals it has been difficult to demonstrate either deficiency or toxicity. The homeostatic mechanism is strong, using the skeleton as a store.

Total daily intakes up to 700 mg are associated with good health, and approximately half this amount would be expected to be acquired from a European diet without supplements.

In dietary excess, particularly in single doses, there can be severe (but reversible) gastric disorder, but the lowest level associated with an irreversible adverse effect has not been established.

Trace Elements

Chromium

The biologically active form of chromium is trivalent and is not toxic. The form found in metallic dust is hexavalent and is highly toxic. Chromium (trivalent) has the ability to potentiate the action of insulin. It is thought that this action is carried out by chromium as part of one or more organic complexes. It is also postulated that chromium (trivalent) is involved in DNA synthesis and in gene expression.

There is no evidence of toxicity from orally ingested trivalent chromium. Long-term use, especially in diabetic patients, has focused on daily supplementary amounts of 200 μg. There are no published values for mean or median dietary intakes of chromium in Europe.

Copper

Because copper is one of the elements that has two different states of oxidation (monovalent and divalent), it can take part in oxidation and reduction reactions. Consequently copper is involved in some of the fundamental processes of the body through its association with enzymes that facilitate electron transfer. These include cytochrome oxidase, copper-zinc dismutase and amino acid oxidases.

Copper homeostasis is achieved through a combination of an intestinal block on the absorption of excessive amounts and regulation through biliary excretion. The intestinal block can be overcome and acute toxicity can follow. More commonly, concern relating to high dietary intakes relates to the interaction between copper and zinc.

Sensitivity to copper is rare and supplementary amounts as high as 7.5 mg daily for 90 days have been consumed without adverse effects. Approximately 1.5 mg can be expected to be obtained from European diets that have not been supplemented.

Iodine

Three-quarters of the iodine normally present in an adult is found in the thyroid, the gland which is primarily involved in regulating metabolism. Iodine is an essential constituent of both thyroxine and tri-iodothyronine, the regulatory hormones produced in the thyroid gland.

Toxic effects are not observed in humans until daily intakes have exceeded 10 mg. Taking account of the likely consumption from foods, including those that have been fortified, it is considered that supplementary intakes should not exceed 500 μg.

Iron

Iron, as a component of the blood pigment haemoglobin, is responsible for carrying oxygen from the lungs to the body tissues. Iron is also present in the equivalent pigment of muscle, myoglobin, where it is again associated with the transport of oxygen. In the plasma iron is stored organically as ferritin. Iron is a functional component of the cytochrome enzymes, which are essential in the sequence of reactions through which energy is obtained from food. There is a relationship between a mild deficiency of iron and disturbance of thermoregulation, and also of some neurotransmitter systems in the brain where dopamine and serotonin are involved.

For adults, concerns relating to safety are more indirect than direct. Harm from overdose is primarily a problem of infants and young children having acquired excessive amounts of iron by accident, often from medicines prescribed for adults. In pregnancy, daily intakes of up to 60 mg have been consumed safely. For general use, excluding the special conditions of female puberty and pregnancy, it is desirable that total daily intake does not exceed 20 mg and that daily supplements do not exceed 15 mg.

Manganese

Metallic manganese, as a dust or particulates in air, is toxic; manganese as a salt or in organic form is not toxic and it is in this condition that it occurs physiologically. There is an interaction between zinc, manganese and iron, and manganese is one of several trace minerals that can interact with enzymes. It is also the specific active component of three enzymes: arginase, pyruvate carboxylase and manganese-superoxide dismutase. Through these activities, manganese is involved in fundamental metabolic processes including antioxidant activities.

Molybdenum

Molybdenum is able to facilitate electron exchange and hence take part in oxidation–reduction reactions, including those in which riboflavin takes part. In particular, molybdenum is a cofactor for the enzymes sulfite oxidase and xanthine dehydrogenase.

The results of animal studies suggest that intakes of molybdenum in excess of 10 mg per day are likely to disturb metabolic systems involving copper. There is little published data relating to daily intakes in humans in excess of 300 mg, at which level there appears to be no adverse effect.

Selenium

The increasing evidence that excessive activity of free radicals is associated with the occurrence of some chronic diseases, particularly those relating to the heart and some forms of cancer, has led to growing interest in the use of selenium as a supplement, because of its sparing action on vitamin E and its direct involvement in the enzyme glutathione peroxidase.

Selenium deficiency has undesirable consequences, chiefly associated with myopathies. The best known of these is Keshan disease, a cardiomyopathy first identified in a province of China. Although the complete aetiology has not been elucidated, it is established that deficiency of selenium is a major factor. The cause of the deficiency is the low content of selenium in the soil, and hence in the crops that are grown locally. Selenium-deficient soils are not confined to China and have been identified in many regions, including Finland, where fortification of soils through selenium addition to fertilizer is government policy.

Supplementary selenium has been consumed in Western environments for many years at low levels of supplementation (50 μg daily), and for shorter periods (up to 1 year) at higher levels of supplementation (200 μg daily).

Zinc

Physiologically, zinc is associated with reproduction and with the integrity of the epidermis. More recently, zinc has been shown to be involved in the immune system and to be necessary for the development and functioning of the nervous system. Zinc is a component of more than 200 enzymes. These include alkaline phosphatase, carbonic anhydrase, cytosolic superoxide dismutase and alcohol dehydrogenase. Although studies in animals and *in vitro* support the hypothesis that zinc possesses antioxidant properties, attempts to demonstrate this in humans have so far failed.

In dietary excess, zinc can induce a deficiency of copper and can also interact with iron.

When zinc is regularly consumed as part of the diet, most data on long-term consumption have been associated with daily supplementary levels of 15 mg or less, with a comparable amount from other dietary sources.

See also: **Ascorbic Acid**: Physiology, Dietary Sources and Requirements. **Biotin**: Physiology, Dietary Sources and Requirements. **Calcium**: Physiology. **Carotenoids**: Chemistry, Sources and Physiology. **Cholecalciferol and Ergocalciferol**: Physiology, Dietary Sources and Requirements. **Chromium**: Physiology, Dietary Sources and Requirements. **Cobalamins**: Physiology, Dietary Sources and Requirements. **Copper**: Physiology, Dietary Sources and Requirements. **Fatty Acids**: Health Effects of n-6 Polyunsaturated Fatty Acids; Health Effects of n-3 Polyunsaturated Fatty Acids. **Fish**: Nutritional Value. **Folic Acid**: Physiology, Dietary Sources and Requirements. **Iodine**: Physiology, Dietary Sources and Requirements. **Iron**: Physiology, Dietary Sources and Requirements. **Magnesium**: Physiology, Dietary Sources and Requirements. **Manganese**: Physiology, Dietary Sources and Requirements. **Niacin**: Physiology, Dietary Sources and Requirements. **Pantothenic Acid**: Physiology, Dietary Sources and Requirements. **Phosphorus**: Physiology, Dietary Sources and Requirements. **Potassium**: Physiology, Dietary Sources and Requirements. **Retinol**: Physiology. **Riboflavin**: Physiology. **Selenium**: Physiology, Dietary Sources and Requirements. **Sodium**: Physiology. **Thiamin**: Physiology. **Tocopherols**: Physiology. **Vitamin B$_6$**: Physiology. **Vitamin K**: Physiology. **Zinc**: Physiology.

Further Reading

Abdulla M (1994) Hälsokostbranchens Leverantörförening, oktober Positive responses, side effects and toxicity symptoms after the ingestion of large doses of

Alhadeff L, Gualtieri CT and Lipton M (1984) Toxic effects of water-soluble vitamins. *Nutrition Reviews* 42:33–40.

Apports Nutritionels Conseilles pour la Population Française, 1992, 2nd edn. Paris: Lavoisier.

Bender DA (1992) *Nutritional Biochemistry of the Vitamins*. Cambridge University Press.

Bendich A and Chandra RK, eds (1990) Micronutrients and immune functions. *Annals of the New York Academy of Sciences* **587**:1–320.

Brubacher GB (1989) Scientific basis for the estimation of the daily requirements for vitamins. In: Walter P, Brubacher GB and Stäkelin H (eds) *Elevated Dosages of Vitamins – Benefits and Hazards*, pp 3–11. Berne: Hans Huber.

Consell Supérieur d'Hygiène Publique de France: Section de l'Alimentation et de la Nutrition (1996) *Les Limites de Sécurité dans les Consommations Alimentaires des Vitamines et des Mineraux*. Paris: Lavoisier.

Counsell JN and Horning DH, eds (1991) *Vitamin C (Ascorbic Acid)*. London: Applied Science.

Dictary Reference Values for Food, Energy and Nutrients for the United Kingdom, 1991. Report on Health and Social Subjects 41. London: HMSO.

Diplock AT (1994) Antioxidants and diseases prevention. *Molecular Aspects of Medicine* **15**:293–376.

Empfehlungen für die Nahrstoffzufuhr, 1991, 5th edn. Frankfurt: Deutsche Gesellschaft für Ernährung.

Fairweather-Tait SJ (1993) Optimal nutrient requirements: important concepts. *Journal of Human Nutrition and Dietetics* **6**:411–417.

Flodin NW (1990) Micronutrient supplements: toxicity and drug interactions. *Progress in Food and Nutrition Science* **14**:277–331.

Food and Nutrition Board, Institute of Medicine (1994), *How Should the Recommended Dietary Allowances be Revised?* Washington DC: National Academy Press.

Gibney MJ (1991) Food policy – implications for the nutritional sciences. In: Deelstra H, Fondu M, Ooghe W and van Havere R (eds) *Food Policy Trends in Europe*, pp 19–32. New York: Ellis Horwood.

Hathcock JN, ed. (1982) *Nutritional Toxicology*. New York: Academic Press.

Hathcock JN (1993) Safety limits for nutrient intakes: concepts and data requirements. *Nutrition Reviews* **51**:278–285.

Hathcock JN (1996) Safety limits for nutrients. *Journal of Nutrition* **126**:2386S–2389S.

Hathcock JN (1997) Vitamins and minerals: efficacy and safety. *American Journal of Clinical Nutrition* **66**:427–437.

Horwitt MK (1991) Data supporting supplementation of humans with vitamin E. *Journal of Nutrition* **121**:424–429.

Lindemann J (1990) Biotechnologies and food: a summary of major issues regarding safety assurance. *Regulatory Toxicology and Pharmacology* **12**:96–104.

Mertz W (1993) Essential trace metals: New definitions based on new paradigms. *Nutrition Reviews* **51**:287–295.

Mertz W (1995) Risk assessment of essential trace elements: new approaches to setting recommended dietary allowances and safety limits. *Nutrition Reviews* **53**:179–185.

Proceedings of a Workshop on Future Recommended Dietary Allowances (1993) Rutgers University, Cook College, Office of Continuing Professional Education.

Recommended Dietary Allowances, 10th edn. Washington: National Research Council.

Reports of the Scientific Committee for Food, 31st series (1993) *Nutrient and Energy Intakes for the European Community*. Luxembourg: Office for Official Publications of the European Communities.

Savory J and Wills MR Trace metals: essential nutrients or toxins. *Clinical Chemistry* **38**:1565–1573.

Scientific Considerations for the Development of Measures on the Addition of Vitamins and Minerals to Foodstuffs (1996) SCOOP Task 7.1.1 Working Group. Brussels: European Commission.

Shrimpton DH (1993) A conceptual approach to the determination of upper safe limits for the consumption of micronutrients. *Proceedings of the Nutrition Society* **52**:59A.

Shrimpton DH (1997) *Vitamins and Minerals: A Scientific Evaluation of the Range of Safe Intakes*. Thames Ditton: Council for Responsible Nutrition.

Snodgrass SR Vitamin neurotoxicity. *Molecular Neurobiology* **6**:41–73.

Whitehead RG Recommended dietary amounts for the United Kingdom. *British Journal of Nutrition* **61**:123–124.

Ziegler EF and Filer LJ, eds (1996) *Present Knowledge in Nutrition*, 7th edn. Washington: ILSI Press.

Heart disease *see* **Coronary Heart Disease**: Lipid Theory of Coronary Heart Disease.

HEAVY METALS

Toxicology

C Reilly, Chipping Norton, UK

Copyright © 1998 Academic Press

The term 'heavy metal' is usually used to describe a group of metallic elements of high density which are toxic. It is not a scientific definition and there is disagreement as to which elements should be included in the group. The *Food Chemical Codex* of the US Food and Drug Administration includes 'all common metallic impurities that are coloured by hydrogen sulfide', namely lead, mercury, cadmium, copper, nickel, silver and tin, as well as the two metalloids, arsenic and antimony. The term is usually used by nutritionists in a more restrictive sense for metals with a relative density greater than about 8, which are not essential nutrients and produce adverse physiological effects if consumed. These are listed in **Table 1** and will be considered here.

The article will discuss the toxic properties of heavy metals in general and their public health significance. Each will be considered individually, with reference to dietary sources, overall intakes and health implications.

Toxicology of the Heavy Metals: General Considerations

It is not always possible to draw a distinction between toxic and nontoxic, or even essential metals. All metals are possibly toxic if ingested in sufficient amounts. It is, moreover, difficult to consider the toxicity of a particular metal in isolation. Many interact with other metals when consumed together. Their effects may be modified by the presence of other food components. There are, however, some metals which cause toxic symptoms even at low concentrations and have no obvious beneficial effects. Lead, mercury and cadmium are three of these.

Table 1 Toxic heavy metals

Metal	Atomic no.	Atomic wt	Density (kg m^{-3})
Lead (Pb)	82	207.19	11.34
Mercury (Hg)	80	200.59	13.55
Cadmium (Cd)	48	112.40	8.65
Nickel (Ni)	28	58.71	8.90
Bismuth (Bi)	83	208.98	9.78

A characteristic of heavy metals, in contrast to those of lower density, is strong attachment to biological tissues and slow elimination from the body. This accounts for the cumulative effect of long-term ingestion, even at low intakes. What the outcome of this will be depends on the particular metal, its chemical form, the species of organism affected and the presence of possible modifying factors.

Public Health Significance of Heavy Metals

The toxic metals are usually distributed in low concentration in soil and water and enter the food chain in small amounts. Living organisms have learned how to deal with such intakes. Some metals are of low bioavailability and little is absorbed. For others a variety of detoxification mechanisms have been evolved which are effective, provided the dietary load remains low. If not, tolerance can break down.

Overloading can be the result of natural causes, but often it is due to human activities. Metals which were once rarely encountered, and then in small amounts, are now widely distributed, often in high concentrations, and the possibility of ingestion is increased.

The public health implications of heavy metals in the diet are well recognized. Most countries have legislation to deal with the problem. Since 1961 the UK has had *Lead in Food Regulations* and limits for certain other metals are also in force. Similar, though not identical, regulations exist in other countries. International harmonization of metals in food standards is promoted by the FAO/WHO Codex Alimentarius Commission and the European Community.

Lead

Lead is ubiquitous. It is in all animal and plant tissues, in all foods and beverages, usually at levels ranging from barely detectable to about 2 mg kg^{-1} (**Table 2**). These levels can be exceeded, especially in processed foods, as shown in **Table 3**. Adventitious lead in foods comes from many sources such as lead solder used to seal containers. This was once a widespread problem, but is now less common since modern canning technology uses lead-free seals. The use of aluminium to replace tinned steel in can-making has also reduced lead uptake. Tin plate contains a

Table 2 Lead content of foods

Food	Lead content (mg kg⁻¹, fresh wt) Mean	Range
Cereals	0.17	< 0.01–0.81
Meat and fish	0.17	< 0.01–0.70
Vegetables	0.22	< 0.01–1.5
Fruit (fresh)	0.12	< 0.01–0.76
Milk and dairy products	0.03	< 0.01–0.08

After Reilly (1991).

Table 3 Uptake of lead by food from processing/storage equipment

Food	Lead content (mean) (mg kg⁻¹, fresh wt)
Blackcurrants	10.00
Cabbage (cooked in tinned saucepan)	0.79
Cabbage (cooked in aluminium pan)	0.18
Orange juice (canned)	2.00
Orange juice (bottled)	0.35
Vegetable salad (canned)	20.00
Vegetable salad (fresh)	0.27
Wine (lead capped bottle)	102.00 (μg l⁻¹)

After Reilly (1991).

small amount of lead which can be leached out, especially by acidic foods. A similar problem can arise in food cooked in utensils surfaced with tin plate.

There are many other uses of lead-containing materials which cause uptake of the metal by foods which come into contact with them, such as plastics, printing inks and pottery glazes. Fragments of lead-based paint which accidentally get into food, or are ingested from painted surfaces, are still recognized as a health hazard, especially for children, though the use of lead in paints is now restricted.

Domestic water can be a major source of lead ingestion where lead pipes and fittings are used. Data in **Table 4** illustrates the problem, which can be particularly acute in soft water areas. Such water is acidic and strongly plumbosolvent. Even in systems without lead pipes, pick-up can occur from other fittings, such as heating coils and storage tanks.

Table 4 Lead in domestic water

WHO Standard for Drinking Water	50 μg l⁻¹
Cold tap, lead-free pipes	< 5 μg l⁻¹
Cold tap, lead pipes	> 100 μg l⁻¹
Hot tap, lead-free pipes	20 ± 10 μg l⁻¹
Moorland water at source (Scotland)	25 μg l⁻¹
Domestic water, lead pipes (Glasgow)	> 100 μg l⁻¹

Data from Reilly (1991).

Lead in food is usually in inorganic form, though its alkyl compounds, which are used as additives in 'leaded' petrol, may be present as a result of contamination. Total daily intake for an adult is normally about 20–200 μg per day (**Table 5**) and meets the 3 mg Provisional Tolerable Weekly Intake (PTWI) recommended by FAO/WHO. In recent years, following efforts made by government authorities and the food industry to reduce levels of lead in food, daily intakes of the metal have been decreasing in most countries, in some cases quite dramatically. In the USA, for instance, daily lead intake by adolescent males fell from 60–90 μg in 1972, to 38 μg ten years later, and, in 1991, to 3 μg.

Differences in lead intake are related to differences in dietary consumption pattern in various countries, as shown in **Table 6**. The data indicates that both Germany and Japan have higher levels of lead contamination in food than does Finland.

About 10% of the body's total lead is found in blood. Levels are related to intake and are used to monitor exposure to the metal. A level of 100–250 μg l⁻¹ (0.5–1.2 μmol l⁻¹) in an adult is considered acceptable. **Table 7** summarizes guidelines used to monitor lead intake in children.

Up to 95% of the body's lead is stored in skeleton, where its half-life is about 20 years. This store can be mobilized as a result of stress, such as injury or pregnancy, and thus can cause poisoning even when current intake is low.

Though there is some evidence that lead may be a requirement for certain animals, this has not been shown to be so in humans. When lead enters the cells of the body, it can bind to active sites of enzymes and block their function. Particularly sensitive to this effect are enzymes involved in porphyrin metabolism, such as δ-amino laevulinic acid dehydrase (δ-ALAD). Measurement of δ-ALAD activity, as indicated by levels of ALA in urine, is used to monitor lead exposure. Lead also interferes in cells with ion

Table 5 Dietary lead intake in different countries

Country	Mean intake (μg per day)
Belgium	96
Canada	36
Finland	66
Germany	123
Japan	165
Netherlands	25
Spain (Basque Country)	40
UK	60
USA	41

After Louekari and Salminen (1986), Reilly (1991) and van Dokkum (1995).

Table 6 Intake of lead by food groups in three countries

Food group	Lead intake, μg per day (Food intake, g per day)		
	Finland	Germany	Japan
Cereals	7.7 (267)	10.9 (254)	25.4 (503)
Roots and tubers	3.6 (238)	17.2 (221)	6.2 (72)
Vegetables, green	1.3 (87)	39.6 (188)	26.4 (299)
Fruits	18.0 (219)	40.0 (287)	9.8 (178)
Meat and offals	4.9 (169)	12.5 (268)	16.0 (82)
Eggs	0.3 (29)	5.1 (47)	6.1 (45)
Sea foods	2.2 (78)	3.0 (27)	41.1 (239)
Milk	8.8 (711)	3.4 (329)	5.8 (136)
Alcoholic beverages	3.5 (180)	23.3 (489)	8.8 (160)
Total:	50.3 (1978)	155　(2110)	145.6 (1714)

Data from Loukari and Salminen (1986).

Table 7 Interpretation of children's blood tests and follow-up activities

Blood lead (μg dl^{-1})	Comment/action required
≤ 9	Normal level – no action
10–14	Rescreen
15–19	Nutrition and educational intervention
20–44	Environmental and medical evaluation and possible treatment
45–69	Medical and environmental intervention: possible chelation treatment
≥ 70	Immediate medical and environmental management

After Centres for Disease Control (1991) *Preventing Lead Poisoning in Young Children*. Washington, DC: US Department of Health & Human Services, Public Health Service.

transport, plasma membrane function, cellular respiration and macromolecule synthesis.

Symptoms of lead poisoning are varied and depend on levels of intake. At first they may be vague, such as lassitude, appetite loss and pallor. Classical symptoms of serious lead poisoning are colic, stomach pain and paralysis. 'Devonshire colic' was the name once given to the result of drinking cider that had been made in lead-lined vats. With increasing intake, anaemia, peripheral neuropathy, encephalopathy and kidney damage are seen.

There is increasing evidence of adverse effects on children of even low levels of lead. Chronic exposure to environmental lead may delay neurophysiological development and cause behavioural and performance problems in school. How much dietary ingestion contributes to these outcomes is not clear.

Mercury

Mercury, like lead, is one of the ancient metals. In spite of its peculiarity as a liquid metal, useless for implement making, it has been in use for many hundreds of years. It was formerly valued largely for its medicinal properties and now is used as an industrial catalyst, as well as in pigments, paints, chemicals, electrical equipment, and numerous other applications. Its toxicity has long been recognized. Medieval mercury miners suffered from 'quicksilver disease'; its use in felt making was responsible for 'mad hatter' disease. Today mercury poisoning still occurs, usually due to food contaminated as a result of industrial pollution.

Mercury released from natural sources, such as volcanoes, or by industry, is normally in inorganic form. However, the element can undergo chemical transformations of toxicological significance. Aerobic bacteria in sediments at the bottom of lakes and seas transform it into organic compounds, such as methyl and ethyl mercury. These compounds are then taken up by plankton, and via plankton feeders and their predators to carnivorous fish and eventually the human diet.

Food contains both organic and inorganic mercury. Absorption, distribution in tissues, retention and toxicity are all related to the chemical form of the element. Metallic mercury, seldom found in food except as a result of accidental or deliberate contamination, is poorly absorbed and quickly eliminated. Its vapour, however, can be absorbed rapidly through the lungs. Inorganic mercury compounds are highly toxic. Though absorption in the gastrointestinal tract is initially low, at about 10%, some compounds, such as mercuric chloride (also known as

Table 8 Mercury content of food

Food	Total mercury ($\mu g\ kg^{-1}$, fresh wt)
Cereals	4–22
Dairy products	< 1–5
Fish (not deepsea)	40–250
Vegetables	1–10
Meat	
Beef muscle	1–16
Beef liver	2–40
Beef kidney	1–136
Other foods	< 1–5

After Reilly (1991).

Table 10 Dietary intake of mercury in different countries

Country	Total mercury intake (μg per day)
Belgium (adults)	6.5
Brazil (adults)	9
Denmark (adult males)	26
Germany (adult males)	16
Germany (adult females)	13
Italy (total diet)	29
Spain (total diet)	4
Sweden (pensioners)	4
Sweden (adult females)	7
Switzerland (adults)	< 5
UK (total diet)	3
USA (total diet)	3

Data from Parr et al. (1991), Reilly (1991) and van Dokkum (1995).

corrosive sublimate) can cause intestinal damage which leads to increased absorption. Most of the mercury that enters the blood is carried to the organs, especially the kidney, where it accumulates. Poisoning is painful and usually fatal, as a result of kidney failure.

Organic mercury compounds are efficiently absorbed and distributed to the different organs where they can be retained for a long time. Brain has a special affinity for them. In pregnant women alkyl mercury can cross the placenta and accumulate in the brain of the fetus, causing encephalopathy.

Clinical symptoms of organic mercury poisoning include sensory disturbances of the limbs, the tongue and around the lips. With increasing intake, symptoms become more severe. The central nervous system is damaged irreversibly, resulting in ataxia, tremor, slurred speech, tunnel vision, blindness, loss of hearing and, finally, death.

The total amount of mercury in any food, in the absence of gross contamination, is normally very low, ranging from trace amounts to about $50\ \mu g$ kg^{-1}, with the exception of seafoods (**Table 8** and **Table 9**). Daily intake is normally about 10–50 μg, and meets the FAO/WHO PTWI (**Table 10**).

Table 9 Mercury in fish/seafood

Fish/seafood	Mean total mercury ($mg\ kg^{-1}$ fresh wt)
Cod	0.17 (0.04–0.40)[a]
Lobster	0.07 (0.01–0.24)
Marlin, blue	4.78 (0.35–14.0)
Salmon	0.04 (0.00–0.14)
Shark	0.62 (0.20–1.14)
Sole	0.10 (0.00–0.23)
Swordfish	1.15 (0.05–4.90)
Tuna, bluefin	0.68 (0.46–0.91)
Tuna, canned	0.47 (0.03–0.58)

[a]Range in parenthesis.
[b]After Margolin (1980).

A diet high in contaminated fish was the cause of the notorious Minimata Bay tragedy in Japan. The bay was grossly contaminated with mercury released from a nearby industrial plant. Levels of up to 30 mg kg^{-1} of methyl mercury were found in fish caught there and consumed in large amounts by local people. Their mercury intake was as much as 10 mg per day and many suffered debilitating and even fatal poisoning.

In contrast to the Minimata community, Greenland Eskimos and Faroe Islanders, who also eat large amounts of mercury-rich fish, do not normally suffer from mercury poisoning. It has been suggested that this immunity is due to the fact that toxicity only occurs from eating mercury in fish when the natural protective system of the body has been overwhelmed by pollution. When mercury is accumulated by fish under natural conditions through the food chain, a surplus of antagonistic elements, especially selenium, is present which counteracts the effects of the mercury. While selenium levels are high in seafoods consumed in Greenland and the Faroe Islands, this is not believed to have been the case in Minimata. The protective role of selenium against methylmercury (the main form of mercury in fish) is believed to be brought about by the formation of a selenite complex which is less toxic than the methyl compound.

Several incidents of poisoning through ingestion of mercury in cereals have been caused by the accidental use of wheat treated with mercury-containing fungicides, and intended for use only as seed, to make flour. Hundreds were poisoned in this way in Iraq in 1960. As a result of this, and similar tragedies elsewhere, mercurial seed dressings have been replaced by safer fungicides for agricultural use.

Cadmium

Unlike lead and mercury, cadmium has only come into wide industrial use in the twentieth century. It is used mainly in electroplating, in steel and in specialist alloys, as well as in the manufacture of pigments and plastics. Cadmium has won for itself a high profile as a food contaminant.

Cadmium is found in food in inorganic form. About 6% of ingested cadmium is absorbed, though the presence of other substances, including calcium and protein, can increase absorption. It is bound mainly to the low molecular weight protein metallothionein, synthesized in response to cadmium, zinc and other metals, mainly in liver. Metallothionein can bind more than 10% of total metals in the body.

Most of the absorbed cadmium is retained very efficiently and has a biological half-life of up to 40 years. Newborn infants have very little cadmium in their tissues. By the age of 50, the body store will be 30–100 mg, mainly in the kidneys. Clinical monitoring of cadmium accumulation is difficult. Blood levels reflect recent intake. Levels in urine may indicate accumulation in the kidney.

Ingestion of cadmium at first causes nausea, vomiting and abdominal cramp, followed by renal damage and disturbances in calcium metabolism. This can lead to osteomalacia, with resulting skeletal brittleness and fracturing. These were the symptoms seen in the notorious incident of cadmium poisoning in Japanese peasants who consumed contaminated rice. Their cries of *itai-itai* (ouch-ouch) as they suffered multiple bone fractures has been taken as the name of the disease.

Normally most foods and beverages contain <0.001–0.050 mg kg^{-1} of cadmium (**Table 11**). Where industrial and other pollution occurs, levels can be higher. Rice implicated in *itai-itai* disease contained 1 mg kg^{-1}, more than 20 times the levels in rice elsewhere in Japan. More than 3.5 mg kg^{-1} were found in fish in polluted waters in the USA. In the Netherlands kidneys from cattle whose fodder was contaminated with cadmium contained up to 2 mg kg^{-1} of the metal.

In most countries the average intake of cadmium does not exceed the FAO/WHO PTWI of 400–500 μg (**Table 12**). Differences in intakes between countries are related to differences in dietary patterns as well as to levels of local contamination, as indicated in **Table 13**. The considerably higher intake of seafoods in Japan, as well as of vegetables and offal in Germany, account for the higher levels of cadmium intakes in these two countries compared with Finland.

Intake of cadmium has on occasion been markedly increased by use of domestic water which has come through zinc-coated (galvanized) pipes and tanks. Zinc nearly always contains a significant amount of cadmium, and this is readily leached from zinc plate by hot, and especially acidic, water. Water in boilers in some Scottish hospitals was found to contain up to 21 μg l^{-1} of cadmium, more than twice the WHO standard of 10 μg l^{-1}.

Agricultural land can be contaminated with cadmium, with resultant high levels in cattle and crops produced on it, by the use of cadmium-containing fertilizers. Some superphosphates are rich in cadmium, as is sewage sludge sometimes used as a top dressing on farm land. Cadmium pollution can also result from horticultural use of rehabilitated mining land, as occurred in the English village of Shipham, in Somerset. There are reports of high levels of cadmium in vegetables, in areas of eastern Europe where former mining and manufacturing activities have left a legacy of soil contamination.

Nickel

Nickel, unlike the other heavy metals considered here, is a *transition metal*, similar in atomic structure

Table 11 Cadmium in foods

Food	Cadmium content (range, μg kg^{-1}, fresh wt)
Apples	<2–19
Beef	<2–28
Bread	<2–43
Cabbage	<2–26
Fish	89–770
Kidney, sheep	13–2000
Potatoes	<2–51
Poultry	2–69
Prawns	17–913

Data from Reilly (1991).

Table 12 Dietary cadmium intakes in different countries

Country (type and year of survey)	Cadmium intake (mean, μg per day)
Japan (MB[a]; 1975)	46
USA (MB; 1978–1979)	32 ± 4.7
Denmark (MB; 1980)	32
France (MB; 1976–1978)	29
Australia (MB; 1977)	22
UK (MB; 1982)	15
Sweden (Prepared diet; 1981)	10
China (DD[b]; 1980)	5

[a]Market Basket Survey.
[b]Duplicate Diet Survey.
After Morgan and Sherlock (1984).

Table 13 Intake of cadmium by food groups in three countries

	Cadmium intake, µg per day (food intake, g per day)		
Food group	Finland	Germany	Japan
Cereals	6.6 (267)	11.0 (254)	17.6 (503)
Roots and tubers	2.4 (238)	10.4 (221)	2.1 (72)
Vegetables, green	1.4 (87)	15.4 (188)	10.3 (299)
Fruits	0.3 (219)	3.0 (287)	0.9 (178)
Meat and offals	2.0 (169)	4.3 (268)	1.0 (82)
Eggs	0.1 (29)	0.6 (47)	0.5 (45)
Seafoods	0.7 (78)	1.2 (27)	21.4 (239)
Milk	1.1 (711)	1.2 (329)	0.7 (136)
Alcoholic beverages	0.2 (180)	1.5 (489)	0.5 (160)
Total:	14.8 (1978)	48.6 (2110)	55 (1714)

After Loukari and Salminen (1986).

to chromium, manganese, iron and copper. Their atoms have valence electrons in more than one shell and thus have more than one oxidation state. As a result they are highly active and are able to take part in many metabolic activities, particularly as components of metalloenzymes. In contrast, lead, mercury and cadmium belong to the *representative metals*, with their valence electrons all in one shell, and lack oxidative flexibility.

Nickel occurs in small amounts in soils. It usually occurs in association with other metals. It is widely used industrially, particularly in high-quality alloys. Nickel steel is highly corrosion resistant and for this reason is often used to make food processing equipment. Another food-related use is as a catalyst in the hydrogenation of edible oils.

Nickel ingested in food is poorly absorbed, with 3–6% retained in the body. It does not appear to be stored in any particular organ, but is evenly distributed among tissues. The absorbed nickel is rapidly and efficiently excreted through the kidneys as low molecular weight complexes. The essentiality of nickel for a number of animal species has been established and it is likely that it will be shown to be required by humans. Nickel-containing enzymes, such as urease, occur in bacteria and plants. Several animal enzymes, including carboxylase, trypsin and acetyl coenzyme A, can be activated by nickel.

Industrial exposure to nickel is a recognized cause of cancer of the respiratory tract, and, less seriously, of contact dermatitis. Intake of as little as 0.6 mg of a soluble zinc salt can cause a positive skin reaction in people with nickel allergy. Nickel in food may be responsible for a form of persistent eczema in some people. This may be an indirect effect of antagonism between nickel and zinc in tissues since the eczema has been shown to be caused by zinc deficiency. In

certain animals high doses of dietary nickel can cause growth depression and anaemia.

Nickel levels in food are generally low, as shown in **Table 14**. Certain foods contain unusually high levels of the metal, including cocoa powder, with up to 8.5 mg kg⁻¹. Foods stored in steel cans and prepared in stainless-steel utensils can also have higher than average levels of nickel as a result of leaching from the steel. Daily intakes of nickel from normal diets are generally low, as is seen in **Table 15**.

Bismuth

There has been concern in recent years at the possible toxic effects of ingested bismuth as use of the metal, especially in pharmaceutical preparations, has been increasing. It is not a common metal and its natural distribution is limited. It is obtained mainly as a by-product of refining of lead and copper. It is used

Table 14 Nickel in foods

	Nickel content (mg kg⁻¹, fresh wt)	
Food	Mean	Range
Cereals and cereal products	0.16	0.10–0.30
Meat and poultry	<0.14	<0.05–1.1
Offal	<0.05	<0.05–0.10
Fish	<0.11	<0.05–0.30
Vegetables, green	0.11	0.05–0.30
Potatoes	<0.07	<0.05–0.28
Other vegetables	0.14	0.10–0.20
Canned vegetables	0.25	0.10–0.45
Fruit	<0.06	<0.05–0.30
Beverages	0.04	0.03–0.06
Milk	<0.02	<0.02

Data from Smart and Sherlock (1987).

Table 15 Intake of dietary nickel in different countries

Country	Mean nickel intake (μg per day)
Denmark	130
Finland	130
Germany (women)	111
Germany (men)	123
UK	160
USA	117

After Reilly (1991) and Anke *et al.* (1993).

industrially in certain alloys and in nuclear reactors. A growing use is in the pharmaceutical industry, in cosmetics, ointments, as a therapeutic agent for gastrointestinal disturbances, and other applications. A recent application has been in the treatment of peptic ulcers, especially those caused by *Helicobacter pylori*.

Absorption of bismuth and its compounds from food appears to be low. A specific transport mechanism across the intestinal mucosa has been postulated. The element accumulates at low levels in most organs, with the highest level in kidney and lowest in liver. Excretion is rapid, mainly in urine. Tissue retention is apparently directly related to dietary zinc levels. It appears that metallothionein is involved in this relationship. Both bismuth and zinc induce metallothionein formation and thus intake of one may increase retention of the other.

There is no evidence that bismuth plays an essential metabolic role in the human body. High intakes of water-soluble bismuth compounds can cause renal damage and encephalopathy, as well as less serious problems of skin irritation and pigmentation. An increased intake of zinc can reduce bismuth toxicity. Poisonings have occurred as a result of oral intake of large amounts of bismuth-containing pharmaceuticals.

Little information is available about bismuth in foods. Levels appear to be very low, between 1 and 10 μg kg^{-1}. Dietary intakes are estimated to be about 5 μg per day. In the absence of deliberate or accidental contamination, poisoning by the ingestion of bismuth in food is highly unlikely to occur.

See also: **Aluminium**: Occurence and Toxicity. **Chro-** **mium**: Physiology, Dietary Sources and Requirements. **Copper**: Physiology, Dietary Sources and Requirements. **Food Contaminants**: Pesticides. **Magnesium**: Physiology, Dietary Sources and Requirements. **Potassium**: Physiology, Dietary Sources and Requirements. **Sodium**: Physiology. **Zinc**: Physiology.

Further Reading

Anke M, Angelow M, Müller M and Glei M (1993) Dietary trace element intake and excretion in man. In: Anke M, Meissner D and Mills CF (eds) *Trace Elements in Man and Animals – TEMA 8*, pp. 180–188. Gersdorf, Germany: Verlag Media Touristik.

Elsenhans B, Beck R, Strugala G and Forth W (1993) Oral doses of bismuth, dietary zinc supply and trace metal levels in the rat. In: Anke M, Meissner D and Mills CF (eds) *Trace Elements in Man and Animals – TEMA 8*, pp. 928–932. Gersdorf, Germany: Verlag Media Touristik.

Loukari K and Salminen S (1986) Intake of heavy metals from foods in Finland, West Germany and Japan. *Food Additives and Contaminants* 3:355–362.

Margolin S (1980) Mercury in marine seafood: the scientific medical margin of safety as a guide to the potential risk to public health. *World Review of Nutrition and Diet* 34:182–265.

Morgan H and Sherlock JC (1984) Cadmium intake and cadmium in the human kidney. *Food Additives and Contaminants* 1:45–51.

Nielsen FH (1990) Other trace elements. In: Brown ML (ed.) *Present Knowledge in Nutrition*, 6th edn, pp. 294–307. Washington, DC: International Life Sciences Institute.

Parr RM, Abdulla M, Aras NK, Byrne AR, Camara-Rica C, Finnie S, Gharib AG, Ingrao G, Iyengar GV, Khangi FA, Krishnan SS, Kumpulainen J, Liu S, Schelenz R, Srianujata S, Tanner JT and Wolf W (1991) Dietary intakes of trace elements and related nutrients in eleven countries: preliminary results from an IAEA research programme. In: Momcilovic M (ed.) *Trace Elements in Man and Animals – TEMA 7*, pp. 13/3–13/5. Zagreb: Institute for Medical Research.

Reilly C (1991) *Metal Contamination of Food*, 2nd edn. London: Elsevier Applied Science.

Smart GA and Sherlock JC (1987) Nickel in foods and the diet. *Food Additives and Contaminants* 4:61–67.

van Dokkum W (1995) The intake of selected minerals and trace elements in European countries. *Nutrition Research Reviews* 8:271–302.

Height *see* **Nutritional Status**: Anthropometric Assessment.

HIV DISEASE

Nutritional Management

C J Green, Nutricia Corporate Research, Zoetermeer, The Netherlands

C Summerbell, Royal Free Hospital School of Medicine, London, UK

Copyright © 1998 Academic Press

HIV infection affects host immunity, resulting in secondary opportunistic infections and an increased susceptibility to certain neoplasms. Acquired immunodeficiency syndrome (AIDS) is an illness characterized by one or more 'indicator' diseases, depending on the status of laboratory evidence of HIV infection. The term HIV disease is used in this article to describe all persons with HIV infection, both asymptomatic and symptomatic.

Persons with HIV disease are at risk of nutritional deficiencies as a result of many factors. This article aims to describe the nutritional status in this population and to discuss the mechanisms that lead to malnutrition, including the many factors that can affect appetite and eating behaviour. The objectives of nutritional support are outlined, and the different methods of providing nutritional support are described. Finally, some discussion is given to the use of unproven dietary therapies in HIV disease.

Nutritional Status

Body weight and composition

The fact that weight loss is a significant problem in HIV disease is reflected by the fact that loss of greater than 10% of usual body weight associated with either chronic diarrhoea or fever (the 'HIV wasting syndrome') is an AIDS-defining illness. Cross-sectional studies have confirmed that weight loss occurs in a high percentage of cases of HIV infection, the effect becoming more distinct with advancing illness. It should be noted, however, that some groups at high risk of HIV infection, such as drug abusers, are likely to be at risk of depletion irrespective of HIV status.

Prospective studies have shown however that weight loss in HIV infection is not inevitable and can be reversed, at least to a certain extent. Two patterns of weight loss are seen: acute severe weight loss associated with systemic infections, and chronic progressive weight loss, in general associated with gastrointestinal disease. Periods of weight stability and weight gain primarily associated with recovery from opportunistic infections also occur.

Little is known about the relative proportions of body fat and body cell mass (BCM) lost and gained over the course of HIV infection, although it is thought that BCM is depleted to a greater degree and may occur early and independently of changes in body fat. Shifts in fluid occur, with a relative decrease in intracellular water volume and increase in extracellular water. In total, this resembles the depletion associated with stress and injury rather than uncomplicated starvation. The decreases in plasma albumin, iron-binding capacity and retinol-binding protein that have been observed at various stages of HIV disease are also characteristic of cachexia (profound loss of lean tissue and fat associated with disease particularly cancer and HIV disease) and an acute-phase response. Death from wasting has been related to the magnitude of tissue depletion and may even be independent of the underlying cause of wasting.

Micronutrient status

Data describing micronutrient status in HIV disease are conflicting. Biochemical deficiencies of many micronutrients have been described at different stages of disease, in some cases in spite of seemingly adequate intakes. These deficiencies are, however, not apparent in all subjects; plasma levels of many micronutrients within the normal range or above normal have also been reported.

HIV disease can affect micronutrient status in a number of ways. Appetite and dietary intake for all nutrients can be reduced as a result of a number of factors, including the side effects of certain drugs. Malabsorption is common and can result in losses of carotenoids and vitamins A, D and E. Increased requirements of the antioxidant nutrients during infection, owing to increased free radical production, may lead to a decline in their levels, and some drug therapies may also increase requirements for some micronutrients.

Under certain circumstances micronutrient status may appear to be abnormal, but it is not. Metabolic changes occurring as a result of acute and chronic infection, such as the release of cytokines and interleukin-1, cause shifts in the levels of acute-phase transport proteins such as retinol-binding protein, transferrin and albumin. Consequently, tissue distribution of nutrients which use these acute-phase proteins for transport occurs, resulting in changes in plasma levels of these nutrients. Furthermore, some drugs used in the management of HIV disease may compete with these nutrients for binding sites on transport proteins thus reducing available sites and therefore measurable levels of nutrients in plasma.

·Some groups who are at high risk of HIV infection may have low levels of some micronutrients irrespective of HIV status. For example, homosexual men have been shown to have higher rates of enteric infection compared with heterosexual males regardless of HIV status (the 'gay bowel syndrome'), thus possibly resulting in malabsorption. Finally, self-supplementation of single or combinations of micronutrients occurs frequently and may be associated with high plasma levels (see Unproven Dietary Therapies below).

Mechanisms of Malnutrition

Reduced food intake is an important mechanism of malnutrition in HIV disease. Malabsorption and altered metabolism also play an important part. The possible interrelationships between HIV infection,

immune function, gut function and undernutrition are shown in **Fig. 1**.

Reduced food intake

Many factors serve to reduce food intake in HIV disease, as discussed below. However, there is a relatively large body of data which suggests that energy intake in clinically stable persons with HIV disease is comparable with or even higher than in control subjects. In contrast, individuals who are losing weight associated with overt opportunistic infection have significantly decreased food intake. Apart from reducing energy intake, reduced food intake will also result in impaired intake of protein and micronutrients. Nutritional status has been discussed above.

Malabsorption and diarrhoea

Chronic weight loss that occurs in spite of apparently adequate energy intake may be attributed to gastrointestinal disease, malabsorption and diarrhoea, which are widespread and distressing problems occurring in the majority of individuals with HIV disease. Malabsorption and diarrhoea may occur for a number of reasons. The gastrointestinal tract is vulnerable to opportunistic pathogens which include bacteria (e.g. *Mycobacterium avium-intracellulare*,

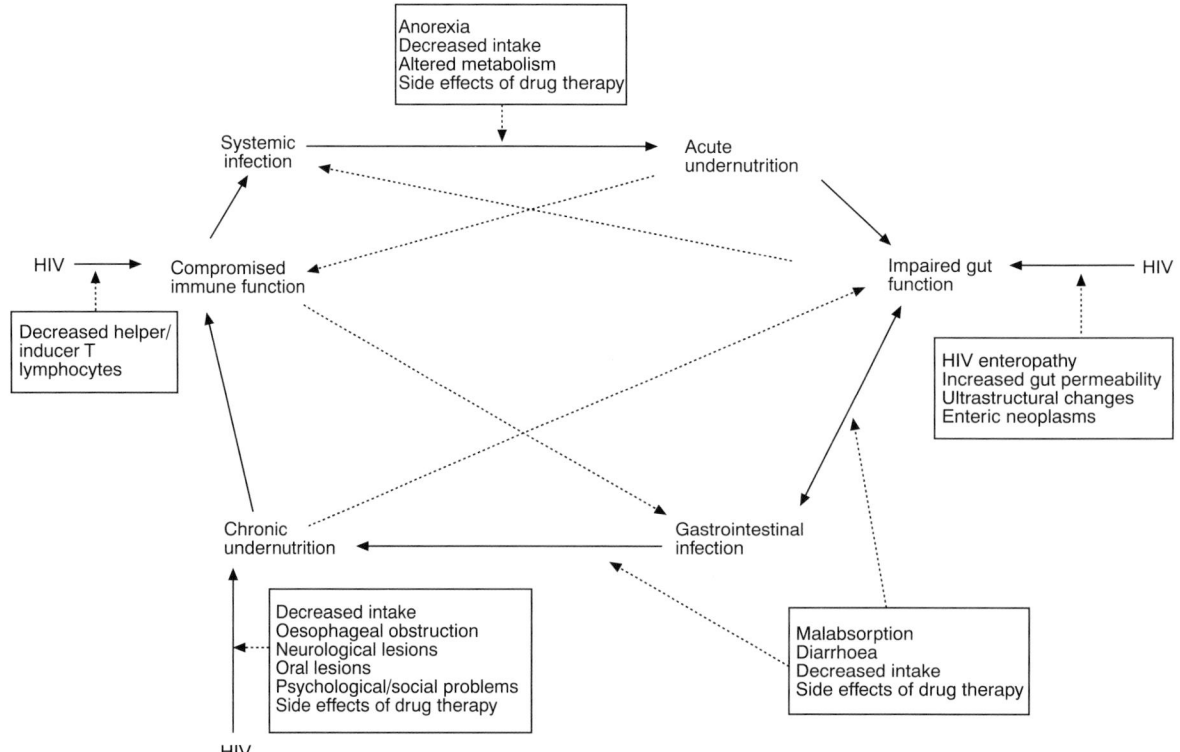

Figure 1 Proposed schematic illustration of interrelationships between HIV infection, immune function, gut function and undernutrition. Reproduced from Green CJ (1995) Nutritional support in HIV infection and AIDS. *Clinical Nutrition* **14**:157–212.

Salmonella, Clostridium difficile), protozoa (e.g. *Cryptosporidium, Microsporidium, Isospora*), and viruses (e.g. cytomegalovirus, herpes simplex virus). *Cryptosporidium* is the most common infection, causing secretory diarrhoea which is refractory to treatment. Enteric neoplasms are also relatively common and include Kaposi's sarcoma and gastrointestinal lymphoma. Intestinal fistulas may occur, leading to protein and electrolyte losses. In addition, drug therapy may cause diarrhoea and other side effects or nutritional interactions. Many patients with gastrointestinal symptoms have no identifiable cause, which could be related in part to inadequate diagnostic techniques. However, lymphoid tissue along the gastrointestinal tract is a main target of HIV infection, leading to HIV enteropathy, i.e. villous atrophy, crypt hyperplasia and lymphatic infiltration in the jejunum. Increased intestinal permeability and ultrastructural changes in the duodenal mucosa are also features of HIV disease which may contribute to gastrointestinal symptoms.

Malabsorption of nutrients will lead to losses in the stool, as well as contribute to diarrhoea. A trend towards decreased D-xylose absorption, an index of intestinal absorptive area, has been reported at various stages of disease, but is not a consistent feature. Malabsorption of lactose will cause fluid accumulation in the lumen, abdominal cramps and watery diarrhoea. Absolute lactase deficiency and decreased lactase activity have been demonstrated, even in the absence of identifiable enteric infection.

Little is known about protein digestion and absorption in HIV infection, although protein hydrolysates and elemental diets are often recommended on the empirical basis that they are better absorbed and tolerated. From an energy balance point of view, fat malabsorption is particularly significant. Steatorrhoea is apparent in some HIV-positive individuals, particularly in those with chronic diarrhoea. It is thought to be less of a problem in constitutionally well patients without intercurrent infections.

Chronic weight loss is associated with gastrointestinal symptoms or malabsorption although quantitatively significant malabsorption may not be a consistent feature. Fat malabsorption will impair absorption of the fat-soluble vitamins. Fatty acid and bile salt malabsorption will contribute to diarrhoea by interfering with absorption and secretion of water and electrolytes, thus increasing bowel motility. Patients with poor ileal function may also malabsorb vitamin B_{12}. Assessment of gut function should form an important part of individual assessment in HIV disease.

Altered metabolism

A number of metabolic aberrations have been observed in HIV infection, including relative loss of body cell mass compared with fat (see above), elevated resting energy expenditure (REE), abnormally elevated triglyceride levels, raised free fatty acid turnover, raised fat oxidation rates unrelated to counter-regulatory or thyroid hormone increases, and various endocrine abnormalities. Insulin sensitivity is increased, which is in contrast to that seen in other catabolic states. Cytokines such as tumour necrosis factor and interleukin-1 are released during infection and have been implicated in many of these abnormalities.

It has been suggested that raised REE (approximately 10% in asymptomatic individuals and 30% during secondary infection despite a reduction in energy intake in the latter case) may contribute to accelerated weight loss. However, weight loss episodes are associated with a decrease in total EE, mainly due to a decrease in activity-related EE. Thus the reduction in energy intake during episodes of infection by far outweigh any increases in REE.

Despite the metabolic abnormalities observed and some reports of poor results with repletion studies, patients without systemic illness are able to mount a normal anabolic response to an adequate nutritional stimulus. The situation in HIV disease compounded by systemic infection can be compared with other situations of sepsis and catabolism, whereby nutritional repletion is unlikely to occur until the underlying infection has been adequately treated.

Effects on Appetite and Eating Behaviour

Many factors serve to reduce food intake in HIV disease. Anorexia is a common feature which may result from a number of causes, including emotional stress, fever and infection, and side effects of drug therapy or other medical interventions such as chemotherapy or radiotherapy. A reduced food intake may be self-imposed because of early satiety, pain, nausea, vomiting, diarrhoea or fear of these. Restricted diets may be self-imposed in the belief that they may be beneficial and, in some cases, there may be voluntary attempts to lose weight.

Lesions in the mouth, pharynx and oesophagus caused by fungi, viruses and Kaposi's sarcoma cause pain and obstruction and can make chewing and swallowing uncomfortable and difficult. Oral candidiasis is particularly common and can also lead to changes in taste perception. Neurological problems can result in dysphagia, apathy and depression.

Extreme tiredness, confusion, dementia and blindness will also contribute to inability to obtain and prepare food. Finally, social factors such as lack of money, storage and cooking facilities should not be overlooked as contributary causes of reduced food intake.

Objectives of Nutritional Support

The objectives of nutritional support and the most appropriate dietary intervention will depend on individual clinical and social circumstances, and age (i.e. child or adult). An early dietary evaluation should be completed, preferably during the asymptomatic period before weight loss has occurred. Although it has not been proven that early dietary advice and maintenance of nutritional status will improve survival, it is thought that malnutrition could be a cofactor in disease progression.

It is generally recommended that dietary advice in asymptomatic individuals should be tailored to maintain body cell mass and provide adequate levels of all nutrients in order to preserve immune function and prevent weight loss. In patients with more advanced disease or who are already depleted, energy intake should be assessed and underlying causes of nutritional depletion should be diagnosed and treated if possible. The goals of nutritional support in these circumstances include those stated above, as well as minimizing symptoms of malabsorption, providing symptomatic relief, optimizing nutritional repletion following infection, and enhancing quality of life.

There is no single nutritional therapy that is applicable for all persons with HIV disease. The type of intervention depends on the clinical situation, absorptive and digestive capacity, weight variation following nutritional intervention, patient acceptance, feasibility and cost. Possible therapies include simple dietary advice and counselling, oral supplements, enteral nutrition and parenteral nutrition. Combining dietary advice with exercise education, appetite stimulants and other pharmacological methods of promoting BCM may be applicable in the future, but as yet remain to be fully investigated.

Dietary advice

A regular and well-balanced diet with adequate intake of all nutrients according to individual needs should be promoted. There is no evidence that asymptomatic HIV-positive individuals have differing requirements from those of the healthy population. If food intake is less than optimal, the aetiology of inadequate food intake should be explored. Practical information and culinary tips to prevent or correct weight loss and overcome typical problems such as decreased appetite, painful mouth and oesophagus, chewing and swallowing problems, taste alteration, diarrhoea, nausea and vomiting should be given. An individual approach is essential and food preferences in particular should be taken into account. Dietary advice should be given in the context of knowledge of lifestyle and socioeconomic circumstances. Lack of money, storage and cooking facilities, skills, energy and motivation may all influence food choices. Information on food safety and reducing risk of food-borne infection should be given.

Oral supplements

If a patient does not succeed in preserving nutritional status and body weight in spite of dietary advice for improving oral intake, or if it is clear that a person will not be able to achieve adequate energy, protein and micronutrients from conventional foods alone, then oral supplements are indicated. The preparations can be categorized as shown in **Table 1**.

Energy, protein and combined nutrient supplements Oral supplementation of the diet is often the simplest way to increase nutrient intake. The feasibility and benefits are well established in a wide variety of patient groups. Use of nutritional supplements in HIV disease can result in improvements in intake and nutritional status. However, most published studies have included small numbers of patients, often at different disease stages and for

Table 1 Types and characteristics of oral supplements

Type of supplement	Characteristics
Energy	Carbohydrate (e.g. maltodextrin), liquid or powder form, can be added to other foods
Protein	Skimmed milk powder for adding to other foods
Micronutrients	Single or multivitamin and mineral complexes, in the form of tablets, capsules or liquids
Combination of nutrients	Products for use as dietary supplements or as partial substitution of diet, usually containing energy, protein and micronutrients, in the form of liquid or powder
	Nutritionally complete products for use as dietary supplements or as partial or complete substitution of diet, containing all nutrients in balanced amounts, in the form of liquid or powder

short periods of time. Compositional aspects are discussed below in the section on Enteral Nutrition.

Micronutrient supplements Micronutrients are important for the function of various components of the immune system and can influence resistance to infection. Associations have also been noted between certain micronutrients and mood as well as neurological and cognitive functions.

Status of some micronutrients may be low or deficient in HIV disease (see section above on Nutritional Status). Retrospective and epidemiological studies support the view that deficits of some micronutrients, in particular vitamin A, are associated with advancing HIV disease, and that use of a daily multivitamin preparation may be beneficial in reducing disease progression. However, no prospective intervention studies have been performed, except with β-carotene, which did result in improvements in some parameters of immune function. Interest is also growing in the role of the antioxidant nutrients, such as vitamin E, vitamin C and other dietary components such as cysteine, as it is becoming apparent that advancing HIV disease may be linked to poor antioxidant status.

The consensus view is that a multivitamin and mineral supplement at levels equivalent to recommended daily amounts is appropriate. Furthermore, modest daily supplements of β-carotene may be beneficial. Depending on individual circumstances, in particular in relation to malabsorption, supplements of specific micronutrients, e.g. fat-soluble vitamins due to fat malabsorption or vitamin B_{12} due to ileal disease, may be necessary (see also section below on Unproven Dietary Therapies).

Enteral nutrition

Enteral nutrition (tube feeding) is an important means of nutritional support for patients who are not able to consume sufficient energy and protein via the oral route and should be considered if a patient has an adequately functional gut. Provision of nutrition in this way, rather than intravenously, is thought to have benefit in terms of maintaining the integrity of the gut. Nasogastric or nasoduodenal feeding is the method of choice for short-term use. A gastrostomy or jejunostomy should be considered if longer-term support is anticipated. Nocturnal feeding may be used to supplement oral intake.

There are relatively few studies that have specifically examined the efficacy of enteral nutrition in HIV disease. Most are small, retrospective or prospective evaluations at various stages of disease. However, enteral nutrition is feasible in patients who are free of serious small intestinal disease and in spite of systemic infection.

No single oral supplement or enteral formula is suitable for all persons with HIV disease. The most appropriate formula will depend on the clinical circumstances and objectives of nutritional support, and on assessments of nutritional status and gut function. If gut function is adequate, intact nutrients should be provided. A standard polymeric diet should thus be the first choice of formula. Anecdotally, hydrolysed or elemental formulae are said to be useful if intact protein formulae are not well tolerated. In those with established exocrine pancreatic insufficiency, hydrolysates may be indicated, although use of pancreatic enzyme supplements in conjunction with whole protein feeds may be equally beneficial.

In the case of fat malabsorption, low-fat formulae and/or products containing medium-chain triglycerides (MCT) may be beneficial, but there is little justification in use of extremely low-fat diets in patients with normal gut function. If possible, fat intake should be adjusted according to tolerance, and preferably some assessment of gut function should be made. Despite the theoretical advantages relating to digestion and absorption, MCT may reduce palatability and increase costs of formulations. In addition, formulae with a high MCT content will be at risk of failing to provide adequate essential fatty acids (linoleic and α-linolenic) to meet current public health guidelines either in terms of absolute amount or ratio of n-6 : n-3 fatty acids.

Carbohydrate is a valuable energy source, particularly if fat restriction is genuinely necessary. In certain cases, such as bowel diseases resulting from gastrointestinal infections and nonspecific enteropathies, a low-lactose or lactose-free diet is appropriate. Most enteral formulae are clinically lactose free.

Reduction in fibre intake is often recommended in cases of gastrointestinal disease and diarrhoea, and most oral and enteral formulae are fibre free. There are some anecdotal reports that fibre may be useful in terms of stool bulking, but little attention has been focused on soluble, fermentable fibre as a method of alleviating diarrhoea by its fermentation to short-chain fatty acids (SCFA) in the colon. The potential benefit of this will depend on the cause of diarrhoea (e.g. fibre is unlikely to be of value in cases of steatorrhoea or bile salt malabsorption), and the use of concomitant antibiotic therapy, which may inhibit SCFA production. Soya polysaccharide is commonly used in fibre-containing enteral formulae, but further research is required to establish whether this, or alternative sources of fibre, are beneficial in reducing diarrhoea associated with HIV infection. However, the fact that fibre may have other valuable effects on gut morphology and barrier function suggest that in the future, fibre may be regarded as a standard component of all enteral formulae.

There is at present insufficient evidence to support the addition of micronutrients at levels greatly in excess of dietary reference values to oral or enteral formulae. There is some evidence that immune function can be manipulated by altering the lipid or amino acid composition of the diet. Diets low in linoleic acid content (e.g. coconut oil) or high in eicosapentaenoic acid (e.g. fish oil) may blunt inflammatory responses. Requirements for the amino acids glutamine and arginine appear to be raised during stress and infection. However, since there is some suggestion that immune activation could contribute to disease progression, the existing data on safety and efficacy are not yet strong enough to make recommendations on such changes.

Parenteral nutrition

There is a general consensus that when the gut is functioning, it should be used as the first route of choice for nutritional support. As in other situations, intravenous nutrition (IVN) is indicated in cases of bowel obstruction, severe refractory diarrhoea, intractable vomiting or intolerance to enteral feeding. In some cases, IVN may be used as an adjunct to enteral feeding, since it is thought preferable to use the gastrointestinal tract wherever possible, even if only small volumes can be tolerated, or it may be necessary to use IVN to meet all nutritional requirements.

A peripheral line may be appropriate if IVN is anticipated to last for 7–10 days. If longer-term IVN is expected, then a central line is indicated. Usual measures (i.e. sterile technique) should be taken to ensure that the infection risk associated with IVN is kept to a minimum. Standard or high-nitrogen formulae with sufficient lipid to prevent essential fatty acid deficiency should be used, in conjunction with monitoring to assess lipid tolerance.

Unproven Dietary Therapies

The individual with an incurable disease often focuses on the possibility that by consuming a certain type of diet or nutrient, they may extend the period of time when they are well. Although the use of unproven dietary strategies is particularly high in HIV disease, the evidence on which these practices are based is mostly poor. The safety of most alternative therapies is unknown, and thus their use should be carefully monitored by the physician since they may be harmful when taken in excess or in combi-

nation with prescribed drugs. Unrecognized toxicity or resulting weight loss could be mistaken for symptomatic disease. In addition, nonprescribable products may utilize limited financial resources. Nevertheless, their use may have psychological value and until proper studies have been performed, possible benefits cannot be ruled out.

Vitamins and minerals

Micronutrient status in HIV disease and guidelines for supplementation have been described above. Despite the relatively cautious recommendations, many HIV-positive individuals believe that vitamin and mineral supplements are particularly important for their health. Self-supplementation with vitamins and minerals (e.g. vitamins E, C, B_{12} zinc and iron) occurs frequently, often at levels ten times or more higher than dietary references values. Megadose intakes can lead to deleterious effects, e.g. high doses of vitamin C can cause kidney stone formation and rebound scurvy, and excess zinc and iron can suppress immune function. High intakes of zinc and vitamin A have been associated with increased risk of disease progression.

Special diets

There are a number of 'special' diets which are purported to improve health and well-being. Many of these diets emphasize the consumption of wholegrain cereals, fresh fruit and vegetables with little or no meat or sugar, e.g. macrobiotic diets and Maharishi Ayurveda. The 'anti-candida' diet which excludes all carbohydrate-rich and yeast-containing food is also popular. These diets are restrictive and not energy dense. In their extreme form they will lead to weight loss and other nutrient deficiencies.

Special foods

The consumption of certain foods which are thought to reduce the rate of viral replication, inhibit infections or boost immune function is popular in HIV disease. These foods include lipids from egg yolk (AL 721), lecithin, garlic, specific amino acids, glandular enzymes/extracts, bee propolis and live yogurt. As with other unproven dietary therapies, safety may be an issue, either in terms of the food itself (e.g. safety of live microorganisms in situations where a compromised gut barrier may occur is unknown) or in relation to the method of preparation (such as salmonella risk from uncooked eggs). In addition, some foods are thought to be most beneficial if consumed before or after fasting for several hours, which may restrict intake of other foods, resulting in deficiencies.

Herbal remedies

The use of Chinese herbs, often drunk as tea, has been advocated as an alternative treatment strategy for HIV infection. Other herbal remedies include Glycyrrhizin (derived from liquorice), Hypericin (extract from the St John's wort plant) and Compound Q (a purified protein extract from the root of the Chinese cucumber). These herbs are usually expensive and overdose may lead to toxicity.

See also: **Appetite**: Physiological and Neurobiological Aspects. **Body Composition**: Determination and Physiological Significance. **Diarrhoeal (Diarrheal) Diseases**: Nutritional Factors. **Malnutrition**: Definition, Classification and Epidemiology. **Nutritional Support**: Enteral Feeding; Parenteral Nutrition. **Vitamin Supplementation**: Role.

Further Reading

Coodley GO, Loveless MO and Merrill TM (1994) The HIV wasting syndrome: a review. *Journal of AIDS* 7: 681–694.

Gorbach SL, Knox TA and Roubenoff R (1993) Interactions between nutrition and infection with human immunodeficiency virus. *Nutrition Reviews* 51:226–234.

Green CJ (1995) Nutritional support in HIV infection and AIDS. *Clinical Nutrition* 14:197–212.

Henderson RA and Saavedra JM (1995) Nutritional considerations and management of the child with human immunodeficency virus infection. *Nutrition* 11:121–128.

Jariwalla RJ (1995) Micronutrient imbalance in HIV infection and AIDS: relevance to pathogenesis and therapy. *Journal of Nutritional and Environmental Medicine* 5: 297–306.

Kotler DP (ed.) (1991) *Gastrointestinal and Nutritional Manifestations of the Acquired Immunodeficiency Syndrome.* New York: Raven Press.

Macallan DC and Griffin GE (1995) Nutrition support in human immunodeficiency virus infection. In: Payne-James J, Grimble G and Silk D (eds) *Artificial Nutrition Support in Clinical Practice*, chap. 34, pp. 493–509. London: Edward Arnold.

Moorwessel M, Hopkins B, and Mueller Buzby K (1993) *Human Immunodeficiency Virus Infection.* In: Gottschlich MM, Matarese LE and Shronts EP (eds) *Nutrition Support Dietetics, Core Curriculum*, 2nd edn, chap. 13, pp. 261–274. Maryland: ASPEN.

Peck K and Johnson S (1990) The role of nutrition in HIV infection. A report of the working party of the AIDS interest group of the BDA. *Journal of Human Nutrition and Dietetics* 3:147–157.

Summerbell CD (1994) Appetite and nutrition in relation to human immunodeficiency virus (HIV) infection and acquired immunodeficiency virus syndrome (AIDS). *Proceedings of the Nutrition Society* 53:139–150.

Summerbell CD (1994) Nutritional advice and support for individuals with incurable diseases. *British Journal of Biomedical Sciences* 51:271–277.

Task Force on Nutrition Support in AIDS (1989) Guidelines for nutrition support in AIDS. *Nutrition* 5: 39–44.

Thomas B (ed.) (1994) AIDS and HIV disease. In: *Manual of Dietetic Practice*, 2nd edn, chap. 4.32, pp. 567–584. Oxford: Blackwell Scientific Publications.

Timbo BB and Tollefson L (1994) Nutrition: A co-factor in HIV disease. *Journal of the American Dietetic Association* 94:1019–1022.

Watson RR (ed.) (1994) *Nutrition and AIDS.* Boca Raton: CRC Press.

HUNGER

Overview

A J Hill, University of Leeds, Leeds, UK

John E Blundell, Department of Psychology, University of Leeds, UK

Copyright © 1998 Academic Press

Hunger is a familiar but commonly misunderstood and mistrusted part of our eating behaviour. This article will clarify the meaning of the term, describe the common procedures for measuring hunger, the ways in which hunger and satiety are interrelated, and the adaptability of hunger experience in a learning framework. The relationship between hunger and eating behaviour will be examined at both a methodological and conceptual level, and putative disorders of hunger will be briefly examined.

Definition

The term hunger is used in more than one sense by both scientists and the lay public. World hunger is a widely used phrase to describe the shortage of food and state of malnutrition experienced by a substantial proportion of the world's population. Its use is emotive and largely descriptive. It is in the study of motivation that the term takes on a more precise and individual definition. In this context, hunger describes the drive or the motivational force that urges us to seek and consume food. It is the expression of a biological need to sustain growth and life. Hunger is therefore a purposeful experience that possesses a clear biological function.

There are two ways in which the term hunger is used within nutritional science. One is its use as a motivational construct in a scientific theory. Here, hunger is inferred from directly observable and measurable events. In this way, inferring increased or high levels of hunger from a long period of food deprivation or an increased willingness to expend effort in order to obtain food, hunger becomes a mediating concept or intervening variable. However, a more familiar use of the word is that collection of conscious feelings or sensations that are linked to a desire to obtain and eat food. This is the sense in which lay people understand the term hunger, and is what researchers attempt to capture by means of rating scales and other measurement devices.

The first serious investigation of the everyday experience of hunger used a questionnaire in which people were asked to note the presence of physical sensations in a number of bodily areas, together with moods, urges to eat, and preoccupation with thoughts of food. It was found that the observation, 'I feel hungry', is typically based on the perception of bodily feelings which at times are very strong. Gastric sensations, a hollow feeling or stomach rumbling, are frequent indicators of hunger, although people also report sensations in the mouth, throat and head. These accompany more diffuse feelings of restlessness and excitability as well as an urge to eat. The consumption of food changes both the pattern of physical sensations and the accompanying emotional feelings, with unpleasant and aversive sensations becoming replaced by more pleasant ones. So, for example, an aching stomach becomes relaxed and the feeling of excitement and irritability is replaced by one of contentment.

Subsequent research has confirmed these general patterns of characteristic premeal sensations and feelings, particularly with regard to the salience of gastric sensations. However, it has also noted a great deal of variability both within and between individuals. In other words, hunger demands neither the consistent presence of single sensations prior to every act of eating, nor in every person sitting down to eat. Despite this variability people are able to, and frequently do, make judgements regarding their state of hunger, partly through reference to these sensations.

The Measurement of Hunger

The process of measuring hunger is not as straightforward as it might seem. One reason is the frequently raised mistrust of subjective reports. Critics point to the variability in response between individuals and the absence of any objective 'standard' by which internal experience can be calibrated. However, as argued below, this issue of 'validity' is more complex than this criticism suggests. A second reason is the failure to appreciate the distinction made above between an individual's assessment of their disposition to eat, and inferring hunger from the amount of food consumed or from some part of the act of eating (e.g. eating speed). While in many circumstances they will be in accord, the subjective report and inferred construct can as easily diverge.

The two most common methods for quantifying hunger are fixed-point rating scales and visual analogue scales (**Fig. 1**). Fixed-point scales are quick and simple to use, and the data they provide are easy to analyse. Past examples of these scales show they vary greatly in complexity. In considering the appropriate number of points to be included in this type of scale, the freedom to make a range of possible responses must be balanced against the precision and reliability of the device. Research seems to indicate that scales with an insufficient number of fixed points can be insensitive to subtle changes in subjective experience. In addition, the fixed points themselves are important determinants of the way people use the scales and distribute their ratings.

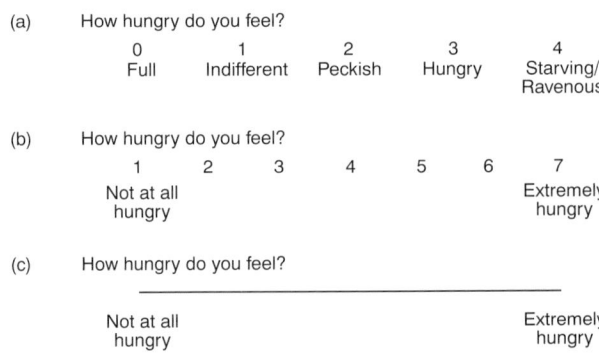

Figure 1 Examples of different types of scales used in the assessment of hunger: (a) fixed-point scale with points defined, (b) fixed-point scale, (c) visual analogue scale.

One way of overcoming some of these failings is to abolish the points completely. Thus, visual analogue scales are horizontal lines (often 100 or 150 mm long), unbroken and unmarked except for word anchors at each end. The user of the scale is instructed to mark the line at the point that most accurately reflects the intensity of the subjective feeling at that time. The researcher measures the distance to that mark in millimetres from the negative end (no hunger), thus yielding a score of 0–100 (or 150). This is done either by hand or automatically if presented by computer screen. By doing away with all of the verbal labels except the end definitions, visual analogue scales retain the advantages of fixed-point scales, while avoiding many of the problems with uneven response distributions.

An important aspect of these methods concerns the interpretation of differences between the fixed-points or intervals on a visual analogue scale. So for example, it should not be assumed that the difference between 20 and 30 mm on a hunger scale is perceptually the same as the difference between 80 and 90 mm. Nor can a hunger rating of 80 mm be said to represent a feeling of hunger that is twice the intensity of that rated at 40 mm. Related to this is the problem of 'end effects'. This refers to the reluctance of a minority of subjects to make ratings away from the upper or lower end points of the scale, despite clear instructions. Despite these limitations, data from such scales are often analysed using parametric statistical procedures, such as analysis of variance, and in general this appears to be a satisfactory approach.

Hunger and Satiety

If hunger is that feeling that reminds us to seek food, then eating relieves hunger, albeit until the next snack or meal. The capacity of a food to reduce the experience of hunger is called 'satiating power' or 'satiating efficiency'. This power is the product of the body's handling of the nutritional composition and structure of the food eaten. It follows that some foods will have a greater capacity to maintain suppression over hunger than other foods.

The distinction between hunger and satiety is both conceptual and technical. As hunger diminishes, satiety rises. But it is useful to further separate those events that occur across the course of a meal from those between meals. In this way the process of satiation can be clearly distinguished from the state of satiety. Satiation can be regarded as the process that develops during eating and that eventually brings a period of eating to an end. Accordingly, satiation can be defined in terms of the measured size of an eating

episode (such as its energy, weight or volume). Hunger declines as satiation develops and usually reaches its lowest point at the end of a meal. Satiety is defined as the state of inhibition over further eating that follows at the end of a meal and that arises from the consequences of food ingestion. The intensity of satiety can be measured by the duration of time until eating starts once more, or by the amount consumed at the next meal. The strength of satiety is also measured by the time that hunger is suppressed. And as satiety weakens, then hunger is restored.

In examining the mechanisms responsible for suppressing hunger and maintaining its low state, it is clear that they range from those that occur when food is initially sensed, to the effects of metabolites on body tissues following the digestion and absorption of food (across the wall of the intestine and into the bloodstream). By definition, satiety is not an instantaneous event but occurs over a considerable time period. The different phases of satiety and their associated mechanisms are shown in **Fig. 2**. Sensory effects are generated through the smell, taste, temperature, and texture of food, and it is likely that these factors have effects on eating in the very short term. Cognitive influences represent the beliefs held about the properties of foods, and these factors may also help inhibit hunger in the short term.

The category identified as postingestive processes includes a number of possible actions such as gastric distension and rate of emptying, the release of hormones such as cholecystokinin, and the stimulation of certain receptors along the gastrointestinal tract. The postabsorptive phase of satiety includes those mechanisms arising from the action of metabolites after absorption into the bloodstream. These include the action of glucose and amino acids, which act directly on the brain after crossing the blood–brain barrier, and which influence the brain indirectly via neural inputs following stimulation of peripheral

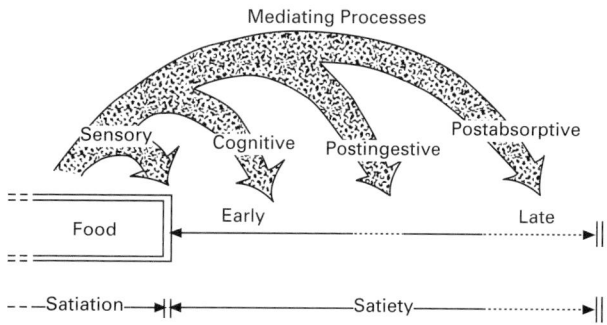

Figure 2 A representation of the satiety cascade showing the different phases of satiety and their associated mechanisms.

chemoreceptors. The most important suppression and subsequent control of hunger is brought about by postingestive and postabsorptive mediating processes.

It follows from this framework that foods of varying nutrient composition will have different effects on the mediating processes and will therefore differ in their effects on hunger, satiation and satiety. There is considerable interest, for example, in whether protein, fat and carbohydrate differ in their satiating power.

The balance of evidence shows that per unit energy, protein (within normal dietary limits) has the greatest satiating efficiency of all the macronutrients. This is particularly true in short-term studies, and is observed in lean and obese subjects alike. Longer-term evidence of this effect is currently lacking. However, of great practical and theoretical interest is the comparative effect of carbohydrate and fat, since they form the majority of our routine energy intake. Research shows that carbohydrates are efficient hunger relievers. A variety of carbohydrates, including glucose, fructose, sucrose and maltodextrins, all suppress later test meal energy intake. This suppression is roughly equivalent to their energy value, although the time course of this effect varies according to the rate at which they are metabolized. In contrast, high-fat foods appear to stimulate energy intake (in contrast to low-fat, high-carbohydrate foods), or at least have a disproportionately weak action on satiety. The mechanisms responsible for this may include the effect of fat promoting food palatability, the high energy density of fat, and the absence of inhibitory feedback from body fat stores. Taken together, these findings show why diets high in fat can promote weight gain and lead to obesity.

Conditioned Hunger

One of the essentials for an omnivore faced with a variety of new and different foods is the capacity to learn. It is not possible for an inborn preference or aversion to guide the choice of every possible food. Therefore, we learn which foods are beneficial (and which are not), by eating them. This learning involves the association between the sensory and the postabsorptive characteristics of foods. In this way the sensory characteristics of foods act as cues and come to predict the impact that foods will later have. Consequently, these cues should suppress hunger according to their relationship with subsequent physiological events.

It is possible to demonstrate experimentally how human beings adapt their eating to a food's energy content. A distinctively flavoured food which contains 'extra' hidden energy, presented on several occasions, will result in a change in eating and in preference. When deprived of food, subjects' preference for the taste increases with gained experience. If presented when satiated, preference for the taste decreases. This process is also observable in young children, who eat smaller meals following a taste previously associated with a high-energy snack, and larger meals following a taste previously associated with a low-energy snack.

The idea that we can have conditioned hunger for specific nutrients is far more contentious. The concept of conditioned hunger suggests that the organism, faced with a diet deficient in a single important nutrient, will seek an alternative food source that contains the missing nutrient. However, earlier evidence from animals has largely been reinterpreted from the standpoint of conditioned aversions. Indeed, conditioned aversions are far more potent examples of the impact of learning on eating behaviour than any examples of conditioned hunger. A conditioned aversion that will be familiar to many readers is the profound dislike that occurs in response to a food or drink that was eaten prior to vomiting or illness. An example of a conditioned taste aversion was famously described by learning theorist Martin Seligman. Steak with sauce Béarnaise was Seligman's last meal before a bout of gastric flu. Yet knowing that it was the flu rather than the food that made him sick did not prevent the subsequent aversion to sauce Béarnaise. In fact, surveys show that conditioned taste aversions are commonplace and reported by 40–60% of people.

Conditioned taste aversions are important in the present context not because they represent a special form of one-trial learning that we are biologically pre-prepared to acquire. Rather, they show that the strength of cue–consequence learning in the area of food intake depends on the stability and reliability of the relationship between tastes (sensory cues) and physiological effects (metabolic consequences) of food. When there is distortion, variation, or extreme complexity in the relationship between sensory characteristics and nutritional properties, then the conditioned control of hunger is weakened or lost. In many respects, the variety of foods available to us represents a cacophony of different sensory characteristics, and has the added complication of ingredients that preserve the sensory qualities while altering their nutritive value. Learned hunger therefore is a relatively less important factor when the food supply contains many food items with identical tastes but differing metabolic properties.

Hunger and Eating Behaviour

If hunger is biologically useful and a subjective experience that indicates a depleted nutritional state, then a close correspondence between hunger and eating would be expected. So hunger should be either a necessary or sufficient condition for eating to occur. However, this is not invariably the case. Instances of people deliberately refraining from eating in spite of hunger (fasting for moral or political conviction) show hunger not to be a sufficient condition. And examples in research and daily experience, of eating a tempting food when otherwise satiated, show hunger not to be necessary for eating to take place. But while the relationship between hunger and eating is not based on biological inevitability, in many circumstances they are closely linked.

Unfortunately, the lack of a one-to-one correspondence between hunger and eating has been used as another way to question the validity of hunger ratings. But should a high correlation between hunger ratings and subsequent food intake be expected in all circumstances? The examples above show that in certain circumstances the two can be disengaged. So, for example, eating can occur when hunger is low (such as when highly palatable food is offered unexpectedly), and not at other times when hunger is high (when food is unavailable, or other activities have priority). In addition, many experimental analyses of the correlational relationship between hunger and food intake report the relationship only when subjects are hungry. In other words, the correlation is only examined for a small portion of the available scale. Very few studies have looked at the association between hunger and food intake when hunger has been represented in all its possible degrees.

It is clear that hunger ratings cannot be used simply as a proxy measure for food intake. Equally, there is good evidence that in most circumstances self-report ratings of hunger correlate statistically and meaningfully with eating. This association exists not simply across single meals, but across the entire day as shown in **Fig. 3**. The rhythmic oscillation of hunger is tied closely to the overall pattern of food intake in this group of individuals. As such it presents an elegant and experimentally useful way of examining diurnal variations in the experience of hunger.

In questioning the relationship between hunger and eating, we are also forced to place the action of hunger within a broader context of social and psychological variables that moderate food choice and eating behaviour. Eating patterns are maintained by enduring habits, attitudes and opinions about the value and suitability of foods and an overall liking

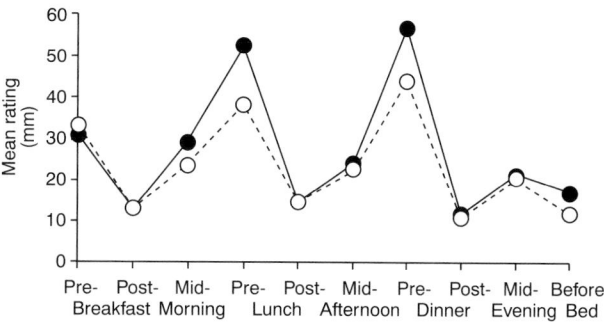

Figure 3 Ratings of hunger made across the day by a group of obese women taking an appetite suppressant drug (dotted lines) or placebo (solid lines).

for them. These factors, derived from the cultural ethos, largely determine the range of foods that will be consumed and sometimes the timing of consumption. The intensity of hunger experienced may also be determined, in part, by the culturally approved appropriateness of this feeling, and by the host of preconceptions brought to the dining table. Hunger is therefore only one portion of the range of determinants of eating in any given situation.

Disorders of Hunger

The clinical eating disorders, anorexia nervosa and bulimia nervosa, are commonly believed to encompass major disturbances of hunger. Yet the role that hunger may play is not entirely clear. Contrary to the literal meaning of the term, 'anorexia' is not experienced as a loss of appetite. Rather, clinicians recognize that anorexics may endure intense periods of hunger during their self-restricted eating. For some, their strength in resisting intense episodes of hunger provides a feeling of self-mastery and control that is absent in other areas of their lives. Research suggests that restricting anorexics (compared with those who binge) have the greatest blunting of hunger response, and that this disturbance in hunger is not a product of other areas of perceptual confusion.

There is some evidence that in conditions of total starvation hunger may become temporarily diminished. This circumstance is extremely rare and obviously relatively brief. Once eating is recommenced, hunger returns rapidly and with extreme intensity. The accounts of the male volunteers who submitted to a 6-month period of semistarvation during World War II (the 'Minnesota Experiment') are a testament to the extreme power of hunger. Referred to as semistarvation neurosis, these men's activities were shaped by their need for food. And their hunger experience was extreme. Nearly two-thirds reported feeling hungry all the time and a similar proportion experienced physical discomfort due to hunger. Participants described a marked increase in what was referred to as 'hunger pain'. For some this was mildly discomforting and vaguely localized in the abdomen. For others, it was extremely painful. This account is especially useful in reminding why energy-reduced diets aimed at achieving weight loss are often difficult to maintain, and easy to abandon.

Like anorexia, bulimia finds its literal meaning in changed hunger – 'ox hunger'. Again, however, the term is imprecise. Close analysis of the precursors of binge episodes show hunger to be lower than it is prior to a normal meal. In addition, while the urge to eat may be strong during a binge, the large amount of food consumed implies some defect in satiation rather than in hunger. And bingeing is often a well-practised behaviour that develops and changes with time. As with anorexics, it is likely that a stable eating pattern is necessary in order to normalize the experience of hunger, a process that may take a long time to establish.

The question of whether obesity reflects a disorder of hunger is now regarded as largely redundant. Obesity is strictly a disorder of weight, and as such reflects potentially long-term failure in the regulation of energy balance. There is hardly any evidence of heightened levels of hunger contributing to excessive energy input. However, an exception to this is the rare disorder Prader–Willi syndrome. Genetically determined and characterized mainly by intellectual disability, obesity is a well-recognized feature of the syndrome. Emerging research suggests that the excessive levels of food intake are associated with both a delayed reduction in hunger while eating, and a more rapid return to premeal states when eating has finished. Clearly, a better understanding of the biological events that accompany such aberrant eating patterns will strengthen understanding of the psychobiological framework that supports hunger.

See also: **Appetite**: Physiological and Neurobiological Aspects; Psychobiological and Behavioural Aspects. **Carbohydrates**: Requirements and Dietary Importance. **Eating Disorders**: Anorexia Nervosa; Bulimia Nervosa. **Famine**: Population Responses. **Food Choice**: Factors Influencing Food Choice. **Obesity**: Definition, Aetiology and Assessment. **Starvation and Fasting**: Biochemical Aspects. **Weight Management**: Approaches.

Further Reading

Birch LL and Deysher M (1985) Conditioned and unconditioned caloric compensation: evidence for self-regulation of food intake in young children. *Learning and Motivation* **16**:341–355.

Blundell JE (1980) Hunger, appetite and satiety – constructs in search of identities. In: Turner M (ed.) *Nutrition and Lifestyles*, pp. 21–42. London: Applied Sciences Publishers.

Booth DA (1977) Satiety and appetite are conditioned reactions. *Psychosomatic Medicine* **39**:76–81.

Cornell CE, Rodin J and Weingarten H (1989) Stimulus-induced eating when satiated. *Physiology and Behaviour* **45**:695–704.

de Graff C (1993) The validity of hunger ratings. *Appetite* **21**:156–160.

De Castro JM and Elmore DK (1988) Subjective hunger relationships with meal patterns in the spontaneous feeding behaviour of humans: evidence for a causal connection. *Physiology and Behaviour* **43**:159–165.

Halmi KA and Sunday SR (1991) Temporal patterns of hunger and fullness ratings and related cognitions in anorexia and bulimia. *Appetite* **16**:219–237.

Hill AJ, Rogers PJ and Blundell JE (1995) Techniques for the experimental measurement of human eating behaviour and food intake: a practical guide. *International Journal of Obesity* **19**:361–375.

Keys A, Brozek J, Henscher A, Mickelson O and Taylor HL (1950) *The Biology of Human Starvation*. Minneapolis: University of Minnesota Press.

Kissileff HR (1984) Satiating efficiency and a strategy for conducting food loading experiments. *Neuroscience and Biobehavioural Reviews* **8**:129–135.

Lawton CL, Burley VJ, Wales JK and Blundell JE (1993) Dietary fat and appetite control in obese subjects: weak effects on satiation and satiety. *International Journal of Obesity* **17**:409–416.

Logue AW (1991) *The Psychology of Eating and Drinking*, 2nd edn. New York: WH Freeman.

Mattes RD and Friedman MI (1993) Hunger. *Digestive Disease* **11**:65–77.

Monello LF and Mayer J (1967) Hunger and satiety sensations in men, women, boys and girls. *American Journal of Clinical Nutrition* **20**:253–261.

HYPERACTIVITY

Dietary Issues

M Wolraich, Vanderbilt University, Nashville, Tennessee, USA

Copyright © 1998 Academic Press

To discuss the issues of hyperactivity and diet, it is first important to understand the issues related to the diagnosis of hyperactivity, or what is now called the 'attention deficit/hyperactivity disorder' (ADHD). Since most of the recommendations for dietary changes have been for children who have been diagnosed with ADHD, this article will first review the historic and current changes in the diagnosis of ADHD and then review the diets that have been recommended for treatment and the evidence as to their efficacy.

Diagnostic Issues

Hyperactivity, or ADHD, is a condition that has been recognized for many years and has been quite extensively researched, but the diagnostic criteria and treatment continue to be controversial. The symptoms of ADHD were first described by a German physician, Heinrich Hoffman, in a children's book written in 1848. The symptoms were represented by two children, Harry who looks in the air (inattention) and Fidgety Phil (hyperactivity). In 1902, George Still presented a lecture in England about 20 children who were aggressive, defiant, excessively emotional and lacking inhibitory volition, and who were also noted to have impaired attention and overactivity. A more aetiological conceptualization of the condition did not occur until after World War I.

Symptoms of hyperactivity and inattention were suspected to be caused by the influenza epidemic occurring after World War I, when postencephalitic behaviour manifestations in children included extreme examples of hyperactivity and inattention. This led to the suggestion that these symptoms were due to organic brain damage. The concept of inattention and hyperactivity being part of a spectrum with less intense manifestations secondary to subtle injuries became known as the syndrome of 'minimal brain damage' in the 1960s. However, the lack of clear evidence for brain damage eventually resulted in a shift to a more descriptive labelling of the disorder. This is reflected in the American Psychiatric Association classification system (DSM) defining the 'hyperkinetic reaction of childhood'. The same disorder was similarly described in the UK, as reflected in the World Health Organization (WHO) classification. However, the conditions described differed in that the British disorder included more severe symptomatology and required that the symptoms had to be present in all settings.

In 1980, the US characterization of inattention and hyperactivity was changed in several ways. It was conceptually defined by three symptom dimensions: inattention, impulsiveness and hyperactivity, with inattention playing a more prominent role. In addition, to address the heterogeneity within the disorder, two subtypes ('attention deficit disorder with hyperactivity' and 'attention deficit disorder without hyperactivity') were defined. Again, different from the British criteria, the symptoms were only required to be present in one setting such as school. Retaining the concept that the major contribution to the symptoms were related to innate characteristics in the child rather than to environmental influences, the symptoms were required to have been present before the age of 7 years and to have lasted for at least 6 months. The British system continued to use the term 'hyperkinetic syndrome of childhood' and to include the pervasive nature of the symptoms.

The most recent changes in diagnostic criteria used by the American Psychiatric Association (DSM-IV) and the WHO have moved the definitions closer to agreement. Considering the most recent studies, there is evidence to support two dimensions. In DSM, the first dimension, inattention, is characterized by the 'often' occurrence of at least six of nine of the inattentive behaviours presented in **Table 1**. The second dimension consists of both hyperactivity and impulsiveness and is characterized by the 'often' occurrence of at least six of nine of the hyperactive and/or impulsive behaviours presented in Table 1. The WHO definitions are similar but do not attempt to quantify the specific behaviours and do not include impulsiveness in the hyperactivity dimension.

In DSM, the two dimensions define three subtypes. These are: *predominantly inattentive type* (meeting criteria on the inattentive dimension); *predominantly hyperactive/impulsive type* (meeting criteria on the hyperactive/impulsive dimension); and *combined type* (meeting criteria on both dimensions). In addition, there are other general criteria including

Table 1   DSM-IV behaviours for ADHD

Inattention
- careless mistakes
- difficulty sustaining attention
- seems not to listen
- fails to finish tasks
- difficulty organizing
- avoids tasks requiring sustained attention
- loses things
- easily distracted
- forgetful

Hyperactivity
- fidgeting
- unable to stay seated
- moving excessively (restless)
- difficulty engaging in leisure activities quietly
- 'on the go'
- talking excessively

Impulsiveness
- blurting answers before questions completed
- difficulty awaiting turn
- interrupting/intruding upon others

the onset of symptoms before 7 years of age, the presence of symptoms for at least 6 months, the presence of symptoms in two or more settings (e.g. home, school or work), and evidence that the symptoms cause significant clinical impairment in social, academic or occupational functioning. The WHO condition has been renamed 'disturbances of activity and attention'.

Treatments Other Than Diet

In considering dietary interventions, it is important to note that there are two other forms of treatment with proven efficacy. These are stimulant medications and behaviour modification. Considerations about dietary interventions have to be considered in the context of these other interventions. The nature of the main beneficial treatments, stimulant medication and behavioural interventions, makes the issue of diagnostic criteria for ADHD extremely important. Both of these treatments are not specific for the disorder so that the determination about which children are treated is very dependent on who is diagnosed.

The stimulant medications consist of methylphenidate (Ritalin), dextroamphetamine (Dexedrine) and pemoline (Cylert). They are particularly popular in the USA because they represent safe, effective and low-cost treatment. A review of numerous studies has shown that stimulants improve the core behaviours of inattention, impulsiveness and hyperactivity for the duration of action of the medication, as well as providing temporary improvement of associated features including aggression, social interaction and academic productivity. The margin of safety is very high, and the side effects on appetite, sleep and, infrequently, tics or bizarre behaviour, are all reversible when the medication is stopped. The concern about growth has proved to be insignificant and, although abused by adults, the stimulants are rarely abused by the children who take them because they usually do not find taking the medication pleasurable. While there is no long-term evidence that the use of stimulant medication or behavioural interventions on their own have any long-term benefits, there is suggestive evidence of long-term benefits when they are used in combination.

Effective behavioural interventions have generally consisted of direct contingency management programmes (e.g. point or token programmes, or a response cost programme) and social skills training. Like stimulant medication, these interventions are not specific to ADHD and have no proven long-term benefit when used in isolation. Other approaches such as traditional psychotherapy and play therapy have not been found to be effective with this group of children. Likewise, cognitive behavioural techniques, where a therapist teaches a child to control his or her behaviour, have usually not been effective for children with ADHD because of the difficulty these children experience in generalizing the techniques beyond the therapeutic sessions.

Dietary Interventions

The concept that specific dietary components may adversely affect behaviour have rested on three hypotheses:

1   oligoallergenic diet
2   sugar restriction
3   Feingold diet.

The idea that food might have an adverse effect on behaviour was first raised in 1922 by Shannon. This concept was further elaborated in 1947 by Randolph in his description of the 'tension fatigue syndrome', a behavioural extension of the vomiting reaction to milk proteins, and was also promoted by Speer. Their theory suggested that some children have atypical allergic reactions to various foods, consisting of subtle and behavioural effects. Their treatment entailed placing a child on a restricted diet and then adding foods one at a time to determine which foods caused an adverse reaction. This has been referred to as the oligoallergenic diet by one of the more recent clinical/research groups.

A specific focus on sugar as a nutrient adversely affecting behaviour first appeared in the 1970s, with a study reported by Langseth and Dowd. Among 271 hyperactive children, these authors found a large number of children who, during glucose tolerance tests, had patterns of blood glucose levels similar to the pattern seen in adults with functional reactive hypoglycaemia. Similar results have also been found in aggressive criminal offenders. A subsequent study showed that the patterns that Langseth and Dowd found can be normal variations in childhood, but the Langseth and Dowd study was followed by two correlational studies which suggested an association between sugar intake and hyperactivity. The hyperactive children who consumed more sugar displayed more hyperactive and aggressive behaviour.

The third dietary intervention suggested to improve behaviour was proposed by Dr Benjamin Feingold in 1975. He reported that at least 50% of hyperactive and learning-disabled children improved when placed on diets which were salicylate and additive free. Over time, the three dietary interventions have been combined so that proposed dietary restrictions now tend to incorporate all three in their recommendations. However, it is useful to examine the scientific evidence for each of these three dietary interventions.

Objective Standards

In discussing the evidence for the efficacy of dietary interventions in improving behaviour in children, it is first important to review the concepts important to prove efficacy. The major point to emphasize is that it is impossible to prove the null hypothesis. It is virtually impossible to prove definitively that no relationship exists between dietary constituents and behaviour or cognitive function. This is because it is impossible to test every possible variation or type of child. Therefore, a realistic approach needs to be similar to that taken by the US Food and Drug Administration for the criteria it requires to license a new medication. Basically, pharmaceutical companies are required to demonstrate that a new medication is both efficacious and does not cause significant harm. It is not the role of the FDA to disprove the efficacy of a drug treatment. With dietary interventions, they should not be recommended as a primary intervention for behavioural problems until there is clear evidence of their efficacy.

The main criteria required to evaluate objectively the efficacy of psychotropic medications are presented in **Table 2**. It is useful to use these criteria to evaluate the scientific merit of any studies on interventions affecting behaviour. It is also important to examine the pattern of results of multiple studies from different research groups. Ideally, where other

Table 2 Objective study criteria

- Uniformity of subjects
- Standard doses
- Objective verifiable dependent measures
- Control group
- Placebo
- Double-blind

efficacious therapies are available (e.g. stimulant medication and behaviour modification for children with ADHD), the proposed therapy should be compared with those existing therapies. This latter examination, by and large, has not been undertaken with any of the three dietary interventions.

Study Designs

There are two designs that can be employed to study the effects of nutrients on behaviour. The most commonly employed design is the challenge study. This first places the children on the diet under study for a period of time, and then challenges them with a food containing the offending agent (e.g. sucrose or tartrazine) or a food that does not contain the offending agent but looks and tastes identical to the offending agent, referred to as a placebo. This is the most commonly employed design because it is the easier and less expensive type to complete. The other design develops diets which appear similar, but the diets differ in what they contain (e.g. sugar or artificial sweeteners). In both designs the children, their families and the researchers need to be blind about which diet or challenge food the children receive at any given time. In most studies, the children are used as their own controls (crossover studies). They are able to receive both diets or challenges in a sequence because the diets are not believed to result in permanent changes lasting once the diet is stopped.

The measures used to assess the effects (dependent measures) are then completed within the few hours after a challenge, or repeatedly while the children are on diets. While parents, clinicians and teachers are utilized as observers (completing behaviour rating scales), ideally multiple measures are employed including some that are by independent observers or include objective assessments (e.g. performance on a continuous performance test, measuring activity level, etc.). Finally, it is important not to base results on one study. There need to be multiple studies performed by different groups of researchers, and a clear pattern of effects should emerge. When a number of studies have been completed, it is possible to combine them statistically with such techniques as meta-analysis to gain a more definitive picture.

Oligoallergenic Diet

While this is the oldest of the three dietary interventions, few controlled studies meeting the objective criteria outlined above have been undertaken. Five investigations have studied the effects of placing children on restricted diets. These studies all included restricting the dietary intake of additives and simple sugars. The studies found beneficial effects from placing children on restricted diets compared with a placebo diet, or they found worsening behaviours in children on the restricted diets when they were challenged with offending foods compared with placebo challenges. In all but one of the studies, the only successfully completed dependent measure was behaviour rating scales completed by the parents. While these are important measures and are collected in most studies, the raters are not independent of the children's behaviours. One study had multiple measures, but only those of the parents and physician found a significant difference between the offending agent and placebo challenges. More extensive research by additional research groups and additional independent measures are required to document the efficacy of this intervention before a decision can be made about its efficacy. Since the initial diet is extremely restrictive, care must be taken to make sure that the diet is adequately balanced and contains adequate nutrition.

Sugar Restriction

Sugar restriction usually refers to limiting the amount of sucrose in the diet. While most of the studies examined sucrose restriction, some also examined restriction of fructose or glucose. The artificial sweetener employed as a placebo was most frequently aspartame, but several studies used saccharin or both aspartame and saccharin as separate conditions. The type of sweetener used did not seem to affect the results.

Sugar restriction has been studied as a treatment for children since 1982. There have been a total of 23 appropriate objective studies contained within 16 reports employing a wide variety of types of children including children with ADHD and aggression as well as normal children, and varying in age from preschool children to adolescents. All of the studies with two exceptions were challenge crossover studies where children were challenged with drinks containing either sugar (sucrose in most studies) or an artificial sweetener (mostly aspartame). The other two studies consisted of giving the children diets which were high in sucrose content or low in sucrose and sweetened with aspartame or saccharin. A recent meta-analysis of the 23 studies did not find any significant behavioural or cognitive effects from sugar. There were not enough studies to reach a definitive conclusion, and there was insufficient statistical power to detect small effects or to detect effects on a small subset of children. To date there is not enough evidence to warrant the recommendation to restrict a child's sugar intake for the purpose of improving the child's behaviour or cognitive functioning.

Feingold Diet

The Feingold diet restricts foods with dyes, preservatives and salicylate compounds. Investigations of this diet, which were reviewed in 1986, generally involved children with ADHD. In most of the studies the children were kept on an additive-free diet and then challenged with a food containing an additive or an additive-free food as placebo. Two studies used additive-containing and additive-free diets. A problem in comparing studies was the variation in type and dose of additives used. There were a total of 13 controlled studies. The summation of the findings found little, if any, effect. At best there was some suggestion that a small percentage of children (1%) were adversely affected by additives. However, a recent study found that 24 of 34 children referred for hyperactivity (no formal diagnosis was established) who responded in an open clinical trial to an additive-free diet, responded adversely to challenges with varying doses of tartrazine compared with placebo, while all except two of 20 in a comparison group did not. The dependent measures were two behaviour rating scales completed by the parents. There appeared to be a dose response which would be contrary to a usual allergic response. This is a much higher rate of response than found in any previous study including those using tartrazine. Further study is required to substantiate these results since they run contrary to most of the previous research. Overall, the evidence to date does not confirm the efficacy of the Feingold diet to warrant its promotion as a treatment for most children with behavioural problems. In addition, if the diet is strictly maintained including foods containing salicylate compounds, the diet may be deficient in vitamin C.

Potential Side Effects of Diets

With all the diets, maintaining compliance may be difficult. Children who have behavioural problems are generally less likely to be compliant, and it can require a major effort to maintain the diet, detracting from efforts to control other areas of behaviour.

Diets are also problematic because they require the children to eat foods different from their peers. In children who are already singled out as different, this can further reduce their self-esteem. Care has to be taken to weigh the benefits of diets with as yet objectively unproved effects against the potential harm and difficulties in administering them.

Conclusions

In conclusion, ADHD is a mental disorder and its diagnosis is based on a child manifesting the symptoms of inattention, hyperactivity and impulsiveness to the extent that the symptoms impair the child's ability to function. The main beneficial treatments are two nonspecific treatments, stimulant medication and behavioural interventions. While neither alone has any proven long-term benefits, there is suggestive evidence that the combination of both treatments does have some long-term benefits.

Dietary interventions have included (1) restriction of allergenic foods starting with a generally restricted diet and adding those foods that do not worsen the child's behaviour, (2) restriction of food additives and preservatives referred to as the Feingold diet, and (3) restriction of sugar. These dietary interventions have not been proved to be efficacious and more study is required to determine their effects.

See also: **Food Allergies**: Diagnosis and Management. **Sucrose**: Nutritional Role, Absorption and Metabolism.

Further Reading

American Psychiatric Association (1994) *Diagnostic and Statistical Manual of Mental Disorders*, 4th edn. Washington, DC: American Psychiatric Association.

Baumgaertel A, Copeland L and Wolraich ML (1996) Attention deficit hyperactivity disorder. In: Wolraich ML (ed.) *Disorders of Development and Learning*, 2nd edn. St Louis: Mosby-Yearbook Inc.

Egger J, Stolla A and McEwen LM (1992) Controlled trial of hyposensitisation in children with food induced hyperkinetic syndrome. *Lancet* 339:1150–1153.

Pelham WE and Sams SE (1992) Behavior modification. *Child and Adolescent Psychiatric Clinics of North American* 1:505–517.

Sprague RL and Werry JS (1971) Methodology of psycho-pharmacological studies with the retarded. *International Review of Research into Mental Retardation* 5:147–157.

Swanson JM, McBurnett K, Wigal T, Pfiffner LJ, Lerner MA, *et al.* (1993) Effects of stimulant medication on children with ADD: A review of reviews. *Exceptional Children* 60:154–162.

Wender EH (1986) The food additive-free diet in the treatment of behavior disorders: A review. *Journal of Developmental and Behavioral Pediatrics* 7:35–42.

Wolraich ML, Lindgren SD, Stumbo PJ, Stegink LD, Appelbaum MI, Kiritsy MC (1994) Effects of diets high in sucrose or aspartame on the behavioral and cognitive performance of children. *New England Journal of Medicine* 330:301–307.

Wolraich ML, Wilson DB and White JW (1995) The effect of sugar on behavior or cognition in children: A meta-analysis. *Journal of the American Medical Association* 274:1617–1621.

World Health Organization (1992) *The ICD-10 Classification of Mental and Behavioural Disorders*. Geneva: World Health Organization.

HYPERLIPIDAEMIA (HYPERLIPIDEMIA)

Contents
Overview
Nutritional Management

Overview

T R Trinick, The Ulster Hospital, Belfast, Northern Ireland, UK

Copyright © 1998 Academic Press

Normal Lipid Metabolism

Lipids are a heterogeneous group of substances soluble in organic solvents, but insoluble in water. They are largely intracellular, but circulate in blood as lipoprotein particles. There are four general functions for lipids:

Table 1 Physicochemical characteristics of the major lipoprotein classes

Lipoprotein	Density (g ml^{-1})	Molecular weight (Da × 10^6)	Diameter (nm)	Triacylglycerol (% lipid)	Cholesterol (% lipid)	Phospholipid (% lipid)	Source
Chylomicrons	0.95	> 400	75–1200	80–95	2–7	3–9	Intestine
VLDL	0.95–1.006	10–80	30–80	55–80	5–15	10–20	Liver
IDL	1.006–1.019	5–10	25–35	20–50	20–40	15–25	Catabolism of VLDL
LDL	1.019–1.063	2.3	18–25	5–15	40–50	20–25	Catabolism of IDL
HDL	1.063–1.21	1.7–3.6	5–12	5–10	15–25	20–30	Liver, intestine

- structural component of membranes
- storage forms of metabolic fuel
- transport forms of metabolic fuel
- protective function as an outer coating of the organism.

Lipids consist of cholesterol and its derivatives, fatty acids, triacylglycerols, phospholipids and apolipoproteins. The lipoprotein particle has a core of neutral lipids (cholesterol esters and triacylglycerol) and a surface coat of polar lipids (unesterified cholesterol and phospholipids) and apolipoproteins. They are classified in terms of density. The main lipoproteins are:

- chylomicrons
- very low-density lipoprotein (VLDL)
- immediate-density lipoprotein (IDL)
- low-density lipoprotein (LDL)
- high-density lipoprotein (HDL).

Synthesis of lipoproteins occurs in the intestine or liver. They are then modified by enzymes and taken up by cell surface receptors in processes largely regulated by the apolipoproteins. The physicochemical characteristics of the main lipoprotein classes are shown in **Table 1**.

Interest in lipids lies in circulating lipid concentrations and their relationship to atherosclerosis, in particular coronary heart disease, stroke and peripheral vascular disease.

Cholesterol

Cholesterol is a sterol with the structure shown in **Fig. 1**. Daily cholesterol intake is 0.5–1.0 g, half of which is absorbed. It occurs largely as free cholesterol in membranes but in the plasma is two-thirds esterified, mainly as cholesterol linoleate and cholesterol oleate. Free cholesterol in plasma exchanges freely with cholesterol in membranes. The major route of cholesterol excretion is through the bile, directly as cholesterol or after conversion to bile salts, some of which are reabsorbed from the terminal ileum in the enterohepatic circulation.

Triacylglycerol

Triacylglycerols are glycerol molecules esterified with three fatty acid molecules (**Fig. 2**). Diacylglycerols and monoacylglycerols have two and one fatty acid molecules, respectively. Triacylglycerols constitute the main energy storage form in mammals and are the main storage form of fatty acids.

Fatty acids

Fatty acids can be present as triacylglycerol, as part of lipoprotein particles and as free fatty acids (bound to albumin). Common fatty acids and their sources are listed in **Table 2**.

Fatty acids are straight-chain compounds of differing lengths, connecting a hydrocarbon group to a

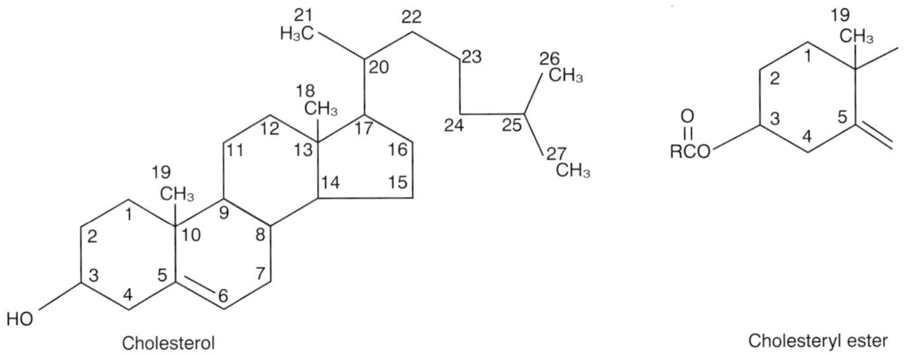

Figure 1 Structure of cholesterol and cholesteryl ester.

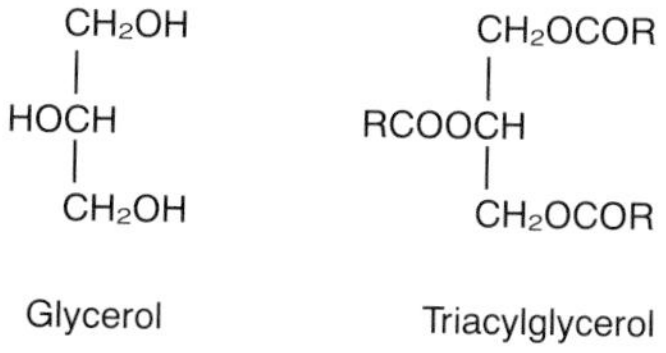

$$CH_2OH \qquad\qquad CH_2OCOR$$
$$| \qquad\qquad\qquad |$$
$$HOCH \qquad\qquad RCOOCH$$
$$| \qquad\qquad\qquad |$$
$$CH_2OH \qquad\qquad CH_2OCOR$$

Glycerol   Triacylglycerol

Figure 2 Structure of glycerol and triacylglycerol. R denotes the position of a fatty acid within the triacylglycerol.

hydroxyl group. With only single bonds in the straight chain, the fatty acid is saturated; with one or more additional double bonds, the fatty acid is unsaturated. Fatty acids with only one double bond are said to be monounsaturated (e.g. oleic acid, $C_{18:1}$), while fatty acids with two or more double bonds are said to be polyunsaturated (e.g. arachidonic acid, $C_{20:4}$). The presence of a double bond allows there to be two isomers, depending on whether the hydrogen atoms attached to the carbon atoms either side of the double bond lie on the same side (*cis*) or opposing sides (*trans*). *Cis* isomers are the only naturally occurring isomer and form kinks in the fatty acid chain. *Trans* isomers occur as part of food processing and maintain the straight direction of fatty acid chains.

The common saturated fatty acids are palmitic ($C_{16:0}$) and stearic ($C_{18:0}$) acids.

Phospholipids

The common phospholipids in plasma are derived from glycerol and consist of triacylglycerol containing phosphate and a nitrogenous base (glycerophospholipids). The phosphate group is usually attached at position 3 of the glycerol molecule and the nitrogenous base is usually an amino acid or an alcohol. The phosphatidyl cholines (lecithins) are the commonest phospholipid and are found in plasma and in cell membranes. Lecithin–cholesterol acyl transferase (LCAT) catalyses the transfer of a fatty acyl group at position 2 on glycerol to cholesterol to produce cholesteryl ester and leaving monoacyl glycerophosphate (lysolecithin). Another class of phospholipids, the cephalins, includes phosphatidyl ethanolamine, phosphatidyl serine and phosphatidyl inositol.

Phospholipids are able to bridge nonpolar lipids and water and act to allow lipids to mix with water in an emulsion. The nonpolar hydrocarbon end of the phospholipid is attracted to lipid, while the polar phosphate group is attracted to water. In a lipid droplet, the inner oily centre is surrounded by phospholipid which has its outer phosphate group attracted to the surrounding water environment, to form a micelle.

Apolipoproteins A, B, C and E

The lipoprotein particle (VLDL, LDL, HDL) is made up of lipid and protein molecules. Among the protein molecules are a group of proteins found at the surface of the lipoprotein particle called apolipoproteins. Their function is integral to the metabolism of lipoproteins. They interact with phospholipids to solubilize cholesterol esters and triacylglycerol, they regulate the reaction of enzymes (LCAT, lipoprotein lipase and hepatic lipase) with lipid and bind with cell surface receptors to determine the metabolism of lipoproteins.

Table 2 Fatty acids and their sources

Fatty acid	Structure	Source	Melting point (°C)
Saturated			
Lauric	$C_{12:0}$	Coconut oil, palm kernel oil	44
Palmitic	$C_{16:0}$	Palm oil, milk, butter, cocoa, butter, beef, pork, lamb	63
Stearic	$C_{18:0}$		69
Behanic	$C_{22:0}$	Some seed oils, especially peanut	80
Lignoceric	$C_{24:0}$		84
Unsaturated			
Oleic	$C_{18:1}$	Oliver oil, most commonly occurring fatty acid	11
Linoleic	$C_{18:2}$	Corn oil, soya bean oil, sunflower oil and sunflower seed oil	−5
Linolenic	$C_{18:3}$	Linseed oil	−11
Arachidonic	$C_{20:4}$	Fish oils	−50
Eicosapentaenoic	$C_{20:5}$	Cod, salmon, pilchard, mussel, oyster	−54
Docosahexaenoic	$C_{22:6}$		

From Durrington (1989).

Apolipoprotein A This is the chief protein of HDL and has two forms – apo A-I and apo A-II. Apo A-I is the main protein component in HDL. It acts as an activator of LCAT, which is responsible for esterification of free cholesterol in plasma, and allows the binding of HDL to many cell surfaces. Apo A-II is a structural component of HDL.

Apolipoprotein B Apo B-100 is the main protein component of LDL and is synthesized in the liver. It is also found in chylomicrons and VLDL. Apo B-48 is synthesized from the intestine and is the amino terminal half of apo B-100 synthesized from the same gene. Apo B-100 is the receptor ligand for the LDL receptor.

Apolipoprotein C Apo C is made up of three separate apolipoproteins. Apo C-I is mainly found in VLDL, but also in chylomicrons and HDL. Apo C-II is present in a circulating reservoir of HDL, transferring to chylomicrons and VLDL where it acts as an activator of lipoprotein lipase, allowing the lipolysis of triacylglycerols from circulating triacylglycerol-rich lipoproteins. Apo C-III is the most abundant form of apo C and may act as a modulator of lipoprotein lipase.

Apolipoprotein E Apo E is present in VLDL, IDL and HDL (mainly HDL$_2$). Apo E facilitates chylomicron remnant metabolism through the remnant receptors of the liver. It also facilitates metabolism through the LDL receptor. A large number of tissues express mRNA for apo E including the brain, although the reason for this is unclear.

Apolipoprotein (a) Apo (a), joined together with one LDL particle, which contains apolipoprotein B, constitutes a lipoprotein called Lp(a). Interest in Lp(a) arose because apo (a) shows close sequence homology with plasminogen, suggesting that a high level of Lp(a) would impair thrombolysis.

Lipoproteins

The main function of the lipoproteins is to transport lipids from one organ to another. Their main characteristics are set out in Table 1.

Chylomicrons This is the largest lipoprotein, consisting mainly of triacylglycerol with apo B-48, apo A, C and E. Triacylglycerol is hydrolysed with endothelial bound lipoprotein lipase, changing the chylomicron into a chylomicron remnant, rich in choles-

teryl ester. These remnants are removed from the circulation by interaction with the remnant receptors mainly present on hepatocytes. Peak chylomicronaemia occurs 3–6 h after a meal, with a half-life of under 1 h, and are cleared from the circulation after a 12 h fast.

Very-low Density Lipoproteins (VLDL) These triacylglycerol-rich lipoproteins are secreted mainly by the liver, with apo B-100 and apo E on their surface, while some VLDL is synthesized by the gut. They are transformed into mature VLDL by accumulating cholesterol ester, apo C and apo E from HDL. They then either interact with lipoprotein lipase to convert into IDL, which can be taken up by the liver, or convert to LDL by interacting with hepatic triglyceride lipase.

VLDL particles vary in size. Small VLDL is converted into LDL, via IDL, to a greater extent than large VLDL, which is converted to a form of IDL that appears to be removed from the plasma before conversion to LDL.

Intermediate-density lipoproteins (IDL) IDL are intermediate particles formed from the conversion of VLDL to LDL. Also known as VLDL remnants, some are removed directly from plasma while some convert into LDL.

Low-density lipoproteins (LDL) LDL is the major cholesterol carrying particle in the plasma. The core is cholesterol ester and has one apolipoprotein – apo B-100. There are different sizes of LDL. About one-third of the intravascular pool is catabolized per day and three-quarters of the circulating LDL is cleared through the liver, mainly through the LDL receptor. Small dense LDL is more common in some dyslipidaemias and may be more easily oxidized than larger LDL.

Normal LDL does not cause foam cell formation, but lipid peroxidation of LDL makes the LDL a ligand for certain receptors (the scavenger receptor and perhaps a specific receptor for oxidized LDL) and results in the formation of cholesterol-laden foam cells. In addition, oxidized LDL in the cell wall stimulates the production of cytokines and growth factors, resulting in monocyte recruitment and the proliferation of smooth muscle cells. This mechanism underlies one model of atherogenesis.

High-density lipoproteins (HDL) Nascent HDL is secreted by the liver and gut. It acquires unesterified cholesterol in the circulation, catalysed by LCAT to cholesteryl ester. HDL can pass cholesteryl ester to

VLDL in exchange for triacylglycerol, facilitated by CETP (see **Fig. 5**), or HDL can be taken up by the liver directly.

Enzymes and transfer proteins

Lipoprotein lipase (EC 3.1.1.34)   Lipoprotein lipase and hepatic triglyceride lipase are endothelial bound enzymes which remove triacylglycerol from lipoproteins. Lipoprotein lipase is activated by apo C-II and is involved in catabolism of chylomicrons and VLDL. Hepatic triglyceride lipase is involved in chylomicron, VLDL and HDL metabolism.

Lecithin–cholesterol acyltransferase (LCAT, EC 2.3.1.43)   LCAT mediates the esterfication of cholesterol by transferring a fatty acid from lecithin to cholesterol to form cholesteryl ester.

Cholesterol ester transfer protein (CETP)   CETP mediates the exchange of cholesteryl ester from HDL with triacylglycerol from VLDL or chylomicrons.

Receptors

A large number of lipoprotein receptors have been identified. Some of the more important receptors are discussed below. Lipoprotein uptake at the cell membrane may be non-receptor-mediated, perhaps by pinocytosis, where 'binding' is of low affinity, but is not saturable.

LDL receptor   The LDL receptor is a glycoprotein present on most cell surfaces. Free cholesterol, building up in the cell through the receptor, reduces both cell synthesis of cholesterol and cell uptake of more LDL cholesterol.

Scavenger receptors   These receptors are found on macrophages and hepatic endothelium. They bind and degrade chemically modified LDL such as oxidized or acetylated LDL. They are not downregulated by intracellular cholesterol accumulation.

LDL receptor-related protein (LRP)   This is a multifunctional receptor (binding VLDL/chylomicron remnants and other nonlipid ligands such as bacterial toxins) present in nearly all tissues. It has a high affinity for apo E and a low affinity for apo B-100.

VLDL receptor (VLDLR)   This receptor binds VLDL, β-VLDL and IDL. It recognizes apo E and is located mainly in adipose tissue and muscle.

Other remnant receptors   The lipolysis-stimulated receptor (LSR) found on fibroblasts recognizes surface apo E and takes up VLDL, chylomicrons and LDL. Two membrane-binding proteins (MBP 200 and MBP 235) have been described on macrophages and appear to bind VLDL. Remnants from both chylomicrons and VLDL (after hydrolysis of over 70% of their triacylglycerol content) appear to be removed by both the LDL and the LRP receptors.

Exogenous (dietary) lipid pathways

Ingestion of food containing fat (triacylglycerol) and cholesterol results in absorption into the enterocyte of fatty acids, monoacylglycerols, free cholesterol and lysolecithin. In the enterocyte, re-esterification of fatty acids into triacylglycerol and cholesterol into cholesteryl ester occurs to form chylomicrons, to which is added, a surface layer of apo B-48, A-I, A-II, A-IV, phospholipid and free cholesterol. This allows secretion of the chylomicron into the intestinal lymphatics. Apo B-48 is required for secretion of the chylomicron.

Chylomicrons in the circulation take up apo C from HDL (releasing it back to HDL later) and acquire apo E. Apo C-II allows the chylomicron to activate lipoprotein lipase on capillary endothelial cells of muscle and fat. This allows hydrolysis of triacylglycerol, releasing glycerol and fatty acids to be taken up by local tissue. Surface phospholipids, free cholesterol and apo C transfer to HDL as the particle shrinks. This small chylomicron is called a chylomicron remnant and is catabolized through the LDL receptor and other remnant receptors on the liver.

This transport of dietary lipid from the intestinal to the peripheral tissues is shown in **Fig. 3**.

Endogenous lipid pathways

The liver is the main source of endogenous lipid (**Fig. 4**). In particular, the liver secretes the triacylglycerol-rich lipoprotein VLDL. Triacylglycerol, which is formed from fatty acids either newly synthesized or taken up from plasma, together with free cholesterol, synthesized from acetate or delivered to the liver in chylomicron remnants, joins with apo B and phospholipids to form VLDL. Apo C and apo E are added in the circulation. Triacylglycerol is progressively removed from VLDL in the same way as occurs with chylomicrons. Free cholesterol transfers to HDL and is esterified with LCAT and transferred back to VLDL, using a protein called cholesteryl ester transfer protein (CETP), in exchange for triacylglycerol transfer from VLDL to HDL. In this way, VLDL becomes smaller and transforms to become IDL, although some small VLDL may be removed directly. IDL is further changed through interaction with hepatic lipase to LDL. In this way, most VLDL is transformed to LDL.

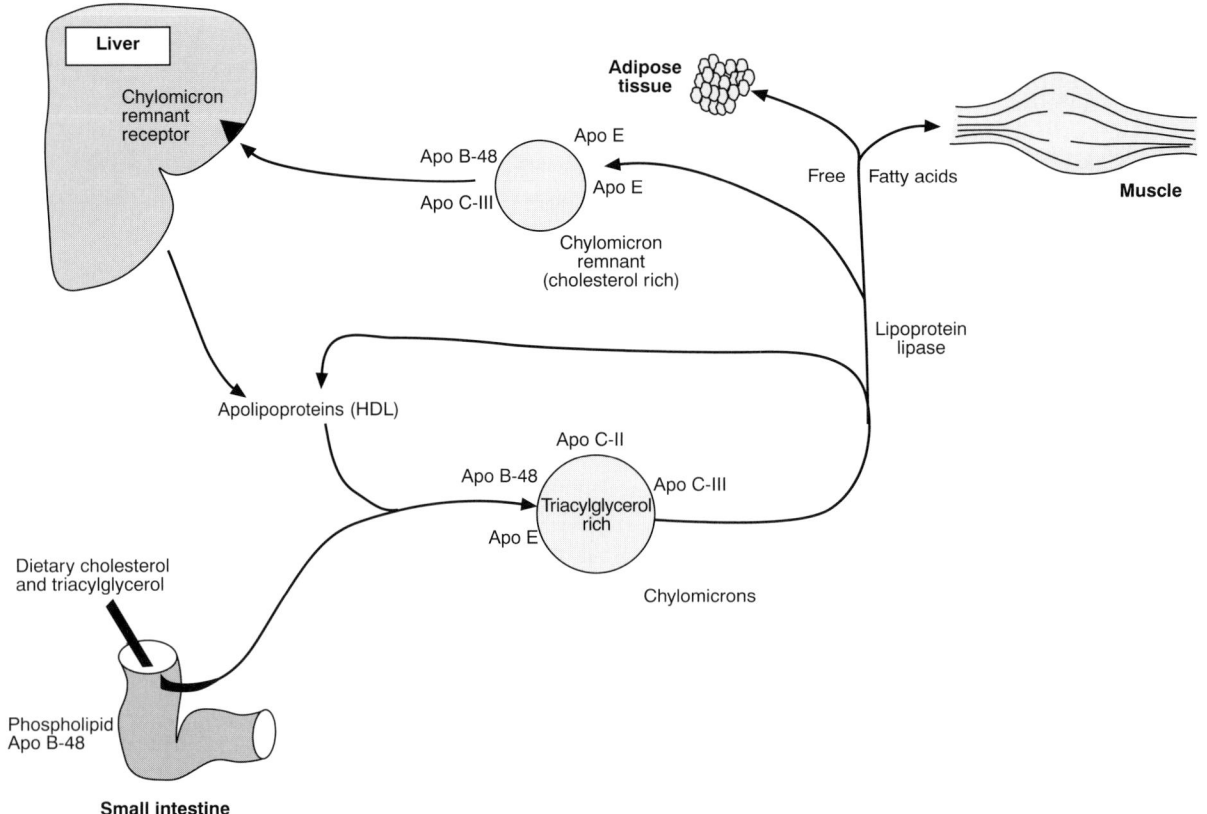

Figure 3 Exogenous (dietary) lipid pathway showing the transport of dietary lipid from intestine to peripheral tissues and liver. Movement of apolipoprotein between HDL and chylomicrons is shown from Ginsberg (1994).

Reverse cholesterol transport

Lipids are transported to the peripheries from the gut and the liver. They return to the liver via HDL in a process known as reverse cholesterol transport (**Fig. 5**). HDL particles arise in the liver and gut from a coalescence of apo A-I and phospholipid to form cholesterol-deficient bilayered discs in the form of HDL_3. Circulating HDL particles, in particular a subset of HDL_3 called pre-β HDL, come into contact with cells and act to accept free cholesterol from the cell surface. This cholesterol is converted by LCAT to cholesteryl ester and moves into the core of the HDL. After accumulating cholesterol, the HDL starts to accept other apolipoproteins and becomes HDL_2. In turn, HDL_2 appears to pass cholesteryl ester to chylomicrons and VLDL under the influence of CETP. The cholesterol then finds its way back to the liver in the form of chylomicron remnants, IDL and LDL. Some of the HDL_2 particles may lose cholesterol directly to the liver and some may be taken up directly by the liver.

Consequences of Hyperlipidaemia

Clear evidence exists to show that, as serum cholesterol rises, the risk of coronary heart disease (CHD) rises, and as serum cholesterol falls, the risk of developing CHD falls. The epidemiological evidence comes from within-country studies, between-country studies and migration studies. Support comes from animal studies and there is now evidence of the beneficial effects of decreasing serum cholesterol in both primary and secondary prevention of heart disease.

The within-country studies include the Multiple Risk Factor Trial Intervention (MRFIT) study, which included 360 000 middle-aged men screened and followed up for CHD mortality. This trial showed a strong positive correlation between cholesterol levels at initial screening and later death from CHD. The Framingham Heart Study, started in 1949, was another prospective survey which followed a large cohort of Americans and looked at lipid levels and risk of CHD, in particular the relationships between lipoprotein fractions and CHD. It showed a strong association between elevated LDL cholesterol and

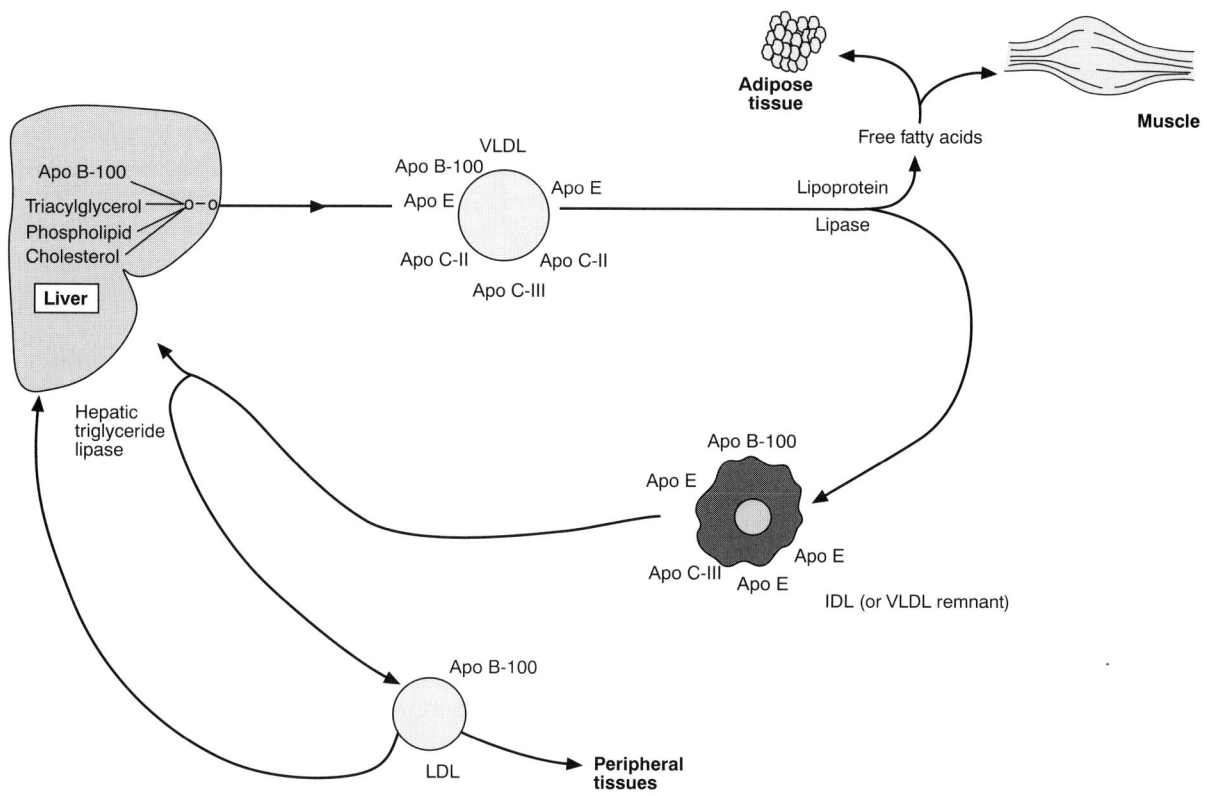

Figure 4   Endogenous lipid pathway showing transport of lipids produced in the liver and interconversion from VLDL through IDL to LDL. From Ginsberg (1994).

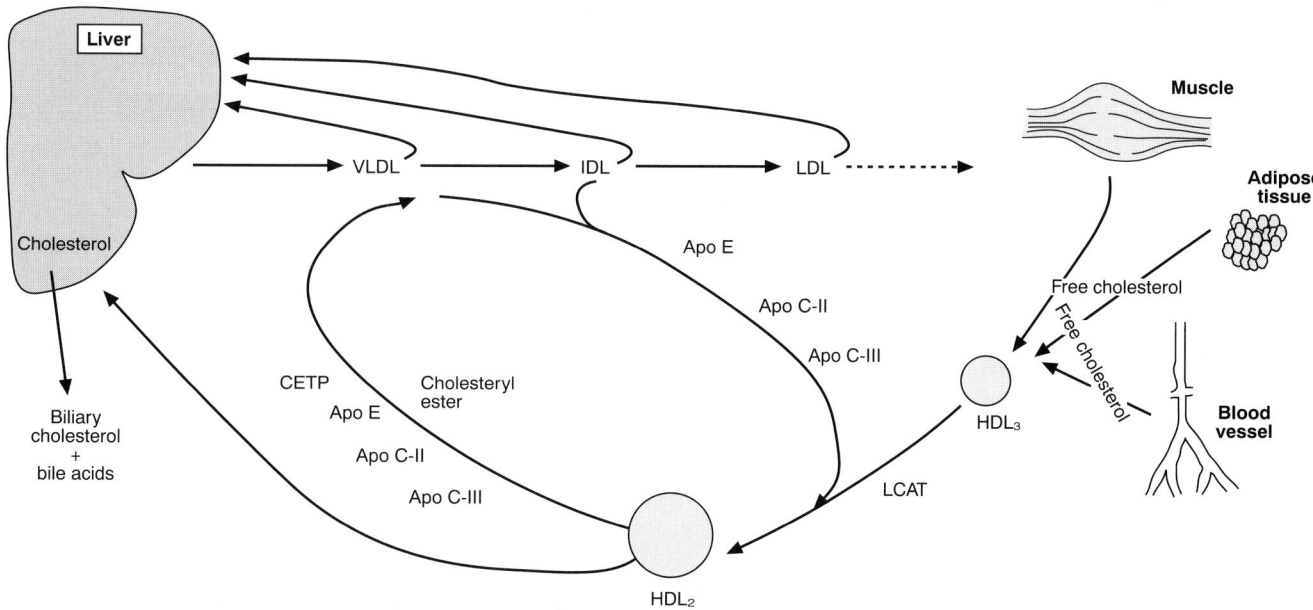

Figure 5   Reverse cholesterol transport. Nascent HDL (HDL$_3$) picks up free cholesterol from the peripheries to become HDL$_2$. CETP influences the transfer of lipid between HDL$_2$ and VLDL/IDL to maintain a cycle within HDL, and IDL/LDL deliver cholesterol from the peripheries to the liver. HDL may deliver cholesterol directly to the liver. From Ginsberg (1994).

increased incidence of CHD and an inverse association between HDL cholesterol and CHD risk. More recently, Framingham has drawn attention to the value of the ratio of total cholesterol to HDL cholesterol, where a ratio of three and below suggests the disease is static, while values of four and above suggest the disease is progressive. Framingham also drew attention to the incremental effect of additional risk factors in the development of CHD such as hypertension, hyperglycaemia and smoking. Combinations of risk factors come together in the plurimetabolic syndrome where insulin resistance appears to be the common denominator.

The best known between-countries study is the Seven Countries Study by Ancel Keys, linking diet, hypercholesterolaemia and CHD. He showed that a plot of each country's median total cholesterol against deaths from coronary heart disease was highly correlated. The variations in serum cholesterol were highly correlated with the ratio of saturated to unsaturated fats in the diet.

Studies of migration and CHD include the Ni-Hon-San Study, where cholesterol levels and CHD rates were compared in Japanese living in Japan, Honolulu and San Francisco. There was a rise in both cholesterol levels and CHD rates across these three groups, suggesting that as Japanese adopted a Western lifestyle their cholesterol rose and their risk of CHD increased.

Evidence that treatment of hyperlipidaemia influences CHD is substantial. The methods of treating hyperlipidaemia have varied through diet, drugs, surgery, meditation and multiple risk factor reduction. The conclusion is that treatment of hyperlipidaemia improves CHD morbidity and mortality. The Lipid Research Clinics Coronary Primary Prevention Trial (LRC-CPPT), started in the 1970s, looked at 4000 men, without evidence of CHD but with hypercholesterolaemia, randomized to receive cholestyramine or placebo. After 7 years, despite a relatively small difference in cholesterol levels, there was a 20% decrease in coronary heart disease in the drug-treated group.

In the Oslo study, high-risk Norwegian men were given antismoking and dietary advice with a signifi-cant reduction in the incidence of CHD. The effect of partial ileal bypass surgery has been studied in patients who had experienced a myocardial infarction and were hypercholesterolaemic (POSCH study). This surgical procedure improved blood lipids and reduced morbidity caused by CHD. More recently, in the Scandinavian Simvastatin Survival Study (4S study), patients with CHD and hypercholesterolaemia were randomized to receive the HMG-CoA reductase inhibitor simvastatin or placebo. After a 5.4-year follow-up period, both morbidity and mortality were significantly reduced in the treatment group. This secondary prevention study was followed by a primary prevention study using pravastatin in men with hypercholesterolaemia. This study (WOSCOPS study) randomized men, without evidence of CHD, to treatment with the HMG-CoA reductase inhibitor pravastatin or to placebo, and followed them up for 4.9 years. Treatment with the drug significantly reduced the incidence of myocardial infarction and death from cardiovascular causes.

Studies such as the Cholesterol Lowering Atherosclerosis Study (CLAS), where patients were allocated to drug therapy or placebo, use coronary angiography to follow the effect of drugs on the disease. A small decrease in cholesterol results in a disproportionately larger reduction in cardiovascular events.

These studies show that it is possible to arrest progress of the disease and, in some cases, bring about regression of atherosclerosis. The extent to which this happens seems to depend on underlying disease and the degree of cholesterol lowering.

Classification of Hyperlipidaemia

There are a number of classification systems available. In 1967 Fredrickson, Levy and Lees introduced the first classification as a method of reporting which lipoproteins were raised. The World Health Organization (WHO) adopted this classification (**Table 3**).

In 1987 the European Atherosclerosis Society (EAS) recommended a five group classification of primary hyperlipidaemia (**Table 4**).

Clinically, the most important step is to determine

Table 3 Fredrickson/WHO classification of hyperlipoproteinaemia

Type	Lipids increased	Lipoprotein increased
I	Triacylglycerol	Chylomicrons
II-a	Cholesterol	LDL
II-b	Cholesterol and triacylglycerol	LDL and VLDL
III	Cholesterol and triacylglycerol	Chylomicron remnants and IDL
IV	Triacylglycerol	VLDL
V	Cholesterol and triacylglycerol	Chylomicrons and VLDL

Table 4 European Atherosclerosis Society classification of hyperlipoproteinaemia

Group	Total cholesterol (mmol l⁻¹)	Triacylglycerols (mmol l⁻¹)
Normal	< 5.2	< 2.3
A (mild hypercholesterolaemia)	5.2–6.5	and < 2.3
B (moderate hypercholesterolaemia)	6.5–7.8	and < 2.3
C (isolated hypertriglyceridaemia)	< 5.2	and 2.3–5.6
D (combined hyperlipidaemia)	5.2–7.8	and 2.3–5.6
E (severe hypercholesterolaemia and/or hypertriglyceridaemia)	> 7.8	and/or > 5.6

Table 5 Lipid changes in some common conditions

Condition	Total cholesterol	HDL cholesterol	Triacylglycerol
Diabetes mellitus	Normal or ↑	↓	↑
Hypothyroidism	↑	↑	Can be ↑
Chronic renal failure	Normal or ↑	↓	↑
Nephrotic syndrome	↑	Often ↓	Often ↑
Cholestasis[a]	↑	↓	Can be ↑

[a]An abnormal lipoprotein called LpX is present.

if the lipid abnormality is primary or secondary to another condition. **Table 5** shows the lipid changes seen in some common conditions. In practice, it is often easiest to classify lipid abnormalities into three categories:

- raised total cholesterol
- raised triacylglycerol
- mixed hyperlipidaemia.

It is becoming clear that certain lipoprotein patterns are particularly atherogenic. Elevated IDL with increased small dense LDL particles and low HDL is one such pattern. Classifications based on these patterns may emerge.

Causes of hypercholesterolaemia

Serum cholesterol at birth does not exceed 2.5 mmol l⁻¹ and is rarely above 4.0 mmol l⁻¹ in children. The values for adults are given in Table 4.

A raised cholesterol, with little or no elevation of triacylglycerol, is usually a result of raised LDL level. Occasionally a raised HDL is responsible for a high cholesterol, as seen in the familial condition of primary hyper-α-lipoproteinaemia. Secondary causes given in Table 5 include hypothyroidism, nephrotic syndrome, some cases of diabetes mellitus and cholestasis. Primary causes include polygenic familial hypercholesterolaemia, in which several gene

Table 6 AHA dietary recommendations

	Recommendations (% of total calories)	
Nutrient	AHA step one	AHA step two
Total fat	< 30%	< 30%
Fatty acids		
Saturated fat	< 10%	< 7%
Polyunsaturated fatty acid	< 10%	< 10%
Monounsaturated fatty acids	10–15%	10–15%
Carbohydrates	50–60%	50–60%
Protein	10–20%	10–20%
Cholesterol	< 300 mg per day	< 200 mg per day

Reduce total calories to achieve and maintain desirable weight

From Denke (1994).

Table 7 Intermediate and ultimate nutrient goals for Europe

	Intermediate goals		Ultimate goals
	General population	Cardiovascular high-risk group	
Percentage of total energy[a] derived from:			
Complex carbohydrates[b]	> 40	> 45	45–55
Protein	12–13	12–13	12–13
Sugar	10	10	10
Total fat	35	30	20–30
Saturated fat	15	10	10
P:S ratio[c]	≥ 0.5	≥ 1.0	≥ 1.0
Cholesterol (mg per day)	< 300	< 300	< 300
Fibre (g per day)	30	> 30	> 30
Salt (g per day)	7–8	5	5

[a]All values given refer to alcohol-free total energy intake.
[b]The complex of carbohydrate figures are implications of the other recommendations.
[c]The ratio of polyunsaturated to saturated fatty acids.
From Pyorala et al. (1994).

abnormalities, together with environmental effects, serve to raise serum cholesterol. Much less common, but more clearly defined, are the two autosomal conditions of familial combined hyperlipidaemia (FCH) and monogenic familial hypercholesterolaemia (FH). In FCH there appears to be an increase in apo B production and so an increase in serum LDL. Serum VLDL levels are raised in one-third of these subjects with an associated triacylglycerol increase, one-third show increases in LDL and one-third show increases in LDL and VLDL. Monogenic FH is caused by a defect in the LDL receptor. The consequent decreased LDL uptake by cells, in particular in the liver, results in raised LDL and cholesterol levels.

Predominant hypertriglyceridaemia may result from raised VLDL or chylomicron levels. Secondary causes include excess alcohol ingestion, obesity and excess carbohydrate intake, diabetes mellitus, renal failure and pancreatitis. Primary hypertriglyceridaemia can be a result of familial combined hypertriglyceridaemia, familial endogenous hypertriglyceridaemia or hyperchylomicronaemia.

Familial endogenous hypertriglyceridaemia results from increased hepatic triacylglycerol production with increased VLDL production. It is associated with obesity, glucose intolerance and hyperuricaemia. Hyperchylomicronaemia is a result of inherited or acquired impairment of lipoprotein lipase activity.

Reduced insulin levels in diabetes mellitus impair the activity of lipoprotein lipase and hyperchylomicronaemia can occur. Inherited deficiency of the lipase enzyme is seen rarely, as is deficiency of the apolipoprotein (apo C-II) required to activate the enzyme.

Mixed hyperlipidaemia is often a secondary condition. Primary causes include familial combined

hyperlipidaemia and type III hyperlipidaemia (dys-β-lipoproteinaemia or broad β disease). Type III hyperlipidaemia is associated with the apo E 2/2 phenotype, resulting in impaired recognition of the apo E by hepatic receptors and an accumulation of IDL.

Dietary Effects

Principles of treatment

Treatment of hyperlipidaemia is part of the management of CHD risk. This encompasses lifestyle changes such as stopping smoking, increasing exercise, and modifying diet, as well as management of hypertension. Diet is the cornerstone of treating hyperlipidaemia, best delivered by qualified dietitians, involving the whole family.

The main aims of diet are to correct excess calorie intake and to decrease the cholesterol and saturated fat content. Patients with hyperlipidaemia can expect to see benefits from diet after 6 weeks and are reviewed every 4 months.

Diet can decrease total cholesterol 8–12% with between 60 and 80% of this change attributed to decreases in saturated fatty acid intake. The remaining change comes from decreased dietary cholesterol and changes in the intake of fibre, monounsaturated and polyunsaturated fatty acids. Dietary modification may not be successful in some primary hyperlipidaemias. The diet and re-infarction trial (DART) and the Mediterranean diet study, in postmyocardial infarction survivors, showed that dietary modification, not necessarily accompanied by plasma cholesterol lowering, can improve short-term prognosis.

Fat Most of the saturated fats in the diet come from just four fatty acids – lauric acid ($C_{12:0}$), myristic acid ($C_{14:0}$), palmitic acid ($C_{16:0}$) and stearic acid ($C_{18:0}$). The first three fatty acids (but not stearic acid) decrease LDL receptor activity, raising LDL and total cholesterol by approximately 0.25 mmol l^{-1} per 10 g of saturated fat ingested.

Monounsaturates are now being recommended more often. The most common is oleic acid ($C_{18:1}$), found in the Mediterranean diet as olive oil. Animal fats are rich in monounsaturates but are also rich in saturated fats. The *trans* optical isomers of monounsaturates may raise total and LDL cholesterol, and are best avoided.

In both type I and type V hyperlipidaemia the dietary management is to decrease fat intake to between 20–40 g per day. Medium-chain triacylglycerols are used and fish oils can be tried, but the mainstay of therapy is decreased fat intake.

Dietary β-sitosterol can block cholesterol absorption to a limited extent but is not used therapeutically.

Carbohydrate and calories Obesity is a common cause of hypertriglyceridaemia, owing to raised VLDL levels in the obese subject. This may be because of an increase in insulin resistance resulting from obesity with concomitant hyperinsulinaemia and elevation in hepatic VLDL synthesis. Some hypertriglyceridaemic patients experience a further rise in triacylglycerol levels with an increase in carbohydrate intake – known as carbohydrate induction. This situation is accompanied by a rise in serum insulin levels. With weight reduction, the hypertriglyceridaemia improves and HDL cholesterol rises after 2–4 months.

Mild alcohol ingestion raises HDL cholesterol. Excess alcohol ingestion can precipitate hypertriglyceridaemia of a type IV phenotype owing to increased hepatic synthesis and secretion which, in subjects who cannot clear triacylglycerols efficiently, can progress to a type V phenotype. Serum LDL levels are usually low in alcoholics, although in occasional individuals they can be elevated.

Protein Changes in dietary protein intake have minimal effects on lipid levels. Vegetarians have lower serum lipids than nonvegetarians, but it is not clear how much of this is the result of a change from animal to vegetable protein.

Fibre Soluble fibre such as oat bran and guar lower cholesterol levels, perhaps by reducing bile acid absorption.

Recommendations

The British diet typically has 40–50% of calories from fat, of which 15–20% come from saturated fat, with a cholesterol intake of 500 mg per day. The American Heart Association (AHA) has recommended a two-step approach to dietary change, outlined in **Table 6**, and recent European recommendations for the diet of the population are shown in **Table 7**. The central approach of dietary therapy is to decrease cholesterol-raising fatty foods, decrease cholesterol intake and to achieve a desirable body weight. The AHA step one diet can decrease total cholesterol by 0.5–1.0 mmol l^{-1} and the step two diet can add a further 0.2–0.4 mmol l^{-1} reduction. Saturated fat in the diet is best replaced by increasing complex carbohydrates, with modest increases in monounsaturated and n-6 polyunsaturated fatty acids. Increased fish oil intake giving additional n-3 fatty acids will reduce triacylglycerol levels (but increase LDL cholesterol in certain patients). Fresh fruit, vegetables and fibre are encouraged.

See also: **Adipose Tissue**: Structure, Function and Metabolism of Adipose Tissue. **Antioxidants**: Observational Epidemiology. **Carbohydrates**: Requirements and Dietary Importance. **Cholesterol**: Sources, Absorption, Function and Metabolism; Factors Determining Blood Cholesterol Levels. **Coronary Heart Disease**: Lipid Theory of Coronary Heart Disease; Haemostatic Factors and Coronary Heart Disease; Aetiology; Prevention. **Exercise**: Beneficial Effects. **Fats and Oils**: Nutritional Value. **Fatty Acids**: Metabolism; Health Effects of Saturated Fatty Acids; Health Effects of Monounsaturated Fatty Acids; Health Effects of n-6 Polyunsaturated Fatty Acids; Health Effects of n-3 Polyunsaturated Fatty Acids; Health Effects of *trans* Fatty Acids. **Hyperlipidaemia (Hyperlipidemia)**: Nutritional Management. **Insulin Resistance**: Aetiology and Association with Disease. **Lipids**: Chemistry and Classification; Composition and Role of Phospholipids in the Body. **Lipoproteins**: Physiology. **Stroke**: Nutritional Management. **Sucrose**: Dietary Sucrose and Disease. **Vegetarian Diets**: Nutritional Adequacy.

Further Reading

Denke MA (1994) Diet and lifestyle modification and its relationship to atherosclerosis. In: Hunninghake DB (ed.), *The Medical Clinics of North America: Lipid Disorders*, vol. 78, pp. 197–223. Philadelphia: WB Saunders.

Durrington PN (1989) *Hyperlipidaemia: Diagnosis and Management*. London: Wright.

Ginsberg HN (1994) Lipoprotein metabolism and its relationship to atherosclerosis. In: Hunninghake DB (ed.), *The Medical Clinics of North America: Lipid Disorders*, vol. 78, pp. 1–20. Philadelphia: WB Saunders.

Grundy SM (1992) Etiologies and treatment of hyperlipidemia. In: Willerson JT (ed.), *Treatment of Heart Disease*, chap. 4, pp. 4.1–4.79. London: Gower Medical Publishing.

Pyorala K, De Backer G, Graham I, Poole-Wilson P and Wood D (1994) Prevention of coronary heart disease in clinical practice. Recommendations of the Task Force of the European Society of Cardiology, European Atherosclerosis Society and the European Society of Hypertension. *European Heart Journal* 15:1300–1331.

Scandinavian Simvastatin Survival Study Group (1994) Randomised trial of cholesterol lowering in 4444 patients with coronary heart disease: the Scandinavian Simvastatin Survival Study (4S). *Lancet* 344:1383–1389.

Shepherd J, Cobbe SM, Ford I, Isles CG, Lorimer AR, MacFarlane PW, McKillop JH and Packard CJ (1995) Prevention of coronary heart disease with pravastatin in men with hypercholesterolaemia. *New England Journal of Medicine* 333:1301–1307.

Steinberg D, Parthasarathy S, Carew TE, Khoo JC and Witztum JL (1989) Beyond cholesterol. Modifications of low-density lipoproteins that increase its atherogenicity. *New England Journal of Medicine* 320:915–924.

Thompson GR (1989) *A Handbook of Hyperlipidaemia*. London: Current Science Ltd.

Nutritional Management

A H Lichtenstein, Tufts University, Boston, Massachusetts, USA

Copyright © 1998 Academic Press

The relationship between intake of dietary fat and cholesterol, and levels of blood lipids was first identified at the beginning of the twentieth century. It is now generally accepted that there is a positive relationship between intakes of saturated fat and levels of both total and low-density lipoprotein (LDL) cholesterol, as well as between intake of carbohydrates and alcohol, and levels of triacylglycerol. Similarly, evidence now suggests a positive relationship between total and LDL cholesterol levels and risk of cardiovascular disease (CVD), and a negative relationship between high-density lipoprotein (HDL) cholesterol levels and CVD. Also, there is a strong negative correlation between triacylglycerol and HDL cholesterol levels. Recommendations regarding the nutritional management of hyperlipidaemia focus on limiting saturated fat and cholesterol intakes with respect to elevated total and LDL cholesterol levels, and on limiting intakes of carbohydrates (especially simple carbohydrates) and alcohol with respect to elevated triacylglycerol levels.

Increasing knowledge of the relationship between diet and hyperlipidaemia has been followed by the process of debating and defining dietary recommendations. The aim of maximizing the lowering of LDL while minimizing the lowering of HDL has remained constant, and the resulting recommendations have primarily focused on decreasing the intake of total and saturated fat as well as cholesterol. Current debate surrounding the management of hyperlipidaemia centres on refining such recommendations with regard to the balance of the diet, i.e. the relative benefits of diets high in monounsaturated fatty acids (MUFA) or polyunsaturated fatty acids (PUFA), n-6 or n-3 PUFA, and *cis* or *trans* fatty acids with respect to blood cholesterol levels, as well as the relative benefits of moderate-fat diets or very low-fat, high-carbohydrate diets with respect to blood triacylglycerol levels.

Dietary Fat

Studies in the mid 1960s demonstrated that changes in dietary fat intake alter blood lipid concentrations in most individuals. Since then a plethora of studies have confirmed these original observations. Inconsistent findings among studies are not rare and should not detract from the basic observations; the inconsistencies, when they do occur, are attributable to variations in the experimental diet, such as the magnitude or type of dietary perturbation, length of study period, habituation to nutrient intakes prior to the start of the study period and the background diet on which the dietary variable was superimposed, as well as to differences among experimental subjects, such as in age, sex, genetics, rate and efficiency of intestinal absorption, and initial blood lipid concentrations.

Current guidelines recommend that the fat content of the diet should be only 30% or less of total energy intake. This goal can be achieved by first identifying the major sources of fat in the diet and then finding acceptable alternatives to or reducing portion sizes of such foods. The proliferation of low-fat and fat-free products should facilitate this end. However, not all types of fats or individual fatty acids elicit the same response in blood lipid levels.

Saturated fatty acids

Early evidence demonstrated that the consumption of foods relatively high in saturated fatty acids (SFA) increased blood total cholesterol levels, but that not all SFA had identical effects. Subsequent work refined the hypercholesterolaemic effect of SFA and established that dietary SFA results in an increase in both LDL and HDL cholesterol levels.

Short-chain fatty acids ($C_{6:0}$ to $C_{10:0}$) and stearic acid ($C_{18:0}$) produce little or no change in blood cholesterol levels, whereas SFA with chain lengths of C_{12} to C_{16} appear to be the most potent in increasing blood cholesterol levels. It has been postulated that stearic acid (18:0) is not absorbed or is rapidly converted to oleic acid (18:1), and for this reason has a relatively neutral effect on blood cholesterol levels. The underlying mechanism by which fatty acids with 10 or fewer carbon atoms have different effects from those with 12–16 carbons is unknown.

Current recommendations regarding dietary SFA both for the general population and for hyperlipidaemic individuals are to limit consumption initially to less than 10% of total energy intake, and if an inadequate effect on blood cholesterol levels is observed, to reduce intake to less than 7% of total energy. Foods relatively high in SFA include meat and full-fat dairy products. Saturated fatty acids tend to be solid at room temperature. Notable exceptions are the tropical oils (palm, palm kernel and coconut) which are liquid at room temperature yet have high levels of short chain SFA. Efforts to reduce SFA intake should include use of lean meat, the trimming of excess fat and skin off poultry, and the substitution of fat-free and low-fat dairy products for their full-fat counterparts. Judicious use of ingredient listings and nutrient labels on processed foods will also help achieve the goal of reducing the SFA content of the diet. Frequently, when the total fat content of the diet is decreased, so is the SFA content.

Monounsaturated fatty acids

In the past more emphasis was placed on the SFA and PUFA intakes or PUFA/SFA ratios of the diet than on the MUFA intake. This occurred, in part, because of early work suggesting that consumption of MUFA had a neutral effect on blood cholesterol levels relative to the consumption of carbohydrates. More recently, a number of investigators have specifically studied the effect of substituting MUFA or PUFA for SFA. Most report that replacement of SFA with either class of fatty acids results in a hypocholesterolaemic effect.

The advent of more refined methodology to monitor individual lipoprotein concentrations raised additional issues with respect to the differential effects of MUFA or PUFA beyond total cholesterol levels. Initial reports suggested that the decrease in total cholesterol levels resulting from a decreased consumption of SFA and increased consumption of PUFA was attributable to decreases in both LDL and HDL cholesterol levels. Some, but not all work, suggests that diets relatively high in MUFA compared with those high in PUFA have the advantage of selectively decreasing LDL cholesterol levels. Discrepancies in the effect of MUFA on HDL cholesterol levels may be related to the total levels of fat in the diet.

Current recommendations for the general population and hyperlipidaemic individuals are that MUFA consumption should make up between 5% and 15% of the total energy intake of the diet. The major MUFA in the diet is oleic acid (18:1). Foods relatively high in oleic acid are canola (rapeseed) and olive oils and foods made with these oils. Oils relatively high in MUFA should be used as a substitute for, not in addition to, SFA.

Polyunsaturated fatty acids

Substitution of PUFA for SFA results in a decrease in total, LDL and HDL cholesterol levels. The magnitude of change for LDL and HDL tends to be proportional. The absolute fall in HDL cholesterol levels has raised questions about the physiological value of such a dietary change with respect to lipoprotein profiles. However, there is no evidence that decreasing HDL cholesterol levels as a result of the substitution of PUFA for SFA puts an individual at increased risk for CVD. Additionally, societies with low total and HDL cholesterol levels tend to have low rates of CVD.

Recent food disappearance data from the USA have suggested that there has been an overall downward trend in total fat intake (percent of calories), but with a relative upward trend in PUFA intake at the expense of SFA. During this same period, there has been a downward trend in blood cholesterol levels. Evidence suggests that the downward trend is related, in part, to this change in dietary source of fatty acids.

Classified as dietary PUFA are a wide range of fatty acids differing in chain length, degree of saturation, position of the double bonds (positional isomers) and configuration of the double bond (geometric isomers). Two positional isomers of interest with respect to diet and CVD are n-6 and n-3. The distinction is made on the basis of the location of the first double bond relative to the methyl end of the fatty acyl chain: the sixth carbon for n-6 and the third carbon for n-3. Additionally, each double bond in the fatty acyl chain exists as one of two geometric isomers, *cis* or *trans*. The two hydrogen atoms attached to the carbon atoms making up the double bond are on the same side in the *cis* configuration and are on opposite sides in the *trans* configuration.

Effects of n-6 PUFA The major n-6 PUFA in the Western diet is linoleic acid (18:2). Other important n-6 PUFA are γ-linolenic acid (18:3 n-6) and arachidonic acid (20:4). Vegetable oils with the exception of the tropical oils are the primary source of n-6 PUFA. Consumption of PUFA, relative to SFA or carbohydrate, has consistently been shown to lower blood cholesterol levels. The current recommendation for the general population and hypercholesterolaemic individuals is for PUFA intake to contribute up to 10% of total energy intake.

Effects of n-3 PUFA   Early in the study of dietary fat and blood lipid levels, it was noted that oils derived from fish and marine mammals had hypocholesterolaemic effects similar to those derived from vegetable oils high in PUFA. However, it was not until reports of low rates of CVD among the Greenland Eskimos and an inverse relationship between fish consumption and mortality from CVD were published that the topic received serious attention. Interestingly, the advantage of n-3 PUFA in decreasing risk of developing CVD is not attributable to the lowering of blood cholesterol levels. In contrast with studies on n-6 PUFA, consumption of n-3 PUFA does not result in total or LDL cholesterol lowering. The n-3 PUFA have been demonstrated to alter other factors which result in decreased risk of developing CVD. These factors include lowering triacylglycerol levels in hypertriacylglycerolaemic individuals, decreasing platelet aggregation, lowering blood pressure and decreasing vulnerability to ventricular fibrillation. A more recent report has raised some concern by suggesting that high levels of fish consumption can result in decreased parameters of the immune response; however, the clinical significance of this observation is still unclear.

The major n-3 PUFA in the diet are, from plant sources, α-linolenic acid (18:3 n-3); and from marine sources, eicosapentaenoic acid (EPA, 20:5 n-3) and docosahexaenoic acid (DHA, 22:6 n-3). No specific recommendations regarding n-3 PUFA consumption have yet been made, although general recommendations range from 3% to 5% of total energy intake. The n-3 PUFA content of the diet should be added to the n-6 PUFA content of the diet when calculating total PUFA intake. At present, it would seem prudent to recommend a moderate intake of foods containing high levels of n-3 PUFA. Good sources of n-3 PUFA are marine products, especially fatty fish, and oils high in α-linolenic acid, such as soya bean and canola (rapeseed). In addition to these foods being rich sources of n-3 PUFA, the substitution of fish for meat or of vegetable oil for animal fat can result in a decrease in the SFA content of the diet, which will have independent beneficial effects on blood cholesterol levels.

MUFA, PUFA and susceptibility of LDL to oxidation

Recent interest regarding the PUFA and MUFA content of the diet has centred on the differential effect of these classes of fatty acids on the susceptibility of LDL to oxidation. The atherogenicity of LDL has been reported to be increased by the postsecretory oxidation of the particle. Antibodies to oxidized LDL have been reported to circulate in patients with established CVD. Diets rich in MUFA compared with diets rich in PUFA have been repeatedly shown to decrease the susceptibility of LDL to oxidation *in vitro*, a result probably attributable to the lesser total number of double bonds in the MUFA molecule. Dietary supplementation with vitamin E, an antioxidant vitamin, but not with β-carotene or ascorbic acid, has been demonstrated to decrease the susceptibility of LDL to oxidation. Epidemiological evidence had previously suggested that individuals who consume a relatively high level of vitamin E found in dietary supplements, but not in food, have a decreased risk of developing CVD. More recent work, however, suggests that dietary, rather than supplemental vitamin E, may also be related to decreased risk of developing CVD. Complicating the picture further, a recent report in African Green monkeys suggested that substituting dietary MUFA for PUFA offers no advantage in terms of reducing atherosclerotic lesion formation, although the predicted differences in susceptibility *in vitro* of LDL to oxidation were observed. The issue of the relationship of diet, LDL oxidizability and CVD development may be important; however, more data are needed before more specific guidelines regarding the management of hyperlipidaemia can be given.

Trans fatty acids

Trans fatty acids, by definition, contain at least one double bond in the *trans* configuration. Dietary *trans* fatty acids occur naturally in meat and dairy products as a result of anaerobic bacterial fermentation in ruminant animals. *Trans* double bonds are also introduced into the diet as a result of the consumption of hydrogenated vegetable or fish oils. Oils are hydrogenated to increase their plasticity and chemical stability, thus expanding their potential use in food products. Currently, the major source of dietary *trans* fatty acids is from hydrogenated fat. When assessing the effect of *trans* fatty acids on blood lipid levels, it is important to take into consideration that hydrogenation results in a number of changes in the acyl chain of the fatty acid moiety: the conversion of *cis* to *trans* double bonds, the saturation of double bonds, and the migration of double bonds along the acyl chain, resulting in multiple positional isomers. Elaidic acid, a fatty acid containing 18 carbons and one double bond at C-9, along with its isomers, contributes the majority of *trans* fatty acids to the diet.

Most early studies demonstrated that consumption of dietary *trans* fatty acids or hydrogenated fat resulted in higher blood cholesterol levels than consumption of the native oil, but also lower blood cholesterol levels than consumption of equal amounts of saturated fat. Effects on triacylglycerol levels are equivocal. These results have persisted despite variability among study designs, levels of *trans* fatty acids consumed by study subjects, and sources of *trans* fatty acids.

More recent work focused attention on the effects of *trans* fatty acids on specific lipoprotein fractions. These studies suggested that consumption of relatively high levels of a *trans* fatty acid, elaidic acid, resulted not only in increased LDL cholesterol levels but decreased HDL cholesterol levels; however, subsequent observations have been inconsistent. Variations in the absolute level of *trans* fatty acid intake as well as differences in source are likely explanations for such inconsistencies. Some research has also suggested that *trans* fatty acids may increase lipoprotein(a) (Lp(a)) levels. Levels of Lp(a) tend to be positively correlated with risk of developing CVD. The absolute magnitude of potential changes in Lp(a) levels needs further clarification as does the physiological significance of such changes within the range reported.

Epidemiological data on the relationship between *trans* fatty acid intake and CVD risk have been conflicting. Data estimating *trans* fatty acid intake obtained from food frequency questionnaires support a positive relationship between intake of *trans* fatty acids and risk of developing CVD. Unfortunately, such estimates of *trans* fatty acid intake are hampered by the lack of a complete data base. In contrast, data estimating *trans* fatty acid intake derived from more objective measures, such as blood or adipose tissue levels, do not support an association between *trans* fatty acid intake and increased CVD risk. However, the accuracy of estimating long-term *trans* fatty acid intake from tissue levels awaits further confirmation.

No formal recommendations for *trans* fatty acid intake currently exist. With respect to lowering plasma lipid levels, current evidence suggests that when using hydrogenated products, it is preferable to use the softer (less hydrogenated fat) and 'diet' (low-energy) varieties and, when possible, to choose products that list oil, not hydrogenated fat, as the predominant fat on the ingredient label.

Dietary Cholesterol

The observation that dietary cholesterol increased blood cholesterol levels and was associated with the development of arteriosclerosis was originally made in animals. In humans, a positive correlation has been repeatedly confirmed between dietary cholesterol intake and both blood cholesterol levels and CVD risk, although interpretation of these findings is complicated by variations among study designs. The two major factors apparently affecting responsiveness to dietary cholesterol are the basal intake of cholesterol to which extra cholesterol is added, and genetic variability among study subjects. An additional factor may be the tendency for responsiveness to vary over a wider range than reported for other dietary fat variables. The majority of evidence supports the premise that increased dietary cholesterol results in increased blood cholesterol levels. Whether the magnitude of response is linear or curvilinear with increasing dietary cholesterol intake, or whether there is a break point or threshold/ceiling relationship beyond which individuals are no longer responsive, remains to be determined.

The current recommendations for the general population and hyperlipidaemic individuals are that the upper limit of dietary cholesterol should be 300 mg per day, and if inadequate response is seen in the latter group, the limit should be 200 mg per day. The major sources of dietary cholesterol are eggs, meat and dairy products. Since dietary cholesterol is frequently found in foods also relatively high in SFA, reducing the SFA content of the diet, as discussed above, should reduce the cholesterol content of the diet.

Very Low-fat, High-carbohydrate Diets

When considering diets very low in fat and high in carbohydrates ('very low-fat' diets), it is important to separate the effects of the composition of the diet from confounding factors associated with potential weight loss. It is also important to define the term 'very low-fat' diet. For the purposes of this discussion, a very low-fat diet will have 15% or less of energy as fat.

Consumption of a very low-fat diet without a decrease in energy intake or body weight frequently results in a decrease in blood total, LDL and HDL cholesterol levels and an increase in triacylglycerol levels. The reduction in lipoprotein levels may be a reflection of the decrease in SFA intake. Alterations in the metabolism of the triacylglycerol-rich lipoprotein particles probably contribute to the increased blood triacylglycerol and decreased HDL cholesterol levels observed.

Short term weight loss is frequently associated with consumption of very low-fat diets. It has been speculated that the weight loss observed may be attributable to the lower energy density of the food, and hence lower total energy intake. Weight loss itself has been associated with an improvement in blood lipid profiles. Coupled with a very low-fat diet, weight loss has been reported to dampen the increase in blood triacylglycerol levels and decrease in HDL cholesterol levels normally observed. Populations that normally consume very low-fat diets generally have lower blood lipid concentrations and rates of CVD than those consuming higher-fat diets. In such populations, energy intake tends to be lower and fibre intake and levels of physical activity higher than in populations consuming relatively high-fat diets, and obesity is not generally a public health problem.

The value of recommending a very low-fat diet for the general population is questionable at this time from the point of view of physiological benefit and implementation. Such diets should be approached cautiously, especially in individuals with hypertriacylglycerolaemia or compromised glucose metabolism. Specific recommendations should be used in selecting the source of carbohydrate energy. Simple carbohydrates, i.e. foods high in mono and diacylglycerols, should be avoided to minimize triacylglycerol elevations. Similarly, alcohol use should be restricted, since it can also result in an increase in blood triacylglycerol levels. Emphasis should be placed on including sources of fat that will ensure consumption of adequate amounts of essential fatty acids.

Fibre

Dietary soluble fibre has been reported to have a modest independent effect on decreasing blood total and LDL cholesterol levels. It appears that the soluble fraction, especially β-glucan, is at least partially responsible for this effect. Most evidence suggests that soluble fibre exerts its hypocholesterolaemic effect via binding bile acids and cholesterol in the intestine, resulting in an increased faecal loss and altered colonic metabolism of bile acids. The fermentation of fibre polysaccharides in the colon yields short-chain fatty acids. Some evidence suggests that these compounds have hypocholesterolaemic effects via alterations in hepatic metabolism. At this time there is no evidence to suggest that insoluble fibre has an effect on blood lipid levels.

Diets relatively high in fibre are associated with lower intakes of total fat and SFA. Such diets are relatively high in fruits, vegetables and whole grains. The value of displacing total fat and especially SFA from the diet via increasing the use of fibre-rich foods should be exploited. Limited evidence also suggests that high-fibre diets may blunt the hypertriacylglycerolaemic effect frequently seen after consumption of very low-fat, high-carbohydrate diets.

Conclusions

The relationship between diet and blood lipid levels has clearly been established. Current recommendations for the general population and hyperlipidaemic individuals are to limit total fat intake to 30% or less of total energy and saturated fat to less than 10% (and if inadequate response is observed in hyperlipidaemic individuals, to less than 7%); to consume up to 10% as PUFA; and to consume less than 300 mg cholesterol per day (and if inadequate response is observed in hyperlipidaemic individuals, less than 200 mg cholesterol per day). At present there are no formal recommendations for intakes of n-3 fatty acid, *trans* fatty acid and fibre. However, given the current evidence for *trans* fatty acids, it appears appropriate to suggest that hyperlipidaemic individuals consume soft and 'diet' (low-energy) margarines, and minimize the use of hydrogenated vegetable shortenings and foods made with these products. With respect to fibre, individuals should be counselled to include adequate amounts of fruits, vegetables and whole-grain products. Also, hypertriacylglycerolaemic individuals should be counselled to restrict simple carbohydrate and alcohol intake. Attainment or maintenance of optimal body weight should be emphasized. Since the latter recommendation is a balance between energy consumption and energy expenditure, individuals who would benefit from weight loss should be encouraged not only to reduce energy intake but also to increase levels of physical activity.

The current dietary recommendations are the culmination of nearly a century of work. They have evolved slowly. No doubt this evolution, frequently accompanied by debate, will continue for many years. It is important for nutrition scientists to implement current recommendations aimed at optimizing blood lipid levels, hence reducing the risk of developing CVD, and to reassess these recommendations as new findings present themselves.

See also: **Cholesterol**: Factors Determining Blood Cholesterol Levels. **Coronary Heart Disease**: Lipid Theory of Coronary Heart Disease; Prevention. **Dietary Fibre (Fiber)**: Role in Nutritional Management of Disease. **Fatty Acids**: Health Effects of Saturated Fatty Acids; Health Effects of Monounsaturated Fatty Acids; Health Effects of n-6 Polyunsaturated Fatty Acids; Health Effects of n-3 Polyunsaturated Fatty Acids; Health Effects of *trans* Fatty Acids. **Lipoproteins**: Physiology.

Further Reading

American Heart Association (1996) Dietary guidelines for healthy American adults: a statement for physicians and health professionals by the Nutrition Committee, American Heart Association. *Circulation* **94**:1795–1800.

ASCN/AIN Task Force on *Trans* Fatty Acids (1996) Position paper on *trans* fatty acids. *American Journal of Clinical Nutrition* **63**:463–470.

Denke B (1995) Review of human studies evaluating individual dietary responsiveness in patients with hypercholesterolemia. *American Journal of Clinical Nutrition* **62**:471S–477S.

Glore SR, van Treeck D, Knehans AR and Guild M (1994) Soluble fiber and serum lipids: a literature review. *Journal of the American Dietetic Association* **94**:425–436.

Grundy SM (1983) Absorption and metabolism of dietary cholesterol. *Annual Review of Nutrition* **3**:71–96.

Grundy SM and Denke MA (1990) Dietary influences on serum lipids and lipoproteins. *Journal of Lipid Research* **31**:1149–1172.

Hopkins PN (1992) Effects of dietary cholesterol on serum cholesterol: a meta-analysis and review. *American Journal of Clinical Nutrition* **55**:1060–1070.

Lichtenstein AH, Ausman LM, Carrasco W, Jenner JL, Ordovas JM and Schaefer EJ (1994) Short term consumption of a low fat diet has a positive impact on plasma lipid concentrations only when accompanied by weight loss. *Arteriosclerosis and Thrombosis* **14**:1751–1760.

Mensik RP and Katan MB (1989) Effect of a diet enriched with monounsaturated or polyunsaturated fatty acids on levels of low density and high density lipoprotein cholesterol in healthy women and men. *New England Journal of Medicine* **321**:436–441.

NCEP (1993) Summary of the second report of the National Cholesterol Education Program (NCEP) Expert Panel on Detection, Evaluation, and Treatment of High Blood Cholesterol in Adults (Adult Treatment Panel II). *Journal of the American Medical Association* **269**:3015–3023.

Reiser R, Probstfield JL, Silvers A et al. (1985) Plasma lipid and lipoprotein response of humans to beef fat, coconut oil and safflower oil [published erratum appears in *Am J Clin Nutr* (1986) 43(6):978]. *American Journal of Clinical Nutrition* **42**:190–197.

Ripsin CM, Keenan JM, Jacobs DR *et al.* (1992) Oat products and lipid lowering. *Journal of the American Medical Association* **267**:3317–3325.

World Health Organization (1990) *Diet, Nutrition and the Prevention of Chronic Diseases.* WHO Technical Report 797. Geneva: WHO.

HYPERTENSION

Contents
Physiology
Nutritional Management
Interrelationships Between Hypertension and Diabetes

Physiology

T Morgan, University of Melbourne, Parkville, Australia

H Brunner, Centre Hospitalier Universitaire Vaudois, Lausanne, Switzerland

Copyright © 1998 Academic Press

Blood pressure (BP) is determined by cardiac output (CO) and total peripheral resistance (TPR).

$$BP = CO \times TPR$$

These variables are controlled in turn by the activity of the autonomic nervous system, regulated by a variety of nuclei in the brain. There is a complex interaction between plasma volume, blood pressure and a variety of humoral and neural mechanisms that determine the blood pressure.

Blood pressure is not, however, a static value. It varies markedly in response to a variety of stimuli. Change of posture activates a variety of controls which keep the pressure relatively constant. Physical and mental activity may be associated with alterations in blood pressure, and there is a marked fall in blood pressure during sleep. Thus there is no such value as a normal blood pressure based on a single measurement, as blood pressure needs to be related to the circumstances under which it is measured. Likewise, there is no single blood pressure level that means a person is hypertensive. The present convention is that a blood pressure greater than 140 mmHg systolic or 90 mmHg diastolic on clinic recording makes a person hypertensive. However, blood pressure has a marked circadian variation (**Fig. 1**), and an individual could have a blood pressure of 160/92 mmHg at 09:00 h and be classified as hypertensive, while at 14:00 h it might be 148/83 mmHg and would be classified as normotensive. Thus in a normal person blood pressure may vary markedly during a day associated with reactive events, but in some people the baseline blood pressure eventually rises to a level that is defined as 'hypertension'. In this person with hypertension there will be fluctuations in blood pressure associated with the same controls as in normal people, but the fluctuations may be exaggerated, leading to exceedingly high blood pressure levels.

The aetiology of essential hypertension is unknown; however, the condition is believed to result from an interaction of environmental and genetic factors. Environmental factors are undoubtedly of major importance, because in certain communities hypertension is virtually nonexistent; however, when such a community alters its life style, hypertension becomes common and may exist in 30% of the population. Not all people develop hypertension, and the ones who do are determined by their genetic composition (**Fig. 2**). Investigations are under way to attempt to determine which individuals are more likely to develop hypertension and its complications, so that life style and environmental alterations can be initiated to prevent the disease occurring in such people. Certain specific genetic abnormalities have been identified and these cases are then removed from the classification of essential hypertension. It is

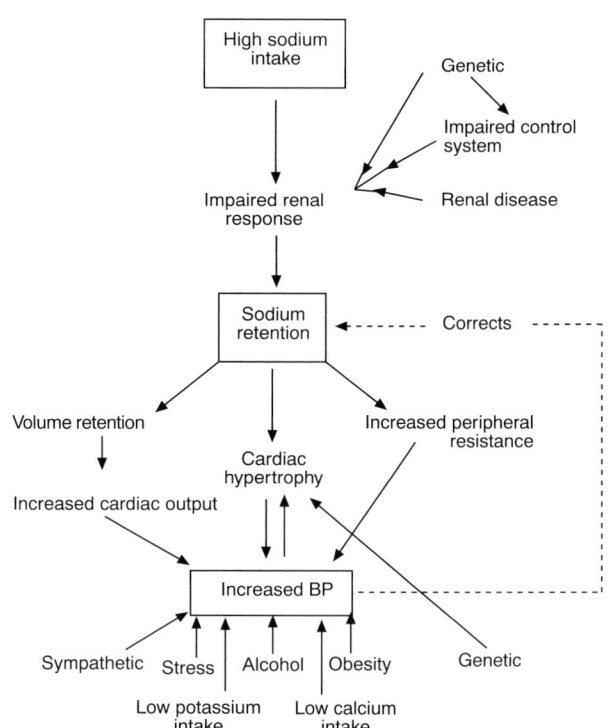

Figure 2 The interrelationships between sodium intake, renal function, hormonal control systems and genetic inheritance in the aetiology of hypertension and cardiac hypertrophy. BP, blood pressure.

of interest that the disorders that have been found in general alter sodium handling by the body. Hypertension is not seen in hunter-gatherer communities where sodium intake is low and potassium intake is high, and thus the genetic abnormality is not expressed phenotypically even though the genotype is probably present.

When hypertension is established the defect is an increased peripheral resistance rather than an increased cardiac output. However, in people with minor blood pressure elevations and prehypertensive people cardiac output is increased, and it has been postulated that increased cardiac output in response to the retention of sodium is the initial haemodynamic change that leads to hypertension (Fig. 2). However, experimentally hypertension can be produced without a stage of increased cardiac output, and increased peripheral resistance can result without an antecedent high cardiac output. It is likely that there is heterogeneity in the way that people respond. The concept of an increased cardiac output leading to hypertension has been extensively developed by Guyton in a variety of computer and experimental models. However, in carefully conducted studies in which blood volume was measured in hypertensive patients, blood volume was decreased rather than increased, making this theory probably

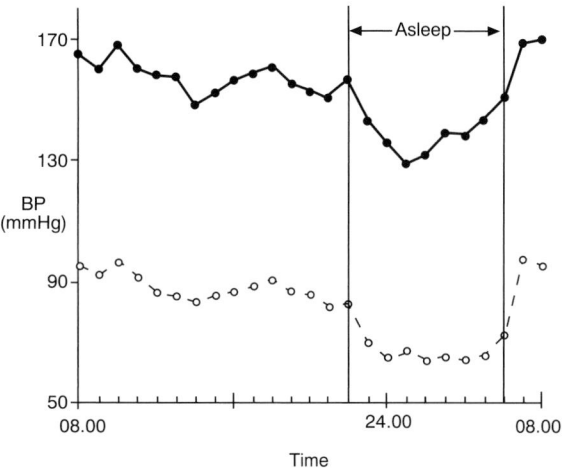

Figure 1 Hourly ambulatory blood pressure (BP) measurements in a 58-year-old man with borderline hypertension. Solid circles, systolic pressure; open circles, diastolic pressure.

not applicable to all people. The relationship with sodium is also complicated. In young hypertensive subjects there is a better inverse correlation with body potassium total rather than a direct correlation with total body sodium content. In older people the correlation with body sodium content becomes more pronounced. The lack of a direct correlation between body sodium and hypertension in the young casts doubt on the absoluteness of the link between sodium and hypertension, and clearly potassium has an important effect modulating the response.

It has been suggested that the prime defect leading to increased peripheral resistance is the presence of a circulating factor that inhibits (Na^+-K^+)-ATPase activity, thereby increasing the sodium content of cells (**Fig. 3**). This increased sodium content decreases the rate at which calcium can be removed from the cell by the Na^+-Ca^{2+} countertransport. In skeletal and cardiac muscle cells the contractile response is triggered by a small influx of Ca^{2+} that

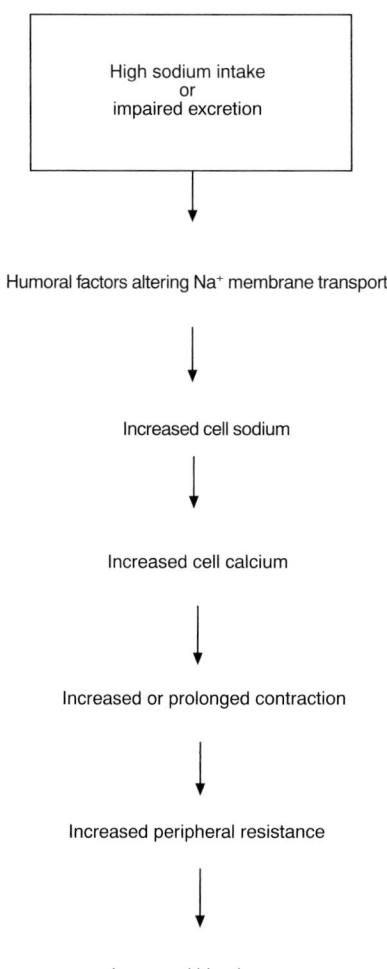

High sodium intake or impaired excretion

↓

Humoral factors altering Na^+ membrane transport

↓

Increased cell sodium

↓

Increased cell calcium

↓

Increased or prolonged contraction

↓

Increased peripheral resistance

↓

Increased blood pressure

Figure 3 Mechanistic approach indicating how at the cellular level a high sodium intake may initiate the series of events leading to increased peripheral resistance and a high blood pressure.

releases Ca^{2+} from the endoplasmic reticulum. The response is terminated by reuptake of Ca^{2+} into the endoplasmic reticulum and thus the Na^+-Ca^{2+} countertransport is not of critical importance, though in all cells the basal level and total content of calcium may be increased. In smooth muscle cells, including the arteriolar (resistance vessels) cells, contraction is initiated by entry of calcium across the cell membrane at least in part by the Na^+-Ca^{2+} countertransport. If there is a defect in calcium removal contraction will be prolonged, and if the basal level of cellular calcium is higher contraction may be more intense. Thus peripheral resistance rises and hypertension results. All the physiological factors to support the above have been identified. However, despite intensive research it is unclear if a true circulating physiological factor capable of inhibiting (Na^+-K^+)-ATPase has been identified. Claims have been made for an ouabain-like factor in plasma and the hypothalamus, but there is scepticism whether this is the important physiological variable. In hypertensive patients cell sodium levels are elevated. This elevation need not necessarily be due to inhibition of (Na^+-K^+)-ATPase but could result from an increased entry of sodium into the cell down its electrochemical gradient by a variety of channels or transporters. There is evidence that abnormalities of these exist and are more prevalent in hypertensive people. There is also evidence that the rate of entry of Na^+ can be increased by a high sodium intake and that a circulating but unidentified factor may be increased. The signal for release of such a factor is unclear and does not appear to be plasma sodium concentration and probably not total plasma volume. It may be modulated by the kidney and be related to 'turnover' of sodium.

The body can control plasma sodium concentration (by antidiuretic hormone) and plasma volume and total body sodium within well-defined limits, despite large variations (20–400 mmol) in daily sodium chloride intake. This control involves a variety of humoral factors (**Table 1**). Renin-angiotensin, aldosterone, atrial natriuretic peptide, sympathetic activity and other variables are all altered by changes in sodium chloride and/or potassium intake. The capacity of these systems to respond maintains blood pressure in the 'normal' range. It is only when this capacity is exceeded that blood pressure becomes elevated. The increase in blood pressure will also correct the body sodium because the kidney has a sensitive 'pressure natriuresis response'. Thus in most people as blood pressure rises sodium is excreted; this self-correction ensures that blood pressure does not rise to excessive levels. It has been suggested that in addition to high sodium intake and abnormalities

Table 1 Factors altering sodium balance

Variable	Site of action
Increases Na+ retention	
Angiotensin II	Proximal tubule
	Increases aldosterone
Aldosterone	Distal nephron
Sympathetic	Proximal tubule
	Haemodynamics
Increases Na+ excretion	
Atrial peptide	Proximal tubule
	Distal nephron
Parathyroid hormone	Proximal nephron
Natriuretic hormone (?)	Loop of Henle, plus others
Elevated blood pressure	Haemodynamics

of sodium handling by cells there must be a defect in the pressure natriuresis response. This could be due to excessive amounts of circulating hormones (aldosterone) or defective control systems in the kidney. The pressure natriuresis response may also be defective owing to reduction in nephron number following developmental problems or disease, or associated with the ageing process. An association has been found between the weight of children at birth and subsequent development of hypertension and cardiovascular disease. The low birthweight could be due to defective nutritional intake of the mother or to diseases that affect fetal and placental growth. It has been suggested that the total nephron number is reduced, and that this alters sodium handling and causes hypertension.

Much research has focused on the importance of dietary sodium chloride, but there needs to be an associated genetic defect which may be a subtle defect in the systems controlling sodium excretion. Thus the defect may be an inability of the renin-angiotensin-aldosterone system to suppress adequately or appropriately for that level of sodium intake. There is evidence from twin studies that the suppressibility of renin secretion is genetically determined and thus in some people there are inappropriate levels of angiotensin II for their level of sodium intake, resulting in hypertension. There are changes in secretion or response of renin, aldosterone, adrenaline, sympathetic activity, atrial peptide and nitric oxide with increase in sodium intake. In most cases these responses are appropriate and prevent the unfettered rise in blood pressure. However, the ability to respond may be exceeded and blood pressure then rises.

Haemodynamics

As discussed above, it is unlikely that all people go through an increased cardiac output stage. There is major variability. Well-established hypertensive patients have high peripheral resistance and a normal cardiac output, but there are exceptions. The hypertension process itself causes significant alterations in haemodynamics affecting both the heart and the blood vessels, and reversal of these effects may be as important as reducing blood pressure (**Fig. 4**).

Early in the hypertensive process there is an increase in the thickness of the arteriolar muscle wall. This is probably a compensatory process which returns the wall tension to normal. Contrary to expectations, compliance of larger arteries is normal or increased in young hypertensive patients. However, the thickening of the resistance vessels, depending on the way it takes place, has certain consequences, and for a similar degree of muscle contraction there is a greater increase in vascular tone and thus peripheral resistance rises more, leading to a higher blood pressure, greater wall tension and a further increase in vessel thickness. This is a positive feedback response and a vicious cycle may result (Fig. 4). In the early hypertensive process the systolic and diastolic blood pressures rise more or less in parallel. However, in the older hypertensive patient the pulse pressure widens, due probably to increased stiffness of the arteries. This increased stiffness, which is associated with a loss of elastin and an increase in collagen, has important effects on the heart.

The endothelium of blood vessels is a major regulator of vascular tone and an important mechanism in the production of nitric oxide. If nitric oxide is removed, peripheral resistance rises and hypertension results. However, it is unlikely that defects in nitric oxide production are the cause of high blood pressure. In fact in early hypertension the nitric oxide production may be increased as a compensatory event modulating the rise in pressure, and this may explain why dynamic compliance is normal (**Fig. 5**). However,

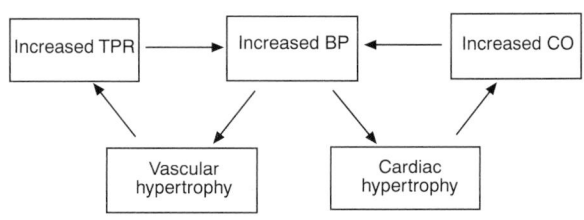

Figure 4 Interaction between the various parameters that control blood pressure, showing how they set up a positive feedback leading to worsening blood pressure. BP, blood pressure; CO, cardiac output; TPR, total peripheral resistance.

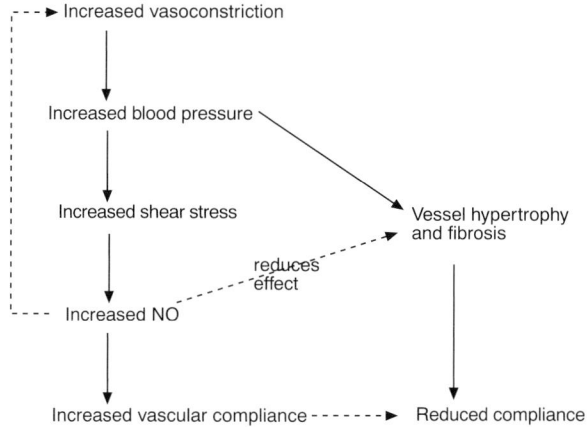

Figure 5   An outline indicating how the initial response of the endothelium is to prevent the rise of blood pressure by releasing nitric oxide (NO). This increases vessel compliance, reducing the adverse effects. If this system's capacity is exceeded the arterial damage process is accelerated. The dotted lines represent negative feedback attempting to restore the status quo.

when hypertension is established and there is vessel disease the nitric oxide response and the endothelial control become impaired, and this is probably an important factor leading to stiffness of the arteries and atherosclerosis.

The stiffness of blood vessels that develops in older hypertensive patients has a number of important consequences. The pulse wave velocity is increased and thus reflected waves arrive back at the heart while the ventricle is still contracting, thereby augmenting the central systolic pressure (**Table 2**). In normotensive people the place at which the reflected wave and the oncoming flow meet is near the brachial artery, and thus central systolic pressure is lower than brachial artery systolic pressure (**Fig. 6**). This increased central systolic blood pressure means that the heart contracts against a greater load and thus performs more work, leading to hypertrophy greater than might be predicted from the brachial artery pressure. The extent of the augmentation due to the pressure wave depends upon the degree of reflection, which is controlled in part by the peripheral resistance. The site at which augmentation is highest depends on the pulse wave velocity. The deterioration in the elastic properties of the large blood vessels with loss of elastin and more collagen leads to increased pulse pressure, increased augmentation of

Table 2   Factors determining extent of reflection and site where the reflected wave meets the flow wave

Poor arterial compliance	Increased pulse wave velocity
	Reflected wave closer to heart
Arterial branch points	Reflective site
Peripheral resistance	Increased reflection

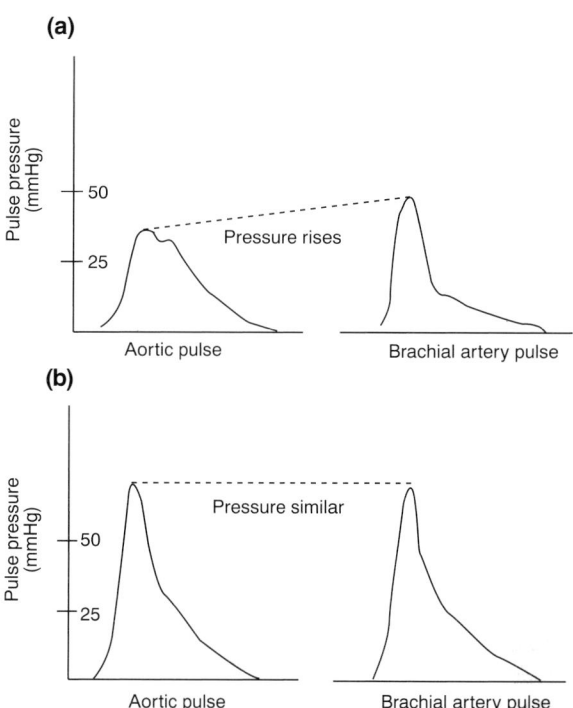

Figure 6   The central aortic and brachial artery pulse wave forms in normotensive (a) and hypertensive (b) subjects. In (b) the heart pumps blood out against a higher pressure leading to cardiac hypertrophy. See O'Rourke (1995) for discussion of how central aortic pressure is higher than brachial artery pressure due to reflected waves.

the central systolic pressure and a decrease in the peripheral diastolic pressure, all of which are common in the elderly hypertensive patient.

The Heart

In hypertensive patients the left ventricle is frequently enlarged and this is associated with an increased risk of cardiovascular death. When assessed by electrocardiography left ventricular hypertrophy (LVH) is relatively uncommon, but if assessed by echocardiography LVH is present in up to 50% of mild hypertensive patients and in adolescents not classified as hypertensive, but in the upper 10 percentile of blood pressure there is a 10–15% prevalence of LVH (**Table 3**). The cause of the LVH is not certain (**Table 4**).

Table 3   Prevalence of left ventricular hypertrophy

Subjects	Prevalence (%)
Normotensive	1–2
Adolescent, upper 10%	10–15
Borderline hypertensive	
by echo	20–50
by ECG	3–5
Severe hypertensive	90

ECG, electrocardiogram; echo, echocardiogram.

Table 4 Factors affecting cardiac hypertrophy

Factors leading to hypertrophy	Factors reducing or preventing hypertrophy
24 h cardiac work	Nitric oxide
Ventricular wall stress	Bradykinin
Sodium intake	
Sympathetic activity	
Angiotensin II	
Insulin-like growth factor	
Growth hormone	
Genotype	

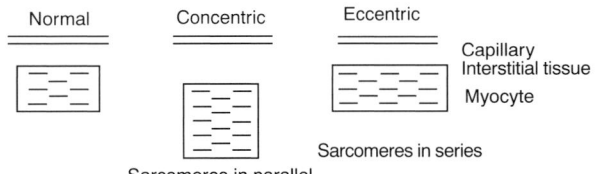

Figure 7 The diffusion distance in normal and eccentric hypertrophy is not increased. In concentric hypertrophy there is often associated fibrosis; this leads to a longer extracellular diffusion distance as well as a longer interacellular pathway. Thus oxygen delivery to mitochondria is poor, the reuptake of calcium (an energy-dependent process) is sluggish, and 'functional' relaxation is slow, leading to impaired diastolic filling.

There is a better correlation with 24 h blood pressure than with clinic values, but the *r* value is about 0.14 indicating considerable variability. It is possible that acute elevations of blood pressure sustained for 1–2 h may have a potent effect by increasing wall stress and activating the processes that lead to myocyte hypertrophy. This may be of particular importance if it occurs at a time when plasma levels of potential growth factors such as angiotensin II and growth hormone are elevated. These hormones are elevated during sleep and thus blood pressure elevation at that time may be particularly detrimental. This is supported by observations that people who do not have the usual night-time (sleep) fall in blood pressure are more likely to have cardiac and renal complications. There is a significant genetic influence on cardiac hypertrophy and it has been proposed that cardiac enlargement may be antecedent to and the cause of hypertension. High blood pressure can undoubtedly cause cardiac enlargement, but independent of blood pressure elevation angiotensin II and salt can probably enlarge the heart.

The strongest predictor in some studies of cardiac size was the salt intake. In animals a high salt intake can cause cardiac hypertrophy and a low salt intake can cause resolution. The increased size of the heart is a response that decreases the wall stress of the ventricle and is a compensatory phenomenon. The cardiac hypertrophy with hypertension is concentric in nature, with sarcomeres laid down in the myocytes in parallel (**Fig. 7**). In cardiac hypertrophy associated with exercise the sarcomeres are laid down in series, and with this 'eccentric' hypertrophy there is no increased mortality. The increased thickness of the myocytes together with associated fibrosis of the interstitium means that the oxygen diffusion pathway is increased and this may lead to precipitation of arrhythmias and sudden death.

In addition to cardiac hypertrophy in hypertensive patients there is significant impairment of diastolic relaxation. This may result from poor oxygen delivery to the mitochondria and thus a retarded reuptake of calcium into cell organelles. Thus there is a dynamic aspect to diastolic dysfunction which may potentially be reversible. However, in addition the laying down of fibrous tissue in the heart contributes to stiffness and poor diastolic filling. The poor diastolic function may occur prior to any increase in cardiac size. The poor diastolic filling due to reduction in left ventricular compliance may explain the subnormal stroke volume seen in hypertensive patients during exercise. In these circumstances the increased pulse rate means that there is insufficient time for a stiff left ventricle to fill adequately.

Early in the development of hypertension in spontaneously hypertensive rats and in humans total peripheral resistance is elevated. In rats changes in the resistance vessels are seen early. In borderline and mild hypertension in humans there may be little increase in total peripheral resistance at rest, but the total peripheral resistance does not fall to normal levels during conditions when maximal vasodilatation would be expected (e.g. exercise, heating, autonomic blockade). This probably indicates that structural changes occur early in the disease and the failure to dilate adequately may in part explain the excess rise in blood pressure seen in hypertensive patients during exercise.

Increased peripheral resistance is not evenly distributed across all regional vascular beds and the resistance in the kidney frequently appears to be increased, resulting in a reduction of about 10% in renal blood flow. In contrast, in prehypertensive people an increase has been reported in renal blood flow. Whether this has any pathogenic significance is not known. However, the reduced blood flow could result from activation of the tubuloglomerular feedback response due to altered sodium reabsorption in the proximal tubule.

The coronary flow in hypertensive patients is of importance. These people already may have an increased oxygen demand. The flow at rest is usually normal but even in patients with no evidence of coronary artery disease the flow reserve is impaired. In normal people the coronary artery rapidly dilates to meet the increased oxygen demand but in hypertensive patients this dilation is sluggish and does not reach the same maximal flow. The reason is complex and is possibly a combination of structural change and an impaired endothelial response.

The Sympathetic Nervous System

Many investigators have postulated that hypertension may result from impaired central control and this is mediated via the sympathetic nervous system. The increased cardiac output and heart rate seen in many people with early or incipient essential hypertension could be explained by excess sympathetic activity. However, it has been difficult to demonstrate that there is increased sympathetic activity because many of the techniques are relatively crude. It has been reported that plasma noradrenaline levels correlate with cardiac index and peripheral resistance in mildly hypertensive patients. It is difficult to know if increased sympathetic activity is primary, but in adolescents who later develop hypertension there is an increased blood pressure rise associated with mental or physical stress, which supports the concept of a dysregulatory neurogenic component. Sympathetic activity may also be altered by changes in sodium or potassium intake, and thus the 'prime' cause of hypertension remains to be elucidated.

Renal Function

There are undoubtedly subtle abnormalities in renal function in most hypertensive people. It is unclear if this is a cause or effect of hypertension. In spontaneous hypertensive rats (SHR) early in life the proximal tubule cells are very responsive to angiotensin II and this could cause sodium retention and initiate the development of the hypertensive process. However, in mature rats the responsiveness to angiotensin II of the proximal tubule is lost.

In hypertensive patients there is a reduced renal blood and plasma flow associated with an increased filtration fraction and hence a normal glomerular filtration rate. These changes would result in an increased fractional absorption of sodium by the proximal tubule and potential difficulty in excreting sodium by a pressure natriuresis. The pressure natriuresis curve is shifted with less sodium being excreted for a given pressure at rest, but exaggerated when pressure is acutely increased. It is not clear what is cause or effect, but it is tempting to assume that resetting of the pressure natriuresis response takes place, because if it operated normally the increased pressure should cause salt loss and correct the hypertensive process.

In some but not all people blood pressure falls with sodium restriction. Patients with salt-sensitive hypertension tend not to have a nocturnal fall in blood pressure; they have a greater prevalence of cardiac hypertrophy, microalbuminuria and a worse prognosis.

Conclusions

Hypertension is not a disease but a sign of some underlying disturbance in the usual control systems for blood pressure. It is thus difficult to have a single description of the physiology of essential hypertension as it will depend upon the cause. There are, however, certain features common to many people. It appears that in people with certain (at present unknown) abnormalities in their genotype, exposure to a high-sodium, low-potassium diet together with other alterations in their life style leads to an elevation in blood pressure. In some people there is an initial stage of high cardiac output, but when this is established the peripheral resistance is elevated and is the explanation for the high blood pressure. The genetic abnormalities may relate to impairment of the control systems for excreting sodium chloride or a deficit in the ability of the kidney to excrete sodium. There are associated abnormalities in the sympathetic nervous system and the central regulation of blood pressure. When blood pressure is elevated a series of compensatory events are activated, particularly cardiac and vascular hypertrophy, which are initially appropriate responses but lead to the creation of a positive feedback loop which eventually becomes a vicious cycle leading to malignant hypertension.

Essential hypertension in some ways is a misnomer. It is caused by alterations in nutrition and life style in people with a susceptible genotype. The challenge is to identify such people and remove the appropriate environmental factor.

See also: **Coronary Heart Disease**: Aetiology. **Hypertension**: Nutritional Management. **Potassium**: Physiology, Dietary Sources and Requirements. **Renal Function and Disorders**: Nutritional Management of Renal Disorders. **Sodium**: Physiology.

Further Reading

Avolio AP, Deng FQ, Li WQ *et al.* (1986) Improved arterial distensibility in normotensive subjects on a low salt diet. *Arteriosclerosis* 6:166–169.

Barker DJ, Winter PD, Osmond C, Margetts B and

Simmonds SJ (1989) Weight in infancy and death from ischaemic heart disease. *Lancet* **ii** (8663):577–580.

Dampney RAL (1994) Functional organisation of central pathways regulating the cardiovascular system. *Physiological Reviews* **74**:323.

Draaijer P, Kool MJ, Maessen JM *et al.* (1993) Vascular distensibility and compliance in salt-hypertensive and salt-resistant borderline hypertension. *Journal of Hypertension* **11**:199–1207.

Folkow B (1982) Physiological aspects of primary hypertension. *Physiological Reviews* **62**:347–504.

Guyton A (1980) *Arterial Pressure and Hypertension*. Philadelphia: WB Saunders.

Hayoz D, Rutschmann B, Perrett F *et al.* (1992) Conduit artery compliance and distensibility are not necessarily reduced in hypertension. *Hypertension* **20**:1–6.

Lund-Johansen P and Omvik P (1990) Haemodynamic patterns of untreated hypertensive disease. In: Laragh J and Brenner BM (eds) *Hypertension: Pathophysiology, Diagnosis and Management*, pp 305–327. New York: Raven Press.

O'Rourke M (1995) Mechanical principles in arterial disease. *Hypertension* **26**:2–9.

Nutritional Management

G A MacGregor St George's Hospital Medical School, London, UK

Copyright © 1998 Academic Press

Importance of Blood Pressure

The level of blood pressure is the most important predictor of life expectancy that is known. The higher the pressure, the more likely is the development of premature vascular disease (atherosclerosis) with consequent death from heart attacks and strokes. Atherosclerosis now accounts for six out of ten deaths in Europe and the USA, and is rapidly increasing in countries that are adopting a Western life style. High blood pressure also has direct effects, independent of its accelerating effect on atherosclerosis. It can cause cerebral haemorrhage with direct bleeding into the brain, causing stroke; aortic aneurysm; dissecting aneurysm; and through the increased work that the heart has to do, there can be enlargement of the left ventricle and eventually heart failure.

High blood pressure can be pragmatically defined as pressure that is worth investigating and treating because outcome trials have shown that this level of blood pressure when lowered reduces both strokes and heart attacks. On this entirely arbitrary basis, a systolic pressure above 150 mmHg and a diastolic pressure above 90 mmHg are considered to be high. In most developed countries this represents approximately 10% of the population. The risk of stroke and heart attack in this group is much greater and is compounded by the other well-known risk factors for premature vascular disease:

- high fat intake, leading to high blood lipids concentrations;
- cigarette smoking;
- diabetes or glucose intolerance.

However, the majority of strokes and heart attacks in the population occur in subjects whose blood pressure is in the upper range of normal; this is because, although the risk in these individual subjects is less, there are a far more individuals exposed to this lesser risk and the number of events is greater than among the hypertensives.

When dealing with the problem of blood pressure in a population, a three-fold strategy is required:

1. Reduction of blood pressure when raised in individual patients. Nutritional management, particularly salt restriction, has a major role to play in all patients with high blood pressure and may control the blood pressure without the need for drugs; however, studies have shown that the effect of nutritional management is additive to that of antihypertensive drugs.
2. Reduction of other associated risk factors for atherosclerosis. Dietary and drug management will include in all patients advice to lower fat intake in order to reduce blood cholesterol levels, as well as advice to reduce weight and excess alcohol intake. It is vital that all subjects stop smoking.
3. Reduction of the whole population's blood pressure; small reductions in population blood pressure will be immensely beneficial. Nutritional advice, therefore, should not be directed solely at those with high blood pressure, but at the whole population.

Nutritional Advice in Hypertension

Nutritional advice to individuals to lower blood pressure can be summarized as follows:

1. Reduce salt intake to the lowest practicable level.
2. Increase potassium intake to more than 100 mmol per day.
3. Reduce fat intake, particularly saturated fat, and if necessary substitute monounsaturated fats.
4. Eat more fruit and vegetables.
5. Avoid excessive alcohol intake – limit intake to 3 units a day (1 unit = 10 ml or 8 g alcohol).

Although dietary advice is immensely important to

the individual patient with high blood pressure, it is also essential to ensure that the whole population eats a more healthy diet to prevent or delay the development of atherosclerosis.

Salt intake

There is now strong evidence that a high salt intake has an important role in blood pressure regulation. Evidence for this comes from six different sources.

Epidemiological studies Comparisons between different countries and within the same country suggest that the amount of salt in the diet plays an important part in determining population blood pressure levels.

Intervention studies Intervention studies involve altering the salt intake of a large group of subjects who are then followed for a reasonable length of time to see if there is any change in blood pressure. The best-known of these is a well-controlled study from Holland on newborn babies, which clearly showed that babies on a lower salt intake for 6 months had a significantly lower blood pressure than those on a normal salt intake; follow-up of a subgroup after 15 years showed that this difference in blood pressure was maintained. A further study compared two villages in Portugal; the population of the village that reduced salt intake had a significantly lower blood pressure at the end of the observation period than the village that did not.

Migration studies Such studies include observations of populations who have moved from one environment to another. The best-known of these studied rural Kenyans after migration to the town, and it was found that there was a large rise in blood pressure which was associated with the increase in salt intake and the fall in potassium intake.

Evidence in animals Almost all of the genetic and experimental animal models of hypertension are either caused or exacerbated by an increase in salt intake.

Human genetic studies All of the genetic causes of high blood pressure so far described in humans involve either a direct genetic defect in the kidney's ability to excrete sodium or an imposed defect on the kidney's ability to excrete sodium and a worsening of the high blood pressure.

Studies of salt restriction The effects of salt restriction are discussed below.

Salt restriction

Many experiments in animals, including humans, have shown that once blood pressure has been raised, removing the cause does not necessarily lower the blood pressure to normal. Nevertheless, it has been known for many years that reducing the amount of salt in the diet does cause a fall in blood pressure. The first report was in patients with renal disease from the early 1900s. This study showed a fall in blood pressure when patients were put on a reduced-salt diet. Interestingly, as only chloride excretion could be measured, the fall in blood pressure was attributed not to a reduction in sodium, but to a reduction in chloride intake. This study, undertaken in France, was largely ignored, as were the much more carefully controlled studies by Allen and Sherrill in the early 1920s, despite the fact that there was no effective treatment for high blood pressure at that time, and patients with severe hypertension were known to die within a few months. It was not until the 1940s when Kempner, working on a rather obscure concept unrelated to salt, decided to give patients with severe hypertension a rice and fruit diet. On this diet patients experienced regression of the eye changes of malignant hypertension, reduction in the size of the heart, and in some cases the prevention of progressive kidney impairment. Kempner originally did not attribute the fall in blood pressure to the reduced salt intake, but further well-controlled studies showed that the major factor in lowering blood pressure was the reduction of salt intake rather than the reduction in protein or fat intake. The usual reduction in salt intake was to around 10 mmol sodium per day; for reasons that are not clear the diet consisted entirely of boiled rice and fruit which, unsurprisingly, was somewhat tedious for most patients. With the advent of diuretic drugs in the mid 1950s salt restriction was largely abandoned by many physicians.

However, more recent work has shown that a reduction of sodium intake from 160 mmol (10 g salt per day) to 80 mmol (5 g salt per day) reduces blood pressure. These initial studies were dismissed as they were not well controlled. However, in the late 1970s a double-blind study of salt restriction was conducted in patients with mild to moderate essential hypertension. Patients were instructed on how to reduce salt intake from approximately 10 g to 5 g a day. Once they had adjusted to this diet they were entered into a double-blind, randomized, crossover study, where salt tablets in the form of 'slow sodium' (a wax-encapsulated form of salt that is well tolerated and absorbed) were then given in an amount calculated to bring their salt intake back to their usual intake. This was compared with 1 month of giving placebo tablets that contained no salt. This short-term study, and subsequent studies including a large study from Australia, clearly demonstrated that salt restriction causes a fall in blood pressure in patients with essential hypertension. There is a dose response to salt restriction: in a study of three sodium intakes – 200 mmol, 100 mmol and 50 mmol per day – there was a stronger lowering effect on blood pressure as salt intake was reduced. Indeed, the reduction of daily sodium intake from 200 mmol to 50 mmol was associated with a greater fall in blood pressure than that seen in double-blind studies of a single antihypertensive drug (**Fig. 1**). Patients were then followed up for a year on the 50 mmol diet and it was shown that the blood pressure remained at its reduced level after 1 year of salt restriction.

These studies clearly show the efficacy of salt restriction in patients with high blood pressure who are not receiving drug treatment. However, many studies have now demonstrated that salt restriction not only lowers blood pressure on its own, but is also additive to antihypertensive drugs, in particular drugs that block the renin-angiotensin system, i.e. beta-blockers, the angiotensin converting enzyme (ACE) inhibitors and the angiotensin II antagonists (**Fig. 2**). This is perhaps not surprising as part of the mechanism whereby salt restriction lowers blood pressure is mediated through the response of the renin-angiotensin system.

The effects of salt restriction have been compared with diuretic therapy when patients are receiving an ACE inhibitor. In a double-blind study of patients treated with captopril the effect of salt restriction was directly compared with the addition of a thiazide diuretic. Salt restriction was found to be as effective as adding a diuretic to the ACE inhibitor, with the advantage that with the salt restriction there was no fall in plasma potassium levels, whereas with the diuretic there was a significant fall (**Fig. 3**).

The mechanism for the fall in blood pressure with salt restriction is not clear, but appears to be due in part to suppression of the renin-angiotensin system as blood pressure rises. When salt intake is reduced there is less rise in renin and therapy in angiotensin II levels than would occur in subjects with normal blood pressure. This lack of the normal compensatory rise in angiotensin II seems to be why the blood pressure falls, and this has been directly demonstrated both with angiotensin II antagonists and converting enzyme inhibitors. These findings also explain why some subjects with high blood pressure have a greater fall in blood pressure with salt restriction than others, in a similar fashion to that occurring with diuretics. In particular, there is some evi-

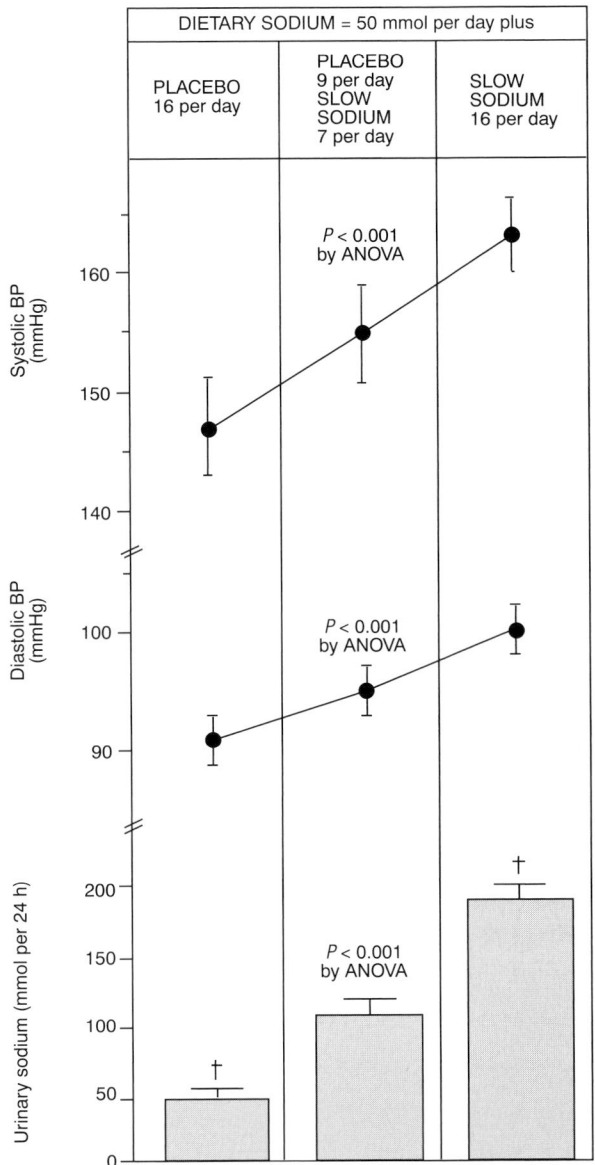

Figure 1 Blood pressure (BP) and urinary sodium excretion in 20 patients randomized in a double-blind, crossover trial of three salt intakes: 200 mmol, 100 mmol and 50 mmol per day for 1 month each. Note the progressive fall in blood pressure with increasing salt restriction; the fall in systolic pressure is 16 mmHg and in diastolic pressure is 9 mmHg when intake is reduced from 200 mmol to 50 mmol per day. ANOVA, analysis of variance.

dence that black patients and older patients are more sensitive to the effects of salt restriction alone because they have a more suppressed renin system. However, once the renin system is blocked, e.g. with a converting enzyme inhibitor, all subjects irrespective of age, race or blood pressure have large falls in blood pressure with salt restriction.

When all studies of salt restriction are included in a meta-analysis it is clear that a modest reduction in salt from the current Western intake of

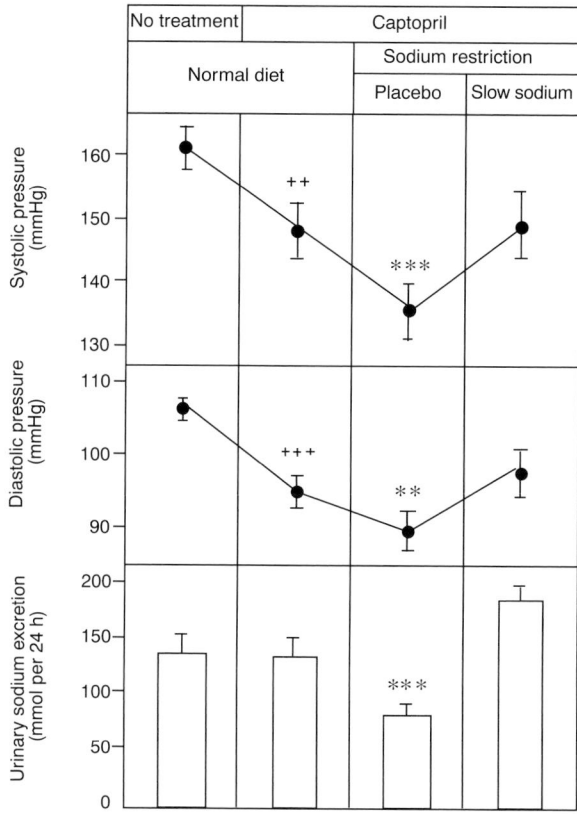

Figure 2 Average supine systolic and diastolic blood pressure and urinary sodium excretion after 1 month's observation and no treatment; after 1 month's treatment with captopril 50 mg twice daily; and at the end of each month of randomized crossover trial of slow sodium tablets compared with matching placebo. During the crossover trial patients moderately restricted their sodium intake. Note the antihypertensive activity of captopril is effectively doubled by moderate salt restriction. Comparing measurements on slow sodium with placebo, **P <0.01, ***P <0.001; comparing no treatment with captopril alone, ++P <0.01, +++P < 0.001.

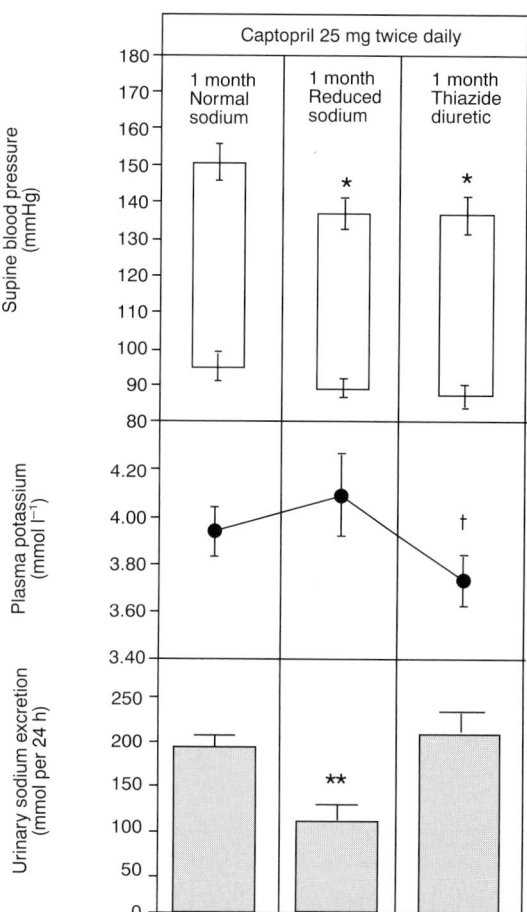

Figure 3 Moderate salt restriction is as effective as diuretic drug treatment when patients with essential hypertension are receiving an ACE inhibitor. Values are shown for 24 h urinary sodium excretion, blood pressure and plasma potassium in subjects with essential hypertension at the end of 1 month's treatment with (1) 25 mg captopril twice daily, (2) 25 mg captopril twice daily and moderate salt reduction, and (3) 25 mg captopril twice daily and 25 mg hydrochlorothiazide once daily. *P < 0.5 versus captopril alone; †P < 0.5 versus captopril alone and versus captopril combined with moderate reduction in salt intake; **P <0.1.

approximately 9 g to 6 g a day is an effective way of lowering blood pressure in most patients with high blood pressure. However, in the normotensive population, while there are significant falls in blood pressure, the absolute falls in both systolic and diastolic blood pressure are less, although a meta-analysis in normotensive subjects showed that the salt restriction in these studies only lasted for an average of 10 days. It would seem likely from a variety of different sources of evidence that the mechanism whereby salt restriction lowers blood pressure is not the same as the mechanism whereby exposure to a high salt intake over a lifetime may result in a gradual increase in blood pressure. To address, therefore, the problem of salt causing high blood pressure, longer-term studies need to be done.

The longest study of salt restriction so far comes from Holland, where around 500 newborn babies were randomized into a double-blind study: half the babies were put on a reduced salt intake and the others were maintained on their normal salt intake for a period of 6 months. During this time there was a gradual and progressively increasing difference in systolic blood pressure; by the end of 6 months the babies on the reduced salt intake had a systolic pressure 2.1 mmHg lower than those on the usual salt intake ($P < 0.001$). At this time the difference in diets was discontinued. However, a subgroup of these babies were followed up at the age of 15 years. After correction for factors that might alter blood pressure, there was a continuing and if anything slightly greater difference in blood pressure between subjects who in the first 6 months of life had been on the lower salt intake, compared with those on the normal salt intake.

This study demonstrates the importance of salt intake early in life in determining blood pressure levels subsequently. These results, and the fact that some young children may have diets that are high in salt, indicate that we should be considering dietary changes much earlier in life than we have previously in the prevention of cardiovascular disease.

Potassium intake

Much epidemiological evidence suggests that potassium intake is directly related to blood pressure levels both within communities and between communities. The INTERSALT study clearly demonstrated the importance of potassium, which appeared to be independent of salt intake. Evidence from animal models of high blood pressure suggest that increasing potassium intake will lower blood pressure and in particular will prevent the effect of an increase in salt intake on blood pressure. There are no intervention studies with potassium but a growing body of evidence suggests that increasing potassium intake does result in reduction of blood pressure.

The concept that increasing potassium intake might cause a fall in blood pressure goes back to the 1930s when it was found that if potassium chloride was given to patients with heart failure there was a reduction in body weight with a loss of sodium in the urine; the potassium seemed to act as a diuretic. In spite of this knowledge and the fact that the Kempner rice and fruit diet increased potassium intake, it was not until the early 1980s that a controlled study of potassium supplementation was performed in patients with high blood pressure to see if there was any fall in pressure. This study from Japan clearly demonstrated that for patients with high blood pressure on a normal Japanese diet (i.e. with a high salt intake), increasing potassium chloride resulted in a fall in blood pressure. This was followed by a double-blind study of potassium chloride supplementation in patients with untreated essential hypertension who were on a more moderate intake of sodium, the equivalent of what is normally consumed in the UK, i.e. around 9 g sodium chloride or 144 mmol sodium per day. Patients who had been off treatment for some months and were used to the measurements, were entered into a double-blind, randomized, crossover study, involving 1 month of 8 slow potassium tablets (64 mmol potassium chloride daily) and 1 month of placebo. The increase in potassium intake of 64 mmol per day was calculated to approximately double potassium intake. This increase in potassium intake caused a significant fall in blood pressure, both systolic and diastolic (**Fig. 4**).

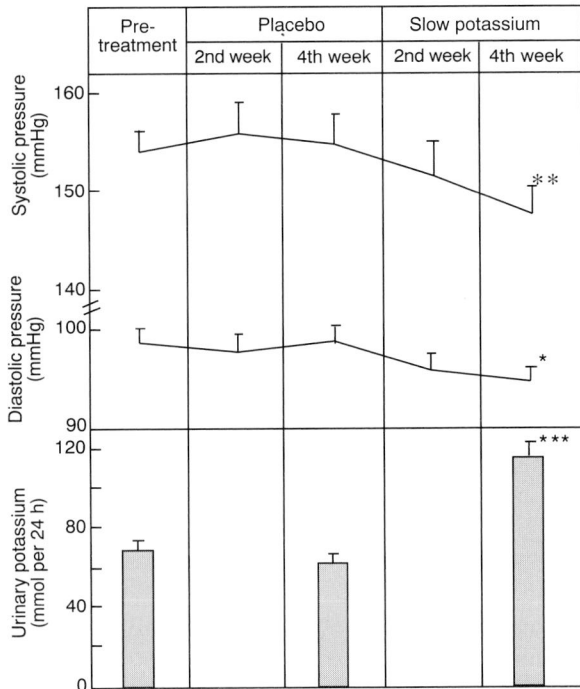

Figure 4 Average systolic and diastolic blood pressures and urinary potassium excretion before and during treatment with potassium and placebo. *$P < 0.05$, **$P < 0.025$, ***$P < 0.001$.

A number of similar studies have all confirmed that an increase in potassium intake results in a fall in blood pressure.

There are a variety of different ways in which potassium could lower blood pressure, although the mechanism is not yet clear. Increasing potassium intake causes an increase in sodium excretion and a small reduction in total body sodium. Some studies have suggested that increasing potassium intake might inhibit the expected increase in renin release with this loss of sodium. If this is so, it is not surprising that blood pressure falls. There is also some evidence to suggest that increases in potassium intake might inhibit sympathetic function and also inhibit the sodium-potassium pump, both of which might reduce blood pressure. Animal studies suggest that the higher the salt intake, the greater the effect of potassium chloride on blood pressure. This was tested in humans by studying the effect of potassium supplementation in patients who were already restricting their salt intake; disappointingly, the increase in potassium intake seemed to cause no fall in blood pressure, though it is possible that a larger study with a greater power to detect a difference might have found a fall in pressure. A recent study using a mineral salt with a mixture of sodium and potassium as a substitute for salt used in cooking and also in the processed foods provided, did show that with a small reduction of sodium intake and a small increase in potassium intake there was a fall in blood pressure in a population of elderly hypertensive subjects.

The role of chloride

There has been some controversy in the studies where salt and potassium chloride have been used as to whether the fall in blood pressure is attributable to the reduction in sodium, the reduction in chloride or the increase in potassium. It is now clear that the combined reduction of both sodium and chloride, both extracellular ions, is responsible for the blood pressure changes. In studies where sodium citrate, phosphate or bicarbonate have been added when patients with high blood pressure are on a low sodium intake there is no increase in blood pressure, but there is a rise when the same amount of sodium is given in the form of sodium chloride. It seems that only a manoeuvre that decreases extracellular volume, such as occurs when both sodium and chloride intake are reduced, will cause a fall in pressure.

In relation to potassium, few supplementation studies have looked at ions other than chloride; however, in a carefully controlled study, increasing potassium intake by eating more fruit and vegetables resulted in a highly significant fall in blood pressure, suggesting that it is the potassium *per se* and not the potassium chloride that produces the fall in blood pressure. This finding is of some importance because it suggests that increasing potassium intake by eating more fruit and vegetables, which would be recommended as part of an antiatherosclerotic diet, would have the added benefit of causing a fall in blood pressure.

In relation to sodium intake the above is of little consequence currently, as 95% of our sodium intake is in the form of sodium chloride. Only very small amounts of other sodium salts are consumed. However, it may be of importance to the food industry and in societies where it is common to drink mineral water containing large amounts of sodium bicarbonate, as it is possible that these other salts of sodium do not have the same effect on blood pressure. It is important to realize that if a nonchloride sodium salt is consumed and there is potassium chloride in the diet it is likely that the body will sense this as sodium chloride.

The practicality of reducing salt intake and increasing potassium intake

Partly as a result of the unimaginative Kempner rice and fruit diet and its lack of acceptance by many patients, reducing salt intake has been considered difficult to achieve. This concept is erroneous and it is possible for people to reduce salt intake; the majority of people find that after a period of a few weeks food tastes better without the addition of large amounts of salt. When instructing individual subjects how to reduce salt intake, it is vital to learn the main sources of salt in their diet. The first step in doing this is to assess their salt intake. While to some extent this can be estimated from taking a dietary history, this method is notoriously inaccurate, particularly as the amount of salt added in cooking and at the table may be variable and difficult to quantify, and the amount of salt in processed foods also varies widely. The best way of assessing the amount of salt in the diet is to obtain two 24 h consecutive urine collections and measure the sodium and potassium excreted. These values will accurately reflect the salt intake over the preceding 2 days. The 24 h urine collection must be done accurately, and urinary creatinine excretion is measured in order to give some index of the completeness of the urine collection. Many individuals claim that they are not eating salt but are unaware that large amounts of salt can be added to the food in the form of stock cubes, soya sauce or (particularly in the Afro-Caribbean community) dried salted fish. Individuals are also unaware of salt added to processed foods, bread being a major source of salt in the UK, as are commercially prepared soups, instant noodles and ready-prepared meals. It is vital, both in assessing salt intake and in advising how to reduce salt intake, that whoever cooks in the household is also involved in these discussions.

How to reduce salt intake

Individuals who wish to reduce their salt intake should be advised:

- not to add any salt to the food at the table;
- not to add salt to food that is being cooked at home.

It is important to inform patients that initially the food will taste bland, particularly if they are used to eating heavily salted food. However, after about a month on a lower salt intake the salt taste receptors become much more sensitive, and a much lower sodium concentration gives the same salty taste. It is important that patients and their families are warned of this, otherwise they may be put off in the first few weeks. Once they have become adjusted they will find that they prefer food without the addition of salt and indeed the highly salted foods that they used to eat may become unpalatable. This can be a strong reinforcing factor in maintaining a reduced salt intake. A useful analogy for patients is that of sugar in tea and coffee; giving up sugar may be difficult at first, but eventually tea or coffee with sugar added becomes very distasteful. Exactly the same applies to salt.

While not adding salt at the table and in cooking may result in a reduction in salt intake, particularly if patients cook and eat at home, problems arise where households consume large amounts of processed food, or where individuals eat outside the home, particularly in canteens or restaurants.

Processed food   Estimates in the UK have suggested that about 70–80% of salt intake comes from processed food. A major source of salt in most developed countries is bread, where each slice contains approximately half a gram of salt. Other major sources of salt are some breakfast cereals, ready-prepared meals and instant food. The difficulty for individuals is compounded by the fact that not all food is labelled with the sodium content, and such information is difficult to interpret. In the UK the food label states the number of grams of sodium per 100 g of food. It is difficult to explain to patients how sodium relates to salt, and how to calculate the amount of salt from eating a particular food product. For those who wish to calculate the salt content the sodium value should be multiplied by 2.5. Not only is the sodium concentration important, but the amount of that particular food eaten will determine its contribution to total salt intake; an advantage of the American food labelling system is that one serving of the food is labelled with a percentage of the recommended daily proportion of each nutrient. For example, a packet of crisps will have not only the sodium concentration per 100 g, but also the percentage that the packet of crisps represents in the daily recommended intake of sodium.

If the patient is prepared to give up adding salt to food at the table, using salt at home in cooking, and eating processed foods that contain high amounts of salt, it is easy to reduce salt intake from the average intake of around 9 g salt (144 mmol sodium) per day to around 6 g salt (96 mmol sodium) per day. To reduce salt intake further requires the provision of a reduced-salt or salt-free bread. Most bread varies between 0.5 g and 0.7 g of sodium per 100 g of bread. Foods containing below 0.3 g sodium per 100 g will be found to be not too salted and a useful marker is that this is approximately the concentration of sodium in our own body fluids.

For patients who do not eat at home, or who eat out frequently, it is much more difficult to restrict salt intake. Most fast foods contain large amounts of salt, e.g. pizza and hamburgers. Meals in canteens and restaurants vary in their salt content. Most restaurants now, with or without warning, will be prepared to produce foods with less salt. The most awkward situation can be when eating with friends. It is important for patients who wish to reduce salt intake to realize that one highly salt meal does not matter; what matters is the salt intake over a long period.

Mineral salts or salt substitutes   Mineral salts usually contain a mixture of sodium chloride and potassium chloride in varying amounts, sometimes with added magnesium and lysine. Many people do not like the bitter aftertaste of the potassium chloride. However, people who have difficulty in giving up salt in their food may find that this is acceptable, and it is certainly better than using pure sodium chloride. Indeed, as mentioned above, studies have shown that using mineral salts does lower blood pressure in elderly patients with high blood pressure, and a more recent study in diabetic patients showed a fall in blood pressure when they switched to using a mineral salt.

Other dietary factors that may modulate blood pressure

Evidence that other nutrients may alter blood pressure is not substantial and most of the studies are of poor quality, or show little or no effect.

Magnesium   There is some evidence in animal models of high blood pressure that when the animals are deprived of magnesium, increasing magnesium intake may lower blood pressure. However, there are few studies in humans and these studies show contradictory results. One carefully controlled double-blind study of magnesium supplementation showed that in spite of an increase in plasma magnesium and an increase in urinary magnesium there was no fall in blood pressure in patients with essential hypertension who were not on any other treatment (**Fig. 5**). The consensus is that if magnesium does play a role it is only important in those who have a low magnesium intake. As magnesium is widely distributed in most foodstuffs this is unlikely to occur in most developed countries, at least for those who eat a varied diet.

Calcium   There has been widespread publicity from the Dairy Council in the USA about the possibility that an increase in calcium intake may lower blood pressure. This claim was based on poorly controlled studies, and more carefully controlled studies that have now shown no fall in blood pressure with calcium supplementation in patients with essential hypertension (**Fig. 6**).

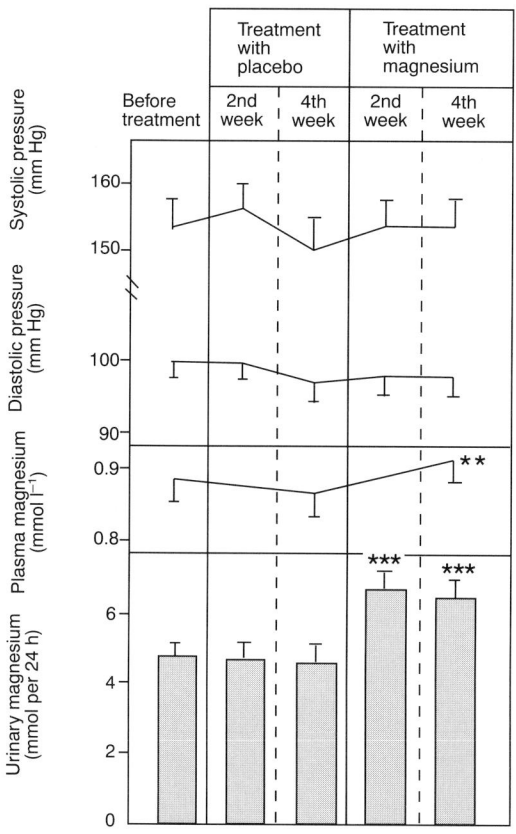

Figure 5 Systolic and diastolic blood pressures, plasma magnesium concentrations, and urinary excretion of magnesium before and during treatment with magnesium and placebo. **P < 0.02; ***P < 0.001 for differences between treatment with magnesium and placebo.

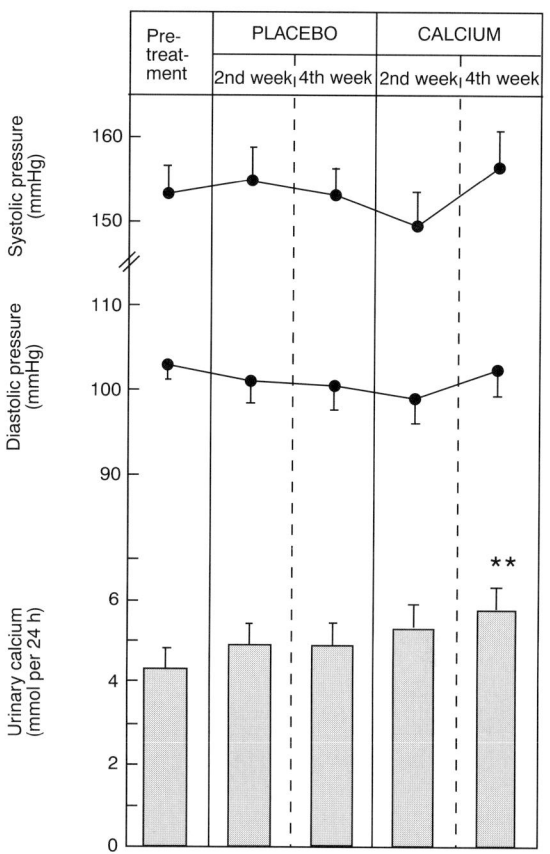

Figure 6 Average systolic and diastolic blood pressures and urinary excretion of calcium before and during treatment with calcium and placebo. Results are means ± SEM. **P < 0.025 for difference between treatment with calcium and placebo.

Garlic Garlic has always been felt to have a beneficial effect on health, and it was suggested for many years that it might lower blood pressure. However, there is considerable confusion about what are the active ingredients of garlic and how garlic is best consumed, with considerable disputes amongst the makers of most forms of garlic as to whether their particular preparation has more of the active ingredients. It seems at present that the best way to take garlic is freshly crushed. However, the evidence that it lowers blood pressure is poor and comes from badly designed and badly controlled studies. There is therefore a need for a carefully controlled study of garlic to determine whether it has any effect on blood pressure.

Fat Some early studies suggested that reducing fat intake might lower blood pressure. Disappointingly, more carefully controlled studies have shown no effect on blood pressure of reducing fat intake. Other studies also suggested that supplementing the diet with fish oil might have an antihypertensive effect, but again better-controlled studies have not substan-

tiated this claim. Nevertheless it makes sense for all patients with high blood pressure to reduce their saturated fat intake, to lower their blood cholesterol, in order to reduce their risk of developing vascular disease.

Alcohol There is good epidemiological evidence to suggest that alcohol intake relates to blood pressure – the higher the average alcohol intake, the higher the blood pressure in the population. However, this effect of alcohol seems to be short-lived; if individuals stop drinking alcohol, their blood pressure initially rises and then falls. Experimental evidence also suggests this is correct. It seems therefore that alcohol does not cause sustained hypertension, but merely transient rises in blood pressure. This concept supports the epidemiological finding that moderate alcohol consumption does not predispose to vascular disease, but if anything has a protective effect. Moderate consumption of alcohol seems to have little effect on blood pressure and may have a small protective cardiovascular effect; patients with high blood pressure should be counselled not to drink excessively, i.e. to drink no more than 3 units per day and in particular to avoid binge drinking, because when they stop drinking alcohol there may be large rises in blood pressure.

Hypertension and Other Conditions

Obesity

Epidemiological evidence suggests that obesity predisposes to high blood pressure, and several studies have shown that when obese subjects lose weight there is a fall in blood pressure. However, this fall in blood pressure has in part been associated with the fall in salt intake that occurs with a reduction in food intake, and may also be due to problems of measurement of blood pressure in obese patients with large arms, which tend to give artificially high blood pressure readings unless large cuff sizes are used. Epidemiologically, abdominal obesity (particularly in men) seems to increase the risk of vascular disease, whereas in women fat distributed around the hips does not seem to cause any increase in risk for premature cardiovascular disease. Nevertheless, it makes sense for overweight subjects with high blood pressure to lose weight.

Diabetes and glucose intolerance

Diabetes and glucose intolerance are major risk factors for the development of premature vascular disease. Diabetic patients tend to have high blood pressure and there is increasing evidence that patients with diabetes should have their blood pressure well controlled. These people are particularly sensitive to the effects of salt restriction, and in many cases their blood pressure can be controlled by a reduction in salt intake.

Atherosclerosis

The aim of lowering blood pressure is to prevent the damaging effects of high blood pressure. By far the most important of these is the effect on the development of vascular disease. However, there is no sense in reducing one risk factor alone, and there is good evidence that by reducing all of the risk factors there is a greater protective effect. In the Western world and increasingly in countries that are becoming developed, consumption of a high-fat diet is thought to be a prerequisite for the development of atherosclerosis. In Japan fat intake was characteristically low and salt intake was high; the Japanese generally had high blood pressure and a high mortality rate from the direct effects of blood pressure such as cerebral haemorrhage, but vascular disease and in particular coronary heart disease were uncommon

because of the low fat intake. However, in Japanese who migrated to the USA and increased their dietary fat intake, the mortality rate from vascular disease also increased.

There is growing evidence that oxidation of low-density lipoproteins that carry cholesterol may play an important role in the development of premature vascular disease. Free radical scavengers can inhibit this oxidation. These substances are mainly present in fruit and vegetables. Therefore when advising patients with high blood pressure about their diet it is clearly important not only to focus on the salt and potassium intake, but also to encourage a greater consumption of fresh fruit and vegetables. This will result in an increase in potassium and antioxidant intake, with no increase in salt or fat. It is also important to encourage patients to reduce their fat intake.

Other Adverse Effects of Salt

While high blood pressure is the most important adverse effect of a high salt intake, there is increasing evidence for other adverse consequences, independent of the effect of salt on blood pressure. Salt intake determines the amount of extracellular fluid present in the body, and this can be illustrated in subjects who switch from a high-sodium diet (200 mmol) to one containing 50 mmol sodium – there is a loss of extracellular fluid of about 1.5 litres or weight loss of 1.5 kg. Salt intake therefore plays an important part in conditions where there is retention of sodium and water such as occurs in heart failure and nephrotic syndrome, and can also exacerbate premenstrual or cyclical oedema and idiopathic oedema. Many women find that these symptoms virtually disappear if they reduce their salt intake. Salt intake has been shown in animals to have a direct effect on stroke independent of its effect on blood pressure, and evidence suggests this may be true in humans as well. Interestingly, potassium may have the opposite effect. Salt intake is an independent determinant of the size of the left ventricle in patients with high blood pressure. A high salt intake has been shown to play an aggravating role in asthma, and this is perhaps not surprising as a high salt intake leads to greater reactivity of smooth muscle, both arterial and bronchial. A high salt intake has also been associated with cancer of the stomach; the most likely mechanism is through the irritant effect of salt on the stomach lining, making infection with *Helicobacter pylori* more likely.

Preliminary evidence that suggests that salt is a major aggravating factor in the development of bone demineralization, leading to osteoporosis. It has been known for many years that salt is the most important determinant of urinary calcium excretion, more important than calcium intake itself. Until recently it was thought that when urinary calcium excretion increased with salt intake, it was matched by an increase in absorption from the gastrointestinal tract. However, evidence particularly in postmenopausal women has shown that when salt intake is increased there is an increase in calcium excretion, with an increase in absorption but also evidence of mobilization of calcium from the bone. A study in postmenopausal women who had measurements of hip bone density and were then followed for 2 years showed that the most important factor determining the change in hip bone density was the salt intake, i.e. the higher the salt intake, the greater the loss of hip bone density. Patients with high blood pressure have been known for many years to have an increase in calcium excretion and evidence of mobilization of calcium from bone. Rats with inherited hypertension develop severe osteoporosis if they are allowed to live long enough. It is possible that patients with high blood pressure are at greater risk from developing osteoporosis than normotensive subjects, although this is likely to be confused by the fact that it has been shown that diuretic drugs reduce calcium excretion, cause a positive calcium balance and reduce the numbers of hip bone fractures. Salt restriction is also known to reduce calcium excretion and cause a positive calcium balance, but as yet no studies have looked at whether it reduces the number of fractures that occur. Nevertheless, it seems prudent that hypertensive patients and the public should reduce salt intake in the expectation that this will have a beneficial effect on osteoporosis, although other factors known to be important in osteoporosis should also be addressed as well.

See also: **Calcium**: Physiology. **Coronary Heart Disease**: Lipid Theory of Coronary Heart Disease. **Diabetes Mellitus**: Secondary Complications and Their Prevention. **Hypertension**: Physiology. **Magnesium**: Physiology, Dietary Sources and Requirements. **Obesity**: Complications of Obesity. **Potassium**: Physiology, Dietary Sources and Requirements. **Salt**: Epidemiology. **Sodium**: Physiology.

Further Reading

Allen FM and Sherril JW (1922) The treatment of arterial hypertension. *Journal of Metabolic Research* 2:429–545.

Ambard L and Beaujard E (1904) Causes de l'hypertension arterielle. *Archives of General Medicine* 1:520–533.

Antonios TF and MacGregor GA (1996) Salt – more adverse effects. *Lancet* 348:250–251.

Australian National Health and Medical Research Council Dietary Salt Study Management Committee (1989) Fall in blood pressure with moderate reduction in dietary salt intake in mild hypertension. *Lancet* i:399–402.

Cappuccio FP, Elliott P, Allender PS, Pryer J, Follman DA and Cutler JA (1995) Epidemiologic association between dietary calcium intake and blood pressure: a meta-analysis of published data. *American Journal of Epidemiology* 142:935–945.

Forte JG, Pereira Miguel JM, Pereira Miguel MJ, de Padua F and Rose G (1989) Salt and blood pressure: a community trial. *Journal of Human Hypertension* 3:179–184.

Geleijnse JM, Hofman A, Witteman JCM, Hazebroek AAJM, Valkenburg HA and Grobbee DE (1996) Long-term effects of neonatal sodium restriction on blood pressure. *Journal of Hypertension* 14:S210.

Geleijnse JM, Witteman JC, Bak AA, den Breeijen JH and Grobbee, DE (1994) Reduction in blood pressure with a low sodium, high potassium, high magnesium salt in older subjects with mild to moderate hypertension. *British Medical Journal* 309:436–440.

Hoffman A, Hazebroek A and Valenburg HA (1983) A randomised trial of sodium intake and blood pressure in newborn infants. *Journal of the American Medical Association* 250:370–373.

Iimura O, Kijima K, Kikuchi K, Ando T, Nakao T and Takigami Y (1981) Studies on the hypotensive effect of high potassium intake in patients with essential hypertension. *Clinical Science* 61:77s–80s.

INTERSALT Cooperative Research Group (1988) Intersalt: an international study of electrolyte excretion and blood pressure. Results for 24 hour urinary sodium and potassium excretion. *British Medical Journal* 297:319–328.

Kempner W (1948) Treatment of hypertensive vascular disease with rice diet. *American Journal of Medicine* 4:545–577.

MacGregor GA and Dawes PM (1976) Angiotensin II blockade in normal subjects and essential hypertensive patients. *Clinical Science and Molecular Medicine* 51:193s–196s.

MacGregor GA, Markandu ND, Best FE et al. (1982) Double-blind randomised crossover trial of moderate sodium restriction in essential hypertension. *Lancet* i:531–535.

MacGregor GA, Markandu ND, Singer DRJ, Cappuccio FP, Shore AC and Sagnella GA (1987) Moderate sodium restriction with angiotensin converting enzyme inhibitor in essential hypertension: a double blind study. *British Medical Journal* 294:531–534.

MacGregor GA, Smith SJ, Markandu ND, Banks RA and Sagnella GA (1982) Moderate potassium supplementation in essential hypertension. *Lancet* ii:565–570.

Poulter NK, Khaw KT, Hopwood BEC et al. (1990) The Kenyan Luo migration study: observations on the initiation of a rise in blood pressure. *British Medical Journal* 300:967–972.

Singer DRJ, Markandu ND, Cappuccio FP, Miller MA, Sagnella GA and MacGregor GA (1995) Reduction of salt intake during converting enzyme inhibitor treatment compared with addition of a thiazide. *Hypertension* 25:1042–1044.

Interrelationships Between Hypertension and Diabetes

P McKeigue and **G Davey**, London School of Hygiene and Tropical Medicine, London, UK

Copyright © 1998 Academic Press

Non-insulin-dependent diabetes mellitus and impaired glucose tolerance are consistently associated with hypertension, independently of obesity. These associations form part of a cluster of physiological disturbances associated with insulin resistance and central obesity in the general population. The mechanisms by which hypertension is related to glucose intolerance are poorly understood. This article reviews the epidemiological and physiological studies of the relationship between hypertension and glucose intolerance, and examines the implications for management of these disorders in practice.

Association of Hypertension with Glucose Intolerance and Obesity

When people with non-insulin-dependent diabetes are compared with people with normal glucose tolerance, the prevalence of hypertension is generally around twice as high, average systolic pressures are about 10 mmHg higher, and average diastolic pressures are about 3 mmHg higher. In most studies blood pressures are as high in people with impaired glucose tolerance as in people with diabetes. This makes it unlikely that the hypertension in diabetic patients develops as a complication of long-standing hyperglycaemia. The associations of raised blood pressure with glucose intolerance are not explained by adjusting for body mass index. Body mass index is only a crude measure of obesity, and it is possible that adjusting for percentage body fat (measured by techniques such as densitometry) would account more fully for the association of glucose intolerance with raised blood pressure. Even if the association between glucose intolerance and raised blood pressure could be accounted for by obesity and body fat distribution, we would still have to explain why obesity leads to raised blood pressure. Understanding the relationship of hypertension to glucose intolerance is therefore likely to depend on understanding the effects of obesity on blood pressure. As both glucose intolerance and obesity are associated with resistance to insulin-mediated glucose uptake, researchers have focused on the relationship of hypertension to raised insulin levels and insulin resistance.

Hypertension and Insulin Resistance

Associations of hypertension with raised insulin levels and insulin resistance

The first study to show that serum insulin levels were higher in hypertensive subjects than in normotensive ones was reported in 1966. Subsequent studies showed that the association of raised fasting or postload insulin levels with hypertension persists after controlling for body mass index or for obesity and body fat distribution measured by computed tomography. Insulin levels are higher in the adult offspring of hypertensive parents than in weight-matched controls.

Although differences in insulin levels are generally found in comparisons between hypertensive and normotensive individuals, in cross-sectional population surveys the correlations between resting blood pressures and fasting or postload insulin levels are usually weak (0.2 to 0.3), and are no longer statistically significant after adjusting for weight for height. This applies both in populations of European descent and in non-European populations such as Tanzanians. In several populations of non-European descent – Pima Native Americans, African-Americans and Afro-Caribbeans – cross-sectional associations between insulin levels and blood pressure have been reported to be weak or absent. In Pimas not receiving antihypertensive medication, there was an inverse correlation between 2 h insulin and diastolic blood pressure.

Plasma insulin levels have been found to predict hypertension in some prospective studies. Two Swedish studies have shown significant associations between raised fasting or postload insulin levels and the subsequent development of hypertension in men and in women. The association in women persisted after adjusting for body mass index, waist-hip ratio and weight gain. In contrast, a study of Mexicans and Europeans in Texas found that although raised fasting insulin levels predicted hypertension in univariate analyses, this association did not persist after adjusting for obesity.

Resistance to insulin-mediated glucose uptake can be measured directly by the euglycaemic hyperinsulinaemic clamp technique, in which high plasma insulin levels are maintained by continuous infusion of insulin, and an infusion of glucose is adjusted to maintain blood glucose within the normal fasting range. In individuals with normal glucose tolerance, the high insulin levels are sufficient to suppress hepatic glucose production completely, and thus the rate of glucose infusion required to maintain euglycaemia is a measure of insulin-mediated glucose uptake. Insulin sensitivity is expressed as the rate of glucose infusion divided by the plasma insulin level. Studies using the clamp technique have generally found that nonobese hypertensive individuals of European descent are more insulin-resistant than weight-matched normotensive controls: mean glucose uptake during the hyperinsulinaemic clamp is typically about 20% lower in the hypertensive group. For comparison, when obese glucose-intolerant individuals are compared with lean normoglycaemic individuals, mean glucose uptake is typically about 50% lower in the glucose-intolerant group. Measurement of glucose oxidation by indirect calorimetry during the clamp study has been used to quantify the contribution of oxidative glucose disposal and nonoxidative glucose disposal (mainly storage as glycogen) to total insulin-mediated glucose uptake. Lower nonoxidative glucose disposal in hypertensive individuals appears to account for most of the difference in total glucose disposal between hypertensive and normotensive individuals. As with the association between blood pressure and insulin levels, the relationships between blood pressure and clamp-derived measures of insulin resistance that were detected in US whites were found to be weak or absent in Pima Native Americans and African-Americans.

Can insulin resistance account for the associations of obesity and glucose intolerance with hypertension?

Although the associations of hypertension with glucose intolerance and obesity are strong and consistent, the associations of hypertension with raised insulin levels and insulin resistance in epidemiological and clinical studies are generally weak and less consistent. Thus it is difficult to account for the association of hypertension with glucose intolerance by assigning a primary role in both disorders to insulin resistance. One reason for the weakness of the association between insulin resistance and blood pressure may be that neither of these two variables are measured accurately enough to rank individuals according to their usual level of insulin resistance and blood pressure. Ambulatory blood pressure measurements may be more valid than a single resting blood pressure measurement. In a study of 149 middle-aged subjects with essential hypertension, inverse correlations of ambulatory blood pressure measurements with insulin levels at 2 h postglucose load were found to be statistically significant

even though there were no significant correlations between insulin levels and resting blood pressure. Although insulin resistance is measured more reliably by the clamp technique than by fasting or postload insulin levels, correlations with blood pressure are not consistently stronger in studies that have used clamps compared with studies that have relied on insulin levels only. Although in people with impaired glucose tolerance a high proportion of the material detected by insulin assays may be proinsulin or split proinsulin, raised proinsulin levels are in any case highly correlated with insulin resistance. Another possible explanation for failure to detect associations between raised insulin levels and raised blood pressure is confounding by recent alcohol consumption. Alcohol intake is inversely correlated with insulin levels, possibly because it increases peripheral glucose utilization. Alcohol also has a pressor effect, causing raised blood pressure levels for up to 24 h after alcohol drinking. Recent alcohol intake is thus associated both with lower insulin levels and raised blood pressure levels, confounding the underlying association between insulin and hypertension in studies that do not adjust for it. This confounding is likely to be present in populations such as Japanese men or Native Americans where heavy alcohol consumption is common, but not in groups such as Afro-Caribbean women, where alcohol consumption is low.

Attenuation of the association of hypertension with insulin resistance in obese individuals

Several studies have suggested that the association between raised blood pressure and insulin resistance or raised insulin levels may be stronger in lean individuals than in the obese; this has been reported in a cross-sectional study of Italians and in a prospective study of Mexican-Americans. In contrast, a study of civil servants in Paris found that the correlation between fasting insulin levels and systolic blood pressure was statistically significant only in obese men with elevated plasma glucose concentration. Although associations between insulin resistance and blood pressure are not consistently seen in older adults of Native American or African-American origin, such relationships have generally been detectable when younger individuals who are less obese are studied. Thus when borderline hypertensive African-Americans were compared with normotensive African-Americans, after adjustment for body mass index, the correlations between blood pressure and clamp-derived measurements of insulin resistance were statistically significant only in subjects whose body mass index was less than 28. In Pima Americans relationships between insulin and blood pressure have been detected in childhood but not in adult life.

Haemodynamic effects of insulin

Indirect evidence for a blood pressure-raising effect of insulin has come from experiments demonstrating that short-term infusions of insulin induce renal sodium retention in humans. This effect of insulin infusion is similar in obese and nonobese subjects, despite large differences in insulin-mediated glucose uptake between these groups. Resistance to insulin-mediated glucose uptake is not accompanied by any impairment of the antinatriuretic effect of insulin. However, studies in experimental animals have yielded little support for the idea that hyperinsulinaemia raises blood pressure. In dogs with reduced kidney mass, insulin infusions maintained for up to 28 days do not increase blood pressure or plasma catecholamine levels; in contrast, when dogs are made obese by feeding them high-fat diets, their insulin levels and blood pressures increase. This effect is dependent on maintaining adequate sodium in the diet, and is attenuated by denervation of the kidneys. When Sprague–Dawley rats are made insulin resistant by high-carbohydrate diets, their mean systolic blood pressures increase by about 20 mmHg. Thus blood pressures can be raised in dogs and rats by experimental manipulations that induce insulin resistance, even though chronic hyperinsulinaemia without insulin resistance does not raise blood pressure. Clues to a resolution of this paradox may come from studies of the haemodynamic effects of insulin. Insulin has two opposing haemodynamic effects: it increases sympathetic nervous activity, and it acts as an endothelium-dependent vasodilator.

Effects of insulin on sympathetic nervous activity The associations of hypertension and obesity with sympathetic overactivity have been recognized for some time. Subjects with essential hypertension have enhanced pressor reactivity to noradrenaline infusions. Central obesity is associated both with higher insulin levels and with higher 24 h urinary noradrenaline excretion. Weight loss reduces both blood pressure and plasma noradrenaline concentration.

The effects of obesity on sympathetic activity may be mediated through the effect of raised insulin levels. In humans, euglycaemic hyperinsulinaemia produced by insulin–glucose infusions is accompanied by increased heart rate and increase in plasma noradrenaline levels. This increase in plasma noradrenaline, however, requires plasma insulin levels of 700–1400 pmol l^{-1}, which are unlikely to occur physiologically except in highly insulin-resistant individuals. Plasma noradrenaline is an insensitive measure of sympathetic nerve activity: it represents a mixture of secretion from the adrenal medulla and spillover from sympathetic nerve endings. Direct recording of muscle nerve sympathetic activity by microneurography has shown that euglycaemic infusions of insulin evoke a marked increase in activity. The dose–response curve for insulin and muscle nerve sympathetic activity is flat above insulin levels of about 500 pmol l^{-1}. Thus in contrast to the increase in plasma noradrenaline, which requires supraphysiological levels of insulin, increased muscle nerve sympathetic activity is evoked at physiological plasma insulin levels. Obese subjects with insulin resistance have increased basal muscle sympathetic nerve activity and a blunted response of muscle sympathetic activity to insulin.

One mechanism relating insulin resistance to raised blood pressure could thus be that hyperinsulinaemia increases muscle nerve sympathetic activity and thereby raises peripheral vascular resistance. Somatostatin infusions, which lower insulin levels, reduce blood pressure in obese, hyperinsulinaemic, hypertensive patients.

Insulin as an endothelium-dependent vasodilator Acute intravenous insulin administration leads to vasodilatation in skeletal muscle, mediated by release of nitric oxide from the vascular endothelium. Although infusion of insulin may precipitate profound hypotension in diabetic patients with autonomic neuropathy, it does not lower blood pressure in subjects whose sympathetic nervous system is intact, presumably because the increased sympathetic nervous activity in other vascular beds compensates for the action of insulin as a vasodilator in vascular beds that are insulin- sensitive. Local or systemic elevation of plasma insulin concentration causes increased blood flow and decreased peripheral vascular resistance in the limbs. Insulin decreases leg vascular resistance more than systemic vascular resistance. Insulin thus amplifies its own action on glucose uptake by redistributing blood flow to insulin-sensitive tissues.

Impairment of the vasodilator action of insulin in obesity and hypertension

The sensitivity of blood flow in skeletal muscle to insulin infusion in humans is closely related to the sensitivity of glucose uptake to insulin infusion. In healthy, normotensive volunteers there is an inverse relationship between mean arterial pressure at baseline and the percentage increase in leg blood flow induced by a high-dose insulin infusion. This relationship is independent of adiposity. The vasodilator response to acute elevation of plasma insulin level is blunted in obese individuals, non-insulin-dependent diabetic subjects and those with blood pressures at the upper end of the normal range.

Obesity is thus associated both with raised basal sympathetic activity and with impairment of the action of insulin as a vasodilator. The impairment of insulin-mediated vasodilation can be demonstrated in an oral glucose tolerance test, as well as in eugly-caemic clamp studies. This alteration of the balance between the action of insulin as a vasodilator and the counteracting action of insulin as a vasoconstrictor could lead to chronic elevation of blood pressure, and eventually to structural changes in the vessel wall. It has been suggested that failure of insulin to increase skeletal muscle blood flow may account for at least some of the impairment of insulin-mediated glucose uptake associated with hypertension. More recent evidence, however, suggests that the impairment of insulin-mediated vasodilation in obesity may be only one manifestation of a more general impairment of endothelial nitric oxide release which could affect both vascular tone and sodium balance.

Impairment of endothelial nitric oxide release in obesity and hypertension

Vascular tone and renal sodium handling are regulated by nitric oxide, and inhibition of nitric oxide synthesis produces hypertension in experimental models. The effects of nitric oxide on renal sodium handling are mediated through formation of cyclic guanidine monophosphate (cGMP) as the second messenger. Short-term administration of nitric oxide synthase inhibitors raises blood pressure in humans. Although endothelium-dependent vasodilation is impaired in hypertension, this has generally been considered to be a consequence rather than a cause of hypertension. Blood pressure is likely to depend more directly on nitric oxide release in resistance vessels and the kidney than on nitric oxide release in large arteries. It has been reported that whole-body nitric oxide synthesis is markedly lower in hypertensive than in normotensive individuals. Urinary cGMP excretion, an index of renal nitric oxide production, has been found to be lower in hypertensive than in normotensive individuals after amino acid infusion. No studies of the relationship of whole-body nitric oxide synthesis to obesity or glucose intolerance have been reported, but it has been shown that obesity is associated with impairment of endothelium-dependent vasodilator responses to stimuli such as methacholine. The impairment of insulin-mediated vasodilation in obese or glucose-intolerant individuals could thus be one manifestation of a more general impairment of endothelial nitric oxide release.

Effects of nonesterified fatty acids on glucose uptake and nitric oxide production

The mechanism by which obesity is associated with resistance to insulin-stimulated glucose uptake in muscle is not understood. Recent studies support an old hypothesis that resistance to insulin-stimulated glucose uptake may be caused by lipolysis of triacyl-glycerol stores in muscle cells. Triacylglycerol stores in muscle maintain a supply of nonesterified fatty acids (NEFA) in muscle even when lipolysis in adipocytes (the main source of NEFA in plasma) is suppressed by insulin. Excess supply of NEFA from tri-acylglycerol stores in muscle could cause resistance to insulin-mediated glucose uptake through substrate competition between NEFA and glucose within the muscle cell. In obese individuals, triacylglycerol stores in skeletal muscle cells are increased and hyperinsulinaemia fails to suppress oxidation of intracellular lipid. Insulin resistance in rats can be induced or reversed by dietary or pharmacological interventions that increase or deplete muscle triacylglycerol stores. In obese women insulin resistance correlates with measurements of the triacylglycerol content of thigh muscle by computed tomography, and this relationship is independent of obesity and body fat pattern. Preliminary studies using proton magnetic resonance spectroscopy to measure lipid signals from human calf muscle suggest that insulin resistance is related to the level of triacylglycerol stores in muscle cells, rather than to the level of tri-acylglycerol stores in adipocytes within the muscle mass.

Excess supply of NEFA from local triacylglycerol stores could account also for the impairment of endothelial nitric oxide release in obese individuals. Non esterified fatty acids inhibit nitric oxide synthase activity in endothelial cells in vitro. Excess supply of NEFA from triacylglycerol stores in skeletal muscle could thus lead both to impairment of insulin-mediated glucose uptake through substrate competition between NEFA and glucose, and to impairment of endothelium-dependent vasodilation through the action of NEFA on nitric oxide production. Excess supply of NEFA from local triacyl-glycerol stores in other tissues could lead to a more general impairment of nitric oxide production. Hypertension would result, especially if renal nitric oxide production also was impaired. **Fig. 1** shows the pathways by which glucose intolerance is linked with hypertension according to this hypothesis.

Effects of glucocorticoids

The supply of NEFA from local triacylglycerol stores will depend both on the level of the stores and on

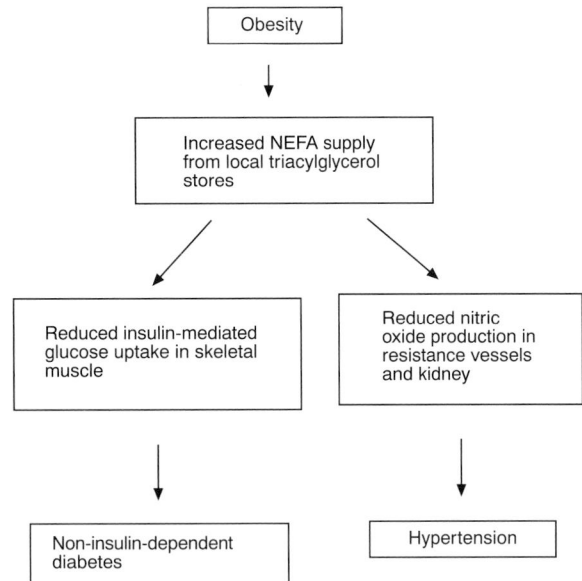

Figure 1 Possible pathways of association between obesity, glucose intolerance and hypertension. NEFA, nonesterified fatty acids.

the activity of hormone-sensitive lipase. In skeletal muscle as in adipocytes, this enzyme is regulated by insulin and adrenaline. Adrenaline is synthesized in skeletal muscle and other tissues by the glucocorticoid-dependent enzyme phenylethanolamine N-methyltransferase. Increased glucocorticoid levels or increased tissue sensitivity to glucocorticoids will thus increase adrenaline levels in muscle and stimulate lipolysis of triacylglycerol stores by hormone-sensitive lipase. This increased NEFA supply would lead to impairment of both insulin-mediated glucose uptake and endothelial nitric oxide production. Glucocorticoid sensitivity, measured by a skin patch test, has been found to vary markedly between individuals and to correlate with both hypertension and insulin resistance. Increased glucocorticoid sensitivity could thus give rise to associations between glucose intolerance and hypertension that are independent of obesity.

Implications for the relations between insulin, obesity and blood pressure

This model can reconcile some of the inconsistencies in epidemiological and experimental studies of the relationships between insulin levels, insulin resistance and blood pressure. Where raised insulin levels occur without impairment of nitric oxide production, as in insulinoma, one would not predict that blood pressure would be raised. In populations where most individuals are lean, a positive association between insulin resistance and hypertension could arise simply because both disorders are conse-

quences of increased supply of NEFA from local triacylglycerol stores. In populations where most individuals are obese and insulin-resistant, this association could be weak or absent because insulin levels in the most insulin-resistant individuals are high enough to overcome the impairment of nitric oxide production.

Relation of Hypertension and Diabetes to Fetal Growth

One explanation that has been advanced to account for the association of hypertension with glucose intolerance resistance is that both these disturbances result from impaired fetal growth. The association of reduced size at birth with hypertension and glucose intolerance in adult life has now been established in several different populations. Although the association between hypertension and glucose intolerance does not disappear with adjustment for birthweight, low birthweight is only an imperfect marker of impaired fetal growth and it is possible that there is still residual confounding by the effects of impaired nutrition *in utero*. More recent studies have suggested that raised insulin levels and insulin resistance in adult life are related more strongly to reduced weight for length at birth than to low birthweight. This does not appear to be the case for blood pressure, which is specifically associated with reduction of both birthweight and birth length. Thus it is unlikely that a single pattern of reduced fetal growth can account for the relationships between raised blood pressure and glucose intolerance. As reduced fetal growth does not predict obesity in adult life, it cannot account for the component of the association between raised blood pressure and glucose intolerance that is attributable to obesity

Implications for Therapy

Nonpharmacologic measures that improve glucose tolerance and reverse insulin resistance – control of obesity and greater physical activity – are generally effective in lowering blood pressure also. The decline in blood pressure with exercise is greater in individuals who are initially sedentary than in those who are initially physically active. In contrast, both diuretics and beta-blockers worsen insulin resistance in hypertensive patients, reducing insulin-mediated glucose disposal by 20–30%. Many patients with hypertension are already insulin-resistant, so one would predict that the risk of developing diabetes would be increased after long-term treatment with diuretics or beta-blockers. In two longitudinal studies in Sweden, treatment for hypertension was associated with increased risk of diabetes at 10-year follow-up. Similar associations were found in a Finnish study in which the risk of developing diabetes between baseline and 4-year follow-up was higher in hypertensive individuals who were treated with beta-blockers or diuretics than in untreated hypertensive individuals at 4-year follow-up.

Other agents such as calcium-channel blockers, angiotensin converting enzyme inhibitors and α_1-adrenergic blockers are neutral or may even alleviate insulin resistance. The effects of different antihypertensive drugs on insulin resistance may relate to their action on systemic vascular resistance: thus beta-blockers and thiazides increase vascular resistance while angiotensin converting enzyme inhibitors and α_1 antagonists increase peripheral blood flow. Experience with newer drugs that alleviate insulin resistance suggests that they may be effective in lowering blood pressure also. Benfluorex, originally developed as a lipid-lowering agent, has been shown to increase insulin sensitivity and also to lower blood pressure in hypertensive men. Thiazolidinediones, developed for their action in reducing insulin resistance, act on a receptor concerned with lipid storage (peroxisome proliferator activator gamma). Pioglitazone, one drug of this class, has been shown to attenuate diet-induced hypertension in rats. The mechanisms by which these two classes of drugs alleviate insulin resistance are not understood; it is at least possible that they act by depleting local triacylglycerol stores in skeletal muscle and other tissues.

Conclusions

Understanding the relationship between hypertension and diabetes is likely to depend on understanding the mechanism by which obesity leads to both raised blood pressure and resistance to insulin-mediated glucose uptake. Epidemiological and experimental evidence does not support the hypothesis that associations of obesity and glucose intolerance with hypertension are mediated through effects of raised insulin levels on blood pressure. Associations between insulin levels and blood pressure are weak or absent in some populations, and experimental studies have failed to demonstrate that chronic hyperinsulinaemia raises blood pressure. Insulin acts both as a vasoconstrictor through its action on the sympathetic nervous system, and as a vasodilator by causing endothelial nitric oxide release. The relationship between insulin levels and blood pressure is likely to depend upon the balance between these two effects. The vasodilator response to insulin and other endothelium-dependent vasodilators is impaired in hypertension, glucose intolerance and obesity. This may be one manifestation of a more general impairment of nitric oxide production that has been found in hypertensive individuals.

The associations of insulin resistance with obesity are most easily explained by the effects of NEFA produced by lipolysis of local triacylglycerol stores. Obesity is associated with increased trigacylglycerol stores in muscle cells as well as adipocytes. Increased NEFA supply in skeletal muscle could cause impaired insulin-mediated glucose uptake through substrate competition. As NEFA have been shown to inhibit nitric oxide production *in vitro*, increased NEFA supply could also underlie the impairment of endothelium-dependent vasodilation in glucose intolerance and obesity and could account for the association of these conditions with hypertension. Interventions that deplete triacylglycerol stores in muscle are likely to reverse both hypertension and insulin resistance. This may be relevant to the effects of drugs such as benfluorex and thiazolidinediones on blood pressure and insulin resistance.

See also: **Alcohol**: Absorption, Metabolism and Physiological Effects; Disease Risk and Beneficial Effects. **Carbohydrates**: Regulation of Carbohydrate Metabolism. **Exercise**: Physiology of Skeletal Muscle. **Fetal Origins of Disease**: Fetal Development and Later Disease. **Glucose**: Metabolism and Maintenance of Blood Glucose Level; Glucose Tolerance. **Hypertension**: Physiology. **Insulin Resistance**: Aetiology and Association with Disease. **Obesity**: Complications of Obesity.

Further Reading

Anderson EA, Balon TW, Hoffman RP, Sinkey CA and Mark AL (1992) Insulin increases sympathetic activity but not blood pressure in borderline hypertensive humans. *Hypertension* 19:621–627.

Barker DJP, Godfrey KM, Osmond C and Bull A (1992) The relation of fetal length, ponderal index and head circumference to blood pressure and the risk of hypertension in adult life. *Paediatric and Perinatal Epidemiology* 6:35–44.

Baron AD (1993) Cardiovascular actions of insulin in humans. Implications for insulin sensitivity and vascular tone. *Baillière's Clinical Endocrinology and Metabolism* 7:961–987.

Baron AD, Brechtel-Hook G, Johnson A and Hardin D (1993) Skeletal muscle blood flow: a possible link between insulin resistance and blood pressure. *Hypertension* 21:129–135.

Bonora E, Zavaroni I, Alpi O *et al.* (1987) Relationship between blood pressure and plasma insulin in non-obese and obese non-diabetic subjects. *Diabetologia* 30:719–723.

Forte P, Copland M, Smith LM, Milne E, Sutherland J and Benjamin N (1997) Basal nitric oxide synthesis in essential hypertension. *Lancet* 349:837–842.

Hall JE, Coleman TG and Mizelle HL (1989) Does chronic hyperinsulinemia cause hypertension? *American Journal of Hypertension* 2:171–173.

Julius S (1991) Autonomic nervous dysfunction in essential hypertension. *Diabetes Care* 14:249–259.

Kennedy B, Elayan H and Ziegler MG (1993) Glucocorticoid induction of epinephrine synthesizing enzyme in rat skeletal muscle and insulin resistance. *Journal of Clinical Investigation* 92:303–307.

Landsberg L, Troisi R, Parker D, Young JB and Weiss ST (1991) Obesity, blood pressure, and the sympathetic nervous system. *Annals of Epidemiology* 1:295–303.

Lithell HO, McKeigue PM, Berglund L, Mohsen R, Lithell U and Leon DA (1996) Relationship of size at birth to non-insulin-dependent diabetes and insulin levels in men aged 50–60 years. *British Medical Journal* 312:406–410.

Steinberg HO, Chaker H, Leaming R, Johnson A, Brechtel G and Baron AD (1996) Obesity/insulin-resistance is associated with endothelial dysfunction – implications for the syndrome of insulin-resistance. *Journal of Clinical Investigation* 97:2601–2610.

Vanhoutte PM (1996) Endothelial dysfunction in hypertension. *Journal of Hypertension* 14 (supplement): S83–93.

Vollenweider P, Randin D, Tappy L, Jequier E, Nicod P and Scherrer U (1994) Impaired insulin-induced sympathetic neural activation and vasodilation in skeletal muscle in obese humans. *Journal of Clinical Investigation* 93:2365–2371.

Walker BR, Best R, Shackleton CHL, Padfield PL and Edwards CRW (1996) Increased vasoconstrictor sensitivity to glucocorticoids in essential-hypertension. *Hypertension* 27:190–196.

HYPOGLYCAEMIA (HYPOGLYCEMIA)

Dietary and Metabolic Aspects

V Marks, University of Surrey, Guildford, UK

Copyright © 1998 Academic Press

Hypoglycaemia, defined as a blood glucose concentration of 2.2 mmol l^{-1} or less, is nothing more, nor less, than a low blood glucose concentration: its definition is therefore necessarily arbitrary. It owes its importance to the fact that it produces brain dysfunction through neuroglycopenia – or the nonavailability of glucose to the neurons.

However, in the minds of many people the word has come to have a totally different meaning that has very little to do with blood glucose concentration but a lot to do with feelings of well-being, of disease and attitudes to life but, above all, with the role of diet in the achievement and maintenance of good health. And while no discussion of the dietary treatment of hypoglycaemia can be meaningful without reference to this concept – referred to, for want of a better term, as 'nonhypoglycemia' – hypoglycaemia will, throughout this article, be used only to describe a measured low blood glucose concentration.

Brain function and hypoglycaemia

The brain malfunction to which hypoglycaemia gives rise will be referred to as neuroglycopenia.

Although the brain is usually spoken of as though incapable of using metabolites other than glucose as sources of energy, it has been known for more than 30 years that the brain is able to utilize the so-called ketone bodies, β-hydroxybutyrate and acetoacetate, almost exclusively, providing their concentration in the blood is high enough such as occurs after prolonged fasting. Under these circumstances both the need for glucose and its supply through gluconeogenesis are drastically reduced. This has immense survival value since it enables fat stores rather than structural muscle and other tissue proteins to be utilized for the maintenance of vital processes. Only when fat stores have become completely exhausted and plasma ketone levels fallen to below normal fasting levels does the brain's demand for glucose rise above the ability of gluconeogenesis to provide it. At this point hypoglycaemia intervenes and portends death from starvation (see later).

The blood glucose concentration

The concentration of glucose in arterial and venous blood, though similar in the fasting subject, may differ by as much as 2.5 mmol l^{-1} for up to 2 h following ingestion of a meal. Consequently it is necessary to define hypoglycaemia in terms of its concentration in arterial (or, failing that, free-flowing capillary) rather than in venous blood, since it is arterial blood glucose that determines glucose supply to the brain, regulates the secretion of insulin and other hormones, and is itself homeostatically controlled.

Failure to appreciate the differences between arterial and venous blood glucose is a major cause of the confusion that has surrounded the recognition and diagnosis of hypoglycaemia and been responsible for 'nonhypoglycemia' becoming a common diagnosis amongst those whom Singer and coworkers refer to as the 'folk sector'.

Mechanism of Hypoglycaemia

Glucose pool in fasting subjects

Glucose is confined within the body to the extracellular fluid where it is referred to as the glucose pool: as soon as glucose enters cells it is phosphorylated and joins the intracellular metabolic pool. In the fasting state glucose enters the glucose pool almost exclusively from the liver and does so at the rate of about 100 mg per kg body weight per hour: it leaves by entering non-insulin-dependent tissues – almost exclusively neural and erythropoietic tissues – at

exactly the same rate. The result is a remarkable homeostasis wherein the blood glucose concentration is kept within the range 3.5–6.0 mmol l^{-1} (see **Fig. 1**).

Insulin release in response to eating and fasting

Evidence for a 'cephalic phase' of insulin secretion in humans is both scanty and conflicting. Most observers have found a minimal, if any, response to the prospect of eating, or the reality of drinking, a noncalorigenic sweet drink except in obese individuals or when the osmolality of the drink was so high as to suggest a direct enteric effect.

After a carbohydrate-containing meal, glucose derived from food enters the portal vein. From here it is conveyed to the liver where much of it is extracted and converted to glycogen. What remains unabsorbed passes into the systemic circulation, producing a small and variable rise in arterial, capillary (and initially venous) blood glucose concentrations. The modest rise in arterial blood glucose concentration perfusing the pancreas, augmented by

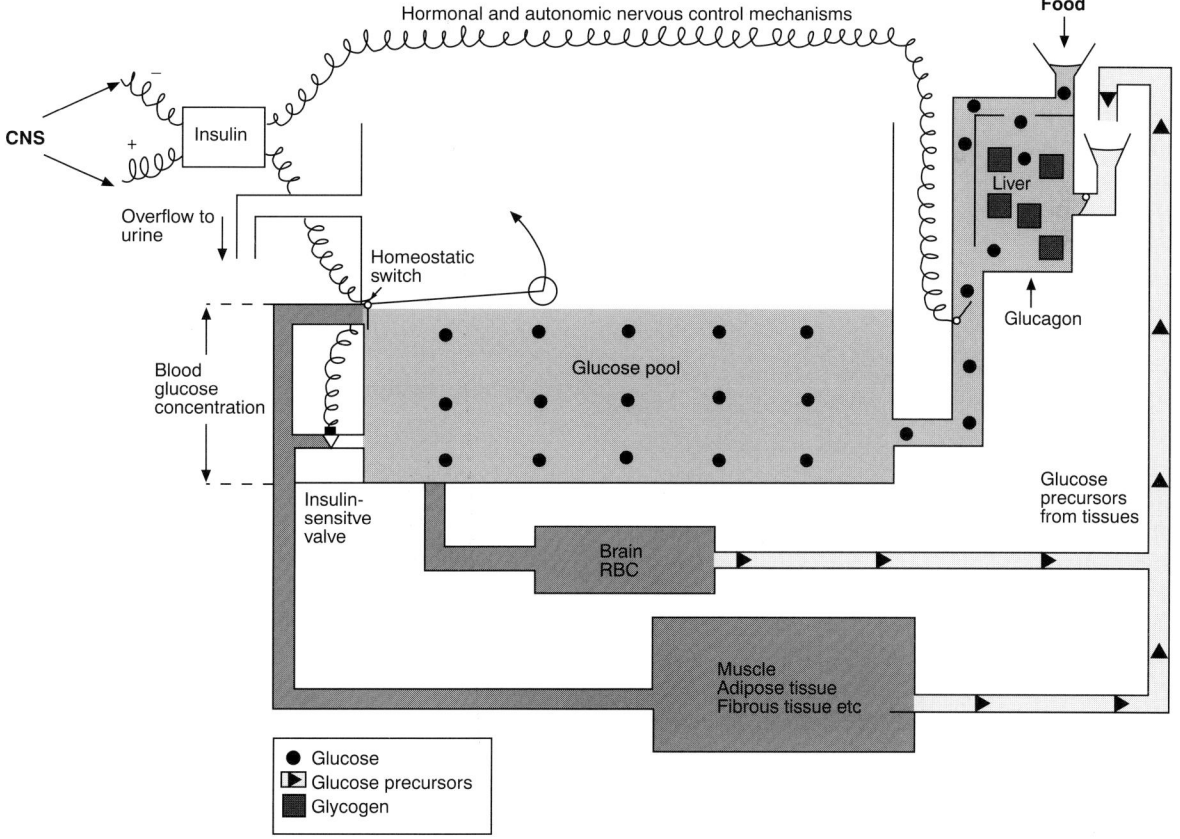

Figure 1   Schematic representation of homeostatic control of blood glucose level and mechanism of hypoglycaemia. Hypoglycaemia results whenever inflow of glucose from the gut and/or the liver fails to meet the outflow of glucose from the glucose pool, which consists of glucose dissolved in the extracellular water only. Imbalance arises from (1) excessive outflow into the tissues due to insulin (or very rarely IGF-II) overproduction or activity; or (2) in the fasting state, an inability of the liver to liberate or produce glucose at a rate sufficient to meet the non-insulin-dependent, and obligatory, requirements of the brain and red blood cells for glucose.

nervous stimuli and insulinotrophic hormones (predominantly GIP and GLP-1) released from the gut in response to meals containing carbohydrate and/or fats, leads to prompt secretion of insulin in greater amounts than that occasioned by the rise in blood glucose concentration alone.

In the postprandial period, as the blood glucose concentration fall towards its homeostatically controlled level, insulin secretion declines to a level that is barely sufficient to suppress unbridled lipolysis and which, in patients with absolutely no capacity to secrete insulin, is the cause of diabetic ketoacidosis.

The role of the liver in glucose homeostasis

The liver, under the influence of insulin reaching it in high concentration in the portal vein after ingestion of a meal, switches from being a net exporter to net importer of glucose from the glucose pool. Any insulin not extracted and degraded by the liver passes through the heart and lungs to reach peripheral tissues, notably muscle, adipose tissue and skin, where – providing the concentration of insulin in blood is sufficiently high – it promotes glucose uptake.

Except in disease the glucose pool, amounting to only some 5–15 g, rarely expands by more than 100% even after ingestion of a meal providing up to 300 g of carbohydrate as starch or glucose. Nor does it shrink to less than 4 g even after many days of fasting. Insulin is the main but not sole agent in achieving this remarkable degree of homeostasis.

The inflow of glucose into the glucose pool is limited only by the rate at which it can be absorbed from the intestine, which is normally in the region of 25–50 g h^{-1} Venous blood glucose generally returns to overnight fasting values within 2 h of eating a meal in people free of impaired glucose tolerance, regardless of how much carbohydrate the meal contains. Arterial blood glucose levels take somewhat longer to return to preingestion levels but they too are always within the normal fasting range by 3 h, even though the evidence provided by measurement of gut hormones, especially GIP, indicate that absorption is still continuing. There is evidence from plasma insulin, C-peptide and GIP measurements that absorption of glucose from the gut is still actively taking place more than 5 h after ingestion of 200 g of liquid glucose (hydrolysed starch) by normal healthy subjects, even though both their venous and arterial blood glucose levels have returned to normal.

The outflow of glucose into the tissues, on the other hand, depends upon many factors; the two most important are the plasma insulin concentration and the blood concentration itself. Under maximum insulin stimulation – and at 'normal' blood glucose levels – glucose typically disappears from the glucose pool at a rate of about 40–50 g h^{-1}.

Onset of insulin action is almost instantaneous and persists for as long as insulin remains bound to insulin receptors. This is generally slightly longer than insulin levels in the blood themselves remain elevated. In other words glucose continues to enter insulin-dependent cells for up to 30 min after plasma insulin levels have returned to 'fasting' levels. During this time the glucose pool may shrink sufficiently to produce hypoglycaemia unless replenished by glucose continuing to enter from the intestine (or experimentally/therapeutically by intravenous infusion) or from the liver – once it has switched from the glycogenic to glycogenolytic mode.

Temporary imbalance between the rate at which insulin action declines and glucose enters the glucose pool is quite common in healthy subjects after ingestion of a large dose of glucose in solution on an empty stomach, but only very rarely following the ingestion of ordinary mixed meals except in people who have undergone gastric surgery.

A slight delay in stimulating insulin release, rather than a reduction in total quantity released in response to a meal, is the earliest and most characteristic abnormality observed in patients with non-insulin-dependent diabetes mellitus (NIDDM) who suffer from hyperglycaemia. It might be expected, therefore, that early and/or exaggerated release of insulin in response to a meal might cause hypoglycaemia. This does occur – though only in exceptional circumstances which will be considered later.

Hypoglycaemic Syndromes

Brain malfunction from hypoglycaemia

The brain ordinarily requires a regular and plentiful supply of glucose. Reduction of supply to below critical limits causes the brain to malfunction and this manifests itself subjectively as symptoms and objectively as neurological deficit. The blood glucose level at which impairment occurs varies, but is generally higher in older and diabetic subjects than in younger and nondiabetic people.

Symptoms are unusual at blood glucose levels above 3.0 mmol l^{-1}, except in diabetic and elderly healthy subjects, although objective evidence of cerebral impairment can often be discerned by an investigator at blood glucose levels around 3.5 mmol l^{-1}.

Causes of neuroglycopenia other than hypoglycaemia, i.e. normoglycaemic neuroglycopenia, are currently thought to be exceedingly rare and include congenital or acquired reduction in glucose transporter activity across the blood–brain barrier and/or neuron cell membranes. The possibility that at least some cases of 'nonhypoglycemia' are due to normoglycaemic neuroglycopenia cannot be dismissed at the present time and would help explain why, under research conditions, sufferers from this condition may develop symptoms at higher blood glucose levels than control subjects.

Neuroglycopenic syndromes

Four, more or less distinct, neuroglycopenic syndromes (one of which is so rare that it will not be considered further here) can be recognized. They are not mutually exclusive, nor do they depend upon the ultimate cause of the hypoglycaemia.

Acute neuroglycopenia This syndrome comprises a collection of vague symptoms such as feelings of alternating hot and cold, feeling unwell, anxiety, panic, inner trembling, unnatural feelings, blurring of vision and palpitations, any or all of which may be accompanied by objective signs of facial flushing, sweating, tachycardia and unsteadiness of gait. There is no particular order in which these features occur, nor are they constant. Nevertheless patients on insulin therapy for diabetes, in whom they are common, usually come to recognize them as prodromal features of more severe neuroglycopenia that may culminate in loss of consciousness and soon learn to abort their progression by eating carbohydrate.

Many of the features of acute neuroglycopenia resemble those produced by adrenaline and consequently are often referred to as adrenergic.

Subacute neuroglycopenia This syndrome is more insidious and may go completely unrecognized unless or until the patient loses consciousness. Often, however, there is loss of spontaneous activity, impairment of cognitive function and the onset of somnolence that is more discernible to the bystander than to the patient and which, when it occurs in an insulin-treated diabetic, is often referred to as 'hypoglycaemia unawareness'.

Both acute and subacute neuroglycopenia can progress to stupor or coma unless relieved by food or injection of glucagon. Even when this is not done, however, full recovery – under the influence of endogenous counter-regulatory mechanisms – is almost invariable.

Chronic neuroglycopenia The third syndrome is exceedingly rare. It occurs only when the blood glucose concentration remains low – either due to the presence of an insulin-secreting tumour of the pancreas or overzealous treatment of diabetes with insulin – for many weeks or months. It is characterized by mental dysfunction resembling clinical depression, schizophrenia or dementia, the symptoms of which are not relieved by restoring the blood glucose level to normal. Partial recovery may, however, take place over the ensuing few months or years if the cause of the hypoglycaemia is remedied.

This condition might be confused with 'nonhypoglycemia' were it not for the fact that the blood glucose concentration is invariably low (3.0 mmol l^{-1}) while the patient is fasting, does not rise normally in response to food, and evidence of underlying disease can always be found.

Diagnosis

Causes of hypoglycaemia

There are something in the region of 100 causes of hypoglycaemia but all, apart from exogenous (or iatrogenic) insulin overdose, are rare. Some of the most important causes of recurrent hypoglycaemia are listed and briefly described in **Table 1**. Diagnosis is seldom simple and **always** rests heavily upon the results of laboratory data. Simultaneous occurrence of symptoms and a measured low blood glucose concentration is a *sine qua non*.

Endocrinological and other anatomico-pathological causes of hypoglycaemia have been discussed elsewhere and will not be considered further. Nor will toxic or iatrogenic causes of hypoglycaemia, of which alcohol-induced fasting hypoglycaemia is easily the most common. Instead attention will be given exclusively to those conditions (including 'nonhypoglycaemia') that have a mainly or exclusively dietary aetiology and which respond partially or completely to dietary measures.

Spontaneous Reactive Hypoglycaemia

Within a year of the discovery of insulin, and the symptoms to which hypoglycaemia can give rise, Seale Harris, an American physician, had proposed that spontaneous overproduction of endogenous insulin might produce a similar condition. Confirmation of this hypothesis soon followed but it was not until the seminal work of Whipple on the diagnosis of insulinoma, and of Conn on diet-induced postprandial reactive hypoglycaemia, both in 1936, that a clear distinction was drawn between fast-induced (fasting) hypoglycaemia and that which occurred only in response to feeding or the administration of large doses of glucose in solution (postprandial reactive hypoglycaemia).

Table 1 Characteristics of main types of recurrent spontaneous hypoglycaemia

Descriptive name	Mechanism	Diagnostic features	Dietary consideration
Fasting hypoglycaemia Insulin-secreting tumour, etc.	Abnormal B cells with failure to suppress insulin secretion in response to hypoglycaemia	Inappropriately high plasma insulin (>30 pmol l^{-1}) and C-peptide (>100 pmol l^{-1}) in presence of hypoglycaemia (BG <2.2 mmol l^{-1}): Suppressed β-hydroxybutyrate levels (<500 μmmol l^{-1})	High carbohydrate intake orally or intravenously until curative surgical ablation or effective hyperglycaemic therapy with diazoxide plus chlorothiazide can be instituted.
IGF-II secreting tumours	Abnormal tumour cells secreting big IGF-II	Low plasma insulin and C peptide levels: low plasma IGF-I, normal or raised IGF-II levels; abnormal IGF-I : IGF-II ratio. Suppressed β-hydroxybutyrate levels (<500 μmmol l^{-1})	High carbohydrate intake orally or intravenously until curative surgical ablation of effective hyperglycaemic therapy with growth hormone and/or prednisone can be instituted.
Endocrine disease, e.g. 1. Hypopituitarism 2. Addison's disease	Reduced availability of diabetogenic or hypoglycaemia counter-regulatory hormones	Clinical features of primary disease with subnormal levels of appropriate counter-regulatory hormones, e.g. cortisol, growth hormone. Appropriately raised β-hydroxybutyrate levels (>500 μmmol l^{-1}) during hypoglycaemia	High carbohydrate intake orally or intravenously until effective hormone replacement therapy has been established
Inborn errors of metabolism 1. Glycogen storage diseases	Inability to release glucose from liver during fasting	Usually present in childhood: low blood glucose, high β-hydroxybutyrate levels, low insulin and C-peptide; high lactate; impaired or absent glucose response to glucagon	Avoid fasting: a constant intake of slowly absorbed carbohydrate may be required day and night in infants.
2. Disorders of mitochondrial β-oxidation	Defective utilization of fat as fuel in tissues: compensatory increase in glucose utilization	Occurs in infancy: low glucose, low insulin and C peptide, high FFA, normal lactate, low β-hydroxybutyrate, increased urinary organic acids. Hypocarnitinaemia in some cases	Avoid fasting: frequent high carbohydrate low fat feeding.
Fasting alcohol-induced hypoglycaemia	Alcohol-impaired hepatic gluconeogenesis	Low blood glucose, raised blood alcohol, lactate and usually β-hydroxybutyrate; low plasma insulin and C-peptide	Avoid drinking alcohol whilst fasting or whilst on a low energy diet.
Accelerated fasting (ketotic) hypoglycaemia of childhood	Varied: but always due to exhaustion of hepatic glycogen stores faster than cerebral adaptation to ketosis can occur	Low blood glucose: high plasma fatty acids and β-hydroxybutyrate; low insulin and C-peptide	High carbohydrate feeding; avoidance of prolonged abstinence from food especially during intercurrent illness such as infections.

Table 1 Continued

Descriptive name	Mechanism	Diagnostic features	Dietary consideration
Stimulative hypoglycaemia Inborn errors of metabolism, e.g. hereditary fructose intolerance: galactosaemia	Impaired release of glucose from liver in response to hepatotoxicity of food constituent	Hypoglycaemia evoked by ingestion of foods containing appropriate noxious stimulus: galactose in galactosaemia; fructose in hereditary fructose intolerance and fructose 1–6 bisphosphatase deficiency	Avoid foods containing provocating sugars.
Autoimmune insulin syndrome	Delayed release of insulin from antibody binding after all of meal has been absorbed	Profound hypoglycaemia from 3–12 h after last eating: total plasma insulin high; C-peptide high, normal or low; proinsulin normal or high. Antibodies to insulin present. Common in Japan, infrequent elsewhere	Frequent small mixed meals rich in dietary fibre.
Postgastrectomy and rapid gastric emptying	Accelerated deposition of nutrients into duodenum and increased release of insulinotrophic hormones, e.g. GIP, GLP-1	Normal blood glucose during fasting: hypoglycaemia only follows [1–3 h after] eating. History of gastrectomy or objective evidence of rapid gastric emptying. Exaggerated insulinaemic response to food	Frequent small mixed meals rich in dietary fibre. May benefit from treatment with acabose or miglitol (α-glucosidase inhibitors).
Idiopathic (essential or functional) postprandial reactive hypoglycaemia	Unknown: probably heterogeneous including increased insulin sensitivity	Normal blood glucose during fasting: low capillary (arterial) blood glucose during spontaneous symptomatic neuroglycopenic episodes. All other objective tests of glucose homeostasis normal	Frequent small mixed meals rich in dietary fibre high and slowly absorbed complex carbohydrates. May benefit from treatment with acabose or miglitol (α-glucosidase inhibitors).

Glucose load test

The observation that glucose taken in solution on an empty stomach produces a 'rebound hypoglycaemia' in a large percentage of normal healthy subjects was made even before the discovery of insulin. This discovery attracted little attention, being considered to have only curiosity value and little pathological significance.

The situation changed dramatically during the early 1950s and subsequently, particularly in the USA, with the appearance of books written for lay consumption attributing a vast array of common symptoms to hypoglycaemia, whether the blood glucose concentration was low at the time or not. Belief in the importance and prevalence of 'hypoglycaemia' grew amongst fashionable medical practitioners and the general public alike to such an extent that, by the early 1970s, alarm bells began to ring amongst consumer action groups and the scientific medical community.

With the passage of time the original, well-defined syndrome of postprandial reactive hypoglycaemia had become so distorted, and the diagnostic criteria for its diagnosis so blurred, that anyone with vague symptoms could be, and often was, described as suffering from 'hypoglycemia', whether their blood glucose concentration was actually low or not.

Not until a consensus *Statement on 'Post Prandial' or 'Reactive' Hypoglycemia* was issued by the Third International Symposium on Hypoglycemia and generally recognized by medical practitioners throughout the world did scientific criteria for the diagnosis of reactive hypoglycaemia gain universal acceptance.

Definition

It is now accepted that some people exhibit, in the course of their everyday life, symptoms similar to those caused by acute neuroglycopenia and may, if accompanied by a capillary or arterialized venous blood glucose concentration of 2.8–2.5 mmol l^{-1} or less, justify description as being of postprandial reactive hypoglycaemic origin.

Reactive hypoglycaemia may itself be a consequence of any one of a large number of well-recognized but generally uncommon conditions, and it is only after all of them have been excluded by appropriate laboratory investigations that a diagnosis of essential, functional or dietary reactive hypoglycaemia is justified.

Specifically the prolonged oral glucose load (tolerance) test is deemed not appropriate for the diagnosis of postprandial or reactive hypoglycaemia since the incidence of false positive results with this test is so high as to make it meaningless, especially if, as is so often the case, venous rather than arterial blood is sampled.

The postprandial syndrome

Typically the patient is a normal-weight woman of 20–50 years whose main complaint is of vague feelings of distress occurring predominantly mid morning, about 11–12 a.m., but occasionally mid afternoon or evening – never before breakfast. In between attacks, characterized by feeling of faintness, anxiety, nervousness, irritability, inner trembling, rapid heart beat, headache and sweatiness, either alone or in combination, they may be completely well. More often they describe themselves as suffering from increased tiredness, lacking in zest for life and apathetic much, or all, of the time.

Patients seldom notice any fixed relationship to food unless, as so often happens nowadays, they have diagnosed themselves, on the basis of articles they may have read, as suffering from 'hypoglycemia'. Almost without exception they reject the possibility that their symptoms might have a large, or even contributory, psychogenic element.

Symptoms wax and wane during middle life but often remit completely for years or may never recur. They are not progressive and never cause severe neurological dysfunction such as coma, psychosis or dementia. Hypoglycaemia cannot be demonstrated during spontaneous symptomatic episodes in most people with the postprandial syndrome and some other explanation should be sought for them.

Differential diagnosis

Studies using fingerprick blood sampling during spontaneous symptomatic episodes have shown that only a very small proportion of sufferers from the postprandial syndrome have hypoglycaemia at the relevant time (**Fig. 2**). Of those who do, a substantial proportion have an identifiable cause for it, such as partial gastrectomy, rapid gastric emptying, insulinoma, the presence in their blood of autoantibodies against insulin or the insulin receptor, or even rarer disorders.

In some people reactive hypoglycaemia occur only in response to a specific dietary indiscretion: for example ingestion of large amounts of gin (alcohol) and tonic (sugar and quinine) on an empty stomach.

After all identifiable causes of spontaneous hypoglycaemia have been eliminated there remains a hard core of subjects for whom no satisfactory pathogenic mechanism can be identified. It is justifiable to describe them as suffering from (idiopathic, essential or functional) postprandial, reactive hypoglycaemia.

Dietary management

Treatment of attacks   Because of their short duration and modest severity, acute spontaneous neuroglycopenic episodes require no specific treatment beyond ingestion of a rapidly assimilable form of carbohydrate (e.g. a lump of sugar), exactly as for iatrogenic hypoglycaemia. There is no evidence that this ever produces rebound hypoglycaemia and should it do so the grounds for making a diagnosis of essential reactive hypoglycaemia should be reviewed.

Prevention   Dietary prevention of reactive hypoglycaemia, whether of the 'idiopathic', alimentary, or secondary varieties, e.g. autoimmune insulin syndrome, is based on the premise that it is a consequence of a transient interruption of normal glucose homeostasis caused by imbalance between the timing and amount of insulin secreted and the disposal of glucose absorbed in response to the ingestion of a meal. Evidence for this supposition is small and disputed but currently provides the best explanation for the apparent breakdown in glucose homeostasis in patients with idiopathic reactive hypoglycaemia.

Frequent small meals, rich in poorly absorbed complex carbohydrates and containing, at most, only modest amounts of sugars (glucose and sucrose) and refined starches have replaced the diets rich in proteins (and fats) previously advocated, but evidence of their unique efficacy is lacking. Avoidance of drinks rich in sucrose or glucose, especially with alcohol, may be helpful in subjects who are highly susceptible to this combination. There is no evidence that

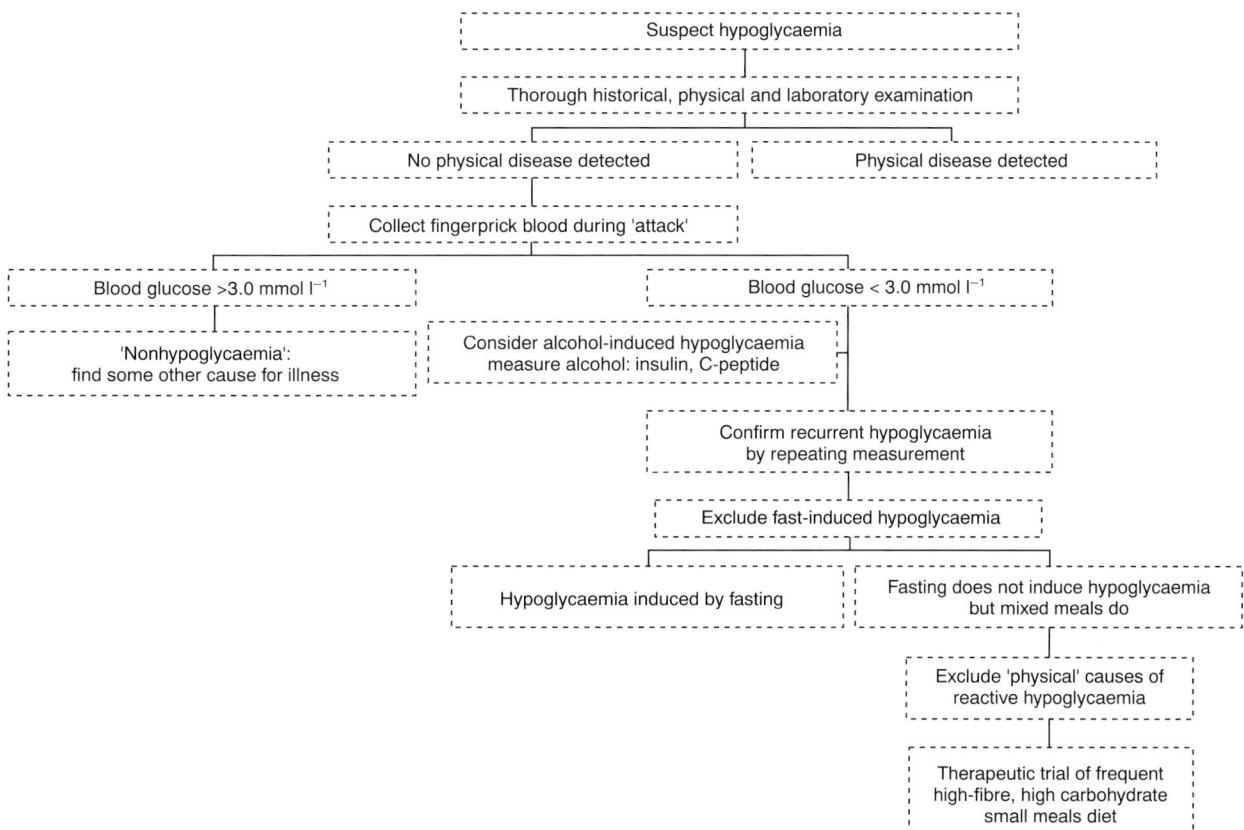

Figure 2 Steps in the diagnosis of hypoglycaemia.

confectionery eaten in moderation is uniquely detrimental, though excessive use should be discouraged on general health grounds.

The long-term outcome of such dietary advice in patients in whom strict criteria for diagnosis were adopted are not available and most published studies on the subject have drawn attention to the need for supplementary pharmacological methods in order to achieve a satisfactory therapeutic outcome.

Pharmaceutical agents that have been used include guar, acarbose and miglitol, all of which slow glucose absorption and decrease the insulinaemic response to food, while others including phenytoin and propranolol do not. Paradoxically, diazoxide, which inhibits insulin secretion by direct action, has not been found effective except in patients with proven endogenous hyperinsulinism

Nonhypoglycemia

No account of dietetic treatment of hypoglycaemia would be complete without a brief description of 'nonhypoglycemia,' which has been described as a controversial illness and epidemic in the USA.

Clinically the illness is indistinguishable from (idiopathic) reactive hypoglycaemia, except that the blood glucose level is never pathologically low during symptomatic episodes. Moreover, although transient 'turns' are often a major feature of the illness, only rarely, if ever, does the patient consider their health, between turns, as normal.

The attribution of these patients' illness to hypoglycaemia had its origins in the early 1950s with the appearance, in the US, of a book by Drs Abrahams and Pezet entitled *Body, Mind and Sugar*. Espousement of its message by other American practitioners, notably John Tintera, founder of the Hypoglycemia Foundation Inc., Stephen Gyland, Harry Saltzer and many others – including the medical writer Carlton Fredericks – led to 'hypoglycemia' being held responsible, by a large section of the public, for such diverse diseases as coronary artery disease, allergy, asthma, rheumatic fever, and susceptibility to viral infections, epilepsy, gastric ulcer, alcoholism, suicide and even homicide, as well as for a whole galaxy of symptoms.

'Hypoglycemia' was treated as though it were a disease entity and asserted by its advocates to be 'one of the most common illnesses in the United States' and that because of it 'thousands of Americans have forgotten, or perhaps never known, what it is like to feel completely healthy'.

Diagnosis of 'nonhypoglycemia' generally depends upon the results of the 6-h oral glucose tolerance test, using venous blood, although some have dispensed even with this discredited formality in favour of purely clinical criteria.

The appearance in the *New England Journal of Medicine* of an article entitled 'Non-hypoglycemia is an epidemic condition' first drew international attention to the illness in 1974. It had previously been almost unknown outside the US and Australia, though known to a few fashionable medical practitioners in Britain.

Many patients with 'nonhypoglycemia' undoubtedly derive some benefit – probably through a powerful placebo effect – from restrictive dietary regimes. Although differing in details most of the diets emphasize the purported specifically detrimental effects of sugar (sucrose), salt, alcohol and caffeine.

While the cause of illness in people with 'nonhypoglycemia' remains unknown, and unlikely to be the same in all cases, in a very small proportion it is due to caffeine intoxication that can be confirmed by a dietary history and, above all, by measurement of plasma caffeine levels. Such patients do benefit specifically from reducing their intake of caffeinated beverages, though not necessarily from avoiding them completely.

Ironically, and possibly significantly, caffeine has recently been shown to restore hypoglycaemia awareness to diabetic patients on insulin who have become insensitive to it. The possibility exists, therefore, that a combination of reasonable or normal caffeine intake occurring in combination with the normal rebound in arterial blood glucose to just below fasting levels, that sometimes occurs 3–5 h after a meal, in someone with an unusually low threshold for neuroglycopenia, might precipitate symptoms.

This explanation of 'nonhypoglycemia' must, however, be considered no more than speculative. On the other hand such diverse illnesses as hyperventilation, panic attacks, unadmitted alcohol or drug abuse and genuine food intolerances are all established as capable of producing the 'nonhypoglycemia' syndrome and should always be considered in the differential diagnosis.

Hepatic and Renal Failure

Considering the importance of the liver and kidney in the maintenance of blood glucose levels during fasting by virtue of their ability to produce new glucose molecules by gluconeogenesis, hypoglycaemia is remarkably rare in both liver and kidney disease.

In liver disease hypoglycaemia is virtually confined to patients with acute toxic hepatic necrosis, whether due to overwhelming viral infection or specific hepatotoxins such as paracetamol. Its appearance always portends an extremely poor prognosis. The association of hypoglycaemia with primary cancer of the liver is comparatively common and due to over-expression and secretion of aberrant, or big IGF-II and not, as was once supposed, due to nonspecific destruction of hepatic tissue. Hypoglycaemia is very rarely due to hepatic secondaries.

Kidney failure is an even rarer cause of hypoglycaemia, probably reflecting the smaller contribution of the kidneys to gluconeogenesis. It does not carry as grave a prognostic significance and responds to appropriate dietary and other supportive treatments for end-stage kidney disease.

Inborn Errors of Metabolism

Hypoglycaemia is a manifestation of many inborn errors of metabolism (see Table 1) but is especially important in some of the varieties of the group known as liver glycogen storage diseases, especially types I and III.

Type I liver glycogen disease is due to a defect in glucose-6-phosphatase activity and produces an especially severe form of fasting hypoglycaemia. Fortunately this responds to dietary therapy in the form of continuous transnasal or gastrostomy feeding with slowly absorbed starch solution during the night when the body has to resort to glycogenolysis to maintain the supply of glucose to the brain. Hypoglycaemia in untreated type I patients produces low plasma insulin levels and, as a consequence, high to very high plasma ketone levels which can partially compensate for the lack of glucose in the brain. This is however an adaptive process which can be impaired if hypoglycaemia is prevented by nocturnal feeding. In the unfortunate event that this is unknowingly or accidentally interrupted the ensuing hypoglycaemia may not be compensated for by hyperketonaemia, resulting in permanent or more severe brain damage than if nocturnal feeding had never been introduced and even death.

Type III glycogen storage diseases is generally much milder and attention to proper dietary habits with a plentiful supply of slowly absorbed carbohydrate strategically distributed throughout the 24 h is generally sufficient to prevent serious brain damage.

Starvation

Although average fasting blood glucose levels are lower in victims of famine than in well-fed populations, overt hypoglycaemia is rare. Even in patients suffering from kwashiorkor hypoglycaemia is uncommon and is usually associated with infection, hypothermia and coma. Patients with anorexia nervosa develop hypoglycaemia only as an agonal phenomenon and its appearance generally portends imminent death. The characteristic clinical biochemistry findings are of low or undetectably low plasma insulin, proinsulin, C-peptide and IGF-I levels, grossly depressed plasma nonesterified fatty acids (NEFA) and β-hydroxybutyrate and elevated growth hormone and cortisol levels. Relief of hypoglycaemia by refeeding is the only measure carrying any chance of preventing death, but it is rarely successful.

Conclusions

Symptoms due to spontaneous hypoglycaemia, an unusual consequence of many different rare diseases, are sometimes the primary reason for a patient seeking medical help. In a tiny minority of patients no pathological cause can be found to account for the hypoglycaemia and no specific curative or palliative therapy can be instituted. Amongst these are a group of patients who only experience neuroglycopenic symptoms 3–5 h after eating a meal. They may benefit from eating small, frequent, slowly absorbed carbohydrate-rich meals but usually require an α-glucosidase inhibitor as well.

Patients with self-diagnosed hypoglycaemia in whom blood glucose levels are never pathologically low in everyday life and do not have any other known cause for their symptoms may also derive some benefit from a high-fibre, high complex carbohydrate diet, but how much of this is due to a placebo rather than specific dietary effect is still unknown.

See also: **Glucose**: Chemistry, Dietary Sources and Glycaemic Index; Metabolism and Maintenance of Blood Glucose Level; Glucose Tolerance. **Inborn Errors of Metabolism**: Classification and Biochemical Aspects; Nutritional Management of Phenylketonuria. **Liver Disorders**: Nutritional Management. **Renal Function and Disorders**: Nutritional Management of Renal Disorders. **Starvation and Fasting**: Biochemical Aspects.

Further Reading

Editorial (1974) Low blood sugar: Fact and Fiction. *Consumer Reports USA* 36:444–446.

Fishman RA (1991) The glucose-transporter protein and glucopenic brain injury. *New England Journal of Medicine* 325:731–732.

Fonseca V, Ball S, Marks V and Havard CWH (1991) Hypoglycaemia associated with anorexia nervosa. *Postgraduate Medical Journal* 67:460–461.

Goldberg NJ, Wingert TD, Levin SR and Adachi RI (1980) Augmentation of insulin secretion buy a non-nutrient drink. *Gastroenterology* 78:1485–1462.

Hofeldt FD (1989) Reactive hypoglycemia. *Endocrinology and Metabolism Clinics of North America* 18:185–201.

Kerr D, Sherwin RS, Pavalkis F, Fayad PB, Sikorski L, Rife F, Tamborlane WV and During MJ (1993) Effect of caffeine on the recognition of and the responses to hypoglycaemia in humans. *Annals of Internal Medicine* 119:799–804.

Lefebvre PJ, Andreani D, Marks V and Creutzfeldt W (1988) Statement on postprandial hypoglycemia. *Diabetes Care* 11:439–440.

Lefebvre PJ and Scheen AJ (1994) The use of Acabose in the prevention and treatment of hypoglycaemia. *European Journal of Clinical Investigation* 24 (supplement 3):40–44.

Marks V (1976) The measurement of blood glucose and the definition of hypoglycemia. In: Andreani D, Lefèbvre PJ, Marks V (eds) *Hypoglycemia*. Proceedings of the European Symposium, Rome: *Hormone and Metabolic Research*, supplement 6, pp 1–6. Stuttgart: Georg Thieme.

Marks V (1987) Functional hypoglycaemia: fact or fancy. In: Andreani D, Marks V and Lefebvre PJ (eds) *Hypoglycaemia: Serono Symposia Publications 38*, pp 1–17. New York: Raven Press.

Marks V (1992) Minimal hypoglycaemia and normoglycaemic neuroglycopenia. In: Andreani D, Lefebvre PJ, Marks V, Tamburrano G (eds) *Recent Advances on Hypoglycaemia: Serono Symposia Publications*, pp 241–243. New York: Raven Press.

Marks V and Rose FC (1981) *Hypoglycaemia*, 2nd edn. Oxford: Blackwell Scientific Publications.

Palardy J, Havrankova J, Lepage R, Matte R, Bélanger R, D'Amour P and Ste-Marie L-G (1989) Blood glucose measurements during symptomatic episodes in patients with suspected postprandial hypoglycemia. *New England Journal of Medicine* 321:1421–1425.

Service FJ (1989) Hypoglycemia and the postprandial syndrome. *New England Journal of Medicine* 321:1472–1473.

Singer M, Arnold C, Fitzgerald M, Madden L and Voight von Legat C (1984) Hypoglycemia: a controversial illness in US society. *Medical Anthropology* 8:1–35.

Snorgaard O, Lassen LH, Rosenfalck AM and Binder C (1991) Glycaemic thresholds for hypoglycaemic symptoms, impairment of cognitive function, and release of counterregulatory hormones in subjects with functional hypoglycaemia. *Journal of Internal Medicine* 229:343–350.

Tamburrano G, Leonetti F, Sbraccia P, Giaccari A, Locuratolo N and Lala A (1989) Increased insulin sensitivity in patients with idiopathic reactive hypoglycemia. *Journal of Clinical Endocrinology and Metabolism* 69:885–890.

Yager J and Young RT (1974) Sounding board: non-hypoglycemia is an epidemic condition. *New England Journal of Medicine* 291:907–908.

I

Immune system *see* **Immunity**: Physiological Aspects; Role of Iron and Zinc.

IMMUNITY

Contents
Physiological Aspects
Role of Iron and Zinc

Physiological Aspects

B M Hannigan, University of Ulster, Coleraine,
Northern Ireland, UK

Copyright © 1998 Academic Press

The immune system of every individual is biologically unique. Its special features derive both from genetic factors that control immune responses and from the person's history of encounters with the surrounding environment, especially with microorganisms. The presence of malnutrition, poor living or working conditions or certain illnesses can compromise the ability to mount effective immune responses. The past two decades of research in immunology have seen the rapid accumulation of knowledge that can provide new perspectives on many infectious diseases, cancer and human ageing. The cells and molecules that participate in immune responses have now been characterized and their functions in health and disease can be studied using a range of *in vivo* and *in vitro* techniques. Immune cells and molecules may be exploited for current and future human diagnostics and therapeutics.

The Immune System

Since the evolution of multicellularity it has been necessary for cells and molecules within individual organisms to be able to identify each other as parts of the 'self'. Anything that does not belong to that self is 'nonself', or foreign. This self/nonself discrimination is fundamental to a defence system, the immune system. The human immune system is complex but highly organized, capable of protecting the individual against many forms of nonself that occur in the environment (**Table 1**).

Physical barriers

Initial interactions between self and nonself are regulated by physical barriers. These barriers are listed in **Table 2** and exist primarily at the self/nonself interface. Clearly, this first line of defence is not impenetrable, for example wounds in the skin or gastrointestinal tract lesions allow foreign material direct access to self tissues.

Table 1 Forms of nonself against which the immune system provides a defence

Bacteria
Viruses
Parasites
Fungi
Yeasts
Worms
Foreign bodies, e.g. splinters
Transplanted tissues or organs
Chemicals, poisons, drugs
Foodstuffs
Malignant tumours
Fetuses

Table 2 Physical barriers between self and nonself

Skin
Mucous membranes, mucus transport and cilia (lining gastrointestinal tract, respiratory tract and genitourinary tracts)
Acid pH of stomach
Normal bacterial flora of skin and intestine
Enzyme (lysozyme) in tears
Antibacterial components of sweat and other secretions

Inflammation

The evolution of circulatory systems permitted specialized cells within the organism to move to, and interact with, the body's tissues and cells as required. Many of these specialized cells and molecules comprise a second wave of defence, known as natural immunity or inflammation.

Effector cells are mononuclear phagocytes and polymorphonuclear leucocytes and originate in the bone marrow. The principal mononuclear phagocytes are monocytes, which initially circulate in the bloodstream before being attracted into tissues to differentiate into macrophages. The polymorphonuclear leucocytes include neutrophils, basophils and eosinophils. Other cells of natural immunity are natural killer (NK) cells. The occurrence of each cell type varies within different tissues and organs and depends upon the level of inflammatory activity.

A series of noncellular factors, predominantly proteins and glycoproteins, are essential for intercellular communication (the cytokines) and for contributing to inflammatory activity (cytokines and acute-phase proteins). Some of these molecules are produced in low levels by many tissues throughout the body, and in higher levels during responses, principally by the liver but also by inflammatory cells. The approximately 30 plasma proteins which constitute the complement system comprise one important group of acute-phase proteins.

Acute inflammatory responses are rapid, nonspecific and normally cause no lasting adverse effects. If the nonself is not eliminated, however, chronic inflammation may ensue and last for many years. This results in pathology.

Acquired immunity

The final phase of a normal immune response comprises the specific reactions mediated by mononuclear leucocytes known as lymphocytes and their protein/glycoprotein products (cytokines, immunoglobulins). This is termed adaptive, or acquired, immunity and its hallmarks are specificity and immunological memory. The two principal types of lymphocytes are T cells and B cells. Both types arise from bone marrow stem cells. B cells complete their maturation within the bone marrow while T cells undergo differentiation and selection within the thymus. Other cell types that are essential for acquired responses, specifically for the activation of T cells, are termed accessory cells. Accessory cells include antigen presenting cells (APC), which often are macrophages or macrophage-like cells found throughout the body. B cells may also act as APCs.

It is not possible to distinguish between the many different cell types that are involved in immune and inflammatory responses solely on the basis of cell morphology. Instead they may be identified according to the molecules that predominate on their cell surfaces. These cell surface markers have been classified according to an internationally recognized system of 'CD' numbers, where CD stands for 'cluster of differentiation'. For example, mature T cells carry CD3 and either CD4 (CD4+ cells) or CD8 (CD8+ cells).

Lymphoid tissues

The bone marrow and thymus are known as primary lymphoid tissues and appear to be at their peak of activity shortly after birth. Cells and molecules of the immune system tend to congregate and interact at particular locations within the body (**Table 3**). It may be noticed that these secondary lymphoid tissues lie in areas where contact between self and nonself is most likely, e.g. in the spleen, where there is extensive interaction with the contents of the bloodstream; in the lymph nodes, where lymph is filtered; and within the gut walls, where ingested nonself is encountered. Many secondary lymphoid tissues contain specialized foci, germinal centres, where lymphocytes undergo further maturation.

Table 3 Secondary lymphoid tissues

Spleen (white pulp)
Lymph nodes
Mucosa-associated lymphoid tissue (MALT)
Gut-associated lymphoid tissue (GALT) including:
    Tonsils
    Adenoids
    Appendix
    Peyer's patches

Coordination

For successful, beneficial responses the immune system must work in concert with the other systems of the body. The area of study termed psycho-neuro-endocrine immunology illustrates the interdependence of immune responses and the body's hormonal and neurological regulatory systems. Both cell–cell interactions and soluble mediators are necessary for this level of coordination. The lymphoid tissues and blood vessels within which leucocytes occur have a nerve supply and so are under the direct control of the nervous system. Leucocytes have cell surface receptors for many endocrine hormones, notably the corticosteroids, which have a generally suppressive effect on immune responses.

Functions of the Immune System

Inflammation

When the physical barriers separating self and non-self are breached an inflammatory response begins. At this stage the cells necessary for the response must be attracted from the bloodstream into the infected tissue. Endothelial cells that line postcapillary venules respond to tissue signals by changing shape so that gaps appear, they become 'sticky' by expressing adhesion molecules on the luminal surface, and they secrete cytokines which stimulate leucocytes within the bloodstream also to express adhesion molecules. Interactions between complementary adhesion molecules allows endothelial cells to 'capture' leucocytes and to guide them through the newly formed gaps in the endothelial layer and into the tissue. Neutrophils are the first cell types to respond.

Leucocytes migrate to the infected area (by chemotaxis) where they are activated to carry out phagocytosis. Phagocytosed (engulfed) cells (e.g. bacteria) are eliminated by a combination of a respiratory burst and lysosomal enzyme activity (acid hydrolases). The respiratory burst involves oxygen consumption and its enzymatic reduction to a series of reactive oxygen species which are toxic to living cells. The respiratory burst also yields an increased H^+ concentration (decreased pH) which activates the acid hydrolases to degrade the killed organisms.

Complement proteins are activated through contact with nonself, especially with bacteria. Activated complement proteins can assemble to form membrane attack complexes (MAC). The structure of a MAC resembles a hollow cylinder. When large numbers of MAC are inserted into the outer wall of a cell or microorganism lysis of the cell occurs, leucocytes are attracted to the site and the action of phagocytes is promoted.

Acquired responses

An acquired response begins when lymphocytes migrate to the site of infection, also attracted through specific adhesion molecules. T lymphocytes are the principal regulatory cell types of the immune system. T cells are activated by recognizing fragments of nonself (antigens) bound to self major histocompatibility complex (MHC) protein on the surface of a host antigen presenting cell (APC). There are two types of MHC protein, class I and class II. Class I MHC molecules are expressed by all nucleated cells and platelets while class II occur only on APCs. The two MHC classes present different types of antigen to T cells. In general terms, class I MHC presents antigens that have been expressed intracellularly, e.g. viral antigens. Class II MHC presents extracellular antigen, e.g. bacteria or soluble proteins. The different modes of presentation allow the tailoring of specific responses. Type I MHC with non-self antigen is recognized by CD8+ T cells which proliferate to form a clone of cytotoxic T lymphocytes (CTL). These CTL can directly lyse virally infected cells, tumour cells and cells in mismatched transplanted tissue. If the antigen has been presented by class II MHC it is recognized by a CD4+ T cell which proliferates and activates B lymphocytes. These B cells proliferate and form a clone of plasma cells that secrete antibody capable of binding specifically to the antigen which originally stimulated the T cells. A minority of, mostly carbohydrate, antigens can activate B cells directly. Cytokines, especially interleukins, contribute to all stages in the response. **Fig. 1** summarizes the most important cell–cell and cytokine-mediated events at the early stages of acquired responses.

Nonself antigen is finally destroyed by a combination of complement-mediated lysis and phagocytosis. Activated complement proteins are anchored to the target antigen surface by binding to the antibody molecules. Antigen with attached antibody and complement presents a very strong target to phagocytes which carry surface receptors specific for antibody (Fc receptors) and for complement.

Antibodies (Immunoglobulins)

Antibody-mediated responses are referred to as humoral immunity. Antibodies are glycoproteins that not only have antigen specificity, but also have particular characteristics (isotypes) which make them appropriate for specific responses. The five principal isotypes are IgG, IgM, IgA, IgD and IgE. The isotypes vary in structure (**Table 4**) and consequently in function.

IgG is the principal immunoglobulin of secondary

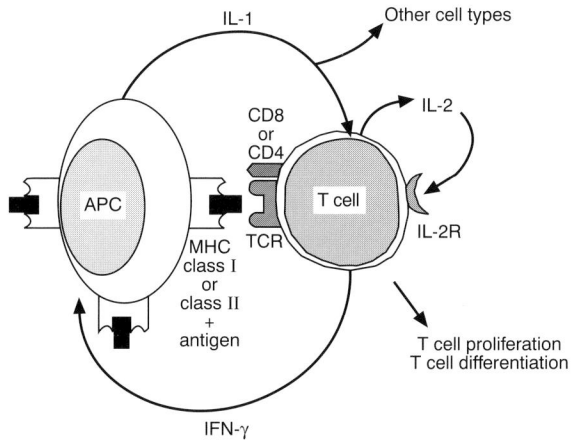

Figure 1 If nonself antigen is presented in association with MHC class I antigen on the APC, a CD8+ T cell will be activated and a cytotoxic response will ensue. Presentation of nonself in association with MHC class II antigen on the APC will lead to CD4+ T cell activation, B cell activation and an antibody-mediated response. Key: APC, antigen-presenting cell; IFN-γ, interferon γ; IL-1, interleukin 1; IL-2, interleukin 2; IL-2R, interleukin 2 receptor; MHC, major histocompatibility complex antigen; T cell, T lymphocyte; TCR, T cell receptor for antigen.

Table 4 Characteristics of immunoglobulin isotypes

Isotype	Mol. wt. (kDa)	Structure	Normal serum conc. (mg/ml)
IgG	150	Monomer	14
IgM	900	Pentamer	1.5
IgA	160/390	Monomer/dimer	0.5/0.05
IgD	190	Monomer	0.03
IgE	190	Monomer	$< 0.05 \ \mu g \ ml^{-1}$

responses, readily infiltrates tissues, activates complement and crosses the placenta. IgM predominates in primary responses and efficiently activates complement. IgA occurs on mucosal surfaces and in secretions more frequently than in the serum. Its principal role is in preventing antigen from attaching to epithelial surfaces. IgD is mostly found only on B cell surfaces. IgE is normally found in trace amounts but is increased during hypersensitivity (allergic) reactions. It is involved in the release of vasoactive amines, e.g. histamine, which promote the symptoms of allergy.

Immunological memory

During T cell activation cell proliferation occurs, giving rise to daughter cells. Not all daughter cells participate immediately in the response; some are destined to remain as memory cells which can be reactivated on any subsequent encounter with the same antigen. This is the basis of memory and sec-

ondary responses are more efficient than the primary response.

Termination of the response

On elimination of antigen macrophages interact with fibroblasts and cytokines to form new tissue. This is known as healing.

Clinical Indices of Immune Function

Frequently our best windows on immune function are patients presenting with illnesses where disordered immunity is a contributory factor. The family histories of these patients can assist in understanding the genetic basis of immune responses. The patient's age, sex, race and lifestyle factors including diet, anorexia or weight loss, medication, alcohol consumption and the presence of potential allergens, infectious agents or toxins in work and home environments are also relevant when interpreting immunological test results.

Physical examination

Changes in lymph nodes may be visible or detectable on palpation. Enlarged nodes may indicate the presence of inflammation as the number and size of cells present is increased. Generalized lymphadenopathy is indicative of systemic disease, e.g. autoimmune diseases such as systemic lupus erythematosus (SLE) where the host is mounting a response against self. Splenomegaly may be caused by immune disorders in which there is increased cell destruction and splenic tenderness is associated with infections. Hepatomegaly may accompany many immune disorders and changes in the bowels may be associated with some autoimmune diseases.

Quantitative and qualitative tests of immune function

Tests on leucocytes Counts of total leucocytes and a differential leucocyte count are simple procedures that provide information on bone marrow function and on the relative proportions of different cell types. In general, increased numbers indicate an ongoing immune or inflammatory response. The use of antibodies specific for cell surface features allows estimation of individual cell types. The most common cell types that are enumerated in this way, either by microscopy or FACS (fluorescence-activated cell sorter) analysis, are CD4+ and CD8+ T cells. The absolute number of CD4+ cells and the ratio of CD4+ to CD8+ cells are used to monitor the progress of patients with HIV infection, a significant decline in CD4+ numbers accompanying the onset of AIDS.

In vitro tests of lymphocyte function involve stimulation of isolated cell populations with mitogens or antigens. The cells respond by *de novo* DNA synthesis, the extent of which can be measured by the addition of radioisotope-labelled nucleotide precursors, usually tritiated thymidine (^{3}H-dT). The amount of label incorporated is proportional to the responsiveness of the cell population. This test is subject to considerable day-to-day and interindividual variation. Depressed responsiveness may indicate primary or secondary immune deficiency, illness, chronic inflammatory disease, recent trauma, malnutrition or pregnancy.

Phagocyte activity may be assessed as the cells' ability to undertake functions such as migration through millipore filters, production of a respiratory burst, cytokine release or the killing of test organisms. Abnormal results may indicate primary disorders of phagocytes however the defects may be secondary to other diseases or to impaired lymphocyte function.

Tests on blood serum or plasma   Molecules secreted from immunocompetent cells are usually measured in blood but are also detectable in other body fluids, e.g. saliva, synovial fluid, cerebrospinal fluid (CSF) or bronchial washings. The most important tests are for immunoglobulins, complement and cytokines.

Immunoglobulins   The different antibody isotypes are easily measured by radial immunodiffusion, nephelometry or serum protein electrophoresis in combination with specific antisera. Their overall concentration and the distribution of the different types provide a rapid assessment of the humoral immune system; however, their levels may vary considerably and no individual result, apart from absence (agammaglobulinaemia) of the antibody is diagnostic. The investigation of hypersensitivity reactions may involve measuring the amount of IgE directed against a specific antigen (allergen) in a radioallergosorbent test (RAST).

Immunoglobulins produced by B cell malignancies such as multiple myeloma, non-Hodgkin's lymphoma or chronic lymphocytic leukaemia are detectable as abnormal patterns on serum electrophoresis and often may be found in the urine (Bence Jones proteins). Autoantibodies may be detected by investigating their binding to cells or tissue sections. These include the antinuclear antibody characteristic of the autoimmune disease SLE.

Complement proteins   Complement assays are based either on the overall ability to lyse red blood cells in the presence of antibody or on levels of individual components. Low complement levels are likely to be more clinically relevant than high levels and indicate either deficient production of the proteins or increased utilization *in vivo*, e.g. in the case of autoimmune diseases which involve antigen–antibody complex formation.

Cytokines   The measurement of cytokines is complicated by several factors including their low concentrations in blood and their short half-life. Cytokines should be measured in plasma rather than in serum. The most commonly used technique for estimating the levels of individual cytokines is the enzyme-linked immunosorbent assay (ELISA), while cytokine activity may be assessed by their effects on target cells in a range of bioassays.

In vivo **tests**   The delayed type hypersensitivity (DTH) test assesses overall immune function as the patient's ability to respond to an antigen introduced under the skin. The most common DTH test uses PPD (purified protein derivative) prepared from the organism *Mycobacterium tuberculosis*. If the patient was previously exposed to the organism the sensitized cells and antibodies still present would cause a visible skin reaction within 48 h. Immunocompromised patients do not react. Confirmation of a person's anergic (nonreactive) status involves testing with a panel of other intradermal antigens. The presence of other infections, e.g. influenza, measles, mumps, scarlet fever or typhus, would also lead to anergy. Similar skin test procedures may be used to identify which allergen may be responsible for a patient's hypersensitivity. Where a patient is suspected of allergy to a food component, tests could involve removal of that item from the diet to observe whether symptoms decreased, and its later reintroduction as a challenge. Great care is needed in the conduct of challenge tests to avoid the risk of anaphylactic shock.

Tumour Immunity

Are tumours 'self' or 'nonself'? The currently favoured response is that tumour cells appear immunologically identical to the host in which they arise except for their expression of what are termed tumour specific antigens. Some tumour specific antigens are normally expressed only on embryonal cells, termed differentiation antigens, while others occur because of the presence of viruses.

If the tumour is predominantly self, is there an antitumour immune response? The theory of immune surveillance would argue that immunogenic (response inducing) tumour cells will be destroyed.

Any surviving tumours would then consist of non-immunogenic, or weakly immunogenic, cells. Disappointingly, while many tumours induced by oncogenic viruses or ultraviolet irradiation in experimental animals are strongly immunogenic, most spontaneously arising animal tumours induce little or no response.

Apparently contrary to this is the finding that most human tumours contain infiltrates of leucocytes, predominantly lymphocytes and macrophages. Information on the function of these tumour-associated cells is confused and some researchers would argue that, instead of destroying the tumour, they can contribute to its development, e.g. by secreting factors that promote tumour cell growth or by encouraging the development of a tumour blood supply.

Studies on immunosuppressed patients would support the idea that not all cancer types may be limited by immune responses. Patients with AIDS or those on posttransplant immunosuppressive drugs show increased susceptibilities only to certain skin cancers and lymphomas. Conversely, diminished immune responsiveness is commonly found in patients with cancers; this occurs most frequently with lymphoid malignancies but also in many patients with solid tumours.

Where responses to tumour cells are present, they are most likely to involve cytotoxicity by T cells, NK cells and cytokines, e.g. tumour necrosis factor α (TNF-α). Cytokines can also contribute to cancer morbidity because they promote cachexia.

Immunotherapy

An aim of immunologists for several decades has been to augment antitumour responses. Immunotherapy for cancer patients is now emerging as an effective adjunct to chemotherapy and radiotherapy. The conventional treatment regimes may be used to diminish the patient's tumour load, allowing the smaller remnants to be dealt with by a stimulated immune system.

Initial attempts to destroy tumours by administering large doses of cytokines to patients induced life-threatening side effects. Cytokine therapy in combination with *ex vivo* leucocyte activation has been more successful, particularly with renal cell carcinoma. In this procedure some of the patient's own leucocytes are extracted and incubated *in vitro* with IL-2. A proportion of these cells develop into lymphokine-activated killer (LAK) cells which are then returned to the patient's body together with a low dose of IL-2. This technique has limited the toxicity associated with high-dose cytokines and further refinements are being explored. These include the insertion of cytokine genes into patient tumour cells

and the use of leucocytes that have been isolated from the tumour which should 'home' onto the tumour upon reintroduction into the body. Interferons α and β (IFN-α/β) may be useful in a range of cancer types, particularly hairy cell leukaemia where a response rate of up to 90% has been reported.

Antibodies may also contribute to cancer management. Antibodies are raised to bind preferentially to tumour-specific antigens. By conjugating a cytotoxic drug or radioisotope to the antibodies these can be delivered more specifically to the tumour target to eliminate many of the side effects of routine chemotherapy or radiotherapy. For many reasons this 'magic bullet' approach has, as yet, failed to realize its potential for cancer treatment.

Cancer diagnosis

Antibodies conjugated to radioisotopes can be administered to patients and their binding visualized by radionuclide imaging. This can be exploited either to locate tumour masses prior to high-risk surgery or to detect residual tumour tissues following surgery. In the laboratory, antibodies are used to detect tumour cells present in tissue biopsies, blood films or other samples.

Ageing and Immune Function

At both ends of the human age spectrum immune function may be compromised. Both older people and infants suffer increased frequency of, and increased morbidity and mortality associated with, infectious diseases. Elderly people also have increased susceptibility to cancer.

Neonatal immunity

Newborn infants experience a period of transient immune deficiency. This is compensated for, in part, by maternal antibodies (IgG) which crossed the placenta during the last trimester of pregnancy and also by antibodies, predominantly IgA, found in colostrum and breast milk. Premature infants have an enhanced susceptibility because they may have missed some of the important *in utero* transfer and may also have difficulties in feeding. Within 2 years normal infants should have adult levels of all antibody isotypes.

Immunosenescence

A simple relationship between ageing and declining immunocompetence (immunosenescence) is the reduced amount of active primary lymphoid tissue. By age 50 the thymus is only about 15% of its maximum size and active bone marrow is found only in the sternum and pelvis, the remainder being replaced by adipose tissues. Clinically relevant deficiency is unlikely to occur, however, until over the age of about 65.

Studies on humans, mice and rats have documented age-associated decreases in both cellular and humoral responses accompanied by increased auto-immunity. These observations would indicate reduced overall control of immune function. Prospective studies on individuals would suggest a strong positive association between maintenance of *in vitro* T cell function and longevity. There is a progressive quantitative and qualitative decline in antibody production.

Several studies have indicated that it is possible to reverse apparent age-associated immune deficiencies by nutritional supplementation with, for example, vitamin B$_6$ and vitamin E. Owing in part to the confounding effects of nutritional status and general health, the precise cellular and molecular basis of immunosenescence is far from being resolved. Certainly, chronic disease and nutritional deficiencies, combined with immune dysfunction, can make a person appear rather older than his or her chronological age.

Environmental Factors and Immune Function

The interactions of the immune system with the host environment are many and various and each one is tailored to deal most effectively with the particular type of nonself being encountered.

Bacteria

The many physical barriers effectively limit access of bacteria to the body. Those that do gain entry are rapidly targeted by natural immunity. Most bacteria are killed by phagocytes but some can escape such responses. These include *Mycobacterium leprae* and *Mycobacterium tuberculosis*, which live within host macrophages. Their replication leads to the diseases of leprosy and tuberculosis, respectively. The host macrophages may, however, be stimulated by the cytokine interferon γ (IFN-γ) from T cells and the mycobacteria are killed.

The acquired response is predominantly antibody-mediated. Antibody can neutralize the toxins produced by several pathogenic bacteria, e.g. diphtheria toxin. It also activates complement which is particularly effective against Gram-negative bacteria.

Immune responses to bacterial infections may be potentially lethal to the host in the condition known as septicaemia. The organisms release powerful stimulants of TNF-α, IL-1 and IL-6. Massive amounts of these cytokines cause excessively high fever, diffuse intravascular coagulation, circulatory collapse and haemorrhagic necrosis. The patient dies from multiorgan failure.

Fungi and yeasts

The precise mechanisms involved in fungal immunity are poorly defined. There may be some neutrophil activity and T cells secrete cytokines to activate macrophages which kill the fungi. Infections with *Candida albicans* are common in immunosuppressed patients

Parasites

Parasitic infections are a major problem, especially in tropical countries where the effects may be exacerbated by malnutrition. Malaria is one of the most widespread of diseases killing up to 2 million people annually. Where parasitic worms are endemic stunted growth and mental retardation in children may occur.

Both antibody and cell-mediated responses may be stimulated, depending upon the particular infecting organism. In general terms, organisms that invade the bloodstream, e.g. malaria, trypanosomiasis, induce antibody production, while those that live in tissues are associated with cell-mediated responses. Helminthic infections involve elevated IgE levels and increased recruitment of eosinophils.

Many parasites may escape from killing by macrophages and live within those cells; these include *Toxoplasma gondii*, *Trypanosoma cruzi* and *Leishmania* spp. As with intracellular bacteria, IFN-γ from T cells is essential to activate the macrophages and so overcome the infection. The possession of genes for certain MHC proteins appears to favour effective antiparasite responses accounting, in part, for different racial susceptibilities. Many parasitic infections are not cleared but enter a chronic phase that may extend over many years. The host response continues throughout this time, causing damage to the host.

Viruses

The earliest responses to viruses involve NK cells, IFN-α and IFN-β. The cytokines induce an antiviral state in which adjacent cells are resistant to infection. NK cells are further stimulated by IFN-γ. Viral antigens are presented in association with class I MHC on cell surfaces so cytotoxic responses can be targeted against virally infected cells.

The most significant effectors in the acquired response are cytotoxic CD8+ T cells, although CD4+

cells also contribute by releasing cytokines to activate macrophages and by producing antibodies. Some antibodies, with complement, may neutralize viruses. Phagocytes also engulf extracellular virus particles. This phenomenon would contribute to the large numbers of HIV particles found within macrophages in infected patients. Macrophages, unlike T cells, are not killed but act as reservoirs of HIV even when the virus is undetectable in the circulation.

Responses to some tumours and to cells in mismatched transplants or transfusions are thought to be the same as those directed against viruses. Although fetal tissues may appear to be nonself, specific immunosuppression normally prevents rejection of the fetus. Breakdown of this system may contribute to many spontaneous abortions (miscarriages).

Responses to ingested antigens

The gut provides a significantly larger area for interaction between self and nonself than does the skin and is more likely to absorb than to exclude nonself. An understanding of the structures and functions of the complex arrangement of lymphoid tissue associated with the gastrointestinal tract is now rapidly emerging. Within Peyer's patches antigen is presented such that antigen-specific suppressor T cells are generated. These cells can recirculate throughout the body and tolerance (nonresponsiveness) to antigens presented in the gut becomes systemic. IgA in the gut lumen is important in preventing microorganisms from binding to the gut wall and so gaining access to tissues.

The question of the importance to human health of unwanted reactions against foods, i.e. food allergy, is unanswered. A possible simplistic interpretation is that unwanted responses to food antigens happen only when antigen is presented inappropriately, e.g. when the gut wall is damaged.

See also: **Ageing**: Biological Aspects. **Arthritis**: Dietary Aspects of Aetiology and Nutritional Management. **Caffeine**: Chemistry and Physiological Effects. **Children**: Nutritional Problems of Preschool Children; Nutritional Problems of School Children. **Coeliac Disease**: Aetiology and Nutritional Management. **Cytokines**: Nutritional Aspects. **Food Allergies**: Aetiology; Diagnosis and Management. **Food Intolerance**: Types and Incidence. **Gastrointestinal Tract**: Structure and Function of the Small Intestine. **HIV Disease**: Nutritional Management. **Immunity**: Role of Iron and Zinc. **Infection**: Nutritional Interactions. **Malnutrition**: Definition, Classification and Epidemiology. **Microflora of the Intestine**: Role and Effects. **Older People**: Physiological Changes; Nutritionally Related Problems. **Pregnancy**: Role of Placenta in Nutrient Transfer.

Further Reading

Brostoff J, Scadding GK, Male DK and Roitt IM (1991) *Clinical Immunology*. London: Gower Medical Publishing.

Hannigan BM (1994) Diet and immune function. *British Journal of Biomedical Science* 51:252–259.

Heatley RV (ed.) (1994) *Gastrointestinal and Hepatic Immunology*. Cambridge: Cambridge University Press.

Holliday R (1995) *Understanding Ageing*. Cambridge: Cambridge University Press.

Male D, Cooke A, Owen M, Trowsdale J and Champion B (1996) *Advanced Immunology*, 3rd edn. London: Mosby.

Roitt IM (1994) *Essential Immunology*. Oxford: Blackwell Scientific Publications.

Roitt IM, Brostoff J, Male DK and Gray A (1994) *Case Studies in Immunology*. London: Mosby.

Roitt IM, Brostoff J and Male DK (1996) *Immunology*, 4th edn. London: Mosby.

Rosenberg SA (1992) *The Transformed Cell*. London: Chapmans Publishers Ltd.

Springhouse Professional Care Guide (1995) *Immune Disorders*. Springhouse, Pennsylvania: Springhouse Corporation.

Thompson AW (ed.) (1991) *The Cytokine Handbook*. London: Academic Press.

Role of Iron and Zinc

G T Keusch, New England Medical Center, Boston, Massachusetts, USA

Copyright © 1998 Academic Press

Dramatic changes in mineral distribution occur at the outset of infections, with particularly striking shifts of extracellular iron and zinc to the intracellular compartment. Similar alterations have been documented in a wide range of species, suggesting that these changes probably have some survival value for the host. Because iron and zinc are essential for growth and replication of microorganisms, it is possible that the rapid decrease in circulating iron and zinc during infections could limit the supply of these essential minerals for the invading pathogens. The hypothesis that the acute response to shift nutrients from the circulation to the intracellular compartment represents a withholding strategy to deprive the invading pathogens of the essential divalent cationic factors they need to thrive, termed 'nutritional immunity', has been controversial. However, whether or not nutritional immunity really constitutes a host strategy for survival is of much more than scientific interest, as decisions regarding both acute care and public health interventions may depend on the answer.

Iron

Two observations underlie the concept of nutritional immunity with respect to iron. The first is the well-documented decrease in circulating iron levels during acute infections, as iron is rapidly taken up into tissue stores, and the second is the apparently heightened susceptibility to infection of patients with iron overload syndromes, suggesting that excess iron promotes infections. These clinical observations have been supported by studies in vitro in which the rate of microbial growth diminished when iron was removed from culture media.

Iron is a reactive transition metal and in its free state readily catalyses oxidative and peroxidative reactions to form unstable, toxic reactive oxygen intermediates that will damage cell membranes and degrade DNA. To limit this oxidative tissue damage, iron is highly protein-bound in metalloproteins and enzymes used in oxygen transport, energy metabolism and DNA synthesis, as well as being tightly bound to transport and storage proteins. As a consequence, humans represent a highly restricted environment for free iron. To be successful, however, pathogens need to obtain iron, and they have developed mechanisms to accomplish this in the face of the limiting amount of free iron in their target hosts. One common solution for pathogenic organisms is the production of high-affinity iron chelators (siderophores) able to strip iron from host iron-binding proteins such as transferrin, even when the binding affinity for iron is high.

Siderophores are not produced when free iron is available, as in the external environment or in artificial culture systems, but they are rapidly synthesized when the organisms encounter limiting iron availability, as in their mammalian host. Free iron concentration itself is the critical signal of this biological sensor system, commonly through a negative transcriptional regulatory system called Fur (ferric uptake regulator). In this system the product of the *fur* gene, the Fur protein, binds iron if it is available and in this form recognizes and binds to a consensus sequence in the promoter region of Fur-regulated genes. The binding of Fe-Fur prevents the transcription of that gene and its product is not made. However, in the absence of free iron Fur falls off the iron box region of the promoter allowing it to become active and functional in transcription and make its gene product. There are, however, several genes required for iron utilization and microbial growth. Because nature frequently opts for parsimony, the whole set of iron regulatory genes, including those regulating uptake and utilization, are all controlled by the Fur system. In addition, low free iron concentration signals to the organism that it is within a mammalian host, and other proteins needed by the pathogen to survive host defence are turned on as well. In this manner the *fur* gene acts as a master switch, controlling not only the whole process of iron acquisition, uptake and utilization, but also a number of other genes, many of which are virulence genes involved in disease pathogenesis. This ability to acquire iron under adverse conditions of iron availability and the use of low iron levels as a signal to make microbial virulence factors raises serious questions whether infection-mediated hypoferraemia has any significant 'nutritional immunity' function.

Iron is also required for the synthesis of DNA, which, in turn, is obligatory for the proliferation of lymphocytes involved in immune responses. The rate-limiting enzyme for DNA synthesis is ribonucleotide reductase, an iron metalloenzyme which must be continuously synthesized and is therefore dependent on a continuous supply of iron. This may be the physiological reason for the expression of transferrin receptors on lymphocytes activated by interleukin 2. Iron deficiency, then, may lead to impaired lymphocyte proliferative responses because transferrin iron, essential for DNA synthesis, is in limiting concentrations. Diminished expansion of lymphocyte clones involved in the immune response in iron deficiency states could underlie the defects in immune function that have been reported. For example, in a number of studies assessing skin test reactions to recall antigens in vivo or incorporation of [³H]thymidine by mitogen-stimulated cells in vitro, the response was diminished in iron-deficient hosts compared with iron-sufficient hosts and improved in the former following iron therapy. The results of mitogen stimulation assays have been somewhat more variable, but still abnormal in the majority, consistent with a defect in DNA synthesis.

Other iron-dependent host defence mechanisms may be affected by iron deficiency. For example, the neutrophil iron metalloenzyme myeloperoxidase is clearly inhibited in iron deficiency states. This enzyme catalyses generation of bactericidal reactive halide radicals during the oxidative burst initiated by phagocytosis by neutrophils. While myeloperoxidase may contribute to host defences by this mechanism it turns out not to be necessary, since patients with congenital deficiency of the enzyme do not exhibit an increased susceptibility to infection. Iron also catalyses the production of bactericidal oxygen radicals by other mechanisms, and a defect in this pathway may explain the reduced ability of neutrophils from iron-deficient subjects to reduce the dye nitroblue tetrazolium under conditions of cell activation. Consistent with this, some but not all studies have shown a modest decrease in bacterial killing capacity by iron-deficient neutrophils, although other iron-independent functions such as chemotaxis, phagocytosis and degranulation are normal.

The other component of the nutritional immunity argument is that iron excess leads to increased infections; ergo, iron withholding may protect the host. Indeed, studies *in vitro* have shown that as iron content of the medium increases from zero to higher levels, microbial growth is enhanced. Moreover, the growth inhibitory effect of adding iron-binding proteins to these cultures is reversed by adding free iron. When *Vibrio vulnificus*, a highly iron-dependent, siderophore-negative organism that will not grow in normal human serum, is inoculated in the presence of serum from haemochromatosis patients, it grows well. Clinical studies have also shown an increase in infection morbidity in patients with iron overload states such as β-thalassaemia, sickle-cell anaemia with a history of multiple transfusions, idiopathic haemochromatosis or so-called 'Bantu' haemosiderosis resulting from grossly excessive oral iron intake. In all of these conditions, transferrin is fully saturated with iron, and the excess free metal circulates as low molecular weight loose complexes with albumin which are readily available to pathogens lacking an iron acquisition system. Both experimental and clinical iron overload states are associated with increased susceptibility to infection, but when more carefully examined this is predominantly susceptibility to organisms that lack an effective iron acquisition system, for example *Yersinia enterocolitica*. Such strains are of low virulence and do not grow well *in vivo* unless iron transport proteins are saturated and free iron becomes available. *Yersinia enterocolitica* may also obtain iron from iron–deferoxamine chelates *in vitro*, and this may explain the reported association between deferoxamine chelation therapy used for iron overload states and *Yersinia* sepsis. Furthermore, careful review of infection deaths in thalassaemia patients shows a highly significant association with splenectomy and not with transfusion siderosis, suggesting it is splenectomy and not iron excess that impairs host defence.

Iron excess states are also associated with impaired immune function, for example diminished neutrophil superoxide and hydrogen peroxide production, diminished nitroblue tetrazolium reduction, and reduced bactericidal activity. Cells from thalassaemic patients are reported to show reduced chemotaxis and random migration, and peripheral blood monocytes show diminished capacity to kill *Candida pseudotopicalis* or *Staphylococcus aureus*. These defects are probably due to the membrane-damaging oxidative and peroxidative reactions associated with iron excess.

Thus, the relationship between iron and infection depends very much on the identity of the causative organism, the ability of that organism to acquire iron, and the state of iron nutriture of the host. Both iron deficiency and iron excess exert adverse effects on immune responses, and alter the metabolism and growth of the pathogens and the mechanisms by which they obtain the iron they require. The balance of these various effects ultimately determines clinical outcome. Population-based morbidity studies have not produced clear-cut results, probably because the design is often flawed, the sample size is too small to analyse statistically or no attempt is made to control for relevant confounding factors. There are differences in the age of subjects, the route, form and dose of iron administered, the adequacy of controls employed and the presence of other nutritional abnormalities that affect host defence; and iron status is often poorly documented, infections are not confirmed, and there is neither a correlation between the severity of the deficiency and the frequency of infections, nor an effect of iron supplementation.

Zinc

The hypozincaemia of infection is, like iron, part of the acute-phase response mediated by cytokines such as interleukin 1, which in this case induces the synthesis of the intracellular zinc-binding protein metallothionine. As a result, zinc is rapidly removed from the circulation and taken up by cells in the liver, thymus and bone marrow. The physiological role of this acute transfer of zinc from the extracellular to the intracellular compartment is not clear but it may be related to the dependency of DNA transcription and RNA translation on zinc metalloenzymes. Because of this, shifts of zinc to the intracellular compartment of lymphocytes could help increase the proliferative efficiency of lymphocytes involved in the immune response to infections and thus enhance host defence. Zinc deficiency, on the other hand, might be expected to diminish the lymphocyte proliferative response and impair host defence.

Severe zinc deficiency has significant clinical and biological effects, including growth retardation, delay in sexual and skeletal maturation, skin lesions and anorexia. In addition, defects in cell-mediated immunity and increased susceptibility to infections are well described in the human disease acrodermatitis enteropathica, and a similar syndrome exists in Friesian cattle. In both examples, zinc deficiency is results from a defect in intestinal absorption of zinc, and the associated abnormalities are reversed by providing increased oral zinc. Experimental zinc deprivation in animals results in thymic involution, splenic atrophy and lymphopenia. As a consequence the proliferative response to both T dependent and T independent mitogens is reduced. In addition to the inhibitory effect of zinc deficiency on DNA synthesis, the depressed lymphocyte proliferative response may be related to altered cytokine metabolism. Whatever the mechanism, zinc deficiency leads to depression of delayed hypersensitivity responses.

Zinc also plays a role in regulating the activation of acute-phase genes via its ability to bind to RNA finger loop domains known as 'zinc fingers' involved in the conformational stabilization of transcription factor proteins that allow sequence-specific DNA recognition and gene expression. If zinc deficiency blocks these regulatory signals as well, host responses may be altered as the translation of genes normally activated during the acute-phase reaction is impaired. Another essential role of zinc in the immune response is its binding to certain thymus-derived peptides that appear to function as hormones in the differentiation of T cells. Reversible inhibition of thymulin function has been described in human zinc deficiency. Several studies have reported that the synthesis of thymic peptide hormones is decreased in protein–energy malnutrition (which is almost always accompanied by zinc deficiency), suggesting that this defect may underlie the decreased number of mature T cells and increased number of immature T cells found in the circulation of these patients. Similar mechanisms may lead to the depletion of mature T cells observed in other zinc deficiency states, and heighten susceptibility to infection.

A few studies have suggested that zinc status may affect the production and/or membrane binding of certain cytokine regulators of immune responses, including interleukins 1 and 2, and interferon. Systematic studies of zinc status, cytokines and immune function will help to unravel these interactions.

Although zinc plays an essential role in biology and immunology and there is a relatively large amount of zinc in the body, there is no physiologically regulated store of the metal. Continuous ingestion of zinc is necessary to sustain zinc-dependent functions at normal levels. Although not yet systematically examined, periodic bolus administration of zinc in the face of zinc-poor diets is not likely to be as effective in preventing or treating zinc deficiency as is the case for vitamin A, which is stored in the liver. Approximately 60% of the 2 g of body zinc is in skeletal muscle and less than 0.1% is in the circulation, the compartment most often sampled to assess zinc status. Interestingly, muscle catabolism releases zinc, but whether this is taken up and used in the acute response to infection is not certain.

Because of the consistent finding of the dependency of normal immune function on adequate zinc availability, the association of zinc deficiency with increased infection morbidity is explicable. Experimental confirmation of this relationship has been accomplished by the challenge of zinc-deficient animals with bacteria (*Francisella tularensis*), protozoa (*Trypanosoma cruzi*), helminths (*T. spiralis*) and fungi (*Candida albicans*) and the demonstration of increased susceptibility and severity of infection. Attention has recently turned to the possibility of using zinc supplements to reduce the incidence or severity of infection in malnourished children. The studies have been interventional trials for children with protein–energy malnutrition in developing countries, in whom there is evidence of limiting zinc in their diet and zinc deficiency as assessed by hair, nail clippings or plasma zinc content. Community-based prospective zinc supplementation of poorly nourished infants and children, and therapeutic trials in acutely ill children, suggest a decrease in susceptibility to diarrhoea, respiratory infection and possibly malaria in the former studies, and a more rapid improvement in patients in some of the latter studies.

Some of the variability in results may be related to the fact that zinc absorption is influenced by a number of factors, among the most important of which are the amount of zinc in the diet, and the presence of phytates (derived from some grains and vegetables) which bind the metal and inhibits its uptake. Many complex interactions occur as well between zinc and other dietary constituents, including proteins, amino acids and calcium, some enhancing and some inhibiting zinc uptake; thus the overall effect can be difficult to predict. Requirements for zinc also increase during catch-up growth when protein–energy malnutrition is treated, and therefore zinc uptake may be the limiting factor during nutritional rehabilitation. There is, however, some danger of toxicity from excessive zinc intake. A study of zinc supplementation in the treatment of protein–energy malnutrition has reported a zinc dose-related increase in mortality ($P = 0.03$; relative risk 4.5, confidence interval 1.09 to 18.8). It is clearly necessary to continue to study the effects of zinc in these patients in order to determine optimal dosage and duration of treatment strategies and define the safety of the intervention.

See also: **Infection**: Nutritional Management. **Iron**: Physiology, Dietary Sources and Requirements. **Zinc**: Physiology.

Further Reading

Allen JI, Kay NE and McClain CJ (1981) Severe zinc deficiency in humans: association with a reversible T-lymphocyte dysfunction. *Annals of Internal Medicine* 95:154–157.

Bandari N, Bahl R, Hambidge KM and Bhan MK (1996) Increased diarrhoeal and respiratory morbidity in association with zinc deficiency – a preliminary report. *Acta Paediatrica* 85:148–150.

Beisel WR (1975) Metabolic response to infection. *Annual Review of Medicine* 26:9–20.

Bhutta ZA (1997) The role of zinc in health and disease: relevance to child health in developing countries. *Journal of the Pakistan Medical Association* 47:68–73.

Brummerstedt E (1977) Animal model of human disease. Acrodermatitis enteropathica, zinc malabsorption. *American Journal of Pathology* 87:725–728.

Bryan CF and Stone MJ (1993) The immunoregulatory properties of iron. In: Cunningham-Rundles S (ed.) *Nutrient Modulation of the Immune Response*, pp 105–126. New York: Marcel Dekker.

Chandra RK and Saraya AK (1975) Impaired immunocompetence associated with iron deficiency. *Journal of Pediatrics* 86:899–902.

Doherty C (1997) Protein-energy malnutrition and zinc supplementation. In: *Zinc and Health in South Asia* (abstracts) p 24. Dhaka: ICDDRB Centre for Health and Population Research.

Driessen C, Hirv K and Rink L (1994) Induction of cytokines by zinc ions in human peripheral blood mononuclear cells and separated monocytes. *Lymphokine and Cytokine Research* 13:15–20.

Fenwick PK, Aggett PJ, McDonald D, Huber C and Wakelin D (1990) Zinc deficiency and zinc repletion: effect on the response of rats to infection with *Trichinella spiralis. American Journal of Clinical Nutrition* 52:166–172.

Guerinot ML (1994) Microbial iron transport. *Annual Review of Microbiology* 48:743–772.

Keusch GT (1994) Nutrition and infection. In: Shils ME, Olson JA and Shike M (eds) *Modern Nutrition in Health and Disease*, 8th edn, pp 1241–1258. Philadelphia: Lea & Febiger.

Mocchegiani E, Santarelli L and Muzzioli M (1995) Reversibility of the thymic involution and of age-related peripheral immune dysfunctions by zinc supplementation in old mice. *International Journal of Immunopharmacology* 17:703–718.

Moynahan EJ (1975) Zinc deficiency and cellular immune deficiency in acrodermatitis enteropathica in man and zinc deficiency with thymic hypoplasia in fresian calves: a possible genetic link. *Lancet* ii:710.

Ninh NX, Thissen JP, Collette L, Gerard G, Khoi HH and Ketelslegers JM (1996). Zinc supplementation increases growth and circulating insulin-like growth factor I (IGF-I) in growth-retarded Vietnamese children. *American Journal of Clinical Nutrition* 63:514–519.

Prasad AS (1993) *Biochemistry and Zinc*. New York: Plenum Press.

Prasad AS (1996) Zinc: the biology and therapeutics of an ion. *Annals of Internal Medicine* 125:142–144.

Prasad AS, Meftah S and Abdallah J (1988) Serum thymulin in human zinc deficiency. *Journal of Clinical Investigation* 82:1201–1210.

Rosado JL, Lopez P, Munoz E, Martinez H and Allen LH (1997) Zinc supplementation reduced morbidity, but neither zinc nor iron supplementation affected growth or body composition of Mexican preschoolers *American Journal of Clinical Nutrition* 65:13–19.

Roy SK, Tomkins AM, Akramuzzaman SM *et al.* (1997) Impact of zinc supplementation on clinical outcome of malnourished Bangladeshi children with acute diarrhea. *Archives of Disease in Childhood*.

Salvin SB and Rabin BS (1984) Resistance and susceptibility to infection in inbred murine strains. IV. Effects of dietary zinc. *Cell Immunology* 87:546–552.

Sazawal S, Black RE, Bhan MK, Bhandari N, Sinha A and Jalla S (1995) Zinc supplementation in young children with acute diarrhea in India. *New England and Journal of Medicine* 333:839–844.

Sazawal S, Black RE, Bhan MK *et al.* (1996) Zinc supplementation reduces the incidence of persistent diarrhea and dysentery among low socioeconomic children in India. *Journal of Nutrition* 126:443–450.

Schwabe JWR and Rhodes D (1991) Beyond zinc fingers: steroid hormone receptors have a novel structural motif for DNA recognition. *Trends in Biochemical Sciences* 16:291–296.

Winchurch RA (1988) Activation of thymocyte responses to interleukin-1 by zinc. *Clinical Immunology and Immunopathology* 47:174–180.

Wooldridge KG and Williams PH (1993) Iron uptake mechanisms of pathogenic bacteria. *FEMS Microbiological Review* 12:325–348.

INBORN ERRORS OF METABOLISM

Contents

Classification and Biochemical Aspects

J Coutts and **J E Wraith**, Royal Manchester Children's Hospital, Manchester, UK

Copyright © 1998 Academic Press

The inborn errors of metabolism are a family of genetic disorders in which an enzyme deficiency usually results in the accumulation of a 'toxic' intermediary compound. In addition, for certain disorders, an essential end product is not produced in adequate amounts. For some disorders, amplification of enzyme activity can be achieved by the administration of the appropriate cofactor, usually a vitamin; in others, supplying the missing product is the only treatment required. For many conditions, specific dietary restriction is the only effective method of treatment and the prescribed diets are often complex and exacting for the affected individuals and family. These latter disorders form the basis of this article.

Detection and Diagnosis

In most developed countries newborn screening for phenylketonuria is well established. Depending on the method employed in the screening laboratory a number of other amino acid disorders, e.g. homocystinuria, may be detected. Modifications of the basic screening procedures have been adopted in some areas to detect other diseases, e.g. galactosaemia. For other conditions, e.g. organic acidaemias, selective screening of populations at risk, such as the sick newborn, may lead to early diagnosis.

Some individuals avoid detection in the neonatal period and present in later infancy or childhood with developmental problems or an encephalopathic illness. The key to diagnosis in this situation is a high index of suspicion on the part of the clinician and ready access to a laboratory specializing in the diagnosis of metabolic disorders. Expert dietetic help and specialized laboratory facilities are essential for follow-up and for these reasons referral to a regional centre specializing in the management of such children is in the best interests of the patient and family.

Galactosaemia

Galactosaemia caused by galactose 1-phosphate uridyl transferase deficiency ('classical galactosaemia') is associated with a severe systemic illness after the introduction of milk feeds in the newborn period.

Characteristically, the infant is normal at birth and the following symptoms appear towards the end of the first week: jaundice, vomiting, lethargy, oedema, ascites and hepatomegaly. Cataracts develop after days or weeks and there is a particular susceptibility to infection. If the infant survives the severe neonatal illness, mental development is retarded. Early diagnosis and institution of a galactose-free diet prevents or reverses the severe neonatal illness, but there are still some late complications. Despite early treatment and good biochemical control, the majority of patients have significant intellectual impairment as adults, with a mean intelligence quotient (IQ) of between 60 and 80. Acquisition of speech is often significantly delayed. In addition, girls are at particular risk from hypergonadotrophic hypogonadism which occurs in 80% of affected females.

Dietary treatment

The diet for galactosaemia is essentially milk-free. All mammalian milks and their products must be completely eliminated from the diet. Although galactosides, which are found in many fruits and vegetables, and nucleoproteins, found in organ meats (e.g. liver) and egg, are potential sources of galactose, the α-galactosidases necessary to release the galactose are not present in the human intestinal mucosa. However, some practitioners still advise that these foods should not be included in the diet of children under the age of 2 years. An important source of galactose is the lactose used as an extender in some pharmaceutical preparations and in flavourings. A soya protein isolate infant formula or a feed based on cow's milk from which the lactose has been removed may be used for babies with galactosaemia.

Table 1   Characteristics and treatment of various inborn errors of metabolism

Disorder	Enzyme deficiency	Clinical features	Dietary treatment
Homocystinuria	Cystathionine synthase	'Marfanoid' habitus, mental retardation, eye lens dislocation, osteoporosis, premature arteriosclerosis	Similar in principle to that for phenylketonuria using protein supplements which are free from methionine and with added cystine
Tyrosinaemia	Fumarylacetoacetate hydrolase	Liver cirrhosis, failure and hepatoma Renal tubular dysfunction	As for phenylketonuria using a protein supplement free from both phenylalanine and tyrosine and in some forms of the condition also free from methionine
Maple syrup urine disease	Branched-chain ketoacid dehydrogenase	Recurrent metabolic acidosis, encephalopathy, mental retardation	In principle, the same as for phenylketonuria with a protein supplement free from leucine, valine and isoleucine. Natural foods are measured in portions containing 50 mg leucine. Small additions of valine and/or isoleucine as pure amino acids may be necessary
Organic acidaemia	Various	Similar to maple syrup urine disease	A low-protein diet with amino acid supplement free from methionine, valine, threonine and isoleucine. May need to be fed by nasogastric tube because persistent anorexia conflicts with the high energy requirement. Protein-free diet during infections causing catabolism
Urea cycle defects	Various	Vomiting, feeding difficulties, encephalopathy, mental retardation	Low-protein, high-energy diet. Protein-free diet during infections causing catabolism
Hereditary fructose intolerance	Aldolase B	Hypoglycaemia, vomiting, hepatomegaly, jaundice, renal tubular dysfunction on exposure to fructose	Fructose- and sucrose-free diet
Glycogen storage disease (hepatic)	Various	Hypoglycaemia, hepatomegaly Severity of symptoms depends on the exact enzyme defect	Type I glycogen storage disease requires a diet with 60–70% energy from carbohydrate, normal protein and low fat (15–20%). Maintaining a normal blood glucose level throughout the 24 h requires frequent daytime feeding and a continuous nasogastric feed overnight. Children over the age of 4 years can be given some of their carbohydrate as raw corn starch at mealtimes and before bed; being slowly digested and absorbed this maintains the blood glucose between meals and overnight.
Familial hyper-cholesterolaemia	Deficiency of low-density lipo-protein receptors	Tendon xanthomas, coronary artery disease	A minimal-fat diet with polyunsaturated oils in moderation
Adreno-leucodystrophy	Very long-chain fatty acid ligase	Neurodegeneration, adrenal failure	Minimal-fat diet with 20% energy supplied by Lorenzo's oil (mixture of 4 parts glycerol trioleate oil and 1 part glycerol trierucate oil); extra glycerol trioleate oil may be used for cooking. Minimal requirements for essential fatty acids should be met with a small supplement of safflower oil

Other Inborn Errors of Metabolism

The natural history of many other inborn errors of metabolism can be influenced by dietary treatment and these are summarized in **Table 1**. In general, the prescribed diet is *specific*, e.g. in inborn errors of essential amino acid metabolism such as homocystinuria or maple syrup urine disease, or *nonspecific*, e.g. a general restriction of dietary protein intake in conditions such as urea cycle defects. Other conditions, e.g. fatty acid oxidation defects, are not influenced by dietary protein intake, but are responsive to manipulations in dietary fat and carbohydrate intake.

The principles of a low-protein and a low-fat diet are described briefly below.

Low-protein diet

The diets for organic acidaemias and urea cycle defects are very similar. The protein must be limited to what the individual can tolerate, which may be from 0.5 g to 1.5 g per kg of body weight per day. Ample energy must also be provided from fat and carbohydrate to spare the protein for synthesis of new tissue as well as vitamins and minerals. Infants may be fed a regular whey-based formula up to their protein tolerance with additional glucose polymer and fat emulsion to make up the energy requirement. An amino acid mixture containing all amino acids except methionine, valine, threonine and isoleucine may be used to provide extra nitrogen in the diet for organic acidaemias such as methylmalonic acidaemia. During periods of metabolic stress caused by infection, the protein intake should be stopped and extra carbohydrate given as high-carbohydrate drinks.

Low-fat, high-carbohydrate diet

Such a diet may be needed for the treatment of fatty acid oxidation defects or some forms of glycogen storage disease. In these conditions frequent feeds rich in carbohydrate and low in fat are needed. For infants a formula made up of 25–50% regular baby milk with additional skim milk powder and glucose polymer provides approximately 2 g protein and 70 kcal (294 kJ) per 100 ml. The amount of regular milk will depend on the individual tolerance of fat. A supplement of fat-soluble vitamins will be necessary. Older children should be kept on a low-fat diet using skimmed milk and between-meal carbohydrate snacks such as drinks of skimmed milk, or fruit juice with added glucose polymer. Advice on dental hygiene and fluoride supplements should be given.

See also: **Fatty Acids**: Metabolism. **Galactose**: Absorption and Metabolism. **Hyperlipidaemia (Hyperlipidemia)**: Nutritional Management.

Further Reading

Francis D (1987) *Diets for Sick Children*, 4th edn. Oxford: Blackwell.

Scriver CR, Beaudet AL, Sly WS and Valle D, eds (1990) *The Metabolic Basis of Inherited Disease*, 6th edn. Maidenhead: McGraw-Hill.

Nutritional Management of Phenylketonuria

P B Acosta, Ross Products Division, Columbus, Ohio, USA

L J Elsas, Emory University School of Medicine, Atlanta, Georgia, USA

Copyright © 1998 Academic Press

Definition and Aetiology

Phenylketonuria (PKU), discovered in 1933, is a group of inherited disorders of phenylalanine metabolism resulting from impaired phenylalanine hydroxylase activity (**Table 1**). The disorder is expressed at 3–6 months of age and is characterized by developmental delay, microcephaly (small head circumference), abnormal electroencephalogram (EEG), eczema, musty odour and hyperactivity. If not treated before 3 weeks of age, the resulting metabolic imbalance produces irreversible mental retardation. The defect in metabolism in classic PKU is associated with less than 2% activity of phenylalanine hydroxylase, which is expressed primarily in liver. Considerable heterogeneity exists for mutations affecting this apoenzyme. Heterozygous parents for 'classic' PKU have 50% enzyme activity but are clinically normal.

The essential amino acid phenylalanine is utilized for tissue protein synthesis and hydroxylation to form tyrosine. The hydroxylation reaction requires phenylalanine hydroxylase, oxygen, tetrahydrobio-

Table 1 Enzyme classification (EC) number for enzymes

Enzyme name	EC number
Dihydropteridine reductase	1.6.99.7
Guanosine triphosphate cyclohydrolase	3.5.4.16
Phenylalanine hydroxylase	1.14.16.1
6-Pyruvoyltetrahyrobiopterin synthase	No number
Tryptophan hydroxylase	1.14.16.4
Tyrosine hydroxylase	1.14.16.2

pterin (H_4 biopterin), dihydropteridine reductase and NADH + H^+ (**Fig. 1**). In the growing normal child, 60% of the phenylalanine required is used for new protein synthesis and 40% is hydroxylated to form tyrosine. In the normal adult, only 10% of the recommended intake for phenylalanine is required for new protein synthesis, whereas approximately 90% is hydroxylated to form tyrosine. Alternative pathways, available for phenylalanine metabolism as outlined in Fig. 1, are minor in the metabolism of phenylalanine at 50 μmol l^{-1} concentration in the plasma of normal persons. However, by-products become apparent when phenylalanine is not hydroxylated to tyrosine and accumulates to over 500 μmol l^{-1}.

Tyrosine is the normal immediate product of phenylalanine and is essential for synthesis of protein, catecholamines, melanin pigment and thyroid hormones (Fig. 1). Tyrosine also provides energy when catabolized through p-hydroxyphenylpyruvate to fumarate and acetoacetate.

The gene for disorders of phenylalanine hydroxylase has been localized to chromosome 12q22–q24. The gene has 90 kilobases, 13 exons and 12 introns. More than 250 mutations have been found in the gene that codes for phenylalanine hydroxylase. At least eight different mutations have been identified that cause the 'PKU phenotype'; these involve deletions in coding frames, missense mutations and intron splice site mutations. Ethnic variation occurs in the type and frequency of phenylalanine hydroxylase mutations.

Other forms of PKU may result from defects in enzymes involved in the overall reaction. Dihydropteridine reductase (Table 1) is an enzyme normally present in many tissues. It reduces the quininoid form of dihydrobiopterin (H_2 biopterin) to H_4 biopterin (Fig. 1). The gene for dihydropteridine reductase is located on chromosome 4p15.1–p16.1. Hyperphenylalaninemia (blood phenylalanine concentration greater than the upper limit of normal, 100 μmol l^{-1}) also results from defects in the synthesis of H_4 biopterin (Fig. 1) because of defects in guanosine triphosphate cyclohydrolase (GTP-CH) (Table 1) and 6-pyruvoyltetrahydrobiopterin synthase (no EC number assigned). In addition to functioning as coenzyme for phenylalanine hydroxylase, H_4 biopterin is required by tyrosine hydroxylase and tryptophan hydroxylase (Table 1).

Incidence

Newborn screening for PKU has been conducted for about 30 years in developed countries. In the mid 1960s, mass screening of newborn infants for PKU was initiated. Blood specimens collected on filter paper are placed on a phenylalanine-free agar base that has been seeded with *Bacillus subtilis* spores. An inhibitor is added to suppress the growth of the organism. Action of the inhibitor is overcome by the

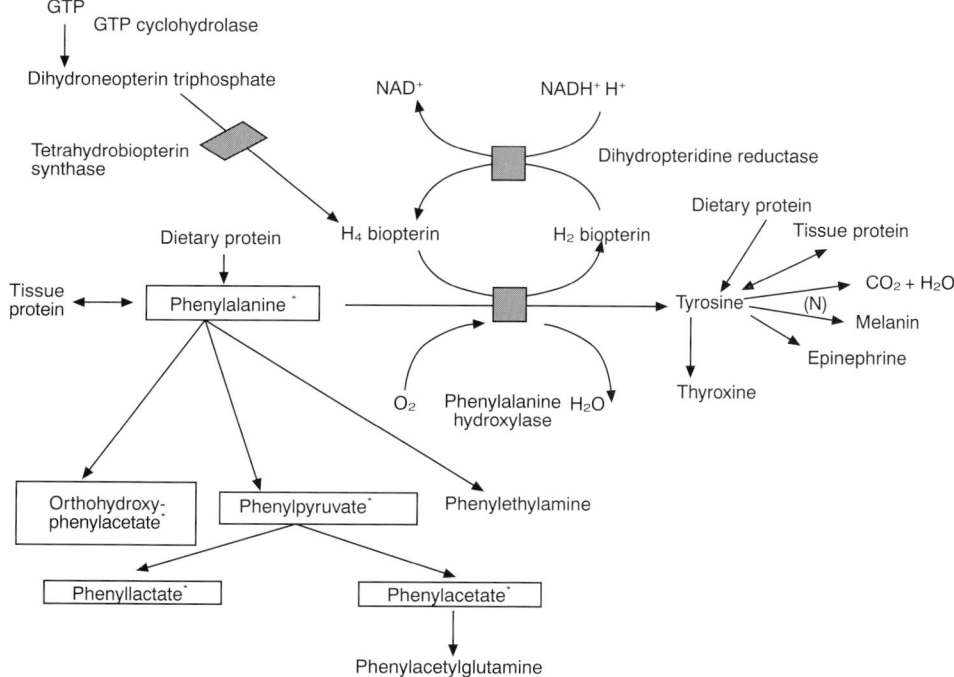

Figure 1 Phenylalanine metabolism in phenylketonuria. Shaded areas indicate sites of possible enzyme defects. Substances marked * accumulate in untreated PKU. GTP, guanosine triphosphate; (N), several steps involved.

presence of phenylalanine, which promotes the growth of *B. subtilis* around the filter paper disc containing the blood. The size of the growth around the disc depends on the amount of phenylalanine in the blood. Incidence of PKU is described in **Table 2** and varies from about 1 in 4500 live births in Ireland to about 1 in 24 000 live births in Greece.

Clinical Features

Untreated PKU

The clinical features of untreated PKU include mental, neurological and extraneural symptoms. Retarded intellectual development is the most important clinical feature. Psychotic behaviour with hyperactivity, destructiveness, self-mutilation, impulsiveness and uncontrolled attacks of rage is common. Schizophrenia-like manifestations, autism and unpredictable behaviour are frequent. About 25% of the patients have grand mal-type seizures. Abnormalities of the EEG are observed in 78–95% of untreated patients. Increased muscle tone is apparent in more than half of the patients. Eczema occurs in 20–40%. A peculiar musty, mousy, or barn-like odour is present. Mild microcephaly may be observed.

Early treated PKU

Children with elevated blood phenylalanine concentration detected by routine neonatal screening and who, after diagnosis of PKU, start phenylalanine-restricted nutrition management soon after birth, generally have intelligence within the normal range if the blood phenylalanine concentrations do not exceed 300 μmol l^{-1}. In addition to the influence of parental IQ and the age at which treatment was initiated, the age at which blood phenylalanine concentrations consistently exceed 300 μmol l^{-1} (5 mg dl^{-1}) is the best predictor of intellectual deficits in children with PKU.

Table 2 Incidence of PKU

Country	Incidence per live birth
Ireland	1 in 4500–7700
Scotland	1 in 6000
Belgium	1 in 6000–8100
Austria	1 in 8200
Australia	1 in 9000
USA	1 in 10 000–25 000
New Zealand	1 in 16 000
Netherlands	1 in 17 000
England	1 in 19 000
Canada	1 in 22 000
Greece	1 in 24 000

Chemical Pathology

Although the precise pathogenesis of mental retardation in classic PKU is not known, the accumulation of phenylalanine or its catabolic by-products, a deficiency of tyrosine or its products, competitive interactions between phenylalanine and other amino acids, or all five circumstances will produce central nervous system damage if phenylalanine accumulates in blood above normal concentrations during critical periods of brain development. The pathological consequence varies with the time in brain development at which the chemical insult occurs. Deficient myelination and abnormalities in brain proteolipids or proteins occur in late gestation and during the first 6–9 months of life. During this period, oligodendroglia (one of the types of cells in the central nervous system) migration may be impaired, resulting in irreversible brain damage later in childhood. Protein synthesis in the brain is depressed, probably owing to the effect of competitive inhibition by high phenylalanine concentrations on blood–brain barrier transport, with consequent imbalance in intraneuronal amino acid concentrations. In the mature brain, neurodegeneration, behavioural difficulties and prolonged performance times may result from depressed neurotransmitter synthesis. Impairment of these functions in the mature brain may be reversible when phenylalanine returns toward normal concentrations in cells and blood.

Nutritional Management

Patients with blood phenylalanine concentrations of greater than 300 μmol l^{-1} and plasma tyrosine concentrations below 50 μmol l^{-1} require treatment beginning prior to the third week of life with phenylalanine-restricted, tyrosine-supplemented nutrition management. The objective of nutrition management of the child with classic PKU is to maintain blood phenylalanine concentrations that will allow optimum growth and brain development by supplying adequate energy, protein and all other nutrients, while restricting phenylalanine and supplementing tyrosine intake.

Although the effects of moderately elevated concentrations of blood phenylalanine are not yet known, optimum concentrations should be as close to normal as possible. This objective is met through use of a combination of medical and natural foods. Some investigators have supplemented the phenylalanine-restricted diet with isoleucine, leucine, valine, tyrosine and tryptophan, and have found unsustained improvement in behaviour and decreased blood phenylalanine concentrations. This may be related to inhibition of phenylalanine transport by competition at either the intestinal or blood–brain barrier uptake steps.

Therapy of the child with H_4 biopterin-deficient forms of hyperphenylalaninaemia requires administration of H_4 biopterin and use of phenylalanine-restricted, tyrosine-supplemented nutrition management in combination with L-dopa (3,4-dihydroxyphenylalanine) and carbidopa. Serotonin that is derived from tryptophan may also improve behaviour if tryptophan hydroxylase is secondarily impaired by the absence of H_4 biopterin.

Initiation of nutrition support

Rapid decline of blood phenylalanine concentration at the time of diagnosis may be obtained by feeding the infant a 68 kcal dl^{-1} (286 kJ dl^{-1}) low phenylalanine or phenylalanine-free formula. Within a mean of 4 days (SD $\pm$ 3), blood phenylalanine concentration should drop to treatment range. Treatment should be initiated in hospitalized infants to enable adequate parental information transfer and to monitor blood amino acid concentrations daily. Laboratory results should be available promptly to prevent precipitation of phenylalanine deficiency and to enable rapid replacement of phenylalanine and tyrosine to optimum blood concentrations.

If the infant or child is not hospitalized for initiation of nutrition support, or if only weekly blood phenylalanine concentrations are obtained, then a maintenance formula containing adequate phenylalanine from an appropriate source should be prescribed. Blood phenylalanine concentration may fall to treatment range within a mean of 10 days (SD $\pm$ 5) with this approach. Choice of initial nutrition support must be predicated on producing controlled blood phenylalanine concentrations no later than the third week of life.

Chronic care

Long-term care of the patient with classic PKU dictates that medical and natural foods provide all nutrients in required amounts to maintain normal nutrition status.

Nutrient requirements **Table 3** shows the suggested amounts of phenylalanine, tyrosine, protein, energy and fluid needed to introduce nutrition management

Table 3 Recommended daily nutrient intakes (ranges) for infants, children and adults with PKU

	Nutrient				
Age	Phenylalanine[a,b] (mg kg^{-1})	Tyrosine (mg kg^{-1})	Protein (g kg^{-1})	Energy (kcal kg^{-1})	Fluid[c] (ml kg^{-1})
Infants					
0 to <3 months	25–70	300–350	3.50–3.00	120 (145–95)	160–135
3 to <6 months	20–45	300–350	3.50–3.00	120 (145–95)	160–130
6 to <9 months	15–35	250–300	3.00–2.50	110 (135–80)	145–125
9 to <12 months	10–35	250–300	3.00–2.50	105 (135–80)	135–120
Girls and boys	(mg per day)	(g per day)	(g per day)	(kcal per day)	(ml per day)
1 to <4 years	200–400	1.72–3.00	≥30	1300 (900–1800)	900–1800
4 to <7 years	210–450	2.25–3.50	≥35	1700 (1300–2300)	1300–2300
7 to <11 years	220–500	2.55–4.00	≥40	2400 (1650–3300)	1650–3300
Women					
11 to <15 years	250–750	3.45–5.00	≥50	2200 (1500–3000)	1500–3000
15 to <19 years	230–700	3.45–5.00	≥50	2100 (1200–3000)	1200–3000
≥19 years	220–700	3.75–5.00	≥50	2100 (1400–2500)	2100–2500
Men					
11 to <15 years	225–900	3.38–5.50	≥55	2700 (2000–3700)	2000–3700
15 to <19 years	295–1100	4.42–6.50	≥65	2800 (2100–3900)	2100–3900
≥19 years	290–1200	4.35–6.50	≥65	2900 (2000–3300)	2000–3300

[a]Modify prescription based on frequently obtained blood and/or plasma concentrations and growth in infants and children and frequently obtained plasma concentrations and weight maintenance in adults.
[b]Phenylalanine requirements of premature infants may be greater than highest value noted.
[c]Under normal circumstances, a *minimum* of 1.5 ml of fluid should be offered to neonates for each kcal ingested.
Note: 1 kcal $\approx$ 4.2 kJ.

after the plasma phenylalanine concentration is normalized. A formal prescription must be written that is individualized to the specific genotype, growth rate and consequent nutrient needs of each patient. Weekly adjustments in the nutrition management prescription may be necessary, particularly during the first 6 months of life, based on hunger, growth, development and laboratory analyses of plasma phenylalanine and tyrosine concentrations. The prescribed phenylalanine should maintain the 3- to 4-h postprandial blood phenylalanine concentration between 50 and 300 μmol l^{-1}. Phenylalanine is an essential amino acid and cannot be deleted from the diet without causing death. Excess restriction produces growth failure, eczema, hair loss, bone changes and mental retardation.

Phenylalanine requirements Phenylalanine required for growth by the infant with classic PKU is 20–55 mg per kg of body weight, with the younger infant requiring the larger amount. Phenylalanine requirement declines rapidly between 3 and 6 months of age as growth rates plateau. Requirements for phenylalanine in the 6- to 12-month-old patient with classic PKU may fall to 15 mg per kg per day, but they vary considerably (Table 3). Frequent monitoring of blood phenylalanine concentration and intake is required to prevent excess intake when growth rate decelerates and to prevent inadequate intake when growth rate is at its peak, as in early infancy and during the prepubertal and pubertal growth spurts and during the later half of gestation.

Tyrosine requirements Tyrosine is an essential amino acid for people with PKU. For this reason, blood tyrosine concentrations must be monitored; if they are low, L-tyrosine supplements are given. Food proteins contain, by weight, on average 5.5% phenylalanine and 4.5% tyrosine. The normal individual hydroxylates some 40–90% of phenylalanine to form tyrosine, depending on age. To supply normal tyrosine intakes to patients with PKU, a minimum of 10% of protein fed should be as tyrosine. Tyrosine supplements alone will not prevent mental retardation in classic PKU.

Protein requirements The protein content of the diet, which is the sum of L-amino acids and intact protein, has traditionally been greater than the Recommended Dietary Allowances (RDA) of the National Academy of Sciences (USA). Because of rapid absorption and oxidation of L-amino acids, protein requirements are increased when either an L-amino acid mix or a protein hydrolysate is the primary protein source rather than intact protein. Thus,

recommendations for protein for nutrition support are greater than RDA. Mean protein intake 24% greater than RDA for age was associated with greater phenylalanine tolerance and growth in infants with PKU than was found when mean protein intake was 9% greater than RDA. Recommendations for energy and fluid intake are the same as those for normal persons (Table 3).

Low-phenylalanine and phenylalanine-free medical foods Adequate protein cannot be obtained from natural foods without ingesting excess phenylalanine (intact proteins contain 2.4–9% phenylalanine by weight). Thus, special medical foods low in or free of phenylalanine are used to provide protein. Medical foods for persons with PKU must also supply most ($\geq$80%) of all known nutrient requirements (minerals, trace and ultratrace elements and vitamins) since natural foods are severely restricted in the diet. More than a dozen medical foods are manufactured for persons with PKU.

Natural foods Serving lists are available to simplify nutrition management for families and professional persons guiding them (**Table 4**). The lists are similar to diabetic exchange lists in that low-protein foods of similar phenylalanine content are grouped together and can be exchanged one for another within a list to give variety to the diet. Each clinical centre often develops its own exchange system for natural foods and the system herein given is that used in many centres in the USA.

Management problems

Maintenance of an adequate intake of protein, energy, minerals and vitamins is important for the infant and child with PKU, even though phenylalanine must be restricted. Nutrition management must be aggressive and if intake fails to meet prescription, a nasogastric or gastrostomy tube should be placed in order to achieve anabolism. Protein is obtained from medical foods; therefore, the amount of medical food offered must be varied to provide the protein needed. Nonprotein sources of energy such as corn syrup, glucose polymers, sugar and pure fats can be added to maintain energy intake and to satisfy the child's hunger without affecting blood phenylalanine concentrations. Natural foods should be prescribed and introduced at the appropriate ages and in the usual textures as they would be for any child, to supply required phenylalanine. Children should be given a variety of foods at the appropriate age so that these foods may be included in nutrition management later in life. In this way, increasing total phenylalanine requirements may be met.

Table 4   Average nutrient content of serving lists for phenylalanine-restricted diets

Food lists	Phenylalanine (mg)	Tyrosine (mg)	Protein (g)	Energy (kcal)
Breads/cereals[a]	30	20	0.6	30
Fats	5	4	0.1	60
Fruits	15	10	0.5	60
Vegetables[a]	15	10	0.5	10
Free foods A[b]	5	4	0.1	65
Free foods B[c]	0	0	0.0	55

[a]Foods low in protein.
[b]Foods containing very little phenylalanine.
[c]Foods containing no phenylalanine.
Note: 1 kcal ≈ 4.2 kJ.

Elevated blood phenylalanine concentrations   A variety of factors may influence blood phenylalanine concentrations. Those that may produce an elevated blood phenylalanine concentration include acute infections with concomitant tissue catabolism, excessive or inadequate phenylalanine intake, and inadequate protein or energy intake. Infection results in increases in blood phenylalanine concentrations in normal adults. Similar increases in blood phenylalanine concentrations occur in febrile, treated patients with PKU if they are in good nutrition status. Because of this fact, any infection should be promptly diagnosed and appropriately treated. The approach to nutrition support during short-term infections is to decrease phenylalanine intake and increase the intake of fluids and carbohydrates through the use of high-carbohydrate, protein-free beverages and soft drinks that do not contain caffeine.

Excess phenylalanine intake is the most common cause of elevated blood phenylalanine concentration in the older child with PKU. This condition may be due to overprescription, misunderstanding of nutrition management by the caretaker, or 'snitching' of food by the child. Frequent evaluations of blood phenylalanine concentration with accompanying accurate diet diaries for calculation of intake are used to determine the dietary phenylalanine prescription. Diet diaries are also useful in determining parental understanding. Misunderstandings of nutrition management requires additional education of parents.

Phenylalanine deficiency   Phenylalanine deficiency has three specific stages of development. The first stage is characterized by decreased blood and urine phenylalanine concentrations. Clinically, the child may appear lethargic or anorexic. Failure to gain length or weight may occur. In the older child,

increases in blood alanine and mild lactic and β-hydroxybutyric acidaemia occur as a consequence of muscle alanine production and β-lipolysis. In the second state, blood phenylalanine concentration is increased as a result of muscle protein degradation. Increased branched-chain amino acid concentrations with decreases in other plasma amino acids may occur. Aminoaciduria appears as a consequence of renal tubular malabsorption. In this stage, body protein stores are catabolized, energy sources are depleted and 'active' membrane functions are impaired. Eczema is common. In the third stage of phenylalanine deficiency, concentrations of blood phenylalanine and other amino acids are decreased below normal. Accompanying clinical manifestations include failure to gain weight, failure to gain height, osteopenia, anaemia, sparse hair, and finally death if the deficiency is not corrected by supplements of dietary phenylalanine. Low blood phenylalanine concentrations ($< 25 \ \mu\text{mol l}^{-1}$) may lead to depressed appetite, decreased growth and, if prolonged, mental retardation. Low blood phenylalanine concentrations are often due to inadequate prescription of phenylalanine for the affected child. In such cases, the prescription for phenylalanine can be increased by addition of measured amounts of infant formula, milk or natural foods.

Protein deficiency   Insufficient protein intake results in an inadequate supply of essential amino acids and nitrogen for growth. When protein synthesis is decreased, phenylalanine is no longer used for growth and accumulates in the blood and tissues. If catabolism occurs because of prolonged lack of nitrogen or amino acid intake, blood phenylalanine concentration increases because tissue protein contains some 5.5% phenylalanine. In case of protein insufficiency, medical food intake should be increased to supply the required nitrogen and essential amino acids. In some situations, medical food may be diluted to a volume that is too great for the child to consume in the allotted time. The volume will need to be decreased to the amount the child is able to ingest. Concentrated medical foods are frequently used without any untoward side effects. They may be mixed as a paste and spoon-fed, even to the young infant. The practice may begin at 3 to 4 months of age when tongue thrust is no longer evident. Extra fluid must then be offered between feedings to maintain appropriate water balance.

Energy deficiency Energy, the first requirement of the body, is necessary for growth. When energy is provided as carbohydrate and fat, and if adequate nitrogen is available, nonessential amino acids may be synthesized from the ketoacid metabolites. Further carbohydrate ingestion leads to insulin secretion, and insulin promotes amino acid transport into the cell and consequent protein synthesis. When energy intake is inadequate, tissue protein catabolism occurs to meet energy needs. Such catabolism releases phenylalanine, leading to elevated blood phenylalanine concentrations. Provision of sufficient energy through generous use of nonprotein and low-protein foods is important to ensure a normal growth rate.

Assessment of nutrition support

Along with biweekly assessment of growth through measurement of height, weight and head circumference and evaluation of development by appropriate developmental scales, the adequacy of phenylalanine and tyrosine intake is determined by twice-weekly quantitation of blood phenylalanine and tyrosine concentrations. The first year is the period of most rapid growth and of greatest vulnerability to nutrition insult. Therefore, twice-weekly blood tests are suggested during the first 3–6 months and weekly thereafter for life. If blood phenylalanine concentrations are greater than 300 μmol l^{-1} (5 mg dl^{-1}), more frequent determinations should be obtained. Where indicated, the prescription for phenylalanine is decreased and frequent blood tests are obtained until blood phenylalanine concentrations are between 50 and 300 μmol l^{-1}. For blood tests to be of use in adjusting the prescription, laboratory analyses must be both accurate and prompt. Quantitative methods of phenylalanine determination using automated ion exchange chromatography and liquid blood are preferable. This method allows evaluation of all amino acids. Fluorometric methods are quantitative and preferred to the microbiological (Guthrie) test to monitor blood phenylalanine concentrations. If properly instructed, parents may be given responsibility for obtaining the blood specimens on filter paper or in microcapillary tubes and sending them to the laboratory.

A record of food ingested before and during blood sampling for blood phenylalanine measurement is essential and should be kept by the child's caregiver. The correlation between the child's intake of phenylalanine, tyrosine, protein and energy; the child's clinical status; and the blood phenylalanine and tyrosine concentrations is considered when nutrition management is altered.

The success of early nutrition management rests with the parents and depends on their understanding of the disease and their ability to cope with the diet. Later, the child's understanding of nutrition management and ability to assume responsibility for it are critical. These factors are related to the support the parents and patient receive from various professional members of the genetic team.

Prognosis

Results of nutrition management

Early diagnosis and treatment of infants with PKU with nutritionally adequate, phenylalanine-restricted, tyrosine-supplemented nutrition management have promoted normal growth and prevented mental retardation. Mean height, weight and head circumference of 111 children treated from before 120 days of age were the same as those of normal children at 4 years of age. Assessment of mental development in these same children at 4 years of age yielded a mean IQ score of 93 on the Stanford–Binet intelligence scale. Delay in treatment and suboptimal control of blood phenylalanine concentration produced lower IQ than projected from parental IQ. More recent programmes with tighter control of blood phenylalanine concentration have improved overall outlook for normal IQ. When blood phenylalanine concentration was controlled to less than 360 μmol l^{-1}, there was no difference in mean IQ of 9-year-old children who had different genotypes.

The semisynthetic nature of nutrition management has led to questions concerning its adequacy. Lower than normal whole-body protein and nitrogen have been reported in children with PKU undergoing therapy. Mean serum carnitine (total, free, esters) of treated patients was about one-third that of normal children of similar age. Low blood tyrosine concentrations were found in both treated and untreated patients. Following an overnight fast, concentration of blood glycine was elevated while patients ingested two different medical foods, suggesting inadequate protein intake. The elevated concentration of blood glycine occurred even in patients receiving a glycine-free medical food. Treated patients with PKU often have concentrations of transthyretin below normal. Depressed plasma concentrations of total cholesterol have been reported in treated children and untreated adults with PKU. Lower than normal plasma and erythrocyte docosahexaenoic acid concentrations and higher than normal n-6 series fatty acid concentrations have been found in patients undergoing therapy for PKU. The significance of these differences is unclear but they appear to be diet related.

Calculation of intake of major nutrients indicates that the amounts are adequate when compared with RDA. Balance studies of calcium, phosphorus, magnesium and iron in 6- to 8-year-old girls ingesting a casein hydrolysate medical food suggested that magnesium may be inadequate to provide for optimal nutrition. Studies of plasma iron, ferritin and selenium of children with PKU revealed low concentrations. Iron deficiency has been reported in significant numbers of children undergoing nutrition management for PKU despite more than adequate iron intake. Low activity of glutathione peroxidase has been found in treated children with PKU who were receiving medical foods without added selenium, Potentially life-threatening cardiac dysrhythmia was found in one selenium-deficient treated child with PKU. Significantly reduced mitogenesis to optimal concentrations of monoclonal antibody (OKT3) and plant lectin phytohaemagglutinin has been demonstrated in a group of treated patients with PKU with reduced serum selenium concentrations when compared with a normal group. Patients with PKU with low plasma selenium concentrations have elevated concentrations of T4 and rT3 which decreased significantly with selenium supplementation. Inadequate intake may be responsible since patients receiving a medical food with adequate added selenium have normal plasma selenium concentrations. Plasma retinol concentrations of infants and children with PKU undergoing treatment are often below those of normal subjects. The intake of vitamin E is sufficient to provide for normal plasma concentrations in patients ingesting some medical foods. Disturbances in tryptophan metabolism and limited intakes of tryptophan and niacin may lead to niacin deficiency in patients with PKU.

Bone changes noted radiographically were reported as early as 1956 in treated children with PKU. Bone mineral content of treated children was more than one standard deviation below the mean for normal children. Bone osteocalcin, a calcium-binding protein with a high content of γ-carboxyglutamic acid, was considerably below the normal range and 80% of patients had a serum calcium <9.0 mg dl^{-1}. The mean of the three most recent blood phenylalanine concentrations correlated negatively with the bone mineral content and osteocalcin. Bone abnormalities were suggested to be due to lack of control of blood phenylalanine concentration rather than to the disease. Normal bone mineralization was found in preschool children with good control of blood phenylalanine concentration. As blood phenylalanine concentration increased in older patients, values for bone mineral content, bone width and bone density were always lower than control values. Trabecular bone mineral content was recently assessed in young adults with PKU who had been treated from early childhood with nutrition management. Bone mineral content was significantly reduced in patients compared with the normal population. Amino acid imbalances, inadequate protein intakes, and the need for phosphorus to buffer organic acids made from excess dietary phenylalanine could have contributed to bone abnormalities. Mean plasma concentrations of IgA and IgM were significantly lower in patients with PKU undergoing therapy than in normal children.

Diet discontinuation

Studies have shown significant differences in performance and intelligence in children and neurological function in adults between those who discontinued the diet and those who remained on the diet. Severe neurological deterioration has been reported in patients with PKU off-diet for varying periods of time. Reversal of most of the symptoms occurred in the patients who returned to nutrition management. Elevated blood phenylalanine concentration may be concentrated by the blood–brain barrier in neural cells and inhibit L-dopa and serotonin synthesis by competing for tyrosine hydroxylase and tryptophan hydroxylase. Severe agoraphobia (an irrational fear of leaving the familiar setting of home), reversible by a return to nutrition management, has been reported in adults. Vitamin B$_{12}$ deficiency, resulting in haematological changes, occurs in those off-diet patients who refuse foods of animal origin. Because of the detrimental effects of long-term elevation of blood phenylalanine concentrations, the phenylalanine-restricted diet should be continued for life.

Maternal phenylketonuria

Pregnant women with PKU who are untreated at conception and during gestation have offspring with intrauterine growth retardation, microcephaly and congenital anomalies, often severe and incompatible with life, and mental retardation is common. Most investigators attribute these effects to elevated maternal blood phenylalanine that is further concentrated by the placenta.

The pathogenesis of the fetal damage is uncertain, but is believed to be related to an elevated maternal blood phenylalanine concentration, because phenylalanine is actively transported across the placenta to the fetus. Fetal blood phenylalanine concentrations are usually significantly greater than those of maternal blood and interfere with embryonic development, although the mechanism of effect is not yet known. Such elevated fetal blood phenylalanine concentrations may again be concentrated by the fetal blood–brain barrier. Intraneuronal phenylalanine concentrations at 600 μmol l^{-1} interfere with brain development by one or more of the several previously described mechanisms, including abnormal oligodendroglial migration or myelin and other protein synthesis. Thus, it is extremely important to maintain normal blood phenylalanine concentrations in the reproductive female with PKU before and after conception. Offspring of untreated women who survive fail to grow and develop normally. If the fertility of these women is normal and they are not treated with nutrition management of phenylalanine intake, the incidence of PKU-related mental retardation could return to the prescreening level after only one generation.

In 1984, the Collaborative Study of Maternal Phenylketonuria (MPKUCS) was initiated to answer questions related to nutrition management and reproductive outcome. Interim results of the MPKUCS support the premise that nutrition management that lowers blood phenylalanine concentration to the near normal range at an early (< 10 weeks) gestational age has a positive effect on reproductive outcome.

See also: **Amino Acids**: Chemistry and Classification; Metabolism. **Bone**: Composition, Metabolism and Bone Growth. **Energy**: Energy Requirements. **Pregnancy**: Nutrient Requirements. **Protein**: Requirements and Role in Diet; Deficiency.

Further Reading

Acosta PB (1996) Recommendations for protein and energy intakes by patients with phenylketonuria. *European Journal of Pediatrics* 155(supplement 1):S121–S124.

Acosta PB and Yannicelli S (1994) Protein intake affects phenylalanine requirements and growth of infants with phenylketonuria. *Acta Paediatrica* 407(supplement): 66–67.

Acosta PB, Michals-Matalon K, Austin V, Castiglioni L, Rohr F, Wenz E and Azen C (1997) Nutrition findings and requirements in pregnant women with phenylketonuria. In: Platt L (ed.) *Effects of Genetic Disorders on Pregnancy Outcome*, pp. 21–32. London: Parthenon Publishing.

Allen JR, Baur LA, Waters DL, Humphries IR, Allen BJ, Roberts DCK and Gaskin KJ (1996) Body protein in prepubertal children with phenylketonuria. *European Journal of Clinical Nutrition* 50:178–186.

Elsas LJ and Acosta PB (in press) Nutrition support of inherited metabolic disease. In: Shils ME, Olson JA and Shike M (eds) *Modern Nutrition in Health and Disease*, 9th edn. Philadelphia: Lea & Febiger.

Gropper SS, Chaung HC, Bernstein LE, Trahms C, Rarback S and Weese SJ (1995) Immune status of children with phenylketonuria. *Journal of the American College of Nutrition* 14:264–270.

Hanley WB, Feigenbaum ASJ, Clarke JTR, Schoonheyt WE and Austin VJ (1996) Vitamin B$_{12}$ deficiency in adolescents and young adults with phenylketonuria. *European Journal of Pediatrics* 155(supplement): S145–S147.

Hillman L, Schlotzhauer C, Lee D, Grasela J, Witter S, Allen S and Hillman R (1996) Decreased bone mineralization in children with phenylketonuria under treatment. *European Journal of Pediatrics* 155 (supplement):S148–S152.

Koch R, Levy HL, Matalon R, Rouse B, Hanley WB, Trefz F, Azen C, Friedman EG, de la Cruz F, Güttler F and Acosta PB (1994) The International Collaborative Study of Maternal Phenylketonuria: status report 1994. *Acta Paediatrica* 407(supplement):111–119.

Report of the MRC Working Party on Phenylketonuria (1993) Recommendations on the dietary management of phenylketonuria. *Archives of Diseases of Childhood* 68:426–427.

Schoeffer A, Hermann ME, Brosicke HG and Moench E (1994) Effect of dosage and timing of amino acid mixtures on nitrogen retention in patients with phenylketonuria. *Journal of Nutritional Medicine* 4:415–418.

Scriver CR, Kaufman S, Eisensmith RC and Woo SLC (1995) The hyperphenylalaninemias. In: Scriver CR, Beaudet AL, Sly WS and Valle D (eds) *The Molecular and Metabolic Bases of Inherited Disease*, 7th edn, vol. 1, chap. 27, pp. 1015–1075. New York: McGraw-Hill.

Thompson AJ, Smith I, Brenton B, Youl BD, Rylance G, Davidson DC, Kendall B and Lees AJ (1990) Neurological deterioration in young adults with phenylketonuria. *Lancet* 336:602–605.

Trefz FK, Burgard P, König T, Goebel-Schreiner B, Lichter-Konecki B, Schmidt E, Schmidt H and Bickel H (1993) Genotype–phenotype correlations in phenylketonuria. *Clinica Chimica Acta* 217:15–21.

Waisbren SE and Levy HL (1991) Agaraphobia in phenylketonuria. *Journal of Inherited Metabolic Disease* 14:755–764.

INFANTS

Contents
Nutritional Requirements
Milk-feeding and Weaning
Feeding Problems
Low-birthweight and Preterm Infants

Nutritional Requirements

J B Morgan, University of Surrey, Guildford, UK

Copyright © 1998 Academic Press

For the purposes of this article infants are defined as aged from birth to 12 months.

In principle, estimating the nutritional requirements of early infancy has relied to date on data derived from feeding studies and growth patterns on healthy and wholly breast-fed infants. Thus requirements and Recommended Dietary Allowances (RDAs) for most nutrients in infancy are based on food intake data. Requirements for nutrients are invariably expressed as tables of values for a hypothetical infant together with explanatory notes in the text. However, individual variation for nutrient requirements makes the task of estimating and expressing requirements more difficult than it first appears.

The wide individual variation in nutrient intake at any age has been recognized for 40 years. At 1 year of age there are infants at the upper end of the range consuming twice as much food as those at the lower end – some infants at 6 months are consuming energy intakes equivalent to those of young women (**Table 1**). This phenomenon has yet to be fully explained with respect to energy requirements.

Table 1 Energy intake of boys and girls, illustrating average intake, maximum and minimum values

	Age group (years)	Average	Maximum	Minimum
Boys (kJ per day)	1	4824	6466	3390
	2	5877	8063	4009
	3	7068	9781	5225
Girls (kJ per day)	1	4815	6818	3520
	2	5982	8561	4410
	3	6408	9731	4142

Calculated from Widdowson EM (1947) *A Study of Individual Children's Diets*. London: Medical Research Council/HMSO.

The effect of gender is well recognized: boys on average have a greater intake of energy than girls. The recent US RDAs did not distinguish between sexes for energy requirements from birth to 10 years. However, other authorities – Department of Health (DoH). World Health Organization (WHO) – do distinguish between the sexes with regard to nutrient requirements.

In young infants the nutrient requirement for growth is substantial, representing up to 30% of the energy requirement, but there exists a large variation within the normal range in the rate of growth and probably also in the composition of the tissue laid down.

The 'average' composition of human milk has been used as a basis for estimating requirements and also for calculating the composition of infant milk formulae. It is as well to remember, however, that the composition of human milk varies, from mother to mother, and from day to day. It also depends on the stage of lactation and on the mother's diet (particularly the content of polyunsaturated fatty acids). Therefore the greater the difference between milk formula composition and human milk composition, the greater the potential harm. As well as providing nutritional substances, milk contains several growth factors, including epidermal growth factor, various milk growth factors, insulin and insulin-like growth factor 1 (IGF-1). The physiological importance of these substances has not yet been established.

Requirement for Energy

Ideally, energy requirements for infancy should be estimated from data on energy expenditure. However, because of the complexities in interpreting information on basal metabolic rate, activity and growth in infants, the convention has been to estimate energy requirements from observed intakes of healthy infants (**Table 2**).

The 1985 FAO/WHO report on energy requirements in humans based its recommendations for infants on the observed intake of healthy infants

Table 2 Calculated energy requirements of infants from birth to 1 year

Age (months)	Median body-weight (kg)		Total requirement (kJ per day)	
	Boys	Girls	Boys	Girls
0.5	3.8	3.6	1965	1860
1–2	4.75	4.35	2300	2115
2–3	5.6	5.05	2550	2280
3–4	6.35	5.7	2740	2470
4–5	7.0	6.35	2910	2635
5–6	7.55	6.95	3055	2800
6–7	8.05	7.55	3220	3010
7–8	8.55	7.95	3390	3140
8–9	9.0	8.4	3580	3350
9–10	9.35	8.75	3870	3620
10–11	9.7	9.05	4060	3790
11–12	10.05	9.35	4395	4080

From WHO (1985).

growing normally (based on the US NCHS 1977 reference charts). It is recognized, however, that observed and desired energy intake may differ, and that a better estimate of energy needs is provided by energy expenditure. The available database on energy expenditure in infants has greatly expanded since 1985, thanks in large part to the application of the doubly-labelled water technique. This noninvasive method permits a reliable quantification of total daily energy expenditure in infants under normal conditions of everyday life. There are now thousands of data points on energy expenditure in infants obtained with this method. In addition, new data on growth and energy intake of exclusively breast-fed infants became available. Taken together, these data on intake, growth and energy expenditure suggest that the actual energy requirements for breast-fed infants may be 10–40% lower than the 1985 estimates. One explanation for the overestimation of the previous recommendation may be that (a) the data set of observed intakes included a large proportion of formula-fed infants, who consume higher amounts of calories than breast-fed infants, and (b) the reference standard for desirable growth is also based largely on a population of predominantly formula-fed infants.

The fact that healthy, exclusively breast-fed infants grow at a slower rate than the current reference standards is the subject of ongoing research. There is evidence, however, that these infants are no different than infants consuming more energy and growing at a faster rate in terms of morbidity, sleep patterns or physical activity.

As a result of these studies, efforts are under way to develop a growth reference chart for exclusively

Table 3 Average daily intake of protein by breast-fed infants, 0–4 months

Age (months)	Boys (g kg^{-1})	Girls (g kg^{-1})
0–1	2.46	2.39
1–2	1.93	1.93
2–3	1.74	1.78
3–4	1.49	1.53

From WHO (1985).

breast-fed infants, which presumably would reflect a more physiological growth pattern than that of formula-fed infants.

Requirement for Protein

Estimates of protein requirements for infants up to six months of age are based on breast milk intake data; both the WHO (1985) report and the National Research Council (1989) report have utilized this method.

Table 3 shows the reported intake of protein in male and female babies between birth and 4 months (after 4 months little data exists on the growth and nutrient intake of exclusively breast-fed infants). Assumptions have been made regarding the protein content of milk (and complementary foods after 4 months). The figure of 1.15 g of protein per 100 ml (for milk) is generally accepted.

In estimating protein requirements from 6 to 12 months the WHO Committee used the factorial approach (**Table 4**). A grey area of knowledge exists for protein requirements between 4 and 6 months of age. Estimates of protein requirements have been extrapolated from energy requirements, i.e. 1040 ml of breast milk per day is needed to fulfil the theoretical energy needs, and hence protein requirements, of male infants aged 5–6 months. This approach is obviously not ideal.

Table 4 Average daily protein requirements for infants (both sexes)

Age (months)	Average protein requirement (g kg^{-1})	Intake from breast milk (g kg^{-1})
1–2	2.25	1.93
2–3	1.82	1.74
3–4	1.47	1.49
4–5	1.34	–
5–6	1.30	–
6–9	1.25	–
9–12	1.15	–

From WHO (1985).

Table 4 outlines the average protein requirements in the period 1–12 months. A major point of issue is the variation in protein requirements for growth. The uncertainty related to this factor has resulted in the addition of 50% to the theoretical nitrogen accretion in the calculation of protein requirements. In fact, adjustment by 50% may even be too small. This is obviously an area where research is urgently needed, i.e. to investigate the daily variation in growth rate and the constraints in storage of essential amino acids to be available when maximum growth occurs. To adjust for interindividual variation in growth and maintenance, a factor of 12.5% has been incorporated. A theoretical basis for calculating the variability of protein requirement for growth does not exist. Work by Fomon indicates that over a period of one month children vary in their average daily rate of growth, with a coefficient of variation of 37%. This variation in weight gain is much greater than the variability in protein intake.

Human milk contains characteristic nitrogen-containing components. In fact, 25% of the nitrogen is derived from nonprotein sources: free amino acids, small peptides, amino sugars, creatine, creatinine and glycolipids. The content of free taurine is 30 to 40 times higher in human milk compared with cow's milk. Although the nutritional or biochemical role of some of these substances is not fully understood, their presence, like the growth-promoting factors previously mentioned, should not be dismissed.

The specific amino acid requirements of infants are of interest. It appears that besides the eight essential amino acids, three other amino acids (cysteine, taurine and histidine) are essential in the postnatal period. This has implications for one aspect of infant feeding – the provision of total nutrition by intravenous (i.v.) feeding. Only recently have amino acid preparations for i.v. nutrition been tailored to the requirements of infants, including an appropriate amino acid profile.

Requirement for Fats

In the broadest sense, infants have a requirement for fats to provide energy, to provide essential fatty acids, to facilitate the absorption of fat-soluble vitamins A, E and D, and as a precursor of structural lipids and eicosanoids. Triacylglycerols in human milk contain more than 150 different fatty acids, but the origin and role of many of these is largely unknown. The average intake of fat can be calculated for breast-fed infants if the fat content of the breast milk is known (**Table 5**).

The specific requirements of long-chain polyunsaturated fatty acids (PUFA) and cholesterol in infants

Table 5 Average daily intake of fat by breast-fed infants aged 0–4 months

Age (months)	Breast milk consumed (ml)	Weight (kg)	Average fat intake	
			(g)	(g kg⁻¹)
Boys				
0–1	719	3.8	30	8
1–2	795	4.75	33	7
2–3	848	5.6	36	6
3–4	822	6.35	35	5
Girls				
0–1	661	3.6	28	8
1–2	731	4.35	30	7
2–3	780	5.05	32	6
3–4	756	5.7	32	6

Fat content of breast milk 4.2 g per 100 ml.

are not often considered. Infants have a specific requirement for PUFA. In the 1950s and 1970s there were reports of deficiency in long-chain fatty acids in premature infants fed parenterally with no lipid source, and in full-term infants fed on formula devoid of linoleic acid. Breast milk contains 7.2 g of linoleic per 100 g total fatty acids or 285 mg per 100 ml, i.e. 3.7% of total energy. The American Academy of Pediatrics recommends that infant formulae contain 2.7% of energy as linoleic acid.

Breast milk is relatively rich in cholesterol, providing an average 0.42 mmol l⁻¹. The existence of this sterol in breast milk is indicative of a biological role, although no authority to date has made recommendations on desirable intakes in infants not receiving breast milk.

Several studies have suggested a specific role for certain polyunsaturated fatty acids on visual development. Eicosapentaenoic acid (EPA) and docosapentaenoic acid (DPA) have been evaluated in term and preterm infants. These fatty acids are found in high concentration in human milk, but they have not been added to infant formulae until recently. These fatty acids may be required in higher amounts in preterm infants, but their contribution to visual development of the full-term healthy infant is not fully documented at this point. Several commercial infant formulae, however, are now fortified with EPA.

Requirement for Carbohydrate

Eighty per cent of the total carbohydrate in human milk is lactose (approximately 7 g per 100 ml of human milk). In early infancy, when the diet consists wholly of milk, 37% of the energy intake is derived from lactose. As the diet of the infant becomes more varied, the carbohydrate content also varies. **Table 6** provides detailed information on the carbohydrate contribution of foods given to infants.

Requirement for Vitamins and Minerals

In the UK, supplementation of vitamins is recommended for breast-fed infants and young children from 6 months to 5 years unless the child's diet is diverse and plentiful (see DoH, 1994, for details). The daily dose of five vitamin drops provides 7 μg of vitamin D, 200 μg of vitamin A and 20 mg of vitamin C.

Requirement for vitamin D

Only small amounts of vitamin D are secreted in human breast milk, which indicates that a dietary source of this substance is teleologically unimportant; the major source of vitamin D is the action of ultraviolet (UV) light on the skin. The amount of exposure to UV light will differ from infant to infant. Because of this uncertainty, and to safeguard against lack of exposure to sunlight, in the UK the RDA is 8.5 μg of vitamin D per day (from food or supplements) from 0–6 months, and 7 μg per day from 7–12 months.

The more recent US RDA is set at 7.5 μg per day for infants from birth to 6 months of age, and 10 μg per day from 6 months onwards because of increased body mass.

Thus two national authorities recommend a value for vitamin D intake, although there is *no* doubt that healthy, wholly breast-fed infants who are exposed to sunlight do not require oral supplementation. Vitamin D deficiency in the maternal diet, lack of sunlight, adverse social or environmental factors, and infant prematurity indicate the need for supplementation.

There has been an ongoing debate regarding the importance of a finding (some 30 years ago) that the

Table 6 Average carbohydrate content of several foods for infants

Food	Carbohydrate (% energy)
Human milk	37
Cow's milk	29
Strained meat	1
Strained fruits	96
Strained desserts	89
Strained vegetables	80
Strained soups and dinners	56
Strained high-meat dinners	29

Data from Fomon (1974).

aqueous fraction of human milk contains vitamin D sulfate. The amount of vitamin D sulfate was reported to be on average 0.80 μg per 100 ml of mature human milk (compared with 0.01 μg per 100 ml of fat-soluble vitamin). It has been reported, however, that vitamin D sulfate does not have the same biological activity as the fat-soluble form, and therefore its physiological value is doubtful.

Excessive intake of vitamin D is potentially harmful: only five times the RDA (45 μg per day) has been reported to be associated with hypervitaminosis in young children.

Requirement for vitamin A

Dietary requirements for vitamin A in infants are based on and extrapolated from intakes calculated from values obtained from a wholly breast-fed infant receiving milk from a well-nourished mother. The breast milk from women living in the USA and Europe contains 40–70 μg of retinol per 100 ml milk and between 20 and 40 μg of carotenoids per 100 ml of milk. Assuming milk is consumed at 750 ml per day (and the concentration of retinol is 40 μg per 100 ml), the infant would receive about 300 μg of retinol per day. After taking into account factors such as individual variation in retinol content of milk, the US Committee recommend an intake of 350 μg per day up to 1 year. The UK recommendations are set at 350 μg of retinol equivalents per day. In developing countries, vitamin A deficiency is uncommon in the first year of life. A drastic fall in the vitamin A content of milk has to be preceded by the exhaustion of the mother's stores of this vitamin.

Requirement for ascorbic acid (vitamin C)

Scurvy occurs primarily in infants fed diets consisting exclusively of cow's milk; as this mode of feeding is very uncommon, scurvy is rare in infants under one year of age. There are reports that infants receiving as little as 7 mg of vitamin C per day are protected from scurvy. Human milk contains approximately 4 mg of vitamin C (ascorbic acid and dehydroascorbic acid) per 100 ml. An infant receiving 750 ml of human milk per day will receive in the order of 30 mg of vitamin C. The UK recommend a daily intake of 25 mg of vitamin C; the USA recommend a daily intake of 30 mg of vitamin C up to one year of age.

Requirement for iron

A normal healthy fetus stores iron in the last trimester of pregnancy. Because of this, a full-term infant can maintain satisfactory haemoglobin levels, without any other sources of iron, for the first 3 months of life. Breast milk is noticeably low in iron – 76 µg per 100 ml. However, because the iron is well absorbed (50–70%, compared with 10–30% from cow's milk), and because an infant has hepatic haemoglobin stores, a dietary source is unnecessary. After 3 months of age, and in non-breast-fed infants from birth, an iron intake of 1 mg per kg of body weight per day is considered necessary. Infant milk formulae and many infant food products contain added iron, thus ensuring an appropriate dietary intake.

Requirement for calcium

Adequate mineralization of the skeleton occurs in breast-fed infants receiving an intake of calcium as low as 200–300 mg per day. The most important factor governing calcium absorption is the degree of skeletal mineralization, mediated by a feedback mechanism controlled by synthesis of 1,25-dihydroxycholecalciferol (a derivative of vitamin D). Other factors include a high dietary lactose content, the composition and structure of dietary fat, and a low buffering effect – all provided by human milk. Approximately 66% of calcium intake is absorbed. Although the requirement for calcium is probably 250 mg per day, the recommended intake is usually set in the region of 600 mg day^{-1}. The safety margin is necessary to allow for a variance in the absorption rate and to allow for individual variation in requirement.

See also: **Amino Acids**: Metabolism. **Ascorbic Acid**: Physiology, Dietary Sources and Requirements; Scurvy. **Calcium**: Physiology. **Carbohydrates**: Requirements and Dietary Importance. **Cholecalciferol and Ergocalciferol**: Physiology, Dietary Sources and Requirements; Rickets and Osteomalacia. **Energy**: Energy Requirements; Energy Balance; Measurement of Energy Intake and Expenditure. **Fatty Acids**: Metabolism; Health Effects of Saturated Fatty Acids; Health Effects of Monounsaturated Fatty Acids; Health Effects of n-6 Polyunsaturated Fatty Acids; Health Effects of n-3 Polyunsaturated Fatty Acids; Health Effects of *trans* Fatty Acids. **Growth and Development**: Physiological Aspects. **Iron**: Physiology, Dietary Sources and Requirements. **Lactation**: Physiology; Dietary Requirements. **Protein**: Requirements and Role in Diet. **Retinol**: Physiology.

Further Reading

DoH (1991) Dietary reference values for food energy and nutrients for the United Kingdom. Report on Health and Social Subjects, no. 41. London: HMSO.

DoH (1994) Weaning and the weaning diet. Report on Health and Social Subjects, no. 45. London: HMSO.

ESPGAN (1982) Guidelines in infant feeding III. Recommendations for infant feeding. *Acta Paediatrica Scandinavica* (supplement) 302.

Fomon SJ (1974) *Infant Feeding*, 2nd edn. New York: WB Saunders.

National Research Council (1989) *Recommended Dietary Allowances*, 10th edn. Washington DC: National Academy Press.

Nestlé Nutrition Workshop (1988) *Biology of Human Milk*, vol. 15. New York: Raven Press.

Paul AA, Whitehead RG and Black AE (1990) Energy intakes and growth from two months to 3 years in initially breast-fed children. *Journal of Human Nutrition and Dietetics* 3:79–92.

Schurch B and Scrimshaw NS (eds.) (1990) Activity, energy expenditure and energy requirements of infants and children. *International Dietary Energy Consultancy Group*. Lausanne: IDECG/Nestle Foundation.

Scrimshaw NS, Waterlow JC and Schurch B (1996) Energy and protein requirements. *European Journal of Clinical Nutrition* (supplement I): 50.

World Health Organization (1985) Energy and protein requirements. WHO Technical Report Series No. 522 and FAO Nutrition Meetings Report Series No. 724.

Milk-feeding and Weaning

J B Morgan, University of Surrey, Guildford, UK

Copyright © 1998 Academic Press

Feeding patterns in the first year of life alter more than at any other stage of life, reflecting the rapid changes in nutritional requirements and physiological development of an infant. In the first 10 days the infant's diet is dominated by a milk, colostrum, which is unique in its content of immunoglobulins and relatively higher in sodium but lower in fat than mature human milk. The transitional period is completed when mature human milk is fed. Inevitably this milk (and formula milk as well) becomes nutritionally and physiologically inadequate and the next major change occurs in feeding patterns. At this stage, which for the majority of infants is not before 4 months of age, foods other than milk are gradually introduced, initially to supplement milk intake but eventually to become the dominant source of nutrients. In this article milestones of infant feeding will be explored in the context of present day practice and recommendations.

Milk-feeding

History

Up to the early part of the twentieth century infants

who were not breast-fed had a high probability of dying; the milk used to feed those infants originated from animals and was nutritionally inappropriate for human infants. High infant mortality rates forced wealthy women, who could afford to observe the many elaborate rules in their selection, to employ women as wet nurses to feed their infants, but this was not always satisfactory. These women often carried infectious diseases, some diluted their milk and there was a widespread belief that the milk of the nurse transmitted her personality to the baby.

The search for a suitable substitute for human milk posed technical problems, not least because without pasteurization animal milks soured quickly. Success with the development of modified cow's milk formulae became possible with the advances in technical knowledge in four separate areas: (1) the development of a safe water supply; (2) the development of easily cleaned bottles and teats; (3) modifications of the casein and calcium precipitate or curd-tension of cow's milk by acidification, dilution, boiling and homogenization which result in a product that is more easily digested by young infants; and (4) development of roller-dried powdered milk (**Fig. 1**).

From the 1940s onwards women in Britain turned increasingly to feeding their infants modified cow's milk formula. Several studies published in the late 1960s and early 1970s reported a low incidence of breast-feeding in various parts of the UK. A study in Dudley, Worcestershire, published in 1972 found that only 28% of infants received breast milk as the first food and of these most had stopped receiving breast milk by the end of the first month. At the same time the majority of infants were fed modified dried cow's milk powders, reconstituted by the addition of water; a smaller proportion of infants were given unsweetened condensed milk to which vitamin D had been added. Few mothers gave their babies cow's milk as supplied by the dairyman, although in certain areas in Scotland as many as 15% of infants were reported to receive doorstep milk within a month of birth. This shift in infant feeding practices has been attributed to the introduction of the Welfare Food Scheme during World War II and the provision of free or subsidized National Dried Milk (NDM) (requiring the addition of sugar as well as water) at a time when cow's milk was rationed; modified milk powders were heavily advertised and there was a gradual shift towards women working outside the home. It is of interest to note that in 1977 NDM was withdrawn – it contained higher concentrations of protein, sodium and other minerals than breast milk and its withdrawal coincided with the publication of a DHSS report which provided the most comprehensive data on the composition of human milk to date.

In fact the 1970s saw a 'sea change' in attitudes towards infant feeding practices among health care professionals. In 1974 the DHSS published 'Present day practice in infant feeding' and 19 recommendations were made in the general area of infant nutrition; breast-feeding was specifically encouraged and the role of 'artificial' feeding (including guidelines for the composition of infant milk formula) was identified. The early introduction of cereals and other solids was discouraged 'before about 4 months of age'.

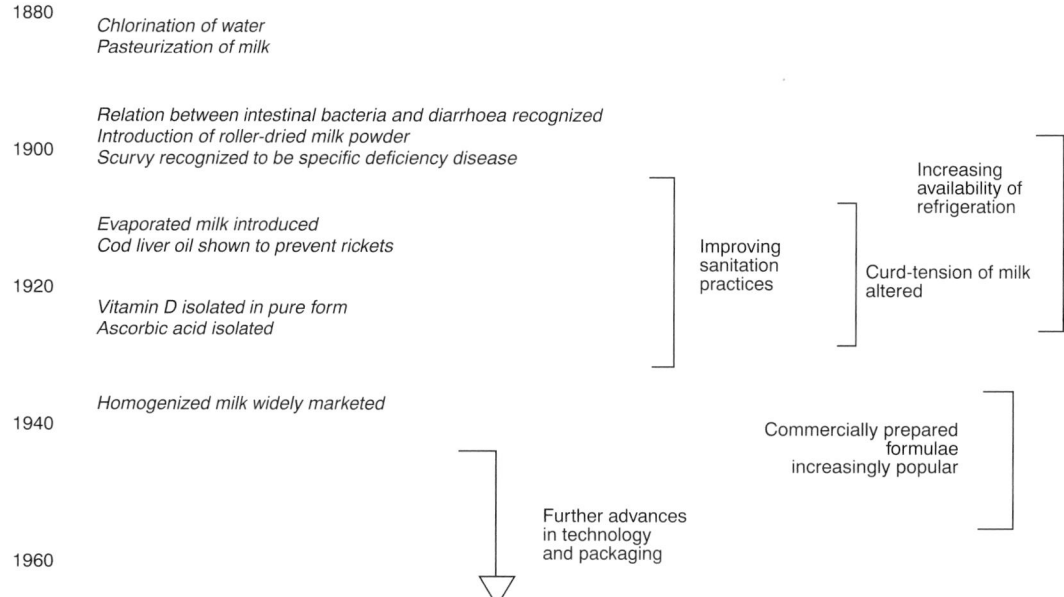

Figure 1   Advances and trends in infant feeding from the late 1860s to the 1960s. Modified from Fomon (1974).

The nutritional value of human milk

Human milk resembles living tissue such as blood, whereas cow's milk formula is an inert multinutrient medium. Human milk contains live cells, a wide range of biologically active factors, a large number of hormones and growth factors, and at least 60 enzymes. Its composition is not uniform and changes during the course of lactation, and even throughout a single feed, showing a diurnal variation with differences from one woman to another.

The greatest change in composition however occurs during the first 10 days postpartum when colostrum, the first milk, changes in composition to mature milk. Colostrum contains a much higher concentration of protein compared with mature breast milk, 50% of which is derived from IgA. It has half the concentration of fat but higher amounts of sodium and vitamins A and B_{12} compared with mature milk (**Table 1**).

From 10 days postpartum milk composition changes, but less markedly so than the earlier changes described above; between 2 weeks and 16 weeks the protein content falls and micronutrients such as calcium, phosphorus and sodium are also lower by 16 weeks.

The energy content of mature breast milk has been the subject of much research. From studies of doubly labelled water it is apparent that breast milk provides not 289 kJ (69 kcal) per 100 ml but about 242 kJ

(58 kcal) per 100 ml at 3 months postpartum. The implication of this finding is still being assessed.

The issue of whether a mother's diet affects the composition and the volume of her milk is a complex one. Certainly the fatty acid composition of breast milk reflects that of the maternal diet. It has been reported that failure-to-thrive in a breast-fed infant could be attributed to reduced milk production because the mother restricted her energy and protein intake. A review of evolutionary and environmental influences on human lactation concluded that:

> ... there must be a threshold of nutritional status probably at quite an extreme level of malnutrition, at which the maternal system can no longer sustain lactation and its own survival.

The implication of this statement for women who live in the developed world and who follow energy-restricted diets while nursing their infant has not been properly evaluated.

Breast milk from a woman who is in good health and nutritional status provides a complete food for healthy infants during the early months of life. Prolonged breast-feeding, practised by such women, may not necessarily result in growth faltering, though the infant's micronutrient status may be compromised.

Nutritional value of infant formula

Infant milk formulae based on cow's milk protein have undergone important changes in their composition but even so we know that human milk is unique and it is not possible to reproduce its exact composition (see above). **Table 2** shows the nutritional composition of human milk, infant milk, follow-on milk and cow's milk based on data from the 1991 European Commission Directive. The Commission of the European Communities (CEC) defines infant formulae as:

> ... foodstuffs intended for particular nutritional use by infants during the first 4 to 6 months of life and satisfying by themselves the nutritional requirements of this category of persons.

Follow-on formulae are defined as:

> ... foodstuffs intended for particular nutritional use by infants aged over four months and constituting the principal liquid elements in a progressively diversified diet of this category of persons.

An alternative milk formula is modified from soya protein and may be useful in the treatment of cow's

Table 1 Energy, macronutrient and selected micronutrient content of colostrum and mature human milk (per 100 g)

Nutrient	Colostrum	Mature human milk
Energy (kJ) (kcal)	236 (56)	289 (69)
Protein (g) (% PER[a])	2.0 (14)	1.3 (9)
Fat (g) (% FER[b])	2.6 (42)	4.1 (55)
Carbohydrate (g) (% CER[c])	6.6 (47)	7.2 (42)
Calcium (mg)	28	34
Sodium (mg)	47	15
Iron (mg)	0.07	0.07
Retinol (µg)	155	58
Carotene (µg)	(135)[d]	(24)[d]
Vitamin B_{12} (µg)	0.1	0.01
Vitamin C (mg)	7	4
Potasium (mg)	70	58
Vitamin D (µg)	N[e]	0.04
Thiamin (mg)	Trace	0.02
Riboflavin (mg)	0.03	0.03
Niacin (mg)	0.1	0.2
Folate (µg)	2	Trace

Modified from Macdonald and Shaw (1993).
[a]PER = protein energy ratio, [b]FER = fat energy ratio,
[c]CER = carbohydrate energy ratio. [d]Estimated amount.
[e]Significant quantities but no reliable information.

Table 2 Energy, macronutrient and selected micronutrient content of mature human milk, infant formula, follow-on formula and cow's milk (per 100 ml)

Nutrient	Mature human milk	Infant formula[a]	Follow-on formula[a]	Cow's milk
Energy (kJ) (kcal)	289 (69)	250–315 (60–75)	250–335 (60–80)	280 (67)
Protein (g)	1.3	1.2–1.95	1.5–2.9	3.2
Fat (g)	4.1	2.1–4.2	2.1–4.2	3.9
Carbohydrate (g)	7.2	4.6–9.1	4.6–9.1	4.8
Calcium (mg)	34	33	54–104	115
Sodium (mg)	15	13–39	26–50	55
Potassium (mg)	58	39–94	66–127	140
Zinc (mg)	0.3	0.33–0.98	0.33–ns	0.4
Iron (mg)	0.07	0.33–0.98	0.65–1.3	0.06
Retinol (μg)	58	39–117	39–117	52
Vitamin D (μg)	0.04	0.65–1.63	0.65–1.95	0.03
Vitamin C (mg)	4	5.2–ns	5.2–ns	1

Data from various sources. NS = not specified.
[a]CEC (1991), based on 270 kJ (65 kcal) per 100 ml.

milk intolerance and for use among certain ethnic groups where cow's milk is unacceptable.

Generally, since the 1950s butterfat from the starting milk, cow's milk, has been replaced with suitable blends of vegetable oils, although this substitution started mainly in the late 1970s and progressed through the 1980s, until now when almost all formulae contain blends based on 100% vegetable oils. The protein content has been decreased, with reductions too in electrolytes (particularly sodium) and phosphate. In whey-dominant formulae the casein : whey ratio has been decreased to 40 : 60 to approximate more closely the ratio of human milk. Carbohydrate levels have been increased by the addition of lactose or glucose syrups or maltodextrins. The use of flour and sucrose as ingredients has been abolished, iron and other micronutrients are added, and the energy density decreased slightly.

Incidence of breast-feeding

In 1975 the proportion of infants in England and Wales receiving breast milk was reported to be 51%; this figure rose in the five subsequent years so that by 1980 67% of women nationally were reported to breast-feed their infants initially. Since then this figure has remained fairly static. By 1986 and 1990 the percentage of mothers who reported that they initially breast-fed their infants was 64% and 63%, respectively. A study of over 1000 respondents where the data was collected in 1992/1993 showed a similar percentage of mothers who initially breast-fed (**Fig. 2**). These proportions vary in different parts of the country. The incidence of breast-feeding in population groups masks the socioeconomic and cultural pressures which affect a woman's desire and opportunities to breast-feed. The woman most likely to

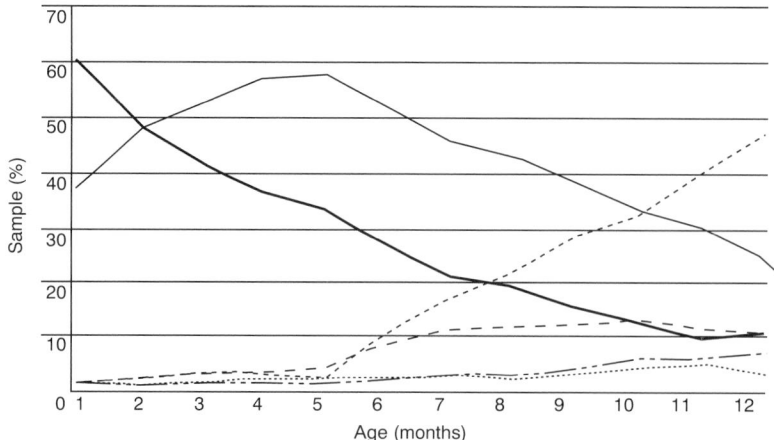

Figure 2 Types of milk fed to the study infants by age. Data presented as percentage of respondents by age (in months) of the infant. Key: —, breast milk; —, infant formula; ---, follow-on formula; —·—·—, normal cow's milk; —··—··—, low-fat cow's milk; ......, other. Modified from Morgan and Stordy (1995).

breast-feed lives in the South East of England, continues education after 19 years of age, is from socio-economic group 1, and is over 30 years of age at the birth of her first child. Other factors relating to breast-feeding are experience with a previous baby, smoking habits, maternal employment status and entry of child into day care.

The trend for mothers to curtail breast-feeding very soon after a baby is born (15% of mothers cease breast-feeding in the first week) is a phenomenon that has been recognized for many years and may in part be related to advice that mothers receive antenatally and postnatally that it is better to feed for a short time than not at all. Women choose to switch from breast-feeding to formula-feeding (usually by 6 months of the infant's life) for complex reasons, but in surveys the usual reasons given are 'insufficient milk' and 'a hungry baby'. A recent study reported that, similarly, the reason for mothers switching brands of milk formula was also related to the perceived 'hungry baby'. There is a widespread belief among mothers and health care professionals that casein-based formulas (e.g. Cow & Gate Plus, Nutricia Ltd.) provide nutritional satisfaction over the predominately whey-based formula (e.g. SMA Gold, Wyeth Ltd.), although there is no scientific evidence to support this.

Current milk-feeding practices

For healthy infants between the age of 6 and 12 months breast-feeding can continue, or an infant milk or follow-on milk may be used. In the UK the use of follow-on milks from 6 months of age is increasing, providing extra iron and vitamin D in some products.

The provision of cow's milk as a main milk drink is not recommended until after the age of 1 year, as infants are more likely to develop iron deficiency anaemia and also because of the possibility of developing an adverse immune response resulting in food sensitivity. However a study in the UK on 488 infants aged between 6 and 12 months found that 76% of all infants aged between 9 and 10 months were receiving cow's milk; 40% of those received it as a main drink, of whom 5% were receiving skimmed milk and 1% semiskimmed milk. Recommendations from the 1994 Department of Health publication *Weaning and the Weaning Diet* include:

> Semi-skimmed cows' milk is not suitable as a drink before the age of two years but that thereafter it may be introduced gradually if the child's energy and nutrient intake is otherwise adequate and if growth remains satisfactory. Fully skimmed cow's milk should not usually be introduced before the age of 5 years.

Marketing of infant milks

The Code of Practice of the Food and Drink Federation (FDF), formerly the Food Manufacturers Federation (FMF), controlled the marketing of milk formulae in the UK until the mid 1990s. In 1991 the European Commission published a directive on infant formula which was implemented in the UK on 1 March 1995. The directive provided nutritional criteria for the composition of infant formula and follow-on formula (see Table 2) in addition to marketing restrictions which have replaced the FDF 1983 Code of Practice. The CEC Directive requires that products made entirely from cow's milk protein will be called 'infant milks' or 'follow-on milks' whereas products made from other protein sources (soya) will be called formulae.

Weaning

History

A review of trends in the feeding of 'beikost' (the German term for semisolid foods other than breast milk or formula milk) revealed that until the 1920s solid foods were seldom offered to young children and until 1911 green vegetables were not recommended before 36 months of age! By the 1940s there were reports of infants receiving fish at 4–6 weeks and solids within the first few days of life. In the 1960s and 1970s in the UK the early introduction of solids (often a wheat-based cereal mix) with milk (inside as well as outside a bottle) was popular. The increased availability of commercial foods coincided with the trend towards the earlier introduction of solids. By the mid 1970s concern for the possible hazards from the early introduction of solid foods (e.g. obesity) resulted in the recommendation that the introduction of cereals and other solid foods should be discouraged before 4 months of age. More recently it has been recommended that solid foods should be introduced between the ages of 4 and 6 months for the majority of infants, whether the infant is being fed human milk or formula milk.

Nutritional and physiological aspects of weaning

Infant feeding is more than breast milk or formula milk alone. In the transition period from an exclusively milk-based diet to a diet based on family meals, special baby foods may be used that are appropriate in both nutritional composition and texture and taste, bearing in mind the physiological limitations of a baby. These foods may be home-made or industrially manufactured and are generally known in the UK as weaning foods. Weaning is defined by the UK Department of Health as: 'the process of expanding the diet to include foods and drinks other than breast milk, or infant formula'.

Weaning represents one of the most crucial dietary events in an infant's life, as either the incorrect timing of introduction of a food or the use of inadequate foods may impair a child's health and development. In poorer countries the introduction of contaminated weaning foods or foods with an inappropriate composition may lead to diarrhoea, disease, growth failure and ultimately death of an infant. In the developed world concern is related to exposure to food allergens which provoke an immune response, or to obesity and to the risk of cardiovascular disease. The avoidance of fat (well-meaning or obsessional) should not be extended to an infant's diet. A reduction in the fat content to 35% of energy (promoted for adults) is undesirable for an infant. At a certain time in a young infant's life the volume of milk (breast or formula) theoretically required to cover an infant's nutritional requirements becomes so great that most mothers cannot produce the necessary quantities and the infant cannot drink them. A semisolid food supplement is then provided to complement the diet but not, at least initially, to replace the milk diet. The time when this is appropriate will vary from infant to infant and is also influenced by other interrelated factors such as the mother's health and nutritional status, the quality and quantity of milk produced, the infant's birthweight, gestational age and health.

In the full-term infant, by 6 months of age (but much earlier in the infant born prematurely) the sources of iron and zinc accumulated *in utero* have become exhausted. As breast milk in particular is a poor source of these trace elements, a readily available dietary source of them, from foods other than breast milk, is vital. Iron deficiency anaemia is common in the preschool child throughout the world. Recent work from Bristol, UK, has shown that up to 25% of infants attending a deprived inner city practice had iron deficiency anaemia at 14 months of age. The aetiology of the anaemia appears to be simply dietary iron deficiency, and mild deficiency can be associated with psychomotor impairment. Meat, particularly red meat, provides a rich source of highly bioavailable iron, copper and zinc.

In a full-term baby, by 9–12 weeks the swallowing reflex is developed; before this age bolus formation, required for controlled swallowing, may not be achieved. From 5–6 months onwards teeth begin to erupt and feeding behaviour changes from sucking to biting and chewing. Children who do not develop these feeding skills at the appropriate age, for whatever reason, may fail to thrive or problems could develop later with the acceptance of lumpy food if this consistency is not introduced at an appropriate age.

In fetal life and during infancy there is a rapid period of accelerated growth. Also the fetus becomes fatter and contains less water in late fetal life. Growth velocity slows in late infancy. Body composition changes with the accretion of protein and minerals and with appearance of teeth. There is evidence that the type of milk fed (i.e. breast versus formula) can alter the body fat content of young infants. There is no similar data on the effect of various weaning diets on body fat content. As there are possible associations between diet in early life and the development of hypertension and cardiovascular disease in adulthood, this area requires further research.

The secretion of gastric and pancreatic enzymes is low in the newborn infant, although this is partly compensated for by enzymes in breast milk which aid the hydrolysis of food in the gut lumen. If starch (cereal) is fed to the young infant there is usually compensation by an increased salivary amylase activity and even digestion in the colon. Infants as young as 1 month are capable of digesting cooked wheat, corn, potato, tapioca and rice starches.

It is well recognized that food antigens are found in the serum of breast-fed infants. These levels tend to be higher in infants born into atopic families where the mothers are eating an unrestricted diet which in turn may sensitize the infant. So, in the case of children born into an atopic family, the UK Department of Health recommends that the introduction of foods traditionally regarded as allergenic (soya protein, gluten, egg, fish and chicken) should be delayed until 6 months of age.

The age of weaning

Because of the different factors involved, the age of weaning varies between populations and individuals (**Fig. 3**). Reports from Australia, the USA and the UK all confirm that formula-fed infants are weaned

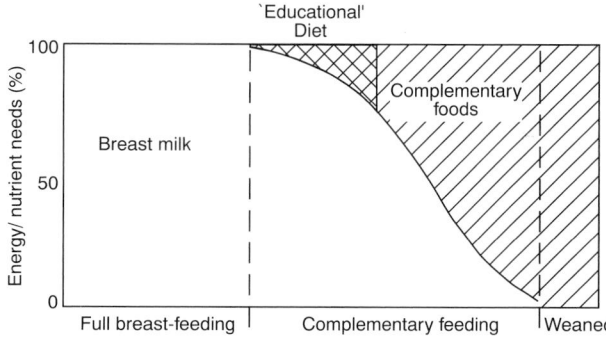

Figure 3   Patterns of infant feeding. Modified from Underwood and Hofvander (1982).

earlier than breast-fed infants. Cereals, particularly baby rice and rusks, used to be the most common foods first offered to infants. The UK Department of Health recommends that 'the majority of infants should not be given solid food before the age of four months, and a mixed diet should be offered by the age of six months'. However, two research studies have reported, respectively, that at 8 weeks 16% and 19% of infants had received solid food; by 3 months 52% and 68%; and by 4 months 84% and 94%. Early weaning may be associated with obesity, infection, adverse reaction to foods and wheezing. Late weaning may be associated with failure-to-thrive and iron deficiency anaemia.

Avoiding micronutrient deficiency

Weaning foods, the types of foods used, nutritional characteristics and methods of preparation have been well reviewed elsewhere. At the outset foods are introduced slowly and are usually cereal based, simply as an addition to the infant's milk intake. Gradually other foods largely replace milk so that by 2 years, or before, the diet is similar to that of the rest of the family. Guidelines on suitability of the introduction of specific foods at various ages have been published. Foods, properly prepared in the home, are often encouraged as suitable weaning foods. However it is only recently that the nutritional composition of home-prepared weaning foods has been studied and in many cases the results revealed that some meals contained surprisingly low amounts of energy, iron, zinc and high amounts of nonstarch polysaccharides, protein and sodium. A national survey of infants aged 6–12 months has demonstrated that infants aged 6–9 months who received predominantly commercial foods had an average iron intake of 10 mg per day compared with 5 mg per day in those infants receiving mainly family foods.

The nutritional status of infants over the age of 6 months is influenced by the type of main milk consumed. Those consuming infant formula or follow-on formula received more appropriate amounts of protein (less), iron (more) and vitamin D (more) when assessed against the reference nutrient intake than those receiving whole cow's milk (**Table 3**).

In another study observing infant feeding trends, manufactured infant foods were given to 95% of 4-month-old infants and 82% of 6-month-old infants. The European Commission has produced a draft directive which was updated in 1994. Annex I contains the nutritional composition of processed cereal-based foods for infants and young children; Annex II gives compositional guidelines for protein, carbohydrate, fat, sodium and vitamins A, C and D in all other commercial baby foods. This directive requires products to comply with these provisions by 31 March 1999.

Conclusion

Mature human milk meets the needs of human babies but they quickly outgrow its provision. Gradual introduction of other foods is essential to meet increasing nutritional requirements. The rate at which this weaning process can occur depends on the coincidental development of the gut and associated structures. Failure to take into account these various considerations can lead to growth faltering, adverse reactions to foods and possibly also diseases later in life.

See also: **Dairy Products**: Nutritional Value. **Infants**:

Table 3 Daily intake of energy and nutrients from all sources (both liquid and solid foods) of infants aged 6–12 months grouped according to main milk consumed

Nutrient	Human milk[a] (n = 48)	Infant formula (n = 267)	Cow's milk (n = 150)	RNI[b] 7- to 9-month infants
Energy (MJ) (kcal)	3.00 (718)	3.64 (871)	3.77 (901)	3.34 (800)
Protein (g)	21.0	26.2	34.8	13.7
Fat (g)	30.9	35.3	37.5	
Calcium (mg)	512	689	880	525
Iron (mg)	6.4	11.3	6.7	7.8
Zinc (mg)	3.6	4.5	4.7	5.0
Retinol (μg)	519	801	462	350
Carotene (μg)	844	961	1250	
Vitamin D (μg)	1.0	9.1	1.0	7
Vitamin C (mg)	76	135	85	25

Modified from Wharton and Morgan (1995).
[a]Note small number; they were younger and therefore smaller than the other two groups.
[b]RNI = reference nutrient intake (estimated average requirement for energy).

Nutritional Requirements; Feeding Problems; Low-birthweight and Preterm Infants.

Further Reading

Barker DJP (1994) *Mothers, Babies, and Diseases Later in Life*. London: British Medical Journal Publishing Group.

Commission of the European Communities (CEC) (1991) Directive on infant formulae and follow-on formulae 91/321/EEC. *Official Journal of the European Community* L175:35–49.

CEC (1994) Draft Commission Directive on processed cereal based foods and baby foods for infants and young children. III/5886/94-EN Brussels/U3/UNICI/04/03/00/BM/dm.

Dewey KG, Heinig MJ, Nommsen LA, Peerson JM and Lonnerdal B (1993) Breast fed infants are leaner than formula fed infants at one year of age: the DARLING study. *American Journal of Clinical Nutrition* 57:140–145.

Department of Health and Social Security (DHSS) (1974) Present day practice in infant feeding. *Report on Health and Social Subjects* 9. London: Her Majesty's Stationery Office (HMSO).

DHSS (1977) The composition of mature human milk. *Report on Health and Social Subjects* 12. London: HMSO.

Department of Health (DoH) (1994) Weaning and the weaning diet. *Report on Health and Social Subjects 45*. London: HMSO.

Fomon SJ (1974) *Infant Nutrition*, 2nd edn. Philadelphia: WB Saunders.

Lovegrove JA and Morgan JB (1994) Feto-maternal interaction of antibody and antigen transfer, immunity and allergy development. *Nutrition Research Reviews* 7:25–42.

Lucas A and Davies PSW (1990) Physiologic energy content of human milk. In: Atkinson SA, Hanson LA and Chandra RK (eds) *Breast Feeding, Nutrition, Infection and Infant Growth in Developed and Emerging Countries*, pp 337–357. St John's, Newfoundland: ARTS Biomedical Publishers and Distributors.

Macdonald S and Shaw V (1993) Breast- and bottle-feeding. In: Macrae R, Robinson RK and Sadler MJ (eds) *Encyclopaedia of Food Sciences, Food Technology and Nutrition*, vol. 4 pp 2507–2511. London: Academic Press.

Mills A and Tyler H (1992) *Food and Nutrient Intakes of British Infants Aged 6 to 12 months*. London: HMSO/MAFF.

Morgan JB and Stordy BJ (1995) Infant feeding practices in the 1990's. *Health Visitor* 68:56–58.

Prentice AM and Prentice A (1995) Evolutionary and environmental influences on human lactation. *Proceedings of the Nutrition Society* 54:391–400.

Sidnell AM (1993) Weaning foods. In: Macrae R, Robinson RK and Sadler MJ (eds) *Encyclopaedia of Food Sciences, Food Technology and Nutrition*, vol. 4, pp 2496–2503. London: Academic Press.

Stordy BJ, Redfern A and Morgan JB (1995) Healthy eating for infants – mothers' actions. *Acta Paediatrica* 84:733–741.

Underwood B and Hofvander Y (1982) Appropriate timing for complementary feeding of the breast fed infant. A review. *Acta Paediatrica Scandinavica* (supplement 294).

Wharton B and Morgan JB (1995) Food for the weanling: have we improved? In: Davies DP (ed.) *Nutrition in Child Health*, pp 33–49. London: Royal College of Physicians.

White A, Freeth S and O'Brien M (1992) *Infant Feeding 1990*. London: HMSO.

WHO/UNICEF (1993) *Baby Friendly Hospital Initiative*. Geneva: WHO/UNICEF.

Feeding Problems

E M Poskitt, Medical Research Council, Keneba, The Gambia

Copyright © 1998 Academic Press

Nutrition is of great importance in infancy. Somatic growth is rapid and will falter in nutritional deficiency. If malnutrition is prolonged, both somatic growth and brain development can be permanently impaired. Malnutrition in infancy is relatively common because of the high nutritional requirements of growth and development. In addition, infants are entirely dependent on others for their nutrition but their carers may have difficulty recognizing their needs. Feeding problems arise from ignorance of infants' needs, from behavioural peculiarities of individual infants, or from underlying pathology.

Failure-to-Thrive

Failure-to-thrive is failure to gain in height and weight at the expected rate. Expected rates of growth are determined from standard growth charts. When successfully treated, failure-to-thrive will be followed by accelerated or 'catch-up' growth (**Fig. 1**a). Without extra nutrition to provide for accelerated growth rates, catch-up growth will be incomplete and affected infants will continue to grow but on lower growth centiles than previously (Fig. 1b).

Some children who present below the third centile (below recognized 'normal' range of height and weight) are labelled as failure-to-thrive although they were low weight for gestational age at birth and have always been small. Their growth velocities may be normal for age, in which case they are not failing to thrive but are constitutionally small (Fig. 1c).

The causes of failure to thrive are numerous and are outlined in **Table 1**. Careful dietary history

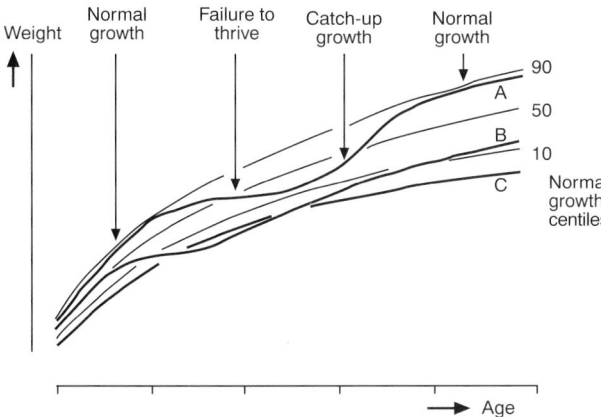

Figure 1 Failure to thrive, catch-up growth and constitutional growth retardation in young children shown against normal growth centiles. A, failure to thrive with complete catch-up; B, failure to thrive with incomplete catch-up; C, constitutional growth retardation.

Table 1 Classification of nutritional problems associated with failure-to-thrive

Basic nutritional problem	Example
Inadequate intake	Poverty; famine; ignorance of child's needs
	Vomiting: all causes
	Feeding difficulties
	Anorexia
Increased losses	Protein-losing enteropathy
	Glycosuria: proteinuria
	Exfoliative skin conditions; Suppuration
Failure to absorb	Cystic fibrosis
	Gluten-sensitive enteropathy
	Giardiasis
	Lactose intolerance
Failure to utilize	Inborn errors of metabolism
	Endocrine problems
	Deficiencies of micronutrients, e.g. zinc
	Chronic renal failure
	Emotional deprivation
Increased requirements	Rapid growth: small-for-dates and premature infants
	Catch-up growth
	Congenital heart disease with left-to-right shunts

should indicate which infants are underfed because of inadequate intakes, inappropriately constituted feeds, or inappropriate weaning practices. Recommended intakes of breast milk or formula are 150 ml per kg per day (441 kJ per kg per day) for full-term normal infants. Intakes increase around 6–8 weeks in many infants but then tend to stabilize despite weight gain. There is tremendous variation in intakes between infants.

In breast-fed infants it may be difficult to determine if failure-to-thrive is caused by inadequate milk intakes. Weighing infants in clean nappies prior to breast-feeding, and then weighing them again after feeding without nappy changes, provides some indication of the weights, and thus the volumes, of milk consumed. 'Test weighing' must be carried out for all feeds over 24 h since infants take different volumes of feed at different times of day. They may consume large feeds early in the morning and in the evening, but relatively small amounts at other times of day.

Where breast milk production seems inadequate, increasing the frequency but not necessarily the duration of suckling, as well as improving maternal nutrition if this seems relevant, may be effective in improving milk secretion. With some breast-fed infants it is necessary to introduce formula milk or to start a weaning diet before 4 months in order to overcome nutritional inadequacy. Breast-feeding failure commonly results from failure to establish feeding owing to infrequent suckling, inappropriate techniques, failure of infants to 'latch on' to the breast correctly, failure to suckle at night, or maternal stress resulting from family and domestic responsibilities.

Where failure-to-thrive is not explained by inadequate feeding, or where inadequate feeding is the result of persistent anorexia or vomiting, medical investigation will be necessary.

In developed countries, where food and medical facilities are readily available, failure to thrive commonly presents with no evidence of clinical disease. These children eat well – sometimes excessively – and seem clinically without abnormality except for small size, apathy, lack of interest in social interaction, and, usually, developmental delay. Their home environment is one of neglect with emotional and/or social deprivation. Although the children receive sufficient food, the stress and lack of love in the environment is such that normal growth is impossible. The importance of the environment to these children's failure-to-thrive is shown by changing the home environment. In emotionally warm, caring and stimulating homes, without change of diet or other treatment, these children show impressive catch-up growth and dramatic changes in affect.

Vomiting

Most normal infants vomit occasionally and some vomit frequently. The most important factor contributing to ready vomiting in infancy is laxity of the gastro-oesophageal sphincter. The sphincter is the spiral area, 2–3 cm in length, at the lower end of the oesophagus. Sphincter competence is poor at birth but increases greatly in infants over 2 weeks old, regardless of gestational age, and is related to the length of intra-abdominal sphincter (which increases with age) and to intragastric pressure. Diet does influence vomiting in infancy since the fluid diet of young infants and the high volumes of liquid that need to be consumed to meet nutritional and fluid requirements produce gastric distension and high intra-abdominal tension. Fluid is readily regurgitated. Infants who vomit excessively may be helped by thickened feeds, which increase resistance to regurgitation, and by smaller volume feeds offered more frequently so that gastric distension is lessened. As infants grow, consume more solid food and adopt upright posture, vomiting ceases to be a problem.

Vomiting can be a symptom of serious gastrointestinal or parenteral disorder. When infants vomit and fail to thrive, vomit bile or blood, or vomit to the extent of causing dehydration, medical investigation is urgently required.

Diarrhoea

The colour, consistency and frequency of stools varies widely both between different infants and in the same infants on different occasions. Breast-fed infants tend to have frequent, watery, yellow stools. Bottle-fed infants have less frequent, greenish, drier looking stools.

Diarrhoea is usually interpreted as frequent, poorly formed and watery, stools. In infancy it is most commonly the result of infection, either gastrointestinal or a generalized viral infection. In such cases onset is acute and associated with other signs of infection: pyrexia, vomiting, anorexia, general malaise. Diarrhoea caused by infection is usually short-lived but may persist with certain infecting organisms (especially rotavirus, *Giardia lamblia* and *Entamoeba histolytica*), in very young infants, and in those who are already malnourished. Frequent episodes of even short-lived diarrhoea can lead to malnutrition because of anorexia and reduced energy intakes. Prior malnutrition predisposes to increased morbidity and mortality from diarrhoeal illness, i.e. the malignant interaction of nutrition and diarrhoeal disease which affects so many children in less developed parts of the world.

Diarrhoea which is persistent and associated with failure-to-thrive, dehydration, bleeding, or other obvious illness requires medical investigation.

Toddler diarrhoea

Some young children who have been weaned persistently produce watery stools with no evidence of infection and no evidence of malnutrition or other ill health. Others have recurrent bouts of loose, watery stools, alternating with periods of relative constipation, for no apparent reason. The stools are usually described as voluminous and watery with bits of 'undigested food' in them, indicating the visible bean husks, tomato skins and other vegetable matter also present, although less obviously so, in normal formed stools. Children with toddler diarrhoea are active and thriving. Their parents are very disturbed by the symptoms.

Toddler diarrhoea probably has multiple aetiology. Whole gut transit time is reduced but there is no evidence of abnormal duodenal or jejunal secretion, nor of malabsorption. In some children diarrhoea is precipitated by minor infections. In others there is a family history of response to stress with diarrhoea. Poor hygiene and low-grade infections caused by constant dummy sucking or prolonged bottle-feeding may contribute to the problem. Milk or sweetened juices kept in feeding bottles for long periods and contaminated after being carried around by the toddlers, hidden in mothers' handbags, dropped on the ground, or offered to the dog, may maintain low-grade gastrointestinal infection in some children.

Many affected children have high intakes of sweetened fruit juices. High fluid intakes with high simple carbohydrate content encourage rapid intestinal transit by the drinks to the extent that small intestinal function is overwhelmed and sugars reach the large intestine unabsorbed. These and their fermentation products in the colon stimulate osmotic diarrhoea. The reduction of fluid intakes, particularly of sweetened juices and 'pop', lessens the symptoms in some toddlers, as do changes to more adult diets with higher concentrations of complex carbohydrates and fats. More mature diets result in higher intakes of lipids. Lipids in the ileum slow duodenal and jejunal transit time (the 'ileal brake') and could modulate mucosal contact time and the absorption of intestinal luminal contents. Discouraging dummies and encouraging maturation to cup-feeding is another important aspect in the management of toddler diarrhoea. Graduating to cup-feeding tends to reduce overall fluid intake and encourages more hygienic feeding practices.

Toddler diarrhoea usually persists for months or years but gradually resolves as the children develop continence and move to more mature diets. It rarely occurs after the age of 6 years.

Dietary Deficiencies in Infancy

Despite the need for carers to be aware of the nutritional needs of infants, significant deficiency of micronutrients other than iron in normal weight, full term, healthy infants is rare. In low birthweight infants and Asian infants, vitamin D deficiency rickets is also a problem.

Iron deficiency

Newborn infants have high haemoglobin levels because of the low oxygen tension *in utero*. After birth, in response to the high oxygen tension of the extrauterine environment, the bone marrow undergoes a period of relative quiescence and haemoglobin levels fall. The bone marrow becomes more active again at 4–6 weeks of age, but by then infants have grown and their blood volumes have expanded. Haemoglobin levels fail to catch up with the increasing blood volumes owing to growth. Haemoglobin levels ($110-120 \text{ g l}^{-1}$) remain below adult levels until late childhood.

Where infants are small and growing very rapidly (e.g. premature and small-for-dates infants) with low total blood volume and low total body iron, the need for iron for new blood formation may exceed the iron stored or the iron absorbable from the diet. Iron deficiency anaemia results. Once body weight has doubled, iron deficiency is likely in all infants since, without good external sources of iron, iron stores of the body will be distributed over twice the blood volume – and haemoglobin levels will have halved. Iron fortification of infant formulae in the UK has reduced the incidence of severe iron deficiency anaemia amongst young children.

Table 2 lists some of the circumstances which predispose to iron deficiency anaemia in childhood. The frequency with which the problem occurs is an indication of the small margin of safety between the quantity of iron a child is likely to ingest and absorb on a nutritionally well-balanced diet and the needs for iron in early childhood. Iron sufficiency is important. There is some evidence that low-grade iron deficiency reduces the body's resistance to infection. Low-grade iron deficiency may also reduce growth rates and affect intellectual function.

Lactoferrin in breast milk binds iron and facilitates iron absorption. This inhibits multiplication of iron-dependent bacterial pathogens. Thus, since lactoferrin is a major anti-infective factor, iron supplementation should be avoided in wholly breast-fed infants unless they show clinical evidence of deficiency.

Vitamin D deficiency: Rickets

Rickets used to be common in weanlings. In the UK the Clean Air Act (1956) probably influenced the prevalence of rickets as much as any medical intervention. Circulating metabolites of vitamin D are predominantly derived from skin synthesis of vitamin D by irradiation of 7-dehydrocholesterol with sunlight of wavelength 300 nm.

Rickets is still seen in newborn Asian infants and mothers in the UK. The mothers have inadequate skin synthesis of vitamin D probably because of their indoor habits and heavy clothing when out of doors. Skin pigmentation increases needs for sunlight exposure when levels of ultraviolet (UV) light of appropriate wavelength are low. Calcium absorption is low owing to low intakes and to the high phytate content of traditional flours. Low calcium intakes may exacerbate the need for vitamin D.

Infants of vitamin D-deficient mothers present with hypocalcaemic tetany and convulsions soon after birth, or with rickets during the weaning period. The incidence of rickets in Asian children is diminishing as Asian women in the UK adopt lifestyles more suited to Northern latitudes.

Vegetarian Diets in Infancy

Infants weaned onto vegetarian diets may become deficient in a variety of nutrients. If infants are not on total vegetarian diets but consume eggs and milk, it is not too difficult to achieve dietary requirements, particularly if feeding infant formula continues beyond the first year of life. Without substantial intakes of milk, riboflavin, calcium and total energy, intakes may not meet requirements. Children should be fed frequently (at least four times a day) to enable them to consume large enough amounts of low energy density vegetarian diets. A variety of vegetable protein sources (e.g. beans, cereals, dark green

Table 2 Classification of problems predisposing to iron deficiency in childhood

Basic nutritional problem	Example
Inadequate intake	Early introduction to cow's milk Prolonged breast-feeding without weaning Poor quality of diet Vegetarian diet
Increased losses	Bleeding disorders Reflux oesophagitis
Failure to absorb	Coeliac disease Pyrexia Iron in ferric form High phytate diet
Failure to utilize	Chronic infection Hypothyroidism
Increased requirements	Rapid growth: previous small-for-dates or premature infants Catch-up growth

leaves, homogenized nut products) should be provided at each meal since essential amino acid requirements can be met only by mixing vegetable proteins which individually do not contain all essential amino acids.

Low-birthweight Infants

The problems of both premature and low-birthweight (for gestational age) infants are similar, although the greater immaturity of the premature infant's gastrointestinal tract and of other organs makes the nutrition of the former more difficult than that of the latter. In both groups there is a need for more nutrients per unit of body weight to cope with the rapid growth to parallel intrauterine growth in premature infants, and with catch-up growth in small-for-dates infants. The smaller stomach volume in these infants means that there are restrictions on the amounts of food that can be administered without causing apnoea, vomiting or necrotizing enterocolitis. Respiratory problems in premature infants may also restrict the amount of enteral food tolerated. Thus there is a conflict between increased nutrient needs, especially for protein, calcium, phosphate, fluid and energy, and the amounts that can be safely administered. Even when small infants are fed parenterally, there are restrictions on the fluid volumes, and thus the nutrient quantities, that can be given when the infants are very young and sick.

Table 3 lists the problems of low-birthweight infants which have been discussed elsewhere in other articles. Small infants should be supplemented with vitamins A, C, D and folate for the first year of life. Iron supplementation is also advisable until the age of one, although iron supplements are usually only administered after 1 month. Earlier iron supplementation risks damage, or encouragement of bacterial infection, by free iron radicals since the iron stores are still replete owing to relative, but temporary bone marrow inactivity because of the high haemoglobin levels at birth. Iron supplements should probably not be given to wholly breast-fed infants unless there is haematological evidence of iron deficiency since iron may counteract the protective effects of lactoferrin in the milk.

Allergy

Cow's milk protein intolerance (CMPI)

Food allergy, particularly CMPI, is widely diagnosed in infants but many of the cases diagnosed as such are not genuine cases of food allergy or intolerance. There is a tendency for infants who vomit, have diar-

Table 3 Nutritional problems of low-birthweight infants

Problem	Precipitating factors
Immediate	
Hypoglycaemia	Limited liver glycogen
	Delay in mobilizing fat stores
	Problems with administering nutrients
Hypocalcaemia	Reaction to loss of high calcium flux across placenta
	Immaturity of calcium homeostasis
	Occasionally maternal vitamin D deficiency
Later	
Poor growth	Nutrient density of breast milk probably not sufficient
	Problems with administering high-energy density, low-birthweight formula
	Poor fat absorption by immature
	Increased needs of bronchopulmonary dysplasia
Bone disease of prematurity	Deficiency of substrate; especially phosphate
	Renal calcium losses: acidosis; diuretics
	Occasionally vitamin D, protein or copper deficiency
Anaemia	Vitamin E deficiency, early
	Folate deficiency
	Iron deficiency

rhoea, have a rash, or cry frequently to be diagnosed as having CMPI. Cow's milk or cow's milk-based formulae are removed from the diet and the infants seem to improve. Improvements might have occurred anyway or might have resulted from mothers feeling reassured that 'something was being done'. If improvements are rapid and dramatic but symptoms recur when cow's milk protein is reintroduced, CMPI is likely to be the cause of the symptoms.

Cow's milk protein intolerance affects between 0.15% and 5% of the population of western Europe. In families in which there is a strong atopic history the incidence may be much higher. Cow's milk protein intolerance most commonly develops in children under 2 months of age, although it may develop at a later age, particularly after gastrointestinal surgery, malnutrition or gastrointestinal infection. Manifestations are varied and nonspecific.

Children with diarrhoea and/or blood loss in association with CMPI may show villous atrophy and increased inflammatory cell infiltrations on jejunal biopsy, or acute colitis on sigmoidoscopy. Those with respiratory symptoms may present with the pulmonary infiltrations of pulmonary haemosiderosis which resolve on removal of all cow's milk-containing products from the diet. When making a diagnosis of CMPI the possibility of lactose intolerance must be excluded. Cow's milk protein-free formulae are also free of lactose, so that removing formula and cow's milk products from the diet does not distinguish the two conditions. Children with lactose intolerance will have acid stools containing reducing substances. If these are not present but the child's symptoms resolve on cow's milk-protein-free diet and recur when milk protein is reintroduced, CMPI is likely. Where symptoms have been dramatic (e.g. angioneurotic oedema; profuse diarrhoea), milk challenges can be dangerous and should be performed with great care and under hospital supervision.

The particular elements of the cow's milk protein causing the allergenic responses vary. At least 18 components that can induce antibody formation have been identified. When purified protein fractions are used as challenges, β-lactoglobulin and casein produce symptoms in over 60% of affected individuals. Antibodies to cows' milk protein are widespread and neither the presence nor the circulating levels of antibody correlate well with reactions to cows' milk.

Breast-fed infants often show circulating cow's milk protein antibodies. Changing from breast-feeding to cow's milk-formula feeding can, very rarely, precipitate dramatic anaphylactic symptoms or angioneurotic oedema. Relevant proteins from the cow's milk consumed by mother are thought to be transferred to affected infants either across the placenta or in breast milk, causing sensitization. The infants are then desensitized by the small amounts of antigen in maternal milk but are overwhelmed when confronted with a large load of antigen from formula feeding.

The management of CMPI involves removal of all cow's milk protein-containing products from the diet. Feeding either soya-protein-based formula or hydrolysed cow's milk-protein-based formula, which renders cow's milk protein no longer allergenic, is appropriate for formula-fed infants. Weaning solids should not contain milk in any form.

Paediatric dietetic advice is required before putting infants on milk-free diets since milk and milk products continue to contribute significant amounts of energy and other nutrients to children's diets even after weaning. Difficulties in meeting nutritional needs on milk-free weaning diets can lead to undernutrition.

Infants with CMPI may also develop soya protein intolerance. Hydrolysed cow's milk protein formulae may be more suitable for treatment of CMPI but are rather unpalatable (to mothers anyway), not available from the supermarkets, and costly.

Infants with CMPI usually develop tolerance to cow's milk proteins in the second or third year of life.

Other food allergens

Other food allergies are quite common in infancy, especially in those with an atopic history. Common precipitants are egg protein, citrus fruits, nuts (not advised for young children anyway) and the food colourants tartrazine and quinoline yellow. Diarrhoea, vomiting, rashes, wheezing and – rarely – behavioural disturbances may occur. (Most behavioural problems are disciplinary rather than allergic.) The pattern of response in each child is usually repeated on subsequent contact with the allergen, but there is great variation in the pattern of individual responses.

Eczema

The role of food intolerance in the development of infantile eczema is an unresolved issue. Some infants with eczema improve when all milk products are withdrawn from the diet. Others only improve when put on very restricted lists of foods. It does seem that diet exacerbates eczema in some children. Studies of infants with a high risk of atopic eczema from family history show that the onset of eczema may sometimes be delayed by giving susceptible infants no food other than breast milk for the first 6 months of life. The interpretation of these studies is open to question and it can be argued that infants who develop eczema despite breast milk only diets, do so because of transfer of foreign proteins in mother's milk.

Colic

Around 3 months of age healthy infants often develop bouts of fractiousness and inconsolable crying, usually in the early evening. Their abdomens become tight and distended, probably because of the air swallowed whilst crying. Infants tend to flex their legs when crying and this is often interpreted as evidence of abdominal pain. 'Three months colic' is an ill-defined problem with a wide range of symptomatology. In the long term, 'colic' resolves without specific treatment and may be a behavioural rather than a medical problem. Nevertheless, it causes parents distress, which probably increases their infants' distress. Removal of cow's milk formula and substitution with nonallergenic formula or soya protein formula has sometimes been associated with improvement. However, it is difficult to know if this has anything to do with resolution of symptoms in a benign self-limiting condition.

Cot Death: Sudden Infant Death Syndrome (SIDS)

Sudden infant death syndrome affects about 1 in 500 infants in the UK and is most common between the ages of 1 and 6 months. Despite enormous efforts in research and many suggestions of causes, no satisfactory explanation for the condition is forthcoming.

It has been suggested that infants who die suddenly and unexpectedly at home, and in whom no cause of death is recognized, die as a result of an hypersensitivity response to cow's milk protein. Where infants die with no pathological findings or clinical history to suggest that they had been ill prior to death, this seems unlikely since true unexplained death in infancy is probably as common in wholly breast-fed infants as in bottle-fed infants. In some infants there is history or postmortem findings to suggest some minor illness prior to death. Bottle-feeding may predominate amongst these infants since breast milk has protective factors against two of the most troublesome infections to inflict young infants: rotavirus and respiratory syncytial virus.

Another nutritional explanation preferred for some forms of cot death is undiagnosed inborn errors of metabolism involving inhibition of breakdown of long-chain fatty acids. There may be evidence for antemortem hypoglycaemia in some cases of SIDS. The child is unable to metabolize fats to cope with the stress of fasting and dies. Postmortem examination reveals acute fatty degeneration of the liver. In such cases, SIDS may be familial since inborn errors of metabolism involving fatty acid breakdown are inherited – usually by autosomal recessive genes.

The explanations and clinical and sociological associations for SIDS are legion. It seems unlikely that one explanation will be found to account for this – sadly – common problem.

Teething Problems

The relevance of tooth eruption to illness and pyrexia in young children is debatable. Between 6 and 30 months teeth are erupting more or less continuously so that it is easy to blame all symptomatology, particularly that associated with grumpiness, mild pyrexia and being 'off colour', on teething.

Those involved in child care vary from those ready to diagnose teething as an explanation for a wide variety of nonspecific symptomatology to those who stick doggedly to the view that teething is never important. The truth is probably somewhere in between these two views. It would seem likely that, if a child is a little unwell with a minor infection, the irritation of tooth eruption may exacerbate the malaise and misery. It would seem wise to avoid attributing significant pyrexia, diarrhoea or vomiting to teething unless clinical examination has excluded other possible causes.

Surprisingly, there is little evidence that the presence or absence of teeth in young children makes much difference to feeding in the first year. Although most children develop their first teeth around 6 months of age, some do not develop teeth until around 2 years, yet these late erupters usually cope well with chewing and should be encouraged to move onto mature diets in the normal way.

Nursing bottle syndrome

Nursing bottle syndrome is less common than it was a few years ago owing to recognition of its main causes. It arises when young children have been allowed to suck dummies sweetened with juices or other sugary solutions, or when they have been put to bed with bottles in their mouths and have sucked juice or formula from bottles through the night.

Constant bathing of the upper incisors with sugary fluids, together with the low level of both salivary secretion and mouth movements at night, leads to development of plaque. Multiplication of cariogenic bacteria and the acid pH under plaque results in carious destruction of teeth, particularly upper incisors. Only discoloured, carious stumps of teeth remain in the front of the upper jaw. Under these circumstances young children often become very faddy eaters as they may have difficulty chewing meat and vegetables and biting fruit.

Protection against caries is provided by fluoridation of water supplies with one part per million of fluoride or by giving fluoride supplements, 0.25 mg per day in infancy and 0.5 mg per day between 1 and 3 years. Regular, at least daily, tooth-brushing should be taught from the first appearance of teeth. It is advisable for adults to load their young children's brushes with toothpaste, since small children may eat toothpaste rather than spit it out after cleaning the teeth. As much as 0.66 mg of fluoride could be consumed per day by small children brushing their teeth inexpertly twice a day with fluoridated toothpaste.

All food, but particularly sweetened drinks, should be discouraged after tooth-brushing at night.

See also: **Anaemia (Anemia)**: Iron-Deficiency Anaemia. **Ascorbic Acid**: Physiology, Dietary Sources and Requirements. **Dental Disease**: Aetiology and Epidemiology. **Folic Acid**: Physiology, Dietary Sources and Requirements. **Food Allergies**: Aetiology. **Food Intolerance**: Types and Incidence. **Inborn Errors of Metabolism**: Classification and Biochemical Aspects. **Infants**: Nutritional Requirements; Milk-feeding and Weaning;

Low-birthweight and Preterm Infants. **Iron**: Physiology, Dietary Sources and Requirements. **Lactation**: Physiology; Dietary Requirements. **Malnutrition**: Definition, Classification and Epidemiology. **Retinol**: Physiology. **Tocopherols**: Physiology. **Vegetarian Diets**: Practice; Nutritional Adequacy.

Further Reading

Cant AJ (1991) Food allergy and intolerance. In: McLaren DS, Burman D, Belton NR and Williams AF (eds) *Textbook of Paediatric Nutrition*, 3rd edn, pp 201–221. Edinburgh: Churchill Livingstone.

Department of Health and Social Security (1980) *Rickets and Osteomalacia*. Report on Health and Social Subjects 19. London: HMSO

Filer Jr LJ (ed.) (1989) *Dietary Iron. Birth to Two Years.* New York: Raven Press.

Poskitt EME (1988) *Practical Paediatric Nutrition*, pp 80–95. Oxford: Butterworth Heinemann.

Simeon DT, Grantham-McGregor SM (1991) Nutritional deficiencies and children's behaviour and mental development. *Nutrition Reviews* 3:1–24

Standing Committee on Nutrition. British Paediatric Association (1988) Vegetarian weaning. *Archives of Disease in Childhood* 63:470–478.

Widdowson EM (1947) Mental contentment and physical growth. *Lancet* i:1316–1318.

Low-birthweight and Preterm Infants

B Caballero, Johns Hopkins University, Baltimore, Maryland, USA

Copyright © 1998 Academic Press

Premature birth has a significant impact on the newborn's ability to metabolize nutrients. Fetal metabolism is optimized for energy accumulation and is adapted to a situation of steady fuel supply from maternal sources, primarily as glucose. Birth causes a dramatic shift in that metabolic steady state: exogenous glucose supply ceases abruptly, and the newborn must rapidly activate enzymatic pathways for gluconeogenesis and for the utilization of fatty acids and ketone bodies as alternative sources of energy. Although many of the key enzymes for fuel utilization increase their activity in response to substrate load, they may still fall short of the large fuel supply needed by the premature newborn.

The newborn's energy stores accumulate in the last trimester of pregnancy. Thus, premature birth deprives the newborn of a significant amount of endogenous energy reserves. It is estimated that, whereas the body energy density of a full-term newborn is around 5 MJ (1200 kcal) per kg, that of a 1.2 kg premature baby may be as low as 1.7 MJ (400 kcal) per kg. The gastrointestinal tract of the premature infant, although anatomically developed, is functionally immature, both in terms of digestive enzymes and motility. Gastric capacity is obviously reduced, particularly relative to the higher energy needs per kg of body weight.

Feeding the premature or low-birthweight infant usually involves a compromise between the high nutrient requirements and the limited capacity to metabolize and utilize these nutrients.

Energy

Energy balance studies on preterm infants are based on feeding formulae of variable energy density. Results yield gross energy intakes ranging from 460 kJ to 750 kJ (110–180 kcal) per kg per day. Infants receiving human milk have usually lower energy intakes, but their rate of weight gain may not necessarily be lower than formula-fed infants. Nevertheless, the lower energy density of human milk relative to premature formulae may limit the total energy intake in some cases.

Glucose utilization is higher in the preterm than the term infant, and has been estimated as 5–6 mg kg^{-1} min^{-1}. Small for gestational age (SGA) infants may have even higher capacity. However, excess glucose administration (usually intravenous) may induce lipogenesis and increase carbon dioxide production, which in turn may compromise respiratory function. The increased phosphorus utilization at high rates of glucose metabolism should also be considered.

Protein

Limitations for protein nutrition in the preterm infant are related to the capacity for nitrogen metabolism and excretion: the urea cycle and kidney function. In addition, several enzymatic steps for amino acid catabolism and conversion may be limiting, potentially causing accumulation of intermediary compounds. Premature newborns have the highest requirements for essential amino acids relative to total amino N needs. This essential amino acid requirement was estimated to be as high as 40% of the total amino acids, and thus makes the premature highly dependent on dietary protein quality.

Protein contributes significantly to the renal solute load through urea synthesis. Urea, potassium and sodium are the major determinants of solute load for the kidney. Thus, an adequate amount of free water and adequate renal function are essential in order to avoid overload. Increased water requirements imposed by other conditions (such as gastrointestinal losses or use of radiant warmers) may limit the infant's ability to excrete the dietary nitrogen load.

Fat

Fat not only provides essential fatty acids, but is also the major form of energy accumulation for the growing premature infant. It is estimated that the preterm infant can oxidize about 1 g per kg per day of fat, depositing the rest in adipose tissue. Thus, fat deposition may be stimulated, to a certain extent, by increasing fat administration. Medium-chain triacylglycerols (MCT), although absorbed better than long-chain fatty acids, are less efficient at sustaining weight gain, and at high intakes may cause gastrointestinal disturbances or diarrhoea. Because of this, it is recommended that MCT should not exceed 30–40% of the total fat administered to the preterm infant.

In recent years there has been increasing interest in defining the role of long-chain polyunsaturated fatty acids. Docosahexaenoic acid ($C_{22:6}$) and eicosapentaenoic acid ($C_{20:5}$) are present in relatively high levels in human milk, but not in infant formulae. In several studies, addition of these fatty acids to formulae fed to premature infants enhances visual development. It is less clear whether full-term infants may benefit as well. Several formulae for premature infants are now enriched with these fats.

Parenteral Nutrition in Premature Infants

Very low-birthweight infants usually require parenteral nutritional support (**Table 1**). A combination of intravenous glucose and fat is better than either alone as energy source. There has been concern about the possible adverse effects of high intakes of lipid emulsions. Some studies have reported impaired immune function and increased incidence of respiratory distress. It is recommended that intravenous fat should not contribute more than 50% of the nonprotein energy, and that serum triacylglycerol levels should not exceed 2.2–2.8 mmol l^{-1} (200–250 mg dl^{-1}). In some cases, intermittent infusion of fat may be better tolerated.

Small for gestational age newborns may exhibit higher energy expenditure than those with adequate weight for gestational age. Although SGA newborns usually gain weight adequately, the hydration of tissue gained may be higher than normal weight infants.

Table 1 Recommended daily intakes for preterm infants

Nutrient	Daily intake
Energy (kcal kg^{-1})	120
Energy (kJ kg^{-1})	500
Protein (g kg^{-1})	3.5–4.0
Essential fatty acids $C_{18:2}$ (g per 100 kcal)	0.3
Vitamins	
Vitamin A (IU)	1400
Vitamin D (IU)	500
Vitamin E (IU)	5–25
Vitamin C (mg)	35
Thiamin (μg)	300
Riboflavin (μg)	400
Niacin (mg)	6
Vitamin B_6 (μg)	300
Folic acid (μg)	50
Vitamin B_{12} (μg)	0.3
Minerals	
Ca (mg kg^{-1})	< 200
P (mg kg^{-1})	< 120
Mg (mg kg^{-1})	8

Minerals

The accumulation of calcium and phosphorus in bone during intrauterine life increases rapidly from 24 weeks of gestation until term. Thus, premature birth is associated with limited bone calcium accretion. The Ca : P ratio of fetal bone is approximately 2 : 1, but the ratio of dietary calcium and phosphorus needs is also determined by body weight gain relative to bone mass accretion, since more phosphorus is present in soft tissues.

Intestinal calcium absorption in the preterm infant is very efficient, and may be as high as 80–90% in some studies. Phosphorus absorption is also high, particularly from human milk, which has a lower phosphorus content than cow's milk formulae.

The optimal calcium and phosphorus intakes for premature infants have not been experimentally established. Requirements are higher than for full-term infants, and several studies have shown that higher intake can enhance bone calcium accretion. A daily intake of 200 mg kg^{-1} of calcium 100–120 mg kg^{-1} of potassium has been recommended, assuming an average retention of 64% and 71% respectively. The duration of this higher intake may be defined by body weight (attainment of a weight of 2 kg) or as 8–10 weeks. Preterm infant formulae are fortified with calcium and phosphorus and can usually provide these amounts when the infant is receiving full feeding. Human milk can be supplemented with these minerals. Infants on parenteral nutrition may receive high amounts of calcium and phosphorus, and should be monitored for rapid shifts in serum levels and urinary excretion.

Calcium and phosphorus deficiency (rickets of prematurity) is a relatively common occurrence, particularly in sick infants, who often are unable to receive adequate intakes and have other concurrent metabolic disturbances. Clinical diagnosis is usually difficult, and factors that increase the risk of calcium, phosphorus and magnesium deficiencies should alert the physician for close monitoring of serum levels. Among these factors are severe sepsis and metabolic stress, use of diuretics (particularly frusemide), and protracted gastrointestinal losses (which may lead to Mg depletion). Deficiency of calcium or phosphorus due to inadequate supply in parenterally fed neonates may also occur, particularly when there are difficulties in delivering the full calculated volume. Conversely, parenteral nutrition is also a common cause

of excess administration of these minerals. The only means of avoiding deficiency or excess is the regular monitoring of serum levels.

See also: **Calcium**: Physiology. **Energy**: Energy Balance. **Fatty Acids**: Metabolism. **Nutritional Support**: Parenteral Nutrition. **Phosphorus**: Physiology, Dietary Sources and Requirements. **Protein**: Requirements and Role in Diet.

Further Reading

American Academy of Pediatrics (1993) *Pediatric Nutrition Handbook*. Chicago: AAP.
Tsang R, Nichols B (1988) *Nutrition During Infancy*. Philadelphia: Hanley & Belfus, The CV Mosby Co.
Williams AF (1991) Low birthweight infants. In: McLaren DS, Burman D, Belton NR, Williams AF (eds), *Textbook of Pediatric Nutrition*. pp 75–104. London: Churchill Livingstone.

INFECTION

Contents
Nutritional Interactions
Nutritional Management
Nutritional Management of Measles and Human Immunodeficiency Virus Infection in Children

Nutritional Interactions

G T Keusch, New England Medical Center, Boston, Massachusetts, USA

Copyright © 1998 Academic Press

In 1968, Scrimshaw, Gordon and Taylor published a classic review of the world's literature on nutrition–infection interactions, including both animal and human studies. In most of the examples reviewed the interaction of malnutrition and infection was detrimental to the host, in some examples there was no effect and in a few examples there was evidence of clinical antagonism, that is malnutrition inhibited the usual progression of the infection and attenuated the host response. The authors concluded that nutrition and infection most often interacted in a manner that adversely affected the host, sometimes by a synergistic interaction, that is the combined adverse effects of the two factors were distinctly greater than additive. Most of the human studies were conducted in young children in developing countries with the complex nutritional disease, protein–energy malnutrition (PEM). The data were interpreted to support a paradigm in which poor diets led to nutritional deficiencies, associated with frequent infections and ultimately with wasting (deficits in weight for age) and/or stunting (deficits in height for age). It was presumed that the malnutrition had a direct and negative effect on the immune system, and this acquired immunodeficiency was responsible for increased morbidity and mortality.

This formulation led to a search for the primary cause of PEM and the choice of single dietary interventions. Most investigations initially focused on dietary protein deficiency because of the poor quality and reduced quantity of protein in the diet of these children, the negative nitrogen balances observed during infection, and the resulting marked loss of muscle mass and visceral protein. The concept was both simple and supported by experimental animal studies: dietary protein deficiency led to malnutrition with adverse affects on the immune system which, in turn, increased host susceptibility to infection. The combination of malnutrition and infection was often deadly. Interventions were tested, for example provision of protein supplements or simply supplementations of the limiting amino acids in the diet, with the goal of improving the quantity or the quality of the protein in the diet. While the hope was that this would prevent severe PEM, the benefits were limited and, in retrospect, unimpressive.

Attention therefore shifted to the limiting energy intake of these children. It was known that there were marked alterations in energy metabolism during infectious episodes, with a shift toward gluconeogenesis, which suggested the importance of energy in the response to infection. Dietary interventions using energy supplements were tried next, much in the same way that protein supplements had been employed. Again, the results were limited in terms of preventing malnutrition and the cycle of malnutrition and infection.

Meanwhile, careful field studies in developing countries began to suggest the importance of infection as a major force in the development of kwashiorkor, the most severe clinical presentation of malnutrition, with marked wasting and oedema. Prospective studies of nutritional status, infection, and food intake and utilization showed that over the first 3 months of life breast-fed infants in poor developing countries grew in parallel to infants in the industrialized nations, even though they were lower in birthweight. However, during the weaning period, infections occurred more commonly, especially diarrhoea, respiratory disease and (in endemic areas), malaria, and each infection correlated with a period of growth faltering. On the typical nutrient-poor diet in this setting, catch-up growth was usually incomplete when the next infection occurred, initiating a cycle of infections, failure to grow and progressive deficits in nutritional status. In many infants, the cumulative deficits from multiple episodes of infection ultimately resulted in kwashiorkor, often culminating in death.

This insight led to a significant alteration in the hypothesis underlying the paradigm for nutrition–infection interactions. The data suggested that not only could malnutrition lead to an increase in infection morbidity, but infection could result in deterioration in the host's nutritional status. The initial causal model therefore had to be modified to a more complex one in which malnutrition was seen to lead to infection and, at the same time, infection also would lead to malnutrition. If this was true then optimal interventions to reduce PEM would require both improved nutrient content of the diets as well as a reduction in the prevalence of infection.

Subsequently many studies focused on defining the effects of infection on host nutrition. It had been known since the early years of the twentieth century that fever of any aetiology caused an increase in basal metabolism. Indeed, in a study of patients with a variety of conditions it was calculated that each degree Celsius increase over basal body temperature resulted in a 13% increase in resting metabolic rate. However, with the new understanding of nutrition–infection interactions, the significance of this observation could be appreciated from a different perspective. Specifically, the concept is that fever increases energy consumption, independent of any other impact of elevations in body temperature on the host–pathogen relationship. In part, this effect of fever on energy stores is related to the biology of enzyme reactions, in which reaction rates increase in a predictable manner as temperature increases. To fuel the increased rate of all enzymatic reactions in the body, energy consumption must increase. In part the increase in energy consumption is also due to the increased production of cells and synthesis of proteins involved in the host defence response to the infection, as well as to repair tissue damaged in the process. The increase in energy consumption during infection has been measured using sophisticated experimental methods, documenting an increase in resting energy expenditure of as much as 30–40% over normal in septic humans.

The logical next question concerned the source of the energy. This was of particular interest because it has long been known that fever initiates a number of 'non-specific' symptoms including anorexia and myalgias. Anorexia, the loss of appetite, obviously results in decreased food intake, making it difficult to obtain the extra energy being consumed by increasing dietary nutrient intake. Careful measurements of food intake of malnourished infants with infection have shown a 25–35% decrease during febrile periods. With such a significant reduction in food intake, coupled with an increase of similar magnitude in nutrient requirements, the host clearly has a need to use endogenous stores of energy in the body.

Ultimately, the consequence of this depletion of body stores is a change in body composition, which is one way of defining acute nutritional depletion states. To restore health, the altered body composition would need to be reversed and corrected in the host, presumably during convalescence when the initiating infection was controlled and no longer driving the host metabolism along an abnormal pathway. It also was clear that if body stores are used to provide for the metabolic needs of infection, then weight loss must occur. This is consistent with the known onset of growth faltering and either reductions in weight gain or sometimes an absolute loss of weight in growing infants and children, and weight loss in adults. The reduction in body mass is not subtle, especially in chronic infections, as the loss of fat and muscle mass is visible to the naked eye. In fact this sort of observation led to the introduction of the lay term 'consumption' to describe tuberculosis, the classic chronic wasting infectious disease. Metabolic studies have shown the reduction in muscle mass is due to catabolism of muscle protein in excess of protein anabolism, with a net release of amino acids to the circulation. The increase in catabolism was ushered in by fever and temporally related to the classic 'nonspecific' symptom, myalgia, suggesting that excessive proteolysis could induce pain.

To clarify the relationship of these metabolic events to fever an experimental model was needed. It also was believed that fever itself was a response to an endogenous mediator induced by the infection, which was therefore known as 'endogenous pyrogen'. A model was established using rabbits injected with bacterial lipopolysaccharide, or subsequently with fractions obtained by activated leucocytes, and changes in rectal temperature were recorded. By standardizing the conditions for inducing and measuring the fever response, reproducible rises in temperature could be produced by specific stimuli. This allowed investigators to carry out careful experimental studies, which soon narrowed the search for the source of this factor to leucocytes that were in some way activated. By the late 1970s, application of the rapidly developing sciences of molecular and cellular biology to the search for this mediator led to the isolation, purification and characterization of a peptide from activated peripheral blood leucocytes with the properties of endogenous pyrogen. This culminated a few years later in the cloning of the endogenous pyrogen gene from both human and mouse macrophages. This peptide was subsequently named interleukin 1 (IL-1) and its discovery initiated a true revolution in biology, that is appreciation of the role of cytokine regulator peptides in biology, and a revolutionary way to look at nutrition–infection interactions as specifically regulated events. According to this view, infections were processes in which microbial products or products of the pathogen–host interaction were able to activate leucocytes to produce cytokine mediators which, in turn, acted as transcriptional regulators of a set of genes whose products initiated and mediated the acute-phase responses during infection.

With this as a framework, it became possible to ask specific questions to define the nature of the regulatory events for the metabolic and immunologic responses to infection, and even to conceptualize the potential to use these regulator molecules at some future time to modulate responses for therapeutic clinical benefit. When purified, the cytokine peptides are generally small, with molecular weights in the range of 15–30 000; some of the cytokines have sequence relationships to one another, allowing their grouping together in families; they bind to specific receptors and cause specific responses; they may interact with one another to mediate and regulate the host responses; and they often have key roles in the immune response in addition to their metabolic effects.

Stimuli for the production of early response cytokines, such as IL-1β and tumour necrosis factor α (TNF-α), include bacterial lipopolysaccharide of Gram-negative organisms, peptidoglycan of Gram-positive organisms, antigen–antibody complexes, products of phagocytosis, virus interactions with host cells, soluble factors such as products of the activation of the complement cascade, as well as some hormones, catecholamines and many others. Some cytokines induce other cytokines; some cytokines function together to cause stereotypical host responses; and some cytokines have the capacity to inhibit the production or function of others. Both IL-1β and TNF-α alter the local production of prostaglandin E_2 within the temperature-regulating regions in the central nervous system and turn up the thermostatic set point, resulting in fever, and in some manner, in anorexia – probably a cytokine-induced response as well. Elevated levels of the proinflammatory cytokines IL-1, TNF-α and IL-6 have been reported in children and elderly subjects with PEM. The two cytokines, IL-1 and TNF-α, probably acting indirectly via the induction of IL-6 rather than by a direct action, induce proteolysis in muscle, the local use of branched-chain amino acids for energy, and the release of the rest of the amino acids to the bloodstream. Increased release of amino acids to the circulation provides substrates needed for the increase in protein synthesis in the liver mediated by these same cytokines. In fact, while many hepatic genes are transcriptionally activated, some others are inhibited. In this manner, not only is there an increase in the overall rate of hepatic protein synthesis in the liver, but there is also a change in the priorities for protein production away from normal export proteins such as albumin and transferrin to secreted acute-phase proteins active in the host response to the infectious process, including the third component of complement, caeruloplasmin, α_1-antitrypsin and many others. This differential effect on hepatic gene activation leads to decreased serum albumin and transferrin levels and the appearance of higher than normal levels of acute-phase proteins, many of which appear to function in host defence against infection.

Increases in protein synthesis are also critical for the necessary increases in the production of immunologically competent cells by the bone marrow and lymph nodes, including B and T lymphocytes, macrophages, neutrophils and other leucocyte types, and their products such as immunoglobulins, various cytokines, interferons, growth factors and many others. The host biosynthetic response, choreographed by the cytokines, provides the substrate amino acids by catabolism of protein stores in muscle needed for translation of the transcriptionally upregulated genes whose products are of immediate high priority for the host, accompanied by the downregulation of genes whose products are less acutely needed.

Protein synthesis requires energy, and in the face of anorexia (so common in infection) it is necessary to find sources other than dietary intake. Unfortunately, the body reserve of carbohydrate, liver glycogen, is insufficient for more than a day at most. The most plentiful source of stored energy is fat; however, in many infections the cytokine and hormonal responses are inhibitory to the efficient use of lipids for energy, as occurs in simple starvation in which visceral protein and muscle are spared, at least for a while. Instead, during infection the regulatory proteins force the body to convert certain amino acids released from muscle as a consequence of proteolysis to glucose via the gluconeogenic pathway in the liver. A marked increase in this pathway during sepsis has been documented; however, the need for a continuing supply of energy is at the cost of further catabolism of muscle contractile proteins. With deamination of amino acids, conversion of the nitrogen to urea, which is excreted in the urine, and oxidation of the carbon skeleton of the amino acid during the consumption of the newly made glucose, with loss of the carbons as respiratory carbon dioxide, the entire amino acid is lost from the body.

In addition to the significant changes in protein and energy metabolism, major shifts in divalent cations occurs, including decreases in circulating iron and zinc and an increase in plasma copper levels. These shifts are also due to cytokine-mediated changes in the binding, transport and storage proteins for these minerals. The apparent rationale for the shift of iron and zinc from the extracellular to the intracellar compartments is to support the cellular proliferative component of the acute-phase response, as both of these metals are critical for the function of a number of the metalloenzymes required for DNA synthesis, without which cellular division cannot occur. Some of the iron taken up into the cell is converted to the long-term storage form, haemosiderin, and is removed from the metabolically active compartment, resulting in a functional iron deficiency state leading to impaired haemoglobin synthesis. Copper levels increase in the circulation because the copper-binding protein, caeruloplasmin, is synthesized in much greater quantities as an acute-phase respondent, and this carries copper from cells into the circulation. The functional significance and possible advantage to the host of this shift in copper is not clear; however, this complex has ferroxidase activity which oxidizes ferrous iron to ferric iron in the transfer to apotransferrin. Hence increased copper-caeruloplasmin levels could assist in the mobilization of iron from ferritin to erythroid precursors in the bone marrow.

The data summarized above indicate the profound metabolic changes that occur during infection. There are major changes in body composition, catabolism of body protein, ultimately depletion of lipid stores, and alterations in mineral metabolism. In growing children, growth ceases and weight may diminish, although not in proportion to the catabolism of visceral and muscle protein as water is retained, sometimes because of an inappropriate antidiuretic hormone secretion initiated by the infectious process. In adults who are no longer growing, weight usually diminishes owing to body composition changes. It is clear that nutrient stores are eroded, as shown by negative balances for nitrogen, energy and minerals. The end of the acute phase of illness and the beginning of convalescence actually represents the nadir of nutritional depletion, a point at which nutritional recovery may begin. Unfortunately, it takes much longer to replete nutrients than it does to create the defects, even when the host has access to an adequate and sufficient diet. It is estimated that the daily energy requirement for growth is 2% of total requirements for a 2-year-old child, while the comparable figure for protein is around 12%. Since catch-up growth under ideal circumstances of care, control of infection and access to energy-dense diets containing high-quality protein is as much as 7 times the normal rate, there is a minimal need for 14% more energy and 84% more protein, and an optimal diet should provide approximately 130% of normal energy and 200% of normal protein requirements for a 2-year-old. This is generally not achieved for most children in the developing world, and the length of time for catch-up may be much increased. However, in settings with a heavy force of infection, nutritional deficits due to the prior infection may not have been repaired at the time a new infection is contracted. The nutritional deficits from the sequential infections then accumulate, and the cycle of infection–malnutrition–infection leads to a downward spiral in host nutrition, sometimes terminating in the severe oedematous form of protein–energy malnutrition, kwashiorkor. Such individuals are highly vulnerable and new infections are frequently superimposed, and so nutritional status deteriorates further and mortality rates climb.

This, then, is the dilemma in nutrition–infection interactions; it is neither a nutritional nor an infection problem in isolation. The two clinical features interact with one another, and initiate the malnutrition–infection cycle, unless broken by attention to both the force of infection and the adequacy of the diet. By and large, we are what we eat.

See also: **Cytokines**: Nutritional Aspects. **Energy Metabolism**: Tricarboxylic Acid Cycle and Oxidative Phosphorylation. **Malnutrition**: Primary Malnutrition. **Protein**: Synthesis and Turnover; Deficiency.

Further Reading

Baggiolini M, Dewald B and Moser B (1997) Human chemokines: an update. *Annual Review of Immunology* 15:675–705.

Beisel WR (1975) Metabolic response to infection. *Annual Review of Medicine* 26:9–20.

Beisel WR and Wannemacher RW Jr (1980) Gluconeogenesis, ureagenesis, and ketogenesis during sepsis. *Journal of Parenteral and Enteral Nutrition* 4:277–285.

Brisco J (1979) The quantitative effect of infection on the use of food by young children in poor countries. *American Journal of Clinical Nutrition* 32:648–673.

Castillo-Duran C, Vial P and Uauy R (1988) Trace and mineral balance during acute diarrhea in infants. *Journal of Pediatrics* 113:452–457.

Cederholm T, Wrelind B, Hellstrom K *et al.* (1997) Enhanced generation of interleukins 1β and 6 may contribute to the cachexia of chronic disease. *American Journal of Clinical Nutrition* 65:876–882.

Cohen MC and Cohen S (1996) Cytokine function: a study in biologic diversity. *American Journal of Clinical Pathology* 105:589–598.

Dinarello CA (1984) Interleukin-1 and the pathogenesis of the acute phase response. *New England Journal of Medicine* 311:1413–1418.

Dinarello CA and Wolff SM (1982) Molecular basis of fever in humans. *American Journal of Medicine* 72:1349–1352.

DuBois EF (1936) *Basal Metabolism in Health and Disease*. Philadelphia: Lea & Febiger.

Jackson AA, Picou D and Reeds PJ (1977) The energy cost of repleting tissue deficits during recovery from protein-energy malnutrition. *American Journal of Clinical Nutrition* 30:1514–1517.

Keusch GT (1979) Nutrition as a determinant of host response to infection and the metabolic sequelae of infectious diseases. In: Weinstein L and Fields BN, (eds) Seminars in Infectious Diseases, pp 265–303. New York: Medical Book.

Keusch GT and Scrimshaw NS (1986) Selective primary health care: strategies for control of disease in the developing world. XXIII. Control of infection to reduce the prevalence of infantile and childhood malnutrition. *Review of Infectious Disease* 8:273–287.

Kunkel SL, Lukacs N and Strieter RM (1995) Chemokines and their role in human disease. *Agents Action* 46:11–22.

Long CL (1977) Energy balance and carbohydrate metabolism in infection and sepsis. *American Journal of Clinical Nutrition* 30:1301–1320.

Manary MJ, Brewster DR, Broadhead RL, Crowley JR, Fjeld CR and Yarasheski KE (1997) Protein metabolism in children with edematous malnutrition and acute lower respiratory infection. *American Journal of Clinical Nutrition* 65:1005–1010.

Mata LJ (1978) *The Children of Santa Maria Cauque: A Prospective Field Study of Health and Growth*. Cambridge: MIT Press.

Michie HR (1996) Metabolism of sepsis and multiple organ failure. *World Journal of Surgery* 20:460–464.

Plata-Salaman CR (1996) Anorexia during acute and chronic disease. *Nutrition* 12:69–788.

Rose D and Martorell R (1990) The impact of protein-energy supplementation interventions on child morbidity and mortality. In: Hill K (ed.) Child Health Priorities for the 1990s. Baltimore: Johns Hopkins Press.

Sauerwein RW, Mulder JA, Mulder L *et al.* (1997) Inflammatory mediators in children with protein-energy malnutrition. *American Journal of Clinical Nutrition* 65:1534–1539.

Scrimshaw NS, Taylor CE and Gordon JE (1968) Interactions of nutrition and infection. Monograph Series 57. Geneva: World Health Organization.

Ye J and Young HA (1997) Negative regulation of cytokine gene transcription. *FASEB Journal* 11:825–833.

Nutritional Management

B Caballero, Johns Hopkins University, Baltimore, Maryland, USA

Copyright © 1998 Academic Press

The Metabolic Effects of Infectious Illness

In the well-nourished host, infection episodes trigger a cascade of adaptive responses, aimed at enhancing immune competence, preserving vital cellular activities and preventing colonization by the infective agent. During the incubation period, major responses of the host include an increase in phagocytic activity and the sequestration of circulating nutrients that are presumed to favour bacterial growth, such as iron, zinc and some amino acids. The hormonal milieu is modified to favour an active defence: deiodination of thyroxine is increased, as well as the release of glucocorticoids and growth hormone. A progressive decrease in the sensitivity of peripheral insulin receptors develops, facilitating fat mobilization and amino acid outflow from peripheral protein breakdown.

The role of cytokines as mediators of systemic responses to infection is becoming more clear. Interleukin 1 (IL-1) causes a significant decrease in appetite in animals, and contributes to the fall in a number of circulating nutrients, particularly iron and zinc. Recombinant tumour necrosis factor (TNF), another cytokine related to infection, causes a marked catabolic state in adipocytes, by suppressing the transcription and translation of key lipogenic enzymes. In experiments *in vitro*, the TNF-induced lipolysis caused a reversal of the differentiation of adipogenic TA1 cells, leading to the formation of fibroblasts. Cachectin or TNF also enhances the transcription of several liver enzymes, resulting in increased rates of gluconeogenesis, ureagenesis and synthesis of acute-phase proteins. It is important to emphasize that this cytokine-induced catabolic state cannot be overcome merely by enhancing substrate availability.

Effects of infection on nitrogen metabolism

Acute infection has a major negative impact on nitrogen balance. Studies in humans show that the infection process is responsible for higher nitrogen losses than can be accounted for by a decreased protein intake. This specific effect of infection varies depending on the causative agent, and on the initial nutritional status of the host. In the well-nourished host, mild infection is associated with an increased protein turnover. The modest rise in protein synthesis, however, is overcome by the marked increase in the rate of protein breakdown, which is also driven by a decreased peripheral amino acid uptake caused by insulin resistance, and by the catabolic action of steroid hormones and catecholamines. Studies using the [^{15}N]glycine end product method suggest that well-nourished children exhibit a more pronounced protein breakdown response to infection than children with mild malnutrition.

Faecal nitrogen losses may contribute significantly to the negative nitrogen balance in children with acute diarrhoea. Nitrogen malabsorption may be substantial during acute diarrhoea, ranging from 40% to 75% of intake. Rotavirus diarrhoea appears to be associated with more marked and prolonged nitrogen losses than *Shigella* or *Escherichia coli* infections. The energy cost of nitrogen losses during acute illness has been estimated at 21–29 kJ kg^{-1} (5–7 kcal kg^{-1}) per day. Chronic diarrhoea, intestinal parasitism and protein-losing enteropathy are all associated with sustained loss of protein through the gastrointestinal tract. It has been estimated that a moderate degree of intestinal hookworm infestation may cause an average loss of 420 kJ (100 kcal) per day.

Effects of infection on energy balance

Dietary intake   Some degree of anorexia is present almost invariably in acute infections. In some cases, this anorexia can be readily explained by the involvement of the gastrointestinal tract, with nausea and vomiting; in others, tachypnoea or oral and oesophageal lesions can also limit oral intake. It has been proposed that cachectin/TNF, a peptide cytokine produced by macrophages, plays a central role in inducing anorexia during acute infections. Similarly, zinc supplementation during recovery from malnutrition has been associated with increased food intake. It should be pointed out, however, that most studies on this topic only measure food intake and assume a direct correlation with appetite, which may not be the case.

Common symptoms of illness in malnourished children under 6 years old cause a reduction of around 20% in energy intake, equivalent to 710–750 kJ (170–180 kcal) per day. It is estimated that fever causes a reduction of 10–40% in dietary intake. Interestingly, the impact of illness appears to be less for breast milk intake. There is good evidence that withholding food during illness does not improve the course of the illness and may contribute substantially to the decreased intake.

Malnourished children (90% or less of weight for age) tend to exhibit larger weight losses during and after infection episodes compared with children of normal weight. Thus, prior nutritional status and age at onset are two important factors in determining the energy imbalance caused by illness.

Energy losses   In well-nourished children, mild episodes of diarrhoea may have little impact on nutrient absorption, but the malnourished child is particularly vulnerable to diarrhoeal disease in terms of nutrient balance. The role of dietary lactose in exacerbating intestinal nutrient loss during acute diarrhoea has been studied, both in well-nourished and malnourished children. The data suggest that in a controlled, clean environment, even severely malnourished children can tolerate progressive amounts of lactose-containing formulae. Identifying true carbohydrate malabsorption may not be practical outside of the hospital setting, given the heterogeneity of signs and symptoms associated with the condition. The reduction in carbohydrate absorption during acute diarrhoea is also dependent on the infective agent: absorption rates of 74% in rotavirus, 77% in *Shigella* and 92% in *E. coli* diarrhoeas have been reported.

Energy expenditure Resting energy expenditure rises by as much as 10–15% for each degree Celsius increase in body temperature. As in the case of appetite, the role of cytokines in the febrile response is being clarified by recent studies. Both interleukin 1 and interleukin 2 appear to play a role in the infection-induced rise in core body temperature. In protein–energy malnutrition cytokine production may be increased or, in severe cases, blunted, which correlates with the clinical picture of infection in moderate or severe cases.

Some decrease in energy expenditure may occur owing to reduced physical activity during illness, but its precise contribution to the energy balance has not been adequately quantified. There is evidence that chronic undernutrition causes an adaptation of energy metabolism in adults and in children. This adaptation is reflected in substantial decreases in whole-body protein turnover, which has an estimated physiological cost of 20–25% of the resting energy expenditure. It should be noted, however, that intense nutrient losses through the gastrointestinal tract can rapidly cause a net negative nutrient balance, regardless of the compensatory response of the host. The decreased physical activity associated with sickness may reduce energy expenditure by around 10%.

Dietary lipids Dietary lipids play an important role in the immune response. The fatty acid composition of cell membranes, including that of lymphocytes, can be modified by dietary fatty acid manipulations. Studies both *in vitro* and *in vivo* have shown that fatty acid content of the diet or the culture medium affects cellular immune responsiveness, possibly by changes in membrane fluidity. Fatty acids also modulate the cytokine-mediated response to infection, possibly by enhancing prostanoid formation, which suppressed the thermic response to experimental infection. Dietary supplementation with n-6 fatty acids also inhibits splenic T cell activity. In a study in human volunteers, 6 weeks of n-3 supplementation caused a significant decline *in vitro* in production of IL-1 and TNF by circulating mononuclear cells.

Nutritional Management of Infection

The general considerations of nutritional management are as follows:

- Emphasis should be placed on the continuation of feeding during mild or moderate episodes of common infections, including diarrhoea.
- Breast-feeding continues to be the most useful and cost-efficient dietary intervention to prevent infections diseases in small children.
- Early supplementary feeding during acute infection can have a significant, positive effect on the course of the disease.
- More important than the net energy deficit caused by one episode of illness, is the cumulative effect of repeated common illnesses that do not allow a full recovery of weight.
- The energy density of habitual diets should be assessed, to determine if they can sustain recovery growth after common illnesses. Enrichment or supplementation using locally available high-energy density staples should be considered when appropriate.
- Repletion of nutrients lost during the acute phase of infection requires high intake levels for extended periods of time. Thus, above-normal nutrient requirements may continue well after normalization of the clinical manifestations of infection. Patients with chronic infections and poor appetite may require supplemental feeding of high-energy formulae, either orally or by tube.

Macronutrient needs

Dietary intake during recovery must be sufficient to sustain rates of growth that may be several times higher than in healthy children of the same age (catch-up growth). Furthermore, in regions where infections are common, as many as 50% of children at certain age ranges can exhibit a reduced body size, known as 'stunting'. A reduced weight for height in childhood is associated with increased mortality and morbidity. When an important weight deficit exists, the rate of weight gain during catch-up growth can be as much as 20 times higher than rates in healthy children of similar age. In stunted children, the rate of weight gain is 2–4 times that of age-matched controls. During the time of recovery from illness, a clear inflection in the weight gain curve can be observed, caused by a significant decrease in weight gain velocity when a normal or almost normal ratio of weight to height is attained.

A major drive for weight gain in children with initial weight deficit appears to be dietary energy. Most studies found little correlation between dietary protein intake (at adequate ranges) and rate of weight gain, while there is a clear association between dietary energy intake and nitrogen accretion, measured by the traditional nitrogen balance method or by stable isotope-labelled amino acid turnover. However, very high energy intakes in the treatment of primary or secondary protein–energy malnutrition may produce a preferential accumulation of fat in newly gained tissue, relative to lean tissue.

The comparison between rates of growth of children receiving similar diets with or without infection may provide a measure of the contribution of infection to the total energy deficit. In the few studies exploring this aspect, surprisingly little difference was found between infected and noninfected children living in rural communities. Alternatively, estimates of nutrient needs for catch-up growth have been derived from the rehabilitation of severely malnourished children. Average values of 21 kJ (5 kcal) per gram of tissue have been proposed. For protein, the rate of new protein deposition is assumed to be 0.16 g per gram of tissue, which with a 70% efficiency yields a dietary requirement of 0.23 g per gram of weight gain. In most circumstances, the protein to energy ratio of catch-up diets will be higher than that of regular diets.

Catch-up of linear growth occurs at a much slower rate than recovery of body weight. The World Health Organization has recommended that estimation of energy and protein requirements of stunted children be made based on their age for height, rather on chronological age. Alternatively, the calculation may use the weight considered normal for the child's age. This approach, however, may provide substantial excess energy above actual energy expenditure, thus potentially leading to obesity. Consistent data from short-term studies on nutritional rehabilitation of children with different degrees of malnutrition show that the additional energy and protein estimated with these approaches can sustain rates of tissue accretion substantially higher than in normal children of similar age. Chil-

dren with secondary malnutrition living in more favourable environments can recover an adequate height in around 1 year of nutritional rehabilitation.

The Food and Agriculture Organization/World Health Organization/United Nations University, (FAO/WHO/UNU) Expert Committee of 1985 considered two possible approaches for the inclusion of catch-up nutritional needs into the overall recommendations for protein and energy intake. One approach would be to double the growth component of the protein-energy recommendations, which would entail the increases above 'normal' shown in **Table 1**. Given that the safe levels of protein intake of the 'normal' recommendations already allow for up to 70% growth rates above the average, it is likely that the usual recommendations for protein intake would provide sufficient amounts for catch-up growth for many children. More importantly, the table shows that the relative increase in protein–energy needs for recovery is higher at younger ages, which relates to the higher vulnerability of this age group to infection and protracted growth failure.

The other approach suggested by the FAO/WHO/UNU committee is based on long-term balance studies on protein requirements in young children. Using the actual balance data and adding an additional allocation for frequent infections, a figure of 1.69 g kg^{-1} of protein per day is derived, equivalent to 114% of the 'normal' recommendations.

The energy needs of adult patients are usually based on estimations of energy expenditure by the Harris–Benedict equation, with the addition of energy losses or increased requirements due to the primary disease. The metabolic effects of drugs should also be considered.

Micronutrient needs

A number of circulating micronutrients and their transport proteins respond to the early phase of infection by exhibiting dramatic changes in their blood concentration. Examples of significant decreases in circulating levels not related to deficiency are those of retinol and iron. Thus, values outside the normal range should be considered with caution, as they may not be indicative of deficiency. Even when there is a preexisting deficiency, administration of large vitamin or mineral doses should not be initiated immediately, since the ability to absorb and utilize these nutrients may be impaired in the acutely ill patient. An exception may be the infected child with severe protein–energy malnutrition and hypovitaminosis A. Such a child is always in imminent danger of irreversible ocular damage due to vitamin A deficiency (xerophthalmia), and should be

Table 1 Recommended nutritional intakes for catch-up growth

Age (years)	Daily weight gain (g kg^{-1})	Percentage increase above normal	
		Energy (%)	Protein (%)
0.5–0.75	1.83	14.5	50
0.75–1	1.15	8.5	45
1–1.5	0.67	5	32
1.5–2	0.51	3.5	25

From WHO Technical Report No. 724 (1984).

treated upon admission with 100 000 IU of retinol, either enterally or parenterally. The dose may be repeated the following day.

The role of vitamin A deficiency in vulnerability to infection was recognized early in the twentieth century. Vitamin A deficiency is associated with decreased T lymphocyte mitogen-induced proliferation, abnormal T cell population, impaired antibody production and decreased epithelial defence against bacterial adhesion. A clear epidemiological link between vitamin A deficiency and infection has emerged following a report of increased risk of diarrhoea and respiratory infections in Indonesian children with mild vitamin A deficiency. Routine administration of large doses of vitamin A in children diagnosed with measles is recommended in areas of the world where hypovitaminosis A is prevalent.

Ascorbate depletion in experimental animals is associated with depressed immune response, loss of integrity of epithelia, and impaired bactericidal capacity of neutrophils. Bacterial phagocytosis and lysis require a massive burst of reactive oxidants, which are highly cytotoxic also for the host. If these oxidants are not rapidly neutralized, they will inhibit chemotaxis, phagocytosis and other key antimicrobial activities. Thus, the likely biological role of ascorbate would be to protect granulocytes by neutralization of hypochlorous acid and other hydroperoxides generated during antibacterial processes. There is no consistent evidence that large doses of ascorbate in nondeficient individuals alter the course of common viral illnesses.

Zinc is a constituent of key enzymes of cell replication, DNA polymerase and RNA polymerase. Thus, its deficiency will greatly affect antimicrobial activities dependent on cellular replication and differentiation. Zinc deficiency is associated with lymphoid tissue atrophy, decreased delayed cutaneous hypersensitivity response, and impaired killer T cell activity. Children with acrodermatitis enteropathica, an inherited defect of zinc absorption, exhibit significantly higher rates of infection than normal controls. Zinc deficiency associated with protein–energy malnutrition appears to enhance the deleterious effects of macronutrient deficiencies on immune function. The impairment in immune response of zinc deficiency is readily reversed by supplementation.

Copper is a component of the superoxide dismutase and cytochrome c oxidase systems, enzymes involved in lymphocyte differentiation and antioxidant activity in granulocytes. Children with Menkes' syndrome, an inherited disorder of copper metabolism, exhibit an impaired T cell antibody response and altered phagocytic activity.

Iron is a component of cytochrome and myeloperoxidase enzymes, which are essential for the bactericidal activity of macrophages. Iron deficiency causes impaired responses both *in vitro* and *in vivo* to tests of immune competence. Bacterial survival was found to be longer in iron-deficient than in control human neutrophils. Although animal studies have shown that excess iron promotes the growth of microorganisms, there is no compelling clinical evidence that this is a common occurrence in adult humans receiving oral iron supplementation. In infants, however, early iron administration may be associated with decreased bactericidal activity, and it is recommended that iron therapy not be started immediately after birth, particularly in premature newborns. Iron supplementation in appropriate enteral doses poses no risk for older infants and children. Parenteral iron administration may be indicated in cases of severe impairment of gastrointestinal function or uncertain compliance.

See also: **Ascorbic Acid**: Physiology, Dietary Sources and Requirements. **Copper**: Physiology, Dietary Sources and Requirements. **Energy**: Energy Balance. **Immunity**: Physiological Aspects; Role of Iron and Zinc. **Iron**: Physiology, Dietary Sources and Requirements. **Malnutrition**: Definition, Classification and Epidemiology; Primary Malnutrition; Secondary Malnutrition. **Nutritional Support**: Enteral Feeding; Parenteral Nutrition; In the Home Setting. **Retinol**: Physiology. **Zinc**: Physiology.

Further Reading

Chandra RK (1990) Micronutrients and immune functions, an overview. *Annals of the NY Academy of Sciences* 587:9–16.

Coutsoudis A, Broughton M and Coovadia HM (1991) Vitamin A supplementation reduces measles morbidity in young African children: a randomized, placebo-controlled, double-blind trial. *American Journal of Clinical Nutrition* 54:890–895.

FAO/WHO (1985) *Energy and Protein Requirements.* Technical Report 724. Geneva: WHO.

Kauffman CA, Jones PG and Kluger MJ (1986) Fever and malnutrition: endogenous pyrogen/interleukin-1 in malnourished patients. *American Journal of Clinical Nutrition* 44:449–452.

Martorell R, Yarbrough C, Yarbrough S and Klein RE (1980) The impact of ordinary illnesses on the dietary intakes of malnourished children. *American Journal of Clinical Nutrition* 33:345–350.

Scrimshaw NS (1991) Effect of infection on nutrient requirements. *Journal of Parenteral and Enteral Nutrition* 15:589–600.

Nutritional Management of Measles and Human Immunodeficiency Virus Infection in Children

G Hussey and **B Eley**, University of Cape Town, South Africa

Copyright © 1998 Academic Press

In developing countries malnutrition and infectious diseases remain major public health problems. WHO estimates that approximately 12 million children die before the age of 5 years. Approximately 70% of these deaths are caused by measles, malaria, pneumonia, diarrhoea and malnutrition.

The synergistic effect of malnutrition and infection is well recognized. Protein–energy malnutrition increases susceptibility to infection and infection has a negative effect on nutritional status. More recently vitamin A has been identified as a key micronutrient influencing host susceptibility to infections, particularly in relation to measles, diarrhoea and acute respiratory tract (ARI) infections. The emergence of human immunodeficiency virus (HIV) infection, especially in the poor nations of Africa, is having a significant impact on child survival. Many of these children succumb as a consequence of the associated malnutrition and opportunistic infections, which are characteristic of HIV infection.

This article focuses on the interaction between vitamin A and infection and reviews the nutritional management of measles and HIV infection.

Synergism between Vitamin A and Infection

It is well known that vitamin A deficiency results in xerophthalmia, which is the leading cause of acquired childhood blindness in developing countries, affecting approximately 0.5 million children annually. Probably of greater significance are the research findings in the last decade that indicate vitamin A to be essential for child health and survival. Subclinical vitamin A deficiency is now known to be associated with reduced immune competence, an increase in the incidence and severity of infections, poor growth, iron deficiency anaemia and excess childhood mortality. Improvement of vitamin A status in children results in the enhancement of growth and iron status, a decrease in infectious morbidity and, most strikingly, a reduction in overall childhood mortality in community studies by the order of 30%.

Vitamin A and infection

The association between xerophthalmia (and, therefore, by implication vitamin A) and infection has been noted for over 100 years. Clinicians observed that common childhood infections frequently precipitated xerophthalmia and that children who presented with the latter frequently developed severe and often fatal infections. In 1928 Green and Mellanby proposed that vitamin A be regarded as an anti-infective agent. Scrimshaw in his review in 1964 stated:

> no nutritional deficiency is more synergistic with infectious diseases than that of vitamin A. One of the first recognized features of hypovitaminosis A, increased susceptibility to infection, has had strong confirmation.

In the last decade there has been a resurgence of research interest in vitamin A and infection, particularly with regards to measles, HIV infection and respiratory and gastrointestinal infections.

Measles

Measles induces a transient hyporetinaemia (biochemical vitamin A deficiency) and frequently precipitates xerophthalmia, especially in situations where pre-existing retinol stores are marginal, as is the case in malnourished children. Low vitamin A levels are associated with increased disease severity and mortality, even in situations where clinical vitamin A deficiency is not a problem, such as in the USA. A number of hospital-based studies have shown that high-dose vitamin A therapy had a significant impact in reducing mortality (**Fig. 1**). A meta-analysis of three studies showed a 55% reduction in measles deaths. Large community-based intervention trials evaluating the effect of vitamin A prophylaxis on overall childhood mortality have also shown a reduction in measles-specific mortality, with an effect similar to that of the hospital-based studies.

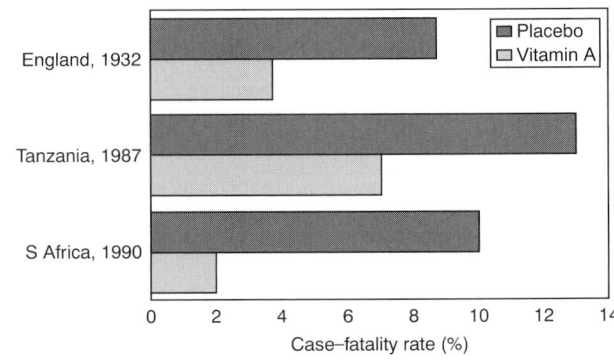

Figure 1 High-dose vitamin A therapy in children hospitalized with measles: randomized placebo-controlled trials.

Studies from South Africa have shown that vitamin A therapy also reduces the rate of complications, particularly related to respiratory and gastrointestinal infections, hospital stay and the need for intensive care.

HIV/AIDS

Over the last few years evidence of a significant association between vitamin A and HIV infection has emerged. Observational and case–control studies have reported significant vitamin A deficiency in HIV-positive adults and children in developed and developing countries. In addition, recent studies from Africa and the USA have suggested that vitamin A deficiency in pregnant HIV-infected women contributes to mother-to-infant transmission of HIV infection. In adults lower retinol levels have been associated with lower CD4+ cell counts and increased mortality risk. Vitamin A supplementation of children has been shown to be associated with significant short-term improvement of immune function and reduced morbidity, particularly in relation to diarrhoeal disease.

Acute respiratory infections and diarrhoeal disease

Vitamin A deficiency is associated with an increased risk for ARI and diarrhoea. In addition, studies have indicated that the mortality rates in vitamin A-deficient children were 3- to 5-fold greater than in vitamin A-sufficient children. Community-based intervention studies have shown vitamin A supplementation to be associated with a 39% reduction in diarrhoeal deaths but no significant impact was noted with deaths due to pneumonia. The morbidity trials assessing impact of vitamin A prophylaxis on diarrhoea and ARI, however, gave conflicting results. One study reported increased incidence of mild ARI and diarrhoea in treated children. Other studies have shown that vitamin A supplementation impacted significantly on reducing severity of disease.

Mechanism for vitamin A deficiency

Retinol homeostasis, particularly during infections, is a complex phenomenon that is not entirely understood. The reason for low retinol levels in acute infections is unclear. The low levels may be related to anorexia, increased utilization of marginal liver stores, increased urinary excretion, impairment of retinol release from the liver as a consequence of decreased synthesis and mobilization of retinol-binding protein, or redistribution of retinol into the extracellular compartment during the acute illness. Reduced liver stores have also been reported to follow infections.

Vitamin A and immunity

The precise mechanisms by which vitamin A exerts its effects are not fully understood. Vitamin A is important in maintaining the integrity of epithelial surfaces and immune function. Experimental studies indicate that vitamin A deficiency results in decreased cellular turnover, stratification of epithelial cells and ultimately squamous metaplasia, keratinization and desquamation of cells. The net effect of these changes is loss of the first line host defence barriers, predisposing the host to infections. Vitamin A-induced immune abnormalities include atrophy of the thymus and spleen, reduced lymphocyte counts and lymphocyte mitogenic responses, and impairment of macrophage function. Antibody affinity, production and responses are also impaired. Vitamin A supplementation in experimental animals has been associated with restoration of the normal epithelium and enhancement of cell-mediated cytotoxicity, natural killer cell activity, macrophage function and antibody production.

Vitamin A-deficient children have been found to have low CD4+ and increased CD8+ levels and a lower CD4 : CD8 ratio when compared with normal children. In addition, vitamin A-deficient children have lower IgG responses to tetanus toxoid than children given vitamin A supplements. High-dose vitamin A supplementation reversed these abnormalities. In measles and HIV infection vitamin A results in enhancement of T cell-dependent antibody production.

Conclusion

Vitamin A deficiency is the micronutrient deficiency that is most commonly associated with infections, immune dysfunction and increased mortality in children. In addition, it is associated with poor growth and defective vision. Improvement of vitamin A status in children results in the enhancement of growth and haematopoesis, a decrease in infectious morbidity, an improvement in immune function and a reduction in childhood mortality.

It is estimated that over 100 million children, predominantly in developing countries, are affected. Strategies to reduce the burden of disease have been identified. These include vitamin A supplementation, food fortification and dietary diversification. Ultimately the control and eventual elimination of vitamin A deficiency will be dependent upon improving the socioeconomic conditions of the affected populations.

Nutritional Management of Measles

Measles remains a leading cause of childhood morbidity and mortality worldwide. The World Health Organization estimates that globally over 40 million cases and one million deaths occur annually, the majority in developing countries. Most of these deaths follow complications such as pneumonia, croup and diarrhoea, and are frequently associated with malnutrition. Recovery following acute measles may be delayed for many weeks and even months and is characterized by failure to thrive and recurrent infections. The survival rate of children during this phase is also significantly reduced.

Effect of measles on nutrition

Measles is recognized as a significant cause of childhood malnutrition. The nutritional status of a child with measles can be adversely affected through a number of mechanisms which include:

- the catabolic effects of the infection;
- associated diarrhoea and vomiting;
- protein-losing enteropathy;
- refusal to take food because of mouth ulcers or poor appetite.

Energy balance studies in children with measles have highlighted significantly increased faecal and urine losses and reduced intake. Serious weight loss is thus the invariable consequence of negative energy balance (estimated to be as much as 184 kJ (773 kcal) per kg per 24 h). The shortfall is compensated by tissue catabolism.

Most children suffer from some degree of acute diarrhoea. Severe symptoms develop in a variable number of children and is responsible for about 20% of measles-related deaths. Prolonged diarrhoea, which has a major impact on nutritional status and subsequent mortality, may follow the acute episode in about 30% of cases.

Diarrhoea in measles is a consequence of a number of interrelated factors. The measles virus causes epithelial damage, which is compounded by the hyporetinaemia that invariably occurs in the acute phase. In addition, both measles and vitamin A deficiency reduce immune competence, resulting in increased susceptibility to gastrointestinal pathogens. The net effect of the gastrointestinal damage is diarrhoeal disease and protein-losing enteropathy. The mean absolute albumin loss in children with postmeasles diarrhoea may be as much as 1 g daily. Measles is thus a common precipitating cause of kwashiorkor.

Herpetic gingivostomatitis is a common complication of measles. Additional secondary bacterial infections may develop, especially if oral hygiene is poor. This may cause difficulty with feeding that may result in dehydration and aggravate malnutrition.

Effect of malnutrition on measles

Data derived mainly from hospital surveys show that children who are significantly malnourished have a higher morbidity and mortality rate (**Table 1**). However, this does not necessarily imply a causal relationship. As mentioned above, measles is an acute catabolic event associated with reduced dietary intake, increased gastrointestinal losses and rapid weight loss. Lower weight may therefore be a reflection of more severe disease.

Management

Children with measles frequently present with a number of interrelated complications, the major ones being pneumonia, diarrhoea, croup and mouth ulcers. All of these may impact negatively on the nutritional status of children. It is thus essential that a comprehensive approach be adopted to the management of measles. One of the reasons for the high mortality associated with measles is delay in instituting effective treatment or providing inappropriate care. Reducing the case–fatality rate from measles through effective case management has been identified as an important strategy by the Expanded Programme on Immunization of the World Health Organization. A policy document on integrated measles case management has thus been developed to assist health workers, particularly in developing countries, in their efforts to reduce measles severity. The basic principles are outlined in **Table 2**.

There is no specific drug therapy for measles except for vitamin A (discussed in previous section). Give 200 000 IU vitamin A (either in liquid or capsule form) at the time of diagnosis and repeat the dose 24 h later. In children aged less than 12 months

Table 1 Association between nutritional status and rate of complications (%)

Regional morbidity and mortality	Percentage of expected weight			
	All	>80%	60–80%	<60%
Morbidity in Jakarta				
Pneumonia	74.9	61.9	84.6	100
Diarrhoea	18.6	13.7	19.9	39.2
Convulsions	7.5	8.2	7.7	2.2
Otitis media	5.9	6.7	5.9	2.2
Mortality				
Jakarta	10.3	5.9	12.7	23.1
Tanzania	8.0	3.6	7.3	24.5
Kenya	1.8	0.8	1.4	4

Table 2 Basic principles of measles case management

- Anticipate complications in high-risk groups
- Admit severely ill children to hospital
- Give paracetamol if the temperature exceeds 39°C
- Treat with high-dose vitamin A
- Encourage breast-feeding
- Provide nutritional support to all children
- Act quickly to treat eye lesions to prevent blindness
- Use antibiotics only when there are clear indications
- Give oral rehydration solution for diarrhoea
- Treat multiple complications such as pneumonia, dehydration and croup at the same time
- Advise regular follow-up for growth monitoring

give half the dose. Children who have clinical evidence of xerophthalmia should receive an additional dose 4–6 weeks later.

Since measles virus infection is a major catabolic event and is associated with significant weight loss, careful attention must be paid to the nutritional needs of children with measles. Encourage the mother to continue breast-feeding an infant. If the child is not breast-fed, then continue feeding even if diarrhoea is present. Increase the energy content of the food by adding a teaspoon of vegetable oil and a teaspoon of sugar to the milk or cereal. Provide additional vitamins and minerals such as multivitamin syrup. If the child refuses to take feeds, then pass a nasogastric tube and give liquid feeds and fluids through the tube.

Give the child more fluids than usual to prevent dehydration. If dehydration is present, then additional fluids should be provided in the form of oral or intravenous rehydration solution. Antimicrobial therapy is recommended if significant pathogens such as shigella are isolated from the stools.

Nutrition education of the mother or carer is important. In many cultures there is the mistaken custom to stop feeding or to reduce feeds in children with measles. The importance of maintaining adequate feeding during the acute and convalescent stage must be stressed. Failure to thrive and recurrent infections are common in the months following measles. The reason for this phenomenon is not fully understood, but is probably related to the combined effects of immune suppression and vitamin A deficiency. It is therefore essential that children are closely monitored and regular clinic attendance is recommended for at least 6 months following recovery from acute measles.

Conclusion

The goal of integrated measles case management is to reduce the morbidity and mortality rate. An important component of care is the provision of optimal nutrition, treatment of complications that may compromise nutritional status, and the provision of vitamin A therapy. The mechanism of action of vitamin A is unclear. However, its effects are probably mediated via improvement in immune function and restoration of epithelial integrity.

It should not, however, be forgotten that measles is a disease that is preventable by immunization and that ultimately the control of measles is dependent upon obtaining and maintaining a measles vaccine coverage that is in excess of 90%.

Nutritional Management of HIV-infected Children

Infection caused by the human immunodeficiency virus (HIV) is a major public health problem. It has been estimated that more than 1 million children have already been infected worldwide; over 80% of these reside in sub-Saharan Africa. Growth failure is a frequent concomitant of HIV infection and is associated with a significantly shorter survival time. A study of HIV-infected children showed that at diagnosis (median age of 6 months) 64% were below 80% expected weight-for-age, and 18.5% were below 60% expected weight-for-age (NCHS growth curves). Postnatal growth failure manifests early in the course of infection and is sustained throughout childhood (**Table 3**).

Several mechanisms are responsible for abnormal growth and malnutrition in HIV infection. These include decreased dietary intake caused by oropharyngeal and oesophageal disease, anorexia, and neuropsychiatric complications; malabsorption, primarily associated with gastrointestinal infections and HIV enteropathy; hypermetabolism; and altered metabolism. Pro-inflammatory mediators including

Table 3 Growth and nutritional changes in HIV infection

- Mean birthweight is lower in infants of seropositive than seronegative mothers
- Growth parameters at birth are similar for infected and uninfected infants born to seropositive mothers
- Mean birthweight is lower in infants born to mothers with AIDS than to seropositive mothers without AIDS
- Postnatal growth is significantly impaired from as early as 3 months of age
- Postnatal growth is compromised throughout childhood
- Preferential muscle wasting over fat wasting occurs
- Somatic and visceral protein depletion
- Essential amino acid depletion
- Multiple micronutrient deficiencies: trace elements, vitamins, electrolytes

cytokines, and endocrine abnormalities have been implicated in these metabolic derangements.

Malnutrition adversely affects immunity and predisposes to opportunistic infections. In protein–energy malnutrition most host defences are breached, particularly cell-mediated immunity. Observed immunological changes resemble those documented in HIV infection. Deficiencies of many micronutrients have been described in HIV-infected patients, including deficiencies of those nutrients that are essential for normal immune function. Furthermore, the concentrations of certain micronutrients correlates with the function of some immune components in HIV-infected patients. Thus well-nourished patients may have a better chance of remaining relatively asymptomatic with a lower tendency to develop opportunistic infections.

Aspects of the nutritional management of HIV-infected children are discussed below.

Prevention of HIV infection

HIV infection can be transmitted postnatally from breast-milk to the developing infant. An analysis of five studies showed that for mothers infected antenatally, the additional risk of transmission from breast-feeding is 14%. Although the accuracy of this meta-analysis has been questioned, a similar estimate has been obtained in a cohort study based on serial polymerase chain reaction testing. Furthermore, it has been shown that the risk of breast-feeding transmission in mothers who become infected with HIV-1 postnatally is 26%. Any strategy to reduce postnatal transmission should form part of a comprehensive prevention campaign targeting all expectant women. HIV-seropositive women should be informed about available methods to reduce vertical transmission. In particular, they should be encouraged to formula-feed their offspring. Seronegative expectant women should be counselled about primary prevention, particularly during pregnancy and breast-feeding.

Treatment of HIV infection

Although specific therapy against HIV is limited, antiretrovirals are able to alter the natural history of paediatric infection. In particular, zidovudine causes appreciable weight gain in HIV-infected children. Current evidence indicate that combination therapy may be superior to single drug administration. Early identification and vigorous treatment of opportunistic infections prevent deterioration of nutritional status. Patients with untreated cytomegaloviral (CMV) infection lose weight, total body protein and fat, and experience progressive decline in serum albumin concentration. In contrast, patients treated with ganciclovir gain weight, replete body cell mass and

body fat, and increase serum albumin concentration. Furthermore, wasting illnesses such as CMV and *Mycobacterium avium-intracellulare* infections cause depletion of body cell mass, which is directly related to the length of survival of patients with AIDS. Although HIV-associated diarrhoea frequently fails to respond to therapy, investigation is necessary to identify those patients with treatable conditions.

Nutritional support

Regular growth monitoring should include a history of feeding problems, gastrointestinal symptoms and intercurrent infections; serial recording of growth parameters; examination for signs of overt malnutrition; and frequent monitoring of haemoglobin and other red blood cell indices to detect anaemia. Children with evidence of growth failure should, in addition, be screened for gastrointestinal infections, malabsorption and micronutrient deficiencies, and have a detailed dietary assessment (**Table 4**).

Table 4 Nutritional assessment of HIV-infected children

Medical history

- Feeding problems: length of each feed; frequency of feeding; coughing, choking and vomiting during feeds
- Attainment of age-appropriate feeding skills
- Gastrointestinal symptoms: nausea, vomiting, diarrhoea, abdominal pain
- Dietary recall: dietary history or 24 h intake recall
- Other: fever, intercurrent infections

Anthropometry

- Serial weight, length or height, head circumference
- Serial arm data: arm circumference, triceps skinfold; calculated muscle arm area and fat arm area
  (These measurements provide information about body composition)

Medical examination

- Features of protein–energy malnutrition and specific micronutrient deficiencies

Laboratory investigations

- Visceral protein: serum albumin, prealbumin, retinol-binding protein, total protein concentrations
- Anaemia: red blood indices; folate, vitamin B_{12} and iron studies
- Micronutrient deficiency: calcium, magnesium; vitamin A, zinc, selenium, other
- Stool microbiology
- Malabsorption: stool pH, reducing substances, faecal fat quantitation
- Gastroduodenoscopy, sigmoidoscopy intestinal biopsies and cultures

Nutritional recommendations for HIV-infected children are largely based on theoretical considerations. Age-related macro- and micronutrient requirements have not been optimized. Recommended daily allowances (RDAs) applicable to normal children are used as guidelines, but those who fail to thrive require additional nutrition for catch up growth. This may be calculated according to the formula: (RDA for age × ideal weight for height)/(actual weight). Additional calories may be provided by glucose polymer, medium-chain triglyceride or vegetable oil preparations. The energy density of food may also be improved with liberal portions of butter or margarine, cheeses, peanut butter and other foodstuffs. A recent study cautioned against widespread use of dietary fish oil as it was associated with a trend towards decline in CD4+ cell numbers. Daily vitamin and trace element supplements are recommended, provided that the dosages do not exceed RDAs. Dietary modifications may be considered in special situations such as lactose-free diets for lactose intolerance, and enteral or parenteral alimentation for patients who fail to thrive despite adequate oral feeds. Enteral alimentation in HIV-infected children causes weight and arm fat area gains, but not height or arm muscle area changes. Intravenous alimentation may be considered, should enteral alimentation prove ineffective. Adult AIDS patients gain weight, body fat and body cell mass in response to parenteral nutrition. Studies have indicated that the risk of infection from central venous catheters is not significantly increased in HIV infection, however practical constraints may prevent widespread use of parenteral nutrition.

Pharmaceutical preparations

Various therapies to improve nutritional status and prevent wasting are being evaluated. Megestrol acetate, a synthetic derivative of progesterone, is able to increase weight by stimulating appetite and increasing calorie intake. Weight gain is primarily due to increased body fat content. The results of a pilot study of seven children with HIV infection showed that significant weight gain occurred in all patients over the first month of therapy and sustained weight gain occurred in five and three patients over 3 and 5 months, respectively. Although therapy appears to improve general wellbeing, it does not prolong survival in adults. Results of clinical trials in children are awaited with interest.

Other drugs that are being considered include dronabinol (Δ^9-tetrahydrocannabinol), the psychoactive substance of marijuana, pentoxyfilline, an inhibitor of tumour necrosis factor production; cyproheptidine, an antihistamine with appetite-stimulant properties; and glucocorticoids. Although short-term therapy with growth hormone (GH) appeared promising, a recent placebo-controlled trial which evaluated the combination of GH and insulin-like growth factor 1 showed that initial improvements are transient and a result of water weight gain.

Nutritional management in developing countries

In developing countries, where the majority of HIV-infected children reside, the burden of malnutrition among infected children is often greater and more severe than in the general paediatric population. A study conducted in Zimbabwe recently showed that of 219 HIV-infected children, 52% were below 80% expected weight for age and 26% were below 60% expected weight for age. In contrast, of 485 uninfected children assessed, 21% were below 80% expected weight for age and 6% below 60% expected weight for age. As antiretrovirals and drugs required to control opportunistic infections are not widely available, the majority of infected children are not treated optimally.

Universal breast-feeding is advocated in most developing countries as it is associated with reduced paediatric morbidity and mortality. Government expenditure needed to implement formula-feeding schemes for all infants of HIV seropositive mothers is prohibitive. Cost considerations include subsidy of formula milk, development of laboratory services to undertake comprehensive HIV antibody testing, provision of test kits, education to promote the service, and counselling facilities. Furthermore, domestic expenditure is appreciable. The cost of formula-feeding a 3-month-old infant with 800 ml per day of formula milk ranges from 27% (Zimbabwe) to 900% (Uganda) of the daily wage of a hospital cleaner. Thus breast-feeding policies are unlikely to change.

Growth assessments are frequently limited to plotting weight for age measurements on longitudinal growth charts and performing a rapid clinical examination. Furthermore, dietary supplements, such as medium-chain triglycerides, and enteral and parenteral feeding are not widely used as they are extremely expensive. Therefore supplements are often limited to multivitamin preparations. The challenge for researchers in these disadvantaged settings is to identify effective, low-cost nutritional supplements that can be administered at community or village level. A study from Zimbabwe indicated that regular use of a commercial substitute that provided protein, energy and micronutrient supplements resulted in appreciable weight gain in HIV-infected children. Furthermore, a study from South Africa showed that vitamin A supplementation resulted in significant short-term increases in total lymphocyte, CD4+ and natural killer cell counts. Whether these and other relatively inexpensive measures are able to produce sustained benefits such as improved quality of life and reduced infectious complications remains to be established in well-designed clinical trials.

See also: **Diarrhoeal (Diarrheal) Diseases**: Nutritional Factors. **HIV Disease**: Nutritional Management. **Immunity**: Physiological Aspects; Role of Iron and Zinc. **Malnutrition**: Definition, Classification and Epidemiology. **Pregnancy**: Nutrient Requirements. **Retinol**: Physiology.

Further Reading

Baum MK, Shor-Posner G, Bonvehi P, Cassetti I, Lu Y, Mankro-Atienza E, Beach RS, Sauberlich HE (1992) Influence of HIV infections on vitamin status and requirements. *Annals of the New York Academy of Science* 669:165–174.

Beaton GH, Martorell R, L'Abbe K, Edmonston B, McCabe G, Ross AC, Harvey B (1992) *Effectiveness of vitamin A supplementation in the control of young child morbidity and mortality in developing counties.* Final report to CIDA, University of Toronto, Canada.

Chandra RK (1991) 1990 McCollum award lecture. Nutrition and immunity: Lessons from the past and new insights into the future. *American Journal of Clinical Nutrition* 53:1087–1101.

Choto RG (1994) Clinical evaluation of nutrition mix – I.A. dietary supplement in sick and undernourished children. *Central African Journal of Medicine* 40:29–32.

Coutsoudis A, Bobat RA, Coovadia HM, Kuhn L, Tsai WY and Stein ZA (1995) The effects of vitamin A supplementation on morbidity of children born to HIV-infected women. *American Journal of Public Health* 85:1076–1081.

Cutting WAM (1994) Breast-feeding and HIV – a balance of risks. *Journal of Tropical Pediatrics* 40:6–11.

Glasziou PP and Mackerras DEM (1993) Vitamin A supplentation in infectious diseases: a meta-analysis. *British Medical Journal* 306:366–370.

Gorbach SL, Knox TA and Roubenoff R (1993) Interactions between nutrition and infection with human immunodeficiency virus. *Nutrition Review* 51:226–234.

Hussey GD and Klein M (1990) A randomized, controlled trial of vitamin A in children with severe measles. *New England Journal of Medicine* 323:160–164.

Hussey G and Klein M (1992) Measles induced vitamin A deficiency. *Annals of the New York Academy of Science* 669:188–196.

McKinney RE, Robertson JW and Duke Pediatric AIDS Clinical Trials Unit (1993) Effect of human immunodeficiency virus infection on the growth of young children. *Journal of Pediatrics* 123:579–582.

Morley D (1969) Severe measles in the tropics–1. *British Medical Journal* 1:297–300.

Nicolas SW, Leung J and Fennoy I (1991) Guidelines for nutritional support of HIV-infected children. *Journal of Pediatrics* 119:S59–S61.

Reddy V (1987) Interaction between nutrition and measles. *Indian Journal of Pediatrics* 54:53–57.

Semba RD, Miotti PG, Chiphangwi JD, Saah AJ, Canner JK, Dallabetta GA, Hoover DR (1994) Maternal vitamin A deficiency and mother-to-child transmission of HIV-1. *Lancet* 343:1593–1597.

Sommer A (1990) Vitamin A status, resistance to infection, and childhood mortality. *Annals of the New York Academy of Science* 587:17–23.

Timbo BB and Tollefson L (1994) Nutrition: A cofactor in HIV disease. *Journal of the American Dietetics Association* 94:1018–1022.

Tomkins A and Hussey G (1989) Vitamin A, immunity and infection. *Nutrition Research Reviews* 2:17–28.

INSULIN RESISTANCE

Aetiology and Association with Disease

J Mann, University of Otago, Dunedin, New Zealand

Copyright © 1998 Academic Press

There is considerable variation amongst individuals within a population with regard to sensitivity to the action of insulin. Both genetic and environmental factors determine the phenomenon of insulin resistance and its clinical consequences. The constellation of metabolic and clinical consequences and insulin resistance play an important role in the aetiology of coronary heart disease, especially in genetically predisposed populations and families.

Definitions

The term 'insulin resistance', a concept first introduced by Himsworth in the 1930s, tends now to be used to describe a wide range of metabolic and clinical situations. On the one hand there is a group of relatively uncommon syndromes, quite distinct from each other, in which extreme insulin resistance is the underlying abnormality. These include the classical type A and type B syndromes characterized by amenorrhoea due to ovarian androgen overproduction, and acanthosis nigricans, respectively; and congenital lipodystrophy, in which body fat distribution is markedly abnormal from a very early age. Leprechaunism in infants (associated with growth retardation, specific physical characteristics and early death) and pseudoacromegaly (associated with gross obesity) are also associated with marked insulin resistance. On the other hand, there is mounting evidence that within the population at large there is wide variation among individuals in their sensitivity to the effects of insulin. Resistance to the effects of insulin may lead to a spectrum of metabolic and clinical responses (**Table 1**). The severity of each of these features may vary. This constellation of biochemical variables and clinical characteristics has been described by several names including 'insulin resistance syndrome' (IRS), 'Reaven's syndrome' (after the person who first described it) and 'syndrome X' (by Reaven himself), though Reaven has always emphasized that obesity is not an essential aspect of the syndrome. None of these names is entirely satisfactory. In cardiological parlance the term 'syndrome X' has been used to describe the clinical condition of microvascular angina; cardiological and endocrinological syndromes with the same name lead to confusion. In the opinion of this author, IRS is the most appropriate term to describe

Table 1 Features of the insulin resistance syndrome

More consistent features
  Hyperinsulinaemia
  Hyperglycaemia, glucose intolerance, non-insulin-dependent diabetes mellitus
  Dyslipidaemia, including hypertriglyceridaemia and low levels of HDL
  Hypertension

Less consistent features
  Obesity
  Hyperuricaemia
  Change in LDL composition
  Increased magnitude of postprandial lipaemia
  Increased levels of PAI-1

HDL, high-density lipoprotein; LDL, low-density lipoprotein; PAI-1, plasminogen activator inhibitor 1.

the collection of abnormalities listed in Table 1, though of course the existence of the rare syndromes of extreme insulin resistance must be acknowledged. Future research may suggest a more appropriate classification.

Diagnosis

For research purposes the most appropriate method for measuring insulin sensitivity is the euglycaemic hyperinsulinaemic clamp technique. In this procedure the plasma insulin concentration is acutely raised and maintained at approximately 718 pmol l^{-1} (100 mU l^{-1}) by a continuous infusion of insulin. The plasma glucose concentration is held constant at basal levels by a variable glucose infusion using the negative feedback principle. Under these steady state conditions of euglycaemia, the glucose infusion rate equals glucose uptake by all the tissues in the body and is therefore a measure of tissue sensitivity to exogenous insulin. The index of sensitivity of peripheral insulin is calculated by dividing the amount of glucose taken up by the mean insulin concentration attained during the last 60 min of the clamp. This technique is too complex for use in large-scale clinical studies and epidemiological investigations. As hyperinsulinaemia is the almost inevitable consequence of insulin resistance (see below), fasting or postglucose load insulin levels are used in epidemiological studies to provide a continous variable which serves as a measure of insulin resistance. For clinical purposes, plasma insulin levels greater than 2 standard deviations above the mean for a control population are used to identify hyperinsulinaemia and, by implication, insulin-resistant individuals. A major limitation of using plasma insulin levels lies in the fact that after a prolonged period of hyperinsulinaemia insulin levels will fall as decompensation occurs. The presence of the clinical and metabolic features listed in Table 1 identifies individuals as having the insulin resistance syndrome.

Aetiology

Under normal circumstances insulin is released from the β cells of the pancreas, enters the circulation and is responsible for the initiation of a range of biochemical events following recognition by membrane receptors. Some of these events occur in all tissues, others are specific to certain groups of cells. Rapid changes in the rates of membrane transport of molecules such as glucose and ions, activation and inactivation of various enzyme systems and changes in the level of gene expression are some of the most important consequences of insulin action. Insulin resistance primarily affects muscle and involves both the oxidative and nonoxidative pathways of glucose disposal. In the syndromes of extreme insulin resistance, the primary abnormality is at the level of the target cell for insulin action. Antireceptor antibodies and mutations of the insulin receptor gene play a major role in the causation of these disorders, but the cause of severe target cell resistance in patients without defects in the receptor locus is still unknown.

The IRS is of greater interest to nutritionists. The coexistence of several metabolic and clinical abnormalities have made it difficult to establish which is cause and which is effect. The fact that in at least two groups – Pima Indians and a Joslin Clinic cohort – insulin resistance has been identified before any abnormality of glucose levels, strongly suggests that insulin resistance leading to hyperinsulinaemia is the initial abnormality. There are many plausible candidate genes for inherited insulin resistance in non-insulin-dependent diabetes mellitus (NIDDM) and other variations of the IRS including genes determining the insulin receptor, the insulin-responsive glucose transporter Glut 4, glucokinase, hexokinase, signalling intermediates in insulin action, enzymes mediating or regulating the pathways of glucose storage and oxidation, and potential regulators of insulin receptor function such as tyrosine phosphatases.

While predisposition to insulin resistance may be determined by one or more genes, life-style factors play an important role in determining whether or not the genetic predisposition will result in metabolic or clinical consequences. Centrally distributed obesity, itself a product of genetic and environmental interaction, has long been known to be a major determinant of decreasing insulin-mediated glucose uptake, whereas weight loss in obese individuals can produce enhanced insulin action. Insulin sensitivity can also be profoundly influenced by exercise training. The results of a study carried out in 55 Pima Indian men and 35 white men with normal glucose tolerance illustrate the effects of obesity and physical activity. *In vivo* insulin action was measured using the hyperinsulinaemic, euglycaemic clamp technique. Body composition was determined by densitometry, and maximal aerobic capacity estimated using a graded exercise test. In both groups there was a significant decline in insulin action with increasing obesity up to a body fat content of 28–30%. The relationship was nonlinear, with further increases in obesity in the Pima Indian group not being associated with significant changes in insulin action. Maximal aerobic capacity was positively linearly correlated with insulin action over the entire range of insulin action in both racial groups. Degree of obesity and maximal aerobic capacity were each independently associated with insulin action and accounted for about half the variability observed in insulin action in the group as a whole. Another study from the same research group carried out in nonobese subjects and using similar methods for expressing insulin sensitivity and physical training states found a strong and highly significant correlation ($r = 0.63$) between these variables. In these nonobese people Vo_2 max as a single measure of physical training accounted for over 40% of the variance in insulin-stimulated glucose utilization.

Individual dietary factors contribute to obesity in varying degrees. If it is accepted that a high fat intake is an important factor in the aetiology of obesity, it is by implication a risk factor for insulin resistance. Peripheral insulin sensitivity may also be influenced by the nature of dietary fat. Saturated fatty acids, and palmitic acid in particular, are associated with increased insulin resistance whereas linoleic acid and n-3 polyunsaturated fatty acids tend to be associated with increased insulin sensitivity. In a population-based study in elderly men, more than 50% of the variation in insulin sensitivity was explained by an equation including body mass index, serum triacylglycerol concentration, and palmitic acid content of skeletal muscle phospholipid. Physical training was not assessed in this study, but it seems reasonable to conclude that quantity and nature of dietary fat and physical inactivity are profoundly important determinants of insulin resistance.

Disease Implications of Insulin Resistance

The metabolic and some clinical consequences of insulin resistance have already been listed. This section considers the mechanism by which insulin resistance may produce those metabolic consequences and the relationship between insulin resistance, NIDDM and coronary heart disease (CHD).

Insulin resistance and compensatory hyperinsulinaemia

The inevitable consequence of insulin resistance is compensatory hyperinsulinaemia, because the pancreatic β cells attempt to secrete whatever amount of insulin may be required to achieve plasma glucose levels of about 5–7 mmol l^{-1}. The more resistant an individual is to insulin-mediated glucose disposal, the greater will be the degree of hyperinsulinaemia. Plasma glucose will remain normal until the β cells can no longer sustain the extent of hyperinsulinaemia to overcome the deficit in insulin action.

Non-insulin-dependent diabetes mellitus

Insulin resistance primarily affects muscle. Hyperglycaemia, glucose intolerance or frank NIDDM only occurs when muscle resistance to insulin-mediated glucose uptake can no longer be matched by the insulin secretion required to overcome this resistance. At the stage at which the β cell starts to fail, insulin secretion first returns to normal or below normal levels. The fall in insulin secretion will also result in an increase in plasma free fatty acids (FFA) which in turn stimulate FFA oxidation, gluconeogenesis and hepatic glucose production. Thus hyperglycaemia is further increased and β cell secreting function further compromised. Whether or not an individual with insulin resistance will go on to develop glucose intolerance or NIDDM again depends upon a combination of genetic and environmental factors.

Hypertension

About half of all hypertensive patients are hyperinsulinaemic when compared with a control population, but this does not prove a cause and effect relationship between insulin resistance and hypertension. However, there are a number of possible mechanisms by which elevated plasma insulin may lead to hypertension. Hyperinsulinaemia can enhance renal retention of sodium and stimulate sympathetic nervous system activity. In addition, there are enhanced fluxes of sodium and calcium into vascular smooth muscle cells, leading to an increased vascular sensitivity to the vasoconstrictor effect of pressor amines. Finally, insulin acting directly or indirectly through the stimulation of insulin-like growth factors (e.g. IGF-I) may also contribute to the development of hypertension by causing hypertrophy of the vascular wall and narrowing of the lumen of the resistance vessels in the regulation of systemic blood pressure.

Dyslipidaemia

The dyslipidaemia of insulin resistance is characterized by an increase in levels of very low-density lipoprotein (VLDL) and consequently of tri-acylglycerol, its principal lipid component; a reduction in high-density lipoprotein (HDL); and an increased proportion of small, dense low-density lipoprotein (LDL) particles. Plasma concentration of VLDL is determined by synthesis in the liver and removal by peripheral tissue. Both processes are regulated by insulin. With hyperinsulinaemia, hepatic VLDL synthesis is increased, and the ensuing hypertriglyceridaemia associated with raised levels of VLDL is enhanced by resistance of lipoprotein lipase (responsible for triacylglycerol clearance from the plasma) to the action of insulin. Higher fasting levels of triacylglycerol are associated with increased postprandial lipaemia, so that in insulin-resistant individuals triacylglycerol levels tend to be higher throughout the day. The close association between plasma insulin and tri-acylglycerol levels has been demonstrated in people with NIDDM and in healthy subjects of normal weight. Concentrations of HDL are inversely associated with triacylglycerol and insulin levels. The mechanism by which insulin might regulate HDL levels, is not clear but in the presence of hyperinsulinaemia the fractional catabolic rate of apoprotein A-I (the major protein component of HDL) is increased, leading to a fall in plasma HDL levels. Increased cholesteryl ester transfer protein activity may also be responsible by promoting the movement of cholesteryl ester from HDL to VLDL. The association between insulin resistance and the diameter of the LDL particle is a more recent observation. Particles of LDL usually have a diameter greater than 255 Å (subclass pattern A). Individuals with a predominance of particles of subclass pattern B (diameter less than 255 Å) tend to have higher triacylglycerol and lower HDL concentrations, and are relatively insulin resistant.

Hyperuricaemia

The association between raised levels of uric acid and glucose intolerance, hypertriglyceridaemia and hypertension has been known to clinicians for many years. In normal volunteers, a significant correlation has been demonstrated between insulin resistance and plasma insulin response to an oral glucose load, and serum uric acid as well as urinary clearance of uric acid. This suggests that the link between hyperuricaemia and insulin resistance may be explained by the renal handling of uric acid.

Plasminogen activator inhibitor

Increased levels of plasminogen activator inhibitor (PAI-1) represent the most recent addition to the collection of metabolic features of the IRS. High concentrations of PAI-1 are associated with reduced fibrolysis and probably increase the risk of CHD by this mechanism. Levels of this risk factor are significantly associated with hyperinsulinaemia, hypertriglyceridaemia and hypertension, though whether the relationship between insulin resistance and PAI-1 is a direct one or simply a consequence of hypertriglyceridaemia is still to be established.

Coronary heart disease

In view of the fact that many of the individual features of the IRS have been shown to be risk factors for the development of CHD (most notably low levels of HDL, high levels of small dense LDL, glucose intolerance and NIDDM, hypertension) it would be inconceivable to suggest that the full-blown syndrome was not of major importance in determining cardiovascular risk. Furthermore, given the high frequency of this clustering of risk factors which constitute the IRS, it seems likely that the syndrome contributes to a considerable extent to the global epidemic of CHD. There are no reliable data comparing frequency in different populations – which is not surprising in view of the complexity of the syndrome and the lack of clear definition – but there is no doubt that it differs from one country to another and therefore its overall contribution to CHD varies. There appears to be a particularly strong predisposition amongst people of Polynesian and Micronesian descent, native North Americans and those from the Indian subcontinent. Manifestation of the full-blown clinical syndrome occurs when such people are exposed to rapid acculturation to the Western way of life, characterized in particular by energy intake in excess of requirements (i.e. high availability of energy-dense foods, especially convenience foods high in fat and sugars and relatively low levels of physical activity). However, the recent demonstration of the syndrome in Chinese people similarly exposed to the Western way of life at home and abroad led to the suggestion that white populations may in some way be protected, rather than other groups being at risk.

There has been an extraordinary amount of rather futile debate as to whether or not hyperinsulinaemia is an independent risk factor for CHD. There is less support for insulinaemia *per se* rather than the entire IRS as an explanation for enhanced cardiovascular risk, but the issue has not entirely been resolved. The matter is of more than theoretical importance when it comes to treating NIDDM patients with insulin. Because of the insulin resistance inherent to the condition, these patients often require large insulin doses to achieve normoglycaemia. If hyperinsulinaemia confers increased risk of CHD, the extremely high risk of cardiovascular disease in NIDDM patients may be further increased by insulin treatment.

Nutritional Management

While genetic factors are clearly responsible for setting the scene for the development of IRS and its consequences in populations and individuals, nutritional modification (**Table 2**) and physical activity can profoundly influence the extent to which the syndrome manifests clinically. Avoiding obesity, reducing fat intake and increasing exercise are the key messages for reducing population risk, the major

Table 2 Principles of nutritional management of the insulin resistance syndrome

Avoid or treat obesity

Decrease intake of saturated fatty acids, especially palmitic acid

Reduce intake of sugars and fibre-depleted carbohydrate foods

Encourage the consumption of foods rich in linoleic and n-3 polyunsaturated fatty acids

Encourage the consumption of cereals, vegetables and fruit, especially those rich in dietary fibre

difficulty being the implementation of such advice in populations at greatest risk. For individuals at high risk because of a family history and for those in whom the syndrome has been clinically diagnosed, the principles of life-style therapy are similar, though individual targets may be set and more specific advice given. For example, reduction of palmitic acid consumption can be achieved by particularly recommending a reduction in butter and other high-fat dairy products as well as in palm oil products. The issue arises as to whether carbohydrate or unsaturated fatty acids should replace the saturated fatty acids removed from the diet. For many individuals there will be no need for replacement energy for the displaced saturated fats, since a reduction in total energy intake is usually required. It has been argued that linoleic acid and long-chain n-3 unsaturated fatty acids may be the most appropriate nutrients when replacement energy is required, because they tend to improve insulin sensitivity. Carbohydrate-rich foods, especially sugars and highly processed complex carbohydrates depleted of dietary fibre, may induce hypertriacylglycerolaemia and hyperglycaemia and aggravate insulin resistance, so their consumption is not advised. On the other hand, fibre-rich foods may enhance satiety and facilitate weight reduction without these adverse metabolic consequences, so a mix of such foods and the beneficial unsaturated fatty acids may be appropriate when replacement energy is required. Conveniently, the dietary advice required to reduce insulin resistance is identical to that recommended to all populations at high risk of CHD and non-insulin-dependent diabetes, and to individuals with hyperlipidaemia and diabetes.

See also: **Coronary Heart Disease**: Aetiology. **Diabetes Mellitus**: Classification and Chemical Pathology. **Glucose**: Metabolism and Maintenance of Blood Glucose Level; Glucose Tolerance. **Hypertension**: Interrelationships Between Hypertension and Diabetes. **Obesity**: Complications of Obesity.

Further Reading

Bogardus G, Lillioja S, Mott DM, Hollenbeck G and Reaven G (1985) Relationship between degree of obesity and in vivo insulin action in man. *American Journal of Physiology* 248:E286–E291.

Borkman M, Storlein LH, Pan DA, Jenkins AB, Chisholm DJ and Campbell LB (1993) The relationship between insulin sensitivity and the fatty acid composition of skeletal-muscle phospholipids. *New England Journal of Medicine* 328:238–244.

DeFronzo RA and Ferrannini E (1991) Insulin resistance: a multifaceted syndrome responsible for NIDDM, obesity, hypertension, dyslipidaemia, and atherosclerotic cardiovascular disease. *Diabetes Care* 14:173–194.

DeFronzo RA, Tobin FD and Andres R (1979) Glucose clamp technique: a method for quantifying insulin secretion and resistance. *American Journal of Physiology* 237(3):E214–E223.

Ferrannini E, Haffner SM, Mitchell BD and Stern M (1991) Hyperinsulinaemia: the key feature of a cardiovascular and metabolic syndrome. *Diabetologia* 34:416–422.

Flier JS (1992) Lilly Lecture: syndromes of insulin resistance: from patient to gene and back again. *Diabetes* 41:1207–1219.

Jarrett RJ (1994) Why is insulin *not* a risk factor for coronary heart disease? *Diabetologia* 37:945–947.

Martin BC, Warram JH, Krolewski AS, Bergman RN, Soeldner JS and Kahn CR (1992) Role of glucose and insulin resistance in development of type 2 diabetes mellitus: results of a 25-year follow-up study. *Lancet* 340:925–929.

Pollare AT, Lithell H, Selinus I and Berne C (1988) Application of prazosin is associated with an increase of insulin sensitivity in obese patients with hypertension. *Diabetologia* 31:415–420.

Popp-Snijders C, Schouten JA, Hein RJ, van der Meer J and van der Meer EA (1987) Dietary supplementation of omega-3 polyunsaturated fatty acids improves insulin sensitivity in non-insulin-dependent diabetes. *Diabetes Research* 4:65–73.

Reaven GM and Laws A (1994) Insulin resistance, *compensatory* hyperinsulinaemia, and coronary heart disease. *Diabetologia* 37:948–952.

Reaven GM (1995) Pathophysiology of insulin resistance in human disease. *Physiological Reviews* 75:473–484.

Rosenthal M, Haskell WL, Solomon R, Widstrom A and Reaven GM (1983) Demonstration of a relationship between level of physical training and insulin-stimulated glucose utilization in normal humans. *Diabetes* 32:408–411.

Stern MP (1994) The insulin resistance syndrome: the controversy is dead, long live the controversy! *Diabetologia* 37:956–958.

Storlein LH, Kraegen EW, Chisholm DJ, Ford GL, Bruce DG and Pascoe WS (1987) Fish oil prevents insulin resistance induced by high-fat feeding in rats. *Science* 237:885–888.

Storlein LH, Pan DA, Kriketos AD and Baur LA (1993) High fat diet-induced insulin resistance. Lessons and implications from animal studies. In: Klimes I, Howard BV, Storlein LH and Sebökova E (eds) Dietary lipids and insulin action. *Annals of the New York Academy of Science* 683:82–90.

Tremblay A (1995) Nutritional determinants of the insulin resistance syndrome. *International Journal of Obesity and Related Metabolic Disorders* 19 supplement 1:S60–68.

Vessby B, Tengblad S and Lithell H (1994) Insulin sensitivity is related to the fatty acid composition of serum lipids and skeletal muscle phospholipids in 70-year-old men. *Diabetologia* 37:1044–1050.

Zavaroni I, Bonora E, Pagliara M *et al.* (1989) Risk factors for coronary artery disease in healthy persons with hyperinsulinaemia and normal glucose tolerance. *New England Journal of Medicine* 320:702–706.

Intensive care management *see* **Therapeutic Dietetics**: Intensive Care Management.

Intestine *see* **Gastrointestinal Tract**: Structure and Function of the Small Intestine.

IODINE

Contents

Physiology, Dietary Sources and Requirements

R Houston, Emory University Rollins School of
Public Health and Department of International Health,
Atlanta, Georgia, USA

Copyright © 1998 Academic Press

A relevant thing, though small, is of the highest importance

MK Gandhi

Iodine is classified as a nonmetallic solid in the halogen family of the Periodic Table of the elements and therefore is related to fluorine, chlorine and bromine. The halogen family lies between the oxygen family and the rare gases. Iodine sublimates at room temperature to form a violet gas; its name is derived from the Greek *iodes*, meaning 'violet-coloured'. Iodine was discovered by Bernard Courtois in Paris in 1811, the second halogen (after chlorine) to be discovered. It took nearly 100 years to understand its critical importance in human physiology. In 1896, Baumann determined the association of iodine with the thyroid gland, and in 1914 Kendall, with revisions by Harrington in 1926, described the hormone complexes synthesized by the thyroid gland using iodine that are so integral to human growth and development.

As the biochemistry of iodine and the thyroid was being established, the scarcity of the element in the natural environment became evident and the link between deficiency and human disease was revealed. Enlargement of the thyroid, or goitre, is seen in ancient stone carvings and Renaissance paintings, but it was not until years later that the link with lack of iodine was firmly established. Even with this knowledge, many years passed before preventive measures were established. From 1910 to 1920 in Switzerland and the USA work was done on the use of salt fortified with iodine to eliminate iodine deficiency, with classic work being done by Dr David Marine in Michigan. Recently the linkage of iodine deficiency with intellectual impairment has brought iodine into the international spotlight.

Recent work has demonstrated that the halogens, including iodine, are involved through the haloperoxidases in enzymatic activity and production of numerous active metabolites in the human body. While the importance of iodine for the thyroid has been known for some time, recent research on halogen compounds in living organisms suggest additional more complex roles including antibiotic and anticancer activity. Yet it is the critical importance of iodine in the formation of the thyroid hormones thyroxine (T_4) and triiodothyronine (T_3) that makes any discussion of this element and human physiology of necessity bound up with a review of thyroid function.

Existence of Iodine in the Natural Environment

The marine hydrosphere has high concentrations of halogens, with iodine being the least common and chlorine the most. Halogens, including iodine, are concentrated by various species of marine organisms such as macroalgae and certain seaweeds. Release from these organisms makes a major contribution to the atmospheric concentration of the halogens. Iodine is present as the least abundant halogen in the Earth's crust. It is likely that in primordial times the concentration in surface soils was higher, but today the iodine content of soils varies and most has been leached out in areas of high rainfall or by previous glaciation. Environmental degradation caused by massive deforestation and soil erosion is accelerating this process. This variability in soil and water iodine concentration is quite marked, with some valleys in China having relatively high iodine concentrations in water, and other parts of China with negligible amounts in soil and water. **Table 1** shows the relative abundance of various halogens in the natural environment, while **Fig. 1** illustrates the cycle of iodine in nature.

Commercial production of iodine occurs almost exclusively in Japan and Chile, with iodine extracted from concentrated salt brine from underground wells, seaweed or from Chilean saltpetre deposits.

Table 1 Relative abundance of halogens in the natural environment

Element	Abundance in oceans (ppm)	Abundance in Earth's crust (ppm)	Abundance in human body (mol)
Fluorine	1.3	625	0.13
Chlorine	19 400	130	2.7
Bromine	67	2.5	0.0033
Iodine	0.06	0.05	0.00013

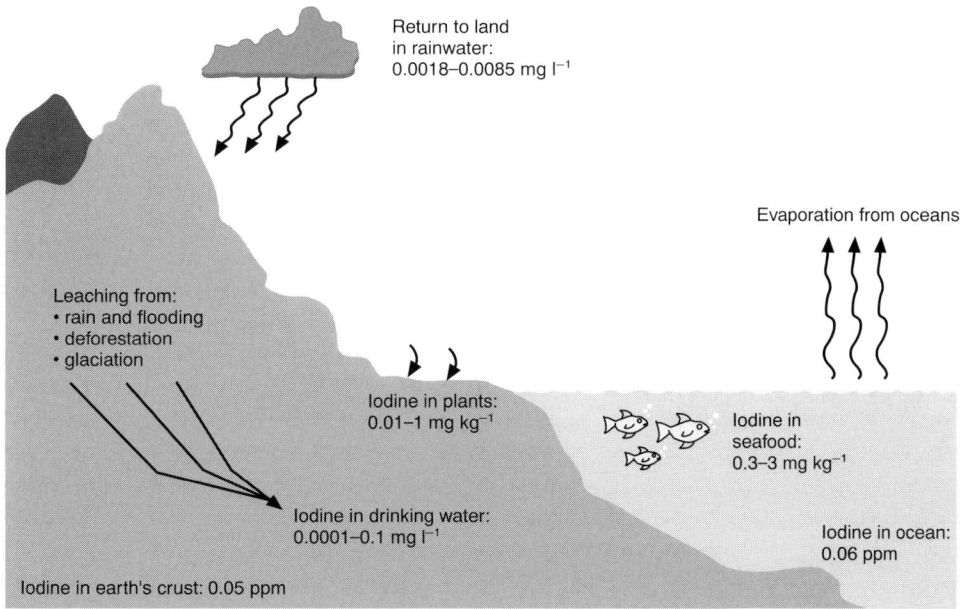

Figure 1 Cycle of iodine in nature.

Absorption, Transport and Storage

Iodine is usually ingested as an iodide or iodate compound, and is rapidly absorbed in the intestine. Iodine entering the circulation is actively trapped by the thyroid gland. This remarkable capacity to concentrate iodine is a reflection of the fact that the most critical physiological role for iodine is the normal functioning of the thyroid gland. Circulating iodide enters the capillaries within the thyroid and is rapidly transported into follicular cells and on into the lumen of the follicle. This active transport is likely to be based on co-transport of sodium and iodine, allowing iodine to move against its electrochemical gradient. Several anions such as thiocyanate, perchlorate and pertechnetate inhibit this active transport. There is evidence that the active transport clearly demonstrated in the thyroid gland is also true for extrathyroidal tissues, including the salivary glands, mammary glands and gastric mucosa.

In addition to trapping iodine, follicular cells also synthesize the glycoprotein, thyroglobulin (Tg), from carbohydrates and amino acids (including tyrosine) obtained from the circulation. Thyroglobulin moves into the lumen of the follicle where it becomes available for hormone production. Thyroid peroxidase (TPO), a membrane-bound haem-containing glycoprotein, catalyses the oxidation of the iodide to its active form, I_2, and the binding of this active form to the tyrosine in thyroglobulin to form mono- or diiodotyrosine (MIT or DIT). These in turn combine to form the thyroid hormones triiodothyronine (T_3) and thyroxine (T_4). Thyroglobulin is very concentrated in the follicles through a process of compaction, making the concentration of iodine in the thyroid gland very high. Only a very small proportion of the iodine remains as inorganic iodide, although even for this unbound iodide the concentration in the thyroid remains much greater than that in the circulation. This remarkable ability of the thyroid to concentrate and store iodine allows the gland to be very rapidly responsive to metabolic needs for thyroid hormones. **Fig. 2** shows the structures of the molecules tyrosine and thyroxine.

Formation of thyroid hormones is not restricted to humans. Marine algae have an 'iodine pump' that facilitates concentration; invertebrates and all vertebrates demonstrate similar mechanisms to

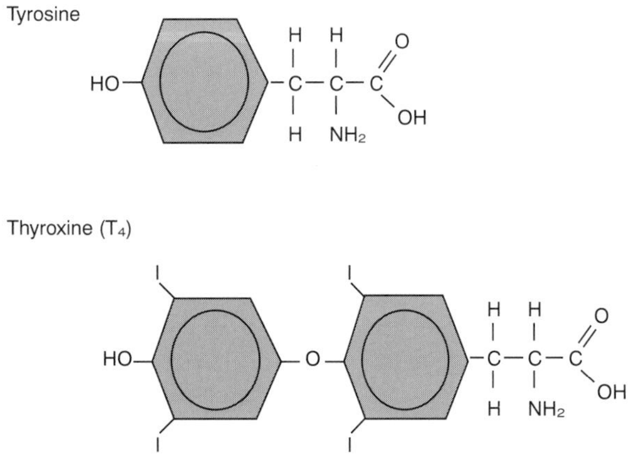

Tyrosine

Thyroxine (T₄)

Figure 2   Structures of tyrosine and thyroxine (T₄).

concentrate iodine and form iodotyrosines of various types. Although the function of these hormones in invertebrates is not clear, in vertebrates these iodine-containing substances are important for a variety of functions, such as metamorphosis in amphibians, spawning changes in fish and general translation of genetic messages for protein synthesis.

Metabolism and Excretion

Once iodine is 'captured' by the thyroid and thyroid hormones formed in the lumen of the follicles, stimulation of the gland causes release of the hormones into the circulation for uptake by peripheral tissues. Both production and release of the hormones are regulated in two ways. Stimulation is hormonally controlled by the hypothalamus of the brain through thyroid releasing hormone (TRH) which stimulates the pituitary gland to secrete thyroid stimulating hormone (TSH), which in turn stimulates the thyroid to release T_3 and T_4. In addition to the regulation of thyroid hormones by TSH, iodine itself plays a major role in autoregulation. The rate of uptake of iodine into the follicle, the ratio of T_3 to T_4, and the release of these into the circulation, among other things, are affected by the concentration of iodine in the gland. Thus, an increase in iodine intake causes a decrease in organification of iodine in the follicles and does not necessarily result in a corresponding increase in hormone release. Recent research suggests that this autoregulation is not entirely independent of TSH activity and that several other factors may contribute. However, regardless of the mechanism, these regulatory mechanisms allow for stability in hormone secretion in spite of wide variations in iodine intake.

When stimulated to release thyroid hormones, thyroglobulin is degraded through the activity of lyso-

somes and T_3 and T_4 are released and rapidly enter the circulation. Iodide freed in this reaction is for the most part recycled and the iodinated tyrosine reused for hormone production. Nearly all of the released hormones are rapidly bound to transport hormones, with 70% bound to thyroxine binding globulin (TBG). Other proteins such as transthyretin (TTR), albumin and lipoproteins bind most of the remainder; with significant differences in the strengths of the affinity for the hormones, these proteins transport the hormones to different sites.

This remarkable ability of the thyroid actively to trap and store the iodine required creates a relatively steady state, with daily intake used to ensure full stores. T_4, with a longer half-life, serves as a reservoir for conversion to the more active hormone, T_3, with a much shorter half-life of 1 day. Target organs for thyroid hormone activity all play a role in the complex interplay between conversion of T_4 to T_3 deiodination, and metabolism of various other proteins involved with thyroid function. The liver, which is estimated to contain 30% of the extrathyroidal T_4, is responsible, through the activity of the liver cell enzyme, deiodinase, for ensuring adequate supply of T_3 to peripheral tissues and degradation of metabolic by-products. The kidney demonstrates a strong ability to take up the iodothyronines. Iodine is ultimately excreted in the urine, with average daily excretion rates of approximately 100 μg per day. This accounts for the vast majority of iodine excretion, with negligible amounts excreted in faeces. **Fig. 3** illustrates a thyroid follicle and summarizes iodine transport.

Metabolic Functions

Separating the role of iodine from the complex and pervasive function of the thyroid gland is difficult since iodine is a critical component of the hormones that mediate these functions, and whatever other roles iodine may have are poorly understood. Thyroid hormones affect a wide range of physiological functions, from liver and kidney to heart and brain. Earlier work supported a role for thyroid hormones in affecting the energy generating capacity of cells through biochemical changes in mitochondria. More recent work has shown, however, that these hormones act on specific genetic receptors in cell nuclei, and perhaps through other extranuclear mechanisms. The nuclear receptors belong to a large family of receptors that bind other extranuclear molecules including vitamins A and D and steroids. Through this interaction, along with a number of other proteins, thyroid hormones modify genetic expression. A great deal of research currently focuses

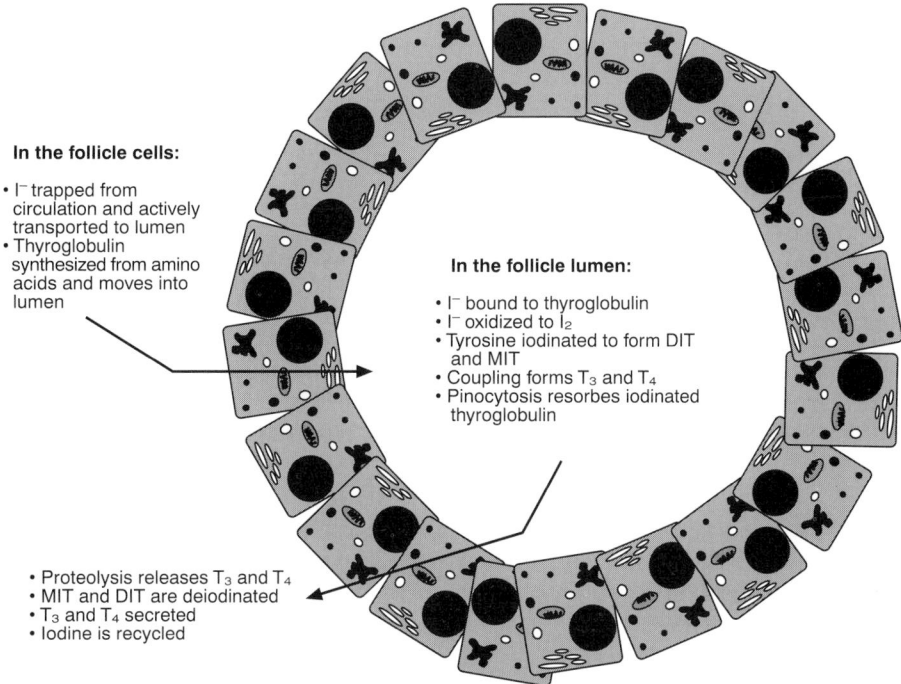

In the follicle cells:

- I⁻ trapped from circulation and actively transported to lumen
- Thyroglobulin synthesized from amino acids and moves into lumen

In the follicle lumen:

- I⁻ bound to thyroglobulin
- I⁻ oxidized to I_2
- Tyrosine iodinated to form DIT and MIT
- Coupling forms T_3 and T_4
- Pinocytosis resorbes iodinated thyroglobulin

- Proteolysis releases T_3 and T_4
- MIT and DIT are deiodinated
- T_3 and T_4 secreted
- Iodine is recycled

Figure 3 Thyroid follicle (courtesy of Kiely Houston).

on these thyroid hormone receptors, and the effect primarily of T_3 on the physiological function of the target organ through genetic transcription. These receptors are present in pituitary, liver, heart, kidney and brain cells.

In the pituitary gland, thyroid hormones, along with many cofactors, regulate the synthesis and secretion of growth hormone by increasing gene transcription. Similarly, as part of the feedback loop for hormone regulation and release, thyroid hormones affect transcription of TSH in the pituitary. In cardiac and skeletal muscle, thyroid hormones affect production of the muscle tissue myosin in a variety of ways, depending on the stage of life and specific muscle tissue affected. In addition, the hormones affect muscle contraction through genetic alteration of calcium uptake within the cell. Carbohydrate metabolism and formation of certain fats (lipogenesis) are affected through hormone-induced changes in gene transcription in liver cells.

In the adult brain, receptors have been identified, but the specific genes affected by thyroid hormones have not yet been located. However, in the developing brain of the fetus and neonate, the effects of thyroid hormones are significant even though the exact mechanisms are still not fully understood. The effects of thyroid hormones on brain development are suggested by failure in development of the nerve elements, failure of differentiation of cerebellar cells,

and reduced development of other brain cells, in hypothyroid states. It is this early effect that has recently elevated the status of iodine from an element whose deficiency caused goitre, to one whose deficiency is the leading cause of mental impairment worldwide.

In addition to these nuclear mechanisms, several alternative pathways have been suggested, some based on earlier historical studies. The thermogenic effects of thyroid hormones were originally felt to be a direct action on mitochondria, though this has recently been questioned. Thyroid hormones stimulate glucose transport, and again though originally attributed to a direct action on the plasma membrane, recent evidence suggests a genetic mechanism. There may also be a direct effect of thyroid hormones on brain enzymatic activity.

The overall effects of these cellular and systemic actions is to stimulate respiratory and other enzyme synthesis, which results in increased oxygen consumption and resultant increased basal metabolic rate. This affects heart rate, respiratory rate, mobilization of carbohydrates, cholesterol metabolism, and a wide variety of other physiological activities. In addition, thyroid hormones stimulate growth and development and, as noted earlier, are critical for the normal proliferation, growth and development of brain cells. **Table 2** shows the estimated iodine concentration in selected organs.

Table 2 Estimated iodine concentrations in selected organs

Total body	Thyroid gland	Brain	Liver	Blood
15–20 mg	8–12 mg (for a 15–25 g gland)	0.02 μg g^{-1} (wet weight)	0.2 μg g^{-1} (wet weight)	0.08–0.60 μg dl^{-1} (plasma inorganic iodide

Iodine Deficiency and Excess

Iodine deficiency

Iodine deficiency is the most common cause of preventable mental retardation in the world. This fact, along with the recognition that iodine deficiency is not limited to remote rural populations, has stimulated agencies and governments to mobilize resources to eliminate this problem. This global effort, focusing primarily on iodization of salt for human and animal consumption, is slowly succeeding in eliminating a hidden set of disorders that have plagued mankind for centuries.

Unlike many nutritional deficiencies that are more directly related to socioeconomic status, insufficient intake of iodine is a geographical disease, related to lack of iodine in the environment. Iodine originally present in soil was subjected to leaching by snow and rain, and while a portion of the iodine in the oceans evaporates and is returned to the soil in rainwater, this amount is small. Thus, many areas have insufficient iodine in the environment, and this is reflected in plants grown in that environment. The diets in many developing countries are limited in variability, and contain few processed foods. This places large populations at risk of iodine deficiency. The World Health Organization (WHO) estimates that at least 1572 million people are at risk in 118 countries, with 43 million affected by 'some degree of mental impairment'.

In the most simplistic physiological model, inadequate intake of iodine results in a reduction in thyroid hormone production, which stimulates increased TSH production. TSH acts directly on thyroid cells, and without the ability to increase hormone production, the gland becomes hyperplastic. In addition, iodine trapping becomes more efficient, as demonstrated by increased radioactive iodine uptake in deficient individuals. However, this simplistic model is complicated by complex adaptive mechanisms which vary depending on the age of the individual affected. In adults with mild deficiency, reduced intake causes a decrease in extrathyroidal iodine and reduced clearance, demonstrated by decreased urinary iodine excretion, but iodine concentration in the gland may remain within normal limits. With further reduction in intake, this adaptive

mechanism is overwhelmed, and the iodine content of the thyroid decreases with alterations in iodination of thyroglobulin, in the ratio of DIT to MIT, and reduction in efficient thyroid hormone production. The ability to adapt appears to decrease with decreasing age, and in children the iodine pool in the thyroid is smaller, and the dynamics of iodine metabolism and peripheral use more rapid. In neonates, the effects of iodine deficiency are more directly reflected in increased TSH. Diminished thyroid iodine content and increased turnover make neonates the most vulnerable to the effects of iodine deficiency and decreased hormone production, even with mild deficiency.

A number of other factors influence iodine balance. Active transport of iodide is competitively inhibited by several compounds, including complex ions such as perchlorate, and by thiocyanate, a metabolic product of several foods. Other compounds, such as propylthiouracil, affect coupling reactions and iodination, doing so regardless of iodine intake, e.g. without blocking iodide transport. Several pharmaceuticals affect peripheral hormone action. Dietary goitrogens, as these compounds have been called, include cassava, lima beans, sweet potatoes, cabbage and broccoli; these contain cyanide compounds that are detoxified to thiocyanate, which may inhibit iodide transport. Cabbage and turnips, and other plants of the genus *Brassica*, also contain thionamide compounds which block iodination. Certain industrial waste products, such as resorcinol from coal processing, contain phenols that cause irreversible inhibition of TPO and block iodination. In some countries the staple diet includes such goitrogens, and iodine deficiency may be exacerbated, as has been well documented for cassava. While this may be a significant problem in some geographical areas, in most instances adequate dietary iodine can reverse the goitrogenic effect.

The most important clinical effect of deficiency relates to the fact that thyroid hormone is required for the normal development of the brain in both humans and other animals. Numerous studies have demonstrated reduced psychomotor skills and intellectual development in the presence of iodine deficiency, and most experts now believe that there is a continuum of deficits, from mild impairment in

IQ to severe mental retardation. Studies in China demonstrated shifts in IQ point distributions in rural communities that were deficient, suggesting an impact of deficiency of 10–15 IQ points. In Europe, where mild deficiency still exists, studies have demonstrated decreased psychomotor, perceptual integrative motor ability as well as lower verbal IQ scores in schoolchildren. Studies in Iran showed similar findings. A recent meta-analysis of 18 studies demonstrated a strong relationship, with an overall 13.5 IQ point difference between deficient and non-deficient populations. These findings, coupled with the high prevalence of deficiency in many countries, have major implications for development.

The most severe effect of iodine deficiency is cretinism, which is rare in areas of mildly endemic deficiency, but may have reached 5–10% or more in areas with severe deficiency. There are general classifications of cretinism, the symptoms of which frequently overlap. Neurological cretinism presents as extreme mental retardation, deaf-mutism, and impaired motor function including spastic gait. Myxoedematous cretinism presents as disturbances of growth and development including short stature, coarse facial features, retarded sexual development, mental retardation and other signs of hypothyroidism. It appears likely that severe deficiency resulting in decreased maternal T_4 may be responsible for the impaired neurological development of the fetus occurring early in pregnancy. The effect of deficiency on the fetus after 20 weeks' gestation may result in hyperstimulation of the developing fetal thyroid, with the extreme manifestation being thyroid failure causing myxoedematous cretinism. Other factors may affect thyroid hormone metabolism. Selenium deficiency, when present with iodine deficiency, may alter the clinical manifestations. Selenium deficiency decreases the activity of the enzyme, glutathione peroxidase (GPX), which, along with thyroid hormone synthesis, reduces hydrogen peroxide (H_2O_2). Combined with iodine deficiency and reduced hormone synthesis, it has been speculated that selenium deficiency may contribute to accumulation of H_2O_2 which may in turn lead to cell damage and contribute to thyroid failure. Selenium is also essential for the deiodinase enzyme activity affecting thyroid hormone catabolism, and deficiency may actually increase serum thyroxine. The balance between these two effects is still not fully understood. The study of cretinism has been critical to the evolution of our understanding of the critical role of iodine for normal mental development.

Iodine deficiency has a number of other effects, including development of goitre, clinical or subclinical hypothyroidism, decreased fertility rates, increased stillbirth and spontaneous abortion rates, and increased perinatal and infant mortality. This spectrum of clinical effects, collectively called 'iodine deficiency disorders', underlines the importance of iodine in human health.

The most effective method to eliminate iodine deficiency in populations is through iodization of salt. The most classic success of salt iodization was demonstrated in Switzerland. Salt is universally consumed, and in most countries the amount consumed is relatively constant between 5 and 10 g per person per day. Iodine is usually added as iodide or iodate (which is more stable) to achieve 25–50 ppm iodine at consumption. This provides about 150–250 μg of iodine per person per day.

The challenge for national iodine deficiency elimination programmes is to mobilize the various sectors that must be involved in a sustainable national programme, including education, industry, health and the political arena. There must be an appropriate regulatory environment, effective demand creation, adequate production to make iodized salt available, and quality assurance of both the product and all programme elements to ensure that the programme is sustained forever. Success in these efforts has the potential to have a greater impact on development than any public health programme to date.

Iodine excess

Iodine is used in many medications, food preservatives and antiseptics with minimal adverse effects on populations. Pure iodine crystals are toxic, and ingestion can cause severe stomach irritation. Iodine is allergenic, and acute reactions to radiographic contrast media are not rare. Yet because of the thyroid's unique ability to regulate the body's iodine pool, quite a wide range in intake is tolerated without serious effects, particularly when the exposure is of limited duration.

When ingestion of iodine in excess of the daily requirement of approximately 150 μg per day, changes in thyroid hormones can occur. A variety of clinical problems can occur, and these differ depending on the dose, the presence of thyroid disease, and whether the individual has been deficient in the past. In iodine-replete individuals without thyroid disease, goitre can result, and rarely, hypothyroidism, although the latter is more common in individuals with other illnesses such as lung disease or cystic fibrosis. The relationship of iodine excess to other diseases such as Hashimoto's thyroiditis remains controversial. In the US iodine levels were quite high from 1960 to 1980, with estimates for adult males as high as 827 μg per day. There was no immediate evidence of an impact on thyroid disease, although longer-term longitudinal data are lacking. Effects usually remain subtle and transient, even with ingestion of up to 1500–4500 µg per day.

In the presence of thyroid disease, and in areas with endemic iodine deficiency, suddenly raising daily iodine intake may precipitate hyperthyroidism, and this has been the subject of some concern as salt iodization efforts proceed with fledgling quality assurance. This effect is felt to be related in part to autonomous nodules in the gland that synthesize and release excess thyroid hormone. The exact prevalence of iodine-induced hyperthyroidism in deficient areas is not clear. Many countries initiating salt iodization programmes have reported increases in the incidence of toxic nodular goitre and iodine-induced thyrotoxicosis, usually in older people. While this may be a significant clinical problem, the risk is estimated to be between 0.01 and 0.06%, and must be considered in the light of the benefit from correction of deficiency.

Assessment of Iodine Status

A standard set of indicators of iodine status has been established by the WHO in response to the need to determine prevalence in countries with endemic deficiency. These indicators reflect iodine status as mediated through the response of the thyroid gland to fluctuations in iodine intake. There are several additional indicators that are used to assess thyroid function, such as T_4 and T_3, but these are less accurate in reflecting iodine status since conversion of T_4 to T_3 and cellular uptake is so responsive to peripheral need.

Urinary iodine reflects iodine sufficiency, and output decreases with diminished intake. Since this indicator reflects the amount of iodine per unit volume of urine, its accuracy is impaired by variable fluid intake and factors affecting the concentration of the urine. Therefore, as a measure of iodine status in an individual, it is less accurate than as a measure of iodine status of a population. Median urinary iodine values are used extensively to assess population prevalence of iodine deficiency.

Thyroid size, either estimated by palpation or using ultrasound volume determination, reflects iodine status since deficiency results in thyroid enlargement, or goitre. Due to the relative ease of palpation, that measure has been a traditional standard to assess populations for iodine deficiency, and has been particularly useful in schoolchildren. In adults, where longstanding thyroid enlargement from iodine deficiency may be minimally responsive to corrected iodine intake, palpation may be misleading and could overestimate the current level of iodine suf-

ficiency. In children, palpation becomes increasingly difficult and significantly less accurate when deficiency is mild. Ultrasound volume determination provides a more accurate estimate of thyroid size. For any measure of thyroid size, other factors besides iodine deficiency can cause enlargement, including iodine excess, carcinoma and infection. In areas of the world where deficiency is a problem, the prevalence of these other diseases compared with goitre from iodine deficiency is negligible.

Thyroid stimulating hormone (TSH) is produced in response to decreased iodine intake and diminished thyroid hormone production and is used as a measure of iodine status. TSH is best measured in neonates – in the developed world for surveillance against congenital hypothyroidism, and in endemic countries to estimate the magnitude of iodine deficiency. Neonatal TSH has been a useful advocacy tool to demonstrate to policy makers that iodine deficiency is not limited to rural remote populations, but affects children born in big city hospitals. However, with the complexity of the interactions between TSH and other hormones, TSH has not been shown to be as useful in older children or adults in estimating prevalence of iodine deficiency. Also, use of iodine containing antiseptics affects TSH distributions in neonates.

Uptake of radioactive iodine isotopes can be used to scan the gland, and determine the affinity of the gland to introduced iodine, and is a measure of deficiency. The most common isotope used is ^{123}I because of its relatively short 13-hour half-life and γ photon emission. Uptake is increased in iodine deficiency. Isotopes can also be used to examine the organification of iodine in the formation of thyroid hormones. This is an impractical method for surveying populations. **Table 3** provides the WHO criteria for defining iodine deficiency as a public health problem.

Requirements and Dietary Sources

The daily requirement for iodine in humans has been estimated based on daily losses, iodine balance and turnover, with most studies ranging from 40 to 200 µg per day, depending on age and metabolic needs, as shown in **Table 4**.

Natural sources of iodine include seafood, seaweeds, and smaller amounts from crops grown on soil with sufficient iodine, or from meat where livestock has grazed on such soil. The contribution of the latter two is small, and in most countries other sources are required. Iodine added to salt, as noted above, is the primary source for many populations.

Table 3   WHO criteria for iodine deficiency as a public health problem in populations

Indicator	Population assessed	Mild deficiency (%)	Severe deficiency (%)
Goitre by palpation	Schoolchildren	5–19.9	≥ 30
Thyroid volume by ultrasound (> 97th percentile)	Schoolchildren	5–19.9	≥ 30
Median urinary iodine (µg l^{-1})	Schoolchildren	50–99	< 20
TSH (> 5 mU l^{-1} whole blood)	Neonates	3–19.9	≥ 40

Table 4   Recommended dietary intake

Age	WHO Recommended intake (µg per day)	US RDA 1989 (µg per day)
0–6 months	40	40
6–12 months	50	60 (at age 1 year)
1–10 years	70–120	60–120
11 years–adult	120–150	150
Pregnancy	175	175
Lactation	200	200

Table 5   Sample iodine content for various sources

Water	Cabbage	Eggs	Seafood	Sugar	Iodized salt
0.1–2 µg l^{-1} in endemic area	0–0.95 µg g^{-1}	4–10 µg egg^{-1}	300–3000 µg kg^{-1}	< 1 µg kg^{-1} in refined sugar	20–50 ppm (at household level, depending on climate, and currently subject to review
2–15 µg l^{-1} in nonendemic area				30 µg kg^{-1} in unrefined brown sugar	

Table 6   Iodine intake from average US and British diets

Country	Milk (µg per day)	Grains (µg per day)	Meat, fish and poultry (µg per day)
US	534	152	103
Britain	92	31	36

Table 5 shows sample iodine content for various sources.

In the US and Britain, as well as in other developed countries, most dietary iodine comes from food processing. Intake can vary, as illustrated in **Table 6**. Iodophors used as antiseptics in the dairy and baking industries provide residual iodine in milk and processed foods. In addition, iodine is present in several vitamin and pharmaceutical preparations.

Iodine as a trace element in low concentrations in most environments plays a critical role in the normal growth and development of many species. In humans, iodine is critical for brain development and correction of global deficiencies is an unparalleled opportunity to improve the wellbeing of our global community.

See also: **Fruits and Vegetables**: Nutritional Value. **Iodine**: Iodine Deficiency Disorders. **Legumes**: Types and Nutritional Value.

Further Reading

Braverman LE and Utiger RD (eds) (1996) *Werner and Ingbar's The Thyroid, A Fundamental and Clinical Text*. Philadelphia: Lippincott-Raven.

Burgi H, Supersaxo Z and Selz B (1990) Iodine deficiency diseases in Switzerland one hundred years after Theodor Kocher's survey: A historical review with some new goitre prevalence data. *Acta Endocrinologica (Copenhagen)* 123:577–590.

Gaitan E (1990) Goitrogens in food and water. *Annual Review of Nutrition* 10:21–39.

Hall R and Kobberling J (1985) *Thyroid Disorders Associated with Iodine Deficiency and Excess*. New York: Raven Press.

Hetzel BS (1994) Iodine deficiency and fetal brain damage. *New England Journal of Medicine* 331(26):1770–1771.

Hetzel BS (1989) *The Story of Iodine Deficiency: An International Challenge in Nutrition*. Oxford: Oxford University Press.

Hetzel BS and Pandav CS (eds) (1994) *SOS for a Billion – The Conquest of Iodine Deficiency Disorders*. Delhi: Oxford University Press.

Mertz W (1986) *Trace Elements in Human and Animal Nutrition*, 5th edn. New York: Academic Press.

Patai S and Rappoport Z (eds) (1995) Supplement D2: *The Chemistry of Halides, Pseudo-halides and Azides*, part 2. New York: John Wiley & Sons.

Stanbury JB (eds) (1994) *The Damaged Brain of Iodine Deficiency*. New York: Cognizant Communication Corporation, The Franklin Institute.

Sullivan KM, Houston RM, Gorstein J and Cervinskas J (1995) *Monitoring Universal Salt Iodization Programmes*. Ottawa: UNICEF, MI, ICCIDD, WHO publication.

Thorpe-Beeston JG and Nicolaides KH (1996) *Maternal and Fetal Thyroid Function in Pregnancy*. New York: The Parthenon Publishing Group.

Todd CH, Allain T, Gomo ZAR, Hasler JA, Ndiweni M and Oken E (1995) Increase in thyrotoxicosis associated with iodine supplements in Zimbabwe. *Lancet* 346:1563–1564.

Troncone L, Shapiro B, Satta MA and Monaco F (1994) *Thyroid Diseases: Basic Science Pathology, Clinical and Laboratory Diagnosis*. Boca Raton: CRC Press.

WHO, UNICEF and ICCIDD (1994) *Indicators for Assessing Iodine Deficiency Disorders and Their Control Through Salt Iodization* (limited publication). Geneva: WHO, UNICEF, ICCID.

Wilson JD and Foster DW (eds) (1992) *Williams Textbook of Endocrinology*. Philadelphia: WB Saunders.

Iodine Deficiency Disorders

Festo P Kavishe, Tanzania Food and Nutrition Centre, Dar es Salaam, Tanzania

Copyright © 1998 Academic Press

Aetiology

The term 'iodine deficiency disorders' (IDD) refers to all the effects of iodine deficiency on growth and development, and it replaces the terms 'endemic goitre' and 'cretinism' which, for many years, have been used to articulate the problem of iodine deficiency. The use of the term 'IDD' emphasizes that the problem of iodine deficiency manifests in a wide spectrum of disorders with far wider and more far reaching effects than endemic goitre and cretinism. The full range of these disorders are discussed on the section on clinical features. The two major aetiological factors for IDD are iodine deficiency and goitrogens.

Iodine deficiency

The central aetiological factor in IDD is a deficiency of dietary iodine. The nutritional value of iodine lies in its essential requirement during the bioformation of thyroid hormones, chiefly thyroxine or tetraiodothyronine (T_4) which is converted into triiodothyronine (T_3) in the tissues. Because it is required in the metabolism of virtually all tissues, thyroxine – and, therefore, iodine – plays an essential role in human and animal growth and development. Although recent evidence indicates that the element iodine affects brain development in its own right, the major effects of iodine deficiency are mediated through a decreased synthesis of thyroxine. The physiological quantitative requirement for iodine is very minute, thus it is referred to as a 'trace element' or 'micronutrient'. It occurs in the human body in very small amounts (15–20 mg) and the essential requirement for normal growth is only 100–150 µg (0.1–0.15 mg) per person per day.

Under normal circumstances about 90% of dietary iodine is derived from food, and the remaining 10% from drinking water. Poor iodine content in food and water is caused by poor iodine content in the soil from which the food or water are derived. People living in areas of iodine-poor soils and relying on locally produced foods will have very low iodine intakes, sometimes below 25 µg per person per day. Such low intakes lead to severe IDD.

In nature, iodine is widely, but sparsely distributed. It occurs in fairly constant amounts in ocean water, but is distributed very unevenly in the earth's crust. Concentrated forms are known to occur as nitrate layers only in some North American and West Saharan soils. Although this ecological distribution of iodine may be due to natural occurrence, there is no doubt that geophysical changes which have taken place over time have played a role in the geographical redistribution of iodine. Leaching of iodine from the soil by rain, glaciers and recurrent floods has concentrated iodine in the ocean waters. Thus people living in mountainous areas or in areas subject to frequent flooding are at the highest risk of IDD, while those near the oceans are least at risk.

Because of the high iodine concentration in oceans, seafoods such as seaweeds and saltwater fish are particularly rich in iodine. However, it is important to clarify that sea salt contains negligible amounts of iodine because the process of evaporation used in the production of sea salt causes loss of iodine as well as water.

Goitrogenic factors

The diet or water may also contain certain substances, called goitrogens, that reduce the bioavailability of iodine. The most well-known are the thiocyanates, which are present in foods like cassava, cabbage and certain types of millets. However, only cassava has been fairly well-implicated as a contributing factor to the goitre which is endemic in Zaire. Excessive intakes of calcium from drinking water may precipitate iodine or increase its renal excretion and thus reduce its bioavailiability, but the ingestion of such goitrogenic factors in amounts capable of producing IDD is probably negligible in practical nutrition. In all cases, goitrogenic factors seem to be superimposed on primary iodine deficiency. This emphasizes the fact that dietary iodine deficiency is the primary, necessary and sufficient aetiological factor in IDD.

Prevalence

The classical IDD endemic regions are mainly found in geologically young mountain ranges such as the Alps, Andes and Himalayas, and the frequently flooding and large river deltas of the Ganges, Yellow River and the Rhine.

The global situation

Iodine deficiency disorders constitute a massive global problem and one of the major health issues of the twentieth century. Over 14% of the world's population, a staggering one billion people, are estimated to live in iodine-deficient areas, and are therefore at risk of IDD. Of these, about 710 million are in Asia, 227 million in Africa, 60 million in Latin America, and 20–30 million in Europe. Those exhibiting a demonstrable consequence of iodine deficiency are estimated to be at least 200–300 million with goitre and 7 million are cretins (**Table 1**).

Europe

Until recently, reports gave the impression that the problem of IDD was no longer significant in Europe. However, a surprise report, published by a special committee of the European Thyroid Association in *The Lancet* in 1985, indicated that IDD still present serious problems in a number of countries. Evidence of IDD of public health significance and requiring national action has been found in Germany, Italy, Spain, Portugal, Romania, Greece and Turkey. None of these countries has a national iodized salt programme.

That said, the brunt of the IDD problem is borne by the developing countries.

Asia

The largest populations suffering from iodine deficiency are found in Asia where three of the world's most populous countries are found – China, India, and Indonesia. Other Asian countries are also affected. The areas most affected are the Himalayan region, the mountain ranges of China, and the river valleys of the Ganges in India and Bangladesh, the Songhua River in northern China, and the Irawaddy in Burma, which are all subject to periodic flooding. Because of their fertility, these river valleys support large populations that are usually totally dependent on local crops. Much progress has been made in the control of IDD in Asia over the past few years, but owing to the large populations involved, there is still a long way to go.

Africa

In Africa a third of the population – over 200 million people scattered over 38 of the continent's 51 countries – are known to be living in iodine-deficient areas. In western Africa, with the possible exception of Mauritania, all countries are affected by IDD.

The ecological zones most affected are the forest zones and Sudanian savannah. The Sahelian and Saharan zones north of the 15th parallel are practically not affected. Central Africa contains some of the

Table 1 The prevalence of IDD in the world

Continent	Population (1991 estimates) ($\times 10^6$)	Population at risk of IDD ($\times 10^6$)	Population with: Goitre ($\times 10^6$)	Cretinism ($\times 10^6$)
Asia	3050	710 (23.3)[a]	130 (4.3)	6.5 (0.2)
Africa	661	227 (34.3)	50 (7.6)	0.5 (0.08)
South America	300	60 (20.0)	30 (10.0)	0.25 (0.08)
Europe	500	20 (4.0)	2 (0.4)	?
World	4511	1017 (14.5)	212 (3.0)	7.25 (0.1)

Data modified from Hetzel BS *et al.* (1987) and from Dunn JT and Van der Haar F (1990).
[a]Percentage of total populations given in parentheses.

most severely affected populations in the world. In most of these areas, cassava is consumed after methods of preparation that do not remove traces of thiocyanate precursors, because of inadequate soaking and washing. This aggravates the existing iodine deficiency in soil, water and food. The eastern and southern African countries are less affected than Central Africa, but there are also large populations affected by IDD at moderate levels.

With the continued leaching of iodine from the soil in heavy rainfall areas, and a greater tendency towards increased consumption of goitrogenic foodstuffs, especially cassava, the prevalance of IDD in Africa would be expected to increase unless preventive measures were vigorously implemented. Fortunately, active preventive measures are under way in at least 10 countries, with the Tanzanian programme usually quoted as the model programme in Africa.

Central and South America

In Central and South America, IDD occur widely. The most severe IDD, however, occur in the Andean region, extending the length of South America from Colombia through Ecuador, Peru, and Bolivia, to Argentina and Chile. Ecuador, Peru and Bolivia are particularly affected, and since 1983 there has been notable progress and impact of IDD control programmes in these countries.

Clinical Features

Complete lack of iodine is probably incompatible with life, but a deficiency produces a wide spectrum of ill effects which depend on the severity of the deficiency and the stage in life at which the deficiency is experienced. The effects are generally more severe and permanent when they occur early rather than later in life. In the adult, the consequences are more serious in women, particularly when pregnant, than in men. The spectrum of IDD is shown in **Table 2** and their clinical features are described below.

Goitre

Goitre is a thyroid gland which is bigger than normal, usually defined as 'lateral lobes of the gland bigger than the terminal phalanx of the subject being examined'. The commonest cause of a large thyroid gland is iodine deficiency.

Conversely, the commonest observable manifestation of iodine deficiency is goitre. Iodine deficiency causes thyroid growth through increased production of a controlling hormone called thyroid stimulating hormone (TSH). The low blood levels of thyroxine (T_4) which occur in iodine deficiency stimulate the

Table 2 The spectrum of IDD according to the life stage at which iodine deficiency occurs

Life stage	Major disorders
Fetus	Abortions, stillbirths, congenital anomalies, fetal hypothyroidism, increased perinatal and infant mortality, psychomotor defects, low birthweight, cretinism – neurological, myxoedematous, cretinoidism
Neonate and infancy	Neonatal hypothyroidism, neonatal goitre, increased neonatal and infant mortality, retarded mental and physical development
Childhood and adolescence	Goitre, juvenile hypothyroidism, impaired mental function, retarded physical development
Adult	Goitre with its complications – hypothyroidism, impaired mental and physical function, iodine-induced hyperthyroidism

Data modified from Hetzel BS *et al.* (1987).

pituitary, a small gland at the base of the brain, to produce TSH, which in turn stimulates the thyroid to work harder in order to produce thyroxine. Chronic adaptive increased TSH production stimulates the thyroid gland to grow, and this produces goitre. Although there may be other causes of goitre, chronic TSH stimulation of the thyroid gland is the leading factor for thyroid growth, and thus for goitre, in areas of iodine deficiency. Clinically, goitre sizes are classified into three grades, as shown in **Table 3**.

Table 3 The classification of goitre

0	No goitre
IA	Goitre detectable only by palpation and not visible even when the neck is fully extended
IB	Goitre palpable and visible only when the neck is fully extended; this stage includes nodular glands even if not goitrous
II	Goitre visible with the neck in normal position; palpation is not needed for diagnosis
III	Very large goitres that can be recognized from a considerable distance

Dunn JT *et al.* (1986).

The grading is done in the reverse order: III, II, IB, IA, 0. Whenever there is doubt between any two of the grades, the lower grade should be recorded. The total goitre rate (TGR) is the prevalence of grades I + II + III, and the visible goitre rate (VGR) that of grades II + III. This classification is appropriate for field studies, but for clinical purposes, more precise information can be obtained by other techniques, including scintigraphy and sonography.

In public health practice goitre becomes endemic, and therefore of public health significance, when its prevalance within any circumscribed area reaches either of the following rates:

1. TGR of 10% or more, or VGR of 1% or more in pre- and periadolescent individuals.
2. A prevalence of grade IA of at least 30% among adults.

Small goitres pose only a cosmetic problem, but very large (monstrous) goitres may compress the windpipe and produce choking. There are stories in Central Africa of people who have died in their sleep as a result of choking caused by monstrous goitres.

Hypothyroidism

Hypothyroidism is a condition in which the body does not receive enough thyroid hormone. In adults, hypothyroidism is clinically manifested by myxoedema, sluggishness, lethargy, dry skin, hoarse voice, cold intolerance and constipation. It is detected by finding low blood levels of thyroid hormones. In young children, in addition to the clinical features described for the adult, hypothyroidism also produces mental and growth retardation. The mental retardation may sometimes be very severe; at other times it may be rather mild and may escape detection unless specifically looked for.

In the newborn the condition is called *neonatal hypothyroidism*. Neonatal hypothyroidism is a well-recognized cause of permanent mental defect. This is because an adequate supply of thyroxine is important for brain development. Since only about one third of normal brain development occurs before birth and the other two thirds is completed in the first 2 years of life, iodine deficiency occurring during the period of brain development will have a serious, irreversible impact on mental development.

Endemic cretinism

The term 'endemic cretinism' refers to the congenital, severe, irreversible mental and growth retardation associated with endemic goitre in iodine-deficient populations. It must be distinguished from 'sporadic cretinism', which refers to congenital hypothyroidism, a condition which occurs in all parts of the world.

There does not seem to be a concise description of an endemic cretin. A person designated as an endemic cretin by one observer may have clinical features sharply different from a subject so designated by another observer. Since there is no objective test which defines an individual as an endemic cretin, and the only common feature in all cretins is perhaps mental deficiency, it has become a rule to define endemic cretinism by three main features derived from epidemiological concepts:

1. Endemic cretinism is associated with endemic goitre and severe iodine deficiency.
2. The clinical manifestations comprise severe to profound mental deficiency and characteristic facies. There are two possible manifestations, either a predominant neurological syndrome (neurological cretinism) including defects of hearing and speech, squint, and characteristic disorders of stance and gait (spastic diplegia) of varying degrees, or predominant features of hypothyroidism and stunted growth (myxoedematous cretinism).
   In some areas, one of the two types may predominate, but usually a combination of the two syndromes occurs.
3. In areas where adequate correction of iodine deficiency has been achieved, endemic cretinism is prevented.

The typical *neurological cretin* has predominantly neuromotor disturbances. Unless contractures prevent him/her from walking, he/she has a shuffling gait, sometimes a squint and often deaf-mutism. There may be difficulties in articulation, and motor disturbances of the arms and legs which are primarily central rather than peripheral. Developmental milestones are severely delayed. Surprisingly, a number of complex functions under neuronal control such as thirst, temperature control, sweating, sleeping and walking are well preserved. The thyroid glands are not always enlarged, and biochemical hormonal levels may be normal or only slightly hypothyroid.

The typical *myxoedematous cretin* has a remarkably short stature with very low bone ages compared to the chronological age. Neuromotor deficits are less profound than in the neurological cretin, and hearing is preserved. The most outstanding features are those of profound hypothyroidism typified clinically be myxoedema, when the skin and subcutaneous tissue are thickened, because of accumulation of mucin, and become dry and swollen. Other features include dry and swollen tongue, deep hoarse voice, apathy, mental deficiency, and slow reflex relaxation time with slow movements; they may also include umbilical hernia. The thyroid glands may be normal or moderately enlarged. Biochemical parameters also indicate profound hypothyroidism, with very low T_4 and T_3 and elevated plasma TSH levels.

The features of the myxoedematous cretin are essentially the same as those of the sporadic cretin, except for the association with severe iodine deficiency. To prevent confusion, the term 'congenital hypothyroidism' is now generally preferred to 'sporadic cretinism'.

In areas where IDD are endemic, iodine deficiency sometimes produces intellectual or growth retardation that is not severe enough to classify the individual as a cretin. Various terms, such as 'cretinoidism' or 'subcretin', have been used to describe the condition, but a better term is '*iodine deficiency developmental retardation*'. This condition is also a result of hypothyroidism caused by iodine deficiency.

Thus it is apparent that endemic cretinism displays a distinct spectrum from the typical neurological and myxoedematous cretin to the intermediate condition of subcretin. In all endemias in which one form dominates, examples of the other types can be found.

Although several explanations have been given for the differences in the clinical pattern of cretinism, none has yet been proven. All types disappear when iodine supplementation in a community reaches women in their reproductive ages, indicating that iodine deficiency is both a necessary and sufficient cause for their occurrence.

Reproductive failure

Compared with women living in iodine-sufficient areas, women in severely iodine-deficient areas experience more abortions, miscarriages, stillbirths and other problems of pregnancy and reproductive failure. They also bear children with higher rates of congenital abnormalities, lower birthweight and lower survival rates, as indicated by a higher perinatal and infant mortality.

Evidence indicates that these varying manifestations of iodine deficiency in the fetus probably arise from lowered T_4 levels in the blood of the iodine-deficient mother, and that the lower the level of maternal T_4, the greater the threat to the integrity of the fetus. All these manifestations can be prevented by iodine supplementation, indicating the serious impact of iodine deficiency on child survival and development.

Variability in clinical features in IDD

An interesting observation in the clinical effects of iodine deficiency is the wide variation in the clinical features, even when the level of iodine deficiency is similar. What causes the differences in manifestations of iodine deficiency among the various endemias is not known.

Also unexplained is the fact that some people exposed to the same level of iodine deficiency develop the manifestations (e.g. goitre) while others do not. Genetic variation, immunological factors, sex, age and growth factors have been mentioned as possible modifiers of expression of the conditions. There is some evidence from China that cyclic or chance availability of iodine around a threshold level may determine the clinical outcome of iodine deficiency in the infant. While questions remain unanswered with regard to pathogenesis and causes of the clinical variability, it is acknowledged that iodine prophylactic programmes prevent the development of the whole spectrum of IDD.

There is now no doubt that iodine deficiency is by far the most widespread cause of preventable retardation of physical, neuromotor and intellectual growth which demand the immediate inauguration of prophylactic programmes.

Biochemical assessment of iodine deficiency

The clinical features of iodine deficiency described above, especially goitre, represent an adaptive challenge to the maintenance of the availability of the thyroid hormone, T_3, for the tissues. Although the thyroid gland produces largely T_4, a substance intrinsically 10 times less active than T_3, most of the T_4 is converted into T_3 in the tissues.

The clinical features of iodine deficiency like goitre and cretinism are indicative of past iodine deficiency and not necessarily the current state of iodine nutriture. A person with a goitre or a cretin may be euthyroid (normal thyroid function).

As it is complicated, or often impossible, to obtain data on iodine intake in most populations, current iodine nutrition is classically evaluated through indirect methods, described below.

Urinary iodine excretion   Since almost all iodine in the body is eventually excreted in the urine, measurement of iodine in the urine remains the most precise index of dietary iodine intake.

Data from the literature indicate that mild IDD are generally associated with a population median daily urinary iodine excretion ranging from 50 to 100 µg; for moderate IDD the range is 25–50 µg; for severe IDD the figure is below 25 µg, which will frequently also be associated with endemic cretinism.

Thyroid hormones   The commonly assessed parameters of thyroid function are the levels of thyroid hormones and TSH. The classical hormonal profile in iodine deficiency is a marked decrease in serum T_4, a normal or slightly elevated serum T_3 and a markedly increased TSH. Serum T_4 directly reflects the iodine content of the thyroid gland and its low level in iodine deficiency stimulates a high level of TSH production. The maintenance of normal or slightly elevated T_3 is the result of a shift from T_4 to T_3 in synthetic activity and secretion of the thyroid gland exposed to iodine deficiency. This constitutes one of the most efficient adaptive mechanisms of the thyroid gland. When serum T_3 falls, this indicates that iodine deficiency must be very severe.

In iodine-deficient areas, screening for congenital hypothyroidism may constitute a most sensitive index for evaluating the severity of iodine deficiency. Definite shifts of TSH levels towards high values and of T_4 levels towards low values in cord blood are indicative of the sensitivity of newborns to iodine deficiency.

Groups at Risk

Every individual living in an iodine-deficient area is at risk of developing IDD. However, as a result of their higher iodine requirements, the following groups are at greatest risk:

1. Women of reproductive age.
2. Young children, particularly under-fives.
3. Periadolescent individuals.

Treatment

The objective of treatment for IDD is first and foremost to restore thyroid function to normal. Treatment is either by replacement thyroid medication or by iodine supplementation, and will depend on the clinical disorder under consideration. Cretinism, with its associated mental deficiency, cannot be reversed through treatment, although for the myxoedematous type both replacement thyroid medication and iodine supplementation are beneficial in reducing the effects of severe hypothyroidism. Treat-

ment of myxoedematous cretins may bring out neurological deficits that were not apparent before.

In some countries, every newborn child is tested for blood thyroxine, usually taken from a prick in the heel at the fourth and fifth day of life (neonatal hypothyroidism screening). If low levels of thyroxine are confirmed after further checking, replacement treatment with daily thyroxine is begun immediately. Provided that treatment is given within the first month of life, and no further exposure to iodine deficiency is experienced, the results are generally excellent.

In older children and adults, treatment is highly beneficial. Iodine administration is known to return thyroid function to normal within a period of 2–8 weeks, and all the clinical manifestations, including mental deficiency, hypothyroidism and goitre, can be reduced or eliminated. Large goitres, however, need surgical removal in addition to iodine supplementation. Mass treatment by iodine supplementation is also preventative.

Prevention

Prevention of IDD is usually achieved by the correction of iodine deficiency through mass iodine supplementation, which is also therapeutic at the individual level. The major items that have been iodized are salt, oil, bread and water. In general, the method of choice will depend on the severity of the IDD endemia, as shown in **Table 4**.

The use of iodized salt, bread or water will depend on the central production or processing system of these items in a particular country and their widespread dietary use. Sudan is experimenting with the use of iodized sugar. However, at a global level, iodized salt and iodized oil are the major methods used in the prevention of IDD.

Iodized salt

Iodized salt has been used effectively in the prevention of endemic goitre since the 1920s, when it was first introduced in Switzerland and the USA,

Table 4 Classification of IDD severity and the need for correction

		Clinical features				Median urinary iodine (I) excretion		
		Goitre rate (%)						
Stage	Severity	Total	Visible	Hypothyroidism	Cretinism	(μg I day^{-1})	(μg I dl^{-1})	Need for correction
I	Mild	10–29	1–4	±	0	50–100	3.5–5.0	Important
II	Moderate	30–49	5–9	++	+	25–49	2.0–3.4	Urgent
III	Severe	50–100	≥10	+++	++	<25	<2.0	Critical

followed by New Zealand in the 1940s and a number of European countries in the 1950s and 1960s. To date, iodized salt is the major prevention strategy in almost all countries where IDD is a problem of public health significance and long-term control measures have been initiated. The advantage of supplementing salt with iodine is that it is used by all sections of the community in fairly constant amounts, irrespective of social and economic status. The level of iodine added to salt must be enough to meet at the consumer level the minimum daily iodine requirement of 150 μg per person, and enough to cover the various losses which occur from the point of production to the point of consumption. In the West, where the risk of hypertension dictates that the recommended salt consumption level is 3–5 g per person per day, the iodate level that will provide the minimum daily intake of 150 μg per person is between 20 and 60 mg per kg of salt. In Africa, as a result of various factors such as humidity, high temperatures, poor packaging, delays in transit and open selling of salt, the level of salt iodation recommended by the World Health Organization/United Nations Children's Fund (WHO/UNICEF) and the International Council for the Control of Iodine Deficiency Disorders (ICCIDD) is 100 mg per kg of salt in order to achieve effective prevention and control of IDD.

Despite the simple technology involved in salt iodation and the proven effectiveness of iodized salt in the prevention of IDD, large populations continue to suffer from IDD, sometimes in the presence of salt iodization programmes operating in their areas. It should therefore be recognized that preparation of iodized salt is only the first stage of the social process by which it eventually reaches the consumer. The salt supply and distribution process in a particular country, the level of iodization and quality control measures, from the point of origin, through retail, to the consumer level, are all important. In addition, an effective salt iodization programme requires legislative and enforcement measures and, above all, public awareness and advocacy to create demand so that national governments are pressured to mobilize and allocate resources for sustained salt iodization.

Iodized oil

Iodized oil is the accepted major alternative to salt iodization for the prevention of IDD, particularly in situations where the problem of IDD is severe or moderate and for various reasons a salt iodization programme cannot be launched immediately. The principal methods for the administration of iodized oil are the intramuscular injection or the oral route. Thus, unlike salt iodization programmes, direct contact must be made with each subject who will receive the iodized oil. This limits the coverage of iodized oil programmes, so that they are often seen as stop-gap measures in severe and moderate IDD endemias before a salt iodization programme is introduced.

Experience with the deep intramuscular administration of iodized oil since the 1970s indicates that a single injection can provide adequate stores of iodine for 3–5 years. The recommended dose is 480 mg of iodine (1 ml) for subjects 1 year or older and 240 mg of iodine (0.5 ml) for infants aged under 1 year. The possible factors responsible for the sustained duration of effect include the high dose, the slow release from the muscle, recycling of iodine by the thyroid gland and its storage in depot fat.

Experience with oral iodized oil is more recent and thus more limited than the intramuscular administration. Although precise guidelines for its optimal dose and duration of effect are not well established, it is recommended that a single dose of 480 mg of iodine (1 ml), which can provide adequate levels of iodine for 1–2 years, should be used.

Most recent programmes have been using a single dose of two capsules of iodized oil, each containing about 190 mg of iodine, which means a dose of about 380 mg of iodine for 1–2 years. The attraction of oral administration is that it is cheaper and simpler to administer than the intramuscular route, since it does not require the medical skill necessary for injections. Moreover, it avoids the risks of the transmission of AIDS and hepatitis B inherent in mass injections.

There are two principal methods of conducting iodized oil distribution programmes, whether by injection or the oral route. The first approach is to distribute the oil through the primary health care system, where health personnel prescribe to target communities or integrate with other programmes such as those of immunization. The second aproach is to organize small teams that travel, campaign-style, within the target area and distribute the oil.

Iodine-induced thyroidism

A few cases of hyperthyroidism (thyrotoxicosis) have been described in places where mass prophylactic iodization programmes using salt, bread or oil have been instituted. The condition, largely confined to those over 40 years of age, can be readily controlled with antithyroid drugs or radioiodine, but in many cases spontaneous remission is likely to occur. Iodine-induced thyrotoxicosis (or Jod–Basedow disease) is caused by elevated levels of thyroid hormones which produce palpitations (rapid heart rate) and other features of a nervous state, such as trembling, excessive sweating, lack of sleep, and loss of weight and strength. The elevated thyroid hormones for those over 40 years with lifelong iodine deficiency is believed to be caused by autonomous thyroid glands that continue to turn over iodine rapidly, despite an increase in intake. Although iodine supplementation should generally be minimized for those over 40 years because of the risk of thyrotoxicosis, the control of iodine deficiency makes the condition disappear, and may thus be classified as an iodine deficiency disorder.

In very rare instances, iodism, which simply means sensitivity to iodine, indicated by a skin rash, may appear in those who are allergic to iodine. Since its occurrence is very rare, and the allergic reaction is usually mild, the slight risk of iodism should not prevent iodine supplementation programmes from being launched.

The Elimination of IDD

Since the formation of the ICCIDD in Kathmandu, Nepal, in March 1986, an international movement, championed by ICCIDD and supported by WHO, UNICEF and other donors, has emerged. The role of ICCIDD in reducing the gap between knowledge and its application in the control of IDD has been so successful that the World Health Assembly in May 1990 and the first World Summit for Children, attended by over 70 heads of state and 80 other government representatives in September 1990, accepted a global goal of the virtual elimination of IDD by the year 2000. The global action plan encompasses advocacy, information and monitoring systems at the global level and a series of IDD working groups at the regional level. At the national level, baseline assessment, planning seminars, development of national IDD control programmes, including laboratory services for monitoring and evaluation, are also included. The ICCIDD believes that the elimination of IDD as a major public health problem by the year 2000 is achievable if the necessary resources are made available.

See also: **Calcium**: Physiology. **Food Fortification**: Importance in the Diet. **Fruits and Vegetables**: Nutritional Value. **Growth and Development**: Physiological Aspects. **Ultratrace Elements**: Physiology.

Further Reading

Dunn JT and Van der Haar F (1990) *A Practical Guide to the Correction of Iodine Deficiency.* ICCIDD/UNICEF/WHO Technical Manual No. 3. Geneva: World Health Organization.

Dunn JT, Pretell EA, Daza CH and Viteri F (eds) (1986) *Towards the Eradication of Endemic Goitre, Cretinism and Iodine Deficiency.* Pan American Health Organization and WHO Scientific Publication No. 502. Geneva: World Health Organization.

Hetzel BS (1989) *The Story of Iodine Deficiency. An International Challenge in Nutrition.* Oxford: Oxford University Press.

Hetzel BS, Dunn JT and Stanbury JB (eds) (1987) The prevention and control of iodine deficiency disorders. ICCIDD Monograph. Amsterdam: Elsevier Science Publishers BV (Biochemical Division).

Stanbury JB (1986) Aspects of the clinical findings in endemic cretinism. In: Medeiros-Neto G, Maciel RMB and Halpern A (eds) *Iodine Deficiency Disorders and Congenital Hypothyroidism*, pp 7–14. São Paulo: Ache.

IRON

Physiology, Dietary Sources and Requirements

S R Lynch, Eastern Virginia Medical School, New York, USA

Copyright © 1998 Academic Press

Iron plays a central role in metabolic processes involving oxygen transport and storage as well as oxidative metabolism and cellular growth. The fact that it readily serves as an electron donor or acceptor accounts both for its critical metabolic role and its potential toxicity. Iron-containing compounds function as carriers for oxygen and electrons and as catalysts for oxidation and hydroxylation reactions. Ionic iron can also participate in reactions that produce toxic free radicals. Free radicals may in turn damage cellular constituents. It is therefore not surprising that body iron content is controlled within narrow limits, and that the metal itself is transported and stored as a component of specific iron-binding proteins rather than as the free cation. This article reviews the functional role of iron in the body, the physiological processes responsible for the control of internal iron exchange and iron balance, and the consequences of iron deficiency and excess. Some aspects of the physiology of iron that are specifically related to impaired iron balance and iron deficiency anaemia are discussed later.

Body Iron Distribution

The normal human body contains 3–4 g of iron (40–50 mg per kg of bodyweight; **Table 1**), 75% (approximately 36 mg kg^{-1}) of which is present in metabolically active compounds. The remainder is contained in a storage pool (approximately 10 mg kg^{-1} in men and 5 mg kg^{-1} in menstruating women) which is readily available if metabolically active iron is depleted for any reason.

Functional iron compartment

Haem proteins   Most of the functional iron in the body is present in the form of haem proteins, i.e. proteins with an iron protoporphyrin IX prosthetic group.

Haemoglobin, which is made up of four globin chains, each with an attached haem group, transports oxygen to the tissues. It is quantitatively the most important haem protein and contains 80% of all functional iron.

Myoglobin is found in the sarcoplasm of muscles. It has a structure similar to haemoglobin but contains only one globin chain attached to a single haem group and accounts for a further 10% of functional iron. Myoglobin functions as an oxygen store, ensuring an adequate oxygen supply during muscle contraction.

Despite its vital metabolic role, all other tissue iron represents only a very small fraction of total body iron. The *cytochromes* are a group of *haem-containing electron transport enzymes* that are essential for the oxidative metabolism necessary to generate adenosine triphosphate (ATP) as well as for the oxidative degradation of drugs and endogenous substrates. *Catalase and peroxidase* are involved in the reduction of endogenously generated hydrogen peroxide.

Nonhaem tissue iron   In mitochondria, nonhaem compounds account for more iron than do those containing haem. This group of enzymes includes the iron sulfur flavoproteins such as xanthine oxidase, NADH (the reduced form of nicotinamide adenine dinucleotide) dehydrogenase and succinate dehydrogenase, as well as other nonhaem enzymes, e.g. ribonucleotide reductase and phenylalanine hydroxylase. In addition, iron is necessary in a loosely bound form for the activity of other enzymes, such as those responsible for the hydroxylation of proline and lysine in protocollagen, during synthesis of collagen.

All functional iron compounds are constantly being degraded and replaced by newly synthesized material. Internal iron exchange therefore plays a crucial role in preserving normal iron-dependent metabolic processes.

Iron transport and storage

Iron entering the plasma is rapidly bound to the specific iron transport protein, *transferrin*. The iron-free protein, apotransferrin, is a single-chain glycoprotein (M_r 79 570) with two nonidentical iron-binding sites that have a high affinity for ferric iron under physiological conditions (effective stability constant, 10^{24} M^{-1}). Plasma apotransferrin is synthesized predominantly in the liver. It exists in the plasma in the iron-free form or as monoferric or diferric transferrin since iron loading at each binding site is a random process.

Iron delivery from plasma transferrin to the tissues is mediated by a specific transferrin receptor which is a glycoprotein dimer composed of two identical subunits (M_r 94 000) linked by a disulphide bond. Transferrin receptors are expressed on the surfaces of all cells in proportion to their iron requirements. Large numbers are present on cells with high iron requirements, e.g. developing red blood cells and placenta.

At the pH of plasma and extravascular fluid bathing cell surfaces, receptors have very little affinity for apotransferrin and the highest affinity for diferric transferrin (2–7 × 10^{-9} M). Once bound, the transferrin–receptor complex, together with its attached iron, is internalized by the cell in an endosome which

Table 1   Distribution of iron in adult human beings

	Men, total body content		Women[a], total body content	
	(mg)	*(mg kg^{-1})*	*(mg)*	*(mg kg^{-1})*
Functional				
Haemoglobin	2300	31	1700	28
Myoglobin	320	4	180	3
Haem enzymes	80	1	60	1
Nonhaem enzymes	100	1	76	1
Storage				
Ferritin	540	7	200	3
Haemosiderin	235	3	100	2

[a]Age range 18–44 years.

then fuses with an acidic vesicle (pH <5.5). The fall in pH results in release of iron from the transferrin. The iron is utilized or stored in the cell. The transferrin receptor remains intact, but acquires a higher affinity for apotransferrin than for mono- or diferric transferrin because of the lower pH. The complex is transported back to the cell surface, where the apotransferrin is released back into the plasma.

Iron that is entering cells and is not immediately used for the synthesis of metabolically active compounds is stored in the form of *ferritin*. Apoferritin is a hollow, spherical protein shell composed of 24 subunits which may be of two types, differing slightly in molecular weight – L (M_r 19 700) and H (M_r 21 100). Each complete apoferritin molecule can store as many as 4500 iron atoms within its central core as ferric hydroxyphosphate. Iron enters and leaves the intact protein shell through channels about 1 nm wide.

Catabolism of cellular ferritin may result in the formation of a second type of iron storage protein, *haemosiderin*, which is water-insoluble and has both a higher iron content and a slower turnover than ferritin.

The maintenance of intracellular iron homeostasis requires the coordinated regulation of iron acquisition, utilization and storage. Enlargement of the intracellular transit iron pool stimulates ferritin synthesis and decreases the expression of transferrin receptors. Intracellular iron depletion has the opposite effect. In most cells regulation occurs primarily at a posttranscriptional level and is mediated by iron regulatory proteins (IRPs) that bind to iron responsive elements (IREs) on the 3^1 or 5^1 untranslated regions of the messenger RNAs (mRNAs) for transferrin receptor and the H- and L-chains of ferritin, respectively. Low cellular iron levels favour increased binding of the IRPs to the IREs repressing the synthesis of ferritin, but stabilizing transferrin receptor mRNA against cellular ribonucleases, thereby increasing transferrin receptor expression and cellular iron uptake. High cellular iron leads to decreased IRP binding with a decrease in iron uptake and increased ferritin synthesis and iron storage.

The above description characterizes iron transport and storage in most cells of the human body. However erythroid cells have very high iron requirements and appear to possess mechanisms for regulating iron uptake at a transcriptional level that can override post-transcriptional control. Iron transport and storage by the macrophages of the spleen, bone marrow and liver are also different. These cells are involved primarily in processing haemoglobin derived from senescent red blood cells, with the return of the iron to the plasma or its storage within the cell for future need. Unlike all other body cells macrophages derive almost no iron from plasma transferrin.

At the end of their lifespan red blood cells are phagocytosed by macrophages, predominantly in the spleen. Haem is separated from the globin and rapidly catabolized by the enzyme, haem oxygenase. Iron is released and either returned to the plasma within a few hours or incorporated into the storage compartment of the cell with a more gradual return to the plasma (half-life about 7 days). Normally, two-thirds of the iron is released immediately, but this fraction may be either increased when demands are high or reduced when less iron is required and the storage pool more abundant.

Internal Iron Exchange

The development of radioiron tracers made it possible to quantify the processes involved in iron exchange described above. Since 80% of the body's functional iron is in the haemoglobin of the circulating red blood cells, measurements of internal iron exchange are dominated by the requirements of this compartment (**Fig. 1**). Complete exchange of the iron in the circulating red blood cell compartment occurs every 4 months. This involves rapid transfer of iron by plasma transferrin. Only 3–4 mg iron is found in the plasma at any one time, but 35 mg is transported through this compartment each day. Most of it comes from haemoglobin catabolism in macrophages. Two-thirds (24 mg per day) is delivered to erythroid precursors in the bone marrow for the synthesis of new haemoglobin. While there is some iron loss owing to ineffective red cell production or the removal of iron not used for haemoglobin synthesis from red cell precursors, most of the iron (70%) is returned to the circulation as haemoglobin in erythrocytes. Erythrocytes have a lifespan of about 120 days. The senescent cells are catabolized in the macrophages of the liver, spleen and bone marrow, completing the cycle.

Most of the iron lost during red cell production and the iron derived from senescent red cells is processed by macrophages. Thus a quantity of iron equivalent to about 1% of the functional haemoglobin in the circulating red cell compartment (22 mg iron) enters the macrophages each day with a corresponding quantity being released to the plasma.

A smaller but quantitatively significant daily exchange occurs between the plasma iron and storage iron in hepatocytes. The rate of exchange and direction of net flow is dependent on serum iron concentration and transferrin saturation. A high serum

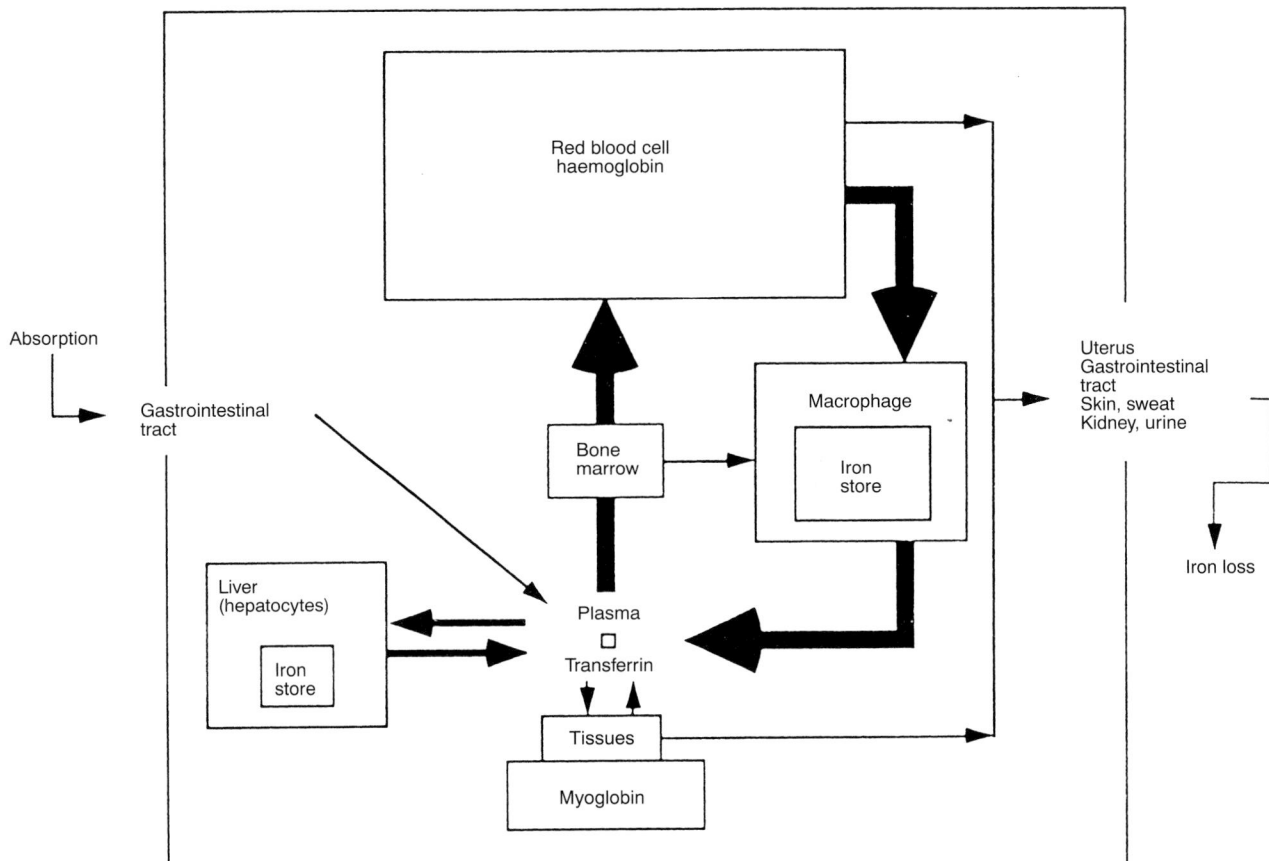

Figure 1   Body iron exchange.

iron concentration favours the accumulation of iron in the liver.

Finally, a minor fraction of the daily iron turnover (about 3 mg per day) is transferred between the plasma and the extravascular transferrin compartment and approximately two thirds of this (2 mg per day) exchanges with the tissues, supplying iron to haem and nonhaem iron-dependent enzymes.

Iron Absorption and Excretion

The body iron content of healthy human beings is held within narrow limits. This is primarily a consequence of the iron being located in tightly regulated functional compartments. Iron stores that usually account for only 15–30% of the total may vary 25-fold without any apparent physiological impairment.

Iron loss

In contrast to the dynamic transfer of iron between body compartments, exchange with the external environment is minimal. No adjustable excretory mechanism exists, but a small obligatory loss occurs with the physiological turnover of skin epithelium and the cells of the gastrointestinal and urinary tracts

(Fig. 1). Low concentrations of iron are also present in sweat, bile and urine. In addition, small quantities of blood are present in the faeces. Finally, menstruation accounts for a significant proportion of the iron lost by women of child-bearing age.

In normal men the loss of iron from the body is about 1 mg per day. This is balanced by an equivalent absorption. Complete iron exchange with the environment in a normal man would therefore be expected to take about 10 years. In women menstrual losses account for an extra 0.5 mg per day, which is again matched by a higher rate of absorption.

Iron absorption

Typical Western diets contain approximately 1.5 mg iron per MJ. From the point of view of absorption, food iron may be considered to exist in one of three forms. Ten per cent or less is present as haem derived chiefly from haemoglobin and myoglobin in meat. Haem iron is readily absorbed and this small fraction of dietary iron may supply a third of the iron requirements of individuals eating a mixed meat-containing diet. The remainder of the iron (90% or more in Western diets and often virtually 100% in the diets of developing countries) must be solubilized for absorption. If solubilized, nonhaem iron derived from all dietary sources enters a common pool in the lumen of the upper small intestine before absorption. A variable proportion of nonhaem iron is insoluble and unavailable for absorption. This iron is generally regarded as contaminant iron. Much of it may enter food products during storage or processing, particularly in developing countries.

Absorption of soluble nonhaem iron from the common pool is quite variable. It is governed both by the body's requirement and the balance between enhancing and inhibiting ligands in the diet which either promote uptake by mucosal cells (increase bioavailability) or render the iron in the pool unavailable for absorption. Enhancing factors include ascorbic acid, meat and fish tissue. Low gastric luminal pH, resulting from hydrochloric acid secretion by the stomach or from the ingestion of acidic foods, also promotes nonhaem iron absorption. The most powerful inhibitors are found in vegetable foods and include phytates, tannates, vegetable proteins and calcium and phosphate.

Absorption of both haem and nonhaem iron is maximal in the upper small intestine, partly because the luminal conditions (particularly lower pH) favour solubilization and absorption of nonhaem iron, but also because cells in this region show the greatest ability to respond to changes in body iron needs. Absorption may be considered to occur in three phases: (1) uptake across the mucosal cell brush border; (2) a phase that involves either rapid tranfer of iron through the mucosal cells or its retention in the cellular ferritin store; (3) transfer from the mucosal cell to plasma transferrin. Most of the iron retained in the cell is lost when the cell exfoliates.

Haem iron enters the mucosal cell through a pathway different from that for nonhaem iron. It is transferred into the cell as the intact haem moiety. Its absorption is relatively little affected by dietary factors. Once within the cell, iron is released from haem by the enzyme, haem oxygenase. It joins an absorption pathway common to both haem and nonhaem iron.

Despite years of research, the precise molecular mechanisms involved in the uptake of iron into mucosal cells and its transfer to the plasma remain a subject of controversy. Nevertheless, there is considerable evidence that the process is tightly regulated, particularly for the larger nonhaem iron pool with control points at the mucosal uptake and cellular transfer steps. Percentage absorption of bioavailable food iron may vary as much as 20-fold. Variations in the percentage absorption of haem iron are much smaller, approximately twofold.

The factors regulating absorption remain obscure but there is overwhelming evidence that the rate of iron absorption is closely regulated by the size of iron stores. In health this is the only important controlling factor yet identified, and there is a close inverse correlation between the size of iron stores and iron absorption. Increased absorption inappropriate to need may occur in the presence of pathologically accelerated erythropoietic activity in conditions such as thalassaemia major.

Iron Deficiency

In Western countries iron deficiency most often occurs when there is a relatively sudden increase in iron requirements or iron losses, e.g. during pregnancy or in association with pathological blood loss.

The physiological importance of both the storage iron compartment and the capacity for the rapid transfer of iron through the plasma in preventing overt functional iron deficiency is illustrated by the effect of blood loss. In response to significant anaemia caused by bleeding, individuals with an iron store of 1000 mg can mobilize 40 mg per day, allowing rapid restoration of the functional deficit. On the other hand, an individual who lacks storage iron and depends on absorption from an average diet for additional iron will increase delivery to the bone marrow by only 2–4 mg per day. Red cell production is increased by a small margin. Thus loss of iron from the major functional compartments is rapidly corrected when stores are adequate, but very slowly replaced by absorption, even when dietary iron bioavailability is relatively high. If meal iron bioavailability is low, positive balance may not be achieved, leading to chronic iron deficiency anaemia.

Negative iron balance leads to a reduction in the iron content of all functional compartments. Anaemia caused by reduced haemoglobin synthesis is the most easily documented. However, iron availability to support metabolic systems in the tissues is reduced concurrently, and the physiological consequences of iron deficiency are related both to impaired oxygen delivery and to reduced metabolic tissue iron. The consequences of anaemia *per se* are dealt with in the section on iron deficiency anaemia.

Tissue iron deficiency

Mucosal and epithelial abnormalities Angular stomatitis, glossitis, postcricoid webbing of the oesophagus associated with painful dysphagia (Patterson–Kelly or Plummer–Vinson syndrome), atrophic gastritis and koilonychia (spoon-shaped fingernails) have all been attributed to tissue iron deficiency. These clinical findings appear to be less common in recent years and a marked geographic variation in prevalence has frequently been noted, suggesting that factors other than iron deficiency may play an important role. A specific role for iron is most likely in patients with gastric mucosal atrophy and for duodenal villous atrophy in children.

Immunity and infection   Several laboratory tests of immune function are abnormal in patients with iron deficiency anaemia. Lymphocyte proliferation in response to the mitogens, phytohaemagglutinin and concanavalin A, are impaired, demonstrating defective T cell immunity. Impaired intracellular bacterial killing by polymorphonuclear leucocytes, and decreased reduction of the dye, nitroblue tetrazolium, have also been documented. These defects appear to result from diminished myeloperoxidase activity. The clinical importance of such findings is uncertain although some studies have suggested that the administration of iron to iron-deficient individuals may reduce the prevalence of enteritis and influenza-like illnesses. Iron deficiency does appear to be an important predisposing factor in chronic mucocutaneous candidiasis.

Skeletal muscle dysfunction   A significant limitation of the ability to perform endurance physical activity has emerged as an important consequence of chronic iron deficiency. Animal studies conducted by Finch and coworkers demonstrated that iron-deficient rats show a marked impairment of running ability which is unrelated to haemoglobin level. It results from impaired oxidative metabolism in iron-depleted muscles. Field studies from many developing countries suggest that a similar disability reduces an iron individual's ability to carry out prolonged physical work.

Behavioural and neurological abnormalities   An intriguing sensory disturbance encountered both in children and adults who are iron-deficient is the perversion of taste leading to the consumption of nonfood items (pica) or compulsive ice eating (pagophagia). The specificity of the association has been confirmed by the study of patients in whom iron deficiency was induced by phlebotomy alone, making the contribution of confounding nutritional and social factors unlikely. It is corrected by iron repletion.

Recently, an increasing body of evidence connecting iron deficiency in early childhood with impaired psychomotor development and cognitive function has accumulated. While the nature and the extent of the problem remains controversial, there is considerable cause for concern. Animal studies indicate that a brief period of iron deficiency in young animals reduces brain iron content. The later administration of iron readily corrects body iron stores but has much less effect on brain iron. Some recent observations suggest that long-term effects on behaviour and cognitive function resulting from iron deficiency in early childhood may not be corrected completely by later iron administration.

Iron Toxicity

Acute iron toxicity

The ingestion of large quantities of elemental iron can cause acute iron poisoning. This occurs most often in young children who may eat iron tablets as 'sweets'. The pathological consequences include a severe necrotizing gastroenteritis as well as disseminated intravascular coagulation, liver and cardiac injury. Death may ensue if the dose is large or treatment not instituted immediately.

Chronic iron toxicity

More important from the nutritional point of view is the gradual accumulation which occurs when the quantity of iron entering the body exceeds requirements by even a small margin. The body has no means of increasing iron excretion significantly, making positive iron balance inevitable if regulation of absorption is impaired, or if the diet contains a quantity of available iron that overwhelms the absorptive control mechanism. Excess iron can also be introduced through the parenteral route (blood transfusion, parenteral iron administration).

Impaired regulation of absorption   *Hereditary haemochromatosis* is the commonest cause of iron overload resulting from the impaired regulation of iron absorption, and the commonest form of iron overload in the USA and western Europe. It is an autosomal recessive disorder with a gene frequency reported to be as high as 1 in 10 in some Caucasian populations. A haemochromatosis gene (HFE) candidate and mutation with structural similarities to MHC class 1 molecules was recently discovered 4 megabases telomeric of HLA-A on the short arm of chromosome 6. Eighty-three percent of unrelated American patients with hereditary haemochromatosis were found to be homozygous for a single gene mutation, Cys282Tyr in this study. However, the mechanistic connection between intestinal iron absorption and the function of Class 1 genes remains to be elucidated. Phenotypic expression occurs only in homozygotes, is much more likely to occur in males, and depends on iron intake.

The clinical disorder is characterized by a rate of iron absorption that is inappropriately high for body iron stores. Downregulation of nonhaem iron absorption is impaired and haem iron absorption virtually unregulated. Equally important to the pathogenesis of the condition is the presence of an abnormally high serum iron and transferrin saturation associated with disordered iron distribution within the body, favouring iron accumulation in the parenchymal cells of organs such as the liver, heart and pancreas. Comparatively less iron is located in the normal macrophage iron store.

Although the defective control of absorption is an inborn error of metabolism manifest from birth, the prevalence of the clinical syndrome is highest in men over the age of 40. Excess iron is accumulated slowly because maximal absorption from the average Western diet is only 3–5 mg per day. Once the total body iron load has increased to 15 g or more (a process which takes 15–20 years), organ damage becomes evident.

The exact mechanism by which the iron damages tissues has not been established, but lipid peroxidation in membranes and subcellular organelles, as well as iron-induced lysosomal disruption are probably involved. The clinical consequences include increased skin pigmentation, cirrhosis of the liver associated with an increased risk of developing liver cancer, congestive cardiac failure and cardiac arrhythmias, diabetes mellitus and hypogonadism owing both to end-organ and pituitary dysfunction. In addition, arthropathy characterized by chondrocalcinosis and involvement of the second and third metacarpophalangeal joints of the hand are common complications of hereditary haemochromatosis.

If hereditary haemochromatosis is identified before significant iron overload has occurred, all of the clinical findings may be averted by iron removal. Therapeutic phlebotomy is usually employed. Unchecked progressive iron overload is associated with severe irreversible morbidity and a significantly shortened lifespan.

Excessive iron absorption from a normal diet may also occur in certain iron-loading anaemias, chronic liver disease and porphyria cutanea tarda.

Dietary iron overload is a form of chronic iron toxicity unique to the indigenous population of several countries in southern Africa. Traditional acidic fermented beverages brewed in containers made from iron become contaminated with iron at concentrations of 15–40 mg l^{-1}. Beer consumption may supply 50–100 mg of available dietary iron per day. Total body iron burdens comparable to those encountered in hereditary haemochromatosis are encountered. However, at least in the early stages of the disorder, iron distribution in the body tends to be different, with more iron accumulating in the normal storage cells (macrophages of the spleen, liver, bone marrow and muscle). While organ damage with progression to cirrhosis and the development of diabetes mellitus does occur, two other conditions are commonly encountered – ascorbic acid deficiency and osteoporosis. Ascorbic acid deficiency results from accelerated catabolism in patients with severe iron overload, often in association with a low dietary intake. The factors responsible for the osteoporosis remain poorly understood.

See also: **Anaemia (Anemia)**: Iron-Deficiency Anaemia. **Ascorbic Acid**: Physiology, Dietary Sources and Requirements. **Bioavailability**: Definition and General Aspects. **Exercise**: Physiology of Skeletal Muscle. **Immunity**: Physiological Aspects; Role of Iron and Zinc. **Meat, Poultry and Meat Products**: Nutritional Value. **Osteoporosis**: Aetiology; Treatment and Prevention.

Further Reading

Bothwell TH, Charlton RW, Cook JD and Finch CA (1979) *Iron Metabolism in Man*. Oxford: Blackwell Scientific Publications.

Bothwell TH, Charlton RW and Motulsky AG (1989) Hemochromatosis. In: Scriver CR, Beaudet AL, Sly WS and Valle D (eds) *The Metabolic Basis of Inherited Disease* 6th edn, pp 1433–1462. New York: McGraw-Hill.

Cook JD and Lynch SR (1986) The liabilities of iron deficiency. *Blood* **68**:803–809.

Dallman PR (1982) Manifestations of iron deficiency. *Seminars in Hematology* **19**:19–30.

Finch CA and Huebers H (1982) Perspectives in iron metabolism. *New England Journal of Medicine* **306**:1520–1528.

Klausner RD, Rounault TA and Harford JB (1993) Regulating the fate of mRNA: The control of cellular iron metabolism. *Cell* **72**:19–28.

Ponka P (1997) Tissue-specific regulation of iron metabolism and heme synthesis: distinct control mechanisms in erythroid cells. *Blood* **89**:1–25.

Ischaemic heart disease *see* **Coronary Heart Disease**: Lipid Theory of Coronary Heart Disease.

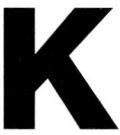

K

Keshan disease *see* **Selenium**: Physiology, Dietary Sources and Requirements.

KETOSIS

Biochemical and Dietary Aspects

D H Williamson, Radcliffe Infirmary, Oxford, UK

Copyright © 1998 Academic Press

The two ketone bodies, acetoacetate ($CH_3COCH_2COO^-$) and D-3-hydroxybutyrate ($CH_3CHOHCH_2COO^-$), are the only freely soluble lipids in the circulation.

The name ketone bodies originates from the German *Ketonkörper* (literally, ketones excreted from the body) and refers to their discovery in the urine of diabetic patients in the latter half of the nineteenth century. In reality, the term is a misnomer because 3-hydroxybutyrate is not a ketone. It arose because the reagent originally used reacted positively with ketones in diabetic urine. Acetone (CH_3COCH_3), the product of the spontaneous decarboxylation of acetoacetate, is also a ketone and is present in blood and urine when the plasma concentration of acetoacetate is elevated. It is excreted via the kidneys and lungs and is responsible for the sweet smell on the breath in ketotic states.

The association of ketone bodies with the pathology of diabetes resulted in the view that they were toxic waste products. It is only in the past 30 years that this view has been convincingly reversed. Two factors led to this change, namely the development of an enzymatic method for the determination of acetoacetate and 3-hydroxybutyrate, which in turn allowed the dramatic finding of Cahill and colleagues in 1967 that adult human brain removed appreciable amounts of ketone bodies from the circulation in prolonged starvation.

The aim in this contribution is to review (a) the formation of ketone bodies in physiological and pathological situations, and (b) the function of ketone bodies as physiological substrates and signals.

Formation of Ketone Bodies

It is well established that in humans and other mammals the only organ that contributes significant amounts of ketone bodies to the blood is the liver; this organ, unlike peripheral tissues, is unable to utilize ketone bodies to any appreciable extent. More recently it has been found that during the suckling period (high-fat diet) the intestine also has the capacity (about 10% of the liver) to produce ketone bodies. Whether ketone bodies are used *in situ* or are transported via the portal blood to supplement the existing hyperketonaemia is an open question.

The main blood-borne substrates for the synthesis of ketone bodies (ketogenesis) are the nonesterified fatty acids; others of lesser importance are the branched-chain amino acids, leucine and isoleucine. In addition, acetate (sources: intestinal fermentation, in vinegar or an oxidation product of ethanol) is a ketogenic substrate.

Long-chain fatty acids contained in dietary lipids do not enter the portal blood directly, but are esterified in the intestinal cells, packaged with proteins and phospholipids to form chylomicrons (large lipoproteins), and transported via the lymphatic system to the thoracic duct where they enter the blood. In contrast, the short- and medium-chain fatty acids (below C_{14}) contained in dairy products or in clinical medium-chain triacylglycerol preparations are directly absorbed as the respective fatty acids and are transported to the liver via the portal blood (**Fig. 1**).

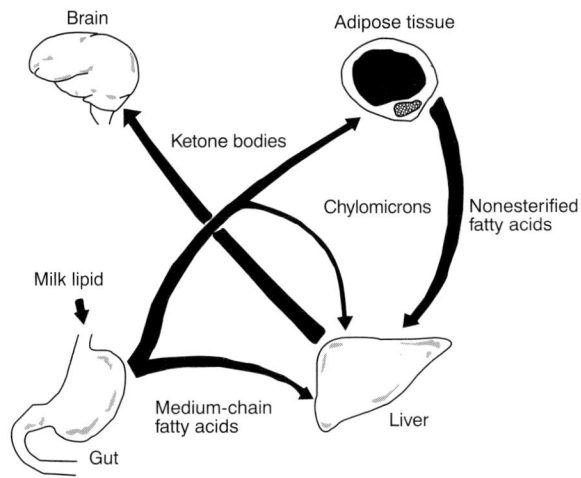

Figure 1   Intertissue fluxes of substrates in the suckling neonate. Thickness of line denotes rate of flux.

The long-chain fatty acids in the plasma are bound to albumin and are released from adipose tissue triacylglycerol stores by the process of lipolysis.

Extrahepatic regulation

A key factor in the regulation of ketogenesis is the availability of nonesterified long-chain fatty acids to the liver, which in turn is controlled by their release from adipose tissue. The enzyme responsible for the initiation of the hydrolysis of stored triacylglycerols to fatty acids is hormone-sensitive lipase. As its name implies, this enzyme is exquisitely sensitive to hormones: adrenaline (in the plasma) and noradrenaline (released from sympathetic nerve endings) are activators, whereas insulin inhibits the activity. In small mammals glucagon is also an activator of the enzyme, but this does not seem to be the case in the human.

Insulin has an additional effect on the net release of long-chain fatty acids from adipose tissue in that it stimulates their reesterification to triacylglycerols. Thus after a high-carbohydrate meal, when insulin secretion and its concentration in the plasma is high, the release of fatty acids from adipose tissue is suppressed and their concentration in the plasma is low (**Fig. 2**). In contrast, during stress, when adrenaline and noradrenaline are elevated, the release of fatty acids is increased and their plasma concentration is high.

In experimental animals increased plasma ketone body concentrations (hyperketonaemia) can inhibit adipose tissue lipolysis (a) indirectly by increasing the secretion of insulin or (b) by a direct effect on the tissue (**Fig. 3**). This can be viewed as a feedback mechanism for controlling the rate of ketogenesis via fatty acid supply to the liver, but whether this is

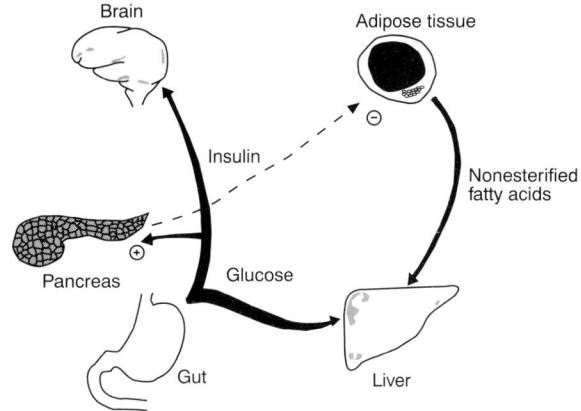

Figure 2   Intertissue fluxes of substrates in the fed state. Thickness of line denotes rate of flux.

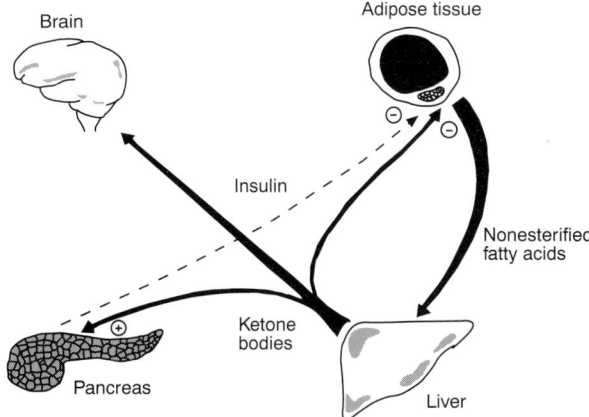

Figure 3   Role of ketone bodies as feedback regulators.

important in the human is not known. In contrast, the supply of short- and medium-chain fatty acids to the liver is mainly dependent on the dietary intake and on the proportion that escapes further metabolism in the intestinal tract; there is no known involvement of hormones in the process.

Intrahepatic regulation

There are situations (e.g. stress) where the supply of fatty acids to the liver may be increased, but there is no necessity to increase the availability of ketone bodies to the peripheral tissues. Consequently, there is a requirement that the rate of hepatic ketogenesis should be controlled independently of the supply of fatty acids. However, it must be stressed that without an increase in the supply of fatty acids the rate of ketogenesis cannot increase.

Much of the current interest is concerned with how the intrahepatic metabolism of fatty acids (**Fig. 4**) is regulated. Long-chain fatty acids entering the liver have three main fates:

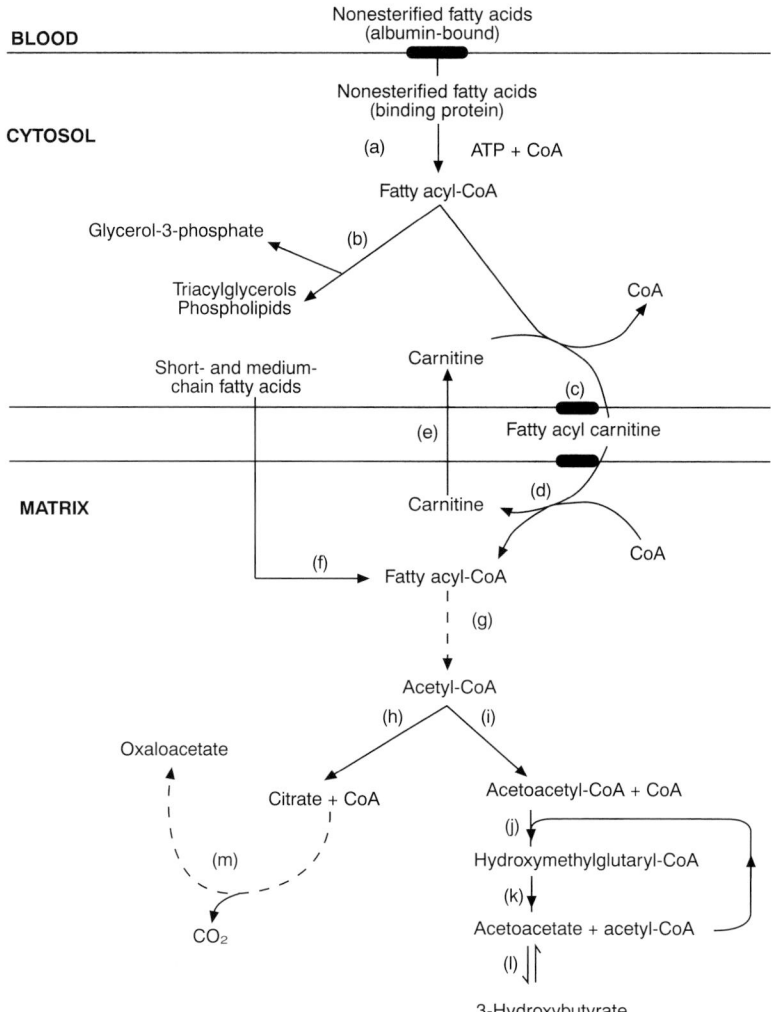

Figure 4 Pathway of fatty acid catabolism in liver. Enzymes involved: (a) long-chain fatty acyl-CoA synthetase; (b) glycerol-3-phosphate acyl-CoA transferase; (c) CAT I; (d) CAT II; (e) carnitine exchange; (f) short- and medium-chain fatty acyl-CoA synthetase; (g) fatty acid oxidation complex; (h) citrate synthase; (i) acetoacetyl-CoA thiolase; (j) hydroxymethylglutaryl-CoA synthase; (k) hydroxymethylglutaryl-CoA lyase; (l) hydroxybutyrate dehydrogenase; (m) tricarboxylate cycle.

1. They can be re-esterified to phospholipids and triacylglycerols and then be secreted as very low-density lipoproteins (VLDL).
2. They can be oxidized via the mitochondrial β-oxidation complex to acetyl-CoA. The latter can combine with another molecule of acetyl-CoA in the reaction catalysed by acetoacetyl-CoA thiolase and then enter the hydroxymethylglutaryl-CoA pathway to form acetoacetate.
3. The acetyl-CoA derived from the fatty acids can be completely oxidized in the tricarboxylate cycle.

The short- and medium-chain fatty acids cannot be re-esterified to any appreciable extent in mammalian liver and therefore they are either metabolized to ketone bodies or are completely oxidized. In addition, unlike the long-chain fatty acids, they are transported directly into the mitochondrial matrix without the need to be converted first to the corresponding acyl-CoA derivatives.

The role of malonyl CoA The entry of free long-chain fatty acids into the hepatocyte is via a specific carrier on the plasma membrane. Once inside the cytosol the long-chain fatty acids are bound to binding proteins, converted to the acyl-CoA derivatives, and then can either be esterified or enter the mitochondria via a complex transport system, the carnitine–acyl-CoA transferase (CAT) system. This consists of two proteins: CAT I located on the outer mitochondrial membrane and CAT II on the inner mitochondrial membrane (**Fig. 5**). The overall action of the two enzymes results in the transfer of a long-chain fatty acyl-CoA to the mitochondrial matrix and the return of free carnitine to the cytosol via an exchange mechanism. Although carnitine is not

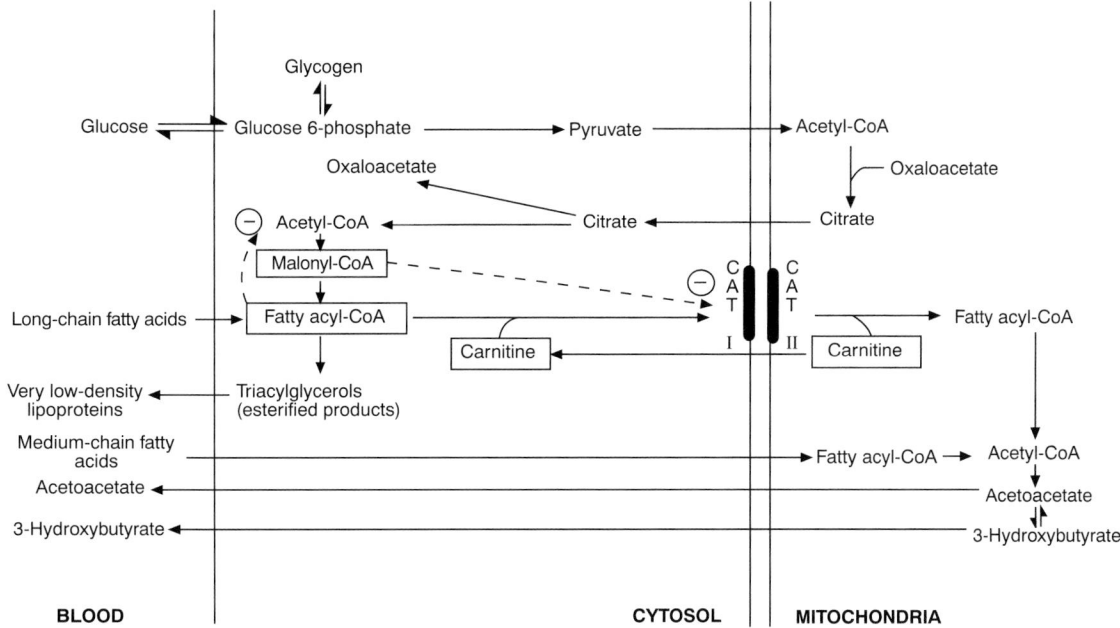

Figure 5 Interrelationship between hepatic carbohydrate metabolism, lipogenesis and ketogenesis. Circled minus signs indicate inhibition by the metabolite.

consumed in the reaction, the available concentration can be critical. In nutritional carnitine deficiency there is impairment of long-chain fatty acid oxidation and ketogenesis.

The activity of CAT I is the key to the intrahepatic regulation of fatty acid metabolism in most situations. Its activity increases in ketogenic situations. More importantly, CAT I is inhibited by malonyl-CoA and the sensitivity of CAT I to this inhibitor changes in various pathophysiological situations such as fasting or diabetes.

As malonyl-CoA is a key intermediate in the synthesis of fatty acids (lipogenesis) from products (pyruvate and lactate) of glucose metabolism, this interaction provides a regulatory link between lipid and carbohydrate metabolism (Fig. 5). Thus on high-carbohydrate diets, when the rate of hepatic lipogenesis, and consequently the cytosolic concentration of malonyl-CoA is high, the activity of CAT I will be inhibited and fatty acids will be diverted to esterified products and secretion as VLDL rather than oxidation and conversion to ketone bodies. Conversely, on high fat diets or in starvation, when lipogenesis is inhibited, malonyl-CoA concentration is low and CAT I is active. The sensitivity of CAT I to malonyl-CoA generally correlates with the prevailing concentration of the latter.

The short- and medium-chain fatty acids do not utilize the CAT I and II system to enter the mitochondrial matrix and therefore their oxidation is not greatly influenced by the prevailing 'carbohydrate status' (amount of glycogen, direction of carbohydrate flux, glycolysis or gluconeogenesis) of the liver (Fig. 5).

Insulin can rapidly depress the rate of ketogenesis *in vitro*. This effect is thought to result mainly from its stimulatory action on a key enzyme of lipogenesis, acetyl-CoA carboxylase, which in turn increases the concentration of malonyl-CoA. Glucagon and the catecholamines have the opposite effect. Thus hormonal effects can be exerted both at the extrahepatic (lipolysis) and intrahepatic (modulation of lipogenesis) levels.

Intramitochondrial regulation Once the fatty acyl-CoA molecule is attached to the mitochondrial β-oxidation complex there appears to be little regulation exerted until release of the acetyl-CoA fragments. As indicated above, the acetyl-CoA can enter the tricarboxylate cycle and be oxidized to CO_2, or can be converted to ketone bodies via the hydroxymethylglutaryl-CoA pathway.

It appears that in most experimental situations the complete oxidation of fatty acids proceeds at a low, but relatively similar, rate and it is the activity of the hydroxymethylglutaryl-CoA pathway that shows larger changes. This has led to the view that the pathway might be regulated by mechanisms other than substrate supply.

Studies on the expression of 3-hydroxy-3-methylglutaryl-CoA (HMG-CoA) synthase have shown that both the mRNA coding for the protein and the amount of protein increase during the onset of keto-genic states (fasting, diabetes) and that these changes are rapidly reversed (refeeding, insulin treatment). However, the finding that rates of ketogenesis from medium-chain fatty acids (CAT I and II) do not alter greatly with change in physiological state, if the rate of fatty acid supply is held constant, would seem to rule out appreciable regulation within the hydroxy-methylglutaryl-CoA pathway. Indeed, current think-ing suggests that the activity of CAT I is the primary intrahepatic site for the regulation of fatty acid oxi-dation and ketogenesis. If there is another important site, particularly during situations associated with the reversal of ketogenesis, it is likely to be proximal to the step catalysed by this protein, e.g. the supply of fatty acids to the liver. Thus *in vivo* there is little doubt that the primary step that controls ketogenic flux is the rate of long-chain fatty acid release from adipose tissue.

Function of Ketone Bodies

The major role of ketone bodies is to supply an alter-native oxidizable substrate to glucose for the brain in situations where the availability of the latter is impaired (e.g. starvation). In addition, ketone bodies can act as precursors for the acetyl-CoA required in neural lipid synthesis (myelin). Other mammalian tissues, including heart, skeletal muscle, kidney and lactating mammary gland, can utilize ketone bodies but, in contrast to glucose utilization, no energy can

be obtained in the absence of oxygen. In these tissues metabolism of ketone bodies results in the inhibition of glucose utilization and inhibition of the oxidation of pyruvate. The net result is a sparing of carbo-hydrate for the brain and the strictly glycolytic tissues (erythrocytes, retina).

Pathways of ketone body utilization

Mitochondrial pathway   The major site of ketone body utilization in peripheral tissues is the mitochon-dria (**Fig. 6**). Although transporters for ketone bodies have been described on the plasma and inner mito-chondrial membranes of some tissues, these do not appear to limit the flux. The initiating enzyme for acetoacetate metabolism is 3-oxoacid-CoA transfer-ase:

Acetoacetate + succinyl-CoA $\rightleftharpoons$ acetoacetyl-CoA + succinate

The resulting acetoacetyl-CoA is cleaved to two mol-ecules of acetyl-CoA by acetoacetyl-CoA thiolase; they are then oxidized in the tricarboxylate cycle

3-Hydroxybutyrate is converted to acetoacetate by 3-hydroxybutyrate dehydrogenase:

3-Hydroxybutyrate + NAD$^+$ $\rightleftharpoons$ acetoacetate + NADH + H$^+$

The ready reversibility of the three enzymes of the mitochondrial pathway (Fig. 6) means that if the overall system is near equilibrium within the cell *in vivo*, the utilization of the ketone bodies will be

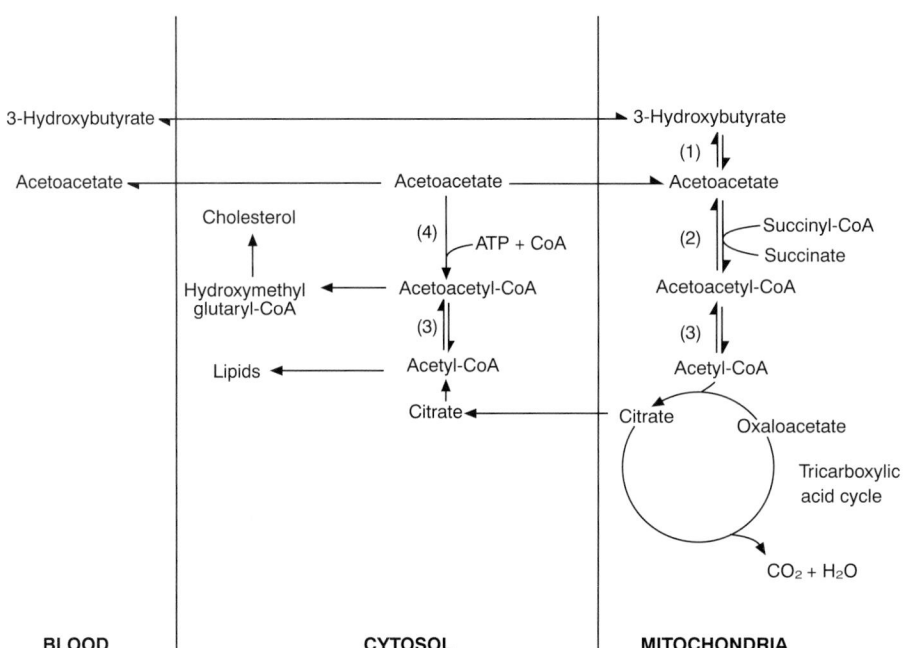

Figure 6   Pathways of ketone body utilization in peripheral tissues. (1) Hydroxybutyrate dehydrogenase, (2) 3-oxoacid-CoA transfer-ase; (3) acetoacetyl-CoA thiolase; (4) acetoacetyl-CoA synthetase.

dependent on their respective concentrations and on the rate of removal of the products. Thus acetoacetate utilization will be promoted when mitochondrial acetyl-CoA is decreased, whereas an increase in the latter will have the opposite effect. Similarly, oxidation of hydroxybutyrate will increase if the concentrations of $NADH_2$ and acetoacetate fall. Unlike the hepatic hydroxymethylglutaryl-CoA pathway for ketogenesis, which is essentially irreversible, the free reversibility of this pathway in peripheral tissues can be viewed as means of buffering the mitochondrial acetyl-CoA pool and hence energy production. Some of the acetyl-CoA can be transported to the cytosol in the form of citrate to act as a precursor for lipogenesis (Fig. 6).

Cytosolic pathway   The cytosol of tissues where active lipogenesis occurs (adipose tissue, developing brain, lactating mammary gland and liver) contains an enzyme, acetoacetyl-CoA synthetase, which converts acetoacetate to acetoacetyl-CoA (Fig. 6):

Acetoacetate + ATP + CoA
  → acetoacetyl-CoA + AMP + pyrophosphate

Its activity is at least an order of magnitude lower than that of the mitochondrial 3-oxoacid-CoA transferase, whereas its affinity for acetoacetate is appreciably higher. The presence of acetoacetyl-CoA thiolase in the cytosol allows the conversion of acetoacetate to acetyl-CoA and then to lipids without the involvement of the mitochondria.

Brain cytosol also contains 3-hydroxy-3-methylglutaryl-CoA synthase, allowing acetoacetate to act as a direct precursor for sterol synthesis. Evidence from *in vivo* experiments with ^{14}C-labelled acetoacetate have confirmed the existence of this pathway in developing brain and liver. The cytosolic route for acetoacetate utilization can be seen as a mechanism for directing this substrate to lipid or sterol synthesis rather than to oxidation.

Ketosis

The concentration of ketone bodies in the blood at any time represents a balance between the rate of hepatic ketogenesis and the rate of utilization by peripheral tissues. It is generally assumed that an increase in ketogenesis leads to a rise in blood ketone bodies, which in turn results in their increased utilization. In rare situations, such as congenital absence of key enzymes involved in ketone body utilization (e.g. 3-oxoacid-CoA transferase) or inhibition of these enzymes by pharmacological agents, blood

Table 1 Range of blood ketone body concentrations in humans

Situation	Ketone body concentration (mmol l^{-1})
Fed normal diet	about 0.1
Fed high-fat diet	up to 3
Fasted: 12–24 h	up to 0.3
Fasted: 48–72 h	2.0–3.0
Postexercise	up to 2
Late pregnancy	up to 1
Late pregnancy: fasted 48 h	4.0–6.0
Neonate: 0–1 days	0.2–0.5
Neonate: 5–10 days	0.7–1.0
Hypoglycaemia	1.0–5.0
Untreated diabetes mellitus	up to 25

ketone bodies may increase without any concomitant increase in ketogenesis.

The concentration of ketone bodies in the blood is exquisitely sensitive to changes in pathophysiological state. It is therefore useful to define *normoketonaemia* in mammals as a concentration of total ketone bodies in blood below 0.2 mmol l^{-1}, *hyperketonaemia* as above this level, and *ketoacidosis* (ketosis; by analogy to the definition of lactic acidosis) as above 7 mmol l^{-1}. In adult mammals there are small but characteristic diurnal variations in ketone body concentrations. Larger increases in concentration occur in man in response to change in pathophysiological state (**Table 1**). The concentrations span a 200-fold range and it is this which underlines the important role of ketone bodies as substrates and signals.

Physiological ketosis

Physiological hyperketonaemia is found in the suckling neonate (high-fat diet of the milk; Fig. 1), postexercise (depletion of hepatic glycogen reserves) and after prolonged fasting (more than 24 h; **Fig. 7**). All

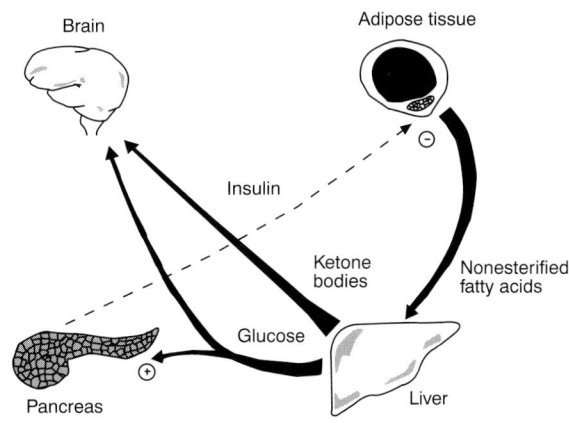

Figure 7 Intertissue fluxes of substrates in the starved state. Thickness of line denotes rate of flux.

these situations have in common a low hepatic carbohydrate status (depletion of glycogen and/or activation of gluconeogenesis) and therefore from a physiological standpoint one would expect an increased rate of ketogenesis. Comparison of the factors which can influence ketogenesis in suckling and fasting (**Table 2**) show the expected broad agreement.

More detailed information on the hierarchy of the regulatory factors during onset and reversal of ketogenesis have been obtained for the fasting state by measurements at short time intervals. The first event after withdrawal of food is a lowering of plasma insulin accompanied by an increase in plasma fatty acids (stimulation of lipolysis). However, for an appreciable period (8–10 h) there is no increase in blood ketone bodies or in the *in vitro* rates of hepatic ketogenesis (measured with saturating fatty acid concentrations). The major increment in ketogenic rate occurs at the nadir of the hepatic malonyl-CoA concentrations and when the sensitivity of CAT I to malonyl-CoA is starting to increase rapidly. This long time lag before a change in sensitivity of the protein to malonyl-CoA inhibition is thought to be due to the time required to bring about alterations to the lipid environment of the outer mitochondrial membrane.

Confirmation of this view is that on refeeding, when insulin rapidly increases and plasma fatty acids decrease with a parallel decrease in blood ketone bodies, there is again a time lag before malonyl-CoA concentrations rise and a longer one before sensitivity returns. In physiological and nutritional terms this delay of return to the normal fed settings of intrahepatic regulation makes excellent sense. It is only when the refeeding consists primarily of large amounts of carbohydrate that the starved liver needs to inhibit the activity of CAT I to prevent the oxidation of newly synthesized fatty acids. If the meal consists mainly of lipid with little carbohydrate the activity of CAT I needs to remain high to allow oxidation of the excess fatty acids. Thus the liver must sense a prolonged increase in plasma insulin before the high activity of CAT I is suppressed.

Table 2 Comparison of factors influencing ketogenesis in suckling and fasted states

Factor	Suckling	Fasted
Plasma nonesterified fatty acids	Increased	Increased
Plasma insulin	Decreased	Decreased
Plasma glucagon	Increased	Increased
Hepatic carnitine	Increased	Increased
Hepatic lipogenesis	Decreased	Decreased
Hepatic malonyl-CoA	Decreased	Decreased
Hepatic CAT I activity	Increased	Increased
Sensitivity to malonyl-CoA	Decreased	Decreased

Pathological ketosis

The major example of pathological ketosis is of course insulin-dependent or type I diabetes. Essentially the changes in this condition are similar to those that occur during fasting, but they are more pronounced. Insulin is absent or very low in the plasma and therefore there is no antagonistic action to restrain the opposing hormones, adrenaline, noradrenaline and glucagon. Consequently, lipolysis in adipose tissue is greatly stimulated and plasma fatty acids increase to high levels.

The lack of insulin and the large flux of fatty acids to the liver means that lipognesis is inhibited at the level of acetyl-CoA carboxylase and there is the expected decrease in malonyl-CoA concentration. In addition, the sensitivity of CAT I to inhibition by malonyl-CoA is considerably decreased. The level of expression of hepatic CAT I and II proteins also increase several-fold in diabetes. Thus the liver is in the ideal mode for producing excessive amounts of ketone bodies.

It has been suggested that diversion of oxaloacetate to hepatic glucose synthesis (which is also increased in insulin deficiency) may also play a role in the increased rate of ketogenesis by diverting acetyl-CoA from the tricarboxylate cycle. However, present evidence suggests that this makes a minor contribution. Although the excessive output of ketone bodies by the liver undoubtedly makes the major contribution to their high levels in the blood, it is likely that there is also a degree of underutilization by peripheral tissues. The net result is ketoacidosis and excretion of large amounts of energy as ketone bodies in the urine.

A rare, but intriguing, example of pathological ketosis (ketone bodies up to $10 \, \mathrm{mmol \, l^{-1}}$) is the inborn error of hepatic glycogen synthase deficiency (**Fig. 8**). Here glycogen is virtually absent from the liver so that after short-term fasting (5–10 h) the glucose falls to hypoglycaemic levels, plasma insulin is decreased, plasma fatty acids increase and ketogenesis is switched on. On consuming a meal the pattern is reversed until the blood glucose falls again. This case illustrates the importance of hepatic glycogen (and its mobilization) in the smooth transition of substrate supply from the fed to the fasted state. Treatment in this case was to recommend the consumption of more frequent high-carbohydrate snacks. It is of interest that this particular child suffered no ill effects from the daily exposure to high concentrations of ketone bodies, underlining their role as normal substrates for the brain when available.

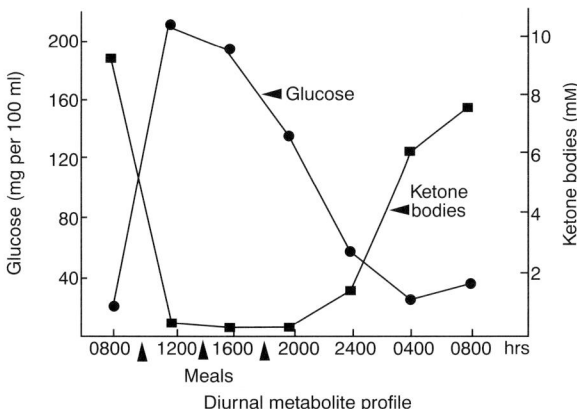

Figure 8 Diurnal blood metabolite profile of a child with glycogen synthetase deficiency. Values taken from Aynsley-Green A, Williamson DH and Gitzelmann R (1977) *Archives of Disease in Childhood* **52**: 573–579. (With permission from BMJ Publishing Group.)

Metabolic Acidosis

The great disadvantage of ketone bodies is that both acetoacetate and hydroxybutyrate are relatively strong acids. When they increase to high concentration there is the expected decrease in the blood pH, the plasma hydrogen carbonate concentration and the partial pressure of carbon dioxide in blood and body fluids. The symptoms of acidosis include malaise, weakness, anorexia and vomiting and these may eventually lead to coma. Treatment of diabetic ketoacidosis is to give insulin as soon as possible, usually as a continuous intravenous infusion. This rapidly decreases the raised plasma fatty acids and more slowly lowers the blood glucose and ketone bodies. Prolonged starvation, where the blood ketone bodies may reach 8–10 mmol l^{-1}, does not usually cause a serious disturbance of the acid–base balance. Loss of ketone bodies via the urine occurs, but is not excessive. The nonenzymic decarboxylation of acetoacetate to acetone and carbon dioxide can be seen as a primitive mechanism for removing the potential acidotic effects of ketone bodies. The fact that acetone can be converted to glucose by the liver at low rates is an extra bonus.

The other common form of metabolic acidosis is lactic acidosis. This can arise because of infection, tissue hypoxia (anaerobic glycolysis), can be drug-induced (ethanol, hypoglycaemic biguanides) or can arise because of a congenital defect (pyruvate dehydrogenase or pyruvate carboxylase deficiency). In addition to the acidosis caused by lactic acid or ketone bodies there is a group of organic acidurias (some 25–30 different types) in which an inborn error results in the accumulation of an organic acid in the blood and urine. However, frank acidosis is not always associated with these conditions. The key investigation is chromatographic identification of the organic acid.

See also: **Adipose Tissue**: Structure, Function and Metabolism of Adipose Tissue. **Carbohydrates**: Regulation of Carbohydrate Metabolism. **Cholesterol**: Sources, Absorption, Function and Metabolism. **Fatty Acids**: Metabolism. **Lactation**: Physiology. **Starvation and Fasting**: Biochemical Aspects.

Further Reading

Bach AC, Ingenbleek Y and Frey A (1996) The usefulness of dietary medium-chain triglycerides in body weight control: fact or fancy? *Journal of Lipid Research* 37:708–726.

Girard JR, Ferré P, Pégorier JP and Duée PH (1992) Adaptations of glucose and fatty acid metabolism during perinatal period and suckling – weaning transition. *Physiological Reviews* 72:507–562.

Krebs HA, Woods HF and Alberti KGMM (1975) Hyperlactataemia and lactic acidosis. *Essays in Medical Biochemistry* 1:81–103.

McGarry JD and Foster DW (1980) Regulation of hepatic fatty acid oxidation and ketone body production. *Annual Review of Biochemistry* 49:395–420.

Nehlig A and de Vasconcelos AP (1993) Glucose and ketone body utilization by the brain of neonatal rats. *Progress in Neurobiology* 40:163–221.

Owen OE, Morgan AP, Kemp HG, Sullivan JM, Herrera MG and Cahill GF (1967) Brain metabolism during fasting. *Journal of Clinical Investigation* 46:1589–1595.

Page MA and Williamson DH (1971) Enzymes of ketone body utilisation in human brain *Lancet* 2:66–68.

Porter R and Lawrenson G (eds) (1982) Metabolic acidosis. *Ciba Foundation Symposium* 87: London: Pitman.

Robinson AM and Williamson DH (1980) Physiological roles of ketone bodies as substrates and signals in mammalian tissues. *Physiological Reviews* 60:143–187.

Williamson DH (1982) The production and utilization of ketone bodies in the neonate. In: Jones CT (ed). *The Biochemical Development of the Fetus*, pp 621–650. Amsterdam: Elsevier Biomedical.

Williamson DH (1987) Brain substrates and the effects of nutrition, *Proceedings of Nutrition Society* 46:81–87.

Zammit VA (1996) Role of insulin in hepatic fatty acid partitioning: emerging concepts. *Biochemical Journal* 314:1–14.

Kidney disorders *see* **Renal Function and Disorders**: Nutritional Management of Renal Disorders.

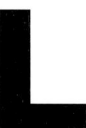

Laboratory Assessment *see* **Nutritional Status**: Biochemical Assessment.

LACTATION

Contents
Physiology
Dietary Requirements

Physiology

M C Neville, University of Colorado, Denver, Colorado, USA

Copyright © 1998 Academic Press

The provision of a specialized maternal body fluid, milk, for neonatal nutrition frees the mother from the necessity of finding appropriate foods for a very young baby. It allows birth to occur at an early stage of development and provides a time of intense maternal interaction with the newborn during early behavioural development. In addition, the nutritional reserves of the mother may be able to sustain the suckling infant through a period of famine. For all these reasons, lactation allows mammals to adapt to a wide variety of environments. It is becoming increasingly clear that breast milk is the most appropriate source of nutrition for human infants at least up to the age of 6 months. Many components of human milk, including (but not limited to) the protein lactoferrin, growth factors, long-chain polyunsaturated fatty acids, bile salt stimulated lipase, and antiinfectious oligosaccharides and glycoconjugates, are not duplicated in formula. These components may be particularly important for the challenged infant (e.g. the preterm infant, infants with feeding problems, infants in homes lacking adequate sanitation) but are increasingly being shown to be beneficial to healthy infants in well-protected environments as well.

Milk Composition

After the first week postpartum the composition of human milk is relatively constant, although some nutrients vary significantly within the feed and with duration of lactation. Breast-feeding can provide adequate nutrition for at least 4 months after birth; whether human milk alone provides sufficient nutrients after this period is a matter of controversy. The major macronutrients in milk are the sugar *lactose* (a disaccharide unique to milk), *oligosaccharides*, *milk fat* (mainly in the form of triacylglycerol), proteins including *casein, lactoferrin, secretory immunoglobulin A* (sIgA), *α-lactalbumin* and many others present at lower concentrations, and *minerals* including sodium, potassium, chloride, calcium and magnesium. The secretion mechanisms for most of these milk components are not as well understood. There are many minor components including enzymes, vitamins, trace elements and growth factors whose function and secretion are less well understood. The concentrations of the major components of human milk are compared with those of bovine milk (used to make infant formulae) in **Table 1**.

The major differences between human and bovine milk can be related to the specific needs of the young of the two species. For example, the concentration of lactose is higher and that of the monovalent and divalent ions lower in human than in cow's milk. The high concentration of lactose and lower content of salts provide a large amount of 'free water', i.e. water

Table 1 Comparison of the macronutrient contents of human and bovine milk

Component	Human milk	Bovine milk
Carbohydrates		
Lactose (g dl^{-1})	7.3	4.0
Oligosaccharides (g dl^{-1})	1.2	0.1
Proteins		
Caseins (g dl^{-1})	0.2	2.6
α-Lactalbumin (g dl^{-1})	0.2	0.2
Lactoferrin (g dl^{-1})	0.2	Trace
Secretory IgA (g dl^{-1})	0.2	Trace
β-Lactoglobulin (g dl^{-1})	0	0.5
Milk lipids		
Triacylglycerols (%)	4.0	4.0
Phospholipids (%)	0.04	0.04
Minerals and other ionic constituents		
Sodium (mM)	5.0	15
Potassium (mM)	15.0	43
Chloride (mM)	15.0	24
Calcium (mM)	7.5	30
Magnesium (mM)	1.4	5
Phosphate (mM)	1.8	11
Bicarbonate (mM)	6.0	5

that does not need to be obligatorily excreted by the kidneys with salts, providing a reserve for temperature regulation by sweating in human infants. The high concentration of casein in bovine milk provides protein and associated calcium and phosphate to support the very rapid growth of the young calf. Generally, casein is removed when bovine milk is used to produce infant formula designed for the much more slowly growing human infant. There are a number of agents in human milk that protect against gastrointestinal and respiratory infections, including the oligosaccharides which have been shown to interact specifically with pathogen receptors, lactoferrin and secretory IgA. These compounds are present in very small concentrations in bovine milk and infant formula.

Anatomy of the Breast

The secretory apparatus of the breast consists of 15–25 ducts extending from the nipple and coursing through the mammary fat pad to terminate in grape-like clusters of alveoli (**Fig. 1**). Each duct serves a specific lobule. The lobules are separated and supported by thick connective tissue septa and, in the nonpregnant, nonlactating breast, by large amounts of adipose tissue. The nipple, which serves as the termination point for the lactiferous ducts, is surrounded by an area of pigmented skin, the areola, containing sebaceous glands and sweat glands. The areola serves as the termination point for the fourth intercostal nerve which carries sensory information

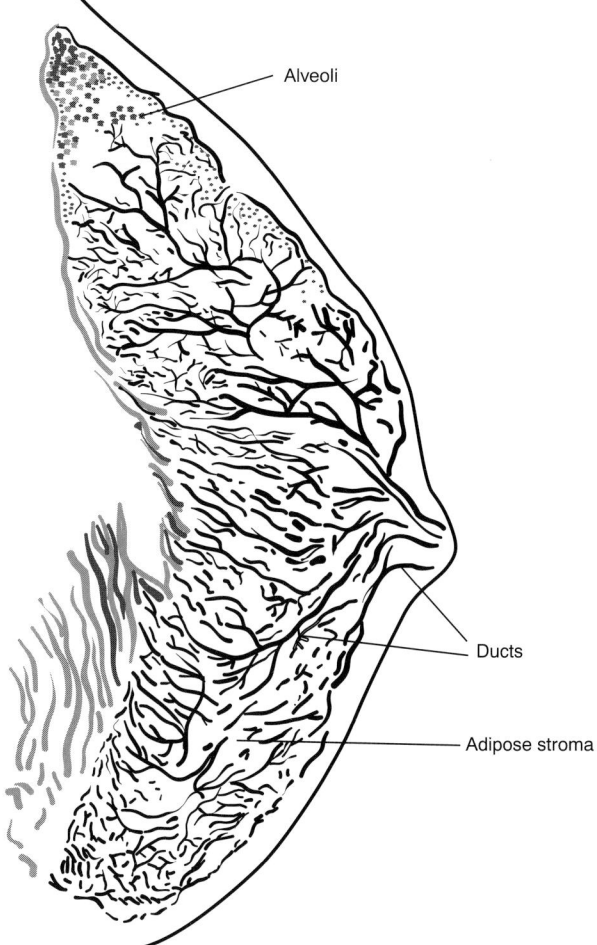

Figure 1 Sagittal section through the breast of a 19-year-old nulligravida. A number of duets terminate on the nipple. They course backward through the stroma, draining the alveoli located near the margins of the gland. From Dabelow A (1941) *Morphol J* **85**:361–416.

about suckling to the spinal cord and brain. This is extremely important in the regulation of oxytocin secretion from the posterior pituitary gland and prolactin from the anterior pituitary. The mammary ducts expand slightly to form sinuses beneath the areola.

Histologically, the secretory compartment of the breast consists of ducts and alveoli. The larger ducts appear to have two layers of cuboidal epithelium. Smaller ductules and alveoli have a single luminal epithelial layer surrounded by a discontinuous layer of contractile cells, the myoepithelium (**Fig. 2**). This latter network of cells forms a basket-like framework around the alveoli and runs longitudinally along the ducts. Myoepithelial cells contract in response to oxytocin, ejecting milk from the alveoli where it is stored after secretion by the luminal epithelial cells. Adipocytes are intimately associated with the glandular elements, as is a prominent blood supply.

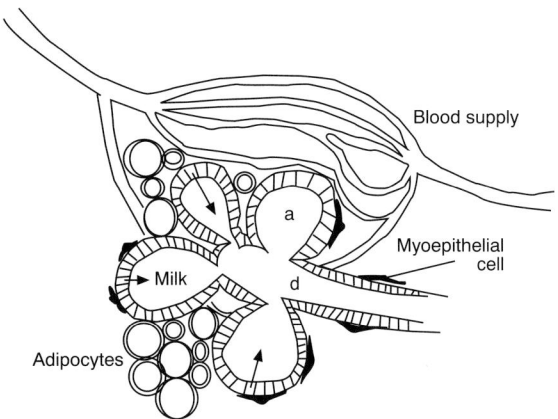

Figure 2 The relation of the mammary epithelial compartment, composed of mammary ducts and alveoli, to the other anatomical compartments of the gland: the myoepithelial cells, the stroma composed of adipocytes and fibroblasts, and the extensive blood supply. Milk secretion by the epithelial cells into the alveolar lumen is indicated by the arrows; a, alveolus; d, ductule.

Although the location and external form of the mammary glands differ from one species to another, the mechanisms of milk production are remarkably similar. Milk is produced and stored in alveolar units as in Fig. 2. Removal of the milk is accomplished by a process called 'milk ejection' during which milk is forced from the alveoli by contraction of surrounding myoepithelial cells. Milk ejection is often called the 'let-down reflex'. The milk exits through ductules into ducts draining several clusters of alveoli. In the human the small ducts coalesce into 15–25 main ducts that drain sectors of the gland. The main ducts dilate into small sinuses as they near the areola where they open directly on the nipple. For milk removal, the entire areola with the underlying milk sinuses is drawn into the infant's mouth and the milk is withdrawn by the stripping action of the tongue.

In comparison with related dermal glands such as the salivary and sweat glands, the rate of milk secretion is slow, about 1.5 ml of milk per gram of tissue per day, and the secretory product is stored in the alveolar spaces until forced out by myoepithelial cell contraction. The larger ducts play a passive role in milk secretion, merely transferring the milk from the alveolar stores to the subareolar sinuses where it is available to the suckling infant. Because the composition of the aqueous phase of milk changes very little during a feed or milking, it is unlikely that reabsorptive processes, like those important in the formation of saliva or sweat, play a significant role in determining milk composition.

Although the mammary epithelial cells are ultimately responsible for converting most precursors into milk constituents and transporting them to the mammary lumen, other cell types are also intimately

involved in milk production (Fig. 2). The myoepithelial cells responsible for milk ejection from the breast have already been mentioned. The mammary ducts and alveoli are embedded in a stroma that contains fibroblasts, adipocytes, plasma cells and blood vessels. Blood flow is greatly expanded during lactation to make available the large amounts of substrate required for milk synthesis. During lactation B lymphocytes 'home' to the mammary gland where they become plasma cells and settle in the interstitial space, producing the immunoglobulins that ultimately find their way into milk. Stromal cells synthesize insulin-like growth factor I (IGF-I), which may promote survival of mammary epithelial cells. The mammary epithelium should, therefore, be viewed as an integrator of the activities of many cells and organs that contribute in a coordinated fashion to the synthesis and secretion of milk and its ejection from the gland.

Mechanisms of Milk Secretion

Fig. 3 depicts a single mammary epithelial cell in a lactating mammary gland. It is positioned on a basement membrane, and processes of myoepithelial cells course along its basal surface. Tight junctions join this cell to its neighbours, and in lactation they prevent the direct transfer of interstitial fluid components to the alveolar lumen.

Secretion pathways

Four major *transcellular* pathways are responsible for the secretion of milk components during lactation. The *paracellular* pathway is open during pregnancy and under certain other conditions allowing movement of interstitial fluid components

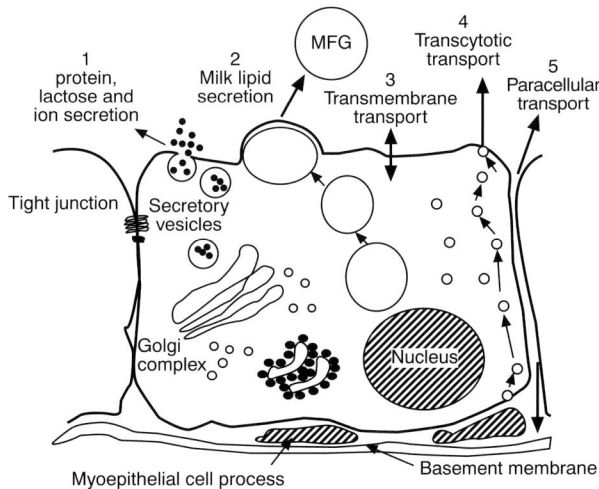

Figure 3 A mammary epithelial cell showing the pathways for the secretion of milk components. MFG, milk fat globule.

into the milk space and the flux of milk components in the other direction.

Pathway 1: exocytosis The exocytotic pathway secretes milk components by a mechanism similar to exocytotic secretion in all endocrine and exocrine glands. Casein and α-lactalbumin are synthesized and secreted via this largely constitutive secretory pathway which is also responsible for the secretion of lactose, calcium, phosphate, citrate and most other components of the aqueous phase of milk. Lactose is synthesized in the terminal portion of the Golgi vesicles from glucose and UDP-galactose by the enzyme galactosyl transferase using α-lactalbumin as an essential coenzyme. Lactose contributes two-thirds of the osmolarity of human milk. Various glycosyl transferases responsible for the formation of the wide variety of complex oligosaccharides present in human milk are also found in the terminal Golgi vesicles.

Pathway 2: lipid secretion The mechanism for the secretion of lipid is unique to the mammary epithelium. Triacyglycerols are synthesized in the mammary alveolar cell from glycerol and free fatty acids. The free fatty acids are derived from the plasma lipid using the enzyme lipoprotein lipase, from plasma free fatty acids carried there on albumin or by synthesis within the alveolar cell from glucose. Free fatty acids synthesized in the mammary alveolar cell are medium-chain fatty acids with 12 or 14 carbon atoms rather than the long-chain fatty acids derived from the plasma. Once synthesized, the triacylglycerols form droplets, merge and gradually move to the apical membrane. When they reach the apical surface of the cell they press on the membrane, gradually becoming enveloped, and eventually pinch off as membrane-bound milk fat globules. The membrane of the milk fat globule prevents coalescence of the fat droplets and serves to deliver both triacylglycerols and phospholipids to the infant.

The composition of milk triacylglycerols depends on the diet. On the high-fat diet usually consumed by American women, the fatty acid composition reflects dietary lipid, with long-chain fatty acids predominating and a fair proportion of unsaturated fatty acids reflecting the consumption of vegetable oils (**Table 2**). In this condition only about 10% of the milk fatty acids are synthesized in the mammary gland itself as medium-chain fatty acids (C_8–C_{14}). On high-carbohydrate, low-fat diets the proportion of fatty acid synthesized in the mammary gland from carbohydrate increases, leading to an increase in the amount of medium-chain fatty acids as can be seen from the data for Nigerian women in Table 2. The milk of the Nigerian women also contained a higher proportion of n-3 long-chain polyunsaturated fatty acids (LC-PUFA). On reducing or low-energy diets, much of the milk fat is derived from adipose tissue; in this case the composition of the triacylglycerols resembles depot fat.

Pathway 3: transmembrane transport There are transport mechanisms for only a few milk components in the apical membrane of the mammary alveolar cell. This membrane is known to be permeable to monovalent ions such as sodium, potassium and chloride as well as to glucose. It is impermeable to divalent cations and disaccharides such as lactose. The mechanisms that control the substantial concentration gradients of monovalent cations across this membrane are not understood.

Pathway 4: the transcytotic pathway Proteinaceous substances from the interstitial space find their way into milk via *transcytotic* pathways. One of these pathways, that for the secretion of IgA, is well understood. An IgA receptor on the basolateral membrane of the cell interacts with dimeric IgA made by plasma cells residing in the interstitial spaces of the mammary gland. The IgA is endocytosed and transported in a vesicle to the apical membrane where it is secreted with a piece of its transporter ('secretory component') into the milk. Secretory component renders the protein resistant to protease and the IgA thus has a reasonable survival time in the infant's intestine where it may contribute to protection from infectious agents. Many other proteins that are not synthesized in the mammary alveolar cell enter milk via transcytosis, e.g. hormones such as insulin and prolactin, growth factors such as IGF-I and even serum albumin.

Pathway 5: paracellular transport During lactation, tight junctions (see Fig. 3) form a seal between alveolar cells closing the paracellular pathway and completely isolating the alveolar lumina from the interstitial spaces. In pregnancy, after involution and during mastitis, these junctions open by mechanisms that are not well understood. At these times even large proteins can be transferred between the milk space and interstitial space. Under these conditions plasma components such as sodium, chloride and albumin enter the milk space directly from the interstitial space, milk components such as lactose enter the bloodstream, and the concentrations of sodium and chloride in milk are high.

Cells from the immune system pass into milk via the paracellular pathway. They appear to be able to squeeze even through the tight junctions of the lactating gland.

Table 2   Major fatty acids of human milk

Fatty acid		Human milk: Western diet (wt %)	Human milk: low-fat diet[a] (wt %)
Structure	Name		
Saturated fatty acids			
Intermediate and medium-chain (formed in mammary gland)			
8:0	Octanoic acid	0.46	–
10:0	Decanoic acid	1.03	0.54
12:0	Lauric acid	4.40	8.34
14:0	Myristic acid	6.27	9.57
Long-chain			
16:0	Palmitic acid	22.00	23.35
18:0	Stearic acid	8.06	10.15
Monounsaturated fatty acids (MUFA)			
16:1 n-7 (*cis*)	Palmitoleic acid	3.29	0.91
18:1 n-9 (*cis*)	Oleic acid	31.30	18.52
18:1 n-9 (*trans*)		2.67	0.86
Polyunsaturated fatty acids (PUFA) (essential fatty acids)			
18:2 n-6	Linoleic acid	10.76	11.06
18:3 n-3	Linolenic acid	0.81	1.41
Long-chain PUFA (n-6)			
18:3 n-6	γ-Linolenic acid	0.16	0.12
20:2 n-6		0.34	0.26
20:3 n-6	Dihomo-γ-linolenic acid	0.26	0.49
20:4 n-6	Arachidonic acid	0.36	0.82
Long-chain PUFA (n-3)			
20:5 n-3	Eicosapentaenoic acid	0.04	0.48
22:5 n-3		0.17	0.39
22:6 n-3	Docosahexaenoic acid	0.22	0.93

Data from Jensen (1995).
[a]Data from Nigerian women whose diet also had a high fish content, as reflected in the n-3 long-chain PUFA values.

Mammary Development

The mammary gland is one of the few organs that undergoes almost the entire cycle of development, differentiation, function and involution in the adult animal. Each of these stages has different control mechanisms, only some of which are understood despite decades of study. The developmental cycle of the mammary gland is usually divided into four stages: (1) *mammogenesis* or development and differentiation; (2) *lactogenesis* or the onset of milk secretion; (3) *lactation*, and (4) *involution*. Mammogenesis takes place in the embryo, at puberty and during pregnancy. Lactogenesis begins in mid-pregnancy and is completed during the first 3–5 days after birth in the human. Lactation lasts as long as milk continues to be removed from the breast after birth of the infant. Involution is the regression of the gland after suckling has been discontinued. Each phase has its own unique control mechanisms.

Embryogenesis

The mammary gland begins to develop in the fourth week of fetal life as a thickening of the epidermis that gradually begins to invade the underlying parenchyma forming an epithelial bud. This bud branches and canalizes, forming about 15–20 rudimentary ducts which consist of a lumen surrounded by a layer of ductal epithelium with an underlying layer of myoepithelial cells. The entire process requires about 28 weeks during which a fully committed epithelial rudiment and an underlying fat pad are formed as well as the nipple. It is becoming clear that interactions between the epithelium and the underlying stroma are critical in determining the morphology of the structures formed. Towards the end of pregnancy the mammary epithelium of the infant may become secretory under the influence of the maternal steroid hormones and at birth many infants secrete a small amount of milky fluid called 'witch's milk'.

Postnatal development

During childhood the mammary gland does little more than keep pace with the general growth of the body.

Pubertal development

One of the earliest signs of puberty in girls is enlargement of the breast. This enlargement involves both the epithelium and the adipose stroma, an obligatory substratum for epithelial growth. Under the influence of oestrogen from the developing ovary the ducts begin to elongate. The most direct evidence that oestrogen is essential for ductal development comes from experiments in which time-release pellets were used to deliver drugs directly into the developing gland. Implantation of oestrogen pellets enhanced ductile development whereas implantation of pellets that released antioestrogens into the local tissue environment inhibited ductal growth. Oestrogen receptors are found in the stroma as well as in scattered epithelial cells.

Pregnancy

During pregnancy the increasing concentrations of sex steroid along with prolactin and placental lactogen bring about maximal development of the breast. Lobular development intensifies until the fat pad is completely filled with epithelial structures. By mid-pregnancy the alveolar cells have differentiated sufficiently to be capable of secreting milk; this point is called stage 1 lactogenesis. However, milk secretion is held in check by the high concentrations of progesterone from the placenta.

Lactogenesis, lactation and involution

With the birth of the young the hormonal support for mammary growth and inhibition of milk secretion are withdrawn and stage 2 lactogenesis begins. This process involves the terminal differentiation of the mammary cells through a carefully programmed series of events that result in copious secretion of milk 4 days after birth. Milk secretion is maintained until regular removal of milk from the gland ceases, at which point involution of the mammary epithelium begins. Many of the alveolar cells undergo apoptosis (programmed cell death) and the gland returns to its prepregnant state.

Lactogenesis

Although the mammary epithelium becomes fully competent to secrete milk some time in mid-pregnancy, the term 'lactogenesis' is normally used to describe the onset of copious milk secretion in the first few days after parturition and will be so used in the rest of this discussion. Withdrawal of progesterone and oestrogen in the presence of sustained prolactin secretion brings about a complex series of well-programmed events that lead to the secretory activity of differentiated mammary cells. Immediately after birth the tight junctions between the cells begin to close and the paracellular pathway is no longer available for the exchange of components between the milk fall and the space and the interstitial space. The concentrations of sodium and chloride in the milk fall and the milk lactose concentration increases (**Fig. 4**). Next, secretion of IgA oligosaccharides and lactoferrin increases, adding large quantities of these protective substances along with high concentrations of lymphoid cells to the mammary secretion, now called *colostrum*. Beginning about 40 h postpartum the alveolar cells increase their secretion of lactose, casein and the other components of mature milk, and milk volume production rises from about 100 ml per day on the second day postpartum to about 500 ml per day on day 5. The corresponding feeling of fullness of the breast is often referred to as the 'milk coming in'. Suckling by the infant is not required to initiate the process; however, milk secretion cannot be maintained if milk is not removed within 3–4 days postpartum.

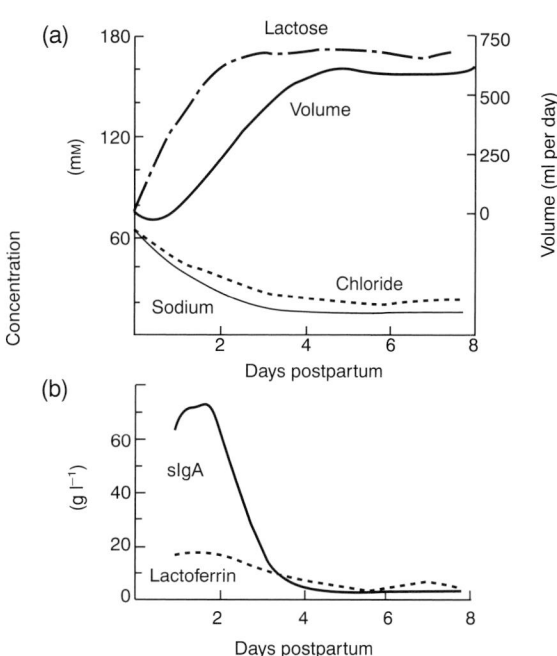

Figure 4 Changes in human milk composition and volume during lactogenesis, the onset of milk secretion sIgA, secretory immunoglobulin A.

Lactation

With the completion of lactogenesis the breast enters into the stage of lactation, sometimes referred to as *galactopoiesis*. This stage persists as long as the infant continues to suckle at least twice a day. The daily milk volume transferred to the infant increases on average from 500 ml on day 5 to about 650 ml at 1 month and about 750 ml at 3 months. Milk volume is largely regulated by infant demand. Infants who are larger at a given age tend to take more milk; if breast milk is supplemented with other foods or formula, milk production decreases. In most women the breast appears to have the capacity to secrete much more milk than is needed for nourishment of a single infant. In fact, wet nurses who removed milk from their breasts using a breast pump have been recorded as producing up to 3500 ml per day, and some women are able to breast-feed triplets!

Regulation of milk secretion

Prolactin is necessary for milk secretion and suckling promotes its secretion. However, the volume of milk secretion is not directly regulated by the concentration of prolactin in the blood. Rather, local mechanisms within the mammary gland related to the amount of milk removed by the infant are responsible for the day-to-day regulation of milk volume. A protein factor called feedback inhibitor of lactation (FIL) is secreted with other milk components into the alveolar lumen. If milk is not removed from the gland, this substance, whose identity is not yet entirely clear, interacts with the mammary alveolar cell and inhibits milk secretion, possibly by altering the sensitivity of the cells to prolactin.

Regulation of milk ejection

Suckling initiates a neuroendocrine reflex essential for removal of milk from the breast. Afferent impulses travel via sensory neurons from the areola to the hypothalamus where they stimulate magnocellular neurons to fire, sending an impulse down their axons into the posterior pituitary where the hormone *oxytocin* is released. This hormone travels through the bloodstream to the breast where it causes contraction of the myoepithelial cells, forcing the milk from the alveoli into the mammary ducts and sinuses from whence it can be removed by the sucking infant. Without an adequate let-down reflex, complete removal of milk from the breast is not possible. The activity of the magnocellular neurons can be profoundly influenced by higher brain centres. For this reason emotional distress can inhibit let-down. Conversely, let-down is subject to conditioning so that a woman often releases oxytocin at the sound of her (or someone else's) infant's cry or in response to a picture of her infant.

Interactions of lactation with maternal conditions

The lactating breast is largely an autonomous organ depending only on permissive levels of prolactin and other hormones such as insulin and hydrocortisone for continued milk secretion. The amount of milk produced is under local control and depends on the rate of milk removal from the breast as discussed above. The gland removes nutrients from the plasma according to its needs for substrate to synthesize milk components and is usually only marginally affected by acute changes in maternal dietary intake and other maternal factors such as fluid intake, body composition, illness and exercise. The limits to which lactation is maintained in starvation are unknown, since experimental observations in this area are difficult. A single case report suggests that 7 days of total fasting does not affect milk secretion. The composition of the diet does, however, affect some milk components – most notably vitamins such as vitamin C, vitamin A, vitamin B_{12}, vitamin D and possibly others. Vitamin B_{12} deficiency has been reported in infants of mothers consuming a vegetarian diet. The milk levels of some trace elements, for example selenium, are also affected by maternal dietary status. The effects of the lipid composition of the diet on milk fat composition have been discussed above. Fluid intake is not directly linked to milk production, as women who take no water during the day during Ramadan produce normal volumes of slightly hypertonic milk. It is likely that hydration severe enough to threaten maternal metabolism would also threaten milk production. The total fat content of milk does not appear to be affected by dietary intake but is inversely proportional to body fat. Diabetic women may have difficulty initiating lactation, but once lactation is established they have no problem nursing an infant. Mastitis alters milk composition by opening the tight junctions between the cells so that the sodium and chloride content of the milk is increased and the protein content decreased. Pregnancy anecdotally reduces milk volume, although there is no reliable evidence on this point. Exercise has not been observed to alter either milk volume or composition.

The impact of lactation on maternal nutritional and reproductive status is more notable. Exclusive breast-feeding inhibits the release of gonadotrophin releasing hormone (GnRH) from the hypothalamus, postponing the return of reproductive function after the birth of the infant. However, even full breast-feeding does not necessarily offer protection against a subsequent pregnancy, particularly in well-nourished women. Bone calcium concentration has been shown to decline during lactation in several studies, probably owing to the lack of oestrogen during the period of postpartum amenorrhoea, but appears to recover to normal values once the menses have resumed. Women with marginal protein nutrition may suffer some deterioration of their protein status. During lactation the folate stores of women with marginal folate status may be depleted of the vitamin, a situation that may adversely affect a subsequent pregnancy. However, compared with other species such as rodents or dairy animals whose body lipid reserves are depleted within a short time after lactogenesis by their copious milk production, metabolic adaptations to lactation in humans are small because feeding a single infant does not impose an enormous metabolic load, in comparison with these animals.

See also: **Adaptation**: Overview of Adaptive Responses to Malnutrition. **Cancer**: Epidemiology of Breast Cancer. **Dairy Products**: Nutritional Value. **Fatty Acids**: Metabolism. **Fertility**: Body Fat, Menarche and Fertility. **Folic Acid**: Physiology, Dietary Sources and Requirements. **Infants**: Milk-feeding and Weaning. **Lactation**: Dietary Requirements. **Nutrition Policies**: In Developed Countries. **Pregnancy**: Energy Requirements and Metabolic Adaptations. **Vegetarian Diets**: Nutritional Adequacy.

Further Reading

Dewey KG and McCrory MA (1994) Effects of dieting and physical activity on pregnancy and lactation. *American Journal of Clinical Nutrition* 59 (supplement 2):446S–452S.

Dils RR (1986) Comparative aspects of milk fat synthesis. *Journal of Dairy Science* 69:904–910.

Jensen RG (1995) *Handbook of Milk Composition*. San Diego: Academic Press.

Lawrence RA (1989) Breastfeeding and medical disease. *Medical Clinics of North America* 73:583–603.

McNeilly AS, Tay CCK and Glasier A (1994) Physiological mechanisms underlying lactational amenorrhea. *Annals of the New York Academy of Sciences* 709:145–155.

Neville MC (1989) Regulation of milk fat synthesis. *Journal of Pediatric Gastroenterology and Nutrition* 8:426–429.

Neville MC (1990) The physiological basis of milk secretion. *Annals of the New York Academy of Science* 586:1–11.

Neville MC and Neifert MR (1983) *Lactation: Physiology, Nutrition and Breastfeeding*. New York: Plenum.

Newburg DS (1996) Oligosaccharides and glycoconjugates in human milk: their role in host defense. *Journal of Mammary Gland Biology and Neoplasia* 1:271–284.

O'Connor DL (1994) Folate status during pregnancy and lactation. *Advances in Experimental Medicine and Biology* 352:157–172.

Peaker M and Wilde CJ (1996) Feedback control of milk secretion from milk. *Journal of Mammary Gland Biology and Neoplasia* 1:307–316.

Prentice A (1994) Calcium intakes and bone densities of lactating women and breast-fed infants in The Gambia. *Advances in Experimental Medicine and Biology* 352:243–255.

Russo J and Russo IH (1987) Development of the human mammary gland. In: Neville MC, Daniel CW (eds) *The Mammary Gland*, pp. 67–96. New York: Plenum.

Sanz AM and Diaz RC (1995) Selenium in human lactation. *Nutrition Reviews*, 53(6):159–166.

Specker BL (1994) Nutritional concerns of lactating women consuming vegetarian diets. *American Journal of Clinical Nutrition* 59 (supplement 5):1182S–1186S.

Telemo E and Hanson LA (1996) Antibodies in milk. *Journal of Mammary Gland Biology and Neoplasia* 1:243–250.

Dietary Requirements

L Houghton and **D L O'Connor**, Ross Products Division, Columbus, Ohio, USA

Copyright © 1998 Academic Press

The total amount of energy required to produce human milk for one month postpartum is equivalent to the total energy cost of pregnancy. Similarly, the nutritive demands made on a lactating women are often considerably greater than those made by pregnancy. Nonetheless, there is very little published data concerning the actual energy requirements and impact of lactation on maternal nutrient status. Most of the recommended dietary intakes for lactating women are derived from the volume of milk produced during lactation, its nutritional content and the amount of nutrient reserves held by the average well-nourished woman. The recommended intakes of specific nutrients during lactation by various authorities are summarized in **Table 1**.

Energy Cost of Lactation

The 1985 Food and Agricultural Organization/World Health Organization/United Nations University (FAO/WHO/UNU) recommended that an additional 2100 kJ (500 kcal) per day be consumed by women to meet the costs of lactation. The 2100 kJ (500 kcal) was derived using the factorial approach which included the following assumptions: (1) that the average breast-milk output of a well-nourished mother is 800 ml per day; (2) that the energy content of breast milk is approximately 294 kJ (70 kcal) per 100 ml; and (3) that the efficiency of conversion of

Table 1 Comparison of FAO/WHO (1957–1989), US (1989), Canadian (1990) and UK (1991) daily recommended intakes for lactating women[a]

	FAO/WHO	USA	Canada	UK
Protein (g)	46	65	70	69
Vitamin A (RE)	1200	1300	1200	1200
Vitamin D (μg)	10	10	5	10
Vitamin E (mg)	–	12	9	–
Vitamin C (mg)	30	95	55	60
Folate (μg)	500	280	285	400
Vitamin B$_{12}$ (μg)	4.5	2.6	1.2	–
Calcium (mg)	1200	1200	1200	1200
Phosphorus (mg)	–	1200	1050	–
Magnesium (mg)	–	355	265	–
Iron (mg)	14–28+	15	13	15
Iodine (μg)	–	200	210	–
Zinc (mg)	150	19	15	–

[a]First 6 months of lactation.

food energy to milk is 80%. Furthermore, the recommendation assumes that the average woman would initiate lactation with an extra 2–4 kg of body fat accumulated during pregnancy that could be partially mobilized to help meet the energy cost of lactation (840 kJ/200 kcal per day). Thus, the average energy cost of lactation over the first 6 months is estimated to be approximately 2940 kJ (700 kcal) per day for women who are exclusively breast-feeding their young.

Milk synthesis is an extremely resilient process in that milk volumes are comparable among women of varying nutritional status, with the exception of overt maternal starvation. In industrialized countries, the average volume of milk produced is 750–800 ml per day in the first 4–5 months, thereby accurately representing the average daily milk volume selected to estimate the 1985 FAO/WHO/UNU energy recommendation. The energy density of breast milk is more difficult to estimate secondary to the variable diurnal and within-feed changes in milk fat content. Using the modified Atwater factors, the average metabolizable energy content of mature breast milk has been reported to be 290 kJ (69 kcal) per 100 ml. An alternative approach has been proposed to assess the energy content of breast milk using measurements of the infant's energy expenditure and analysis of the composition of newly formed tissue in breast-fed infants. Although not yet a validated method, the calculated metabolizable energy in early lactation was estimated to be 240–250 kJ (57–60 kcal) per 100 ml of milk.

The 1985 FAO/WHO/UNU recommendations assumed that the process of converting maternal dietary energy to milk energy occurs with an efficiency of 80%. The remarkable efficacy in human milk synthesis is thought due, in part, to the high-fat diet consumed by humans which minimizes the requirement for *de novo* synthesis of milk fat. More recently it has been proposed that an average efficiency figure of 95% would be more appropriate to calculate the energy cost of lactation.

Maternal fat stores laid down during pregnancy are believed to be deposited to support the energy costs of lactation. Utilization of this storage fat would promote a decline in body weight, with a return to normal (prepregnancy) weight by 6 months of lactation. After this period, energy intake recommendations are increased by 840 kJ (200 kcal) per day, to compensate for depleted fat stores. Not surprisingly, most of the data demonstrate that weight losses do tend to occur during the first 6 months of lactation; however, the losses are very small and may not differ significantly from those found for nonlactating postpartum women. Typically, lactating women experience an average weight loss of 0.6–0.8 kg per month during the first 4–6 months of lactation, averaging 4.4 kg after 1 year of breast-feeding. Breast-feeding alone, however, does not guarantee weight loss. In some instances, a possible gain in body weight has been observed in lactating women. It can be concluded that losses in weight are not obligatory during lactation, particularly in well-nourished women who can support the extra energy costs of lactation by increasing food intake and/or decreasing physical activity.

Usual energy intake during lactation

Healthy normal weight lactating women meet the additional energy requirements of lactation using a combination of increased food intake, mobilization of fat stores and a reduction of physical activity. Energy intakes among nonpregnant, nonlactating women from industrialized countries tend to be lower than those recommended. Likewise reports show that the amount of energy consumed by lactating mothers is not sufficiently increased to accommodate the estimated costs of lactation. There may be several reasons for the low published energy intakes, including underreporting of dietary intake. However, the overestimation of the energy needs of women cannot be ruled out. If, indeed, the recommended energy intakes are too high, the lower than recommended energy intakes may lead to low intakes of several other nutrients including zinc, calcium, folate and possibly vitamin A. Nonetheless, some investigators have shown an increase in energy intake during lactation that closely matched estimated energy needs.

It is possible that the cost of lactation may also be subsidized by mobilization of body fat and/or lower than average energy expenditure. Others have suggested an increased metabolic efficiency during lactation including a decrease in either resting metabolic rate, diet-induced thermogenesis, and/or work-induced thermogenesis; however, there is insufficient evidence to support the theory of any major energy-sparing mechanisms involved during lactation.

Effects of dieting and physical activity

Many women are concerned with weight control, particularly those who retain extra weight postpartum. The practice of dieting and/or physical activity during lactation in well-nourished women appears to be safe if appropriate guidelines are followed. Energy restriction should be moderate and it is recommended that lactating women consume a minimum of 7500 kJ per day (1800 kcal per day) as it is very difficult to obtain adequate intakes of other nutrients (particularly calcium, magnesium, zinc, folate and vitamin B_6) when energy intakes fall below this level. It is probably advisable for lactating women who diet to continue to take calcium and/or supplements used during pregnancy. Intakes below 6300 kJ per day (1500 kcal per day) are not recommended during lactation.

Physical activity is often recommended as an alternative to dieting because of its known benefits for maintaining lean body mass and improving cardiovascular fitness. It has been shown that lactating women can safely undertake a regular exercise programme postpartum without adversely compromising lactational performance. However, lactating women should be cautious and not attempt to lose more than 2 kg per month. It is also important for lactating mothers to maintain an adequate fluid intake as fluid needs during lactation are high.

Dietary Intakes during Lactation and Recommendations

Rationale for recommendations

Dietary recommendations for lactating women are typically determined by estimating the total amount of any given nutrient secreted into milk (milk volume × nutrient concentration in milk) multiplied by a correction factor to account for the bioavailability of that nutrient in the maternal diet. This incremental figure is then added to that amount of the nutrient that is recommended for nonpregnant, nonlactating women. It is extremely difficult, however, in any recommendation to account for the following factors: (1) the varying states of maternal nutrition at the end of the pregnancy; (2) the often huge variability in the woman-to-woman concentration of any given nutrient in her breast milk; (3) the additional requirements of specific nutrients to support the anabolic activities of lactation; and (4) the stage of lactation, as there are considerable temporal changes in the nutrient concentration of breast milk.

The extent and duration of breast-feeding determines the total amount of nutrients secreted in the milk. For adequate lactation, nutrients must be available in sufficient quantities from either the mother's diet or from body stores laid down during pregnancy. If these nutrients are insufficient owing to low energy intake, low nutrient density, or both, the mother will utilize her own body stores to meet her needs and to replace those secreted in her milk. Nutrients at risk of inadequate intake include calcium, zinc, magnesium, vitamin B_6, thiamin and folate. It may also be important to examine more completely the maternal depletion of iron and vitamin B_{12} stores through milk.

Calcium

Calcium is transferred directly from maternal serum to breast milk and breast milk concentrations are relatively independent of maternal intake except in instances where maternal calcium intake is exceptionally low (e.g. < 400 mg per day). The amount of calcium secreted during lactation has shown to be highly variable between women (e.g. in one study values ranged from 166 to 332 mg per day); however, it is estimated that lactating mothers secrete an average of 5 mmol (200 mg) of calcium per day into breast milk. Because of this loss, it is suggested that lactating women increase dietary calcium intake (400 mg) over and above that needed by nonlactating women to offset the calcium secreted into breast milk. If the diet does not provide sufficient calcium for breast milk production, it is believed the maternal skeleton will be drawn upon to provide the calcium needed for milk production. Indeed, women who are lactating, especially those who lactate for an extended period of time, experience a period of bone loss. However, it seems that dietary calcium cannot completely prevent this loss of bone, as even women consuming high levels of dietary calcium still exhibit bone loss during lactation. Although not proven, high prolactin and low oestrogen levels in lactation may be responsible, in part, for the mobilization of bone. Other explanations for the bone loss include decreased activity patterns, altered bone loading due to changes in body weight and regional body composition, and modified bone turnover rates. There is evidence that the bone lost during lactation is recovered after weaning and the re-establishment of menses. However, women who have had several pregnancies followed by extended periods of lactation might be at greater risk for osteoporosis later in life, though the evidence for this is contradictory.

It should also be noted that changes in calcium absorption and excretion, enhanced by alteration in metabolism, could theoretically compensate for these extra needs of milk synthesis without necessitating an increase in dietary calcium. It is known that renal calcium conservation begins during lactation and persists for several months after lactation has ceased. In general, alteration in bone mineral content and in calcium absorption, excretion and metabolism have been observed, but it is not known to what extent these changes are normal physiological modifications of lactation or are merely a response to insufficient dietary calcium intake. Interestingly, some investigators have reported that increased calcium intakes may elevate the risk of kidney stones and urinary tract infections and may reduce the absorption of other minerals, particularly iron, zinc and magnesium. More recent data do not confirm these observations.

Although guidelines for calcium intakes in lactating women differ between countries, most authorities currently recommend 30 mmol (1200 mg) per day, of which 400 mg represents the incremental amount necessary to support lactation. Calcium requirements may be even higher for lactating women less than 25 years of age, as in addition to the elevated calcium requirement to support lactation, these young women are still laying down their own bone calcium to decrease the risk of osteoporosis later in life. Diets of lactating women typically fall short of the recommended guidelines. However, it is also possible that the recommendation of calcium of 1200 mg per day is too high for many women to attain and it may not be necessary for lactating women to consume this level of intake. Current dietary guidance for lactating women should include recommendations for good sources of calcium. It is necessary to educate lactating women on the importance of an adequate intake of specific dairy products or other calcium-rich foods such as fish with edible bones, broccoli, kale and turnip greens.

Folate

Milk folate is quantitatively bound to folate-binding proteins (FBP) and there is a strong correlation between milk folate levels and FBP concentrations. As a result it is hypothesized that the secretion of folate into milk is under the control of FBP. Although not clearly understood, the proposed secretion method includes a critical stage whereby plasma folate entering the mammary gland eventually associates with FBP and the entire complex is then secreted into the milk compartment. It is known that folate is transferred from serum into breast milk against a steep concentration gradient as milk folate concentrations have been reported to be as much as 20 times greater than that of plasma folate among well-nourished women.

The folate content of breast milk has been reported to range from 50 to 320 nmol l^{-1} (20–141 $\mu g\, l^{-1}$) and levels typically increase with the progression of lactation despite declining blood folate concentrations. The nursing infant is thus protected from maternal folate deficiency as the folate content of milk is maintained at the expense of maternal folate reserves. As the average total maternal body stores of folate are between 5 and 10 mg and approximately 50–100 $\mu g\, l^{-1}$ of folate is secreted into milk each day, then theoretically maternal folate stores would be exhausted after 6 months of exclusive breast-feeding without a source of dietary folate.

Most dietary folate recommendations during lactation are based on the average folate concentration of 50 $\mu g\, l^{-1}$ in human milk. However, there is controversy about whether past analytical methods truly measured all available milk folate. It has been suggested that a value of 85 $\mu g\, l^{-1}$ be used to derive the folate requirements of lactating women. Using this higher value, and assuming a 50% dietary absorption factor (from a mixed diet), folate requirements for lactating women would be 320 μg per day (the sum of the maintenance value of 180 μg per day for the nonpregnant, nonlactating adult plus 140 μg per day for lactation). Again, this recommendation does not take into account maternal folate status at the beginning of lactation, or the stage of lactation. In addition, the recommended guidelines do not account for the possible anabolic cost of folate required for milk synthesis or that recent data suggest that the folate recommendation for nonpregnant, nonlactating women should be raised to 400 μg per day. If this higher value of 400 μg per day is added to the incremental amount required for lactation, an average intake of 540 μg per day would be required.

It is apparent that most lactating women do not meet current recommended folate intakes. Using the recommendation of 540 μg per day and calculating the probable folate intakes of an unsupplemented lactating woman ingesting 8400 kJ (2000 kcal) per day, the typical daily intake would be approximately half the needed amount of folate. Maternal folate inadequacy has been implicated in a wide variety of disorders including neural tube defects, low infant birthweight, abruptio placenta, cervical dysplasia, atherosclerosis and colon cancer. Special care should be taken to instruct breast-feeding women to consume folate-dense foods including fruits and vegetables, specifically those which are 'vitamin C rich', e.g. oranges, and 'dark green leafy'. Other excellent sources of folate include many legumes (e.g. lentils, beans and peas), nuts, seeds and super-fortified cereals.

Iron

The mechanism of iron transfer from serum into milk has not yet been determined, but it is known that the iron in human milk is tightly bound to a protein called lactoferrin, which is synthesized in the mammary aveolar cell. The concentration of iron in human milk is low, ranging from 0.2 to 0.9 mg l^{-1}. The amount of iron secreted into milk during the first 6 months of exclusive breast-feeding (~50 mg) is equivalent to approximately half of what would be lost through menstruation during the same period of time. Because the amount of iron secreted into breast milk is small and it is generally accepted that menstrual losses of iron are minimal during lactation, the iron requirements set by most authorities do not differ from those for the nonpregnant, nonlactating woman, and hence range between 14 and 28 mg per day, depending on the availability of dietary iron. However, as many women, even in developed countries, have suboptimal nutrition and may menstrate for several weeks postpartum, the logic of these recommendations can be challenged. In addition, menses does return for many women between 3 and 9 months postpartum, further elevating the need for dietary iron. Upon its return, the combined demands of milk production and menstruation could draw significantly on maternal iron stores if dietary intakes are low.

Dietary surveys of lactating women suggest that intakes of iron may be at risk for inadequacy as compared with recommended values. The significance of lower intakes and the need or the impact of iron supplementation is unknown. To help maintain satisfactory iron status, lactating women should be encouraged to consume cereal products, meat, fish, poultry and vegetables. In addition, iron supplements should be considered for those women who are not able to obtain recommended dietary levels, e.g. complete vegetarians.

Zinc

It is proposed that the zinc present in human milk is preferentially bound to high molecular weight proteins that are saturated at the zinc levels present in milk. Additional zinc then binds with lower affinity to various low molecular weight substances. The mechanism of transfer from plasma to milk has not yet been studied. Zinc concentrations are higher in colostrum (> 10 mg l^{-1}) and decrease significantly during the first 3 months postpartum. For example, in one study the estimated zinc concentrations in milk were 59.4 ± 15.1 μmol l^{-1} and 22.6 ± 9.9 μmol l^{-1} at 0.5 and 3 months postpartum, respectively. The concentration of zinc in milk among well-nourished women is not influenced by either maternal dietary intake or supplementation, although little is known about the impact on milk zinc concentration of extremely suboptimal maternal zinc intakes in developing countries.

To compensate for poor absorption of zinc from dietary sources (~20%), the recommended dietary intake of zinc is four to 13 times higher than the estimated amount secreted in milk. However, there are indications from animal studies that maternal zinc absorption is increased during lactation, independent of maternal zinc status. Renal conservation of zinc during the lactational period may also help retain body stores for the production of milk; however it is unclear whether depressed urinary excretion of zinc is due directly to lactation or secondary to nutritional status. Dietary zinc recommendations vary between 18 and 25 mg per day during the first 6 months of breast-feeding. Surveys have reported actual intakes much lower than recommended dietary zinc intakes, particularly when recommended energy needs are not met. Interestingly, low dietary zinc intakes are often associated with adequate protein and iron intakes, nutrients which are typically found in zinc-containing foods.

To date, there have been no reports of overt zinc deficiency (e.g. health consequences) among lactating women; however, if the lactating woman had inadequate zinc intakes during pregnancy as well as low intakes during breast-feeding, both mother and infant may be at risk of deficiency. Several studies have indicated that in communities where dietary zinc intake is marginal, lactating women exhibit reduced indices of zinc status when compared with non-lactating women. Iron supplements may also inhibit the absorption of zinc, particularly at levels greater than 30 mg per day.

In providing food guidance to ensure adequate intakes of zinc, lactating women should be encouraged to consume meat, poultry, eggs and dairy products – all highly available sources of zinc. Plant-based sources of zinc are absorbed less efficiently and fruits and vegetables contain very small amounts of zinc. Given the impact of adequate zinc status on immunity and other functions, further research on maternal zinc status is recommended.

Vitamin B$_{12}$

Very little is known about the mechanism by which vitamin B$_{12}$ is secreted into milk. Human milk contains two types of vitamin B_{12} protein binders: transcobalamin II (TC-II) and R-type binders (haptocorrin, cobalophilin). It is hypothesized that these binders are located in the mammary gland to trap the vitamin form maternal serum. However, the evidence of TC-II receptors in the mammary cells has not been studied.

Estimates of the vitamin B_{12} output in human milk range from 0.4 to 0.97 $\mu g\ l^{-1}$. To compensate for this loss, it is recommended that lactating women increase their intake of vitamin B_{12} to 1.2–2.5 μg per day. Intakes below this may still prove adequate as low intakes cause increased reabsorption of vitamin B_{12} excreted in the bile. It could take potentially 20 years for vitamin B_{12} stores to become depleted. In a number of reports, however, long-term practising vegan women are shown to have both low serum and milk B_{12} concentrations. Surprisingly, the concentration of vitamin B_{12} in milk has also been reported to be low in women who have been practising vegetarianism for over 30 months. These reports strongly suggest that maternal intake of B_{12} may have a significant impact on breast milk concentrations. Low vitamin B_{12} concentrations in breast milk (less than 0.49 $\mu g\ l^{-1}$) have shown to be inversely related to urinary methylmalonic acid excretion (a functional index of vitamin B_{12} status) of the infant. There are numerous reports demonstrating that breast-fed infants of mothers who severely restrict their intake of animal protein present with anaemia, growth failure and neurological delay.

Animal products are the only significant dietary source of vitamin B_{12} and populations consuming such ingest between 3 and 32 μg per day. Foods of plant origin contain little or no vitamin B_{12}. Lactating women who avoid all animal foods are advised to take a vitamin B_{12} supplement to meet daily recommended intakes.

Vitamin A

The vitamin A content of human milk is composed primarily of retinyl esters which are derived from either plasma retinol-binding protein or chylomicrons and esterfied by the mammary gland. The concentration of this vitamin is high early in lactation and declines thereafter (2000 μg to 600 μg per litre of milk). Concentrations of carotenoids, vitamin A precursors, are reported to vary from 200 to 400 μg per litre of human milk. These amounts could potentially draw upon 50% of maternal stores during the first 6 months of breast-feeding.

To maintain maternal stores, it is recommended that an extra 300 μg retinol equivalent (RE) per day of vitamin A be consumed during the first 6 months of lactation. Chronically inadequate intakes below those recommended must occur to significantly deplete maternal stores. In developed countries, an additional dietary vitamin A intake to support the needs of lactation is easily achieved by regular consumption of fruits and vegetables. Nonetheless, even in these countries, woman from economically disadvantaged communities with lower dietary intakes may potentially exhibit a higher prevalence of inadequate intakes. In contrast, the average intake in developing countries is about two-thirds of the recommended daily intake, significantly less than the average intake of lactating women in developed countries. Preformed vitamin A is obtained exclusively from foods of animal origin, primarily milk products, egg yolks and liver, while carotenoids are widely available from fruits and vegetables. Unfortified cereals contain little, if any, vitamin A.

Conclusions

Lactation is a very demanding process in terms of nutritional requirements. If nutrient intake is lower than the total demand for both maternal nutrient needs and milk production, the mother's body will mobilize available nutrients from body stores. To help maintain optimum nutritional status, lactating women should be encouraged to consume those foods that are major sources of nutrients, such as calcium-rich dairy products, animal products (iron, zinc, vitamin B_{12} and vitamin A), fruits and vegetables (folate and carotenoids) and enriched cereals. Since the recommended increase in energy intake during lactation is proportionately smaller than the recommended increase for many vitamins and minerals, the extra energy required by the lactating woman should come from nutrient-dense foods. Special care should be taken to identify women with restricted eating patterns (e.g. vegetarians, dieters) and women whose diets, on average, have nutrient densities lower than the recommended allowances (e.g. low-income women, adolescent females).

There are many unanswered questions concerning the nutritional status of lactating women and the relationship between maternal nutrition and maternal health. Research is needed to investigate the transfer of nutrients from mother to milk and the effects of lactational performance on maternal nutritional status. In addition, further research is needed to identify groups of lactating women who are at risk of nutritional problems and/or who could benefit from nutrition intervention programmes.

See also: **Infants**: Milk-feeding and Weaning. **Lactation**: Physiology.

Further Reading

Casey CE and Hambidge MK (1983) In: Neville MC and Neifert MR (eds) *Lactation. Physiology, Nutrition and Breast-Feeding*, pp 199–248. New York: Plenum Press.

Gutherie HA and Picciano MF (1995) *Human Nutrition*, pp 509–534. St Louis, MO: Mosby-Year Book, Inc.

Neville MC, Allen JC and Watters C (1983) In: Neville MC and Neifert MR (eds) *Lactation. Physiology, Nutrition, and Breast-Feeding*, pp 49–102. New York: Plenum Press.

Pitkin RM and Hamosh M (1991) In: Nutritional status and usual dietary intake of lactating women. *Nutrition During Lactation*, pp 50–79. Washington, DC: National Academy Press.

Pitkin RM and Hamosh M (1991) In: Maternal Health Effects of Breastfeeding. *Nutrition During Lactation*, pp 197–212. Washington, DC: National Academy Press.

Pitkin RM and Hamosh M (1991) In: Meeting maternal nutrient needs during lactation. *Nutrition During Lactation*, pp 213–235. Washington, DC: National Academy Press.

Prentice A (1994) Maternal calcium requirements during pregnancy and lactation. *American Journal of Clinical Nutrition*, **59** (supplement): 477S–483S.

Prentice AM, Spaaij CJK, Goldberg GR, Poppitt SD, van Raaij JMA, Totton M, Swann D and Black AE (1996) Energy requirements of pregnant and lactating women. *European Journal of Clinical Nutrition*, **50** (supplement 1): S82–S111.

Sowers M (1996) Pregnancy and lactation as risk factors for subsequent bone loss and osteoporosis. *Journal of Bone and Mineral Research* **11**(8):1052–1060.

Todd JM and Parnell JM (1994) Nutrient intakes of women who are breastfeeding. *European Journal of Clinical Nutrition* **48**:567–574.

US National Academy of Science (1991) *Nutrition During Lactation*. Washington, DC: National Academy Press.

LEGUMES

Types and Nutritional Value

A Fehily, HJ Heinz Company Ltd, Wigan, UK

Copyright © 1998 Academic Press

Legumes can provide a valuable contribution to nutrient intakes. This article discusses the types of legumes in the human diet, their nutritional value and their role in the diet.

Types

Legumes (peas, beans and lentils) are seeds of plants of the Leguminosae family (also known as the Fabaceae family). The term 'legume' is derived from a Latin word, *legumen*, meaning seeds harvested in pods. They are also known as pulses, a word derived from the Latin *puls*, meaning a thick paste or pottage. There are about 13 000 species of legumes, but only about 20 of these are commonly consumed by humans. Plants vary in size from tiny wild vetches to large trees. Legumes in the human diet are mainly herbaceous annuals and grow throughout the world. Most legumes are consumed in Central and South America, Africa and Asia.

Peas

The common pea, *Pisum sativum*, also known as the garden pea, green pea, sugar pea or mange tout, has one of the longest histories of the legumes. Remains of peas have been found in the ruins of Troy and in ancient Egyptian tombs. Remains of cultivated peas have been found in Europe which date from 4500 BC. The word *pease* comes from Sanskrit and similar words are found in most Indo-European languages.

Beans

The aduki bean (*Phaseolus angularis*) is a native of Japan, but has also been cultivated for centuries in China and Korea. It was little known in the West until the emergence of the macrobiotic culture, in which it is considered an important staple food.

The blackeye bean (*Vigna unguiculata*) is also known as cow pea, China pea, cowgram, catjang and Southern pea. It came originally from Africa, where it is still an important staple food.

The broad bean (*Vicia faba*) is also known as the faba bean, field bean, horse bean, pigeon bean, trick bean or Windsor bean. It is thought to have originated in Asia Minor and was also grown extensively in ancient Egypt.

The guar bean or cluster bean (*Cyamopsis*

tetragonoloba) is a legume widely used in the food industry as a source of the stabilizer guar gum.

The haricot bean (*Phaseolus vulgaris*) is of Mexican origin and was brought to Europe in the sixteenth century. Also known as navy bean, kidney bean, French bean, Boston bean, pinto bean and string bean, it is grown mainly in the Americas. Navy beans are used to make canned 'baked beans'. Red kidney beans are a well-known ingredient of dishes such as chilli con carne. French beans (*haricot vert*) are haricot beans which have been harvested immature and eaten with the pod.

The Lima bean, butter bean, Madagascar butter bean or Sieva bean (*Phaseolus lunatus*) originates from Peru. It grows only in a hot, humid climate and is a valuable part of the diet of many communities in the tropics.

The locust bean, also known as carob (*Parkia biglobosa*), comes from an evergreen leguminous tree, which originates from the Middle East. It was these beans that gave nourishment to John the Baptist when he lived in the wilderness on 'locusts and wild honey'. The most well-known uses of the locust bean are as a substitute for chocolate (carob) and as a stabilizer in food products (locust bean gum or carob gum).

The runner bean, scarlet runner bean or multiflora bean (*Phaseolus coccineus*) originates from America and was first introduced into England in 1683. At first, the plant was cultivated solely for its ornamental value, and the beans were not regularly eaten as a vegetable until the eighteenth century. The green pods are eaten before the seed matures. For this reason its nutrient composition is closer to that of green vegetables than to that of legumes.

The soya bean (*Glycine max*) is a native of China, where it has been part of the diet for several thousand years. It has also been important in Japan and Korea for almost as long. These beans are used to produce foods which are important components of the diet in the Far East, e.g. fermented soya products such as tofu, miso and tempeh and also soy sauce. More recently, soya beans have become widely used in the Western diet, being used to produce a range of ingredients: soya flour and soya protein, which are used to make foodstuffs such as bread, other cereal products, meat products and vegetarian alternatives; soya oil, which is widely used as a vegetable oil both in domestic cooking and by the food industry and is also used in the manufacture of spreadable fats; soya lecithin, which is used as an emulsifier in many foods; and soya milk, which is a vegan alternative to cow's milk. Soya is also used to produce infant formulae for those infants who are intolerant to lactose or cow's milk protein.

Lentils and similar pulses

Lentils are the seeds of *Lens esculenta*, a plant that originated in the Mediterranean countries. They were one of the first cultivated crops, particularly in the East. There are two main types: Chinese and Indian. The Chinese vary from whitish to green and the Indian are orange-red in colour.

Several similar pulses are widely cultivated in tropical and semitropical countries. In India, these are called dhals. The best known are: red dhal or masur dhal (also *Lens esculenta*); Bengal gram or chick pea (*Cicer arietinum*); black gram, mung bean or urd bean (*Vigna mungo*); green gram or golden gram (*Vigna radiatus*); and red gram, pigeon pea, non-eye pea, Congo pea, Angola pea or yellow dhal (*Cajanus cajan*). The chick pea has become of major importance in Mediterranean countries where it is used to make hummus. Mung bean sprouts, sold as 'beansprouts', are used in many Chinese-style recipes.

Peanuts or groundnuts

Peanuts (*Arachis hypogaea*), also known as groundnuts or monkey nuts, are in fact not nuts but are seeds of a leguminous plant. The plant originated in South America: peanuts have been discovered in Peruvian tombs dating from 950 BC. Peanuts were taken from Brazil to East Africa and to the Philippines in the sixteenth century, where they became an important food. They are called 'groundnuts' because they ripen underground and have to be dug up at harvest. (After flowering, the ends of the flower stalk bend down and the young pods are forced into the ground by the direction of growth.)

Macronutrient Content

The protein, carbohydrate and fat contents of a range of legumes are presented in **Fig. 1**.

Protein

Legumes are a good source of protein. Fig. 1 shows that protein contents for most legumes are generally between 5 and 9 g per 100 g as consumed. This is approximately two to five times more than in most other vegetables and twice that in milk. Soya beans and peanuts contain considerably more protein than other legumes (14 g per 100 g and 25.6 g per 100 g, respectively, as consumed). Beans consumed before the seeds are mature (e.g. French beans and runner beans) and bean sprouts have much lower protein contents than other legumes (1.5–2.5 g per 100 g as consumed).

The amino acid compositions of legumes and other

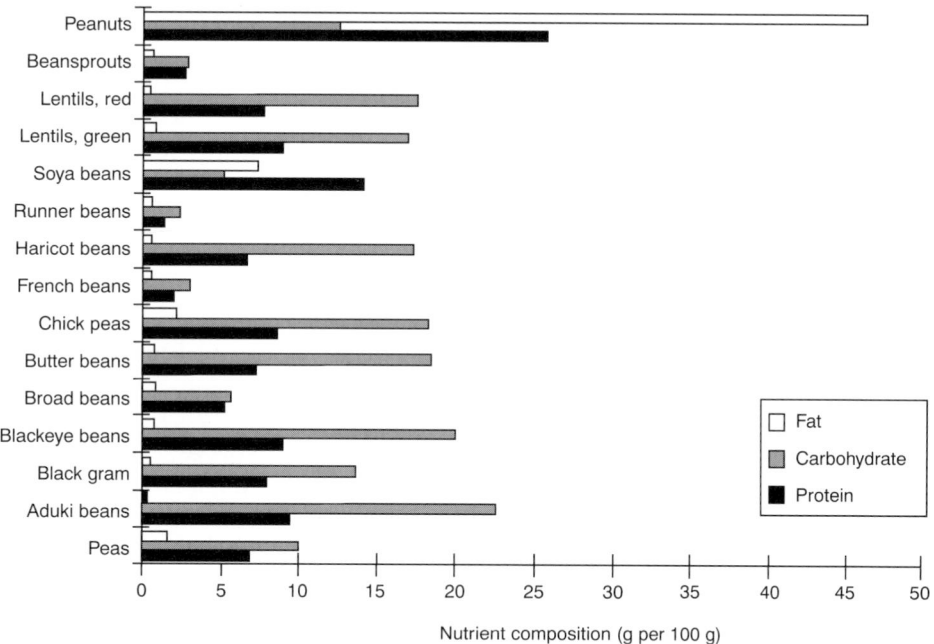

Figure 1 Nutrient composition of legumes (per 100 g as consumed). Data from Holland et al. (1991, 1992). Data from *The Composition of Foods* and supplements are reproduced with the permission of The Royal Society of Chemistry and The Controller of Her Majesty's Stationery Office.

foods are presented in **Fig. 2**, expressed as mg g^{-1} protein. Legume proteins have substantial amounts of most essential amino acids, concentrations generally being higher than in other vegetables. When compared with a reference protein, egg, legumes are deficient in sulfur-containing amino acids (the essential amino acid methionine and the nonessential amino acid cystine) and have a higher content of lysine. Cereals, on the other hand, have adequate amounts of sulfur-containing amino acids but are deficient in lysine. Combining legumes with cereals would, therefore, yield a meal with a high protein quality, e.g. beans canned in tomato sauce served on toast.

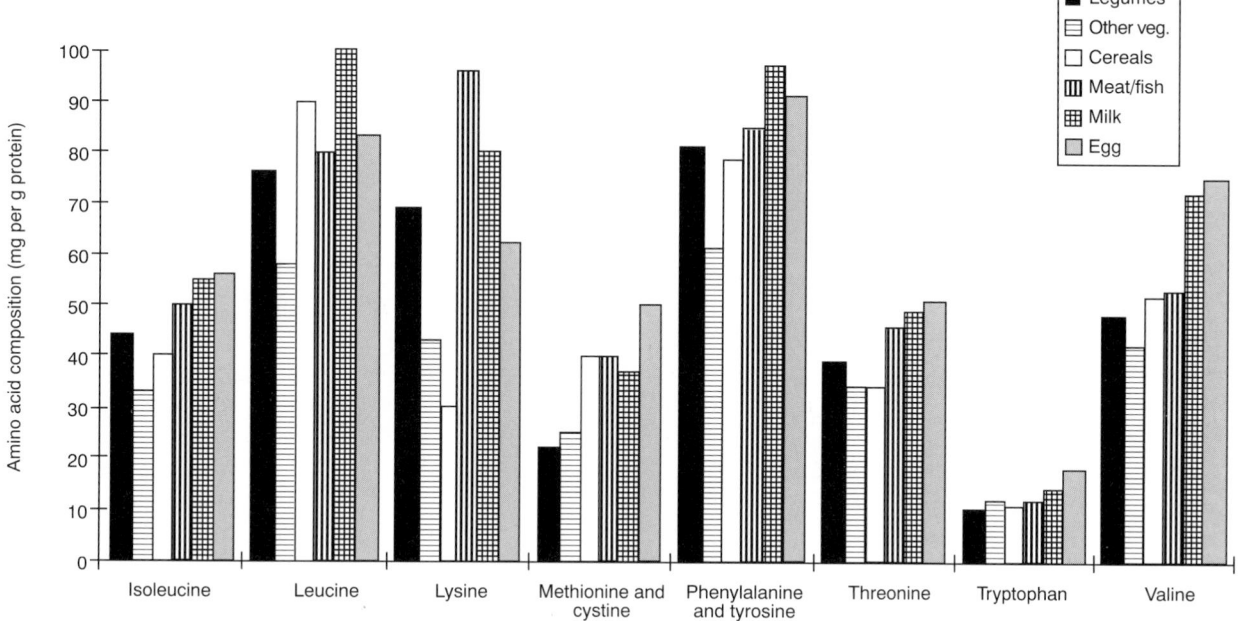

Figure 2 Amino acid composition of foods (mg per g protein). Data from Paul and Southgate (1978).

Carbohydrate

Most legumes provide a source of carbohydrate in the diet (Fig. 1). Contents vary widely across the range of foods: bean sprouts and beans eaten before the seeds mature contain relatively little carbohydrate (2–3 g per 100 g); other legumes vary from 5 to 23 g per 100 g as consumed.

For peas, most beans and lentils, the majority of the carbohydrate is starch (76–96%) and only a small amount is sugars and oligosaccharides. Exceptions to this are beans consumed before the seeds are mature (e.g. French beans and runner beans), bean sprouts, soya beans and peanuts, in which only 13–50% of the total carbohydrate is starch. Of the sugars present, sucrose is the major component for most legumes (60–100% of the total sugars), the remainder being glucose and fructose. Exceptions to this are beans consumed before the seeds are mature and bean sprouts, in which sucrose provides no more than about 25% of the total sugars, the majority being glucose and fructose.

Fat

Most legumes are low in fat, containing 0.2–2.1 g per 100 g as consumed (Fig. 1). The main exceptions are soya beans and peanuts, which contain 7.3 g and 46.1 g of fat, respectively, per 100 g as consumed.

The fatty acid compositions of legumes have a high ratio of unsaturates to saturates. Only 11–38% of the total fatty acids are saturated fatty acids. For most legumes, polyunsaturated fatty acids provide the highest proportion of the total fatty acids (42–71%). The main exception to this is peanuts, in which only 29% of the fatty acids are polyunsaturated. The polyunsaturated fatty acids present in legumes are the essential fatty acids linoleic acid (18:2n-6) and α-linolenic acid (18:3n-3). Peanuts contain a high proportion of monounsaturated fatty acids (48% of the total fatty acids) compared with other legumes (8–33% of the total fatty acids). Most of the monounsaturated fatty acids content of legumes is oleic acid (18:1n-9).

Energy

The energy content of legumes varies widely across the range of foods, from 76 to 590 kJ (18–141 kcal) per 100 g as consumed. Beans consumed before the seeds are mature (e.g. French beans and runner beans) and bean sprouts have lower energy contents than other legumes: 76–104 kJ (18–25 kcal) per 100 g as consumed compared with 204–590 kJ (48–141 kcal) per 100 g as consumed for other legumes.

Micronutrient Content

Minerals

Table 1 shows that legumes contain substantial amounts of several minerals: calcium, iron, magnesium, potassium, phosphorus and zinc. However, there is considerable variation in mineral contents across the range of legumes. The variations in content and richest sources can be summarized as follows.

- Calcium contents vary from 16 to 83 mg per 100 g as consumed; the richest sources are soya beans, haricot beans and peanuts.
- Iron contents vary from 0.8 to 3.5 mg per 100 g

Table 1 Mineral contents of legumes (per 100 g as consumed)

Legume	Calcium (mg)	Iron (mg)	Magnesium (mg)	Potassium (mg)	Phosphorus (mg)	Zinc (mg)
Aduki beans	39	1.9	60	570	180	2.3
Beansprouts	19	2.2	14	46	37	0.3
Blackeye beans	21	1.9	45	320	140	1.1
Black gram	49	2.0	52	260	120	0.9
Broad beans	18	0.8	19	190	100	0.7
Butter beans	19	1.7	38	400	87	0.9
Chick peas	46	2.1	37	270	83	1.2
French beans	34	1.1	16	180	42	0.2
Haricot beans	65	2.5	45	320	120	1.0
Lentils, green	22	3.5	34	310	130	1.4
Lentils, red	16	2.4	26	220	100	1.0
Peas	19	1.5	29	230	130	1.0
Runner beans	22	1.0	14	130	21	0.2
Soya beans	83	3.0	63	510	250	0.9
Peanuts	60	2.5	210	670	430	3.5

Data from Holland et al. (1991, 1992). Data from The Composition of Foods and supplements are reproduced with the permission of The Royal Society of Chemistry and The Controller of Her Majesty's Stationery Office.

as consumed; the richest sources are green lentils, soya beans, haricot beans and peanuts.

- Magnesium contents vary from 14 to 210 mg per 100 g as consumed; the richest sources are peanuts and soya beans.
- Potassium contents vary from 46 to 670 mg per 100 g as consumed; the richest sources are peanuts, soya beans and aduki beans.
- Phosphorus contents vary from 37 to 430 mg per 100 g as consumed; the richest sources are peanuts and soya beans.
- Zinc contents vary from 0.2 to 3.5 mg; the richest sources are peanuts and aduki beans.

Vitamins

Table 2 shows that legumes contain a number of water-soluble vitamins: thiamin, riboflavin, nicotinic acid, vitamin B_6 and folate. However, as for other nutrients, there is considerable variation in vitamin contents across the range of legumes. Most legumes contain only a trace of vitamin C. The exceptions to this are bean sprouts, beans eaten before the seeds mature, peas and broad beans. Of these, the richest sources are peas and broad beans, which contain approximately 16 mg and 20 mg of vitamin C respectively, per 100 g as consumed. Legumes, in common with other vegetables, do not contain vitamin B_{12}.

Since most legumes are low in fat, they are also low in fat-soluble vitamins. They do not contain retinol or vitamin D. However, a few contain a small amount of β-carotene, and many contain vitamin E. The richest sources of vitamin E among legumes are peanuts (10.09 mg per 100 g) and soya beans (1.13 mg per 100 g as consumed).

Fibre Content

Legumes provide a valuable source of fibre in the diet. Nonstarch polysaccharides (NSP) contents range from 1.3 to 6.2 g per 100 g as consumed. The richest sources are peanuts (6.2 g), soya beans and haricot beans (both 6.1 g).

Of the total NSP, on average 35% is cellulose (range 16–67%). Peas and broad beans have the highest proportions of cellulose (60 and 67%, respectively, of the total NSP). Of the noncellulosic polysaccharides, for most legumes approximately two-thirds is soluble fibre (e.g. peas, bean sprouts, broad beans, butter beans, French beans, haricot beans, soya beans and runner beans). Of other legumes, the proportion of noncellulosic polysaccharides which is soluble fibre ranges from 24 to 45%.

Toxins and Contaminants

Raw legumes contain a number of substances which may have detrimental effects on digestion and other metabolic processes (lectins, goitrogens, cyanogenic glycosides, lathyrogens and digestive enzyme inhibitors). These substances are, however, inactivated by appropriate cooking of the legumes. In the case of goitrogens, these are counteracted by adequate iodine intake (*See:* **Food Contaminants**; Mycotoxins - Occurrence and Toxic Effects).

Table 2 Vitamin contents of legumes (per 100 g as consumed)

Legume	Thiamin (mg)	Riboflavin (mg)	Nicotinic acid (mg equivalents)	Vitamin B_6 (mg)	Folate (μg)	Vitamin C (mg)
Aduki beans	0.14	0.08	2.4	NK	NK	Trace
Beansprouts	0.09	0.05	0.7	0.07	17	2–7
Blackeye beans	0.19	0.05	2.4	0.10	210	Trace
Black gram	0.11	0.09	2.0	NK	33	Trace
Broad beans	0.03	0.06	3.8	0.08	32	20
Butter beans	0.16	0.05	1.5	0.16	NK	Trace
Chick peas	0.10	0.07	1.8	0.14	54	Trace
French beans	0.06	0.04	1.0	0.06	57	11
Haricot beans	0.10	0.04	1.7	0.12	NK	Trace
Lentils, green	0.14	0.08	1.8	0.28	30	Trace
Lentils, red	0.11	0.04	1.4	0.11	5	Trace
Peas	0.70	0.03	2.9	0.09	27	16
Runner beans	0.05	0.02	0.3	0.04	42	10
Soya beans	0.12	0.09	2.7	0.23	54	Trace
Peanuts	1.14	0.10	19.3	0.59	110	0

Data from Holland *et al.* (1991, 1992). Data from *The Composition of Foods* and supplements are reproduced with the permission of The Royal Society of Chemistry and The Controller of Her Majesty's Stationery Office.
NK = not known.

Lectins

Lectins, also known as haemagglutinins, are present in many raw legumes. They are, however, heat-labile and are inactivated when legumes are properly cooked. In experimental animals these polymeric proteins have been shown to cause damage to red blood cells and intestinal mucosa, and thereby impaired nutrient utilization and loss of body weight. In humans, these compounds can result in nausea, vomiting, diarrhoea and abdominal pain. For example, during the 1970s, consumption of red kidney beans resulted in an outbreak of food poisoning in the UK. This was due to inadequate cooking of the beans.

Goitrogens

Goitrogens are found in raw soya beans and in the skin of peanuts. These have been shown to cause enlargement of the thyroid gland in experimental animals. The goitrogenic agent in soya beans is unknown; that in peanut skin is a phenolic glycoside. The goitrogenic effect of these legumes is counteracted by adequate iodine intake, and for soya beans the effect is also counteracted by heat treatment of the beans.

Cyanogenic glycosides

Cyanogenic glycosides are present in some raw legumes, e.g. Lima beans. In the raw beans, cyanide may be released from the glycosides by enzymes in the plant tissue. The effects of these glycosides are counteracted by cooking: glycosides are hydrolysed rapidly, cyanide being lost by volatilization, and the enzymes are also denatured.

Lathyrogens

Lathyrism is a disease caused by peas of the *Lathyrus* genus, e.g. *Lathyrus sativus* (lathyrus pea, grass pea, chickling pea, Indian vetch or khesari dhal). This disease has been reported mainly in India, during periods of drought when these peas have provided a high proportion of the total food intake for several months. There are two types of lathyrism: osteolathyrism and neurolathyrism. Osteolathyrism is characterized by an abnormality of the skeleton and osteoporosis, and is a result of an impairment in collagen metabolism. Neurolathyrism is characterized by muscular rigidity, weakness and paralysis of the leg muscles, and is a result of effects on the nervous system. The lathyrogens have been identified as α-N-glutamyl-β-aminopropionitrile (osteolathyrism) and β-N-oxalyl-β-diaminopropionic acid (neurolathyrism). The disease can be prevented by boiling the peas in water and then discarding the water.

Digestive enzyme inhibitors

Raw legumes contain certain proteins which react with digestive enzymes (trypsin, chymotrypsin or salivary and pancreatic α-amylase) and thereby interfering with the digestion of protein and starch. These inhibitors are inactivated by heat and are therefore not a problem in cooked legumes.

Phytic acid

Phytic acid is present in legumes and is also present in other fibre-containing foods. It has been suggested to reduce the absorption of calcium, iron, zinc and vitamin D from the diet. However, these effects have been observed in *in vitro* experiments, and not in *in vivo* studies, even at fibre intakes at the upper limit of the normal human consumption range. In addition, levels of micronutrients tend to be higher in fibre-rich foods than in fibre-poor foods. Thus, adverse effects of phytic acid on nutrient absorption are likely to be unimportant at the levels of fibre normally consumed in the human diet (*See:* **Dietary Fibre (Fiber)**: Physiological Effects and Effects on Absorption).

Flatulence

Flatulence is a problem associated with many beans. This is due to the presence of indigestible oligosaccharides (raffinose and stachyose). These pass into the large intestine where they are attacked by microorganisms, resulting in the production of hydrogen and carbon dioxide (*See:* **Carbohydrates**; Resistant Starch and Oligosaccharides).

Favism

Broad beans are the cause of favism, a haemolytic anaemia, the symptoms of which (high temperature and jaundice) occur soon after eating the beans or inhaling the pollen of the flower. The condition occurs only in those individuals with a genetic defect in their red blood cells: glucose-6-phosphate dehydrogenase (G6PD) deficiency. Lack of this enzyme results in reduced production of NADPH (reduced nicotinamide adenine dinucleotide phosphate) and thereby a deficiency of reduced glutathione, which is essential for maintenance of the stability of red cell membranes.

G6PD deficiency is almost entirely confined to people of Mediterranean and middle-eastern origin, being very common in Southern Italy and Sardinia, and is associated with a reduced tendency to contract malaria. It has been estimated that there are around 100 million people worldwide who are G6PD-deficient. The condition is rare in North European native populations, although the actual prevalence in these countries will be influenced by migration from other countries.

It has been suggested that the Greek philosopher Pythagoras may have suffered from favism: he forbade his followers to eat beans and met his death at the edge of a field of flowering broad beans (rather than running through the beans, he allowed himself to be captured and killed by his enemies).

Role in the Diet

Legumes have a wide range of uses in the diet: vegetable accompaniments to meat and fish; alternatives to meat and fish in main course dishes; ingredients in soups and hors d'oeuvres; snacks, e.g. beans canned in tomato sauce served on toast, peanuts; and even as an occasional ingredient in desserts, e.g. peanuts. Soya beans are particularly versatile, having a wide range of uses in foods, e.g. soya sauce, soya flour, soya protein, soya oil, soya lecithin.

Legumes are also of agricultural importance, as they increase the nitrogen content of the soil. Although green plants cannot utilize nitrogen in the atmosphere, there are several species of bacteria, fungi and blue-green algae which are able to transform nitrogen in the air into a form that can be used by plants. An important genus of nitrogen-fixing bacteria is *Rhizobium*, which forms nodules in the roots of legumes. These bacteria live symbiotically with the legumes, the bacteria obtaining food from the green plant and the legumes obtaining abundant usable nitrogen compounds from the bacteria.

Legumes can be an important component of a normal healthy diet, since most legumes are low in fat and saturates, and also provide fibre. They can therefore provide lower-fat alternatives to cheeses and meats. In addition, foods such as beans canned in tomato sauce provide more fibre per serving than most other foods.

For vegetarians and vegans, legumes play a very important role in the diet. They provide a valuable source of protein which can be of high quality if legumes are combined with cereals, since the amino acid compositions are complementary. Legumes also provide an important source of water-soluble vitamins and of minerals, especially iron. While, in general, iron from vegetable sources is less well absorbed than that from animal sources, soya beans provide a source of iron which can be absorbed as well as that in meat.

For people with non-insulin-dependent diabetes mellitus, legumes may help in controlling plasma glucose concentrations, avoiding undesirable peaks. For people with high plasma lipid concentrations, legumes, particularly soya beans, may help to reduce cholesterol concentrations, as part of a diet low in fat and saturates. Both of these effects have been suggested to be due to the presence of soluble fibre. For infants intolerant to cow's milk protein or to lactose, soya-based infant formulae can be an invaluable alternative to cows' milk-based formulae.

Recent evidence suggests that some legumes may help protect the body against certain cancers. However, available data are not conclusive, being mainly obtained from animal studies. A great deal of further research is therefore needed. It has also been suggested that some legumes (e.g. soya beans) may reduce menopausal symptoms (hot flushes) and reduce bone loss in menopausal women. Again, more research is needed in these areas.

In conclusion, legumes are versatile foods and can provide a valuable contribution to nutrient intakes, both for those wishing to build a normal healthy diet and for many of those with special dietary requirements.

See also: **Ascorbic Acid**: Physiology, Dietary Sources and Requirements. **Calcium**: Physiology. **Cancer**: Epidemiology and Associations Between Diet and Cancer. **Diabetes Mellitus**: Dietary Management. **Dietary Fibre (Fiber)**: Physiological Effects and Effects on Absorption. **Energy**: Energy Requirements. **Fats and Oils**: Nutritional Value. **Fatty Acids**: Health Effects of Monounsaturated Fatty Acids; Health Effects of n-6 Polyunsaturated Fatty Acids; Health Effects of n-3 Polyunsaturated Fatty Acids. **Folic Acid**: Physiology, Dietary Sources and Requirements. **Food Contaminants**: Mycotoxins - Occurrence and Toxic Effects. **Iron**: Physiology, Dietary Sources and Requirements. **Magnesium**: Physiology, Dietary Sources and Requirements. **Phosphorus**: Physiology, Dietary Sources and Requirements. **Potassium**: Physiology, Dietary Sources and Requirements. **Protein**: Quality and Sources. **Riboflavin**: Physiology. **Therapeutic Dietetics**: Short Bowel Syndrome. **Thiamin**: Physiology. **Vegetarian Diets**: Nutritional Adequacy. **Zinc**: Physiology.

Further Reading

Doughty J and Walker A (1982) *Legumes in Human Nutrition*. FAO Food and Nutrition Paper no. 20.

Holland B, Unwin ID and Buss DH (1991) *Vegetables, herbs and spices. The 5th supplement to McCance and Widdowson (eds) The Composition of Foods*, 4th edn. Cambridge: Royal Society of Chemistry and Ministry of Agriculture Fisheries and Food.

Holland B, Unwin ID and Buss DH (1992) *Fruit and nuts. The 1st supplement to McCance and Widdowson (eds) The Composition of Foods*, 5th edn. Cambridge: Royal Society of Chemistry and Ministry of Agriculture Fisheries and Food.

Passmore R and Eastwood MA (1986) Foods from the vegetable kingdom. In: *Davidson and Passmore Human
Nutrition and Dietetics*, pp 197–200. London: Churchill Livingstone.

Paul AA and Southgate DAT (1978) Amino acid composition. In: *McCance and Widdowson's The Composition of Foods, 4th edn*, pp 279–287. London: HMSO.

Sgarbieri VC (1993) Legumes: dietary importance. In:

Macrae R, Robinson RK and Sadler MJ (eds) *Encyclopaedia of Food Science, Food Technology and
Nutrition*, pp 2726–2730. London: Academic Press.

Uebersax MA and Occena LG (1993) Legumes in the diet.
In: Macrae R, Robinson RK and Sadler MJ (eds) *Ency-
clopaedia of Food Science, Food Technology and
Nutrition*, pp 2718–2725. London: Academic Press.

LIPIDS

Contents
Chemistry and Classification
Composition and Role of Phospholipids in the Body

Chemistry and Classification

E Turley, University of Ulster, Coleraine,
Northern Ireland, UK

Copyright © 1998 Academic Press

Lipids, like proteins, carbohydrates and nucleotides,
are essential components of all living organisms.
Unlike the other types of biomolecules, lipids have
widely varied structures. The term lipids is used to
describe a functionally diverse group of substances
that are all water-insoluble to varying degrees. This
article will outline the classifications of the groups,
their chemistry, metabolism and physiological functions, and the various dietary sources of lipids.

Definition of Lipids

A lipid is defined as a water-insoluble biomolecule
that has a high solubility in nonpolar solvents. The
term lipid includes substances more commonly
known as oils, fats and waxes.

Classification of Lipids

The term lipid encompasses acylglycerols, phospholipids, glycolipids, sterols and other molecules
(**Fig. 1**). Other descriptors commonly used with lipids
include saponifiable, nonsaponifiable, hydrophobic
(nonpolar or water-insoluble) and amphipathic
(containing both nonpolar and polar regions).
Saponifiable lipids yield salts of fatty acids upon
alkaline hydrolysis:

Acylglycerols = glycerol + fatty acid(s)
Phospholipids = glycerol + fatty acids + HPO_4^{2-} +
    alcohol (in some cases)
Sphingolipids = sphingose + fatty acid + polar group
Waxes = long-chain alcohol + fatty acid

Nonsaponifiable lipids (terpenes, steroids, eicosanoids and related compounds) are not usually subjected
to hydrolysis. Amphipathic lipids have both a polar
'head' group and a nonpolar 'tail'. Amphipathic molecules can stabilize emulsions and are responsible for
the lipid bilayer structure of membranes.

Chemistry of Lipid Subclasses

Triacylglycerols

Free fatty acids occur only in trace amounts in cells;
this is fortunate because they are detergents and at
high concentrations could disrupt cell membranes.
They are generally present as triacylglycerols. The
three fatty acids esterified to glycerol in triacylglycerols are not randomly distributed in most natural fats
and oils. There is a tendency for particular fatty acids
to be located at specific positions on the three glycerol carbons (**Fig. 2**). An example of such specific
distribution is that palmitic acid tends to be concentrated in position 1 and oleic acid in positions 2 and
3 of human adipose tissue triacylglycerols. The triacylglycerols vary in composition depending on the
various fatty acids from which they are made.

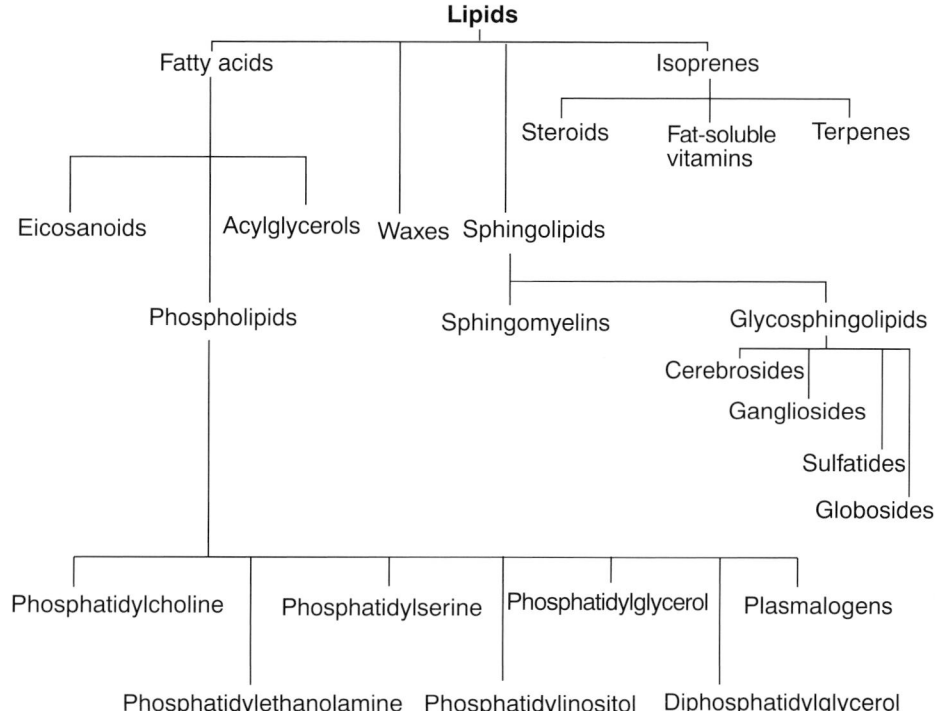

Figure 1 Major classes of lipids. Fatty acids are the simplest lipids. A number of other lipids either contain or are derived from fatty acids.

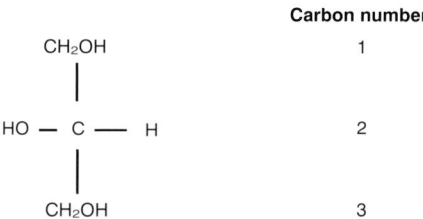

Figure 2 Stereospecific numbering of glycerol.

Phospholipids

Phospholipids are synthesized by the addition of a basic group to phosphatidic acid or 1,2-diacylglycerol. Most phospholipids have a saturated fatty acid on C-1 and an unsaturated fatty acid on C-2 of the glycerol backbone. The major classifications of phospholipids are described below.

Phosphatidylcholines (PC) These phospholipids, also known as lecithins, are the chief phospholipids present in animal cells. They contain primarily palmitic or stearic acid at carbon 1 and primarily oleic, linoleic or linolenic acid at carbon 2. The lecithin dipalmitoyllecithin is a component of lung or pulmonary surfactant. It contains palmitate at both carbon 1 and 2 of glycerol and is the major (80%) phospholipid found in the extracellular lipid layer lining the pulmonary alveoli. This synthesis of dipalmitoyl-lecithin in lung tissue is an example of the modulation of the fatty acid composition of a phospholipid by 'remodelling'. Deacylation–reacylation of phosphatidlycholine occurs in other tissues and provides an important route for alteration of fatty acid substituents at positions 1 and 2.

Phosphatidylethanolamines (PE) These molecules contain primarily palmitic or stearic acid on carbon 1 and a long-chain unsaturated fatty acid (e.g. 18:2, 20:4 and 22:6) on carbon 2.

Phosphatidylserines (PS) Phosphatidylserines are composed of fatty acids similar to the phosphatidylethanolamines. The pathway for PS synthesis involves an exchange reaction of serine for ethanolamine in PE.

Phosphatidylinositols (PI) These molecules contain almost exclusively stearic acid at carbon 1 and arachidonic acid at carbon 2. Phosphatidylinositols exist in membranes with various levels of phosphate esterified to the hydroxyls of the inositol. Molecules with phosphorylated inositol are termed polyphosphoinositides. The polyphosphoinositides are important intracellular transducers of signals emanating from the plasma membrane. One polyphosphoinositide (phosphatidylinositol 4,5-bisphosphate,

PIP$_2$) is a critically important membrane phospholipid involved in the transmission of signals for cell growth and differentiation from outside the cell to inside.

Phosphatidylglycerols   (PG)   Phosphatidylglycerol molecules are found in high concentration in mitochondrial membranes and as components of pulmonary surfactant. The vital role of PG is to serve as the precursor for the synthesis of diphosphatidylglycerols (DPG).

Diphosphatidylglycerols (DPG)   These molecules are found primarily in the inner mitochondrial membrane and as components of pulmonary surfactant.

Plasmalogens   These are glycerol ether phospholipids. Three major classes of plasmalogens have been identified: choline, ethanolamine and serine plasmalogens. Ethanolamine plasmalogen is prevalent in myelin. Choline plasmalogen is abundant in cardiac tissue and may protect cells against the deleterious effects of singlet oxygen. One particular choline plasmalogen (1-alkyl, 2-acetyl phosphatidylcholine) has been identified as an extremely powerful biological mediator, capable of inducing cellular responses at concentrations as low as 10^{-11} M. This molecule is called platelet activating factor, PAF. PAF functions as a mediator of hypersensitivity, acute inflammatory reactions and anaphylactic shock.

Waxes

Waxes are nonpolar esters of long-chain fatty acids and long-chain monohydroxylic alcohols. Waxes are widely distributed in nature. They provide waterproof coatings on the leaves and fruits of certain plants.

Sphingolipids

Sphingolipids also have a polar head group and two nonpolar tails. The core of sphingolipids is the long-chain amino alcohol, sphingosine. The sphingolipids include the sphingomyelins and glycosphingolipids (the cerebrosides, sulfatides, globosides and gangliosides). Sphingolipids are a component of all membranes but are particularly abundant in the myelin sheath, a multilayered membranous structure that protects and insulates nerve fibres.

Sphingomyelins   These are sphingolipids that are also phospholipids. Sphingomyelins are important structural lipid components of nerve cell membranes. The predominant sphingomyelins contain palmitic or stearic acid at carbon 2 of the sphingosine.

Glycosphingolipids   Also termed glycolipids, glycosphingolipids have four principal classes called the cerebrosides, sulfatides, globosides and gangliosides. Cerebrosides have a single sugar group. The most common of these is galactose (galactocerebrosides), with a minor level of glucose (glucocerebrosides). Galactocerebrosides are found predominantly in neuronal cell membranes. By contrast glucocerebrosides are not normally found in membranes; instead they represent intermediates in the synthesis or degradation of more complex glycosphingolipids. The sulfuric acid esters of galactocerebrosides are known as the sulfatides. Globosides represent cerebrosides that contain additional carbohydrates, predominantly galactose and glucose. Lactosyl ceramide is a globoside found in erythrocyte plasma membranes. Gangliosides, so called as they are highly concentrated in the ganglion cells of the central nervous system, particularly in the nerve endings, are very similar to globosides except that they also contain N-acetylneuraminic acid (NANA) in varying amounts. Degradation of glycosphingolipids occurs in a stepwise fashion in lysosomes. Investigations of the degradation process have been stimulated by the occurrence of a number of human genetic diseases, the sphingolipidoses, each of which results in the accumulation of one of these lipids. Sphingolipids have been implicated in the regulation of cell growth, differentiation and programmed cell death, with metabolites serving as second messengers for growth factors and cytokines.

Steroids

Steroids do not contain fatty acids although they contain a hydroxyl group that may be attached to fatty acids to form sterol esters. Cholesterol is the major sterol in animal cells. The bulk of cholesterol in the body is found in cell membranes where it acts as a stabilizing agent. About one quarter of the cholesterol *in vivo* is in the membranes of the nervous system – the brain, the spinal cord and the peripheral nerves. In its precursor role cholesterol provides the molecular skeleton for: (1) the formation of the bile acids, which play a major part in digestion of fats in the intestine; (2) the production of hormones; and (3) the formation of vitamin D.

Terpenes

Terpenes are polymers of two or more isoprene units.

$$CH_2 = C - CH = CH_2$$

Head   CH$_3$ Tail

Isoprene

The terpene limonene is a cyclic lipid chiefly responsible for the distinctive smell of lemons. Squalene, the precursor of cholesterol, is a linear terpene of six isoprene units. The fat-soluble vitamins (A,D,E,K) are also composed of isoprene units.

Digestion, Absorption and Metabolism

Dietary lipids are a heterogeneous mixture consisting of about 93% triacylglycerols, 6% phospholipids, and lesser amounts of sphingomyelins, glycolipids, cholesterol and phytosterols. Lipids are usually fully digested, with less than 5% remaining unabsorbed and excreted in faeces. The absorption of dietary cholesterol varies markedly among individuals. If fat digestion is impaired by pancreatic enzyme deficiency then an oily diarrhoea results, with foamy, floating stools (steatorrhoea). The triacylglycerols are separated from the rest of the ingested food in the stomach into fat globules that float in chyme. In the small intestine they are emulsified by bile and, following enzymatic digestion by pancreatic lipases to glycerol, fatty acids and monoglycerides, the fractions are absorbed into the intestinal microvilli, processed and packaged for export in lymph. Some small lipid fractions can travel directly into capillaries, e.g. fatty acids with shorter chain lengths, as may occur in milk fat, are absorbed straight into the blood and supply the liver.

Following absorption, the fatty acids are reassembled into triacylglycerols and enter the systemic circulation where they are assembled and packaged with cholesterol, cholesteryl esters, phospholipids and apoproteins to form chylomicrons. Chylomicron triacylglycerols are broken down to their constituent fatty acids in the blood capillaries close to adipose tissue by the enzyme lipoprotein lipase. The fatty acids then pass into the adipose tissue and are once again reassembled to triacylglycerols. This sequence of events is called the exogenous transport system because it deals with fats originating from the diet. The endogenous system deals with lipids manufactured in the liver. Lipoproteins rich in triacylglycerols, called very low-density lipoproteins (VLDL), are manufactured in the liver for the transport of triacylglycerols, cholesterol and phospholipids. The blood is the carrier of triacylglycerols in the form of VLDLs and chylomicrons, fatty acids bound to albumin, amino acids, lactate, ketone bodies and glucose.

The fate of dietary phospholipids is similar to that of triacylglycerols. Pancreatic phospholipases secreted into the intestine catalyse the hydrolysis of phospholipids, which aggregate in micelles. The major phospholipase in the pancreatic secretion is phospholipase A_2, which catalyses the hydrolysis of a glycerophospholipid to form a lysophosphoglyceride. These are then absorbed by the intestine and re-esterified to glycerophospholipids in intestinal cells. Unlike other types of lipids, most dietary cholesterol is unesterified. Dietary cholesteryl esters are hydrolysed in the lumen of the intestine by the action of an esterase. Free cholesterol, which is insoluble in water, is solubilized by bile salt micelles for absorption. Most cholesterol reacts with acyl coenzyme A (acyl-CoA) to form cholesterol esters in the intestinal cells.

Besides dietary supply, the second major source of fatty acids for humans is their biosynthesis from small molecule intermediates derived from the metabolic breakdown of sugars, some amino acids and other fatty acids. In the liver the requirements for synthesis of essential membrane components are met before an appreciable amount of triacylglycerol is made. Regulation of synthesis of these lipids is intimately related to the maintenance, proliferation and functions of the plasma membrane and internal cellular membranes such as those of endoplasmic reticulum and the Golgi.

Physiological Functions of Lipid Subclasses

Lipids provide a concentrated energy source, they insulate, carry essential vitamins and prevent dehydration of body surfaces (i.e. skin). Most dietary fatty acids are metabolized by β-oxidation in tissues to provide a source of energy. Some are incorporated into the structure of membranes as parts of phospholipids required for the integrity of intracellular and plasma membranes. Other fatty acids are precursor substrates for additional biologically active metabolites. Fatty acids are usually found in the storage form, triacylglycerols, or as the structurally important phospholipids. Usually, before they can take part in biosynthetic reactions, fatty acids are linked to coenzyme A (CoA).

Lipids as fat stores

In mammals the major reservoir of triacylglycerols is in the cytoplasm of adipose cells. Most of the energy reserve of animals is stored in fat cells. This is not 'dead storage', since they turn over with an average half-life of only a few days. The lipases in adipose tissue are the key enzymes to release the major energy stores and there must be exquisite control of hydrolysis versus synthesis to ensure adequate energy stores and avoid obesity.

The total energy reserve of a standard 70 kg man consists of about 0.17 MJ in glucose, 2.5 MJ in glycogen, 105 MJ in protein and 420 MJ in triacylglycerols. The triacylglycerols constitute about 11 kg of his total body mass. The advantage of triacylglycerols as an energy source is clear – 1 g of fatty acids yields on complete oxidation almost double the energy of 1 g of carbohydrate or protein. Moreover the triacylglycerols are hydrophobic and are stored in nearly anhydrous form, while glycogen is hydrophilic. Consequently 1 g of fat stores more than six times as much energy as does 1 g of glycogen under physiological conditions. If most of the energy of the 70 kg standard man were not stored as triacylglycerols, his mass would be nearly doubled to 125 kg.

The breakdown of fatty acids for energy is via β-oxidation and takes place in the mitochondria. Saturated and unsaturated fatty acids are broken down by the same mechanism except that additional enzymes are required to deal with the double bonds. A normal complement of fat stores will provide sufficient energy to allow several weeks of survival during total food deprivation. The degree of utilization of fatty acids for energy production varies considerably from tissue to tissue and depends on the metabolic state of the body, i.e. fasted or fed. For instance, nervous tissue apparently oxidizes fatty acids to a minimal degree if at all, whereas cardiac and skeletal muscle depend heavily on fatty acids as a major energy source.

Lipid peroxidation

Beta-oxidation is the predominant method of fatty acid breakdown for the generation of energy. There are other ways in which the fatty acids can be oxidized with different consequences – one of these is peroxidation. A problem with polyunsaturated fatty acids (PUFA), both for the body and the food manufacturer, is that PUFA are susceptible to oxidation, producing lipid peroxides which have undesirable biological effects and impart 'off-flavours' in foods. It has been proposed that lipid peroxidation plays a part in the development of atherosclerosis in human blood vessels.

Lipids as precursors of eicosanoids

Peroxidation is not always a haphazard and unwanted reaction. The enzymes that initiate eicosanoid synthesis catalyse a controlled peroxidation to give well-defined products. The long-chain PUFA dihomo-γ-linolenic acid (DHGL), arachidonic acid (AA) and eicosapentaenoic acid (EPA) are the precursors of eicosanoids, which are formed by the action of membrane-bound cyclooxygenase or specific lipoxygenase enzyme systems. Synthesis of eicosanoids occurs in three stages: (1) the release of the 20-carbon fatty acid from cell membrane-bound

phospholipids in response to cellular stimuli (phospholipase A_2 has been shown to be important); (2) the oxidation of fatty acids; and (3) the cell-specific conversion of the oxidized fatty acids to an eicosanoid. More than 20 biologically active eicosanoids have been identified and these include both n-3 and n-6 derived compounds. The eicosanoid family includes prostaglandins, thromboxanes, prostacyclins, leukotrienes, lipoxins and other hydroxy fatty acids. These compounds participate in many physiological and pathological processes and are potent regulators of cell function. They act locally in cells and tissues in which they are formed and are rapidly converted to inactive forms.

Lipids in membranes

Lipid bilayers and membranes are selectively permeable barriers that restrict the free passage of most molecules. A typical biological membrane contains a complex mixture of phospholipids, glycosphingolipids and cholesterol. Cholesterol and some other lipids that do not form bilayers by themselves (~30% of the total) are stabilized in a bilayer arrangement by the other 70% of lipids in the membrane. Cholesterol helps maintain fairly constant fluidity despite fluctuations in temperature or degree of fatty acid saturation. In all instances, glycolipids are oriented asymmetrically in the bilayer of the plasma membrane, facing the outside of the cell. Many observations indicate the glycosphingolipids are more than just structural lipids and have specific cell surface recognition properties that are similar to plasma membrane-bound glycoproteins. Glycosphingolipids are blood group antigens and a person who displays the B blood type has comparable B antigens on both the membrane-bound glycosphingolipids and glycoproteins.

Dietary Sources of Lipids

Lipids perform many functions in food systems and are responsible for much of the appearance, texture and flavour of the food we eat. Dietary lipids are derived mainly from the storage fats of mammals and fish and the seed oils of plants. They occur mainly in the form of triacylglycerols and phospholipids; food sources of the other lipids are relatively minor. Ruminant fats have a low proportion of PUFA because the fats in the animals' diet are hydrogenated by the microorganisms in the rumen. This decreases the degree of unsaturation and results in the formation of some *trans* fatty acids. The storage fats of simple-stomached animals such as pigs and poultry tend to contain a higher proportion of unsaturated fatty acids, depending on the nature of the fatty acids in the animal feed. Fish store fat in the flesh (fatty fish, e.g. herring, mackerel) or the liver (e.g. cod) and fish fats are richer in the n-3 family of PUFA. Seed oils vary widely in fatty acid composition. Oleic acid (olive, rape, palm) or linoleic acid (sunflower, safflower, soya bean) often predominate. Structural lipids generally contain a higher proportion of PUFA than most storage fats. In animal tissue arachidonic acid is the PUFA that predominates while in plant tissue α-linolenic and linoleic acid predominate. As a general rule linoleic and α-linolenic acid are found in foods of vegetable origin, while long-chain PUFA are found in foods of animal origin. Gamma-linolenic acid is found in only a few obscure oils, e.g. evening primrose, borage and blackcurrant.

See also: **Cholesterol**: Sources, Absorption, Function and Metabolism. **Energy**: Energy Requirements; Energy Balance; Measurement of Energy Intake and Expenditure. **Fats and Oils**: Nutritional Value. **Fatty Acids**: Metabolism; Health Effects of Saturated Fatty Acids; Health Effects of Monounsaturated Fatty Acids; Health Effects of n-6 Polyunsaturated Fatty Acids; Health Effects of n-3 Polyunsaturated Fatty Acids; Health Effects of trans Fatty Acids. **Lipoproteins**: Physiology.

Further Reading

Akoh CC (1995) Lipid based fat substitutes. *Critical Reviews in Food Science and Nutrition* 35(5):405–430.

Lands WEM and Pendleton RB (1987) n-3 fatty acids and hydroperoxide activation of fatty acid oxygenases. In: Simic MG (ed.) *Oxygen Radicals in Biology and Medicine*, pp 675–681. New York: Plenum Press.

Sardesai VM (1992) Biochemical and nutritional aspects of eicosanoids. *Journal of Nutritional Biochemistry* 3:562–580.

Spiegel S and Merrill AH (1996) Sphingolipid metabolism and cell growth regulation. *FASEB Journal* 1(12):1388–1397.

Sprecher H, Voss AC, Careaga M *et al.* (1987) Interrelationships between polyunsaturated fatty acids and membrane lipid synthesis. In: Lands WEM (ed.) *Polyunsaturated Fatty Acids and Eicosanoids*, pp 154–168. Champaign: American Oil Chemists Society.

Composition and Role of Phospholipids in the Body

A D Postle, University of Southampton, Southampton, UK

Copyright © 1998 Academic Press

Phospholipids are amphipathic lipids consisting of hydrophobic and hydrophilic regions. This amphipathic nature, which enables phospholipid molecules to assemble into bilayer and hexagonal membrane structures, is critically important for the functional viability of all eukaryote cells. Cellular membranes, composed primarily of phospholipid, separate the intracellular milieu from the extracellular environment and facilitate the formation of specialized intracellular organelles. For many years, phospholipids were considered to be important but relatively inert structural components of the cell. More recently, the central role of membrane phospholipid composition and turnover in the regulation of a wide range of cellular functions has become widely recognized. For instance, all membrane receptor events take place within a phospholipid-rich environment, and it is therefore not surprising that cells have adopted hydrolysis of membrane phospholipids as a major signalling mechanism. Phospholipids have multiple roles which include:

1. providing a structural framework to maintain cellular integrity and to compartmentalize diverse events within the cell;
2. providing the appropriate physicochemical environment to optimize the activities of membrane-associated receptors, enzymes and proteins;
3. acting as substrate molecules for a variety of phospholipase enzymes involved in signalling mechanisms;
4. exerting a physicochemical detergent-like action to facilitate the physiological function of a variety of tissues, including the lungs, stomach and synovial surfaces;
5. regulating the synthesis and secretion of lipoproteins from the liver.

Phospholipid Structures

There are two major classes of phospholipid, depending on whether they contain a glycerol or sphingosyl backbone. Glycerophospholipids are molecules based on phosphatidic acid (3-*sn*-phosphatidic acid); the nature of the esterified group X defines the class of phospholipid (**Fig. 1**). The most common substituent groups include nitrogenous bases such as choline and ethanolamine, and polyalcohols such as *myo*-inositol and glycerol. Sphingophospholipids contain sphingosine (*trans*-D-*erythro*-1,3-dihyroxy-2-amino-4-octadecene). Sphingomyelin is the most abundant sphingophospholipid class, and is the phosphorylcholine ester of *N*-acylsphingosine, otherwise called ceramide. Sphingophospholipids are important components of all cell membranes and are structurally and metabolically closely related to glycosphingolipids such glycosylceramides, gangliosides

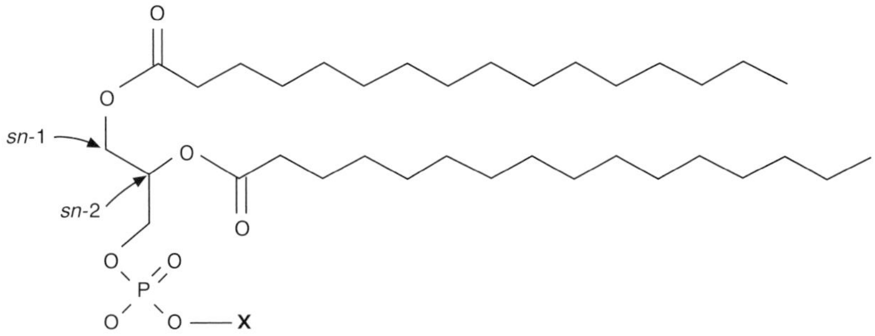

(a) Diacyl species

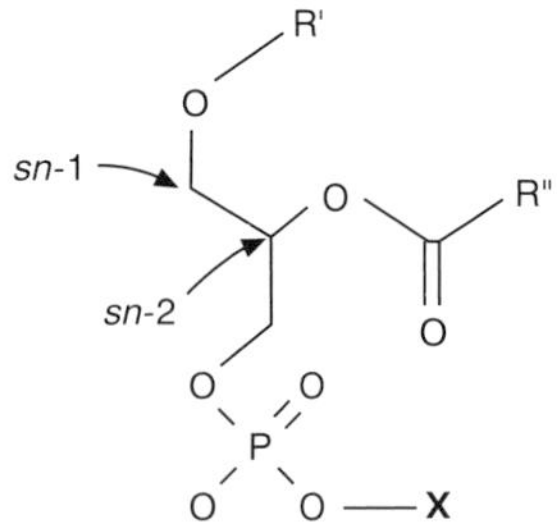

(b) *sn*-1-alkyl-*sn*-2-acyl species

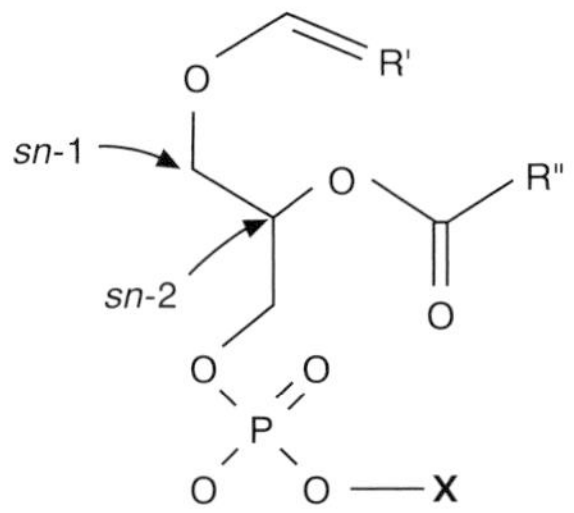

(c) *sn*-1-alkenyl-*sn*-2-acyl species

Phospholipid	Headgroup (X)
Phosphatidylcholine (PC)	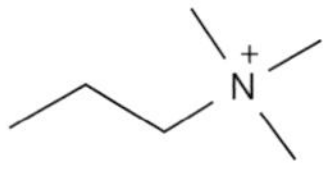
Phosphatidylethanolamine (PE)	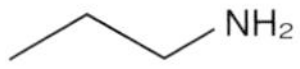
Phosphatidylserine (PS)	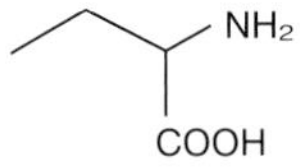
Phosphatidylinositol (PI)	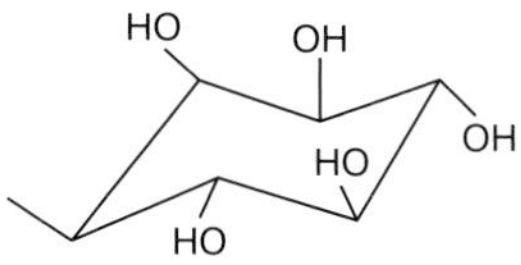
Phosphatidylglycerol (PG)	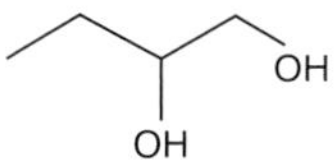
Phosphatidic acid (PA)	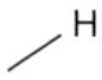

Figure 1 The class of phospholipid is defined by the nature of the nitrogenous base or polyol esterified to the phosphate group (X). The species distribution within any phospholipid class is determined by the fatty acyl substituents at the *sn*-1 and *sn*-2 positions of the glycerol backbone. The dipalmitoyl species shown in (a) would be designated PC16:0/16:0 if X was choline. If arachidonic acid was esterified at *sn*-2, then the molecule would be designated as PC16:0/20:4. In the diacyl species shown above, fatty acids are attached by ester linkages. For *sn*-1-alkyl-*sn*-2-acyl species, the *sn*-1 fatty acid is attached by an ether bond. For *sn*-1 alkenyl-*sn*-2-acyl species, the *sn*-1 fatty acid is attached by a vinyl ether linkage.

and cerebrosides. Sphingomyelin is now recognized as a major substrate for sphingomyelinase enzymes involved in generating intracellular ceramide and sphingosine, which are intimately involved in the regulation of programmed cell death (apoptosis). Sphingophospholipids contain principally saturated and monounsaturated fatty acids; little information is available about nutritional effects on sphingophospholipid composition and sphingomyelin metabolism has been recently reviewed.

Classification and nomenclature of glycerophospholipids

Glycerophospholipid classes are commonly referred to as phosphatidylcholine, phosphatidylethanolamine, etc. They are composed of a spectrum of molecular species defined by the substituent fatty acid groups attached to the sn-1 and sn-2 positions of the glycerol backbone. For example the individual molecular species palmitoyloleoyl phosphatidylcholine can be named formally as either glycerol 1-hexadecanoate 2-9-octadecaenoate 3-phosphocholine or 1-hexadecanoyl-2-octadeca-9-enoyl-3-glycerophosphocholine. One shorthand designation for this molecule, adopted in this article, is PC16:0/18:1, where PC designates the phospholipid class, in this case phosphatidylcholine, and 16:0 and 18:1 designate the fatty acids esterified at the sn-1 and sn-2 positions.

For phospholipids from cell membranes, saturated fatty acids are generally located at the sn-1 and unsaturated fatty acids at the sn-2 position, with notable exceptions. For instance, dipalmitoyl PC (PC16:0/16:0) is a major component of lung and surfactant PC, while significant amounts of didocosahexaenoyl phosphatidylethanolamine (PE22:6/22:6) are present in retinal PE. In addition, PC species with 18:ln-9 at the sn-1 position are minor components of many cells.

In addition to diacyl species, with both fatty acids attached by ester bonds, there are a number of species with ether-linked fatty acids, principally in the sn-1 position. These ether phospholipids include 1-alkyl-2-acyl species, largely present in PC, and 1-alk-1-enyl species (plasmalogens), largely present in PE. These ether lipids are major components of many cell membranes, in particular neuronal and inflammatory cells, and there have been significant recent advances in understanding the biochemical pathways for their synthesis and catabolism. Some alkyl acyl PC species are substrates for the generation of the potent bioactive lipid platelet activating factor (1-alkyl-2-acetyl-sn-glycero-3-phosphocholine, PAF), but the function of most ether lipids is largely unclear. One possibility is that generation of 1-alkyl-2-acyl-glycerol as a second messenger rather than diacylglycerol may contribute to differential regulation of protein kinase C isoforms.

Phospholipid analysis

Phospholipids are extracted from tissues in the organic portion of a chloroform/methanol/sample mixture. Historically, phospholipid composition in such extracts has been determined by isolating classes by thin-layer chromatography, and then analysing total fatty acid composition of each class by gas chromatography after hydrolysis and formation of methyl esters. The bulk of nutritional studies on phospholipid composition have been conducted using variations on this methodology. However, such analysis provides no direct information about the individual molecular species compositions of phospholipids, which are the functional, biologically-relevant molecules. For instance, a fatty acid analysis of a phospholipid mixture as 50% 16:0, 50% 18:1 could represent either 16:0/18:1 or an equivalent combination of 16:0/16:0 and 18:1/18:1, which all have very different physical and functional properties. A variety of techniques have been established to provide such information, including high-performance liquid chromatography (HPLC), NMR and mass spectrometry. Wherever possible in this article compositional data will be provided in terms of individual molecular species.

Many HPLC techniques have been devised for the analysis of intact phospholipid species; gas chromatography techniques are not suitable, given the low volatility and relatively high molecular masses of phospholipids. Reverse-phase HPLC resolution of intact phospholipid species, with addition of suitable ion-suppressant reagents, requires minimal sample preparation but poses significant detection problems. The absorbance response at 195–205 nm is dependent on the degree of acyl unsaturation and is not quantitative for species of different acyl composition. In addition, many HPLC mobile phases absorb strongly at these short wavelengths, causing detector noise and reducing sensitivity. Mass detection by evaporative light detection is insensitive and has limited applicability owing to interactions with non-volatile ion suppressants. Postcolumn fluorescence derivatization with diphenylhexatriene has proved most successful and permits resolution and quantitation of as little as 20 nmol of any phospholipid class.

The alternative approach by HPLC has been to hydrolyse the headgroup with phospholipase C to generate diacylglycerol species, and to synthesize a variety of fluorescent or UV-absorbing derivatives. These techniques have sensitivities in the picomolar range and improved resolution of species, and have been used to define phospholipid compositions of many cultured cell lines. However, they are laborious and prone to error, and have not been applied widely to nutritional studies *in vivo*.

NMR techniques (^{3}H, ^{13}C and ^{31}P) have provided useful structural information, but are relatively insensitive. They have considerable potential for studies of phospholipid metabolism *in vivo*, albeit with limited resolution owing to signals generated by nonphospholipid compounds. HPLC–mass spectrometry techniques have been described for phospholipid analysis, mainly using either fast atom bombardment or thermospray interfaces, and provide both unambiguous characterization and sensitivity of detection in the subnanomolar range. Considerations of flow rate and volatility, however, limit choice of mobile phase compositions and hence restrict HPLC resolutions. Moreover, a variety of disintegration products are generated in the mass spectrometer, leading to complex spectra and some problems with quantitation. Advances in instrument design have very recently introduced the possibility of sensitive and detailed analysis of phospholipid molecular species by electrospray ionization tandem mass spectroscopy. Such technology is now set to revolutionize phospholipid analysis and replace many long-established chromatography-based methodologies.

Phospholipid Composition

The glycerophospholipid composition of most cell types in the body is regulated within relatively restricted limits and is often specialized for the function of the cell involved. These compositions are mediated by interactions between phenotypic expression and cellular nutrition, which determine the specificities of the enzymes of phospholipid synthesis and hydrolysis and of the transfer proteins which exchange phospholipid species between different membranes. Regulation of synthesis is best characterized for formation of PC in rat hepatocytes, where PC synthesis is essential for assembly and secretion of very low-density lipoprotein (VLDL) particles. Phosphatidylcholine species synthesized *de novo* from diacylglycerol by the enzyme cholinephosphotransferase are subsequently modified by acyl remodelling mechanisms involving sequential actions of phospholipase and acyltransferase activities. The rate of PC synthesis is thought to be dependent on the activity of CTP : choline phosphate cytidylyltransferase, which is subject to complex regulatory mechanisms involving phosphorylation and reversible enzyme translocation between cytosol and membrane fractions of the cell.

There is also a considerable diversity of specificity of phospholipase enzymes responsible for phospholipid hydrolysis, both in terms of positional and molecular species selectivity. Phospholipase A_1 activity in rat liver will act selectively to remove *sn*-1 16:0 from PC species containing *sn*-2 18:2, while cytosolic phospholipase A_2 (PLA_2) is specific for species containing *sn*-2 20:4n-6. In contrast,

secretory PLA_2 must be bound to negatively charged phospholipids for activation, but is not acyl specific. Different isoforms of phospholipase C (PLC) act selectively on either phosphatidylinositol-4,5-diphosphate (PIP_2) or PC, agonist-stimulated phospholipase D (PLD) displays some selectivity for PC species containing *sn*-1 18:0, and lysophospholipase D is specific for 1-alkyl-*sn*-glycero-3-phosphocholine. However, although the distribution of phospholipases is tissue specific, the contribution of their activities to the regulation of phospholipid compositions in most tissues has not been well defined.

Phospholipid composition in development

The most extensive changes to phospholipid composition occur during fetal and neonatal development, and have been best characterized for PC in liver, lung and brain. These changes illustrate clearly the limitations of dietary manipulation on phospholipid composition. During human pregnancy, the polyunsaturated fatty acids (PUFA) 20:4n-6 and 22:6n-3 are supplied across the placenta from maternal to fetal circulations in increasing quantities towards term. At birth, the onset of milk feeding is characterized by increased intake of the PUFA precursor 18:2n-6. This sequence of nutritional supply is reflected in fetal and neonatal liver PC composition. Immature fetal human liver contains a high proportion of monounsaturated PC species, particularly PC16:0/18:1, and tends to become enriched with species containing 20:4n-6 and 22:6n-3 towards term (**Table 1**).

Postnatally the content of 18:2n-6 species then increases, and fetal and neonatal plasma PC composition directly mirrors this changing pattern. However, these alterations in development are regulated primarily by metabolic and hormonal rather than by nutritional considerations. The increased supply of PUFA from mother to fetus in later gestation is independent to any change in maternal dietary lipid intake, and instead is a consequence of hormonal effects on the specificity of PC synthesis and lipoprotein export by the maternal liver. Similarly, while switching from placental to enteral feeding is the major factor causing the dramatic changes to plasma PC at birth, this composition is still dependent on the metabolic regulation of the specificity of hepatic PC synthesis. The programmed nature of this regulation is shown clearly by food restriction in newborn guinea pig pups, which still display equivalent postnatal alterations to plasma and liver PC composition as their fed litter mates, even in the total absence of enteral nutrition.

By contrast, immature fetal lung PC also contains a high concentration of PC16:0/18:1 but becomes more rather than less saturated with progression of

Table 1 Phosphatidylcholine molecular species composition of human liver during fetal and postnatal development. Molecular species were analysed by reverse-phase HPLC and quantified by postcolumn fluorescence detection with 1,6-diphenyl-1,3,5-hexatriene

Molecular species	Liver phosphatidylcholine concentration (nmol per g wet wt)		
	Fetal (15 weeks gestation, n = 4)	Stillborn (term, n = 4)	Infant (43–64 weeks old, n = 6)
16:0/16:0	992 ± 156	1004 ± 81	538 ± 121
16:0/18:1	2007 ± 250	2240 ± 173	2353 ± 496
16:0/18:2	466 ± 52	1259 ± 139	2202 ± 273
16:0/20:4	1402 ± 98	1784 ± 38	1062 ± 219
16:0/22:6	431 ± 110	953 ± 82	614 ± 512
18:0/18:2	308 ± 56	443 ± 68	1239 ± 252
18:0/20:4	1298 ± 288	953 ± 89	448 ± 403
18:0/22:6	115 ± 31	210 ± 50	221 ± 267

Concentrations expressed as mean ± SD.

gestation owing to increased synthesis of the disaturated species PC16:0/16:0. PC16:0/16:0 is a major component of pulmonary surfactant which acts to oppose surface tension forces in the lungs and prevent alveolar collapse. Infants who are born preterm with immature surfactant are at high risk of death and disability caused by neonatal respiratory distress syndrome. In contrast to fetal liver, the phospholipid composition of fetal lung is only marginally affected by the changes to lipid nutrition *in utero*. Nevertheless, some nutritional influence is evident, even though PUFA-containing species are minor components of lung PC. Comparison of PC compositions in prenatal human lung show clearly a postnatal increase in the content of PC16:0/18:2, which reflects the increased dietary supply of 18:2n-6. The situation in developing lung reflects that of most other tissues in the body, where dietary lipid modulation causes relatively modest changes to the specificity of phospholipid compositions. Such subtle alterations to membrane composition can, however, exert profound effects on cellular function.

Finally, adult brain PE contains about 50% of 22:6n-3 species, enriched in neuronal synapses and possibly involved in synaptic transmission. Failure to acquire sufficient 22:6n-3 in brain PE during neuronal differentiation in early development can lead to permanent suboptimal neurological function. Many of the changes to maternal lipid metabolism in pregnancy represent adaptations to ensure adequate supply of PUFA to the developing fetal brain. Increased synthesis and secretion of PC16:0/22:6 in livers of pregnant rats and guinea pigs correlates with the period in fetal brain growth of maximal accumulation rate of 22:6n-3 into brain PE. Once incorporated into brain or retinal PE, 22:6n-3 is avidly retained throughout life, even in periods of prolonged nutritional deprivation. Infants who are born

preterm and with inadequate reserves of 22:6n-3 are now recognized to be in danger of nutritional deficiency if fed milk formulae lacking preformed long-chain PUFA. For instance, 22:6n-3 content of brain PE was decreased in infants fed such formulae and who had died suddenly from SIDS (sudden infant death syndrome). For this reason, supplementation of preterm infant milk formula with preformed PUFA has now been recommended by the European Society for Pediatric Gastroenterology and Nutrition.

Phospholipid composition in adult tissues

Information about the detailed molecular species compositions of phospholipids from adult human tissues is surprisingly haphazard. There have been many isolated reports of extensive characterizations of selected phospholipid classes in individual tissues, but such studies have generally measured compositions of bulk preparations from relatively large tissue samples. There have been very few clinical or nutritional studies which have characterized phospholipid compositions in molecular terms. In reality, each cell type contains in excess of 200 glycerophospholipid species, with differential compositions between different membranes in the same cell and even between different regions in the same membrane. Such regions of microheterogeneity may occur either because of the physical properties of the lipids themselves, for instance forming hexagonal rather than bilayer structures, or because of sequestration by membrane proteins. Phase transitions within the membrane can also exert significant effects, and interactions of cytoskeletal components of the cell have been described with relative solid gel-phase phospholipids in the plasma membrane. One additional important factor is the transmembrane phospholipid distribution between the two leaflets of

Table 2 Compositions of diacyl molecular species of human blood cells. Results are presented as mol % of total diacyl species. The abundances of the 10 most significant PC molecular species in human platelet are compared with corresponding species from circulating human mononuclear (lymphocyte) and polymorphonuclear (neutrophil) cells. PC from each cell type comprised over 20 identifiable species. Platelet composition was determined by HPLC, while lymphocyte and neutrophil compositions were determined by electrospray ionization mass spectrometry

Molecular species	Phosphatidylcholine composition (mol %)		
	Platelet[a]	Lymphocyte[b]	Neutrophil[b]
16:0/16:0	3	6	14
16:0/18:1	28	19	28
18:0/18:1	9	8	16
16:0/18:2	12	9	11
18:0/18:2	7	10[c]	11[c]
18:1/18:1	6		
18:1/18:2	1	5[d]	6[d]
16:0/20:3	2		
16:0/20:4	12	7	4
18:0/20:4	10	7	4

[a]Mahadevappa VG and Holub BJ (1984) Relative degradation of different molecular species of phosphatidylcholine in thrombin-stimulated human platelets. *Journal of Biological Chemistry* 259:9369–9373.
[b]Unpublished observations.
[c]18:0/18:2 and 18:1/18:1, and [d]18:1/18:2 and 16:0/20:3, have the same molecular masses and are summed for the lymphocyte and neutrophil results.

the cell bilayer. For practically all cell types, PC is relatively more concentrated in the outer membrane, while PE is located primarily in the inner (cytoplasmic) membrane. Importantly, PS is almost totally restricted to the side of the cell membrane facing the cytoplasm, where it acts as an activator of protein kinase C. Redistribution of PS to the outer leaflet of the plasma membrane is a signal of cell sen-

escence and is a potent activator of the clotting cascade.

Examples of analyses of phospholipid molecular species compositions of a variety of human tissues are summarized in Tables 2–4. Selected species are presented in all these tables for reasons of space and clarity; full information is presented in the original reports. **Table 2** compares the composition of diacyl PC species in human blood platelets, mononuclear cells and polymorphonuclear cells. As for most cell types, the PC composition of these cells is dominated by monounsaturated PC species, especially PC16:0/18:1. The distribution of polyunsaturated species is highly variable between cell types, with neutrophils being relatively depleted in species containing 20:4n-6 and with an increased content of 16:0/16:0. This comparison illustrates an important role for phenotypic expression as one contributor towards the specificity of cell PC composition.

The relative compositions of different phospholipid classes from the same tissue are compared in **Table 3**, which summarizes the molecular species compositions of diacyl PC, diacyl PE, alkenylacyl PE and phosphatidylserine (PS) from the white matter of human brain. While brain PC is highly enriched in monounsaturated species, diacyl PE was enriched in species containing PUFA. The distribution of such species, however, was highly asymmetric with 22:6n-3 and 20:4n-6 species containing 16:0 at the *sn*-1 position being present in much lower abundance than the same species containing *sn*-1 18:0. In contrast, both alkenylacyl PE and PS were characterized by a predominance of monounsaturated species. However, while PC was enriched in PC16:0/18:1, alkenylacyl PE was enriched in PE18:1alk/18:1 and PS was enriched in PS18:0/18:1. This comparison illustrates the tight regulation of the composition of

Table 3 Molecular species composition of human brain phospholipid. Results are presented as mean ± s.e.m. of mol % total PC, PE, alkenylacyl PE and PS of lipid extracts of white matter of human brain

Molecular species	Phospholipid class (mol %)			
	Diacyl PC	Diacyl PE	Alkenylacyl PE	PS
16:0/16:0	7.4 ± 0.2	–	3.9 ± 0.1	–
16:0/18:1	45.4 ± 0.8	5.5 ± 0	15.5 ± 1.5	0.4 ± 0
16:0/20:4	0.9 ± 0.1	1.1 ± 0	1.0 ± 0	–
16:0/22:6	0.3 ± 0.1	2.9 ± 0.1	0.8 ± 0.1	–
18:0/18:1	21.0 ± 0.6	12.3 ± 0.1	10.6 ± 1.7	61.2 ± 2.8
18:1/18:1	6.9 ± 0.1	18.8 ± 0.3	22.9 ± 1.1	8.5 ± 0.2
18:0/20:4	1.9 ± 0	10.4 ± 0.1	2.4 ± 0.1	1.7 ± 0.1
18:1/20:4	0.5 ± 0	5.0 ± 0.1	–	0.3 ± 0.1
18:0/22:6	0.4 ± 0.1	19.3 ± 0.2	2.3 ± 0.1	3.4 ± 0.3

From Wilson R and Bell MV (1993) Molecular species composition of glycerophospholipids from white matter of human brain. *Lipids* **28**:13–17.

individual phospholipid classes, and emphasizes potentially important differences in molecular compositions that could not be predicted from total fatty acid analysis.

Nutritional effects on phospholipid molecular species

Practically all nutritional studies of dietary lipid effects on cellular phospholipid compositions have been reported as fatty acid compositions, with no molecular information. Owing to significant differences in the detailed regulation of their phospholipid composition and metabolism, nutritional data obtained from laboratory animals generally has only a restricted application to human nutrition. The data in **Table 4** come from one study where human volunteers were fed fish oil supplements for 4 weeks, measuring the change to their erythrocyte PE molecular species composition. Two points of interest here are that the extent of increase in species containing n-3 fatty acids was variable, and that the extent of such changes were modest. This comparison illustrates a general observation that, although manipulation of cultured cell phospholipid compositions by medium lipid supplementation is relatively easy, phospholipid compositions of similar cell types *in vivo* are considerably more resistant to dietary manipulation.

Table 4 Dietary lipid and the composition of human erythrocyte phosphatidylethanolamine. Erythrocyte PE species were analysed from six volunteers before and after consumption for 4 weeks of fish oil containing 9 g eicosapentaenoic acid (22:5n-3) and 6 g docosahexaenoic acid (22:6n-3) per day

Molecular species	*Phosphatidylethanolamine (mol %)*	
	Baseline	*Week 4 supplementation*
16:0/18:1	10.81 ± 0.33	10.59 ± 0.25
16:0/18:2	4.05 ± 0.26	4.12 ± 0.19
16:0/20:4	7.03 ± 0.27	6.98 ± 0.28
16:0/20:5	1.38 ± 0.14	2.00 ± 0.16[a]
16:0/22:6	1.63 ± 0.16	2.32 ± 0.19
16:0alk/20:4	5.21 ± 0.16	4.67 ± 0.20
16:0alk/22:4	5.90 ± 0.17	5.04 ± 0.11
16:0alk/22:5	2.37 ± 0.13	3.04 ± 0.07[a]
18:0/18:1	2.92 ± 0.17	3.13 ± 0.07
18:1/18:1	3.90 ± 0.14	4.68 ± 0.21
18:0/20:4	6.81 ± 0.26	6.21 ± 0.31
18:0alk/20:4	12.36 ± 0.23	11.12 ± 0.35
18:0alk/22:5	3.55 ± 0.12	4.05 ± 0.08
18:0alk/22:6	2.77 ± 0.15	3.52 ± 0.14[a]

From Knapp HR, Hullin F and Salem N Jr (1994) Asymmetric incorporation of dietary n-3 fatty acids into membrane aminophospholipids of human erythrocytes. *Journal of Lipid Research* **35**: 1283–1291. Results are mean $\pm$ SEM.
[a]$P < 0.05$.

Functions of Phospholipids

Phospholipid composition is a significant factor in most cellular processes. This section, however, will be restricted to selected examples of the role of molecular species composition on physiological functions.

Membrane fluidity

One frequently addressed role of phospholipids is to maintain an appropriate membrane fluidity for optimal cell function. The term membrane fluidity is rather imprecise, and is generally used to describe the combined effects of lateral and rotational movement of lipids within the plane of the membrane. In this paradigm, alterations to dietary lipid intake may exert their modulatory effect on cell function by changing phospholipid molecular composition, and hence altering these physiochemical properties. While such effects are evident in model systems, extensive measurement of membrane fluidity by fluorescence polarization suggest that processes of homeoviscous adaptation restrict the potential effects of membrane fluidity changes *in vivo*. For instance, increased incorporation of PUFA into membrane phospholipid, which would be expected to have a fluidizing effect, is invariably balanced by compensatory changes to the membrane content of cholesterol and more rigid phospholipid molecules.

The role of membrane fluidity has been most extensively studied in poikilothermic animals in response to temperature variation. For any given membrane phospholipid composition, decreasing body temperature would exert a solidifying effect and decrease membrane fluidity. Direct measurement in comparable animal species acclimated to different temperatures have, however, invariably found similar values for parameters of membrane fluidity. Maintenance of membrane structure is critical for survival, and the molecular composition of membrane phospholipid is rapidly modified at different temperatures to keep the physical state of the membrane relatively constant. For instance, there are dramatic increases in membrane PC and PE species containing 22:6n-3 when fish are transferred from an environment at 20°C to one at 5°C. Temperature effects are obviously less important for homeothermic animals, but the principles regulating membrane function are similar. This is evident in hibernating mammals, where the potential effects on membrane structure in response to the drop in body temperature are compensated for by changes to membrane phospholipid composition.

Lung surfactant

Maintenance of the essential composition of lung surfactant phospholipid is critical for the survival of all mammalian species. Lung surfactant is secreted from specialized type II epithelial cells in the lung alveolus, and forms a continuous lining layer at the air–liquid interface throughout the lungs. To provide adequate gas exchange surface area in the lungs to support respiration, alveolar diameters must be very small, giving a large surface area : volume ratio. One consequence of the small dimensions of the alveolus is that surface tension forces contribute significantly to the dynamics of lung function. Surfactant opposes surface tension in the lungs. It is the absence of adequate surfactant that leads directly to lung collapse and the high incidence of morbidity and mortality associated with neonatal respiratory distress syndrome.

Lung surfactant has a unique phospholipid composition, containing PC16:0/16:0 as 40–60% of total PC, and monounsaturated phosphatidylglycerol (PG) species as 10–15% of total phospholipid. Phosphatidylglycerol is not found at significant concentration in any other membrane of the body. PC16:0/16:0 is the principal surface-active component of lung surfactant, has a gel : liquid crystalline transition temperature of 41°C, and consequently is, in effect, solid at body temperature of 37°C. It has been suggested that the compressed PC16:0/16:0 monolayer at the air–liquid interface survives the high surface pressures within the lungs by forming a solid monomolecular sheet, and thus prevents any surface tension effects. At the same time, PC16:0/16:0 is metabolically inert, and one proposed specialized role for PG is to fluidize PC16:0/16:0 and facilitate its metabolic processing, secretion and adsorption to the air–liquid interface.

This composition of lung surfactant is restricted to air-breathing animals. Comparative studies with reptiles, amphibia and lower vertebrates have shown clearly that concentration of PC16:0/16:0 in surfactant correlates with the ratio of lung : body surface area as a measure of an animal's reliance on lung-mediated respiration. Lung surfactant from amphibia, by comparison, also contain phospholipid, but this is largely cholesterol and unsaturated PC which is thought to serve an antiglue function. By analogy with lung surfactant, phospholipid-rich surfactants have been described for other epithelial surfaces including the stomach, eustachian tube and synovial surfaces, where they are thought to create a protective hydrophobic lining layer. The comparison with lung surfactant is somewhat misleading, however, as the PC fraction of these other epithelial secretions contain minimal PC16:0/16:0 and high contents of mono- and diunsaturated species.

Signal transduction

Phospholipids are substrate molecules for a wide range of lipid-derived signalling molecules, including diacylglycerol (DAG), phosphatidic acid (PA), 20:4n-6, eicosanoid products, PAF and lysophosphatidic acid, generated by the action of PLA_2, PLC and PLD. The activation of these enzymes is complex, partly because of the large number of isoforms present within a cell, and also because of the interdependence and coordination of their regulation. For instance, the bacterial peptide formyl-methionyl leucyl phenylalanine (fMLP) binds to its receptor on neutrophils, and activates the G-protein-regulated $PLC_{\gamma 1}$. $PLC_{\gamma 1}$ hydrolyses PIP_2 to form DAG, an activator of traditional Ca^{2+}-dependent PKC isoforms, and inositol trisphosphate, which stimulates intracellular Ca^{2+} mobilization. Additionally, fMLP also activates PC-specific PLD and cytoplasmic PLA_2. PLD generates PA, which has signalling responses itself including stimulation of NADPH oxidase activity, but which is also readily interconverted with DAG. Alkenyl species of PE are probably the major substrates for cytoplasmic PLA_2, which is specific for molecular species containing 20:4n-6. This multitude of responses to a single agonist is highly coordinated, and is typical of lipid signalling mechanisms in general. The activation of the various phospholipase enzymes is tightly regulated by a variety of protein kinases, phosphatases and regulatory proteins, such that their responses are sequential rather than simultaneous. Recent evidence suggests that phospholipid structure itself contributes to the coordinated regulation of phospholipase activation. PIP_2, the substrate for $PLC_{\gamma 1}$, is an obligate activator of ADP ribosylation factor-dependent PLD; consequently PIP_2 must be regenerated after the transient activation of $PLC_{\gamma 1}$ before maximal activation of PLD can be achieved.

The mechanisms of action of dietary lipid modulation on these signalling pathways are largely unknown. There is good evidence that eating a diet rich in fish oil (containing 22:6n-3 and 22:5n-3) attenuates neutrophil-mediated inflammatory reactions. Part of this anti-inflammatory nutritional effect may be to reduce the content of phospholipid species containing 20:4n-6, and thus decreasing available substrate for synthesis of eicosanoid and leukotriene products derived from 20:4n-6. Alternatively, it may also result in part from the modulation of the spectrum of molecular species of DAG and PA generated by the various PLC and PLD enzymes. In this paradigm, altering the composition of substrate phospholipid will result in formation of different DAG or PA species, which then have differential actions on target kinase enzymes. As inositol phospholipids are generally comprised of the 18:0/20:4 species, activation of PLCγ1 will form DAG18:0/20:4, while hydrolysis of PC will generate predominately monounsaturated DAG species. It has been suggested, for instance, that individual isoforms of protein kinase C can be differentially regulated in response to different molecular species of DAG, hence providing a molecular basis for many nutritional effects on a wide range of cellular functions.

Despite extensive studies since the 1960s, remarkably little is yet understood about the fundamental reasons why cells expend considerable energy in maintaining lineage-specific molecular species compositions of membrane phospholipids. Even for cell lines in culture, which can be grown successfully over many generations with grossly nonphysiological membrane phospholipid compositions, a degree of lineage specificity is maintained. The detailed metabolic processes that control membrane phospholipid composition are slowly being defined, and studies of the specificities and activities in intact cells of acyltransferase and phospholipid synthetic enzymes using gene transfection and sensitive analytical techniques such as electrospray ionization mass spectrometry are set to increase dramatically understanding of the fundamental mechanisms involved.

See Colour Plates 12, 13, 14 and 15.

See also: **Brain and Nervous System**: Biology, Metabolism and Nutritional Requirements. **Fatty Acids**: Metabolism; Health Effects of Saturated Fatty Acids; Health Effects of Monounsaturated Fatty Acids; Health Effects of n-6 Polyunsaturated Fatty Acids; Health Effects of n-3 Polyunsaturated Fatty Acids. **Lipids**: Chemistry and Classification.

Further Reading

Gunstone FD, Harwood JL and Padley FB (1986) *The Lipid Handbook*. London: Chapman & Hall.

Hazel JR and Williams EE (1990) The role of alterations in membrane lipid composition in enabling physiological adaptations of organisms to their physical environment. *Progress in Lipid Research* 29:167–227.

Lee AG (1991) Lipids and their effects on membrane proteins: evidence against a role for fluidity. *Progress in Lipid Research* 30:323–348.

Neuringer ME, Anderson GJ and Connor WE (1988) The essentiality of n-3 fatty acids for development and function of the retina and brain. *Annual Review of Nutrition* 8:517–541.

Zachowski A (1993) Phospholipids in animal eukaryotic membranes: transverse asymmetry and movement. *Biochemical Journal* 294:1–14.

Zeisel SH and Canty DJ (1993) Choline phospholipids: molecular mechanisms for human diseases: a meeting report. *Journal of Nutritional Biochemistry* 4:258–263.

LIPOPROTEINS

Physiology

J M Ordovas, Tuft University, Boston, Massachusetts, USA

Copyright © 1998 Academic Press

Cholesterol and triacylglycerol are transported in blood as lipoproteins. Lipoproteins are generally spherical particles, with a surface layer composed of phospholipid with the fatty acids oriented toward the core of the particle. Included in this phospholipid layer are specific proteins known as apolipoproteins and free cholesterol. The core of the lipoprotein particles is made up of cholesteryl ester and triacylglycerol molecules.

The classification of serum lipoproteins has evolved historically through several phases corresponding with the development of different laboratory methodologies, including electrophoretic, ultracentrifugal and immunological techniques. By using these techniques, lipoproteins can be classified based on their electrophoretic mobility, hydrated density and protein content.

Classification of Lipoproteins

Classification of serum lipoproteins according to their electrophoretic mobilities

With the development of techniques to separate proteins according to their electrophoretic behaviour, it could be demonstrated that most of the lipid present in serum was associated with proteins migrating with α_1- and β-globulin mobilities. This resulted in the first classification of lipoproteins as α_1- and β-lipoproteins. The ratio of lipid to protein on the α_1-lipoproteins was approximately 1:1, whereas the β-lipoproteins had a greater relative content of lipids. Application of more advanced electrophoretic techniques resulted in further discrimination among the lipoprotein classes and for many years lipoproteins were classified as β-, pre-β- and α-lipoproteins. Careful observation of the electrophoretic lipoprotein profiles in normals and subjects with familial lipoprotein disorders gave rise to the first classification of lipoprotein disorders by Fredrickson and colleagues. The equivalence between electrophoretic and ultracentrifugal separation is presented in **Table 1**.

Several electrophoretic supports have been used to separate plasma lipoproteins. These include paper, cellulose acetate, agarose and polyacrylamide. Agarose gel electrophoresis remains the most commonly used for easy and rapid assessment of lipoprotein patterns in the clinical laboratory. This technique is especially useful for identifying the presence of a broad β band in the diagnosis of type III hyperlipidaemia. Gradient agarose-polyacrylamide gel electrophoresis under nondenaturing conditions has been an essential tool to analyse low-density lipoprotein (LDL) and high-density lipoprotein (HDL) subclasses, providing a greater resolution than ultracentrifugation. LDL subfractions have been resolved by nondenaturing polyacrylamide gradient gel electrophoresis (2–16%) in up to seven LDL subclasses with densities ranging from 1.020 to 1.063 g ml^{-1} and diameters ranging from 22.0 to 28.5 nm. Usually a major subpopulation and several (one to four) minor

LDL subpopulations are found in most subjects examined. A predominance of smaller, more dense LDL, versus larger, more buoyant LDL particles in plasma has been associated with increased coronary heart disease (CHD) risk. There is evidence supporting the genetic origin of the distribution of LDL subfractions; however, age, gender and environmental factors strongly influence the penetrance. HDL subfractions have been resolved using a similar technique, with a polyacrylamide gradient ranging from 4–30%, into five subclasses (HDL$_{3c}$, HDL$_{3b}$, HDL$_{3a}$, HDL$_{2a}$ and HDL$_{2b}$). More recently 11–14 subclasses have been described, including β-migrating particles, using an improved electrophoresis technique. The clinical importance of these subfractions is still under investigation.

Classification of serum lipoproteins according to their ultracentrifugal characteristics

The presence of lipids within the lipoprotein particles confers these macromolecular complexes with a lower density compared with other serum proteins. With the arrival of the analytical ultracentrifugation in the 1940s, this characteristic allowed its initial separation as a discrete peak using this technique. During the following years, it was demonstrated that this fraction was made up of a wide spectrum of particle sizes and densities (d) ranging from 0.92 to 1.21 g ml^{-1}.

Lipoproteins were classically separated into four major classes designated as chylomicrons (exogenous triacylglycerol-rich particles of $d < 0.94$ g ml^{-1}), very low-density lipoproteins (VLDL, endogenous triacylglycerol-rich particles of $d = 0.94$–1.006 g ml^{-1}), LDL (cholesteryl ester-rich particles of $d = 1.006$–1.063 g ml^{-1}), and HDL (particles containing approximately 50% protein of $d = 1.063$–1.21 g ml^{-1}). With subsequent improvements to the ultracentrifugation techniques, further heterogeneity was detected within each of those major lipoprotein classes; this resulted in the need for further subdivision into several density subclasses such as HDL$_{2a}$

Table 1 Classification of plasma lipoproteins

Lipoprotein	Diameter (nm)	Density (g ml^{-1})	Electrophoretic mobility	Major lipids	Major apolipoproteins
Chylomicrons	80–500	<0.95	Origin	Dietary triacylglycerols, cholesteryl esters	A-I, A-II, A-IV, B-48, C-I, C-II, C-III, E
Remnants	>30	<1.006	Origin	Dietary cholesteryl esters	B-48, E
VLDL	30–80	<1.006	pre-β	Endogenous triacylglycerols	B-100, C-I, C-II, C-III, E
IDL	25–35	1.006–1.019	pre-β and β	Cholesteryl esters, triacylglycerols	B-100, E
LDL	18–28	1.019–1.063	β	Cholesteryl esters	B-100
HDL$_2$	9–12	1.063–1.125	α	Cholesteryl esters, phospholipids	A-I, A-II
HDL$_3$	5–9	1.125–1.210	α	Cholesteryl esters, phospholipids	A-I, A-II

$(d = 1.10–1.125\,\mathrm{g\,ml^{-1}})$, $\mathrm{HDL_{2b}}$ $(d = 1.063–1.10\,\mathrm{g\,ml^{-1}})$ and $\mathrm{HDL_3}$ $(d = 1.125–1.21\,\mathrm{g\,ml^{-1}})$.

There is no doubt that the separation of lipoproteins by ultracentrifugation has been esential for the advances in this field; however, this technique is very labour intensive and the isolated lipoproteins are usually modified due to the high g force and salt concentrations used in this process. The development of new vertical and near vertical rotors has shortened considerably the runs and thus diminished some of these negative effects.

Classification of serum lipoproteins according to their apolipoprotein composition

Recent interest on the study of lipoprotein subfractions has resulted in an increased use of methods of separation based on affinity chromatography, specially those using immunoaffinity. By using columns containing antibodies against specific apolipoproteins (**Table 2**), a large number of HDL subpopulations have been resolved. Similarly, this technique allows the separation of several triacylglycerol-rich lipoproteins subfractions.

Lipoproteins containing apo A-I can be separated into two major species: those containing both apo A-I and apo A-II, known as LpAI:AII, and those containing apo A-I but not apo A-II (LpAI). Small numbers of particles containing apo A-II, but not apo A-I, have been detected in normal subjects; however, these particles could become predominant in the presence of rare genetic disorders associated with HDL deficiency. Another HDL species containing apo A-I and apo E is important in reverse cholesterol transport by transporting cholesterol from the cell membranes to the liver for elimination from the body.

Lipoproteins containing apo B consist of four lipoprotein families. Lipoproteins containing apo B only (Lp(B)) are cholesteryl ester-rich and are found primarily within the LDL density range, but they have been also detected within the VLDL range. Particles containing both apo B and apo C (LpB:C); apo B and apo E (LpB:E); and all three apolipoprotein groups (LpB:E:C), are triacylglycerol-rich and are found within the VLDL and IDL density range. The apo C and apo E content decreases as density increases.

More recently, the affinity for lectins of Lp(a), a lipoprotein containing apo B-100 as well as an anti-

Table 2 Classification and properties of apolipoproteins

Apolipoprotein	Amino acids	Tissue expression	Chromosomal localization	Functions
apo A-I	243	Liver Intestine	11	Major structural component of HDL Ligand for HDL binding Activator of LCAT Reverse cholesterol transport
apo A-II	77	Liver	1	Structural component of HDL Activator of hepatic lipase
apo A-IV	377	Intestine Liver	11	Regulator of LPL activity Activator of LCAT Intestinal lipid absorption
apo B-48	2152	Intestine	2	Structural component of TRL Secretion of chylomicrons
apo B-100	4536	Liver	2	Structural
apo C-I	57	Liver Intestine	19	Activator of LCAT Inhibitor of the LRP
apo C-II	79	Liver Intestine	19	Activator of LPL
apo C-III	79	Liver Intestine	11	Inhibits LPL
apo D	169	Most tissues	3	Radical scavenger Reverse cholesterol transport Binding of haem-related compounds
apo E	299	Liver Macrophage	19	Ligand for the LDL receptor Ligand for the LRP Reverse cholesterol transport
apo(a)	Variable	Liver	6	?

genically unique apolipoprotein [apo(a)], has been used to develop a new technique to measure the levels of this lipoprotein in plasma.

Synthesis and Catabolism of Lipoproteins

Metabolism of lipoproteins carrying exogenous lipids

Dietary fats absorbed in the intestine are packaged into large, triacylglycerol-rich chylomicrons for delivery through the bloodstream to sites of lipid metabolism or storage. These lipoproteins interact with lipoprotein lipase (LPL) and undergo lipolysis, forming chylomicron remnants. The major sites of LPL activity are adipose tissue, skeletal muscle, the mammary gland and the myocardium. In these sites, the fatty acids from the trcacylglycerols are used for storage, oxidation or secretion back to the circulation. The triacylglycerol-depleted particles resulting from the lipolysis, known as chylomicron remnants, pick up apo E and cholesteryl ester from HDL, and are rapidly taken up by the liver via a process mediated by the apo E receptor. This is a fast process and chylomicron particles are not usually present in the blood after a prolonged fasting period. The occurrence of chylomicronaemia can be easily detected by the presence of a creamy supernatant floating on top of the plasma or serum kept several hours at 4°C.

Transport of endogenous lipids

The liver cell secretes triacylglycerol-rich VLDL, which can be converted first to intermediate-density lipoprotein (IDL) and then to LDL through lipolysis, by a mechanism similar to that described for chylomicrons. The excess surface components are usually transferred to HDL, and the triacylglycerol-depleted VLDL becomes an IDL. Some of these particles may be taken up by the liver via an apo E receptor, whereas others are further depleted of triacylglycerols, becoming cholesteryl ester-enriched particles known as LDL, which contain apo B as their only apolipoprotein. Consumption of fat-rich meals or glucose enhances VLDL production.

Some primary causes of elevated VLDL or IDL levels are familial endogenous hypertriglyceridaemia (type IV according to Fredrickson's classification) and familial dysbetalipoproteinaemia (type III hyperlipidaemia). Genetic mutations at the apo E gene locus are responsible for the type III phenotype. Some secondary causes for elevated VLDL levels are obesity, diabetes mellitus, alcohol consumption, as well as the use of high doses of certain drugs (e.g.

thiazide diuretics and oestrogens). The presence of elevated levels of IDL has been associated with an increased atherosclerotic risk.

LDL particles are major carriers of cholesteryl ester in the blood. An LDL receptor that recognizes apo B-100 and apo E, but not apo B-48, allows the liver and other tissues to catabolize LDL. High-fat and high-cholesterol diets can decrease the activity of the LDL receptor, leading to increased levels of circulating LDL. These particles supply cholesterol to cells in the periphery for synthesis of cell membranes and steroid hormones. Modified or oxidized LDL can also be taken up by the scavenger receptor on macrophages in various tissues, including the arterial wall. This process is a potential initiator of foam cell formation and atherosclerosis.

Several LDL subclasses have been identified using gradient gel electrophoresis. Large, less dense LDL particles are commonly found in premenopausal women and men at low risk for CHD, whereas the small, more dense particles have been associated with a significant increased risk for myocardial infarction. The distribution of these particles appears to have a significant genetic component modulated by age and environmental factors.

Reverse cholesterol transport

HDL is synthesized by both the liver and the intestine. Its precursor form is discoidal in shape and matures in circulation as it picks up unesterified cholesterol from cell membranes, and other lipids (phospholipid and triacylglycerol) and proteins (A-I, E and C apolipoproteins) from triacylglycerol-rich lipoproteins (chylomicron and VLDL) as these particles undergo lipolysis. The cholesterol is esterified by the action of the lecithin–cholesterol acyltransferase (LCAT) and the small HDL_3 particle becomes a larger HDL_2 particle. The esterified cholesterol is either delivered to the liver or transferred by the action of cholesteryl ester transfer protein (CETP) to other lipoproteins (such as chylomicron, VLDL remnants or LDL) in exchange for triacylglycerols. This cholesterol may then be taken up by the liver via receptors specific for these lipoproteins, or it can be delivered again to the peripheral tissues. The triacylglycerol received by HDL_2 is hydrolysed by hepatic lipase and the particle is converted back to HDL_3, completing the HDL cycle in plasma. In the liver, cholesterol can either be excreted directly into bile, converted to bile acids, or reutilized in lipoprotein production.

Several genetic disorders have been identified associated with low levels or total deficiency of HDL.

Effects of Dietary Fats and Cholesterol on Lipoprotein Metabolism

The cholesterolaemic effects of dietary fatty acids have been extensively studied. The saturated fatty acids $C_{12:0}$, $C_{14:0}$ and $C_{16:0}$ have a hypercholesterolaemic effect, whereas $C_{18:0}$ has been shown to have a neutral effect. Monounsaturated and polyunsaturated fatty acids in their most common *cis* configuration are hypocholesterolaemic in comparison with saturated fatty acids. The effects of *trans* fatty acids on lipid levels are under active investigation. Our current knowledge shows that their effect is intermediate between saturated and unsaturated fats. The effect of dietary cholesterol on lipoprotein levels is highly controversial. This may be due in part to the dramatic interindividual variation in response to this dietary component. Specific effects of dietary fats and cholesterol on each lipoprotein fraction are the focus of other articles and they are only briefly summarized below and in **Table 3**.

Effects of diet on chylomicron metabolism

Diets very high in saturated fat have been associated with increased postprandial chylomicrons and chylomicron remnants compared with diets rich in n-6 polyunsaturated fats; however, human experiments carried out using moderate to high fat intake have not shown significant effects of different types of dietary fat or dietary cholesterol on postprandial lipoproteins.

The effects of dietary carbohydrates on postprandial lipoproteins have been also studied. Most protocols have used diets very high in simple carbohydrates. In general, high carbohydrate intake has been associated with increased levels of fasting triacylglycerols and increased postprandial levels of chylomicrons and chylomicron remnants.

Effects of diet on VLDL metabolism

It is well known that diets high in simple carbohydrate increase hepatic secretion of VLDL. This carbohydrate induction of hypertriglyceridaemia is the source of the current controversy regarding the optimal diet for subjects at high risk for cardiovascular disease. Some authors have demonstrated that the increased hepatic triacylglycerol secretion induced by high-carbohydrate diets was not accompanied by parallel increases in apo B-100 secretion. In other words, the consumption of low-fat, high-carbohydrate diets did not affect the number of particles, but resulted in larger, more triacylglycerol-enriched VLDL particles.

Intake of saturated fat results in an increased secretion of the number of VLDL particles by the liver, whereas the opposite effect is observed with polyunsaturated fat. Of special note are the dramatic effects on VLDL production found following high intakes of n-3 fatty acids. These diets are associated with marked decreases in triacylglycerol secretion by mechanisms not fully understood. It has been speculated that n-3 fatty acids may stimulate intracellular degradation of apo B in hepatocytes. Dietary cholesterol, within the physiological range, appears to play a minor role in hepatic VLDL production.

Effects of diet on LDL metabolism

The effects of dietary fat and cholesterol on LDL metabolism have been extensively studied. However, the effects of dietary cholesterol are still highly controversial. Whereas some studies have demonstrated increased LDL production and decreased catabolism associated with high cholesterol intakes, others have failed to find such associations.

Replacement of saturated by polyunsaturated fats has been associated with decreased LDL apo B production in some studies, whereas in other studies, increased ratios of polyunsaturated to saturated fats resulted in increased LDL apo B catabolism. Unlike the effects described for VLDL metabolism, intake of n-3 fatty acids appears to play a minor role on LDL metabolism.

Effects of diet HDL metabolism

Diets high in simple carbohydrates reduce HDL cholesterol levels. This effect appears to be mediated by increases in the catabolism of apo A-I; however, one study has also demonstrated an additional decrease in apo A-I production.

Table 3 Effects induced on the major lipoprotein fractions by different dietary components following isoenergetic replacement of saturated fatty acids

	MUFA	PUFA n-6	PUFA n-3	trans FA	Simple carbohydrate	Carbohydrate plus fibre
VLDL-C	≈	≈/↓	↓	↑	↑	≈
LDL-C	↓	↓	≈/↓	↑	↓	↓
HDL-C	≈/↑	≈/↓	↓	↓	↓	≈↓

≈ equivalent effect; ↓ concentration reduced; ↑ concentration increased.

Disorders of Lipoprotein Metabolism

For historical reasons the classification of disorders of lipoprotein metabolism will be presented according to the classical Fredrickson's classification (**Table 4**).

Type I or familial chylomicronaemia

This disorder is characterized by greatly elevated levels of exogenous triacylglycerols and it is the result of impaired lipolysis of chylomicrons due to a deficiency of LPL or its activator, the apo C-II. Several genetic mutations at the structural genes for both LPL and apo C-II have been reported. These are autosomal recessive traits. In the heterozygous state, subjects have normal to slightly elevated plasma triglycerides, whereas homozygotes have triacylglycerol levels that may exceed 1000 mg dl^{-1} in the fasting state. The diagnosis of the homozygous state takes place during the first years of life from the presence of recurrent abdominal pain and pancreatitis. Eruptive xanthomas and lipaemia retinalis may also occur.

The recommended treatment includes a diet low in simple carbohydrates and with a fat content below 20% of total energy. The use of medium-chain triglycerides (MCT) has also been reported to be efficacious. Body weight should be maintained within the normal limits and alcohol consumption should be avoided.

Other secondary causes leading to the presence of chylomicrons in the fasting state include uncontrolled diabetes mellitus, alcoholism, oestrogen use and hypothyroidism.

Fasting chylomicronaemia has not been clearly associated with increased risk for atherosclerosis; however there is considerable evidence supporting the atherogenic properties of chylomicron remnants.

Type II or familial hypercholesterolaemia

Familial hypercholesterolaemia (FH) is an autosomal dominant disorder characterized by elevation of plasma LDL cholesterol levels. Mutations at the LDL receptor gene locus on chromosome 19 are responsible for this disorder. Multiple different mutations have been described at this locus resulting in the FH phenotype. In the heterozygous state, subjects develop tendinous xanthomas, corneal arcus and CHD. Elevations of LDL can result from well-characterized genetic disorders such as familial hypercholesterolaemia or familial defective apo B-100.

The ranges of LDL cholesterol levels in plasma of FH subjects are 200–400 mg dl^{-1} in heterozygotes and above 450 mg dl^{-1} in homozygotes. The frequency of defects at the LDL receptor locus is about 1 in 500 for the heterozygous state and 1 in a million in the homozygous state.

Inhibitors of 3-hydroxy-3-methylglutaryl (HMG) coenzyme A are useful in the treatment of hyper-

Table 4 Classification of hyperlipidaemias according to Fredrickson

Type	Plasma cholesterol	Plasma triacylglycerol	Lipoprotein fraction(s) affected	Atherosclerosis risk	Genetic disorder
I	Normal to elevated	Very elevated	Chylomicrons	No	Familial LPL deficiency Apo C-II deficiency
IIa	Elevated	Normal	LDL	High	Familial hypercholesterolaemia Familial combined hyperlipidaemia Polygenic hypercholesterolaemia
IIb	Elevated	Elevated	LDL and VLDL	High	Familial hypercholesterolaemia Familial combined hyperlipidaemia
III	Elevated	Very elevated	IDL	High	Familial dysbetalipoproteinaemia
IV	Normal or elevated	Elevated	VLDL	Moderate	Familial hypertriglyceridaemia Familial combined hyperlipidaemia
V	Normal or elevated	Very elevated	VLDL and chylomicrons	Moderate	Familial hypertriglyceridaemia

cholesterolaemia. Most pharmacological therapies are ineffective in the homozygous state. FH homozygotes may be treated with LDL apheresis, liver transplantation and portacaval shunt. More recently, encouraging results have been obtained using *ex vivo* gene therapy.

The genetic defect(s) associated with a common form of hypercholesterolaemia present in most subjects with cholesterol levels between 250 and 300 mg dl^{-1} has not been elucidated. This disorder may be due to a combination of minor gene defects (i.e. presence of apo E-4 allele) that in combination with the environment (i.e. diet, lack of exercise) predispose individuals to moderately elevated LDL cholesterol levels. This disorder has been also named polygenic hypercholesterolaemia.

Familial defective apo B-100

Familial defective apo B-100 is an autosomal dominant genetic disorder that presents with a phenotype similar to familial hypercholesterolaemia. The frequency of this disorder may be similar to FH; however, it varies considerably depending on the ethnicity of the population studied. The specific mutation responsible for this disorder is a point mutation at amino acid 3500 of the mature apo B. The diagnosis of this disorder requires molecular biology techniques.

Type III or familial dysbetalipoproteinaemia

In this disorder both plasma triacylglycerol and cholesterol are increased. Several mutations within the apo E gene locus have been found to be responsible for this disease; however, in most patients the complete expression of the clinical genotype needs additional interactions such as age, obesity and diabetes, to cite some examples. In addition to the accumulation in plasma of VLDL remnants and chylomicrons, other characteristics of this disorder are tuboeruptive xanthomas and in some cases also planar xanthomas. Therapies include diet and hypolipidaemic agents such as fibrates, statin or nicotinic acid. In most cases, diagnosis can be carried out first by agarose gel electrophoresis, followed by molecular biology techniques to detect the presence of the apo E-2 allele.

Familial type IV and type V hypertriglyceridaemias

These two disorders may have overlapping phenotypes. In type IV or familial endogenous hypertriglyceridaemia, triacylglycerol levels are increased and HDL is usually decreased. This disorder appears to be autosomal dominant and relatively frequent in populations consuming high-fat diets. The precise molecular defect has not been defined; however, the increase in triacylglycerol is associated with overproduction of triacylglycerol by the liver and often with consequent reduced clearance. Diet should be the first step in therapy, followed if necessary by pharmacotherapy using fibrates or nicotinic acid. Premature CHD has been seen in some but not all cases presenting with this phenotype.

Type V hyperlipidaemia is a much more rare disorder. Usually the first signs of this abnormality are abdominal pain or pancreatitis. VLDL levels are high and chylomicrons are present in the fasting state. This abnormality has not been linked to any specific molecular defect. Besides the primary genetic defect, other secondary causes of type V hyperlipidaemia are poorly controlled diabetes mellitus, nephrotic syndrome, hypothyroidism, glycogen storage disease and pregnancy. Recent data indicate increased susceptibility to atherosclerosis.

Familial dyslipidaemia

Familial dyslipidaemia may be a variant of the familial hypertriglyceridaemias described above. It is characterized by hypertriglyceridaemia in combination with low HDL cholesterol. Patients are generally overweight, with male pattern obesity, insulin resistance, diabetes and hypertension. These subjects have both increased hepatic triacylglycerol secretion and increased HDL apo A-I catabolism.

Familial combined hyperlipidaemia

Familial combined hyperlipidaemia (FCH) was initially described as the combination of hypercholesterolaemia and hypertriglyceridaemia within the same kindred, and with kindred members having one of these abnormalities or both. Moreover, most subjects with FCH have HDL cholesterol levels below the 10th percentile. Affected subjects have elevation in VLDL, LDL or both. This disorder has a frequency of approximately 10% in survivors of premature myocardial infarction (less than 60 years of age) and about 14% in kindred with CHD.

It has been reported that affected subjects have overproduction of apo B-100. The precise molecular defect has not been elucidated, although there are already several candidate gene loci, including the LPL. The expression of this disorder may be triggered by other factors such as overweight, hypertension, diabetes and gout. The treatment should include diet and exercise and, if necessary, niacin, HMC CoA reductase inhibitors or fibrates, depending on the major lipid present in excess.

Familial hyperapobetalipoproteinaemia

Familial hyperapobetalipoproteinaemia is characterized by apo B values above the 90th percentile in the absence of other lipid abnormalities; it has been suggested to be a variant of FCH. This disorder is relatively common (~5%) in kindreds with premature CHD. The molecular defect is not known, but metabolic studies suggest overproduction of apo B-100.

Familial hypoalphalipoproteinaemia

Severe HDL deficiency, characterized by HDL cholesterol levels <10 mg dl^{-1}, is rare and may be due to Tangier disease, apo A-I deficiencies, LCAT deficiency or fish-eye disease. The apo A-I deficiency states are due to rare deletions, rearrangements or point mutations within the apo A-I/C-III/A-IV gene complex. Familial hypoalphalipoproteinaemia is relatively common and is characterized by HDL cholesterol levels below the 10th percentile of normal. These subjects have been reported to have either decreased HDL production or increased HDL apo A-I catabolism. This phenotype is present in about 4% of kindred with premature CHD.

The genetic defect or defects are not known; however, it has been suggested that familial combined hyperlipidaemia, familial hyperapobetalipoproteinaemia, familial dysbetalipoproteinaemia and familial hypoalphalipoproteinaemia may be variants of a single disorder. This disorder is characterized by a genetic predisposition in subjects consuming high-fat, high-cholesterol diets to an increased secretion of apo B-containing lipoproteins and an increased catabolism of apo A-I-containing lipoproteins. The expression of the phenotype is usually enhanced by the presence of male pattern obesity.

Familial lipoprotein (a) excess

Lipoprotein (a) (Lp(a)) is an LDL particle with one molecule of apolipoprotein (a) attached to it. Elevated levels of Lp(a) (>35–40 mg dl^{-1} or 90th percentile) have been associated with premature CHD. This increased risk appears to result from two different mechanisms: cholesterol deposition in the arterial wall and inhibition of fibrinolysis.

Lp(a) concentrations are highly variable among individuals; however, they tend to remain constant during a person's lifetime. Between 80 and 90% of the variability appears to be of genetic origin, owing, for the most part, to variations at the structural apo(a) gene locus. Lp(a) concentrations are inversely associated with a size polymorphism of apo(a). This polymorphism is due to differences in the number of a multiple repeat of a protein domain highly homolo-

gous to the kringle 4 domain of plasminogen. Diets and medications used to lower LDL cholesterol levels do not appear to have a significant effect on Lp(a) concentrations; however, niacin has been reported to decrease Lp(a) levels. There have been reports suggesting that diets high in *trans* fatty acids have some raising effects on Lp(a) levels whereas oestrogen replacement lowers Lp(a) in postmenopausal women.

General Guidelines for the Treatment of Lipoprotein Abnormalities for CHD Prevention

There is a clear benefit from lowering LDL cholesterol with diet or drug therapy in patients with hyperlipidaemia or CHD or both. Dietary therapy includes using diets that are restricted in total fat (<30% of calories), saturated fat (<7% of calories) and cholesterol (<200 mg day^{-1}). Pharmacological therapies include anion exchange resins, niacin and HMG CoA reductase inhibitors. The latter agents have been demonstrated also to lower CHD mortality. It should be noted that dramatic interindividual variations have been demonstrated in response to diet and drug therapies. Consequently the efficacy of hypolipidaemic therapies will vary from individual to individual. More information is needed about the benefits of HDL cholesterol raising in patients with low HDL cholesterol levels as well as the benefits of lowering triacylglycerol plasma concentrations, and more specifically the triacylglycerol carried in lipoprotein remnants. This is also true regarding the benefits of Lp(a) lowering using niacin in patients with elevated Lp(a) levels.

See also: **Body Composition**: Determination and Physiological Significance. **Cholesterol**: Sources, Absorption, Function and Metabolism; Factors Determining Blood Cholesterol Levels. **Coronary Heart Disease**: Lipid Theory of Coronary Heart Disease; Haemostatic Factors and Coronary Heart Disease; Aetiology; Prevention. **Fatty Acids**: Metabolism; Health Effects of Saturated Fatty Acids; Health Effects of Monounsaturated Fatty Acids; Health Effects of n-6 Polyunsaturated Fatty Acids; Health Effects of n-3 Polyunsaturated Fatty Acids; Health Effects of *trans* Fatty Acids. **Lipids**: Chemistry and Classification.

Further Reading

Alaupovic P (1996) Significance of apolipoproteins for structure, function, and classification of plasma lipoproteins. In: Bradley WA, Gianturco SH and Segrest JP (eds) *Methods in Enzymology, Plasma Lipoproteins*, part C, vol. 263, pp 32–60. San Diego: Academic Press.

Austin MA, Breslow JL, Henneckens CH, Buring JE, Willett WC and Krauss RM (1988) Low density lipoprotein subclass patterns and risk of myocardial infarction. *Journal of the American Medical Association* 260:1917–1921.

Li Z, McNamara JR, Ordovas JM and Schaefer EJ (1994) Analysis of high density lipoproteins by a modified gradient gel electrophoresis method. *Journal of Lipid Research* 35:1698–1711.

National Cholesterol Education Program (1994) Second Report of the Expert Panel on Detection, Evaluation and Treatment of High Blood Cholesterol in Adults (Adult Treatment Panel II). *Circulation* 89:1329–1445.

Ordovas JM (1991) Molecular biological approaches to the understanding of lipoprotein metabolism. In: Witiak DT, Newman HAI and Feller DR (eds) *Medical, Chemical and Biochemical Aspects of Antilipidemic Drugs*, pp 97–121. Amsterdam: Elsevier.

Ordovas JM (1993) Metabolism of triglyceride-rich lipoproteins: Genetic mutations associated with its pathology. *Cardiovascular Risk Factors* 3:1–8.

Ordovas JM (1994) Genetic and environmental factors: Effects on plasma lipoproteins. In: Serrano Rios (ed.) *Dairy Products in Human Health and Nutrition*, pp 303–307. Rotterdam: Balkema.

Ordovas JM, Civeira F, Genest J and Schaefer EJ (1990) Genetic high density lipoprotein deficiency states. In. Lenfant C, Albertini A, Paoletti R and Catapano A (eds) *Atherosclerosis Reviews. Biotechnology of Dyslipoproteinemias. Application in Diagnosis and Control*, vol. 20, pp 261–274. New York: Raven Press.

Ordovas JM, Lopez-Miranda J, Mata P, Perez-Jimenez F, Lichtenstein AH and Schaefer EJ (1995) Gene–diet interaction in determining plasma lipid response to dietary intervention. *Atherosclerosis* 118:S11–S27.

Schaefer EJ and Ordovas JM (1992) Diagnosis and management of HDL deficiency states. In: Miller NE and Tall AR (eds) *High Density Lipoproteins and Atherosclerosis*, vol. III, pp 235–251. Amsterdam: Elsevier.

Schaefer EJ, Genest Jr JJ, Ordovas JM, Salem DN and Wilson PWF (1993) Familial lipoprotein disorders and premature coronary artery disease. *Current Opinion in Lipidology* 4:288–298.

Schaefer EJ, Lichtenstein AH, Lamon-Fava S, McNamara JR and Ordovas JM (1995) Lipoproteins, nutrition, aging, and atherosclerosis. *American Journal of Clinical Nutrition* 61 (supplement):726S–740S.

Zannis VI, Kardassis D and Zanni EE (1993) Genetic mutations affecting human lipoproteins, their receptors, and their enzymes. *Advances in Human Genetics* 21:145–319.

LIVER DISORDERS

Nutritional Management

Lawrence Feinman and **C S Lieber**, Mount Sinai School of Medicine, New York, USA

Copyright © 1998 Academic Press

Liver in Normal Nutrition

The liver's nutritional role derives from the fact that it produces bile salts and is involved in the intermediary metabolism of protein (amino acids), carbohydrate, fat and vitamins.

Bile salts

Bile salts are synthesized in the liver from cholesterol and are secreted in bile in response to a meal to mix with intestinal contents. In the intestine, they act as detergents in the intraluminal phase of fat assimilation. Triacylglycerols enter the duodenum in the form of an emulsion. The surface of this emulsion is covered by a relatively polar layer of phospholipids and proteins which the bile salts remove before lipolysis via pancreatic lipase can proceed. As a result of clearing these polar substances from the emulsion there is a separation of acylglycerol in the emulsion from lipase in the water phase. Lipolysis thus becomes dependent on the presence of another enzyme, colipase, which is secreted with lipase in the pancreatic juice. By binding to lipase and altering its molecular conformation, colipase attaches lipase to the acylglycerols of the emulsion and exposes the active site of lipase, thereby overcoming the inhibitory actions of bile salts on lipolysis.

Fatty acids, monoacylglycerols and small amounts of lysophospholipids, the products of lipolysis, form mixed micelles with bile salts. The intestinal uptake of long-chain fatty acids depends on these mixed micelles, whereas the absorption of short- and medium-chain fatty acids can proceed in the absence of bile. Following uptake of fatty acids, bile salts are conserved via recycling through an enterohepatic circulation. Bile salts, especially conjugates of the trihydroxy bile acid, cholic acid, are reabsorbed from the distal small bowel by an active, sodium-dependent process, but dihydroxy bile salts are absorbed by passive diffusion from the proximal small bowel. The liver extracts these reabsorbed bile salts from portal vein blood and re-secretes them into the bile. Hepatic synthesis of bile salts replenishes about 5% of the bile salt pool that is lost in the faeces daily.

Intermediary metabolism

Carbohydrates The liver regulates carbohydrate metabolism by the synthesis, storage, and breakdown of glycogen, a polymeric form of glucose. In glycogen form, large amounts of 'glucose units' can be stored within the hepatocyte without major effects on the intracellular osmotic pressure. Glycogen formation is favoured when the intake of glucose (or other gluconeogenic fuels) exceeds energy requirements; glycogen is broken down when intake lags behind energy needs. The principal enzymes controlling glycogenesis and glycogenolysis are glycogen synthase and phosphorylase, respectively, a reciprocal relationship existing between these two enzymes. Stimulation of glycogen synthase is usually accompanied by inhibition of phosphorylase. Conversely, agents that stimulate phosphorylase inhibit glycogen synthase. Controlling factors for these enzymes include intracellular levels of glucose-6-phosphate and the hormones epinephrine, glucagon and insulin. Epinephrine and glucagon raise blood glucose levels by activating phosphorylase whereas insulin lowers blood glucose, in part, by stimulating glycogen synthase.

Hepatocytes, possessing enzymes that enable them to synthesize glucose from various precursors such as amino acids, pyruvate and lactate, engage in gluconeogenesis. Hypoglycaemia promotes gluconeogenesis. Hypoglycaemia is probably linked to gluconeogenesis by the secretion of cortisol from the adrenal medulla. Cortisol is secreted under pituitary control (adrenocorticotropic hormone, or ACTH) and mobilizes glycogenic amino acids from various tissues.

Fat The liver is the organ most responsible for fatty acid breakdown and triacylglycerol synthesis. The breakdown of fatty acids provides a source of energy alternative to glucose when glucose is unavailable during fasting or starvation. Triacylglycerol in adipose tissue is hydrolysed to release fatty acids. Bound to albumin in the blood, the released fatty acids are rapidly removed by the hepatocyte and transported into the mitochondria by a carnitine-mediated process. Mitochondrial enzymes degrade the fatty acid molecule to acetyl CoA fragments, a sequence known as β oxidation. Acetyl CoA then enters the citric acid cycle which generates adenosine triphosphate (ATP) by oxidative phosphorylation. Triacylglycerol synthesis occurs when carbohydrate intake exceeds energy requirements: glucose may overwhelm the glycogen reservoir, and the acetyl CoA which is generated by glycolysis, and which is not needed for oxidative phosphorylation, is conserved by its conversion to fatty acids and, ultimately, triacylglycerols. Synthesis of fatty acids involves repetitive additions of two carbon fragments (derived from acetyl CoA) to malonyl CoA. After reaction with α-glycerophosphate, the resulting triacylglycerols are transported to the adipose tissues as part of lipoproteins, specifically the very low-density lipoproteins (VLDL).

Proteins The liver plays a central role in the synthesis and degradation of protein. It contains the enzymes necessary for the transmination and oxidative deamination of amino acids as well as the enzymes required for urea synthesis. As noted previously, amino acids can also participate in gluconeogenesis. Gluconeogenesis proceeds after conversion of deaminated amino acids to pyruvate and other intermediates of the citric acid cycle. Plasma proteins, including albumin, coagulation factors, transferrin and caeruloplasmin, constitute about one-half of the protein synthesized in the liver. These export proteins are synthesized on the rough endoplasmic reticulum. Protein synthesis by the liver is influenced by the nutritional state and by hormones such as insulin, glucagon and glucocorticoids. Insulin and glucocorticoids stimulate the synthesis of hepatic proteins, whereas glucagon inhibits synthesis and promotes their degradation.

Nutritional Consequences of Liver Injury

Acute liver injury

Regardless of aetiology, acute liver injury is often associated with anorexia, nausea, and vomiting. In alcoholic liver injury these symptoms may be exacerbated by concomitant alcoholic gastritis. Thus, acute liver injury is likely to decrease the oral intake of food. When the illness is short-lived and self-limited, nutritional consequences are minimal. Both alcoholic and nonalcoholic acute liver injury may cause fasting hypoglycaemia. This has been attributed to depleted liver glycogen reserves and a block in gluconeogenesis from amino acids. Severe injury may interfere with the detoxification of ammonia and other amines to the extent that hepatic coma develops; protein intake must then be limited.

Chronic liver injury

Chronic liver injury, particularly cirrhosis, is accompanied by liver function impairment that frequently gives rise to nutritional complications. Regardless of aetiology, cirrhosis is likely to cause patients to have abnormal anthropometric measurements (muscle wasting) and to be anergic to common antigens on skin testing. Circulating levels of both fat- and water-soluble vitamins are low in a high percentage of patients with alcoholic cirrhosis. Low serum levels of fat-soluble vitamins (rather than the water-soluble variety) are more characteristic of non-alcoholic cirrhosis. These nutritional deficiencies may be ascribed to one or several of the following: inadequate dietary intake, maldigestion, malabsorption and defective metabolism.

Dietary intake Inadequate intake of protein is common, especially among alcoholics with cirrhosis. When the alcoholic patient continues to drink despite cirrhosis, protein intake may be low and the bulk of dietary energy may be derived from carbohydrates and alcohol *per se*. Energy derived from alcohol can be considered 'empty' because alcoholic beverages are devoid of proteins, minerals, vitamins and significant amounts of carbohydrate. Furthermore, the actual energy contribution of alcohol has been shown to be less than that of an equivalent amount of carbohydrates. Changes in mental status resulting from hepatic encephalopathy also contribute to the poor intake of patients with advanced liver disease.

Maldigestion and malabsorption Less bile salt secretion and a diminished pool size have been demonstrated in patients with cirrhosis. In view of the role of bile salts in fat digestion (see above), contraction of the bile salt pool would be expected to impair micelle formation and lead to abnormalities of fat assimilation. In the patient with underlying pancreatic insufficiency, which is common in the alcoholic, poor fat absorption is exacerbated in patients with chronic liver failure. Steatorrhoea, in turn, causes deficiencies in fat-soluble vitamins with clinical manifestations such as night blindness, osteoporosis, and easy bruisability or haemorrhage.

Metabolic changes Defects in protein metabolism have been noted in patients with chronic liver failure. Prominent among these are decreased hepatic synthesis of export proteins (albumin, coagulation factors), decreased urea synthesis, and decreased metabolism of aromatic amino acids. The effect of advanced liver disease on protein catabolism is controversial. Using stable isotopes such as ^{13}C leucine,

turnover studies indicate that protein degradation is normal in fasted cirrhotics, but after feeding, protein flux appears to be increased. These alterations have important clinical consequences. Decreased synthesis of plasma proteins may lead to hypoalbuminaemia and exacerbate the formation of ascites in patients with portal hypertension. Depressed levels of coagulation factors may predispose these patients to the risk of gastrointestinal haemorrhage. Inadequate detoxification of ammonia and the abnormal amino acid profile of patients with cirrhosis may, in part, increase the likelihood of hepatic encephalopathy. Despite these abnormalities in intermediary metabolism, overall nitrogen balance can be maintained at positive levels by similar amounts of dietary protein needed by the noncirrhotic individual (35–50 g per day).

Glucose tolerance is frequently abnormal in the cirrhotic patient and has been linked to insulin resistance. High fasting and postprandial insulin levels in these patients may relate to factors such as portosystemic shunting, increased levels of growth hormone, and depleted body stores of potassium. Glycogen stores are often depleted in the cirrhotic liver, and fatty acid oxidation appears to supplant glucose as a source of fuel during fasting. The shift to fatty acid oxidation is apparent when examined by indirect calorimetry, which yields a respiratory quotient (RQ) in stable cirrhotics significantly less than that of normal controls. Energy expenditure in chronic liver injury is comparable to that in controls, making hypermetabolism *per se* an unlikely explanation for weight loss in these patients. The higher-than-predicted energy production rates reported in cirrhotic patients require that energy expenditure be expressed in relation to urinary creatinine excretion. However, the use of urinary creatinine excretion as a measure of active cell mass is not quite valid in patients with cirrhosis because the hepatic production of creatinine is depressed. Isotopic methods involving labelled water and potassium have instead been recommended for estimating the metabolically active body cell mass in patients with decompensated cirrhosis.

The status of water- and fat-soluble vitamins is commonly abnormal in cirrhotic patients. In cirrhosis not due to alcoholism, deficiencies of fat-soluble vitamins are likely to arise from malabsorption. In part, abnormal bile salt metabolism and defective micelle formation limit the uptake of such vitamins in these patients. In the alcoholic, inadequate intake of vitamins, especially those that are water-soluble (thiamin and folic acid), is an important factor.

In addition to inadequate intake and decreased uptake, vitamin metabolism *per se* may be abnormal in chronic liver injury. Defects in the phosphorylation of thiamin by alcoholic cirrhotics, in the synthesis of retinol-binding protein, in the degradation of pyridoxal-5'-phosphate, and in the conversion of vitamin D to its active form have been reported. Hepatic vitamin A levels are depressed by both heavy alcohol consumption and drug use. Perhaps part of the hepatic vitamin A depletion may be due to increased mobilization from the liver since hepatic lipoprotein secretion is increased by chronic alcohol consumption. Hepatic microsome 'induction' in the alcoholic may enhance the degradation of both retinol and retinoic acid. These derangements probably dictate different vitamin repletion strategies in patients with liver failure, as discussed later in this article.

Nutritional Therapy in Liver Disorders with Emphasis on Alcoholic Type

Protein and amino acids

It has been assumed that liver regeneration will be delayed and that muscle wasting will be accelerated when nitrogen balance is negative. However, care must be taken not to give so much protein that hepatic encephalopathy occurs, since only a small margin of safety may exist. The amount of dietary protein that can be tolerated will vary considerably. At times, only minimal amounts of protein can be ingested without altering the mental state; the breakdown of remaining protein stores can be minimized by the provision of energy in the form of fats and carbohydrates.

In acute liver injury, work has focused on the role of protein or amino acid supplementation (both enteral and parenteral routes have been studied) on the outcome of alcoholic hepatitis. In general, these studies have demonstrated that hepatic encephalopathy can usually be avoided by judicious titration of dietary protein, that relatively little dietary protein is needed to yield positive nitrogen balance, and that symptomatic as well as biochemical improvement (if not prognosis) can be expected.

Positive nitrogen balance can be achieved in patients with chronic liver injury (cirrhosis) with 0.74 g per kg per day of dietary protein, similar to that required by normal individuals. Results have conflicted as to whether the source of the dietary protein (animal or vegetable) affects overall nitrogen balance.

Attempts have been made to restore the plasma amino acid pattern of cirrhotic patients to normal. The ratio of branched-chain amino acids (BCAA: isoleucine, leucine, valine and lysine) to aromatic amino acids (phenylalanine, tryptophan and tyrosine) is abnormally low in these patients, especially those who are malnourished. Administration of BCAA has shown no significant advantage to that of standard mixtures in achieving nitrogen balance.

Initial hope that correction of the abnormal amino acid profile in patients with cirrhosis would be beneficial in the treatment of hepatic encephalopathy has not been realized. Mixtures with high ratios of BCAA to aromatic amino acids have been administered, and the source of protein (vegetable-derived protein is relatively lacking in aromatic amino acids) has been varied. Expectation of benefit seemed plausible in light of the false neurotransmitter hypothesis of Fischer and colleagues, which describes the entry of aromatic amino acids into the brain as favoured by low plasma levels of BCAA. In the brain, sympathomimetic amines are generated from these aromatic amino acids, especially phenylalanine, the presence of which hinders neuronal transmission by competitive interactions with bona fide neurotransmitters at the receptor level. Despite the encouraging initial studies in humans involving infusion of BCAA-enriched mixtures, trials which were not fully controlled or randomized, the majority of later studies, using tighter designs, have failed to confirm the efficacy of intravenous or orally administered BCAA-enriched mixtures in treating acute hepatic encephalopathy. Although a recent meta-analysis detected a trend favouring this therapy, the evidence does not support the routine clinical use of these amino acid mixtures in acute encephalopathy. It remains possible that a subset of protein-intolerant patients with chronic encephalopathy (and better liver function) will be identified who will benefit from BCAA.

A degree of success has been reported in treating hepatic encephalopathy using protein derived from vegetable sources. Since improvement in encephalopathy does not correlate with changes in the plasma amino acid profile, it has been suggested that the beneficial effects of vegetable protein are mediated by its fibre content rather than by its amino acid composition *per se*. While fibre increases the elimination of nitrogenous waste, these diets are poorly tolerated.

Dietary restrictions of amino acids or protein are important in a number of inherited liver abnormalities, which will be discussed later.

Methionine and *S*-adenosyl-L-methionine

In humans, methionine supplementation had been contemplated for the treatment of liver diseases, especially the alcoholic variety, but some difficulties have been encountered. Excess methionine was shown to have some adverse effects, including a decrease in hepatic ATP. Furthermore, whereas in

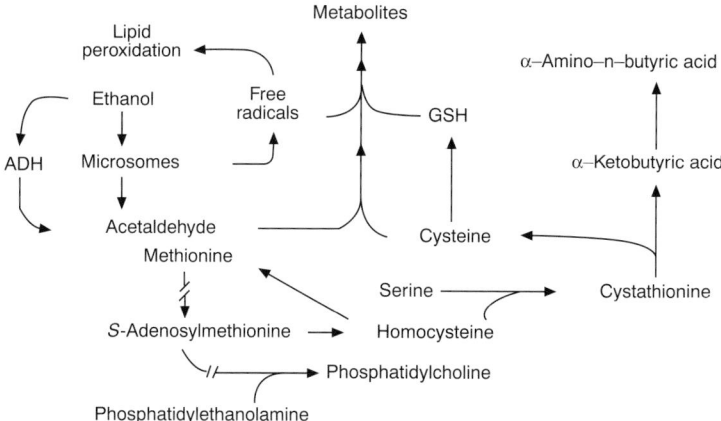

Figure 1 Link between accelerated acetaldehyde production and increased free radical generation by the induced microsomes, resulting in enhanced lipid peroxidation with metabolic blocks due to alcohol, folate deficiency and/or alcoholic liver disease. The possible beneficial effects of GSH, its precursors (including S-adenosylmethionine (SAMe) and phosphatidylcholine are illustrated. ADH, antidiuretic hormone. From Lieber CS (1997), *Digestive Diseases* **15**:42–66.

some patients with alcoholic liver disease circulating methionine levels are normal, the blood clearance of methionine after an oral load of this amino acid was slowed in such subjects. Considering that about half of the methionine is metabolized by the liver, the above observations suggest impaired hepatic metabolism of this amino acid in patients with alcoholic liver disease. Indeed, there are reports of decreases of S-adenosyl-L-methionine (SAMe) synthetase activities in cirrhotic livers. Furthermore, chronic alcohol consumption was found to be associated with enhanced methionine utilization and depletion. As a consequence, one can anticipate SAMe depletion as well as its decreased availability. When the baboon model of alcohol-induced liver injury was used to verify the latter hypothesis and to explore the possibility that SAMe repletion might oppose some of the adverse effects of alcohol on the liver, the study revealed that chronic ethanol consumption is associated with a significant depletion of hepatic SAMe and that SAMe supplementation attenuates ethanol-induced liver injury.

Studies in rats also showed the prevention of fat accumulation in the liver by SAMe. The significant hepatic SAMe depletion after long-term ethanol consumption in primates is partly due to increased GSH utilization secondary to enhanced free radical and acetaldehyde generation by the induced MEOS (**Fig. 1**) as well as to GSH leakage. Under these conditions, increased GSH turnover may ensue, as evidenced by a rise in α-amino-n-butyric acid (**Figs 1 and 2**). However, SAMe synthase activity may become rate-limiting, especially since it is decreased in cirrhosis. As a consequence, methionine supplementation may be

ineffective in alcoholic liver disease and SAMe depletion ensues.

SAMe depletion may potentially have a number of adverse effects. SAMe is the principal methylating agent in various vital transmethylation reactions which are known to be important to nucleic acid and protein synthesis. Methylation is important to cell membrane function, and there is a role for phospholipid methylation in membrane fluidity and the transport of metabolites and transmission of signals across membranes. Thus, decreased SAMe, by being detrimental for methyltransferase activity, may thereby promote the membrane injury which has been documented in alcohol-induced liver damage. SAMe is not only the methyl donor in almost all transmethylation reactions, but it also plays a key role in the synthesis of polyamines and provides one

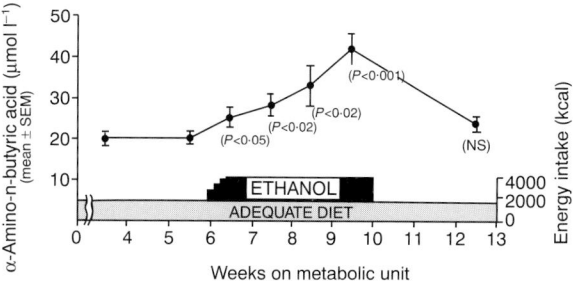

Figure 2 Effect of ethanol consumption on plasma α-amino-n-butyric acid (mean±SEM). Consumption of ethanol (4 g per kg per day) in addition to an adequate diet in three human volunteers resulted in a doubling of plasma α-amino-n-butyric acid after 2–4 weeks which was reversed after cessation of drinking. kcal 14.2 kJ. Data from Shaw S and Lieber CS (1978), *Gastroenterology* **74**:677–682.

of the sources of cysteine needed for glutathione production. Alcohol-induced depletion of glutathione has been prominent in primates.

In rats, chronic alcohol feeding was found to result in decreased methionine formation via the n-5 tetra-hydrofolate pathway, an effect compensated for through an adaptive increase in betaine-homocysteine methyltransferase activity, which maintains hepatic SAMe levels. This adaptive process may be particularly operative in the rodents and much less so in primates. Indeed, rodents contain higher levels of choline oxidase than primates and therefore can produce significantly greater amounts of betaine, which may be one of the reasons why rodents are less susceptible to alcohol-induced liver injury than primates. Therefore, replenishment of methionine, especially in its activated form, SAMe, may be particularly indicated in the primate when subjected to an alcoholic insult.

Administration of SAMe, compared with methionine, has the advantage of bypassing the deficit in SAMe synthesis from methionine already discussed. Indeed, this deficit is due to a decrease in enzyme activity, not in that of substrate, and therefore cannot simply be corrected by excess methionine. Replenishment of the hepatocyte with SAMe is feasible through ingestion of the compound; it has been shown that blood levels of SAMe are increased after oral administration in both rodents and humans. Although it has been claimed that the liver does not take up SAMe from the bloodstream, others have indicated uptake of SAMe by isolated hepatocytes either at pharmacological or physiological extracellular concentrations. The liver SAMe transport system appears to be saturable. Results in baboons also clearly indicate hepatic uptake of exogenous SAMe. Furthermore, in these baboons, the ethanol-induced hepatic SAMe depletion was partially corrected with oral SAMe administration. In addition to uptake of extracellular SAMe, extracellular methionine appears to play a major role in the synthesis of newly acquired intracellular SAMe. Thus, orally administered SAMe may play a precursor role for intracellular SAMe, both as unchanged SAMe and also by the methionine it provides. Since the SAMe transport system does not appear to be saturated under physiological conditions, it is likely that SAMe levels in biological compartments regulate, at least in part, the rate of transport across membranes. Indeed, hepatic levels of SAMe are increased with increasing extracellular levels and the intracellular concentrations reached are above or close to the K_m for SAMe of both phospholipid methyltransferase and catechol-o-methyltransferase. Furthermore, the effective utilization of SAMe both for transmethylation and trans-sulfuration has been demonstrated in vivo.

The therapeutic use of SAMe is a good example of replenishment of a naturally occurring molecule which has been depleted by liver disease, resulting in a beneficial effect. The exact role of SAMe in the treatment of liver disorders has been in part clarified by studies showing that this molecule is beneficial in intrahepatic cholestasis. Treatment with a stable salt of SAMe resulted in both improvement of standard liver function tests and reduction in symptoms such as itch. Consequently, SAMe may become useful for managing pruritus associated with cholestatic liver disease. It has also been successfully used in severe cholestasis of pregnancy, where it has the advantage of few, if any, untoward effects. Recurrent intrahepatic cholestasis and severe jaundice caused by androgens or oestrogens are also conditions in which treatment with SAMe appears to be helpful, perhaps because of changes in membrane phospholipid composition. Experimentally, SAMe prevented total parenteral nutrition-induced cholestasis in the rat. Potentially beneficial clinical effects of SAMe include enhanced bile salt conjugation with taurine in patients with liver cirrhosis. Other observations indicate that administration of exogenous SAMe prevents the glutathione depletion observed in the liver of patients affected by liver disease. Glutathionine and cysteine concentrations have been measured in erythrocytes of alcoholics with (20 subjects) and without (20 subjects) liver cirrhosis. Glutathionine levels were decreased, whereas those of cysteine were increased in all patients. Parenteral treatment with SAMe corrected the erythrocyte thiol alterations. Furthermore, in patients given SAMe, long-term treatment doubles the plasma concentration of the secondary sulfur-containing amino acids cystine and taurine, which were on average low-normal at baseline, without any change in the concentration of methionine, of neutral amino acids or of polyamines. No changes in plasma amino acids were observed in the control group. In experimental animals, SAMe was shown to prevent and reverse erythrocyte membrane alterations in cirrhosis. It also exerted a protective effect against liver damage induced by biliary obstruction in rats, prevented carbon tetrachloride-induced SAMe synthetase inactivation and associated liver injury and improved the histological picture in the liver of rats treated with carbon tetrachloride and ethanol for one month. Betaine administration was reported to have the capacity to elevate hepatic SAMe and to prevent the ethanol-induced fatty liver in rats.

Methionine lack may also result from a deficit in methylation of homocysteine to methionine, mainly by the folate and vitamin B_{12}-dependent enzyme methionine synthase. Since in most alcoholics a disturbed folate metabolism is present (attributable to multiple mechanisms, including an inadequate diet), elevated plasma homocysteine levels in alcoholics could have been anticipated, indeed they have now been noted in a group of alcoholics. Nutrition support was successful in decreasing nutrition-associated complications in patients with alcoholic liver disease. It is now clear, however, that mere nutritional repletion may not suffice, and that 'supernutrients' may be needed, such as SAMe and possibly polyunsaturated phospholipids (see below).

In summary, in chronic liver diseases, a marked reduction in the rate of synthesis and utilization of SAMe has been described as a consequence of a decrease in the activity of the enzyme SAMe-synthetase. Exogenous SAMe may overcome this metabolic block and concomitantly reverse, at least in part, cholestatic and ethanol-related liver injury. The metabolism of exogenous SAMe appears to follow the known pathways of endogenous SAMe metabolism, and the initial data suggest that the process is largely unaffected in patients with chronic liver disease except for a crucial reaction in hepatic phoshatidylcholine synthesis, namely a pathway involving methylation of phosphatidylethanolamine to phosphatidylcholine by SAMe. This reaction may suffer not only from SAMe depletion, but also from decreased activity of the corresponding methyltransferase secondary to severe liver disease (see below). Furthermore, studies in nonhuman primates also clearly indicate hepatic uptake of ingested SAMe. Moreover, it has been shown that blood levels of SAMe are increased after oral administration in rodents and humans.

Carbohydrates

Cirrhotic patients are prone to develop diabetes. As already noted, insulin resistance appears to account for this abnormality of glucose homeostasis. In patients with portal hypertension complicated by portosystemic shunting, an alteration in the metabolism of insulin may contribute to this resistance. Depleted body stores of potassium and elevated levels of growth hormone are probably additional significant factors. As in other patients with diabetes, nutritional management plays an important role in therapy. Specifically, provision of energy in the form of complex carbohydrates is effective in reducing insulin requirements. Increasing the intake of complex carbohydrate may also be advantageous in terms of hepatic encephalopathy because the nonabsorbable fibre found in such foods decreases colonic transit time and lowers colonic pH. Indeed, the effi-

cacy of lactulose, one of the mainstays in the treatment of hepatic encephalopathy, has been related to these same effects. Inherited disorders of carbohydrate metabolism will be discussed below.

Lipids

Fat accumulation in the liver is strikingly affected by the amount and type of dietary triglycerides. With alcohol, the smaller the quantity of dietary triacylglycerols that is present in the diet, the less fat accumulates in the liver (**Fig. 3**), at least down to a level of 10% of total energy. Below that, fat accumulates even when dietary fat is extremely low, probably because of stimulation of lipogenesis.

Dietary phospholipids also have striking effects on liver structure and function. In primates, chronic ethanol consumption results in a decrease of liver phospholipids and of phosphatidylcholine (PC); both can be corrected by PC supplementation. The total phospholipid content of the mitochondrial membranes is decreased, with a significant reduction in the levels of PC and associated striking morphological changes with a corresponding functional counterpart, namely diminished mitochondrial oxidation mainly because of decreased cytochrome oxidase activity. The latter appears to result from alterations in the phospholipid composition of the mitochondrial membranes. Indeed, *in vitro* cytochrome oxidase activity could be restored with phospholipids extracted from normal mitochondria or synthetic ones, PC being the most active.

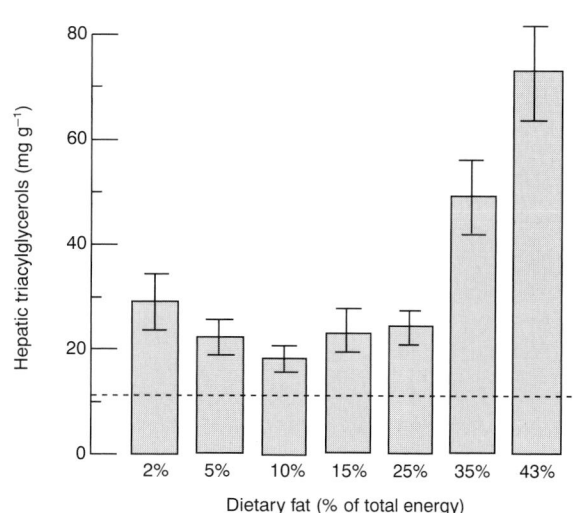

Figure 3 Effect of varying amounts of dietary fat. Hepatic triacylglycerols in seven groups of rats given ethanol (36% of energy) with a diet of normal protein (18% of energy). Average hepatic triacylglycerol concentration in the control animals is indicated by a dotted line. From Lieber CS and DeCarli LM (1970), *American Journal of Clinical Nutrition* **23**:474–478.

The mechanism whereby chronic ethanol consumption alters phospholipids has not been clarified but may be related, at least in part, to decreased phospholipid methyltransferase activity described in cirrhotic livers (Fig. 1). That this is not simply secondary to cirrhosis, but may in fact be a primary defect related to alcohol, is suggested by the observation that the enzyme activity is already decreased prior to the development of cirrhosis. Another mechanism whereby ethanol may affect phospholipids is via formation of phosphatidylethanol, with possible impact on signal transduction, as shown in isolated rat hepatocytes. A third mechanism is increased lipid peroxidation, as reflected by increased F_2 isoprostanes, which could explain the associated decrease of arachidonic acid in phospholipids.

In alcoholic patients, reduction in phospholipid methyltransferase activity together with the decreased activity of SAMe synthetase (see above) may promote the membrane injury which has been documented experimentally in alcohol-induced liver damage. The question then arises as to whether such deficiency can be attenuated, at least in part, by bypassing the enzyme defects through phospholipid supplementation. This was tested by feeding baboons alcohol in a diet supplemented with polyunsaturated lecithin. Administration of phospholipid preparations rich in polyunsaturated phosphatidylcholine (PPC) or virtually pure PPC (**Fig. 4**) was found, in the nonhuman primate, to prevent fully alcohol-induced fibrosis and cirrhosis. Although PPC contains choline, it was found that choline, in the amounts present in PPC, has no protective action against the fibrogenic effects of ethanol in the baboon. PPC is rich in linoleic acid, but this fatty acid *per se* is probably not responsible for the protective effect because the basic diet was supplemented with linoleate and contained large amounts of corn oil, which is rich in linoleic acid. Furthermore, this fatty acid has been incriminated as a permissive rather than as a protective factor in alcoholic liver injury. Thus, the polyunsaturated phospholipids themselves appear to be responsible for protection, perhaps because of their high bioavailability and selective incorporation into liver membranes. Furthermore, PPC directly affects collagen metabolism.

The protection afforded by PC against fibrosis (Fig. 4) was associated with a lesser transformation of stellate cells to transitional cells *in vivo* (48% versus 81%). Thus, to the extent that the transformation of stellate cells in alcohol-fed animals was responsible for the fibrosis, the lesser transformation after PC may be one of the reasons for the decreased fibrosis.

Fibrosis and the associated collagen accumulation does not result simply from enhanced collagen

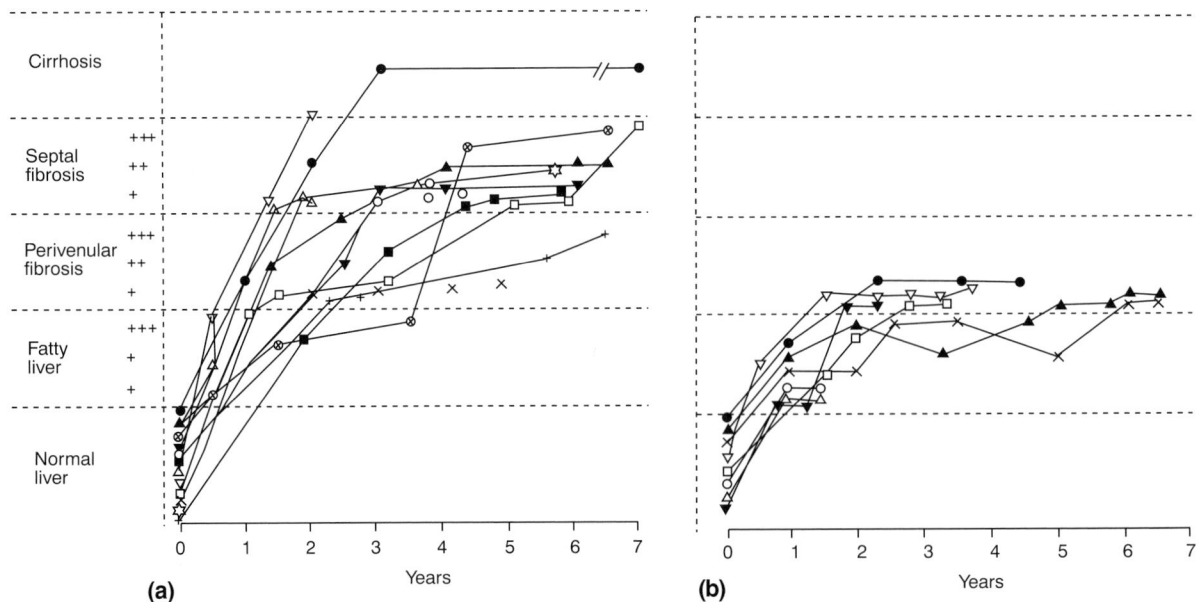

Figure 4 Sequential development of alcoholic liver injury in baboons fed ethanol with an adequate diet (a) and prevention of septal fibrosis and cirrhosis by supplementation with polyunsaturated phosphatidylcholine (PPC) (b). Liver morphology in animals pair-fed control diets (with or without PPC) remained normal (not shown). Data from Lieber CS, Robins SJ, Li J, DeCarli LM, Mak KM, Fasulo JM and Leo MA (1994) Phosphatidylcholine protects against fibrosis and cirrhosis in the baboon. *Gastroenterology* **106**:152–159.

production, but rather from an imbalance between collagen production and breakdown. Breakdown was assessed in cultured rat stellate cells by measuring collagenase activity with different phospholipids, including various species of PC. It was reported before that a mixture of PCs affected the breakdown, but not the synthesis of collagen under those conditions. The PC preparation used contained about 50% 18:2–18:2 PC (DLPC), 25% 16:0–18:2 PC (PLPC) and other minor PC species. We found that pure DLPC stimulates collagenase activity *in vitro*. Increased collagenase activity can be expected to oppose collagen accumulation and the development of fibrosis by promoting the breakdown of collagen. The increase in collagenase activity was observed in both the absence and presence of acetaldehyde, the metabolite of ethanol that has been incriminated in many of its effects. The specificity of the DLPC effect was illustrated by the fact that the other main component of the administered PC, namely PLPC, or other unsaturated or saturated PCs such as dioleoyl-PC, diarachidonoyl-PC, distearoyl-PC, dilauroyl-PC, or another polyunsaturated phospholipid (dilinoleoylphosphatidylethanolamine), or polyunsaturated free fatty acids (linoleic, arachidonic), had no effect on collagenase activity. A similar lack of effect had also been found before with dilauroyl-PC. Choline was inactive *in vitro*, as it had also been found to be ineffective *in vivo*. Taken together, these findings suggest that DLPC is the active agent responsible, at least in part, for the protection afforded by PPC against the development of fibrosis and its ultimate stage of cirrhosis, most likely because of stimulation of collagen breakdown. Collagenase activity is generally increased during the early stage of liver injury. Our previous studies revealed that fibrosis coincides with the stage at which collagen breakdown slackens and stops keeping pace with increased production. Therefore these findings suggest that studies on collagenase activity associated with hepatic injury may be relevant to the elucidation of the pathogenesis of liver fibrosis and its treatment and prevention.

PPC could, of course, also act in some other ways. Phospholipids rich in essential fatty acids have a high bioavailability. More than 50% of orally administered PC is made biologically available for the organism, either by intact absorption (lesser extent) or by reacylation of absorbed lysophosphatidylcholine (greater extent). Pharmacokinetic studies in humans using ^{3}H/^{14}C-labelled phosphatidylcholine showed the absorption to exceed 90%. Similar observations have been made in animals. Indeed, although much of the PC in the diet is degraded by pancreatic phospholipase A_2, the products (l-acyl-lysophosphatidylcholine and fatty acids) are absorbed in the jejunum.

Animal studies show that PCs recovered in intestinal lymph after feeding fat enriched with single fatty acids are highly enriched in both *sn*-1 and *sn*-2 positions with the same acyl groups that were fed. Thus, it can be anticipated that during absorption of a diet enriched with 18:2 fatty acids, new PCs will be formed from dietary 18:2-lysoPC that will have an 18:2–18:2 composition. Various authors have reported PC accumulation in the liver during the first 24 to 48 h after administration. Furthermore, all 18:2 PCs were present in the liver in significantly increased amounts in baboons fed 18:2–18:2PC.

PC has been used before empirically in nonalcoholic liver diseases: beneficial histological effects have been reported in the recovery from kwashiorkor, in HBsAG-positive patients with cirrhosis, and in patients with chronic active hepatitis, in terms of inflammatory parameters. PC was also used for the treatment of alcoholic hepatitis and alcoholic fatty liver, but not as yet for the prevention or treatment of hepatic fibrosis or cirrhosis. As well as exhibiting a lack of toxicity, demonstrated when it was used for these other indications, PC has also been shown to be effective in the prevention of alcoholic fibrosis and cirrhosis in the baboon; this was demonstrated more recently with a virtually pure PC preparation and previously with a less pure extract. Therefore PC or, if possible DLPC, both of which are natural compounds, should now be tried for the control of alcoholic fibrosis and cirrhosis in humans. For the same reasons it may also be useful for the management of fibrosis of nonalcoholic aetiologies. Indeed, fibrosis is a common end stage for most chronic liver diseases. Experimentally, PC attenuated both the carbon tetrachloride and the heterologous albumin produced fibrosis in the rat. Since DLPC promotes the breakdown of collagen, there is a reasonable hope that this treatment may affect not only the progression of the disease, but may also reverse preexisting fibrosis, as demonstrated for carbon tetrachloride-induced cirrhosis in the rat.

Vitamins

Fat-soluble vitamins

Vitamin A It is recommended that the diet of the nonalcoholic with cirrhosis be supplemented with 5000 to 15 000 IU vitamin A. In patients with alcoholic cirrhosis, caution must be exercised in this respect because microsomal induction may increase the toxicity of this vitamin and ethanol can potentiate liver damage caused by excessive vitamin A. Betacarotene, the precursor of vitamin A, is also depressed in patients with severe liver disease such as cirrhosis (**Fig. 5**). It is less toxic than vitamin A, but studies in primates have shown that its toxic

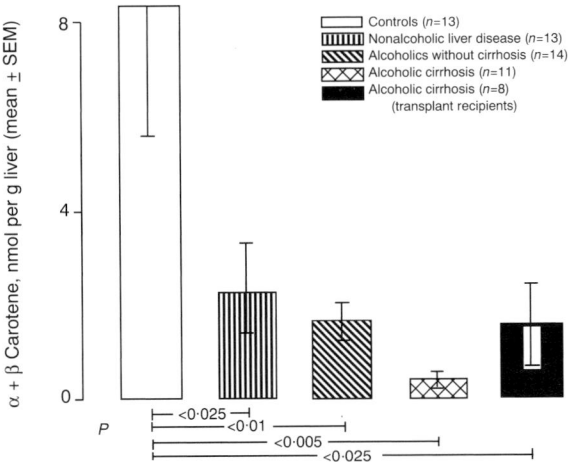

Figure 5 Effects of various liver diseases on hepatic α- and β-carotene. Compared with control livers (transplant donors), those of patients with alcoholic or nonalcoholic liver diseases (with or without cirrhosis, including transplant recipients) had significantly lower α- and β-carotene. From Leo MA, Rosman A and Lieber CS (1993) Differential depletion of carotenoids and tocopherol in liver disease. *Hepatology* **17**:977–986.

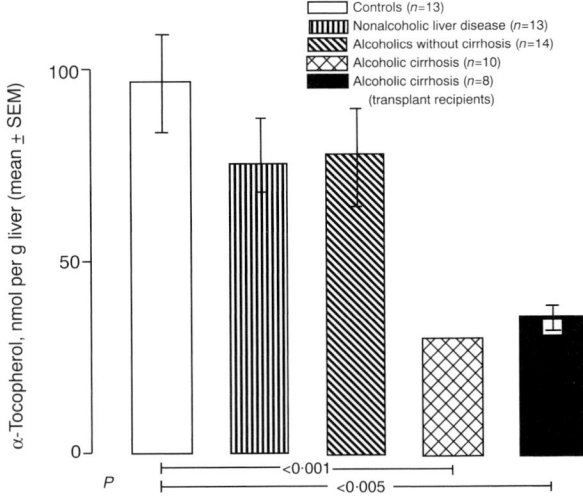

Figure 6 Effects of various liver diseases on total hepatic tocopherol levels. Compared with α- and β-carotene and lycopene, only the two cirrhotic groups had significantly lower α-tocopherol levels. From Leo MA, Rosman A and Lieber CS (1993) Differential depletion of carotenoids and tocopherol in liver disease. *Hepatology* **17**:977–986.

effects are also enhanced by alcohol. Furthermore, β-carotene increases the risk of pulmonary cancer in smokers, an effect related to an interaction between β-carotene and alcohol. Thus, vitamin A or β-carotene supplementation must be used cautiously in alcoholics.

Vitamin D Supplementation of the diet with this vitamin may fail to halt the progression of osteoporosis and osteopenia. However, there appears to be no hazard in recommending ingestion of additional 25-OH D_3 (100–300 nmol (or 40–120 μg per day)) when patients complain of bone pain or demonstrate pathological fractures.

Vitamin E In children with biliary atresia and cholestasis, vitamin E deficiency may be associated with a number of neurological alterations. Although such infants and children may benefit from supplementation, repletion of vitamin E stores in adults with liver injury is of no proven clinical efficacy. In patients with liver disease of various aetiologies, hepatic vitamin E concentrations were normal except in the presence of cirrhosis, both alcoholic and nonalcoholic (**Fig. 6**).

Vitamin K Deficiency of this vitamin leads to easy bruisability and, at times, to overt bleeding from oesophageal varices or haemorrhoids. When the prothrombin time is lengthened, parenteral supplementation of vitamin K (10 mg per day for 3 days) will serve to discriminate between vitamin K deficiency

and failure of the liver to synthesize normal coagulation factors.

Water-soluble vitamins and trace minerals Deficiencies of water-soluble vitamins (folic acid, thiamin and pyridoxine) are most likely to occur in the malnourished alcoholic with advanced liver injury.

Effect of Nutrition on the Liver

In children, protein deficiency (kwashiorkor) is associated with the development of fatty liver. Studies performed during and after World War II indicated that severe malnutrition could also lead to liver injury in adults. These studies did not convincingly prove that malnutrition *per se* caused liver injury. Indeed, a number of other factors including hepatotoxins (e.g. aflatoxin) and parasites (schistosomiasis) prevalent in war-ravaged or underdeveloped countries may have mediated the relationship between poor nutrition and liver injury.

As malnutrition is also common in alcoholics, these early findings were used to foster the argument that malnutrition, rather than alcohol *per se*, explained the pathogenesis of alcohol-induced liver injury. Since the 1970s, however, a more balanced view has evolved. Based on studies in humans, subhuman primates and rodents, it is now established that alcohol can cause liver damage in the absence of dietary deficits. Epidemiological data also support this revised concept. In both France and Germany, a close correlation exists between per capita alcohol consumption and the likelihood of cirrhosis. Moreover, no relationship has been documented between nutritional status and the severity of alcohol-induced liver injury as defined histologically. The above notwithstanding, it is now becoming clear that nutrition and the toxic effects of alcohol are often intertwined at the biochemical level. For example, by inducing microsomal cytochromes, chronic ethanol consumption is known to result in energy wastage, and to promote the breakdown of nutrients including retinol.

Inherited Liver Diseases

Inborn errors of amino acid metabolism

Abnormalities of urea cycle enzymes

Definition Abnormalities of urea cycle function arise from inherited deficiencies of single urea cycle enzyme activity with variable phenotypic expression and are characterized by episodes of hyperammonaemia and hyperglutaminaemia, mental retardation and growth failure. For a full discussion of these entities the reader is referred to the masterful review of Brusilow and Horwich.

Aetiology and prevalence Ornithine transcarbamylase deficiency (OCT) is inherited as an X-linked disorder. The other enzyme deficiencies of the urea cycle are inherited as autosomal recessive traits: carbamylphosphate synthetase deficiency (CPSD), arginosuccinic acid synthetase deficiency (ASD), arginosuccinase deficiency (ALD) and arginase deficiency (**Fig. 7**). Screening programmes in Massachusetts and Quebec have detected an incidence of ALD of 1 in 70 000 and 1.3 in 100 000 new births, respectively. These values are comparable, but in each case represent an underestimate as early deaths in affected cases tend to go unrecorded.

Pathophysiology of disease Impedance of proper functioning of the urea cycle results in failure to synthesize urea from excess nitrogen, accumulation of ammonium and glutamine, and failure to synthesize sufficient arginine (except in the case of arginase deficiency), thereby making it an essential amino acid (Fig. 7). In arginase deficiency symptomatic hyperammonaemia is uncommon and mild.

Hyperammonaemia and hyperglutaminaemia lead to brain swelling, probably mediated in large measure by astrocyte swelling, and neurological deficit. Neuropathological damage is similar in CPS, OTC, AS and AL deficiencies. Patients with adult onset hypercitrullinaemia and fatty liver related to impaired ketogenesis have been described. Although portal fibrosis has been described in OTC deficiency, liver damage is not prominent in any of these disorders and synthetic function is normal.

Clinical features and natural history The urea cycle abnormalities present as episodes of hyperammonaemia and encephalopathy, typically beginning 24 to 72 h after a normal full-term birth. Initial symptoms include vomiting, lethargy, hypothermia and hyperventilation. The episodes tend to recur with consequent mental impairment and shortened life span, especially if inadequately treated. Arginase deficiency is associated with less frequent and prominent episodes of hyperammonaemia, but is characterized by progressive spastic quadriplegia and mental retardation.

Diagnosis, that is attributing acute encephalopathy to these disorders, requires recognition of the hyperammonaemic and hyperglutaminaemic component when confronted with neonatal encephalopathy. Elevated levels of plasma citrulline are found in AS deficiency and elevated arginosuccinate in AL deficiency. CPS and OTC deficiencies lead to increased urinary orotate, since accumulated mitochondrial carbamylphosphate promotes increased pyrimidine synthesis. Prenatal diagnosis can be established by amniotic fluid sampling for abnormal metabolites. DNA analysis of samples from chorionic villi or amniocytes has also been employed, as has enzyme analysis from liver biopsy *in utero*.

Nutritional therapy Nutritional treatment has three goals: provision of dietary arginine to thwart expected arginine deficiency; limitation of dietary protein to that needed for growth in order to minimize the amount of nitrogen which the impaired urea cycle will have to contend with for conversion to urea; and provision of alternate mechanisms for nitrogen excretion (**Table 1**). Limitation of dietary protein is accomplished by providing an amino acid mixture enriched with essential amino acids. The amount of dietary protein and amino acids, as grams per kg per day, lessens as the infant gets older (through childhood and adulthood), as less is needed to sustain growth. It is the excess nitrogen, beyond that needed for tissue synthesis, that becomes a burden for the ureagenic pathway. Provision of sufficient total energy is important to prevent net tissue breakdown.

Phenylbutyrate has proven useful as a medication which promotes an alternative avenue of nitrogen excretion with resultant lessening of hyperammonaemic episodes and very likely prolongation of survival. Phenylbutyrate, which is metabolized to phenylacetate and thereby traps glutamine as phenyl-

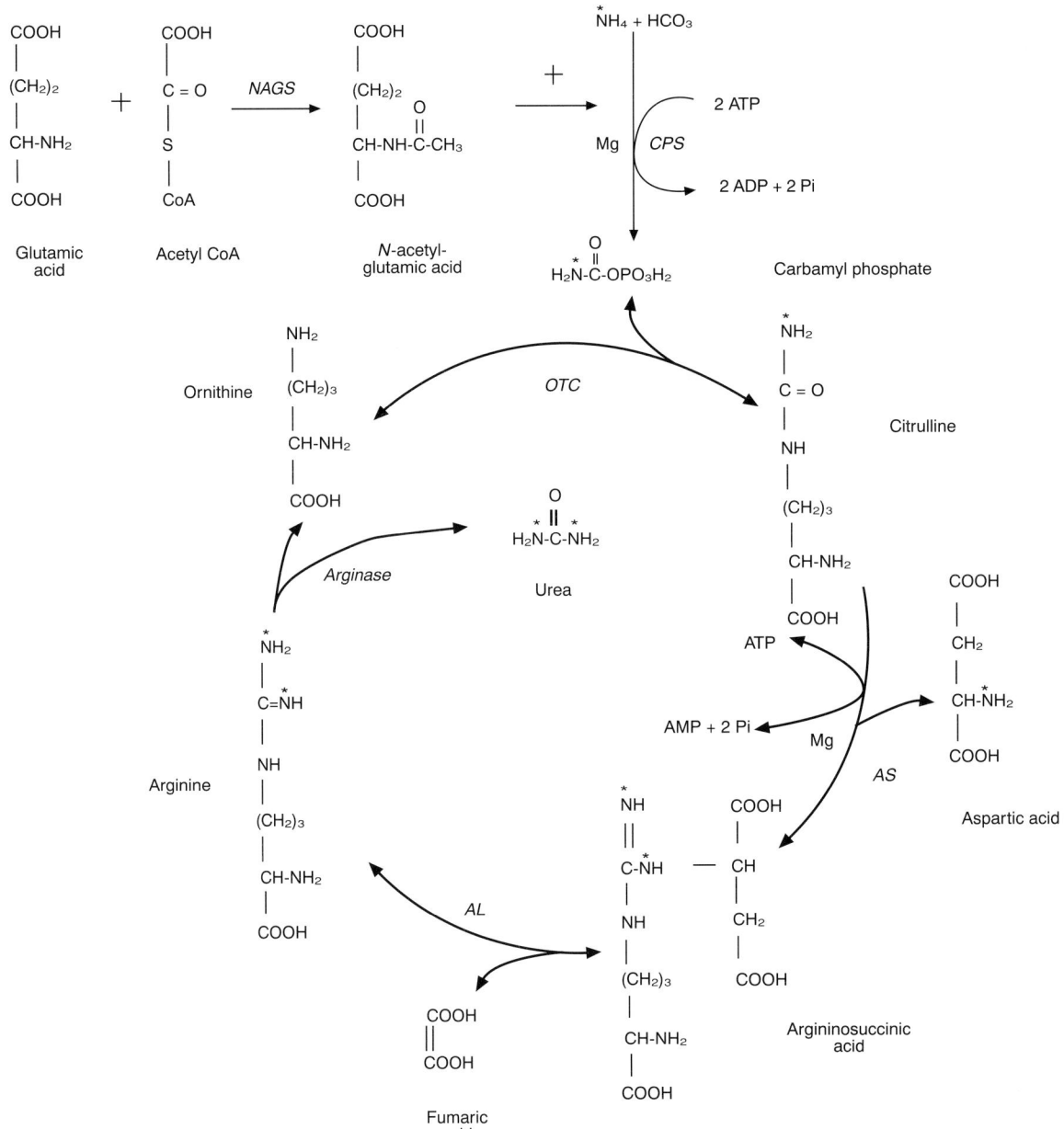

Figure 7 Substrates, products and cofactors required for ureagenesis. The asterisks denote waste nitrogen atoms. AS, argininosuccinic acid synthetase; AL, argininosuccinase; CPS, carbamyl phosphate synthetase; NAGS, *N*-acetylglutamate synthetase; OTC, ornithine transcarbamylase. From Brusilow SW and Horwich AL (1995) In: Scriver C (eds) *The Metabolic and Molecular Basis of Inherited Disease*, 7th edn, chap. 32. New York: McGraw Hill.

acetylglutamine for excretion in the urine, has proven more efficacious than sodium benzoate, which traps nitrogen from glycine as hippurate for urinary excretion. The metabolic pathway is illustrated in **Fig. 8.**

Hyperphenylalaninaemias

Clinical description Hyperphenylalaninaemias are a group of disorders of phenylalanine hydroxylation whereby phenylalanine is not adequately converted to tyrosine and phenylalanine blood levels are elevated to damaging levels. The components of the hydroxylase reaction include L-phenylalanine, oxygen, phenylalanine hydroxylase (PAH), tetrahydrobiopterin (BH_4), and the regenerating system for BH_4, dihydropteridine reductase (DHPR) and reduced pyridine nucleotide. Autosomal recessive inheritance of abnormalities in PAH, BH_4, or the regeneration of BH_4 because of deficiency of DHPR, have been associated with hyperphenylalaninaemia.

Table 1 Recommended management of patients with neonatal onset of urea cycle disorders[a]

Diet	g per kg per day	g per m² per day
Carbamyl phosphate synthetase or ornithine transcarbamylase deficiency		
Diet		
Essential amino acids	0.7[b]	
Protein	0.7[b]	
(Patients with late onset disease including females heterozygous for OTC initially receive a diet containing age-determined minimal daily natural protein requirement which may be increased as tolerated. Essential amino acids are rarely necessary.) Energy supplementation with protein-free powder.		
Medication		
Sodium phenylbutyrate[c]	0.45–0.60	9.9–13.0
Citrulline[d]	0.17	3.8
Argininosuccinic acid synthetase deficiency		
Diet		
Protein	1.25–2.00	
Energy supplementation with Mead Johnson® protein-free diet powder (4.9 kcal per gram)		
Medication		
Sodium phenylbutyrate[c]	0.45–0.60	9.9–13.0
Arginine (free base)	0.40–0.70	8.8–15.4
Argininosuccinase deficiency		
Diet		
Protein	1.25–2.00	
Energy supplementation with Mead Johnson® protein-free diet powder (4.9 calories per gram)		
Medication		
Arginine (free base)	0.40–0.7	8.8–15.4

[a]The goal of therapy is to promote growth and development. To achieve these ends fasting levels of ammonium, branched-chain amino acids, arginine and serum plasma protein should be maintained within normal limits and plasma glutamine at levels less than 1000 μmol l^{-1}. The dose of 0.7 g each of essential amino acids and protein represents an average intake for the average patient with neonatal onset CPS deficiency or OTC deficiency. The degree to which nitrogen intake is partitioned into natural protein and essential amino acids is a function of age, residual enzyme activity and dose of sodium phenylbutyrate. It has become apparent that infants with neonatally expressed disorders may tolerate as much as 2 g per kg per day of natural protein in the first few months of life (plasma ammonium and amino acid levels should be carefully monitored during this period); protein tolerance will decrease as the infant's growth rate decreases and therefore require reduction of nitrogen intake. After 6 months of age the final nitrogen intake for these neonatally expressed disorders is derived from 0.7 g kg^{-1} of natural protein and 0.7 g kg^{-1} of essential amino acids as noted in the table. Some patients may require a lower intake of essential amino acids and protein.
[b]Mixtures containing 80% essential amino acids are available commercially.
[c]The precise dose of sodium phenylbutyrate will depend on clinical circumstances. The highest dose is recommended for all patients, although the lower dose may suffice for patients with significant residual enzyme activity. Because phenylbutyrate on a molar basis is twice as effective as benzoate, the use of oral benzoate is no longer included in this FDA-approved protocol.
[d]In some patients with late onset form of CPS and OTC deficiency arginine (free base) may be substituted for citrulline (whose cost is three to four times that of arginine).

Disease occurs in 100 cases per 1 000 000 live births. When the disorder arises because of problems with BH_4 metabolism, there are concomitant problems, especially significant in the brain, with hydroxylation of L-tryptophan and L-tyrosine to 5-hydroxytryptophan and L-dopa, respectively, which are precursors of serotonin and catecholamines. High phenylalanine levels are probably the major cause of toxicity and result in low cognitive function.

Nutritional management Plasma phenylalanine is kept below toxic levels, normal being 58 ± 15 μmol l^{-1}, by restricting phenylalanine intake to 200 to 500 mg per day in infants and a little more in older children, which corresponds to their requirements. This requires a diet in which phenylalanine content is approximately 25% of the normal diet. Several semisynthetic diets are commercially available. When dietary management has been utilized, loss of IQ has been minimized. Patients should probably restrict ingestion of phenylalanine forever, until the safety of returning to a normal diet is adequately demonstrated. The artificial sweetener *Aspartame*, N-aspartyl-phenylalanine methyl ester, may provide 250–300 mg l^{-1} of beverage, or half the desired daily intake, and should thus be avoided.

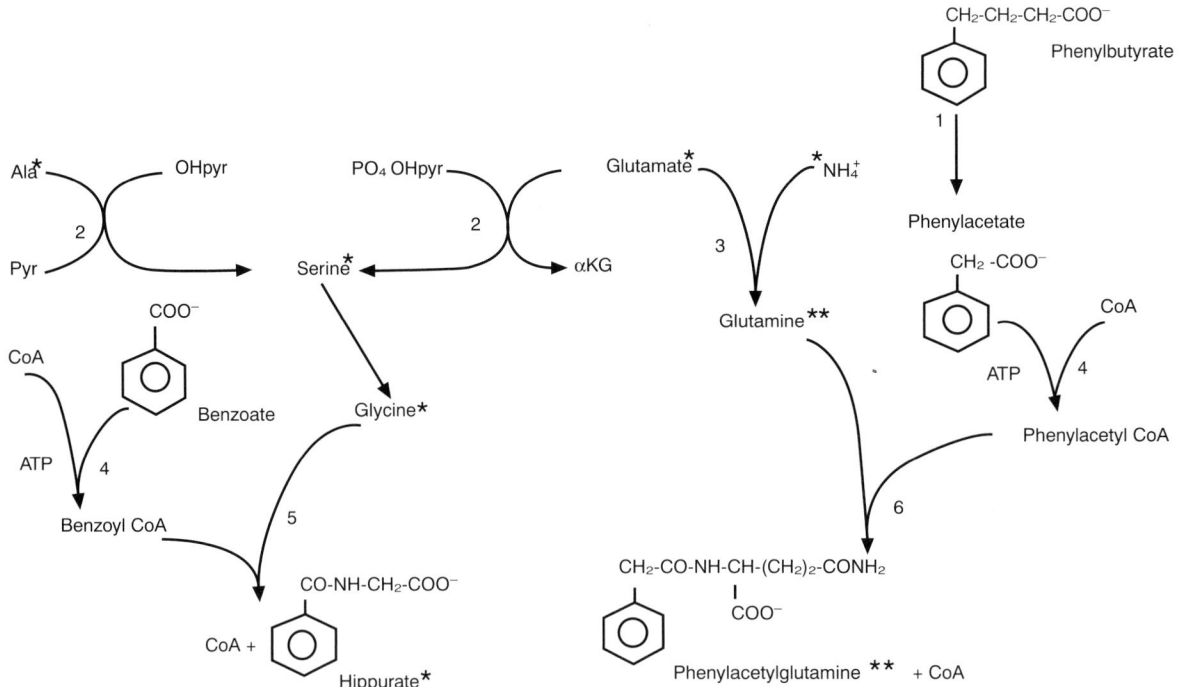

Figure 8 Pathways of waste nitrogen synthesis in patients with CPS, OTC and AS deficiencies. Asterisks denote nitrogen atoms destined for waste nitrogen excretion in hippurate and phenylacetylglutamine. The enzymatic reactions are numbered: 1, β oxidation; 2, transamination; 3, glutamine synthetase; 4, medium-chain fatty acyl CoA ligase; 5, benzyl CoA:glycine acyltransferase; 6, phenylacetyl CoA:glutamine acetyltransferase; αKG, α-ketoglutarate; Ala, alanine; OHpyr, hydroxypyruvate; PO₄OHpyr, pyrophosphohydroxypyruvate; Pyr, pyruvate. From Brusilow SW and Horwich AL (1995) In: Scriver C (eds) *The Metabolic and Molecular Basis of Inherited Disease*, 7th edn, chap. 32. New York: McGraw Hill.

Other inherited enzyme abnormalities

Limitations of space will not permit other than a listing of the disorders and a brief indication of the nutritional treatment (**Table 2**).

Hepatolenticular degeneration: Wilson's disease

Definition, aetiology and prevalence Wilson's disease is an autosomally recessive inherited illness characterized by both greatly impaired ability of the liver to excrete copper, leading to copper overload and organ damage, and by poor incorporation of copper into caeruloplasmin. Poor incorporation of copper into caeruloplasmin provides an elegant, if not generally available, diagnostic test, but the pathogenetic significance of the impairment is not clear. The abnormal gene of Wilson's disease is located on chromosome 13, whereas the gene for caeruloplasmin is on chromosome 3. The carrier frequency of the Wilson's gene has been estimated to be 1 in 90 with disease prevalence varying greatly, from 54 to 144 per million in northern Europe. Prevalence differences worldwide are influenced, in part, by the extent of intermarriage.

Clinical features Patients may present with liver disease, usually chronic and progressive in nature, with fatigue and eventually jaundice and signs of cirrhosis including spider naevi, portal hypertension, ascites, peripheral oedema and oesophageal varices, but also occasionally as acute hepatic failure. Copper-mediated damage to the basal ganglia of the nervous system causes symptoms such as tremors, rigidity, slurring of speech and clumsiness of gait. Characteristic deposits of copper in Descemet's membrane of the cornea appear initially as brown crescents at the periphery, superiorly and inferiorly, near the border with the iris, and eventually take the form of the Kayser–Fleischer ring. Another, somewhat less common manifestation of Wilson's disease, haemolytic anaemia, is probably related to sudden elevation of non-caeruloplasmin-bound copper. Proximal renal tubular damage with aminoaciduria, glycosuria, phosphaturia and renal tubular acidosis is also ascribed to copper overload. Osteomalacia and osteoporosis are associated with Wilson's disease, as is hypoparathyroidism. Typically, Wilson's disease appears in childhood as hepatic illness; after the teenage years neuropsychiatric symptoms are

Table 2 Nutritional therapy of other inherited metabolic disorders

Disorder	Nutritional management
Hypertyrosinaemia	Low phenylalanine and tyrosine diet, ascorbate for some types
Disorders of branched-chain amino acid metabolism, maple sugar urine disease	Low leucine, isoleucine and valine diets, trial of thiamin
Disorders of transsulfuration of amino acids	Low methionine, increased cystine diet, trial of pyridoxine
Branched-chain organic acidurias	Low intake of specific amino acids, e.g leucine, perhaps supplementation with glycine and/or carnitine
Hereditary fructose intolerance (diminished fructose-1-phosphate breakdown)	Diet free of fructose (and sucrose)
'Galactosaemia' (galactokinase or galactose-1-phosphate uridyl transferase, deficiency)	Diet with little or no galactose
Von Gierke's or type I glycogen storage disease (glucose-6-phosphatase deficiency)	Frequent feeding with a high-glucose formula, use of concentrated suspension of uncooked starch
Carnitine deficiency	Avoidance of chronic fasting, oral l-carnitine supplementation

more likely. Of course both may be present. Rarely, Wilson's disease may not be suspected until middle age.

Diagnosis The diagnosis is ideally made in the asymptomatic patient, attention drawn perhaps by family history or abnormal liver function tests obtained inadvertently, since early treatment improves prognosis. The diagnosis must be suspected in any child or young adult with liver dysfunction or liver failure of unexplained cause, in any patient with unexplained haemolytic anaemia, and in any patient with compatible neuropsychiatric symptoms. Low serum caeruloplasm (200–400 mg l^{-1} is normal for adults), low serum copper, 3–10 μmol l^{-1} compared with the normal range of 11 to 24 μmol l^{-1}, and increased urinary copper excretion, 100–1000 μg per 24 h compared with the normal excretion of 40μg per 24 h, are very helpful. Other chronic cholestatic syndromes are also characterized by elevations of hepatic copper, and even by Kayser–Fleischer rings. In addition, it is most desirable to diagnose Wilson's disease before copper retention and damage occur. Decreased incorporation of radioactive copper into

caeruloplasmin serves this purpose well, especially when urinary copper excretion is borderline.

Dietary and pharmaceutical treatment The mainstay of treatment is reduction of body copper by penicillamine treatment. Penicillamine is a chelating agent which binds copper and promotes renal excretion in the range 1000–3000 μg of the metal per day. As D-penicillamine is an antimetabolite of pyridoxine, a daily supplement of 12.5–25 mg of pyridoxine should be provided. For patients who are intolerant to penicillamine it has been shown that oral zinc acetate can promote the faecal loss of copper. The proposed mechanism is the induction of small bowel mucosal cell metallothionein by oral zinc. Metallothionein has a higher affinity for copper than for zinc, and so accomplishes faecal loss as mucosal cells slough. The source of copper is probably salivary and gastric secretions into the gut, estimated at 1.5 mg per day, since biliary copper secretion is much diminished and is usually poorly absorbed.

Dietary management involves the avoidance of food with high copper content. The estimated safe and adequate daily dietary intake, ESADDI, of copper is 0.4 to 0.7 mg for infants under a year, 0.7 increasing to 2 mg for ages 1 to 10 years, and 1.5 to 3 mg for adults. Examples of foods high in copper are: fried beef liver, 2.8 mg per 100 g portion; dry roasted cashews, 0.8 mg per 1/4 cup; black-eyed peas, dried and cooked, 0.7 mg per 1/2 cup; chocolate chips, semisweet, 0.5 mg per 1/4 cup; V-8 juice, 0.5 mg per cup. Shellfish and mushrooms are generally to be avoided also.

Primary haemochromatosis and other iron overload states

Definition and aetiology Disorders of iron overload are characterized by retention of excessive amounts of iron in the body, which may be associated with organ damage such as cirrhosis (haemochromatosis), cardiomyopathy, endocrinopathy (diabetes, anterior pituitary failure, prominent secondary male gonadal failure), and other abnormalities such as arthropathy and grey discoloration of the skin.

Several disorders exist. Primary haemochromatosis is inherited as an autosomal recessive. Homozygosity of a gene very close to the HLA locus on the short arm of chromosome 6 interferes with the intestine's normal function to limit iron absorption. Chronic anaemias, especially those characterized by ineffective erythropoiesis, such as thalassaemia major, but also others such as refractory sideroblastic anaemia, also lead to iron overload by a combination of retained iron from blood transfusions and inappropriately high intestinal iron absorption. Iron overload may also arise from hypertransfusion of blood without a component of inappropriate intestinal absorption of iron. Finally, apparently normal people may occasionally absorb and retain excessive amounts of iron when exposed to chronic, prolonged intake of medicines or other sources of very high iron content.

Prevalence The gene for HLA-linked excessive iron absorption is present in about 10% of the White population, and the homozygous state exists in 3 per 1000. The phenotypic expression depends on homozygosity, the availability of dietary iron and daily iron loss. Heterozygotes do not accumulate harmful amounts of iron. Menstrual blood loss delays iron overload in women and explains the 10-fold greater prevalence in men. Phenotypic expression is quite high in the USA and Australia, for example, where dietary iron is substantial from haem-containing foods like meat from which the metal is absorbed much more efficiently than from vegetables.

Clinical features and prognosis The full-blown clinical syndrome can comprise fatigue and other symptoms of liver involvement, bronze diabetes, cardiac arrhythmia and/or failure, diminished sexual function, loss of body hair, acute crystal synovitis and chondrocalcinosis radiologically. Clinical symptoms of iron overload may appear earlier, but it is most likely to occur after 40 years of age in men and later in women. Death from progressive organ damage, hepatic or cardiac, will ensue if iron is allowed to continue to accumulate, but normal life expectancy can be approximated when accumulation is prevented or reversed. After cirrhosis occurs the high incidence of hepatoma is not avoided despite iron removal.

Diagnosis of homozygosity in a subject of a known kindred is strongly supported upon HLA typing, since the gene associated with hyperabsorption of iron will be passed along with the HLA gene of the affected propositus. HLA typing of suspected sporadic cases yields little useful diagnostic information. The diagnosis of sporadic cases suspected from their compatible clinical features is made by clinical testing: elevated serum ferritin, high saturation of serum transferrin, indication of high hepatic iron content by imaging studies (CT or MRI) when feasible, liver biopsy for histological examination (high stainable iron, parenchymal iron especially, and fibrosis) and quantitative measurement of iron per weight of liver. Diagnosis of the various haematological disorders associated with iron overload need not be reviewed here.

Treatment and prevention The goal of treatment is to prevent accumulation of iron to toxic levels and to reduce body iron levels to normal when they are too high. In a case of hereditary hemochromatosis discovered early in life, periodic phlebotomy will prevent iron overload since each unit of blood removed, 500–600 ml, accounts for 200–250 mg of elemental iron. Symptomatic cases may already have body iron stores expanded, for example, from the normal adult male value of 3.6–4.0 g up to 50 g. Phlebotomy of a unit or more per week for several years may be necessary to achieve normal body iron content. Patients with iron overload secondary to haemolytic and other anaemias, complicated by transfusion siderosis and variable inappropriately high iron absorption, can be managed with combined transfusion of blood to maintain desirable serum haemoglobin levels and iron chelation with parenteral desferoxamine to remove excess iron.

Nutritional therapy is not utilized by most practitioners because low-iron diets are not practical for the prevention of iron accumulation and cannot reverse established iron accumulation. However, given the high gene frequency for hyperabsorption of iron, especially in the White population which often eats a diet rich in efficiently absorbed iron, and given the several other mechanisms for iron overload discussed above, there have been calls for a change of current public policy that fosters acceleration of iron overload by allowing the promiscuous intake of medicinal iron (and vitamin C) and promoting supplementation of many foods with iron.

Primary biliary cirrhosis

Definition and aetiology Primary biliary cirrhosis (PBC) is a liver disease of unknown aetiology, but with prominent immunological features such as lymphoid aggregates in the liver and circulating antimitochondrial antibodies (AMA). Women of middle age are affected predominantly, 51 years being the mean age when first diagnosed, and men representing 10% of those affected. The disease is characterized by chronic cholangitis, involving the middle-sized ductules especially, with progressive destruction of bile ducts, cholestasis, bile ductular proliferation, fibrosis, cirrhosis and liver failure.

Incidence and prevalence PBC is more common in northern compared to southern Europe and higher in first degree relatives of patients with the disease than the prevalence among non-relatives in the area. In Newcastle-upon-Tyne the incidence was 19 with a prevalence of 128.5 per million. Other areas of northern Europe and England had an incidence ranging from about 6 to 15 and prevalence of 40 to 144 per million in the same era.

Clinical features and prognosis The disease typically appears in females between the ages of 40 and 60 years; the patient may be asymptomatic and only have laboratory findings, or may present with pruritus, sometimes accompanied by mild right upper quadrant discomfort, dyspepsia or fatigue. The progression of disease is quite variable. The median survival, in one large series, was 16 years for an asymptomatic group and 7.5 years from the time of symptoms. Cholestasis leads to diminished bile salt presence in the intestine, failure to accomplish micelle-mediated absorption of fat and fat-soluble vitamins, steatorrhoea, fat-soluble vitamin deficiency, osteoporosis and compression fractures of vertebral bodies. Other aspects of the disease are hyperpigmentation, xanthomas, salivary and lachrymal gland pathology (Sjogren's syndrome). Hepatosplenomegaly, jaundice, portal hypertension and liver failure eventually ensue. Median survival is 18 to 24 months when the serum bilirubin reaches $170~\mu mol~l^{-1}$ (10 mg%). Liver transplantation frequently becomes necessary.

Nutritional management Although an increase in stool fat may be documented by quantitative analysis, it is not advisable to restrict dietary fat unless the patient's symptoms can be attributed to steatorrhoea. When the patient may have bloating, postprandial discomfort and diarrhoea secondary to fat malabsorption, dietary fat may be limited to no more than 40 g per day, approximately 1500 kJ (360 kcal), which amounts to 15–20% of daily energy intake. Triacylglycerols comprising fatty acids of medium chain length (MCT) may be used to increase energy intake for patients losing weight, since these fatty acids are absorbed without the need for bile salts to promote micelle formation. MCT oil may be used in cooking and baking, and may be used to dress salads or be mixed with fruit juices. A tablespoon contains 14 g of MCT and provides 115 kcal. Commercial powders afford convenience of handling as they can be reconstituted to aqueous beverages containing high proportions of MCT. Patients are sometimes intolerant to dietary MCT and report mid-abdominal and epigastric distress; gradual introduction of MCT may be necessary.

Deficiency of fat-soluble vitamins A, D, E and K have been diagnosed in patients with PBC. The availability of water-soluble preparations of these vitamins has been of great practical importance. It has been suggested that 100 000 units of parenteral vitamin A be administered when cholestasis is severe, as well as 100 000 units of vitamin D and 10 mg of vitamin K. There is a danger of haematoma formation secondary to intramuscular injection when coagulopathy is already present. In the presence of coagulopathy vitamin K should first be administered intravenously.

See also: **Alcohol**: Absorption, Metabolism and Physiological Effects; Disease Risk and Beneficial Effects; Effects of Alcohol Consumption on Diet and Nutritional Status. **Amino Acids**: Chemistry and Classification; Metabolism. **Carbohydrates**: Regulation of Carbohydrate Metabolism. **Carotenoids**: Chemistry, Sources and Physiology; Epidemiology. **Cobalamins**: Physiology, Dietary Sources and Requirements. **Copper**: Physiology, Dietary Sources and Requirements. **Diabetes Mellitus**: Classification and Chemical Pathology. **Glucose**: Glucose Tolerance. **Inborn Errors of Metabolism**: Classification and Biochemical Aspects; Nutritional Management of Phenylketonuria. **Insulin Resistance**: Aetiology and Association with Disease. **Iron**: Physiology, Dietary Sources and Requirements. **Retinol**: Physiology. **Vitamin K**: Physiology.

Further Reading

Arai M, Gordon ER and Lieber CS (1984) Decreased cytochrome oxidase activity in hepatic mitochondria after chronic ethanol consumption and the possible role of decreased cytochrome aa3 content and changes in phospholipids. *Biochimica Biophysica Acta* 797:320–327.

Brusilow SW and Horwich AL (1995) In: Scriver C (eds) *The Metabolic and Molecular Basis of Inherited Disease*, 7th edn, chap. 32. New York: McGraw Hill.

Bulaj ZJ, Griffen LM, Jorde LB, Edwards CQ and Kushner JP (1996) Clinical and biochemical abnormalities in people heterozygous for hemochromatosis. *New England Journal of Medicine* 335:1799–1805.

Da Costa CM, Baldwin D, Portmann B, Lolin Y, Mowat AP and Mieli-Vergani G (1992) Value of urinary copper excretion after penicillamine challenge in the diagnosis of Wilson's Disease. *Hepatology* 15:609–615.

Inui Y, Kuwajima M, Kawata S, Fukuda K, Maeda Y, Igura T, Kono N, Tarui S and Matsuzawa Y (1994) Impaired ketogenesis in patients with adult-type citrullinemia. *Gastroenterology* 107:1154–1161.

Leo MA and Lieber CS (1982) Hepatic vitamin A depletion in alcoholic liver injury. *New England Journal of Medicine* 307:597–601.

Leo MA and Lieber CS (1985) New pathways for retinol metabolism in liver microsomes. *Journal of Biological Chemistry* 260:5228–5231.

Leo MA, Kim CI, Lowe N and Lieber CS (1992) Interaction of ethanol with β-carotene: Delayed blood clearance and enhanced hepatotoxicity. *Hepatology* 15:883–891.

Leo MA, Rosman A and Lieber CS (1993) Differential

depletion of carotenoids and tocopherol in liver disease. *Hepatology* 17:977–986.

Lieber CS (1992) *Medical and Nutritional Complications of Alcoholism: Mechanisms and Management*. New York: Plenum Press.

Lieber CS (1997) Link between accelerated acetaldehyde production and increased free radical generation by the induced microsomes, resulting in enhanced lipid peroxidation with metabolic blocks due to alcohol, folate deficiency and/or alcoholic liver disease, illustrating possible beneficial effects of GSH, its precursors (including S-adenosylmethionine [SAMe]) and phosphatidylcholine. *Digestive Diseases* 15:42–66.

Lieber CS, Casini A, DeCarli LM, Kim C, Lowe N, Sasaki R and Leo MA (1990) A-adenosyl-L-methionine attenuates alcohol-induced liver injury in the baboon. *Hepatology* 11:165–172.

Lieber CS and DeCarli LM (1970) Effects of varying amounts of dietary fat. Hepatic triglycerides in seven groups of rats given ethanol (36% of calories) with a diet of normal protein (18% of calories). Average hepatic triglyceride concentration in the control animals is indicated by a dotted line. *American Journal Clinical Nutrition* 23:474–478.

Lieber CS, Robins SJ and Leo MA (1994) Hepatic phosphatidylethanolamine methytransferase activity is decreased by ethanol and increased by phosphatidylcholine. *Alcoholism Clinical Experimental Research* 18:592–595.

Lieber CS, Robins SJ, Li J, DeCarli LM, Mak KM, Fasulo JM and Leo MA (1994) Phosphatidylcholine protects against fibrosis and cirrhosis in the baboon. *Gastroenterology* 106:152–159.

Maestri NE, Brusilow SW, Clissold DB and Basset SS (1996) Long-term treatment of girls with ornithine transcarbamylase deficiency. *New England Journal of Medicine* 335:855–859.

Mahan LK and Arlin MT (eds) (1992) In: *Krause's Food Nutrition and Diet Therapy*, 8th edn, chap. 7. Philadelphia: WB Saunders Company.

Myszor M and James OFW (1990) The epidemiology of primary biliary cirrhosis in north-east England: an increasingly common disease? *Quarterly Journal of Medicine. New Series* 75:377–385.

O'Donohue J and Williams R (1996) Primary biliary cirrhosis. *Quarterly Journal of Medicine* 89:5–13.

Shaw S and Lieber CS (1978) Effects of ethanol consumption on plasma α-amino-n-butyric acid (mean ±SEM); consumption of ethanol (4 g/kg/day) in addition to an adequate diet in 3 human volunteers resulted in doubling of plasma α-amino-n-butyric acid after 2 to 4 weeks which was reversed after cessation of drinking. *Gastroenterology* 74:677–682.

Walshe JM (1989) Wilson's Disease presenting with features of hepatic dysfunction: A clinical analysis of eighty-seven patients. *Quarterly Journal of Medicine, New Series* 70:253–263.

Lung diseases *see* **Cancer**: Epidemiology of Lung Cancer. **Therapeutic Dietetics**: Lung Diseases.

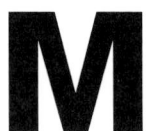

MAGNESIUM

Physiology, Dietary Sources and Requirements

K O'Brien, Johns Hopkins University, Baltimore, Maryland, USA

Copyright © 1998 Academic Press

Magnesium comprises 2.5% of the Earth's crust and is the fourth most abundant cation in the human body. This metal was one of the earliest elements incorporated into primitive life forms, and as such, now plays a key role in over 300 enzymatic reactions. Several key processes such as photosynthesis and oxidative phosphorylation are dependent on magnesium. Magnesium also plays an essential role in the structure of nucleic acids and is required for

DNA replication, transcription and the translation of RNA.

Current research continues to illustrate the importance of magnesium in human health and disease. Roles for magnesium have recently been implicated in several aspects of cardiovascular disease including arteriosclerosis, myocardial damage, arterial hypertension and cardiac arrhythmias.

Increased application of techniques capable of following the *in vivo* physiology of magnesium will continue to expand the breadth of knowledge on the importance and role of magnesium in human health and wellbeing.

Functions of Magnesium

In addition to providing plants with the capability of harnessing light energy, magnesium is essential for oxidative phosphorylation and for all reactions in which adenosine triphosphate (ATP) is required. Processes with enzymatic reactions that require ATP include the synthesis of fat, protein, nucleic acid and coenzymes. Magnesium is also essential for muscle contraction and methyl group transfers.

Many intracellular changes are mediated by second messengers. The formation of the second messenger cyclic adenosine monophosphate by adenylate cyclase is dependent on the presence of magnesium. Magnesium itself may also serve as a second messenger in the insulin stimulation of protein synthesis.

Numerous genetic processes are dependent on magnesium, including the synthesis of the purine and pyrimidine precursors of nucleic acids. Magnesium is also required for enzymes involved in DNA replication, transcription and RNA translation.

Distribution Within the Body

Total body magnesium content increases from approximately 1 g at birth to nearly 23–27 g in adults. The majority of magnesium in the body (approximately 60%) is located in bone. Of this, approximately 30% is freely exchangeable and the remainder is found as an integral part of the bone crystal. The freely exchangeable bone magnesium is believed to serve as a reservoir to maintain extracellular magnesium concentrations within normal ranges.

The remaining body reserves of magnesium (approximately 40%) are located in muscle and non-muscular soft tissues. Only 1% of total body magnesium is present in the extracellular fluid; of this, less than 0.3% circulates in serum.

Dietary Sources of Magnesium

Magnesium is present in virtually all food sources. The largest contribution to daily magnesium intake (45%) is obtained from vegetables, fruits, grains and nuts with slightly lower contributions (29%) from meat, milk and eggs. Fats and sugars do not contribute substantially to dietary magnesium intake. Depending on the geographical area, water can also contribute to daily magnesium intake. It should also be noted that uncertainties currently exist regarding the data available on the magnesium content of food owing to observed discrepancies between published and analysed data.

A substantial amount of magnesium present in various dietary sources may be lost during food processing. For example, the refining of wheat flour, extraction of sugar from molasses and boiling of vegetables all lead to a substantial loss of the original magnesium content of these foods.

Typical daily intakes of magnesium range between 240 and 480 mg. Current recommended magnesium intakes range between 310–320 mg per day for adult women and 400–420 mg per day for adult men.

During pregnancy, an additional 40 mg per day of magnesium are recommended to supply the magnesium needs of the fetus. These account for roughly 1 g over the term of the pregnancy. Recent recommendations do not support the need for increased magnesium intake during lactation because magnesium needs at this time are offset by decreased urinary losses and increased bone resorption. The magnesium content of breast milk typically ranges between 28 and 40 mg l^{-1} such that net daily losses of magnesium into breast milk average 30 mg. The current recommended daily intakes of magnesium are detailed in **Table 1**.

Magnesium Absorption

The primary site of intestinal magnesium absorption in humans is the distal small intestine (jejunum and ileum). Colonic absorption also occurs, as evidenced by the hypermagnesaemia observed following administration of magnesium-containing enemas. The colon may also assist in maintaining magnesium balance in patients with disturbances in magnesium absorption in the small intestine.

To date, no hormone responsible for the control of magnesium homeostasis has been identified. It is known that the efficiency of intestinal magnesium absorption is related to the luminal magnesium concentration in a curvilinear fashion. As dietary intake increases, absorption efficiency decreases (**Fig. 1**). The curved portion of the relationship between

Table 1 Recommended daily intakes of magnesium

	RDA (mg per day)[a]		AI (mg per day)[b]	
Life-stage group	Male	Female	Male	Female
0–6 months			30	30
6–12 months			75	75
1–3 years	80	80		
4–8 years	130	130		
9–13 years	240	240		
14–18 years	410	360		
19–30 years	400	310		
31–70 years	420	320		
>70 years	420	320		
Pregnancy				
≤18 years		400		
19–30 years		350		
31–50 years		360		
Lactation				
≤18 years		360		
19–30 years		310		
31–50 years		320		

Data from National Research Council, 1997
[a]RDA = Recommended Dietary Allowance.
[b]AI = Adequate Intake. AI have been set when insufficient
scientific evidence is available to estimate average
requirements.

magnesium intake and absorptive fraction may
reflect a saturable component of absorption (active
absorption or facilitated diffusion), whereas the linear portion may be indicative of passive diffusion.
The curvilinear component of absorption becomes
saturated at magnesium intakes between 10 and
12 mEq (122–146 mg; 5–6 mmol), and the passive
absorptive component is capable of absorbing 7% of
the ingested magnesium for any given load.

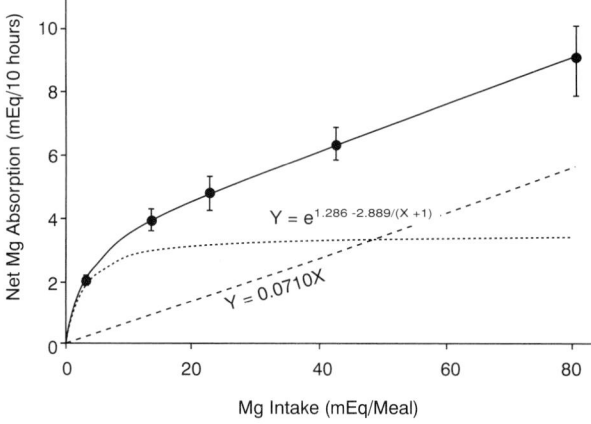

Figure 1 The relationship between net magnesium absorption
versus intake is demonstrated by a nonlinear regression analysis. The equation for net absorption, $y = \exp[1.286 - 2.889/(x+1)]$
$+ 0.0710x$, represents a hyperbolic function plus a linear function.
These separate components and their respective equations are
shown. Reproduced with permission from Fine *et al.* (1991) *J
Clin Invest* **88**:399.

As can be seen from Fig. 1, magnesium absorptive
efficiency varies substantially from 70% to approximately 11% as the magnesium content of the meal
is increased. During periods of rapid growth, absorption efficiency increases to accommodate the
increased physiological demands. The average
absorptive efficiency of magnesium is roughly 85%
in premature infants, 65% in infants, 40% in adolescents, and approximately 25% in adult men and
women. Ageing does not seem to influence significantly the efficiency of magnesium absorption in
women.

A genetic disorder of magnesium absorption has
been characterized in infants. This indicates that
there is a specific intestinal mechanism for absorption, but as yet this mechanism has not been characterized.

Various dietary components such as phytates and
dietary fibre are capable of binding magnesium and
reducing its gastrointestinal absorbability based on
balance data. Few studies have directly examined the
bioavailability of magnesium using either extrinsi-
cally or intrinsically labelled food sources owing to
the lack of suitable radiotracers and the expense and
difficulty associated with the use of stable isotopes
of magnesium. Although magnesium bioavailability
is often assumed to be comparable with that of calcium, this assumption remains to be tested.

Plasma Magnesium Levels

Magnesium circulates in blood in three fashions:
approximately 32% is bound to plasma proteins
(mainly albumin); approximately 13% is complexed
to phosphate, citrate and other small peptides; and
roughly 55% of blood magnesium circulates in the
free state (Mg^{2+}).

Serum levels of magnesium average 0.75–
0.95 mmol l^{-1} in adults, and these concentrations
typically do not vary more than 15% in healthy individuals.

Concentrations of ionized magnesium range
between 0.5 and 0.65 mmol l^{-1} and these levels may
be regulated to a greater degree than are total magnesium concentrations. Erythrocytes have a much
higher magnesium content (1.65–2.73 mmol l^{-1}) in
comparison with serum levels. Serum magnesium
distribution is comparable between men and women
and ageing does not appreciably affect mean serum
levels.

Urinary Excretion

The kidneys are the principal regulator of serum
magnesium levels. Alterations in magnesium intake

can cause urinary magnesium excretion to vary from 10 to 5000 mg day^{-1} in relation to the magnesium load. In adults consuming typical diets, average urinary magnesium excretion ranges from 120 to 140 mg day^{-1} (5–6 mmol day^{-1}). Abnormally low urinary magnesium excretion may be indicative of inadequate magnesium status.

Approximately 95% of ultrafilterable magnesium is reabsorbed by the kidney. The majority of ultrafilterable magnesium is reabsorbed in the thick ascending limb of the loop of Henle (65%); this is where the majority of regulation in response to serum fluctuations is controlled. The remaining 30% of ultrafilterable magnesium is reabsorbed in the proximal tubule.

Endogenous Faecal Losses

During the digestion process magnesium is secreted into the digestive tract via saliva, bile, gastric and pancreatic juice. In contrast to other minerals, the majority of magnesium secreted into the gastrointestinal tract is efficiently reabsorbed and net daily faecal losses of endogenous magnesium only average 25–50 mg in adults. Comparable values of endogenous magnesium secretion have been reported in adolescents.

Dermal Losses

The dermal losses of magnesium are not frequently included in estimations of magnesium balance because they are not believed to be appreciable during typical environmental conditions. However, during exposure to ambient temperatures of 49–50° C, adult men may lose 10–15% of the total magnesium output in sweat. Unlike minerals such as sodium, no acclimatization appears to occur in dermal magnesium losses during prolonged heat exposure.

Ca/Mg Interactions

Recent recommendations have advocated increasing the recommended daily allowance of calcium for both adolescents and adult men and women. In addition, there is an increased availability of calcium-fortified food sources and calcium supplements. One concern associated with increased calcium intake is the potential for high calcium intakes to interfere with magnesium absorption based on early balance data. More recent data involving both adults and adolescent girls have demonstrated that increases in calcium intake to levels of 1500–2000 mg day^{-1} from either diet and/or calcium supplements does not significantly alter magnesium balance.

Although high calcium intakes do not adversely alter magnesium retention, magnesium plays an important role in the metabolism of several calcitropic hormones. Magnesium is required for parathyroid hormone secretion in humans and is also needed for parathyroid hormone to illicit its effects on kidney, bone and gut. Furthermore, magnesium is required for the hepatic 25-hydroxylase enzyme, which converts 25-hydroxyvitamin D into the biologically active form of vitamin D (1,25-dihydroxyvitamin D).

Assessment of Magnesium Status

Balance studies have provided the majority of information on magnesium requirements in humans. Although useful, this technique is limited by the time required for dietary equilibration, the need to correct for the completeness of faecal collections, and by the difficulty and expense of these studies. This technique also underestimates actual magnesium absorption because it does not account for endogenous faecal losses.

Many of the limitations of the balance technique can be eliminated with the use of isotopic tracers. Unfortunately, only one short-lived radiotracer of magnesium exists (^{28}Mg, $t_{1/2}$ = 21.3 h) and its availability is limited. Use of this radiotracer, however, has provided much of the available data on the *in vivo* magnesium metabolism in adults. The limitation to the use of this radiotracer is that it cannot be safely administered to all population groups, especially those who may have increased needs because of growth and increased physiological demands such as infants, children, and pregnant and lactating women.

To overcome limitations associated with the use of radiotracers in human studies, stable isotopes can be administered. Three stable isotopes of magnesium exist (^{24}Mg, ^{25}Mg and ^{26}Mg) at natural abundances of 78.99%, 10.00% and 11.01%, respectively. The high natural abundance of the two minor isotopes also limits the use of these tracers in human studies. Currently, smaller doses of these tracers can be administered if more sensitive mass spectrometric techniques such as magnetic sector thermal ionization mass spectrometry are employed. It is still relatively difficult to measure endogenous faecal magnesium excretion using stable isotopes because the intravenous dose required is relatively high in relation to the initial magnesium distribution volume in children and adults. Despite these limitations, increasing use of stable magnesium isotopes will provide novel information on magnesium physiology and bioavailability in population groups in which other data are limited.

To assess total magnesium levels in biological fluids, atomic absorption spectrophotometry is the method of choice because it is a widely available, sensitive and rapid technique. Colorometric methods are also frequently used to measure magnesium in biological fluids.

It should be noted that serum magnesium levels may not be indicative of overall magnesium status and only 0.3% of body magnesium reserves are found in serum. The concentration of magnesium in mononuclear blood cells or ionized magnesium concentrations in serum may be more sensitive indicators of physiological changes in magnesium status. Both direct (ion-selective electrodes and metallochromic dyes) and indirect methods (ultracentrifugation and equilibrium dialysis) can be used to measure ionized magnesium (Mg^{2+}).

Magnetic resonance imaging and nuclear magnetic resonance are two techniques that are capable of indirectly determining the amount of intracellular ionized magnesium. Fluorescent indicators are also useful in measuring Mg^{2+} in cellular suspensions and individual cells.

One technique that has been used indirectly to assess the magnesium stores of an individual is the magnesium load test. For this test, a parenteral load of magnesium salts is administered (approximately 30 mmol) over a 12 h period. Replete individuals can be expected to excrete virtually all of the magnesium load in a 24–48 h urine collection. Individuals with deficient stores, however, may retain more than 30% of the administered magnesium.

Magnesium Intake and Disease

There is mounting evidence that alterations in magnesium metabolism and conditions of magnesium deficiency can have a negative impact on cardiovascular biology. Dietary magnesium deficiency may lead to elevated arterial blood pressure. Furthermore, patients with ischaemic heart disease may have deficits in ionized magnesium and magnesium administration to patients with ischaemic heart disease may decrease the follow-up death rates in these patients. Epidemiological studies suggest that there may also be an inverse relationship between magnesium in drinking water and cardiovascular and cerebrovascular disease, but not all studies on this association have demonstrated this relationship.

Pharmacological Effects of Magnesium

Well-characterized changes occur when large amounts of magnesium are given either intravenously or intramuscularly. Both vasodilation of the blood vessels and a drop in blood pressure are observed after serum levels are temporarily increased to approximately twice the upper normal values. These physiological changes have been utilized to treat eclampsia during pregnancy by administering large intravenous doses of magnesium sulfate. Comparable doses of intravenous magnesium are also used in the treatment of premature labour. In addition, intravenous doses of magnesium are administered to patients with acute myocardial infarctions to decrease associated complications and mortality.

Magnesium Deficiency and Excess

Because of the efficient renal conservation and the efficiency of intestinal absorption, a magnesium deficiency state does not generally occur in healthy individuals. Magnesium deficiency has been induced in adults following consumption of diets containing less than 0.8 mEq day^{-1} of magnesium. These very low magnesium intakes led to increased intestinal absorption and decreased urinary losses. Plasma and erthryocyte magnesium levels decrease continuously over time and hypocalcaemia, hypophosphataemia and hypocalciuria are also evident. Other symptoms associated with magnesium deficiency include nausea, ataxia, tetany, hallucinations, confusion, depression, anorexia, depression, vomiting, vertigo and muscular weakness. A positive Trousseau sign may also occur during magnesium deficiency. These symptoms can be relieved when magnesium is added back to the diet.

Magnesium deficiency is most often observed clinically in association with other disease processes such as cirrhosis, renal failure, congestive heart failure, and in individuals with malabsorption syndromes or intestinal resections. Chronic alcoholism can also lead to magnesium deficiency. Administration of medications that increase urinary losses such as thiazide diuretics can also be a causal factor in the development of magnesium deficiency. Likewise endocrine disorders including hyperparathyroidism and hyperaldosteronism can deplete magnesium stores and lead to magnesium deficiency.

Genetic conditions have been described in infants that result in altered absorption of magnesium, leading to hypomagnesaemic tetany. This condition is thought to affect carrier-mediated intestinal magnesium absorption while non-carrier-mediated absorption remains unaffected. Large supplemental doses of oral magnesium are required to treat this disorder.

Several clinical conditions can also result in hypermagnesaemia. Conditions of renal failure can lead to hypermagnesaemia when the capacity of the nephron cannot maintain the serum levels. Hypermagnesaemia can occur in individuals receiving excessive antacid therapy, or in infants receiving treatment for neonatal tetany. Hypermagnesaemia has also been reported in neonates born to eclamptic mothers who had been treated with excessive doses of magnesium sulfate.

Symptoms of hypermagnesaemia include hypotension, drowsiness, atonia, vomiting and depression of deep tendon reflexes. At very high levels of serum magnesium (10 times normal) coma, anoxia and death can occur.

Summary

Many recent findings have augmented the significance of magnesium in human health and disease. Despite these advances, there are still questions that remain to be addressed concerning the magnesium needs and normal metabolism in several population groups including healthy infants, children, and pregnant and lactating women. Similarly, many of the mechanisms involved in the intestinal absorption and overall regulation of magnesium homeostasis have yet to be elucidated. Increased research in these areas will expand the knowledge and importance of the role of magnesium in human health.

See also: **Calcium**: Physiology. **Lactation**: Dietary Requirements. **Pregnancy**: Nutrient Requirements.

Further Reading

Aikawa JK (1981) *Magnesium: Its Biological Significance.* Boca Raton: CRC Press.

Elin RJ (1987) Assessment of magnesium status. *Clinical Chemistry* 33(11):1965–1970.

Fine KD, Santa Ana C, Porter JL and Fordtran JS (1991) Intestinal absorption of magnesium from food and supplements. *Journal of Clinical Investigation* 88:396–402.

National Research Council (1989) *Recommended Dietary Allowances*, 10th edn. Washington, DC: National Academy Press.

Shils ME and Rude RK (1996) Deliberations and evaluations of the approaches, endpoints and paradigms for magnesium dietary recommendations. *Journal of Nutrition* 126:2398S–2403S.

Silver L, Robertson JS, Dahl LK, Heine M and Tassinari L (1960) Magnesium turnover in the human studies with Mg^{28}. *Journal of Clinical Investigation* 39:420–425.

Vernon WB (1988) The role of magnesium in nucleic-acid and protein metabolism. *Magnesium* 7:234–248.

Wester PO (1987) Magnesium. *American Journal of Clinical Nutrition* 45:1305–1312.

MALABSORPTION SYNDROMES

Nutritional Management

Aglaia Zellos and **Jose M Saavedra**, Johns Hopkins University, Baltimore, Maryland, USA

Copyright © 1998 Academic Press

The principal function of the gut is to process and absorb the nutrients ingested in the diet. Any condition that alters the intestinal surface area, function or transport results in either global or selective malabsorption of nutrients. The three main foods ingested are fat, protein and carbohydrates. Electrolytes, vitamins and minerals are equally important and any condition that affects the absorption of fat, protein and carbohydrates may result in their deficiency as well.

Physiology of Normal Absorption

Fat absorption

Most lipid consumed in a typical Western diet consists of long-chain triacylglycerols (LCTs), formed of a glycerol backbone attached to three fatty acid molecules, each containing more than 12 carbon atoms. Approximately 10% of ingested triacylglycerols are in the form of medium-chain triacylglycerols (MCTs). In MCTs the three fatty acid chains contain 6–12 carbon atoms. A small amount of lipid is consumed as lecithin and cholesterol.

Lipid digestion begins in the stomach with the action of gastric lipase and continues in the small intestine with pancreatic lipase. Lipases digest triacylglycerols to monoacylglycerols and fatty acids. The stomach further controls the emptying of the fatty contents into the small intestine in order to maximize the surface contact between the water-insoluble lipid and the intestinal mucosa. In the second part of the duodenum, fat encounters the bile acids and the pancreatic lipase.

Bile acids are synthesized in the liver from cholesterol, then are conjugated with either taurine or glycine, and excreted via the biliary tract into the intestine, where they act as detergents. The conjugated bile acids have a polar (water-soluble) end and a nonpolar (lipid-soluble) end, and they aggregate to form a micelle. The nonpolar ends of the bile acids aggregate toward the centre, whereas the polar ends are arranged in a radial orientation making the entire micellar structure water-soluble. Fat molecules are thus solubilized and allow the action of pancreatic lipase. The micelles containing the fatty acids and b-monoacylglycerols are transported through the intestinal cell membrane. Inside the intestinal epithelial cell, the fatty acids are resynthesized into triacylglycerols and are coated by proteins to form chylomicrons. The chylomicrons are taken up by the lymphatic system and then transported into the circulation.

The bile acids are absorbed by the intestinal cells of the terminal ileum and are transported to the liver via the portal vein. This recycling of the bile acids is referred to as the enterohepatic circulation.

In contrast to LCTs, MCTs are taken up directly into the portal venous system, without the use of bile acids. Absorption of MCT occurs even in the absence of pancreatic lipase.

Carbohydrate absorption

The primary carbohydrates in the diet are starches, sucrose, lactose and fructose. Carbohydrates constitute 40–60% of the average energy intake in humans. Sixty per cent of the digestible carbohydrates in adults are ingested in the form of starch, 30% as sucrose and 10% as lactose. The use of high-fructose syrups, in commercial juices, soft drinks, etc., has increased significantly over the past years. A few nondigestible, nonstarch polysaccharides are consumed, mainly from plant cell wall components including cellulose, pectin and hemicellulose, which are categorized as dietary fibres. Additionally, modern diets contain a significant amount of nondigestible sugars, such as stachyose, raffinose and sugar alcohols such as sorbitol and mannitol, also abundant in fruits, juices, soft drinks and prepared foods.

Starch is a glucose polymer. The two major polysaccharides of starch are amylose and amylopectin. Amylose is a chain of $\alpha(1–4)$-linked glucose molecules and typically accounts for 20% of dietary starch. Amylopectin is a chain of $\alpha(1–4)$-linked glu-

cose molecules, but differs from amylose in that every 25 glucose molecules, there is an $\alpha(1–6)$ linkage. Amylopectin accounts for 80% of dietary starch. Glycogen is a polysaccharide found in animal tissues and has a similar structure to amylopectin.

The initial step in the digestion of starch involves the hydrolysis of the $\alpha(1–4)$ linkages by the salivary and pancreatic α-amylases. Little starch hydrolysis is brought about by salivary amylase owing to the short exposure time before gastric acid deactivates the enzyme. However, when food is chewed for a long time, up to 75% of the starch can be digested into disaccharides.

The main step in the digestion of starch occurs in the duodenal lumen by the secreted pancreatic amylase. The pancreatic α-amylase preferentially cleaves the $\alpha(1–4)$ glucose linkages and is incapable of cleaving the $\alpha(1–6)$ branching links of amylopectin and glycogen, and the $\beta(1–4)$ glucose linkages in cellulose. Maltose (a glucose–glucose disaccharide), maltotriose (a trisaccharide) and α-limit dextrins are products of amylase action on amylopectin and glycogen. These products of intraluminal starch digestion, as well as sucrose and lactose, are further hydrolysed by corresponding oligosaccharidases (maltase, α-dextranase, sucrase, lactase) which are an integral part of the brush border membrane. The activity of the mucosal membrane oligosaccharidases is highest in the mid jejunum and lowest in the duodenum and terminal ileum. **Fig. 1** depicts the major pathways for the absorption of carbohydrates.

Maltase is the most active of the oligosaccharidases and hydrolyses maltose and maltotriose into glucose. Sucrase, which is also active against maltose and maltotriose, typically cleaves sucrose into fructose and glucose. Lactase catalyses the hydrolysis of lactose to galactose and glucose.

The final products of hydrolysis are the monosaccharides glucose, galactose and fructose. These monosaccharides are too large to diffuse across the mucosal membrane. Therefore, specific carrier-mediated processes exist. Glucose and galactose are carried across the enterocyte membrane via a sodium–glucose cotransporter located in the brush border. Fructose is absorbed by glucose-independent facilitated diffusion or glucose-dependent cotransport. The rate of fructose absorption is one-sixth to one-third of the rate of glucose absorption.

Protein absorption

The protein content of an average Western diet is 70–90 g per day. Young children require up to 4 g per kilogram of body weight per day in order to grow, compared with 0.6 g per kg per day in adults. The dietary proteins are derived from vegetables, fish

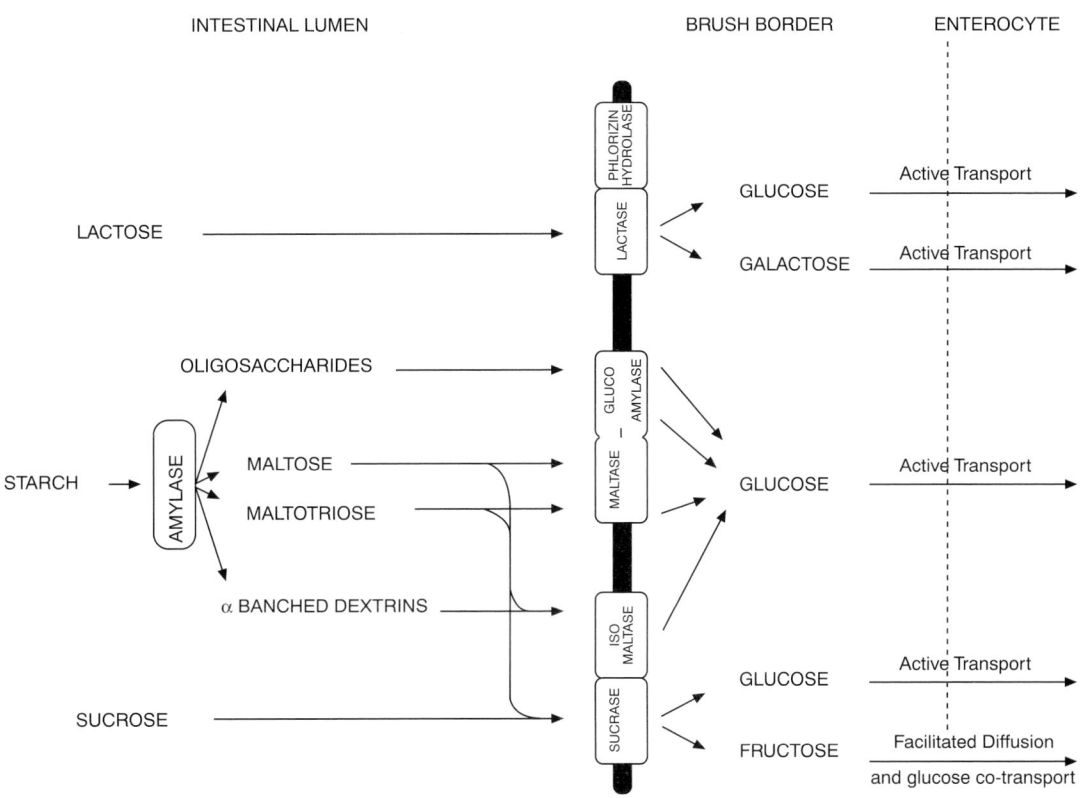

Figure 1 Major pathways for digestion and absorption of dietary carbohydrates. Following ingestion, salivary and pancreatic amylase will begin the hydrolysis of starches into smaller oligosaccharide chains, maltose, maltotriose and alpha-limit dextrins (the branching portions of complex starch polymers). These sugars are further hydrolysed by distinct glycosidases found in three glycosylated protein complexes anchored in the intestinal brush border membrane; and which have their hydrolytic sites facing the intestinal lumen. These are glucoamylase–maltase, sucrase–isomaltase, and lactase–phlorhizin hydrolase. Lactose is hydrolysed to glucose and galactose by lactase and sucrose is hydrolysed to glucose and fructose by sucrase. Maltose is hydrolysed to two glucose molecules by maltase activity. The sucrase–isomaltase complex is responsible for 80% of maltase activity, all of sucrase activity, most isomaltase and some alpha-limit dextrinase activity. The glucoamylase–maltase complex hydrolyses all glucoamylase, most alpha-limit dextrins, 20% of maltase and a small percentage of isomaltase. It is an important alternate pathway for starch digestion in reduced or absent pancreatic amylase activity. The lactase–phlorhizin hydrolase complex is responsible for hydrolysing lactase to glucose and galactose.

and meat. Protein available for absorption in the small intestine is derived not only from food but also from digestive enzymes, mucoproteins, desquamated cells and plasma proteins. Dietary protein is digested in the intestine and absorbed in the form of amino acids, which are used to synthesize the body's own functional and structural proteins. The proteins of the body are synthesized from 20 different amino acids, only half of which can be synthesized in the body. The rest (essential amino acids) must be provided in the diet.

Protein digestion begins in the stomach where pepsin hydrolyses protein into peptones, peptides and polypeptides. The most important part of protein breakdown, however, occurs in the duodenum, where protein is exposed to pancreatic proteolytic enzymes. The pancreatic enzymes are secreted in the duodenum in response to the hormone cholecystokinin. The intraluminal activation of the pancreatic enzymes involves conversion of pepsinogen (inactive precursor) to trypsin (active protease) by enterokinase, an endopeptidase secreted by the enterocyte. The presence of trypsin in the duodenum enhances its own formation from trypsinogen, as well as the formation of other peptidase precursors from the pancreas. The endopeptidases (trypsin, chymotrypsin and elastase) cleave proteins into oligopeptides which are in turn broken down into small peptides and amino acids by exopeptidases (carboxypeptidases A and B).

The oligopeptides are further hydrolysed to free amino acids either at the surface of the brush border membrane or within the cytosol of the enterocyte. Specific carrier mechanisms at the brush border membrane allow di- and tripeptides to enter the cytoplasm of the enterocyte where they are cleaved into free amino acids. Peptides larger than tetrapeptides need to be cleaved to di- or tripeptides by the brush border enzymes in order to be transported into the enterocyte. After all peptides are cleaved into free amino acids inside the enterocyte cytoplasm, they are carried into the portal venous circulation.

Aetiology of Nutrient Malabsorption

The disruption of any of the normal digestive and absorptive mechanisms outlined above may lead to nutrient malabsorption. Depending on the location of the problem, it can be classified as an intraluminal, mucosal or transport phase defect. Intraluminal phase defects refer mainly to macronutrient absorption secondary to inadequate pancreatic digestion. Mucosal phase abnormalities are seen in the context of infections, inflammatory processes, specific enzyme deficiencies and congenital disorders resulting in a decrease in the mucosal absorptive surface area. Transport defects result from either obstruction of the lymphatic system or defective carrier mechanisms across the enterocyte membrane (**Table 1**).

Conditions associated with intraluminal phase defects

Impaired lipolysis The most common cause of impaired intraluminal lipolysis is exocrine pancreatic insufficiency seen in patients with cystic fibrosis, chronic pancreatitis, Shwachman–Diamond–Oski syndrome, Johnson–Blizzard syndrome, Pearson syn-

drome or congenital structural pancreatic anomalies. Cystic fibrosis is an autosomal recessive disease caused by a defect in the chloride transport in epithelial cells, resulting in progressive lung disease and exocrine pancreatic insufficiency; many other organs are also affected. The Shwachman–Diamond–Oski syndrome is an autosomal recessive disorder characterized by cyclic neutropenia, pancreatic insufficiency, metaphyseal dysostosis and failure to thrive. Johnson–Blizzard syndrome presents early in infancy with pancreatic insufficiency, metaplasia of the alae nasi, deafness, hypothyroidism, microcephaly and growth impairment. Pearson syndrome involves pancreatic insufficiency and sideroblastic anaemia.

In these conditions, when pancreatic lipase production falls to levels of 2–10% of normal, massive losses of fat in the stool occur. Faecal loss of 7 g more than 90–95% of ingested fat is termed 'steatorrhoea'. In the colon, bacteria hydrolyse the neutral fats to free fatty acids and glycerol, inducing more diarrhoea. Steatorrhoea also produces malabsorption of the fat-soluble vitamins A, D, E and K, leading to vitamin deficiencies. Patients with exocrine pancreatic insufficiency also malabsorb protein, carbohydrates and electrolytes.

Impaired micellar formation In order to achieve adequate micellar formation, it is important to maintain a critical intraluminal bile acid concentration. Any factors that decrease bile acid synthesis or

Table 1   Aetiology of malabsorption

Intraluminal phase defects	Mucosal phase defects	Transport phase defects

1. Impaired lipolysis
   Cystic fibrosis
   Chronic pancreatitis
   Shwachman–Diamond–Oski syndrome
   Johnson–Blizzard syndrome
   Pearson syndrome
	1. Impaired carbohydrate absorption
	   Adult-onset lactase deficiency
	   Fructose intolerance
	   Glucose-galactose malabsorption
	   Sucrose-isomaltase deficiency
	   Congenital lactase deficiency
		1. Amino acid transport defects
		   Specific amino acid transport defects (cysteine, histidine, lysine, methionine)
		   Group amino acid defects (Hartnup disease, cystinuria)

2. Impaired micellar formation
   Decreased bile acid secretion
   Hepatocellular disease (hepatitis, etc.)
	2. Impaired protein absorption
	   Congenital enterokinase deficiency
	   Protein-losing enteropathy (intestinal lymphangiectasia, Ménétrier's disease)
	   Infections (rotavirus gastroenteritis, HIV, giardiasis)
	   Crohn's disease
	   Protein-sensitive enteropathy
	   Coeliac disease
	   Small bowel bacterial overgrowth
	   Radiation enteritis
	   Microvillous inclusion disease
		2. Congenital chloride malabsorption
		
		3. Trace element and vitamin deficiency
		   Acrodermatitis enterohepatica
		   Menkes' syndrome
		   Vitamin B_{12} deficiency (intrinsic transcobalamin II factor deficiency)

3. Secondary causes of malabsorption
   Decreased bile acid secretion
     Obstructive biliary disease (biliary atresia, choledochal cyst)
   Decreased absorption of bile acids
     Crohn's disease
     Short bowel syndrome
     Small bowel bacterial overgrowth
		4. Lymphatic obstruction
		   Intestinal lymphangiecyasia
		   Lymphoma

4. Impaired carbohydrate digestion Absence of pancreatic amylase (cystic fibrosis, etc.)		

excretion into the intestine, or interfere with bile acid absorption and the enterohepatic circulation, may disrupt proper micellar formation and result in fat malabsorption. Hepatocellular disease and cholestasis from obstructive biliary disease result in bile acid pool depletion. Inflammatory bowel disease (Crohn's disease) with terminal ileal involvement and short bowel syndrome also result in depletion of the available bile acid pool and subsequent loss of fat and fat-soluble vitamins.

In small bowel overgrowth syndrome, excessive concentrations of bacteria in the small intestinal lumen may affect both absorption and digestion of all nutrients, vitamins and electrolytes. Bacteria deconjugate bile acids resulting in poor micellar formation, shortening of the intestinal villi, degrading of brush border enzymes and altering of sugar transport mechanisms. Small bowel bacterial overgrowth can occur in a wide variety of disorders such as intestinal strictures, stagnant loops, prolonged exclusive use of parenteral nutrition, achlorhydria, motility disorders, malnutrition, autoimmune enteropathies and inflammatory bowel disease.

Impaired carbohydrate digestion Pancreatic exocrine insufficiency, in patients with cystic fibrosis, may result in pancreatic amylase deficiency and subsequent starch malabsorption. A developmental deficiency is seen in the newborn, since pancreatic amylase is universally absent in early infancy and develops in the fourth month of life.

Short bowel syndrome is a condition defined as malabsorption following surgical resection of a significant portion of the small bowel. In most children it occurs in the neonatal period after necrotizing enterocolitis (an acute inflammatory condition of the intestine, common in prematurity) or congenital anatomic anomalies (superior mesenteric artery anomalies, gastroschisis, omphalocele), but a smaller number of children present later in life, especially those with conditions such as Crohn's disease, vascular anomalies, radiation enteritis and neoplastic disorders.

The symptoms of malabsorption correlate with the extent and the anatomic level of intestinal resection. Ileal resection can result in vitamin B_{12} and bile acid deficiency, and massive losses of water and sodium. Jejunal resection can result in malabsorption of all macronutrients since the jejunum is the principal site of protein, fat and carbohydrate absorption. After a period of adaptation, the ileum can develop greater absorptive capacity and assume some of the jejunal function, leading to better absorption. Preservation of the terminal ileum and the ileocaecal valve is important to the prognosis following small bowel resection. The ileocaecal valve limits the influx of colonic bacteria into the intestine and controls the exit of fluid and nutrients from the small intestine into the colon.

Conditions associated with mucosal phase defects

Impaired carbohydrate absorption The metabolism of carbohydrates involves a fine balance between absorption, digestion and fermentation. Sugars that are not digested and absorbed in the proximal small bowel exert an osmotic effect in the jejunum, increasing the secretion of water and sodium into the lumen and decreasing the intestinal transit time. Absorption of other nutrients – particularly protein, fat, magnesium, calcium and phosphate – may be affected. Upon entrance into the colon, some unabsorbed sugars are fermented to lactate and acetic acid, as well as to propionic and butyric acids (short-chain fatty acids) which can be absorbed and salvaged as source of energy. In small infants, and in patients with short bowel syndrome or gastrojejunal bypass, acid levels may reach high concentrations, and accumulate in the bloodstream leading to metabolic acidosis. Bacterial flora capable of producing D-lactate can more easily lead to acidosis, since this acid cannot be metabolized by humans. The excessive gas (hydrogen, methane, carbon dioxide) leads to intestinal distension and flatulence. Acid production lowers the stool pH and reduces water absorption leading to diarrhoea. Carbohydrate intolerance resulting from malabsorption is a spectrum of symptoms, from mild abdominal distension cramps and flatulence to severe diarrhoea, dehydration and metabolic acidosis.

The most common cause of carbohydrate malabsorption is adult-onset lactase deficiency, due to the normal decline in lactase activity after weaning which occurs in all mammals. In most adults, lactase levels are 5–10% of the levels present at birth. This ontogenic decline exhibits genetic polymorphism. Lactose absorbers have persistence of lactase activity beyond childhood or adolescence. This phenotype is common in populations of central and northern Europe and in few nomadic milk-dependent populations in North Africa and Arabia. It is hypothesized that this lactase persistence resulted from natural selection, favouring the survival of individuals who could metabolize lactose, during times when milk constituted an important source of nutrition. Lactose malabsorbers (the majority of humans) are homozygous for the recessive allele that determines the decline in lactase activity after weaning. Adult-onset lactase deficiency can induce symptoms as early as 3 years of age in blacks or as late as adolescence in northern

Europeans. Thus, prevalence of malabsorption increases with age.

Ingestion of high levels of fructose in the diet can lead to carbohydrate intolerance. Fructose is abundant in honey and fruits (dates, figs, apples, grapes and berries), but most consumption results from food additives such as the high-fructose syrup used in prepared foods and beverages. Fructose is absorbed at a slower rate than glucose. However, owing to a glucose cotransport system, if fructose is ingested with an adequate amount of glucose, it is better absorbed. In children, drinking excessive amounts of juice results in chronic nonspecific diarrhoea and recurrent abdominal pain. In adults, fructose malabsorption has been associated with irritable bowel syndrome.

Congenital causes of carbohydrate malabsorption are rare. Congenital lactase deficiency is a rare condition in which lactase activity is decreased or absent at birth, and which persists throughout life. The symptoms of diarrhoea begin within the first days of life and may lead to dehydration. When infants are placed on a lactose-free diet, the symptoms disappear.

Glucose-galactose malabsorption (GGM) is a rare congenital disease which occurs when the normal glucose-sodium cotransporter is not present in the brush border. The condition is characterized by severe and acidic diarrhoea in the neonatal period which may result in death. It has been shown that it is mainly the unabsorbed glucose and not galactose that results in secretion of water and electrolytes in the jejunum, generating a large load for the colon which exceeds its absorptive capacity.

Sucrase-isomaltase deficiency is an autosomal recessive condition common in Inuit and native Canadian populations; it is characterized by lack of sucrase and marked decrease in isomaltase activity. Studies suggest that the disease is due to a mutation in pro-sucrase-isomaltase which hampers its homing in the brush border membrane. Osmotic and fermentative diarrhoea and metabolic acidosis become evident with the introduction of sucrose in the infant diet, usually with fruits or juices.

Impaired protein absorption   Congenital enterokinase deficiency is a rare disorder that results in massive faecal protein loss, failure to thrive and hypoproteinaemia. Protein-losing enteropathy may be caused by losses either from intestinal lymphatics or from an inflamed mucosa (Ménétrier's disease, eosinophilic gastroenteritis, inflammatory bowel disease or infections).

Primary or, more commonly, secondary intestinal lymphangiectasia (due to cardiac disease, lymphoma, radiation, chemotherapy or tuberculosis) may result in massive loss of protein in the gut, severe malnutrition and susceptibility to infection.

Secondary causes of generalized malabsorption - Any condition that causes injury to the intestinal mucosa and reduces the functional absorptive surface area will lead to malabsorption of all nutrients. Examples include acute viral gastroenteritis, *Giardia lamblia* enteritis, human immunodeficiency virus (HIV) disease, small bowel bacterial overgrowth, protein-sensitive (allergic) enteropathy, coeliac disease, Crohn's disease and radiation enteritis. In infants, rotavirus gastroenteritis is the most common cause of transient lactose intolerance.

Coeliac disease or gluten-sensitive enteropathy is a condition common in individuals of Irish and northern European descent due to sensitivity to the protein components of gluten such as gliadins, secalins, hordeins and avenins, found in wheat, rye, barley and oats respectively. The pathophysiologic mechanism by which gliadin induces toxicity resulting in flattening of the intestinal mucosa and malabsorption of macronutrients has not been determined. The condition begins in childhood. The classic presentation is anorexia, failure to thrive, and diarrhoea. The younger the child, the more acute the presentation, with oedema, hypotonia and irritability. The older child may have features of chronic steatorrhoea such as vitamin deficiencies, rickets, anaemia and delayed puberty.

Microvillous inclusion disease and tufting disease are congenital disorders which present in the neonatal period with intractable diarrhoea. Microvillous inclusion disease is characterized by absence of normal microvilli in both small and large intestine. Tufting disease involves tufting of the villi of the small bowel and moderate villous atrophy. Both diseases result in malabsorption of all fluid and nutrients, necessitating long-term parenteral nutrition or intestinal transplantation.

Transport phase defects

Protein malabsorption can result from congenital defects in the amino acid transport, involving either specific amino acid transport defects (cysteine, histidine, lysine, methionine, tryptophan) or amino acid group malabsorption (cystinuria, dibasic aminoaciduria, dicarboxylic aciduria, Hartnup disease, iminoglyciduria).

Congenital amino acid transport defects occur in the intestinal epithelial cells and the proximal tubules of the kidney. Since peptides enter the enterocyte either as amino acids or as oligopeptides, if one transport mechanism is not functioning, the other is used. Therefore, these disorders typically present with aminoaciduria and no diarrhoea.

Lymphatic obstruction from lymphoma or intestinal lymphangiectasia also results in protein malabsorption. Intestinal lymphangiectasia is a condition in which the intestinal lacteals are dilated secondary to obstruction of the lymphatic system resulting in intraluminal loss of lymph rich in protein and lymphocytes. Patients present with generalized oedema, hypoproteinaemia, lymphopenia and diarrhoea in the absence of liver or kidney disease.

Congenital chloride diarrhoea is an autosomal recessive disorder characterized by a selective defect in the intestinal Cl^--HCO_3 transport. The disease manifests with lifelong secretory diarrhoea with a high chloride concentration in the stool, severe alkalosis, hypochloraemia, hypokalaemia and dehydration. Maternal polyhydramnios, neonatal abdominal distension and watery diarrhoea are prominent features. Treatment in the neonatal period is geared towards replacement of sodium and chloride intravenously via a continuous infusion. At 3–4 years of age most children become continent for faeces and oral replacement can be implemented.

Acrodermatitis enterohepatica is an autosomal recessive disorder involving a selective defect in the intestinal absorption of zinc at the level of the enterocyte. The symptoms of zinc deficiency develop after weaning in breast-fed infants. A rash over the buttocks, extremities and face precedes the onset of diarrhoea. Alopecia, dystrophic nails, photophobia, conjunctivitis, irritability and failure to thrive are characteristic signs. Oral zinc supplementation with $2 \, mg \, kg^{-1}$ per day in young infants is recommended. Blood levels of zinc and copper should be monitored during replacement therapy.

Menkes' syndrome is an X-linked inherited disorder involving a selective defect in intestinal copper absorption causing accumulation of copper in other cells of the body. The disorder results in abnormal (kinky) hair, progressive cerebral degeneration, hypopigmentation, bone changes, arterial rupture and thrombosis. Vomiting, diarrhoea and protein-losing enteropathy and neurological deterioration can be progressive. Diagnosis is usually made by the age of 2 weeks, when serum caeruloplasmin and copper levels are low. The treatment recommended is parenteral copper up to 600 ng per kg per week.

Vitamin B_{12} deficiency due to transport defects (intrinsic factor deficiency, deficit of transcobalamin II, selective vitamin B_{12} malabsorption), ileal resection and Crohn's disease may result in megaloblastic anaemia.

Clinical Diagnosis and Nutritional Management

When malabsorption is suspected, the diagnostic evaluation (**Table 2**) should begin with a complete history including dietary intake, bowel pattern, type and onset of symptoms and family history. On physical examination, weight, height and head circumference for age and weight for height should be measured. Prior growth and weight data are essential for comparison and further decision-making. Body mass and body fat are also useful for follow-up evaluation. Inspection of skin for cutaneous lesions, stigmata of liver disease and thorough examination of lungs, heart, abdomen, and perianal and rectal areas are important.

Stool studies are fundamental, including looking for occult blood and leucocytes (which suggest an inflammatory or infectious process), bacterial culture, ova and parasites and *Giardia* antigen. A sweat chloride test should be ordered if cystic fibrosis is suspected.

A complete blood count and smear are helpful in evaluating for the chronic anaemia of inflammatory bowel disease, neutropenia of Shwachman–Diamond–Oski syndrome, and lymphopenia of intestinal lymphangiectasia. The erythrocyte sedimentation rate may be elevated in Crohn's disease. Blood chemistry analysis will be useful in assessing protein

Table 2   Diagnosis of malabsorption

General
1. History (including ethnic origin, family history, dietary history)
2. Physical examination
3. Growth chart
4. Screening laboratory tests:
   Complete blood count with differential sedimentation rate
   Electrolytes, total protein, albumin, alanine aminotransferase, γ-glutamic transpeptidase, calcium, phosphorus and cholesterol
   Stool culture, ova and parasites, leucocytes, *Giardia*
   Antigliadin antibodies

Fat malabsorption
1. Stool fat collection vs qualitative stain
2. Fat-soluble vitamin levels (A, D, E), prothrombin time
3. Sweat chloride
4. Serum bile acids

Carbohydrate malabsorption
1. Stool pH, reducing substances
2. Hydrogen breath test
3. Small bowel biopsy for mucosal enzyme determinations

Protein malabsorption
1. Stool α_1-antitrypsin levels
2. Upper gastrointestinal endoscopy with biopsies

status, liver and biliary function, and pancreatic inflammation.

Serum immunoglobulin A (IgA) and IgA antigliadin and IgA antiendomyseal antibodies should be evaluated if there is clinical suspicion of coeliac disease. Small bowel and colonic endoscopy and biopsies are helpful in investigating mucosal infections, allergic and inflammatory bowel conditions.

In general, the management of secondary malabsorption should be geared to that of the primary condition. Specific malabsorptive conditions and their diagnostic and nutritional management are discussed below.

Fat malabsorption

Symptoms and signs of fat malabsorption include fatty, foul-smelling stools that float in the toilet bowl, weight loss or failure to thrive, and deficiencies of fat-soluble vitamins A, D, E and K. Vitamin A malabsorption results in night blindness and xerophthalmia. Vitamin D deficiency results in osteoporosis and osteomalacia leading to bone fractures. Hypocalcaemia may result in tetany with Trousseau's or Chvostek's signs. Vitamin E deficiency results in neuromuscular complications and vitamin K deficiency involves coagulation defects due to decreased synthesis of the vitamin K-dependent coagulation factors and prolongation of the prothrombin time (PT).

Helpful laboratory investigations include a complete blood count, PT and a 72 h faecal fat collection. Excretion of more than 7 g or 90% of ingested fat represents malabsorption. The level of steatorrhoea depends on the underlying condition. Qualitative stool analysis can be done at the clinic, where a small amount of stool is examined under the microscope. Staining with Sudan III shows the presence of fat droplets. A sweat chloride test should be ordered to evaluate for cystic fibrosis.

Treatment depends on the underlying disease. The presence of steatorrhoea *per se* should not lead to limitation of fat in the diet, which can severely curtail energy intake and lead to malnutrition. Pancreatic replacement therapy with meals in a dosage of 500–1500 units of lipase per kilogram is recommended in patients with cystic fibrosis, and other causes of chronic pancreatitis. Doses in excess of 2000 u kg^{-1} may result in colonic strictures. Use of MCT oil in the diet will enhance fat absorption. Nutritional supplementation either orally or via a nasogastric or gastrostomy tube with high-energy formulae containing hydrolysed protein and MCT oil can improve nutritional status and pulmonary disease in patients with cystic fibrosis. Therefore, gastric acid suppression therapy with antacids and H$_2$ blocking

agents which may enhance pancreatic enzyme activity by increasing duodenal pH, and supplementation with vitamins A, D, E and K and monitoring of vitamin levels, are recommended.

Coeliac disease which often results in steatorrhoea is managed with a gluten-free diet for life.

Carbohydrate malabsorption

Mild or severe symptoms of carbohydrate malabsorption may result with the introduction of the offending sugar in the diet. Thus, a history of ingestion of specific sugars, lactose, fructose and sorbitol-containing foods may be helpful. However, since symptoms of intestinal fermentation may occur many hours after ingestion, the association between ingestion and symptomatology may be difficult.

Specific disaccharidase deficiencies can be detected by measuring the levels of the suspected enzyme on a small bowel biopsy. However, this method is invasive and does not reflect the hydrolytic capacity of the entire intestinal mucosa. The most practical and noninvasive tests that are used routinely are stool tests and the breath hydrogen test.

Reducing substances can be detected in the stool after ingestion of the offending sugar (other than sucrose, which is not a reducing sugar) using copper sulfate tablets (Clinitest). A stool pH (tested by nitrazine paper) of less than 5.5 reflects high production of SCFAs from fermentation.

The breath hydrogen test measures the hydrogen excreted in the breath from the portal circulation after its production in the colon by bacterial fermentation of sugars. After an overnight fast, breath samples are obtained at baseline and at 30 min intervals for a minimum of 3 h after the ingestion of the tested sugar in aqueous solution. The most commonly used dose is 2 g kg^{-1} (to a maximum of 50 g) in a 20% solution. The analysis of breath hydrogen samples is accomplished via gas chromatography. A rise of more than 20 parts per million above the baseline indicates a positive test. Many sugars may be tested, such as glucose, lactose, sucrose, fructose and galactose. To avoid a false positive test, ingestion of a protein meal (meat) and an easily fermentable carbohydrate (rice) prior to the morning of the test is recommended. Foods high in fibre and complex fermentable sugars should be avoided. False negative tests may occur after use of antibiotics or result from the existence of non-hydrogen-producing flora, which is rather rare. In general, the treatment of carbohydrate malabsorption requires restriction or elimination of the offending sugar. In children, drinking excessive amounts of juice result in chronic nonspecific diarrhoea and recurrent abdominal pain.

Restriction of juice intake improves symptoms. **Table 3** lists the average sugar content of certain fruits.

In patients with adult-onset lactase deficiency, abdominal pain, bloating, borborygmus and diarrhoea can develop shortly after drinking milk. However, expression of symptoms varies among different lactose malabsorbers and is clearly dose-dependent. Diagnosis is achieved with the lactose breath hydrogen test. Management of lactose intolerance can be accomplished simply by limiting the amount of lactose in the diet. However, in certain populations limitation of lactose-containing dairy products will decrease calcium and vitamin D intake. Other strategies include taking daily products in small doses, with other foods, or as fermented milk products. Many individuals tolerate milk or dairy products with minimal or no symptoms. Overall, digested or fermented milk products, such as yogurt, cultured buttermilk and curds are better tolerated. The fermentation of milk products causes a decrease in the lactose content, and the addition of culture organisms such as *Lactobacillus acidophilus* and *Streptococcus thermophilus* which have lactase activity results in better lactose digestion. Also, the addition of lactase derived from yeast and fungi to commercial milk products or taking oral lactase drops or tablets prior to meals results in better tolerance of lactose.

Infants with congenital lactase deficiency are managed using formulae that contain glucose polymers. Healthy infants with lactose malabsorption secondary to acute gastroenteritis with transient carbohydrate intolerance may benefit from a lactose-free formula for 1–2 weeks until the lactase activity is restored. Older children may be managed by simple restriction of dairy products and high-fructose juices. Breast-fed infants seem better able to tolerate the decrease in lactase activity following gastroenteritis and may be continued on breast milk, with the addition of oral electrolyte rehydration solutions when needed for correction of dehydration.

In GGM, the diagnosis is established by the breath hydrogen test after an oral load of glucose or galactose. Since the only sugar tolerated is fructose, formulae containing glucose and galactose should be avoided. In the neonatal period a glucose-free, galactose-free formula supplemented with iron and vitamins should be given.

In sucrase-isomaltase deficiency, symptoms begin with the introduction of fruit in the diet of previously lactose-fed infants. Symptoms may range from mild to severe diarrhoea depending on the amount of sugar salvaged by colonic bacteria. Therefore, the diagnosis may be missed in children with chronic diarrhoea and normal growth and development. The sucrose hydrogen breath test demonstrates excessive hydrogen excretion in the breath. Treatment in infancy involves the elimination of sucrose, glucose polymers and starch from the diet, including sugars found in medications and syrups. However, by 2–3 years of age starch restriction may be discontinued.

The expression of symptoms in fructose intolerance varies between individuals in the population. Treatment consists simply of decreasing fructose ingestion. Up to 70% of adults have been shown to malabsorb a dose of 50 g of fructose, whereas others develop symptoms with 25 g, the amount of fructose found in 330 ml of a standard carbonated soft drink.

Small bowel bacterial overgrowth syndrome may present with chronic and occasionally explosive diarrhoea, steatorrhoea, abdominal distension and pain, anaemia, weight loss, growth failure, and hypoalbuminaemia. Glucose breath hydrogen tests are used for detection of small bowel overgrowth; a high baseline fasting concentration with an early rise in the first 30 min following sugar ingestion is particularly suggestive of small bowel overgrowth. Duodenal fluid aspiration for aerobic and anaerobic bacterial quantitation and cultures are also helpful but more invasive. Treatment involves the use of oral antibiotics such as oral metronidazole or aminoglycosides in order to reduce bacteria and decrease fermentation by-products.

Protein malabsorption

Protein-losing enteropathy presents with hypoalbuminaemia, anaemia and failure to thrive. The faecal protein loss may be measured by the stool α_1-antitrypsin content. Treatment is geared toward the underlying disease. Intestinal lymphangiectasia is treated with bypassing the intestinal lacteal system by administering MCT oil and limiting the ingestion of LCTs. Eosinophilic gastroenteritis will respond to steroids, whereas Ménétrier's disease is usually self-

Table 3 Average sugar content of selected fruits. The absorptive capacity of fructose is dose-dependent, unless administered with glucose, in which case its absorption is enhanced owing to the glucose-fructose cotransport mechanism. The ingestion of foods, fruits or juices containing equivalent amounts of glucose and fructose (orange and white grape) is better tolerated than those in which fructose content is three times that of glucose (apple, pear)

	Sugar content per 100 g edible portion			
Fruit	Fructose (g)	Glucose (g)	Sucrose (g)	Sorbitol (g)
Apple	6.2	2.7	1.2	0.5
Pear	6.4	2.3	0.0	2.0
White grape	7.5	7.1	0.0	0.0
Orange	2.4	2.4	4.7	0.0

limiting. Supportive care is needed, with intravenous albumin administration in the symptomatic hospitalized patient presenting with severe hypoproteinaemia, abdominal ascites and pleural effusions.

As a general rule, the management of any malabsorptive disorder involves the maintenance of adequate fluid and electrolyte balance as well as an adequate delivery of energy, protein and all essential nutrients so as to maintain a positive nitrogen balance, and adequate weight gain and body composition. In children, the maintenance of adequate growth and development, and the avoidance of subclinical or overt malnutrition is paramount. In situations where the degree of absorption is negligible or where intestinal purging is excessive or intolerable, and weight maintenance (or normal growth in a child) cannot be maintained, parenteral nutrition may be indicated. Intravenous delivery of nutrition is mandatory to maintain body mass. Initially, in cases of severe malabsorption such as short bowel syndrome, the parenteral route will be necessary to maintain hydration and electrolyte balance.

Protein delivery enterally or orally rarely contributes to a significant degree of purging or intolerance. Steatorrhoea when marked can contribute to the volume of stools, but only in a moderate measure. In general, steatorrhoea should not be a reason for drastically decreasing fat in the oral or enterally delivered diet. Use of pancreatic enzymes (if there is pancreatic deficiency) or MCT oil in the diet or enteral formulae is recommended. Carbohydrate malabsorption, on the other hand, can dramatically contribute to stool volume, fluidity and electrolyte loss, owing to its significant osmotic effect. The amount of carbohydrate tolerated can be titrated gradually depending on the severity and progression of the malabsorptive condition. Severe protein malabsorption can be managed using protein hydrolysates or in severe cases amino acid-based formulaes. Maintenance of adequate protein intake, adequate or high-fat intake with a relatively low carbohydrate intake is preferable and generally recommended, particularly in infants and children.

As far as possible dietary modifications should be given orally. When adequate intake is not possible orally, enteral feedings via a nasogastric, gastrostomy or jejunostomy tube may be necessary, depending on the individual circumstances. Tube feedings may be indicated where the delivery of unpalatable formulae such as protein hydrolysates or amino acid formulae is necessary in a protein malabsorptive or allergic condition. Additionally, the delivery of feedings via a continuous drip may facilitate the absorption of nutrients, particularly in individuals with severe malabsorption and chronic diarrhoea. Slow delivery over a long period rather than as bolus feedings may decrease stool volume, enhance absorption and improve tolerance.

An important argument for oral and enteral therapy is the maintenance of an adequate stimulus for intestinal adaptation and improved tolerance and absorption in those malabsorptive conditions, such as short bowel syndrome, where adequate progression to enteral feedings will be the most important factor in gaining independence from parenterally delivered nutrients.

See also: **Amino Acids**: Metabolism. **Anaemia (Anemia)**: Megaloblastic Anaemia. **Carbohydrates**: Regulation of Carbohydrate Metabolism; Requirements and Dietary Importance. **Cobalamins**: Physiology, Dietary Sources and Requirements. **Lipids**: Chemistry and Classification. **Protein**: Digestion and Bioavailability; Requirements and Role in Diet.

Further Reading

Forstner G, Sherman P and Lichtman S (1991) Bacterial overgrowth. In: Walker WA, Durie PR, Hamilton JR, Walker-Smith JA and Watkins JB (eds) *Pediatric Gastroenteral Disease: Pathogenesis, Diagnosis and Management*, pp 812–818. Philadelphia: Decker.

Georgeson KE and Breaux CW (1992) Outcome and intestinal adaptation in neonatal short bowel syndrome. *Journal of Pediatric Surgery*, 27:344–350.

Kien CL, Heitlinger LA, Li BU et al (1989) Digestion, absorption, and fermentation of carbohydrates. *Seminars in Perinatology* 13:78–87.

Lerner A, Branski D and Lebenthal E (1996) Pancreatic diseases in children. *Pediatric Clinics of North America* 43(1):125–156.

Levine JJ, Seidman E and Walker WA (1987) Screening tests for enteropathy in children. *American Journal of Diseases of Children* 141:435–438.

Riley SA and Turnberg LA (1993) Maldigestion and malabsorption. In: Sleisenger MH and Fordtran JS (eds) *Gastrointestinal Disease: Pathophysiology, Diagnosis, Management*, 5th edn, vol. 2, pp 1009–1027. Philadelphia: WB Saunders.

Rosensweig JN and Perman JA (1994) Malabsorption syndromes and celiac disease. *Seminars in Gastrointestinal Disease* 5(2):78–87.

Saavedra JM and Perman JA (1989) Current concepts in lactose malabsorption and intolerance. *Annual Review of Nutrition* 9:475–502.

Shalon LB and Adelson JW (1996) Cystic fibrosis: gastrointestinal complications and gene therapy. *Pediatric Clinics of North America* 43(1):157–196.

Southgate DAT (1995) Digestion and metabolism of sugars. *American Journas of Clinical Nutrition* 62(supplement):2035–2115.

Troncone R, Greco L and Auricchio S (1996) Gluten-sensitive enteropathy. *Pediatric Clinics of North America* 43(2):355–373.

MALNUTRITION

Contents

Definition, Classification and Epidemiology

P S Shetty, London School of Hygiene and Tropical Medicine, London, UK

Copyright © 1998 Academic Press

The causes of malnutrition are multidimensional and its determinants, which include both food and non-food-related factors, often interact to form a complex web of biological, socioeconomic, cultural and environmental deprivations in developing countries. Childhood malnutrition is associated with chronic food deficiencies largely resulting from social, political and economic factors, and responds over the short term to variations in food supply due to seasonal and climatic changes. Although establishing a relationship between these variables and the indicators of childhood malnutrition do not necessarily imply causality, they do demonstrate that, in addition to food availability, many social, cultural, health and environmental factors influence the prevalence of malnutrition. Malnutrition is thus more than a problem of poverty or inadequate food supply. Although, in general, people suffering from inadequacy of food are poor, not all the poor are undernourished. Even in households that are food secure, some of its members may be undernourished. Income fluctuations, seasonal disparities in food availability and demand for high levels of physical activity and proximity and access to marketing facilities may singly, or in combination, influence nutrition. For example, the transition from subsistence farming to commercial agriculture and cash crops may help improve nutrition in the long run; however, they may even result in negative impacts over the short term unless accompanied by improvements in access to health services, environmental sanitation and other social investments. Rapid urbanization and rural to urban migration may lead to nutritional deprivation of segments of society. Cultural attitudes reflected in food preferences and food preparation practices, and women's time constraints including that available for child-rearing practices, influence the nutrition of the most vulnerable, i.e. the women and children. Inadequate housing and overcrowding, poor sanitation and lack of access to protected water supply, through their links with infectious diseases and infestations, are potent environmental factors that influence biological food utilization and nutrition. Inadequate access to food, limited access to health care and a clean environment and insufficient access to educational opportunities are in turn determined by the economic and institutional structures, as well as the political and ideological superstructures within society.

Poor nutritional status of populations affects physical growth, intelligence, behaviour and learning abilities of children and adolescents. It impacts on their physical and work performance and has been linked to impaired economic work productivity during adulthood. Inadequate nutrition predisposes to infections and contributes to the negative downward spiral of malnutrition and infection. Good nutritional status, however, promotes optimal growth and development of children and adolescents. It contributes to better physiological work performance, enhances adult economic productivity, increases levels of socially desirable activities and promotes better maternal birth outcomes. Good nutrition of a population manifested in the nutritional status of the individual in the community contributes to an upward positive spiral and reflects the improvement in the resources and human capital of society.

Malnutrition: Definitions

Malnutrition refers to all deviations from adequate nutrition; it includes both undernutrition and overnutrition, resulting from inadequacy of food or excess of food relative to need, respectively. Malnutrition encompasses specific deficiencies or excesses of essential nutrients such as vitamins and minerals. Conditions such as obesity, though not the result of inadequacy of food, also constitute malnutrition. The terms 'malnutrition' and 'undernutrition' are often used loosely and interchangeably, although a distinction exists and needs to be made.

Malnutrition arises from deficiencies of specific nutrients, or from diets based on wrong kinds or proportions of foods. Goitre, scurvy, anaemia and xerophthalmia are forms of malnutrition, caused by inadequate intake of iodine, vitamin C, iron and vitamin A, respectively.

Undernutrition is the result of insufficient food, of whatever kind, caused primarily by an inadequate intake of dietary or food energy, whether or not any specific nutrient is an additional limiting factor. Undernutrition is defined having a dietary energy intake below the minimum level required to maintain the balance between actual energy intake and acceptable levels of energy expenditure, while taking into account the additional needs in children for growth, and in pregnant and lactating women for maintaining appropriate weight gain associated with fetal growth in pregnancy and sustaining adequate milk production during lactation, respectively. This emphasis on dietary energy as a general measurement of food adequacy seems pragmatically justified: increased dietary energy, if derived from normal staple foods, brings with it more protein and other nutrients, while raising intakes of such nutrients without providing more dietary energy is unlikely to be of much benefit to the individual. Thus, in most situations, increased dietary energy is a necessary condition for nutritional improvement, even if it is not always sufficient in itself.

Malnutrition or undernutrition are terms generally used interchangeably to mean more or less the same thing and refer to nutritional situations characteristic of relatively poorer socioeconomic populations in countries generally considered as belonging to the 'low income' economic groups of developing countries. In practice, the population groups in a developing country suffering from malnutrition or undernutrition as defined in this way are likely to be more or less the same. Although it is possible to arrive at the prevalence (per cent) and the numbers of individuals within a population manifesting signs of specific nutrient deficiency, for instance anaemia as a result of iron deficiency, where signs of vitamin or mineral deficiencies are observed, they are almost always associated with marginal or low dietary energy intakes. The term 'malnutrition' is often used in the broader sense, referring to any physical condition implying ill-health or the inability to maintain adequate growth, appropriate body weight and body composition, or to sustain acceptable levels of economically necessary and socially desirable physical activities, brought about by an inadequacy in food –

both quantity and quality. It thus includes both undernutrition and specific nutrient deficiencies.

Malnutrition: Classification

In order to arrive at reliable estimates in the population, both children and adults, who are malnourished or undernourished, we need reliable but inexpensive techniques to assess the nature of the food shortages and diagnose and categorize the degree of severity of the problem in the community. One generally assesses the nutritional status of the individual in the community using anthropometric characteristics to determine whether the individual appears to be undernourished or not. These methods are more reliable than estimates of how much and what types of food an individual is eating and how adequate they are in terms of the individual's requirements. Thus the most common and reliable measurements of nutritional status are based on growth in children and body weight changes in adults.

Childhood malnutrition

Childhood malnutrition is characterized by growth failure, resulting in a body weight which is less than ideal for the child's age. Hence, in children, assessment of growth has been the single most important measurement that best defines their health and nutritional status. Measures of height and weight are therefore the commonly used indicators of the nutritional status of the child. Classification of childhood malnutrition based on height, weight and age thus continues to be the backbone of nutritional assessment methods for both population and individual assessments.

There are several different classifications of nutritional status in children. According to a WHO Working Group (1986), appropriate *height for age* of a child reflects its linear growth and can measure long-term growth faltering or 'stunting', while appropriate weight for height reflects proper body proportion or the harmony of growth. *Weight for height* is particularly sensitive to acute growth disturbances and is useful to detect the presence of 'wasting'. *Weight for age* represents a convenient synthesis of both linear growth and body proportion and can thus be used for the diagnosis of 'underweight' children. The presence of malnutrition in children is diagnosed using these anthropometric parameters by comparing them with internationally accepted reference standards. If a child has a low weight for age, i.e. below two standard deviations (−2 SD) of the reference population, then such a child is categorized as *stunted*. Similarly a low weight for age is diagnostic of an *underweight* child, while a low weight for height is indicative of *wasting* (**Table 1**). The international 'reference' standard has to be carefully chosen since there is need for universal agreement for what is considered to be an ideal weight or height for a child at any age. In practice, the 50th centiles of the National Centre for Health Statistics (NCHS) values collected for US children between birth and 18 years are used as the reference values. There is increasing evidence of the appropriateness of the NCHS reference values since the growth patterns of well-nourished, uninfected children in the developing world have been shown to be broadly similar to the NCHS data. These standards have now been accepted by the World Health Organization (WHO) as international reference standards.

Adolescent undernutrition

Adolescents comprise a significant proportion of the world's population – some estimates put the numbers of youth at close to 30% of the world population. The proportion of adolescents within a population group is also rising relative to other age groups and an overwhelming proportion of young adolescents live in developing countries. Increases in height as well as weight occur during adolescence. About 25% of an individual's attained height is achieved during adolescence as a result of the adolescent growth spurt and this period marks the end of the growth in height. Variations in adolescent body size and the timing of maturational events is determined genetically in populations whose environment allows full expression of the genotype. Where there are significant environmental constraints including inadequate nutrition, the observed growth and maturation during adolescence reflects environmental rather than inherited growth potential. Although growth differences during adolescence may be attributable to variations in maturational timing, it is clear that growth differences among groups are related to nutritional status, socioeconomic and other factors. Growth in

adolescence may be limited by prolonged undernutrition, infections and chronic disease. *Stunting*, or short stature, in adolescence is not only indicative of past undernutrition during childhood, but is also a cumulative indicator of nutritional status during adolescence. The diagnostic criteria recommended by WHO (1995) for defining *stunting* in adolescents is height for age less than the third percentile of the NCHS/WHO reference data, or below two standard deviations (-2 SD) of the reference population. Undernutrition of thinness in adolescence is said to be indicated by a *body mass index* (BMI, weight in kilograms divided by the square of the height in metres) less than the 5th percentile of the NCHS/WHO reference data. A BMI for age greater than the 85th percentile in adolescence is considered as indicative of risk of overweight.

Adult undernutrition

The simplest way of diagnosing undernutrition in adults, as recommended by the International Dietary Energy Consultancy Group (IDECG) Working Party (1988), is to use the body mass index. This recommendation was based on the observation that BMI was consistently highly correlated with body weight (a proxy for the available energy stores within the body) and was relatively independent of the height of the individual. The appropriate cutoff points suggested were that adults with a BMI of less than 18.5 be considered to be chronically undernourished, with the same criteria being applicable to both males and females. The use of the BMI also enabled categorization or grading of the severity of malnutrition in the adult (Table 1). This definition of chronic undernutrition in adults, using cutoff criteria based on BMI, has been shown to be not only a sensitive and specific index of adult nutritional status, but has also been demonstrated to be responsive to variations in socioeconomic status, dietary intakes and seasonal fluctuations in the availability of food in the community.

Undernutrition in the elderly

Adults aged 60 years of age and older represent the fastest growing segment of populations throughout the world. Decline in height with age is well documented in the elderly. Reduction in weight also occurs with increasing age, although the pattern of change in weight is quite different from that of height and varies with the sex of the individual. The use of anthropometry is relatively recent in the elderly and the anthropometric index of choice is BMI, as for younger adults. Thus height, weight and BMI are good indicators of nutritional status and risk of morbidity and mortality in the elderly population.

Table 1 Diagnostic criteria for malnutrition in children and adults

Childhood malnutrition	
Underweight	Low weight for age[a]
Stunted	Low height for age[a]
Wasted	Low weight for height[a]
Adult undernutrition	
Grade I	BMI 17.0–18.49
Grade II	BMI 16.0–16.99
Grade III	BMI < 16.0

[a]Low is defined as below -2 SD (Z score) of NCHS/WHO reference for age.

Measurement of height can be a problem with the elderly as a result of increasing spinal curvature with age. There are no guidelines regarding the degree of spinal curvature that would invalidate the measurement of height. Height can be estimated preferably from knee height or from arm span in the elderly. The WHO (1995) recommends knee height as being more satisfactory than arm span, and the estimated height can then be used to derive BMIs. The same BMI categories as for younger adults, i.e. a BMI less than 18.5 indicating underweight and a BMI greater than 25 indicating overweight, is currently recommended for the elderly.

Epidemiology of Malnutrition Globally

The WHO global database on child growth has been used to determine the worldwide distribution and magnitude of malnutrition in pre-school children (**Table 2**). This WHO analysis was restricted to nationally representative surveys from developing countries in Asia, Africa, Latin America and Oceania, where the proportion of children covered by these national surveys was >70 or 80% and was obtained between 1990 and 1992. Estimates of under 5-year-old preschool children in these countries were based on data for 1990 obtained from the United Nations Population Division. The numbers of underweight, stunted and wasted children in each geographical region was obtained by applying prevalence estimates to the total population under 5 years old in 1990. This careful analysis of a global database suggests that undernutrition is still very common among preschool children, manifested largely as stunting rather than wasting. It indicates that Latin American countries have low to moderate prevalence of underweight children while countries in Asia have a high or very high prevalence; Africa, on the other hand, demonstrates large regional variations. The exceptions of countries in the Latin American region are Honduras, Guatemala, Guyana and Haiti, which have a high to very high prevalence of underweight children. In Southern Asian and Southeast Asian countries (with the exception of Thailand), the prevalence of underweight children is very high. High to very high prevalence of underweight children is observed in Western and Eastern Africa, while North African countries (Algeria, Egypt, Morocco and Tunisia) appear to be similar to Latin American countries with low to moderate prevalence. The distribution of stunting and wasting among preschool children globally resembles that for the prevalence of underweight children, with low prevalence in Latin America, high prevalence in Asia, and a combination of both in Africa. The most favourable scenario with regard to stunting and wasting, demonstrated by a low/moderate prevalence of stunting and a low prevalence of wasting, is typical of countries in Latin America, while the opposite, i.e. a high/very high prevalence of both stunting and wasting seems to be

Table 2 Global and regional estimates of the prevalence and numbers (in millions) of malnourished children in developing countries

Global regions	Underweight (%)	Numbers ($\times 10^6$)	Stunted (%)	Numbers ($\times 10^6$)	Wasted (%)	Numbers ($\times 10^6$)
Asia	**42.0**	**154.1**	**47.1**	**172.8**	**10.8**	**39.6**
South Asia	60.5	101.2	60.3	100.9	17.3	28.9
Southeast Asia	37.8	21.8	43.2	24.9	7.6	4.4
East Asia	21.3	26.0	32.1	39.2	3.6	4.4
Africa	**27.4**	**31.6**	**38.6**	**44.6**	**7.2**	**8.3**
North Africa	11.3	2.4	25.4	5.5	5.8	1.2
West Africa	32.8	12.2	37.9	14.1	9.5	3.5
East Africa	31.0	11.5	47.0	17.5	6.0	2.2
Latin America	**11.9**	**6.5**	**22.2**	**12.1**	**2.7**	**1.5**
Central America	17.7	2.8	29.8	4.8	4.6	0.7
South America	8.4	2.9	18.1	6.4	1.9	0.7
Caribbean	19.4	0.6	25.9	0.9	2.2	0.1
Oceania	**29.1**	**0.3**	**41.9**	**0.4**	**5.6**	**0.1**
Melanesia	29.5	0.2	42.2	0.3	5.5	<0.1
All developing countries	**35.8**	**192.5**	**42.7**	**229.9**	**9.2**	**49.5**

Adapted from *The Sixth World Food Survey* (1996) Rome: FAO. Prevalence of underweight, stunted and wasted children based on % below -2 SDs (*Z* scores) of the WHO/NCHS reference values for weight for age, height for age and weight for height, respectively.

common for most countries in Asia. In Africa, the prevalence of stunting is similar to that in Latin America, while the prevalence of wasting is more like that in Asia.

Representative data on the current status of adolescent nutritional status on a global basis is lacking. However, data on BMIs of adults are now increasingly available as a result of the initiative taken by the Food and Agriculture Organization (FAO) to consider BMI as an alternative and complementary indicator of nutritional status alongside the standard methodology adopted by FAO to assess energy adequacy. **Table 3** summarizes some of the available data based on nationally representative surveys from different countries of the developing world in different geographical regions. In general, Latin American countries reflect the trends seen in childhood malnutrition; the percentage of individuals with lower than acceptable levels of BMI is small, while there is an increasing tendency for adults to have BMIs greater than 25.0. In Africa, the proportion of individuals undernourished is greater in Sahelian countries than in tropical or subtropical areas. Data on BMI of adults in Asia, in particular South Asia, show that large proportions of their populations have BMIs below 18.5; the proportion varied from 12.5% in China to 48.6% in India in 1989–90. With the use of BMI it is also possible to examine the increasing problem of overweight and obesity among populations.

The problem of overweight and obesity, which is considered as overnutrition or malnutrition, is increasing rapidly on a global basis. Developed, industrialized countries have been showing increasing trends in the prevalence of obesity for several decades, while developing countries are now showing a rise in overweight and obesity among their populations together with economic development and urbanization. The prevalence of obesity (BMI > 30.0) is high in the USA among all ethnic groups (Whites, Blacks, Hispanics and native Americans). Obesity is also relatively common in Europe, especially among women, particularly in Southern and Eastern Europe. Apart from the Netherlands, where the prevalence of obesity has remained stable for some time, in most other countries in Europe the trends are indicative of an increase in obesity in the adult population. Overweight and obesity among children is also on the increase in the Western world. However, the problem of adult and childhood obesity is not confined to the developed world. In several countries of the developing world increasing rates of obesity are already evident (Table 3). The prevalence is highly variable between developing countries and within populations of the same country, although in general the prevalence is higher in women than in men.

See also: **Adolescents**: Dietary Habits and Nutrient Requirements. **Children**: Nutritional Requirements of

Table 3 Prevalence of adult undernutrition and overnutrition assessed by nutritional anthropometry in selected country surveys

Location	BMI categories					
	<16.00	16.00–16.99	17.00–18.49	18.50–24.99	25.00–29.99	≥30.00
Africa						
Congo (women)	0.6	1.8	8.7	73.7	11.8	3.4
Ghana	2.8	3.9	13.3	62.0	17.1	0.9
Ghana (women)	0.8	1.7	8.7	75.9	9.7	3.2
Kenya (women)	0.5	1.3	7.4	76.8	11.5	2.4
Mali	1.9	3.2	11.2	76.5	6.4	0.8
Morocco	0.5	1.1	5.4	69.1	18.7	5.2
Morocco (women)	0.3	0.5	2.8	62.0	23.3	11.1
Senegal	1.4	2.0	10.2	70.4	12.2	3.7
Tunisia	0.3	0.6	3.0	58.9	28.6	8.6
Zambia (women)	0.0	1.1	6.0	70.3	16.9	5.7
Americas						
Brazil	0.5	0.9	4.2	61.7	25.1	8.6
Cuba	0.6	1.3	5.4	56.3	26.9	9.5
Peru	0.2	0.2	2.6	63.2	24.8	9.0
Asia						
China	1.0	3.9	7.4	79.5	7.2	1.0
India	10.2	12.7	25.7	47.9	3.0	0.5
Laos	1.6	2.9	11.4	76.9	6.5	0.7

Adapted from *The Sixth World Food Survey* (1996) Rome: FAO.

School Children. **Lactation**: Dietary Requirements. **Malnutrition**: Primary Malnutrition; Secondary Malnutrition. **Nutritional Status**: Dietary Assessment; Anthropometric Assessment. **Obesity**: Definition, Aetiology and Assessment. **Older People**: Nutritional Requirements.

Further Reading

de Onis M, Monteiro C, Akre J and Clugston G (1993) The worldwide magnitude of protein energy malnutrition: an overview from the WHO global database on child growth. *Bulletin of the World Health Organization* 71:703–712.

James WPT, Ferro-Luzzi A and Waterlow JC (1988) Definition of Chronic Energy Deficiency in Adults, Report of a Working Party of IDECG. *European Journal of Clinical Nutrition* 42:969–981.

Shetty PS and James WPT (1994) *Body Mass Index: A Measure of Chronic Energy Deficiency in Adults*, Food & Nutrition Paper 56. Rome: Food & Agriculture Organization.

WHO (1995) *Physical Status: The Use and Interpretation of Anthropometry*, Technical Report. Geneva: World Health Organization.

Primary Malnutrition

M de Onis and **G A Clugston**, World Health Organization, Geneva, Switzerland

B Underwood, Food and Nutrition Board, Washington DC, USA

Copyright © 1998 Academic Press

The term primary malnutrition, decreased intake of nutrients, is used to refer to a number of diseases, each with a specific cause related to one or more nutrients (e.g. protein, iodine or iron) and each characterized by cellular imbalance between the supply of nutrients and energy on the one hand, and the body's demand for them to ensure growth, maintenance and specific functions on the other. This imbalance can be seen, among others, in situations such as famine; extreme poverty; food faddism; dietary taboos; anorexia, bulimia and adolescent fear of obesity; and low nutrient density diets.

Primary malnutrition in its many forms persists in virtually all countries worldwide in spite of the general improvement in food supplies and health conditions and in the availability of educational and social services. This article focuses on the prevalence, dietary management and prevention of protein–energy malnutrition, a multideficiency state that includes a range of conditions. Other deficiencies of certain nutrients which still plague the world as public health problems, such as iron, iodine and vitamin A deficiencies, are dealt with in separate articles.

Prevalence

The term protein–energy malnutrition (PEM) is used to describe a range of disorders primarily characterized by growth failure or retardation in children. Although PEM and its causes were first recognized early in the twentieth century, with the pioneering work of Cecile Williams in the 1930s, it has only been in the recent decades that a realistic notion has begun to emerge regarding both the spectrum of disability and the vast global dimensions of those affected. Infants and young children are the most severely affected because of their high energy and protein needs and their particular vulnerability to infection. In fact, almost all of the growth retardation documented in studies conducted in developing countries has its origins in the first 2 or 3 years of life. Once present, it remains for life.

The most severe clinical forms of PEM are marasmus, kwashiorkor and marasmic kwashiorkor. In practice, the distinction between these clinical forms is essentially qualitative. However, only 1–2% of the world's children exhibit visible signs of malnutrition. For the majority of affected children the assessment of 'subclinical' PEM or growth impairment in the community must be quantitative and is usually based on weight and height measurements. The most commonly used anthropometric indexes for assessing child growth are weight-for-height, a measure of wasting or thinness, height-for-age, a measure of stunting, and weight-for-age, which is referred to as a measure of 'undernutrition'.

It is estimated that about 170 million children aged under 5 in the developing world are underweight for age (weight-for-age below -2 standard deviations (SD) from the international reference median value), while 206 million are stunted (height-for-age below -2 SD from the international reference median value). The prevalence of protein–energy malnutrition in children under 5 years of age in developing countries worldwide has progressively fallen from 42.6% in 1975 to 31.3% in 1995 (**Table 1**). However, in some regions this fall in percentage prevalence has not been as rapid as the rise in population. The result is that in some regions – such as Africa and Southeast Asia – the actual number of malnourished children has in fact risen. A total of 76% of the world's malnourished children live in Asia (mainly in southern Asia), while 21% are found in Africa and 3% in Latin America. **Fig. 1** presents

Table 1 Global and regional trends in prevalence and absolute numbers of underweight children below 5 years of age

	Prevalence of underweight[a] children (%)				
Region	1975	1980	1985	1990	1995
Africa	30.4 (22.9)[b]	28.0 (24.1)	28.0 (27.9)	26.0 (28.7)	28.4 (34.7)
Asia	47.8 (164.6)	47.0 (150.6)	44.0 (152.9)	37.2 (141.6)	35.6 (129.2)
Latin America	15.6 (7.5)	13.6 (6.9)	12.4 (6.7)	11.4 (6.2)	9.5 (5.2)
Developing countries	42.6 (195.6)	40.4 (181.5)	37.9 (187.5)	32.3 (176.7)	31.3 (169.2)
Global	36.4 (198.6)	34.0 (183.5)	32.5 (188.5)	28.5 (177.6)	27.8 (169.8)

From *WHO Global Database on Child Growth and Malnutrition*, 1997.
[a]Weight-for-age below −2 SD from the international reference median value.
[b]Figures in parentheses are millions of children.

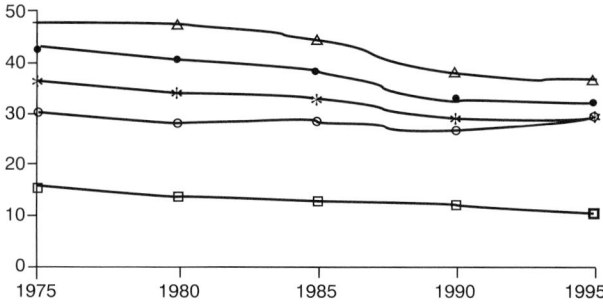

Figure 1 Prevalence trends in underweight children below 5 years of age. Key: ○, Africa; △, Asia; □, Latin America; ●, developing countries; *, all countries. From *WHO Global Database on Child Growth and Malnutrition*, 1997.

trends in prevalence of underweight children from 1975 to date.

Fig. 2 shows the geographical distribution of developing countries according to the prevalence of underweight children based on national data. Prevalences are grouped in four categories that correspond to low, medium, high and very high prevalences. Most countries in Latin America have low or moderate prevalences of underweight children, while most countries in Asia have high or very high prevalences. In Africa, low and moderate prevalences are found in the north, but the situation in sub-Saharan Africa is very serious, with a global prevalence of about 30%. Overall it is estimated that more than half the young children in south Asia suffer from PEM, which is about five times the prevalence in the Americas, at least three times the prevalence in the Middle East and more than twice that of east Asia.

For the affected children the consequences of this situation are very severe in terms of morbidity, mortality and disability. PEM results in poor physical and cognitive development as well as lower resistance to illness. Out of the 12.2 million deaths among children under 5 in 1993 in developing countries, about 6.6 million – or 54% of young child mor-

tality – were associated with malnutrition (**Fig. 3**). In addition, malnutrition, which has a substantial direct effect on the infections disease burden in its own right, is also the single greatest risk factor for death and disability worldwide: in 1990, malnutrition was estimated to have caused 16% of the global burden of disease, considerably more than occupation, tobacco and alcohol, each estimated to have caused about 3% globally (**Table 2**).

Dietary Management

Feeding recommendations for healthy infants and young children

Child growth retardation occurs primarily at the time of introduction of complementary foods, most commonly during the second 6 months of postnatal life, when foods or drinks other than breast milk are added to the diet. Adequate diet and care are crucial during this period because of the high nutritional requirements of infants and young children. The best way to feed a child from birth to at least 4 months of age is to breast-feed exclusively, which means that the child takes only breast milk and no additional food, water or other fluids (with the exception of medicines and vitamins, if needed). Infants at this age should breast-feed as often as they want, day and night. This should be at least eight times in 24 h.

In general, most babies do not need complementary foods before 6 months of age; however, sometimes between the ages of 4 and 6 months, some infants begin to need foods or drinks in addition to breast milk. These foods are often called complementary or weaning foods because they complement breast milk. The mother should only begin to offer complementary foods if the infant appears hungry after breast-feeding, or is not gaining weight adequately. By 6 months of age, all infants should be receiving safe and nutritionally adequate complementary foods. It is important to continue to

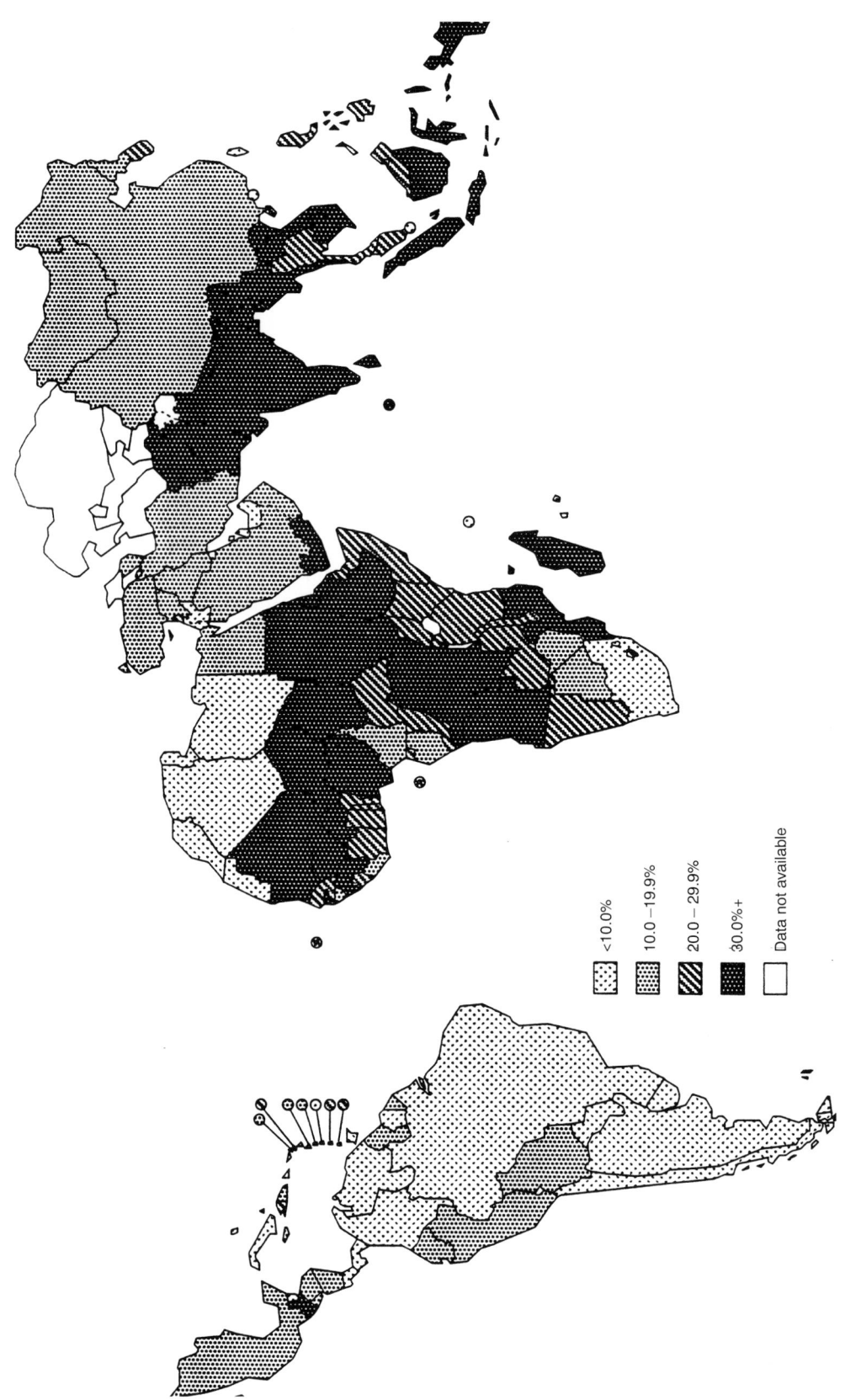

Figure 2 Prevalence of underweight children in developing countries. From *WHO Global Database on Child Growth and Malnutrition*, 1997.

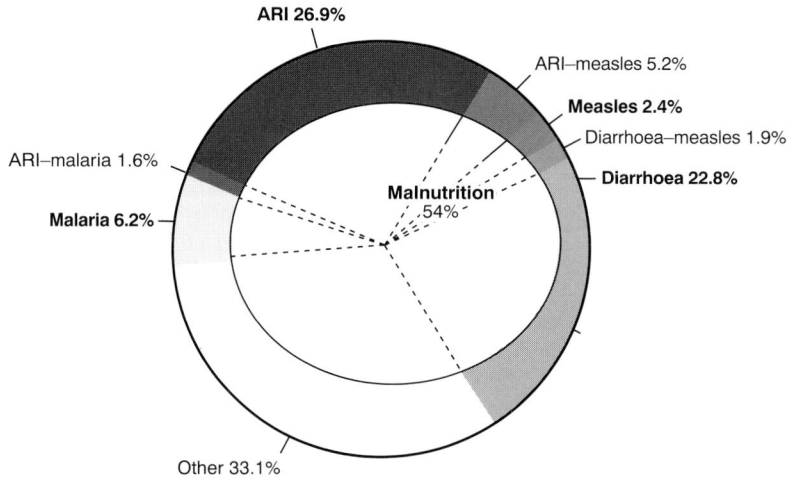

ARI 26.9%

ARI–measles 5.2%

Measles 2.4%

ARI–malaria 1.6%

Diarrhoea–measles 1.9%

Malaria 6.2%

Diarrhoea 22.8%

Malnutrition 54%

Other 33.1%

Figure 3   Distribution of 12.2 million deaths among children less than 5 years old in all developing countries, 1993. Deaths associated with: malnutrition, 54.0%; acute respiratory infections (ARI), 33.7%; diarrhoea, 24.7%; malaria, 7.7%; measles, 9.5%; one or more of these conditions, 71.0%.

Table 2   Risk factor analysis: 1990 deaths and DALYs (disability-adjusted life years) attributable to selected risk factors

Risk factor	Deaths ('000s)	As % total deaths	DALYs ('000s)	As % total DALYs
Drug use	100	0.20	8 389	0.61
Water and sanitation	2 668	5.29	92 531	6.74
Hypertension	2 918	5.78	21 025	1.53
Physical inactivity	973	1.93	13 503	0.98
Malnutrition	5 881	11.65	217 666	15.86
Occupation	1 129	2.24	37 905	2.76
Air pollution	568	1.13	6 624	0.48
Alcohol use	774	1.53	39 603	2.89
Tobacco use	3 013	5.97	35 483	2.59

From *The Global Burden of Disease*, 1996.

breast-feed as often as the child wants; the mother should give the complementary foods 1–2 times daily *after* breast-feeding to avoid replacing breast milk.

From age 6 months up to 12 months, the amount of complementary foods given to the child should be gradually increased; by the age of 12 months, complementary foods should be the main source of energy. If the child is breast-fed, complementary foods should be given three times per day; if not breast-fed, five times per day. Foods that are appropriate will vary from country to country, but in all cases they should be energy-rich, nutrient-rich and locally affordable. In general, a good daily diet should be adequate in quantity and include an energy-rich food, such as thick cereal with added sugar, oil or milk; meat, fish, eggs or pulses; and fruits and vegetables. The flavour, aroma, consistency and variety may affect the intake of complementary foods. If the child receives cow's milk or any other breast milk substitute, these and any other drinks should be given by cup, not by bottle. It is important to feed the child actively until she/he can properly feed herself/himself.

During the second year of life, the child should continue to breast-feed as often as she/he wants, while the variety and quantity of food should be increased (five times a day) and family foods should become an important part of the child's diet. Adequate servings and active feeding (encouraging the child to eat) continue to be important. Children 2 years of age and older should be eating a variety of family foods in three meals per day plus two extra feedings per day. The latter may be family foods or other nutritious snacks which are convenient to give between meals.

Food safety is an essential matter. Each year 1500 million episodes of diarrhoea occur in children below 5 years of age; up to 70% of these are caused by contaminated complementary foods. Sources of contamination are dirty hands, dirty pots and pans, flies, dirty water, cross-contamination during food preparation, as well as storage of cooked food at temperatures that favour bacterial growth. All of these are factors commonly found in poor environments. The control measures are to minimize contamination by using clean utensils and clean (boiled) water and to wash hands, to kill pathogens through proper cooking, to avoid leaving cooked food at ambient temperatures and to cover food.

Feeding recommendations for infants and young children suffering from severe PEM

Treatment phase The treatment of severe PEM involves both intensive medical and nutritional management. **Table 3** outlines ten essential steps in the care of severely malnourished children. During the initial phase, correcting metabolic disturbances as well as infections is crucial. Almost all severely malnourished children are suffering from infection, the most frequent being respiratory tract infections, urinary tract infections, measles, gastrointestinal infections, malaria, skin infections and septicaemia.

Early dietary management of infants and young children suffering from severe PEM should avoid excessive protein and energy intakes. It takes time for the metabolic mechanisms of a severely malnourished child to readjust to food intake. Carefully controlled amounts of protein and energy are therefore needed to avoid overloading the heart, kidney and intestine. Daily consumption of 1–2 g protein per kg body weight and 100 kcal (420 kJ) per kg body weight is recommended. Feeds must be given in small amounts and frequently, throughout the day and night. Mothers should continue to breast-feed, regardless of other foods and treatments.

Two *formula diets* for severely malnourished children are usually recommended. The first, F-75 (75 kcal per 100 ml; 315 kJ per 100 ml) is used during the initial phase of treatment. The second, F-100 (100 kcal per 100 ml; 420 kJ per 100 ml) is used during the rehabilitation phase, after the appetite has

returned. These formulae can be purchased as a powder that is simply mixed with water, or they can be easily made in a hospital kitchen from the basic ingredients: cereal flour, dried skim milk, sugar, oil, *mineral mix* and *vitamin mix* (**Table 4**).

All severely malnourished children have potassium and magnesium deficiencies that adversely affect a number of metabolic functions, including fluid and electrolyte balance. The potassium deficit adversely affects cardiac function and gastric emptying. Magnesium is essential for potassium to enter cells and be retained; in the absence of magnesium, potassium repletion is impaired. Supplements of both these minerals should thus be given routinely. The *mineral mix* described in **Table 5** supplies potassium, magnesium and other essential minerals (e.g. copper and zinc). Multivitamin supplementation is also important for the restoration of depleted tissues. Many malnourished children are deficient in riboflavin, ascorbic acid, pyridoxine, thiamin and the fat-soluble vitamins A, D, E and K. All diets should be fortified with these vitamins by adding the *vitamin mix* (Table 5). Similarly, all severely malnourished children should receive 1 mg per day folic acid orally (5 mg on admission).

In a child with low vitamin A stores PEM predisposes to the development of keratomalacia, which may progress with devastating speed. For this reason vitamin A (200 000 IU) should be given routinely to

Table 4 Composition of liquid diets

(a) F-75 diet

Ingredient	Amount[a]
Dried skim milk	25 g
Cane sugar	60 g
Oil	25 g
Rice flour or other cereal flour	50 g
Mineral mix	20 ml[b]
Vitamin mix	140 mg[c]
Water	to make 1000 ml

(b) F-100 diet

Ingredient	Amount
Dried skim milk	80 g
Cane sugar	50 g
Oil	60 g
Mineral mix	20 ml[b]
Vitamin mix	140 mg[c]
Water	to make 1000 ml

From *WHO* (1998).
[a]Mix milk powder, sugar, oil and flour in 700 ml water. Boil for 5–7 min. Cool, dissolve mineral mix and vitamins, and add water to make 1000 ml.
[b]Or one packet of mineral mix salts per litre.
[c]See Table 5.

Table 3 Ten essential steps in the care of severely malnourished children

1.	Treat/prevent hypoglycaemia (low blood sugar)
2.	Treat/prevent hypothermia (low body temperature)
3.	Treat/prevent dehydration (loss of body fluids)
4.	Correct imbalance of electrolytes (salts in blood and cells)
5.	Treat infection
6.	Correct deficiencies of micronutrients (vitamins and minerals)
7.	Start cautious feeding, *then*
8.	Rebuild wasted tissues (catch-up growth)
9.	Provide stimulation, play and loving care
10.	Prepare for follow-up after hospital discharge

Adapted from Ashworth *et al.* (1996).

Table 5 Composition of mineral and vitamin mixes
(a) Concentrated solution of mineral mix[a]

Ingredient	Amount (g)
Potassium chloride	89.5
Tripotassium citrate	32.4
Magnesium chloride	30.5
Zinc acetate	3.3
Copper sulfate	0.56
Sodium selenate	0.01
Potassium iodide	0.005
Water	to make 1000 ml

(b) Vitamin mix[b]

Vitamin	Amount
Water-soluble	
Thiamin	0.7 mg
Riboflavine	2.0 mg
Niacin	10 mg
Pyridoxine	0.7 mg
Cobalamin	1 μg
Folic acid	0.35 mg
Ascorbic acid	100 mg
Pantothenic acid	3 mg
Biotin	100 μg
Fat-soluble	
Retinol	1.5 mg
Calciferol	30 μg
Tocopherol	22 mg
Vitamin K	40 μg

From WHO (1998).
[a]Twenty (20) ml of the solution should be added to each litre of ReSoMal or liquid feed.
[b]The amounts to be added to 1 l of liquid diet.

Table 7 Typical feeding schedule

Days	Frequency	Vol./kg per feed (ml)	Vol./kg per day (ml)
1–2	2 hourly	11	130
3–5	3 hourly	16	130
6–7+	4 hourly	22	130

is not available. Water-miscible solutions only should be used for intramuscular injections.

It is critical that food be given frequently and in small amounts, day and night, to avoid overloading the intestine, liver and kidney. A typical schedule for feeding is given in **Table 7**. Severely malnourished children have poor appetites when first admitted to hospital. Patience and loving care are needed to ensure the child completes each feed. Feeding bottles should never be used, even in very young infants; the child should be fed from a cup and spoon. It is important that the child is held securely in a sitting position on the attendant's or mother's lap while being fed; under no circumstances should children be left alone in bed to feed themselves. If the child is too weak to eat or if it refuses food, she/he should be fed by continuous nasogastric tube; however, nasogastric feeding should end as soon as possible.

The initial phase of dietary treatment ends when the child becomes hungry. This indicates that infections are coming under control, the liver is able to metabolize the diet, and other metabolic abnormalities are much improved. The child is now ready to begin the rehabilitation phase. This usually occurs after 2–7 days, although it is the child's appetite and general condition that determine the phase of treatment and not the length of time since admission.

Rehabilitation phase A child enters the rehabilitation phase when a good appetite returns. During rehabilitation, for children below 24 months of age F-100 should be given every 3–4 h, night and day (6–8 feeds a day). The amount of diet given at each feed should be increased by 10 ml until the child refuses to finish the feed. Children older than 24 months of

all malnourished children on admission. When clinical signs of vitamin A deficiency are evident, the treatment schedule is given in **Table 6**. Large doses of vitamin A should be given on the first two days with a third dose given before discharge. Oral treatment is preferred except at the beginning in children with severe anorexia, oedematous malnutrition or septic shock. For oral treatment, oil-based preparations are the preferred formulation, but water-miscible formulations may be used if the oily solution

Table 6 Treatment of clinical vitamin A deficiency for children 12 months or older[a]

	Retinyl palmitate	Retinyl acetate	International units
Days 1 and 2	55 mg IM or 110 mg oral	33 mg IM or 66 mg oral	100 000 IU IM[b] or 200 000 IU oral
Discharge	110 mg oral	66 mg oral	200 000 IU oral

From WHO (1998).
IM = intramuscularly.
[a]One-half of the dose should be given to infants aged 6–12 months with xerophthalmia.
[b]Water-miscible preparations *only*.

age can also be treated with increasing quantities of F-100; this has practical value, especially in refugee camps. For most older children, however, it is appropriate to introduce solid food, especially for those wanting a mixed diet. Most traditional mixed diets have a low energy density and are usually deficient in various vitamins and minerals. Thus, local foods should be fortified to increase their content of energy, minerals and vitamins. Oil should be added to increase energy density, and the *mineral and vitamin mixes* used in F-100 should be added after cooking (see Table 5). Other ingredients, such as dried skim milk, may be added to increase protein and mineral content; the mixed diet should contain at least 1 kcal g^{-1} (4.2 kJ g^{-1}). At the beginning of rehabilitation older children should be fed every 4 h, day and night (six times per 24 h); however, as soon as they are growing well, one of the night-time feeds can be omitted.

Nearly all severely malnourished children have anaemia and should be given supplemental folic acid and iron. Iron is never given during the initial phase, but must be added orally to the treatment during the rehabilitation phase (3 mg per kg per day). Similarly, all children must be given folic acid 1 mg per day (5 mg on day 1). The children should also continue throughout rehabilitation to receive the *vitamin* and *mineral mixes* (Table 5) added to their food.

The attitude of those feeding the child is crucial to success. Sufficient time should be allowed for the child to finish each feed and she/he should be actively encouraged to eat while sitting comfortably on the caretaker's lap. During rehabilitation children should take between 150 and 220 kcal per kg per day (630–920 kJ per kg per day); if intake is not at least 130 kcal per kg per day (550 kJ per kg per day), the child is failing to respond. In general, marasmatic children will need higher energy intakes than kwashiorkor cases. F-100 should be continued until the child achieves −1 SD from the reference median weight-for-height value. When this happens the child is ready for the discharge phase of treatment.

Prevention

The causes of chronic malnutrition, the most prevalent form of malnutrition, are deeply rooted in poverty. The prevention of PEM cannot therefore be an isolated objective, separated from more general measures to meet the basic needs of the poor. Understanding the factors most directly influencing nutrition and child growth – namely food, health and care – is a first step in formulating strategies aimed at preventing malnutrition.

Food and nutrition

Stable food availability is a cornerstone of nutritional wellbeing. Household food security depends on an adequate income and assets, including the amount and quality of land owned or to which there is access. Poverty and unemployment, as well as the poor quality of housing, health and education, are important factors affecting nutrition. The degree to which increased income is transformed into improved food consumption and family care depends also on education and sociocultural factors. When the mother has a controlling hand in household expenditures, children's nutrition is generally better. The seasonality of production in developing countries influences access to food. Agricultural practices and technology can significantly affect nutrition through various mechanisms such as employment and income generation, energy expenditures, use of time and effects on the environment and health. Food safety and quality have also an important influence on nutrition.

Health and nutrition

Various infections have a major impact on nutritional status. The interaction of infection and inadequate food consumption causing growth retardation in children leads to a vicious circle: the malnutrition–infection complex. Micronutrient deficiencies, especially of iron and vitamin A, reduce resistance to infections, while infections and parasitic infestations impair micronutrient utilization. It is necessary to improve environmental sanitary conditions to break the malnutrition–infection complex. This includes addressing problems of contaminated water, insanitary disposal of human and household wastes, and poor food and personal hygiene in homes and in places of food processing and marketing. Health services contribute to improved nutritional wellbeing: immunizations prevent disease; curative services shorten disease episodes; and oral rehydration therapy reduces the severity and consequences of diarrhoeal disease. Strengthened health services can more effectively promote breastfeeding, proper weaning practices and home care, as well as the feeding of sick children; provide adequate antenatal care, nutritional counselling and birth attendance services; undertake nutrition education; and develop and support appropriate strategies to prevent micronutrient deficiencies.

Care and nutrition

Care and sound feeding practices are essential elements of good nutrition and health. While adequate incomes, greater food availability and expanded health services are necessary for improved nutrition, these will not bring about improvements unless households are able to take advantage of them. Care consists of the provision in the household and the community of time, attention and support to meet the physical, mental and social needs of the growing child. Of particular importance is child feeding: both breast-feeding and adequate weaning practices are crucial to good nutrition, and success depends on good nurturing and emotional support by caregivers, especially the mother. Maternal education in particular is a crucial factor.

The specific strategies and actions to prevent malnutrition should be developed according to the particular needs and circumstances prevailing in each situation. Nonetheless, most programmes that intend to prevent childhood malnutrition generally include some conventional activities such as the protection and promotion of breast-feeding, attention to appropriate complementary feeding, nutrition education for behavioural change, growth monitoring and promotion, micronutrient deficiency control, nutritional and health support of the sick child, and maternal nutrition. Other activities also include supplementary feeding programmes, immunization campaigns, provision of clean water and sanitary facilities, and family planning and the control of fertility. However, a good technical package has proven not to be sufficient; what often distinguishes successful programmes is that communities are involved in identifying the problems, as well as in mobilizing action and resources. Most successful programmes have strong and well-functioning community organizations and any effort to prevent malnutrition must focus on creating environments for such community programmes to develop, and commiting sufficient human and financial resources to resolving the factors that underline malnutrition.

The international nutrition community has identified a number of priority areas on which to focus in the coming years. These include:

- *Women and adolescent girls:* to date nutrition programmes have largely focused on children; more should be done to ensure good nutritional status of young women before they become mothers and to improve nutrition during pregnancy and lactation.
- *Complementary feeding:* a focus on complementary feeding, combined with continued attention to protection, promotion and support of breast-feeding, will address an important cause of malnutrition. Programmes should put special emphasis on the crucial period from birth to 24 months.
- *Links with micronutrients:* overall malnutrition should no longer be considered without reference to micronutrient status as the two are inextricably linked. Attempting to improve protein–energy status without addressing micronutrient deficiencies will not result in the optimal growth effects and resistance to illness that would follow from a more integrated approach.
- *Emergency prevention and preparedness:* more needs to be done to prevent nutritional emergencies and to design safety nets for infants and young children in case of emergency.

In summary, the problem of malnutrition remains a big challenge to all those concerned with the nutritional wellbeing of individuals and populations. A fundamental need is to focus the attention of policy-makers on nutritional status as one of the main indicators of development, and as a precondition for the socioeconomic advancement of societies in any significant long-term sense. The international community can also make a significant contribution by playing advocacy and supportive roles in promoting efforts to ensure children's fundamental right to healthy growth and development.

See also: **Adaptation**: Overview of Adaptive Responses to Malnutrition. **Anaemia (Anemia)**: Iron-Deficiency Anaemia. **Children**: Nutritional Problems of Preschool Children. **Community Nutrition**: Definition and Approaches. **Diarrhoeal (Diarrheal) Diseases**: Nutritional Factors. **Growth and Development**: Physiological Aspects. **Infants**: Nutritional Requirements; Low-birthweight and Preterm Infants. **Iodine**: Iodine Deficiency Disorders. **Malnutrition**: Definition, Classification and Epidemiology. **Nutritional Status**: Anthropometric Assessment. **Retinol**: Hypovitaminosis A.

Further Reading

ACC/SCN (1996) *How Nutrition Improves*, ACC/SCN State-of-the-art Series, Nutrition Policy Discussion Paper no. 15. Geneva: Administrative Committee on Coordination–Subcommittee on Nutrition.

Anonymous (1993) Treatment of severe child malnutrition in refugee camps. Report of a conference. *European Journal of Clinical Nutrition* 47:750–754.

Ashworth A, Jackson A, Khanum S and Schofield C (1996) Malnutrition: Ten steps to recovery. *Child Health Dialogue* 2nd and 3rd quarter: 10–12.

Berg A (1993) Sliding toward nutrition malpractice: a time to reconsider and redeploy. *American Journal of Clinical Nutrition* 57:3–7.

Golden MHN (1985) Consequences of protein deficiency in man and its relationship to features of kwashiorkor. In: Blaxter K and Waterlow JC (eds) *Adaptation in Man*, pp 169–187. London: Libbey.

Khanum S, Ashworth A and Huttly SRA (1994) Controlled trial of three approaches to the treatment of severe malnutrition. *Lancet* **344**:1728–1732.

Médecins Sans Frontières (1995) *Nutrition Guidelines*. Paris: MSF.

Murray CJL and Lopez AD (eds) (1997) *Malnutrition and the Burden of Disease: The global Epidemiology of Protein–Energy Malnutrition, Anemias and Vitamin Deficiencies*, vol. 8, The Global Burden of Disease and Injury Series. Cambridge, MA: Harvard University Press.

de Onis M, Monteiro C, Akré J and Clugston G (1993) The worldwide magnitude of protein–energy malnutrition: an overview from the WHO Global Database on Child Growth. *Bulletin of the World Health Organization* **71**:703–712.

Pinstrup-Andersen P, Pelletier D and Alderman H (eds) (1995) *Child Growth and Nutrition in Developing Countries – Priorities for Action*. Ithaca: Cornell University Press.

Schofield C and Ashworth A (1996) Why have mortality rates for severe malnutrition remained so high? *Bulletin of the World Health Organization* **74**:223–229.

Waterlow JC (1992) *Protein Energy Malnutrition*. London: Edward Arnold.

WHO (1995) *Physical Status: The Use and Interpretation of Anthropometry*. Report of a WHO Expert Committee no. 854. Geneva: World Health Organization.

WHO (1998) *Management of Severe Malnutrition – A Manual for Physicians and Other Senior Health Workers*. Geneva: World Health Organization.

Young H (1992) *Food Scarcity and Famine: Assessment and Response*. Oxfam Practical Health Guide no. 7. Oxford: Oxfam.

Secondary Malnutrition

N W Solomons, CeSSIAM, Guatemala City, Guatemala

Copyright © 1998 Academic Press

Taken literally 'malnutrition' means *bad nutrition*; this can be interpreted as a nutriture 'outside the limits'. Malnutrition can be either in the direction of deficiency, *under*nutrition, or in the direction of excess, *over*nutrition. For the purposes of this article, we shall restrict our considerations to undernutrition.

Victor Herbert has classified the six possible causes of all nutrient deficiencies (**Table 1**). Primary malnutrition is caused by an insufficient intake of nutrients from the diet – the first cause listed in Table 1. Each of the other causes, and combinations of these, is an example of secondary (also called 'conditioned') malnutrition. Moreover, one can have situations of both primary and secondary malnutrition contributing to a deficiency state.

A straightforward example of a simple combination of a primary and secondary factors would be that of dehydration occurring in a traveller marooned in the desert without food and water. This person has a primary deficiency of water as they have no intake of free water, nor of the water formed in the metabolism of foods. But because of the sweat losses from the heat, there is also excessive wastage of fluids and electrolytes across the skin – a secondary depletion of water.

An example is of multiple mechanisms acting concurrently to precipitate malnutrition is that of an advanced gastrointestinal lymphoid malignancy. The pain, obstruction and anorexia would decrease voluntary intake of food. Past radiation treatments to the abdomen may have produced a radiation enteritis with a concomitant malabsorptive state. Chemotherapeutic drugs often have antinutritional effects decreasing utilization. Fever and the release of cytokine mediators of the acute-phase response produce catabolic loss of nutrients. Finally, with rapid tumour growth of primary or metastatic lesions, increased requirements for nutrients are produced.

Mechanisms of Secondary Malnutrition

Decreased absorption

The efficiency of absorption of each nutrient has a normal range for healthy subjects of a given age. This can range from more than 90% for fats, proteins, carbohydrates, iodine, selenium, sodium, potassium, vitamin C and water, to less than 5% for iron, manganese and chromium. The fractional absorption of some nutrients is regulated homeostatically by the nutritional status of the host individual; in such instances, if the host is depleted, then there is enhanced efficiency of uptake, while if the host has sufficient or is overloaded, then absorption efficiency is reduced. Iron and zinc are two nutrients in which this type of regulation has been documented. Moreover, certain nutrients are absorbed with greater

Table 1 The six possible causes of all nutrient deficiencies

Reduced intake[a]
Decreased absorption[b]
Decreased utilization[b]
Increased destruction[b]
Increased wastage[b]
Increased requirement[b]

From Herbert V and Das KC (1993) Folic acid and vitamin B[12]. In: Shils ME, Olson JA and Shike M (eds) *Modern Nutrition in Health and Disease*, 8th edn, chap. 25, p 413. Philadelphia: Lea & Febiger.
[a]This is the exclusive mechanism of *primary* malnutrition.
[b]These are the various mechanisms of *secondary* malnutrition.

efficiency during pregnancy and lactation than in the nonreproductive phases of a woman's life span.

The normal absorption of a given nutrient can be interfered with by both dietary and host factors, with the potential for causing insufficient uptake of the nutrient to meet nutritional needs. Dietary factors include constituents of unrefined cereal grains, dietary fibre and phytic acid, which inhibit the absorption of charged ions such as iron, zinc and calcium. The polyphenols (tannins) in tea and coffee act in a similar way, especially inhibiting absorption of iron. Oxalic acid is another noted inhibitor of cation absorption. Fibre is suspected of interfering with the absorption of certain vitamins and provitamins, with α- and β-carotene among the candidates. Drugs can directly interfere with nutrient uptake, e.g. sulfazalidine acts against folic acid, or can disrupt the digestive or absorptive physiology, e.g. the resin, cholestyramine, by binding bile salts, can interfere with the absorption of fat and fat-soluble vitamins. A noncaloric fat substitute that has recently been approved in the USA for use in snack foods interferes with absorption of all four fat-soluble vitamins, and compensatory amounts are added to the dietetic products containing this compound.

Nutrients can also block the absorption of other nutrients. For example, calcium interferes with the absorption of iron and zinc; zinc blocks the absorption of copper; and iron interferes with the absorption of zinc. Avidin, a protein in raw egg white, binds biotin in an insoluble complex, preventing its absorption.

Host-related factors are dependent on the gastrointestinal (GI) function of the host. Any disease of the stomach, pancreas or biliary tract that limits the secretion of digestive enzymes will have profound implications for the digestion of foods and the release of absorbable forms of fats, carbohydrates, peptides and amino acids, and even vitamins and minerals. Gastric disease also reduces acid secretion and certain vitamins and minerals are absorbed less efficiently in a neutral-to-alkaline intestinal milieu. Conversely, pancreatic and biliary tract disease reduces bicarbonate secretion into the intestinal lumen, leaving gastric acid unopposed; certain nutrients are poorly absorbed in an acidic microclimate and digestive enzymes cleave their substrates with reduced efficiency at low pH. Small intestinal diseases or damage that affects the extent of surface area, the metabolism or morphology of the mucosal cells, the capillary circulation in the mesenteric portal bloodstream, and/or the lymphatic drainage of the gut, will all produce various grades of malabsorption. Tropical sprue, coeliac sprue, recurrent and persistent infectious gastroenteritis, inflammatory bowel disease, radiation enteropathy and lymphomata are all examples of small bowel diseases in which malabsorption can lead to nutrient deficiency states. Certain genetic conditions may also interfere with the absorption of specific nutrients. Acrodermatitis enteropathica is a congenital disease of inefficient zinc absorption, leading to clinical zinc deficiency in early life. Menkes' kinky hair syndrome blocks absorption of dietary copper. Acquired autoimmune conditions, such as pernicious anaemia, which involves impaired secretion of the gastric intrinsic factor required for absorption of vitamin B_{12}, is another example of absorptive impairment of nutrients.

Decreased utilization

A nutrient may be consumed in adequate amounts and absorbed with normal efficiency, but still the host shows manifestations of nutritional deficiency. This occurs when utilization of the nutrient is blocked; for example, the incorporation of iron into red blood cells is blocked in lead poisoning. In severe protein–energy malnutrition, the body prioritizes the use of protein to the most essential (cerebral, renal, immune) functions, sacrificing oxygen transport and hence the proliferation of red blood cells, with the concomitant decreased utilization of iron.

Inborn errors of metabolism are generally inherited states of decreased nutrient utilization. Menkes' kinky hair syndrome was mentioned above as a condition in which copper is poorly absorbed. In fact, this disease represents a global malutilization of the metal – even if parenteral copper is given, it does not find its way into the cuproenzymes, resulting in overt manifestations of copper deficiency and a fatal outcome. Other inborn errors of metabolism which cause utilization defects are mutations of certain enzymes that have vitamins as cofactors. Massive amounts of vitamins may be used to drive the associated metabolic reaction forward.

Drug–nutrient interactions constitute an important class of decreased nutrient utilization. The 'antifol' (antifolic acid) drugs used in tumour chemotherapy, such as methotrexate, interfere with the metabolic action of folic acid. The warfarin class of anticoagulant drugs acts by antagonizing the normal action of vitamin K in the posttranslational modification of clotting factors. The result is a haemorrhagic condition analogous to extrinsic deficiency of the vitamin. The action of iodine in the thyroid gland can be interfered with by two types of goitrogenic substances. Some of these are commercial drugs, such as thiourea, whereas other are naturally occurring chemicals found in certain water supplies and as plant toxins.

Increased destruction

Only the organic molecules – but not the elemental nutrients – can be destroyed or chemically denatured so that they are no longer able to function in their prescribed roles in metabolism. Vitamin C is susceptible to oxidative destruction. In southern Africa, people afflicted with African-type haemosiderosis develop the signs and symptoms of scurvy owing to accelerated ferrogenic oxidative destruction of the vitamin. Thiamin is susceptible to hydrolysis during its gastrointestinal passage by naturally occurring thiaminases; fermented fish sauces, popular in Thai cuisine, are notorious sources of dietary thiaminase activity. In theory, certain drug–nutrient interactions may also influence oxidative destruction of organic nutrients directly.

Increased wastage

Rivalling impaired absorption as a precipitating secondary mechanism for nutritional deficiency is increased wastage. By this, we mean that the particular nutrient is taken up by the intestine into the body, only to have a shorter than expected retention time. The routes of excessive loss are the same as those of normal turnover, namely the integumentary route (skin, sweat, hair, nails), the renal route (urine) and the faecal route (stool). Excess loss of previously absorbed nutrients into the faeces can come about by their increased transport in bile, pancreatic secretions, or in a reverse direction across the small or large intestinal wall. Three final routes worthy of mention are those of the retrograde gastric route (vomiting, regurgitation, gastric suction), the bronchopulmonary route and the uterovaginal route. A special route of nutrient loss in all mammals, including humans, is through lactation.

Iron, and to a lesser extent other nutrients in blood such as zinc, can be lost to the point of precipitating nutritional deficiency by a haemorrhages that occur from wounds (integumentary) or through any of the mentioned orifices: the gastric retrograde route (varices, gastric and duodenal ulcers), the faecal route (ulcers, tumours, varices, parasites, dysenteries), the bronchopulmonary routes (tumours, vascular malformations), the uterovaginal route (tumours, menorrhagia, abortions, childbirth), and the urinary tract (tumours, vascular malformations, renal trauma, schistosomiasis). Haemoglobinuria produced by *in vivo* haemolysis of red blood cells (drug-induced, copper excess, traumatic or thermal, malarial) is another source of iron loss via the renal route. Dehydration (water loss) and electrolyte wastage, moreover, can occur through sweating across the skin, by hyperventilation by the lungs, and via diatheses of diabetes (mellitus, insipidus) or through gastrointestinal losses in hyperemesis, secretory and osmotic diarrhoeas, and pancreatic hypersecretion.

The gastrointestinal tract can be the site of excess losses of a range of mineral nutrients such as zinc, copper, calcium and magnesium.

The renal route is the most common one for chronic loss of macronutrients and minerals. Glycosuria in uncontrolled diabetes produces a wastage of energy. Catabolic situations, such as severe trauma, thermal burns or sepsis, produce breakdown of visceral and muscular tissue with accelerated loss of protein in the form of nitrogen. The activation of the acute-phase response to injury also results in excess loss of iron, zinc and vitamin A. Finally, the saturation of circulating transport proteins can lead to reduced retention of absorbed nutrients, and their loss in the urine. For instance, chromium is transported on transferrin, the protein that normally carries iron. In haemochromatosis or haemosiderosis, almost all binding sites are occupied by iron, displacing or crowding out chromium and leading to its excessive loss in the urine.

Lactation represents a mechanism for loss of nutrients from the maternal supply. It is dependent upon the frequency and intensity of breast-feeding and the overall duration of lactation. Some of the loss is compensated for by storage during pregnancy, by enhanced absorption efficiency, or – as in the case of iron – by the cessation of menstrual losses (lactation-induced amenorrhoea).

Increased requirement

Increased requirement is sort of a hybrid category in the context of an interaction of primary and secondary malnutrition. If we specify carefully that basal, normal intake recommendations for gender and age are our standard of reference, then an internal demand for more nutrients that is not met by compensatory intake can result in deficiency. Pregnancy is the classical example of a situation of increased nutrient requirements; these nutrients are needed for the growth of the fetus, the energy metabolism of both mother and fetus, deposition into the tissues of the fetus and placenta, and maternal physiological adaptations.

The energy deficiency (weight loss) produced by hypermetabolic conditions such as hyperthyroidism and chronic obstructive pulmonary disease could either be considered excess loss or increased demand, as energy requirement is numerically equivalent to energy expenditure.

Tumours, especially rapidly growing solid tumours, require additional amounts of essential nutrients for cell growth and proliferation. Folic acid and vitamin B_{12} are the classical examples, but tumour growth also results in increased demands for zinc, energy and antioxidant nutrients. This phenomenon raises important therapeutic implications, as discussed below.

Finally, pituitary adenomas producing growth hormone excess either before puberty (gigantism) or in adulthood (acromegaly) stimulate excessive growth, especially of skeletal and connective tissue. This places additional demands for certain nutrients which may be unmet without a compensatory increase in intake.

Epidemiology of Secondary Malnutrition

Clinical dimension

Hospitalized patients represent a population in which undernutrition is common. It is overall a *combination* of primary and secondary malnutrition. Anorexia, the scheduling of procedures, medications and depression and the often unappetizing presentation of 'hospital food' are some of the frequent causes of inadequate intake. However the underlying illnesses, the trauma of surgical, chemotherapeutic and radiotherapeutic interventions, medical–surgical complications and nosocomial infections all contribute to diminishing nutrient stores. Malignancies and other diseases associated with cachexia (chronic pulmonary disease, congestive heart failure) produce the most accelerated and exaggerated forms of wasting of tissue proteins and energy reserves.

The human immunodeficiency virus (HIV) pandemic has been with us since the 1980s. Acquired immunodeficiency syndrome (AIDS) represents a striking example of combined primary and secondary deficiency. Anorexia from ill health and medications and the financial burden and loss of work capacity wrought by the disease, its treatment and its stigma, can all contribute to decreased intake. However, AIDS itself is manifested by opportunistic infections. Some of these, such as cryptosporosis, and other gastrointestinal infections such as *Giardia hominis* or normally nonpathogenic protozoa, *Isospora*, produce diarrhoea and malabsorption. Febrile illnesses can be chronic and unremitting, producing a cachexia owing to the activation of the acute-phase response. *Mycobacteria* infections, such as tuberculosis, a classical example of a wasting infectious disease, is a common concomitant of AIDS.

Public health dimension

It is customary to restrict consideration of secondary malnutrition to the clinical setting. In fact, many of what are *endemic* undernutrition states may be as much – or more – the result of conditioning factors rather than the result of a primary failure to achieve recommended intakes.

Linear growth failure which results in stunting is common in populations of developing countries, particularly in East Asia, Southeast Asia, Central America and the Andean region. It may be as much due to infection as to dietary deficit. Stunting and short stature in later life derive from loss of linear growth before the age of 36 months. Recurrent respiratory and gastrointestinal infections and their varied stresses on the acquisition and retention of nutrients, as well as the simple overwhelming burden of environmental microbes in general, may often activate the acute-phase response so as to disrupt the orderly physiology of growth.

Iron deficiency anaemia, the most common of all deficiency states, may most often be a combination of poor iron bioavailability, gastrointestinal parasites, monthly menstrual blood losses and closely spaced pregnancies. Most low-income populations subsist on diets that are largely devoid of meat and are based on unrefined cereals as the staple, together with other plant-derived foods. Often tea and coffee are the predominant beverages. The iron content of the diet may exceed recommended levels, but the fractional absorption is so reduced by the presence of binders and inhibitors that the body is deprived of the metal. Hookworm disease and schistosomiasis are widely endemic in tropical, lowland regions; both these parasitoses contribute to large losses of blood in the most heavily infested subgroups of the population. Women with the highest constitutional losses of menstrual blood and those with the most frequent succession of pregnancies may lose more iron from their reproductive apparatus than can be taken up and retained from the diet. It is safe to conclude, then, that much of the burden of nutritional anaemia in the world is the result of secondary iron malnutrition.

Decreased bioavailablity of nutrients is a contributing factor in other deficiencies of public health importance. The failure to consume provitamin A carotenoids with sufficient dietary fat, in order to maximize fat absorption with the meal, may be one of the causes of hypovitaminosis A in low-income countries. Moreover, to the extent that zinc deficiency may be endemic in poor societies, it is likely that it is the high-fibre, unrefined cereal-based diet – rather than a dearth of the nutrient in foods – that contributes to poor body stores of the metal.

Therapeutic Considerations

Malnutrition can be the major factor in a patient's debility and proximate cause of death. Whatever the underlying causes and mechanisms for undernutrition, leaving it unredressed sets up the dynamic for death by starvation or by infections associated with malnutrition.

The 'leaky bucket' metaphor has often been used to conceptualize secondary forms of malnutrition. The alternative strategies of: (1) sealing the leaks, (2) delivering nutrients in at a compensatory rate to account for the inefficiency of filling, or (3) doing both, are considered and contrasted. This applies to the issues of decreased absorption, increased destruction and increased losses. Often decreased utilization – if it is *absolute*, as with copper in Menkes' kinky hair syndrome – cannot be overcome by any amount of excess nutrient. If it is *relative*, as in most inborn errors of metabolism involving enzymes, excesses of coenzyme vitamins can drive the defective reaction forward. In theory, sealing the leaks and delivering more nutrients are both strategies that can achieve the common goal of restoring adequate nutritional stores. However, there are practical and ethical dimensions to the decision-making.

If there are curative or palliative procedures that are available to, acceptable to, and accessible to the patient, one is obliged to offer them as therapy; the amelioration of the underlying condition sets the stage for improved retention of nutrients from the diet. However, the rate of recovery of nutritional status will depend upon providing not only the maintenance amounts of nutrients, but also an excess to allow for replenishing depleted reserves. When there is no available or accessible measure that effectively remedies the disease process, provision of enough nutrient flow to cover both basal needs and compensate for inefficient uptake and/or retention is the only option left to provide for adequate nutriture. If the patient is already depleted, the formula must initially provide the three components of nutritional needs: maintenance + compensatory + repletion. Once nutritional status is normalized, the regimen must continue to cover the first two components.

Feed the patient, feed the tumour

Occasionally the dilemma arises as to whether aggressive nutrient therapy will benefit the pathological process *more* than the nutritional status of the patient. This occurs most often with malignancies, in which the 'starve the tumour' approach is a consideration. There is a rich debate in oncological circles as to when nutritional supplementation favours growth of the tumour disproportionately in relation to replenishing host stores.

When eradication is not accessible, compensation is acceptable

The term 'accessible' is important when public health problems, rather than specific clinical illnesses, are at issue. Hookworm disease is estimated to afflict a billion people worldwide. Those with the more intense infections are most susceptible to decompensated iron losses and anaemia. Effective anthelminthics exist to eliminate infections, but they are expensive and cumbersome to deliver. Moreover, if transmission of the infection is not interrupted, people will regress to their original state of infestation after occasional treatments. Confronted with the slight likelihood of pharmaceutical control of hookworm, a strategy of iron supplementation that compensates for iron losses to the worm load and augments intake of the metal beyond usual iron requirements is a more realistic one.

Conclusions

Not all nutritional deficiency can be understood in terms of the simplistic paradigm of not enough food or not enough of the right foods. This paradigm only describes the mechanism of *primary* malnutrition. Even when food is theoretically in sufficient supply in the community, the household and on the plate in the diet, additional (secondary) mechanisms can interfere with access to the nutrients such that nutritional deficiency manifestations occur. Five such mechanisms have been described as part of a generic paradigm for understanding the causality of nutritional depletion. Any reflex association of malnutrition with improper diet can be detrimental to the care of the patient. The presentation of many diseases is often the complaint of symptoms or the recognizing of symptoms related to malnutrition. Cystic fibrosis and juvenile inflammatory bowel disease are diseases that are often diagnosed because the host has a nutrient deficiency syndrome. Iron deficiency anaemia is often the presenting finding for 'silent' peptic ulcers and gastrointestinal malignancies.

It is not only in the clinical setting, but also at the population level in public health, that secondary malnutrition and its mechanisms are of interest. Iron deficiency is widespread not so much because people consume too little iron, but because they absorb too little of what they eat. Hookworms and schistosomes drain many an individual iron reserve in areas of the tropics where these parasitoses are endemic. The reproductive biology of subgroups of women makes them more vulnerable to developing a deficit of body iron.

Whether one has to attack the problem at the level of the pathological state or by providing superabundant nutrients to compensate for interferences and/or losses is the crux of the therapeutic dilemma. Effecting remedial address of the primary problem, where it exists, such as with a gluten-free diet to reverse intestinal damage from coeliac disease, will simultaneously address the nutrient malabsorption. When no effective palliation or cure for the primary pathology exists, attempts to circumvent the effects with additional nutrients can often restore satisfactory nutriture and improve general wellbeing.

See also: **Anaemia (Anemia)**: Iron-Deficiency Anaemia; Megaloblastic Anaemia. **Ascorbic Acid**: Scurvy. **Bioavailability**: Definition and General Aspects. **Biotin**: Physiology, Dietary Sources and Requirements. **Cholecalciferol and Ergocalciferol**: Rickets and Osteomalacia. **Coeliac Disease**: Aetiology and Nutritional Management. **Drugs**: Drug-Nutrient Interactions. **Energy**: Energy Balance. **Folic Acid**: Physiology, Dietary Sources and Requirements. **Gastrointestinal Tract**: Structure and Function of the Small Intestine; Structure and Function of the Colon. **HIV Disease**: Nutritional Management. **Infection**: Nutritional Interactions. **Iron**: Physiology, Dietary Sources and Requirements. **Liver Disorders**: Nutritional Management. **Malnutrition**: Primary Malnutrition. **Microflora of the Intestine**: Role and Effects. **Parasitism**: Effects on Growth and Nutritional Status. **Physical Handicap**: Nutritional Management of Cerebral Palsy. **Protein**: Deficiency. **Retinol**: Hypovitaminosis A. **Selenium**: Physiology, Dietary Sources and Requirements. **Starvation and Fasting**: Biochemical Aspects. **Stroke**: Nutritional Management. **Surgery**: Perioperative Feeding; Long-term Nutritional Management of Patients.

Therapeutic Dietetics: Lung Diseases; Short Bowel Syndrome. **Thiamin**: Beriberi. **Vegetarian Diets**: Nutritional Adequacy. **Vitamin Supplementation**: Role. **Weight Management**: Weight Cycling. **World Health Organization**: Role.

Further Reading

Herbert V and Das KC (1993) Folic acid and vitamin B_{12}. In: Shils ME, Olson JA and Shike M (eds) *Modern Nutrition in Health and Disease*, 8th edn, chap. 25, pp 402–425. Philadelphia: Lea & Febiger.

Keusch GT (1979) Nutrition as a determinant of host response to infection and the metabolic sequelae. *Seminars on Infectious Diseases* 2:265–303.

Keusch GT and Solomons NW (1985) Microorganisms, malabsorption, diarrhea and dysnutrition. *Journal of Environmental Pathology, Toxicology and Oncology* 5:165–209.

Langstein HN and Norton JA (1991) Mechanisms of cancer cachexia. *Hematology and Oncology Clinics of North America* 5:103–128.

Rhead WJ (1996) Inborn errors of metabolism. In: Filer JL and Ziegler E (eds) *Present Knowledge in Nutrition*, 7th edn, chap. 63, pp 623–629 Washington, DC: ILSI Press.

Sandstead HH, Vo-Khactu K and Solomons N (1976) Conditioned zinc deficiency. In: Prasad AS (ed.) *Trace Elements in Health and Disease*, pp 33–49. New York: Academic Press.

Scrimshaw NS, Taylor CE and Gordon JE (1968) *Interactions of Nutrition and Infection*, WHO Monograph Series No. 57. Geneva: World Health Organization.

Solomons NW (1993) Pathways to impairment of nutritional status by gastrointestinal pathogens, with emphasis on protozoal and helminthic parasites. *Parasitology* 107(supplement):S19–S35.

MANGANESE

Physiology, Dietary Sources and Requirements

C L Keen, Jodi L Ensunsa and **Sheri Zidenberg-Cherr**, University of California at Davis, California, USA

Copyright © 1998 Academic Press

The requirement for manganese was established in 1931, when it was demonstrated that a deficit of it resulted in poor growth and impaired reproduction in rodents. It has long been appreciated that a deficiency of manganese can be a practical problem in the swine and poultry industries, and it has been suggested that manganese deficiency may be a problem in some human populations. Here the recent literature related to manganese nutrition, metabolism and metabolic function is briefly reviewed. For additional information the reader is referred to more comprehensive reviews listed under Further Reading.

Chemical and Physical Properties

Manganese is widely distributed in the biosphere: it constitutes approximately 0.1% of the Earth's crust making it the twelfth most abundant element. Manganese is a component of numerous complex minerals including pyroluosite, rhodochrosite, rhodanite, braunite, pyrochroite and manganite. Chemical forms of manganese in their natural deposits include oxides, sulfides, carbonates and silicates. Anthropogenic sources of manganese are predominantly from the manufacturing of steel, alloys and iron products. Manganese is also widely used as an oxidizing agent, as a component of fertilizers and fungicides, and in dry cell batteries. Concentrations of manganese in ground water normally range between 1 and 100 $\mu g\ l^{-1}$, with most values being below 10 $\mu g\ l^{-1}$. Typical airborne levels of manganese (in the absence of excessive pollution) range from 0.05 to 0.10 $\mu g\ m^{-1}$.

Manganese is a transition element located in group VIIA of the periodic table. It can exist in 11 oxidation states ranging from -3 to $+7$, with the most common valences being $+2$, $+4$ and $+7$. The $+2$ valence is the predominant form in biological systems and is the form that is thought to be maximally absorbed. The $+4$ valence occurs in MnO_2, and the $+7$ valence is found in permanganate.

The solution chemistry of manganese is relatively simple. The aquo-ion is resistant to oxidation in acidic or neutral solutions. It does not begin to hydrolyse until pH 10, and therefore free Mn^{2+} can be present in neutral solutions at relatively high concentrations. Divalent manganese is a $(3d)^5$ ion and typically forms high-spin complexes lacking crystal field stabilization energies. The above properties as well as the large ionic radius and small charge-to-radius ratio result in manganese tending to form weak complexes compared with other first-row divalent ions such as Ni^{2+} and Cu^{2+}. Free Mn^{2+} has a strong isotropic EPR signal that can be used to determine its concentration in the low micromolar range. Mn^{3+} is also critical in biological systems. For example, Mn^{3+} is the oxidative state of manganese in superoxide dismutase, is the form in which transferrin binds manganese, and is probably the form of manganese that interacts with Fe^{3+}. Given its smaller ionic radius, the chelation of Mn^{3+} in biological systems would be predicted to be more avid than that of Mn^{2+}. Cycling between Mn^{3+} and Mn^{2+} has been suggested to be potentially deleterious to biological systems since it can generate free radicals. However, it has been argued that at low concentrations Mn^{2+} provides protection against free radicals, and is associated with their clearance rather than their production.

Dietary Sources

Manganese concentrations in typical food products range from 0.4 $\mu g\ g^{-1}$ (meat, poultry, fish) to 20 $\mu g\ g^{-1}$ (nuts, cereals, dried fruit). Teas, which are often listed as an excellent source of manganese, can contain anywhere from 300 to 900 $\mu g\ g^{-1}$ of the element. An important consideration with respect to food sources of manganese, however, is the extent to which the manganese is available for absorption. For example, while tea contains high amounts of the element, the high content of tannin found in tea binds a significant amount of manganese and prevents its absorption from the gastrointestinal tract. Similarly, while the concentration of manganese in cereal grains is significant, the high content of phytates and fibre constituents may bind manganese, limiting its absorption. Therefore, while calculation of intake based on nutrient composition of foods may show that manganese intake is high, the actual amount of manganese absorbed will vary among food sources. Similarly, although meat products contain low concentrations of manganese, absorption and retention of manganese from them is high, making them good dietary sources of the element.

Analysis

Although manganese is widely distributed in the biosphere, it occurs in only trace amounts in animal tissues. Serum concentrations can be as low as 5 nM and typical tissue concentrations are less than 4 μM; tissue concentrations of 4–8 μM are considered high. Owing to the high environmental levels of manganese relative to its concentration in animal tissues, considerable effort must be made to minimize contamination of samples during their collection and handling. As a general precaution, all glassware and plasticware used in the storage or processing of samples should be washed in 20% nitric acid for at least 48 h and then rinsed exhaustively with distilled double-deionized water. Washed glassware and plasticware should be stored under dust-free conditions prior to use. To reduce contamination, tissues containing very low manganese concentrations should be dissected with plastic or quartz knives rather than steel knives.

The most common analytical methods that can sensitively measure manganese (18 $nmol\ l^{-1}$) include neutron activation analysis, X ray fluorescence, proton-induced X ray emission, inductively coupled plasma emission, electron paramagnetic resonance

(EPR), and flameless atomic absorption spectrophotometry (AAS). Currently the most common method employed is flameless AAS. All of these methods, with the exception of EPR, measure the total concentration of manganese in the samples. EPR allows selective measurement of bound versus free manganese.

Physiological Role

Tissue concentrations

The average human body contains between 200 and 400 µmol of manganese, which is fairly uniform in distribution throughout the body. There is relatively little variation among species with regard to tissue manganese concentrations. Manganese tends to be highest in tissues rich in mitochondria; its concentration in mitochondria is higher than in cytoplasm or other cell organelles. Hair can accumulate high concentrations of manganese, and it has been suggested that hair manganese concentrations may reflect manganese status. High concentrations of manganese are normally found in pigmented structures, such as retina, dark skin and melanin granules. Bone, liver, pancreas and kidney tend to have higher concentrations of manganese (20–50 nmol g^{-1}) than do other tissues. Concentrations of manganese in brain, heart, lung and muscle are typically <20 nmol g^{-1}; blood and serum concentrations are about 200 and 20 nmol l^{-1}, respectively. Typical milk concentrations are on the order of 1 fmol l^{-1}. Bone can account for up to 25% of total body manganese because of its mass. Bone manganese concentrations can be raised or lowered by substantially varying dietary manganese intake over long periods of time, but bone manganese is not thought to be a readily mobilizable pool. In contrast to the situation for several other essential trace elements, the fetus does not accumulate liver manganese before birth, and fetal concentrations are significantly less than adult concentrations. This lack of fetal storage can be attributed to the apparent lack of storage proteins and the fact that most manganese enzymes are not expressed prenatally.

Absorption, transport and storage

Absorption of manganese is thought to occur throughout the small intestine. The efficiency of manganese absorption is relatively low and is not thought to be under homeostatic control. For adult humans, manganese absorption has been reported to range from 2% to 15% when ^{54}Mn-labelled test meals are used and 25% when balance studies are conducted; given the technical problems associated with balance studies, the ^{54}Mn data are probably more reflective of true absorption values. Manganese absorption and retention are higher in neonates than in adults. Data from balance studies indicate that manganese retention from human milk and infant formula is elevated during infancy, suggesting that neonates may be particularly susceptible to manganese toxicosis.

The higher retention of manganese in young animals relative to adults may reflect an immaturity of manganese excretory pathways, particularly that of bile secretion which is suppressed in early life. The avid retention of the small amount of manganese from milk, and the postnatal changes in its excretory pattern, underscore the fact that important changes in manganese metabolism occur during the neonatal period.

In experimental animals, high amounts of dietary calcium, phosphorus, fibre and phytate have been shown to increase the requirements for manganese; such interactions presumably occur via the formation of insoluble manganese complexes in the intestinal tract with a concomitant decrease in the soluble fraction available for absorption. The significance of these dietary factors with regard to human manganese requirements remains to be clarified. Studies in avians have demonstrated that high dietary phosphorus intakes decreased manganese deposition in bone by approximately 50%. Given that the average diet of many individuals may be considered marginal in manganese (≤2 mg per day intake) and high in phosphorus (≥2000 mg per day intake), this antagonism may have important implications for human health. For example, the low fractional absorption of manganese from soya formula has been related to its relatively high phytate content. The mechanism underlying this effect of soya protein on manganese absorption/retention has not been fully delineated. However, dephytinization of soya formula with microbial phytase has been reported approximately to double fractional manganese absorption.

An interaction between iron and manganese has been demonstrated in several species. Manganese absorption increases under conditions of iron deficiency in both experimental animals and humans, whereas high amounts of dietary iron can accelerate the development of manganese deficiency in some species. The chronic consumption of high levels of iron supplements (>60 mg Fe per day) has been reported to have a negative effect on manganese balance in adult women. The mechanisms underlying the interactions between iron and manganese have not been identified; however, they probably involve competition for either a transport site or a ligand.

Manganese entering into the portal blood from the

gastrointestinal tract may either remain free or become associated with α_2-macroglobulin which is subsequently taken up by the liver. A small fraction enters the systemic circulation where it may become oxidized to Mn^{3+} and bound to transferrin. Studies *in vivo* suggest that the Mn^{3+} complex forms very quickly in blood, in contrast to the slow oxidation of Mn^{2+}-transferrin complex *in vitro*. Manganese uptake by the liver has been reported to occur by a unidirectional, saturable process with the properties of passive mediated transport. Once entering the liver, manganese enters one of at least five metabolic pools. One pool represents manganese taken up by the lysosomes, from which it is thought to be transferred subsequently to the bile canaliculus. The regulation of manganese is thought to be maintained in part through biliary excretion of the element; up to 50% of manganese injected intravenously can be recovered in the faeces within 24 h. A second pool of manganese is associated with the mitochondria. Mitochondria have a large capacity for manganese uptake and it is thought that mitochondrial uptake and release of manganese and calcium may be related. A third pool of manganese is found in the nuclear fraction of the cell; the roles of nuclear manganese have not been delineated. A fourth manganese pool is incorporated into newly synthesized manganese proteins; biological half-lives for these proteins have not been agreed upon. The fifth identified intracellular pool of manganese is free Mn^{2+}. It is thought that fluctuations in the free manganese pool may be an important regulator of cellular metabolic control in a manner analogous to those for free Ca^{2+} and Mg^{2+}. Consistent with this idea, several studies in pancreatic islets have shown that manganese blocks glucose-induced insulin release by altering cellular calcium fluxes, and that manganese can directly augment contractions in smooth muscle by a mechanism comparable to that of calcium.

The mechanisms by which manganese is transported to and taken up by extrahepatic tissues have not been identified. Transferrin is the major manganese-binding protein in plasma; however, it is not known to what extent tranferrin facilitates the uptake of manganese by extrahepatic tissue. Manganese uptake by extrahepatic tissue does not appear to be increased under conditions of manganese deficiency, suggesting a lack of inducible manganese-transport proteins.

Currently there is limited information concerning the hormonal regulation of manganese metabolism. Fluxes in the concentrations of adrenal, pancreatic and pituitary–gonadal axis hormones affect tissue manganese concentrations; however, it is not clear to what extent hormone-induced changes in tissue manganese concentrations are owing to alterations in cellular uptake of manganese-activated enzymes or metalloenzymes.

Metabolic function and essentiality

Manganese functions as a constituent of metalloenzymes and as an enzyme activator. Manganese-containing enzymes include arginase, pyruvate carboxylase, and manganese-superoxide dismutase (MnSOD). Arginase, the cytosolic enzyme responsible for urea formation, contains 4 mol Mn^{2+} per mol of enzyme. Although the activity of this enzyme can be lower in manganese deficient animals than in controls, the functional significance of the reduction has not been defined; however, reductions in arginase activity owing to manganese deficiency have been shown to result in elevated plasma concentrations of ammonia and lowered plasma concentrations of urea. In addition, it has been found that manganese binding by arginase is critical for the pH-sensing function of this enzyme in the ornithine cycle, suggesting that manganese plays a role in the regulation of body pH. With experimental diabetes, liver and kidney manganese concentrations and arginase activity can be markedly elevated. This manganese effect on arginase has been suggested to be owing to an effect of Mn^{2+} on the conformational properties of the enzyme with a resultant modification of arginase activity. Whether this finding implies an increased manganese requirement for diabetics has not been determined.

Pyruvate carboxylase, the enzyme that catalyses the first step of carbohydrate synthesis from pyruvate, contains 4 mol Mn^{2+} per mol enzyme. Although the activity of this enzyme can be lower in manganese-deficient animals than in controls, gluconeogenesis has not been shown to be markedly inhibited in manganese-deficient animals.

MnSOD catalyses the disproportionation of O_2^- to H_2O_2 and O_2. The essential role of MnSOD in the normal biological function of tissues has been clearly demonstrated by the homozygous inactivation of the SOD2 gene for MnSOD in mice. Mice with this phenotype die within the first 10 days of life with a dilated cardiomyopathy, accumulation of lipid in liver and skeletal muscle, and metabolic acidosis. The activity of MnSOD in tissues of manganese-deficient rats can be significantly lower than in controls. That this reduction is functionally significant is suggested by the observation of higher than normal levels of hepatic mitochondrial lipid peroxidation in deficient rats. It has been shown that this decrease in MnSOD activity after manganese deficiency is owing to the downregulation of MnSOD at the (pre)-transcriptional level, supporting a role for manganese in the control of this enzyme by a mechanism of gene activation. Tissue MnSOD activity can be increased by several diverse stressors including alcohol, ozone, irradiation, interleukin 1 and tumour necrosis factor α, presumably as a consequence of stressor-associated increases in cellular free radical (or oxidized target(s)) concentrations. Stressor-induced increases in MnSOD activity can be attenuated in manganese-deficient animals, potentially increasing their sensitivity to these insults. Transgenic mice have also been produced which overexpress MnSOD; a decreased severity of reperfusion injury has been noted in these animals.

For manganese-activated reactions, the metal can act by binding either to the substrate (such as ATP) or directly to the protein, resulting in conformational changes. In contrast to the relatively few manganese metalloenzymes, there are a large number of manganese-activated enzymes, including hydrolases, kinases, decarboxylases and transferases. Manganese activation of these enzymes can occur as a direct consequence of the metal binding to the protein, causing a subsequent conformation change, or by binding to the substrate, such as ATP. Many of these metal activations are nonspecific in that other metal ions, particularly Mg^{2+}, can replace Mn^{2+}. An exception to the nonspecific manganese activation of enzymes is the manganese-specific activation of glycosyltransferases. Several manganese deficiency-induced pathologies have been attributed to a low activity of this enzyme class. A second example of an enzyme that may be specifically activated by manganese is phosphoenolpyruvate carboxykinase (PEPCK), the enzyme which catalyses the conversion of oxaloacetate to phosphoenolpyruvate, GDP and CO_2. While low activities of PEPCK can occur in manganese-deficient animals, the functional significance of this reduction is not clear.

A third example of a manganese-activated enzyme is glutamine synthetase. This enzyme, found in high concentrations in the brain, catalyses the reaction NH_3 + glutamate + ATP $\rightarrow$ glutamine + ADP + P_i. Brain glutamine synthetase activity can be normal even in severely manganese-deficient animals, suggesting that the enzyme either has a high priority for this element or that magnesium can act as a substitute when manganese is lacking. It should be noted that this enzyme can be inactivated by oxygen radicals; therefore a manganese deficiency-induced reduction in MnSOD activity theoretically could act to depress further the activity of glutamine synthetase.

Manganese Deficiency

Manganese deficiency has been demonstrated in several species, including rats, mice, pigs and cattle. Signs of manganese deficiency include impaired growth, skeletal abnormalities, impaired reproductive performance, ataxia, and defects in lipid and carbohydrate metabolism.

The effects of manganese deficiency on bone development have been studied extensively. In most species, manganese deficiency can result in shortened and thickened limbs, curvature of the spine, and swollen and enlarged joints. The basic biochemical defect underlying the development of these bone defects is a reduction in the activities of glycosyltransferases; these enzymes are necessary for the synthesis of the chondroitin sulfate side chains of proteoglycan molecules. In addition, manganese deficiency in adult rats can result in an inhibition of both osteoblast and osteoclast activity. This observation is particularly noteworthy, given the reports that women with osteoporosis tend to have low blood manganese concentrations and that the provision of manganese supplements might be associated with an improvement in bone health in postmenopausal women.

One of the most striking effects of manganese deficiency occurs during pregnancy. When pregnant animals (rats, mice, guinea pigs, mink) are deficient in manganese, their offspring exhibit a congenital, irreversible ataxia characterized by incoordination, lack of equilibrium, and retraction of the head. This condition is the result of impaired development of the otoliths, the calcified structures in the inner ear responsible for normal body-righting reflexes. The block in otolith development is secondary to depressed proteoglycan synthesis owing to low activity of manganese-requiring glycosyltransferases.

Defects in carbohydrate metabolism, in addition to those described above, have been shown in manganese-deficient rats and guinea pigs. In the guinea pig, perinatal manganese deficiency results in pancreatic pathology, with animals exhibiting aplasia or marked hypoplasia of all cellular components. Manganese-deficient guinea pigs and rats given a glucose challenge respond with a diabetic-type glucose tolerance curve. In addition to its effect on pancreatic tissue integrity, manganese deficiency can directly impair pancreatic insulin synthesis and secretion as well as enhance intracellular insulin degradation. The mechanism(s) underlying the effects of manganese on pancreatic insulin metabolism have not been fully delineated, but they are thought to be multifactorial. For example, the flux of islet cell manganese from the cell surface to an intracellular pool may be a critical signal for insulin release. It is also known that insulin mRNA levels are reduced in the deficient animal, which is consistent with the depressed insulin synthesis observed in these animals. In addition, insulin sensitivity in adipose tissue is reduced in manganese-deficient rats, a phenomenon which may be related to fewer insulin receptors per adipose cell in the deficient animals. Manganese deficiency may also affect glucose metabolism by a reduction in the number of glucose transporters in adipose tissue by an as yet unidentified mechanism. Finally, the effect of manganese deficiency on insulin production may also be owing to the destruction of pancreatic β cells. It is worth noting that constitutive pancreatic MnSOD activity is lower than in most tissues; this, coupled with the observation that most diabetogenic agents function via the production of free radicals with subsequent tissue damage, suggests that an additional mechanism underlying pancreatic dysfunction in the manganese-deficient animals may be free radical mediated.

In addition to its effect on endocrine function, manganese deficiency can affect pancreatic exocrine function. For example, manganese-deficient rats can be characterized by an increase in pancreatic amylase content. The mechanism underlying this effect of manganese deficiency has not been delineated; however, it is thought to involve a shift in amylase synthesis or degradation because secretagogue-stimulated acinar secretion is comparable in control and manganese-deficient rats.

Although the majority of studies concerning the influence of manganese deficiency on carbohydrate metabolism have been conducted with experimental animals, there is one report in the literature of an insulin-resistant diabetic patient who responded to oral doses of manganese (doses ranged from 5 to 10 mg) with decreasing blood glucose concentrations. While this is an intriguing case report, others have reported a lack of an effect of oral manganese supplements (up to 30 mg) in diabetic subjects, and low blood manganese concentrations have not been found to be a characteristic of diabetics.

Abnormal lipid metabolism is also characteristic of manganese deficiency: specifically a lipotrophic effect of manganese has been suggested in the literature. Severely manganese-deficient animals can be characterized by high liver fat, hypocholesterolaemia and low high-density lipoprotein (HDL) concentrations. Deficient animals can also be characterized by a shift to smaller plasma high-density lipoprotein particles, lower high-density lipoprotein apolipoprotein (apo E) concentrations, and higher apo C concentrations. As stated above, tissue lipid peroxidation rates can be increased in manganese-deficient animals, possibly as a result of low tissue MnSOD activity.

There is considerable debate as to the extent to which manganese deficiency affects humans under free living conditions. Manganese deficiency can be induced in humans under highly controlled experimental conditions. In one study, manganese deficiency was induced in adult male subjects by feeding a manganese-deficient diet (≤ 0.1 mg Mn per day) for 39 days. The subjects developed temporary dermatitis, as well as increased serum calcium and phosphorus concentrations and increased alkaline phosphatase activity, suggestive of bone resorption.

Since the late 1980s several diseases have been reported to be characterized, in part, by low blood manganese concentrations. These diseases include epilepsy, mseleni disease, maple syrup urine disease and phenylketonuria, Down syndrome, osteoporosis, and Perthes' disease. The finding of low blood manganese levels in subsets of individuals with the above diseases is significant since blood manganese levels can reflect soft tissue manganese concentrations. The reports of low blood manganese concentrations in individuals with epilepsy are particularly intriguing, given the observations that manganese-deficient animals can show an increased susceptibility to drug and electroshock-induced seizures and a genetic model for epilepsy in rats (the GEPR rat) is characterized by low blood manganese concentrations. Given that Mn^{2+} is implicated in activation of glutamine synthetase, a Mn^{2+}-specific brain ATPase, production of cyclic AMP, altered synaptosomal uptake of noradrenalin and serotonin, glutamate, GABA and choline metabolism and biosynthesis of acetylcholine receptors, it is evident that a deficiency of manganese may contribute to the pathology of epilepsy at multiple points.

Although it is evident from the above that the role of altered manganese metabolism in several disease states needs to be clarified, evidence of widespread manganese deficiency in human populations is still lacking. Typically, manganese intakes are within the US estimated safe and adequate daily dietary intakes (ESADDI), which are as follows: 0.3–1.0 mg per day for infants, 1.0–3.0 mg per day for children, and 2.0–5.0 mg per day for older children, adolescents and adults.

Manganese Toxicity

In domestic animals, the major reported lesion associated with chronic manganese toxicity is iron deficiency, resulting from an inhibitory effect of manganese on iron absorption. Additional signs of manganese toxicity in domestic animals can include depressed growth, depressed appetite and altered brain function.

In humans, manganese toxicity represents a serious health hazard, resulting in severe pathologies of the central nervous system. In its most severe form, the toxicosis is manifested by a permanent crippling neurological disorder of the extrapyramidal system, which is similar to Parkinson's disease. In its milder form, the toxicity is expressed by hyperirritability, violent acts, hallucinations, disturbances of libido and incoordination. The above symptoms, once established, tend to persist even after the manganese body burden returns to normal. While the majority of reported cases of manganese toxicity occur in individuals exposed to high concentrations of airborne manganese (>5 mg m^{-3}), subtle signs of manganese toxicity including delayed reaction time, impaired motor coordination and impaired memory have been observed in workers exposed to airborne manganese concentrations less than 1 mg m^{-3}. Based on the above, an inhalation reference concentration (RFC) range for manganese has been established by the US Environmental Protection Agency to be between 0.09 and 0.2 μg m^{-3}. Manganese toxicity has been reported in individuals who have consumed water containing high levels (≥ 10 mg Mn per litre) of manganese for long periods of time. There has been concern recently that the risk for manganese toxicity may be increasing in some areas because of the use of methylcyclopentadienyl manganese tricarbonyl in gasoline as an antiknock agent, although there is little evidence that air, water or food manganese concentrations have increased where this fuel is used.

In addition to neural damage, reproductive and immune system dysfunction, nephritis, testicular damage, pancreatitis, lung disease and hepatic damage can occur with manganese toxicity, though the frequency of these disorders is unknown. While there is a limited body of epidemiological data which suggests that high levels of manganese can result in an increased risk for colorectal and digestive cancers, most investigators do not consider manganese to be a carcinogen. In contrast to the above, both divalent (MnCl$_2$) and heptavalent forms (KMnO$_4$) of manganese are recognized to be strong clastogens both *in vitro* and *in vivo*; exposure to high concentrations of either form result in chromosomal breaks, fragments and exchanges. In addition to being clastogenic, high concentrations of manganese ions can also induce forward and point mutations in mammalian cells. High levels of dietary manganese have not been reported to be teratogenic in the absence of overt signs of maternal toxicity. High levels of brain manganese have been reported in subjects with amyotrophic lateral sclerosis, and it has been suggested that this increase may contribute to the progression of the disease. Similarly to the cases in humans, chronic manganese toxicity in rhesus monkeys is characterized by muscular weakness, rigidity of the lower limbs and neuron damage in the substantia nigra. Findings from a recent study suggest that iron and aluminium which accumulate in the globus pallidus and the substantia nigra of these animals induce tissue oxidation which may contribute to the damage associated with manganese toxicity. Neural toxicity is a consistent finding in rats exposed to chronic manganese toxicity. Significant manganese accumulation was accompanied by an increase in cholesterol content in the hippocampal region of manganese-treated rats, which was associated with impaired learning; this impairment was corrected by an inhibitor of cholesterol synthesis. Several recent papers have described the development of manganese toxicity in individuals with compromised liver function or compromised biliary pathways or both. Significantly, these individuals may have abnormal magnetic resonance image (MRI) patterns, which can improve following the alleviation of the manganese toxicity. For example, in some cases improvements in brain function have been achieved after liver transplant. The mechanisms underlying the toxicity of manganese have not been agreed upon but may involve multiple aetiologies including endocrinological dysfunction, excessive tissue oxidative damage, and mitochondrial dysfunction caused by manganese inhibition of some pathways of the mitochondrial respiratory chain.

To date, severe cases of manganese toxicity in humans have only been reported for adults, although other groups of individuals who may be vulnerable include children on long-term parenteral nutrition, and parenteral nutrition patients who have cholestasis or other hepatic disease. The above groups of individuals have been reported to be characterized by high brain manganese concentrations based on MRI. Although no known cases have been reported, infants may be at a high risk for manganese toxicity owing to a high absorptive capacity for the element and/or an immature excretory pathway for it. If manganese is taken up by extrahepatic tissues via the manganese–transferrin complex, the developing brain may be particularly sensitive to manganese toxicity owing to the high number of transferrin receptors elaborated by neuronal cells during development, coupled with the putative need by neural cells for transferrin for their differentiation and proliferation. Studies aimed at evaluating the relative sensitivity of the developing brain to manganese toxicity are needed.

Assessment of Manganese Status

At present, reliable biomarkers for the assessment of manganese status have not been identified. Whole blood manganese concentrations have been reported to be reflective of soft tissue manganese levels in rats; however, it is not known whether a similar relationship holds for humans. Plasma manganese concentrations have been shown to decrease in individuals fed manganese-deficient diets, and to be slightly higher than normal in individuals consuming manganese supplements. Lymphocyte MnSOD activity has been reported to be increased in individuals who consume manganese supplements; however, its value as a biomarker for manganese status may be complicated owing to the number of cytokines and disease states which may also increase its expression. Urinary manganese excretion has not been found to be sensitive to dietary manganese intake. With respect to the diagnosis of manganese toxicosis, the use of MRI appears to be promising as the images associated with manganese toxicity are relatively specific. Although it is relatively expensive, the use of MRI to detect cases of manganese toxicity may be particularly useful as a means of identifying susceptible individuals in, or around, manganese-emitting factories. In addition, the method may be useful in the evaluation of patients with liver failure.

See also: **Bioavailability**: Definition and General Aspects. **Caffeine**: Chemistry and Physiological Effects. **Calcium**: Physiology. **Carbohydrates**: Regulation of Carbohydrate Metabolism. **Cereal Grains**: Dietary Significance and Nutritional Value. **Dietary Fibre (Fiber)**: Physiological Effects and Effects on Absorption. **Fatty Acids**: Metabolism. **Glucose**: Chemistry, Dietary Sources and Glycaemic Index; Metabolism and Maintenance of Blood Glucose Level. **Iron**: Physiology, Dietary Sources and Requirements. **Lipoproteins**: Physiology. **Meat, Poultry and Meat Products**: Nutritional Value.

Further Reading

Butterworth RF, Spahr L, Fontaine S and Layrargues GP (1995) Manganese toxicity, dopaminergic dysfunction and hepatic encephalopathy. *Metabolic Brain Disease* 10:259–267.

Cooper WC (1994) The health implications of increased manganese in the environment resulting from the combustion of fuel additives: a review of the literature. *Journal of Toxicology and Environmental Health* 14:23–46.

Davidsson L, Almgren A, Juillerat MA and Hurrell RM (1995) Manganese absorption in humans: the effect of phytic acid and ascorbic acid in soy formula. *American Journal of Clinical Nutrition* 62:984–987.

Fell JME, Reynolds AP, Meadows N, *et al.* (1996) Manganese toxicity in children receiving long-term parenteral nutrition. *Lancet* 347:1218–1221.

Freeland-Graves JH and Turnlund JR (1996) Deliberations and evaluations of the approaches, endpoints and paradigms for manganese and molybdenum dietary requirements. *Journal of Nutrition* 126:2435S–2440S.

Galvani P, Fumagalli P and Santagostino A (1995) Vulnerability of mitochondrial complex I in PC12 cells exposed to manganese. *European Journal of Pharmacology* 293:377–383.

Gravert DJ and Griffen JH (1996) Specific DNA cleavage by manganese (III) complexes. *Metal Ions in Biology* 33:515–536.

Keen CL (1996) Teratogenic effects of essential metals: Deficiencies and excesses. In: Chang LW, Magos L and Suzuki T (eds) *Toxicology of Metals*, pp 977–1001. New York: CRC Press.

Keen CL and Zidenberg-Cherr S (1996) Manganese. In: Ziegler EE and Filer LJ (eds) *Present Knowledge in Nutrition*, 7th edn, pp 334–343. Washington, DC: ILSI.

Li Y, Huang T-T, Carlson, EJ, Medov S, Ursell PC, Olson JL, Nobel LJ, Yoshimura MP, Berger C and Chan PH (1995) Dilated cardiomyopathy and neonatal lethality in mutant mice lacking manganese superoxide dismutase. *Nature Genetics* 11:376–381.

Nasu T (1995) Actions of manganese ions in contraction of smooth muscle. *General Pharmacology* 26:945–953.

Olanow CW, Good PF, Shinotoh H, Hewitt KA, Vingerhoets F, Snow BJ, Bead MF, Calne DB and Perl DP (1996) Manganese intoxication in the rhesus monkey: A clinical, imaging, pathologic, and biochemical study. *Neurology* 46:492–498.

Ono M, Sekiya C, Ohhira M, Namiki M, Endo Y, Suzuki K, Matsuda Y and Taniguchi N (1991) Elevated level of serum manganese-superoxide dismutase in patients with primary biliary cirrhosis: Possible involvement of free radicals in the pathogenesis in primary binary cirrhosis. *Journal of Laboratory and Clinical Medicine* 118:476–483.

Senturk UK and Gulsen O (1996) The effect of manganese-induced hypercholesterolemia on learning in rats. *Biological Trace Element Research* 51:249–257.

US Environmental Protection Agency (1994) *Reevaluation of inhalation health risks associated with methylcyclopentadienyl manganese tricarbonyl (MMT) in gasoline* (final), report no. EPA/600/R-94/062. Washinton, DC: Office of Research and Development.

MEAL SIZE AND FREQUENCY

Effect on Absorption and Metabolism

V Burley, University of Leeds, UK

Copyright © 1998 Academic Press

In the 1970s there was great interest in observations that people who consumed more than three meals per day were leaner and were less likely to suffer from heart disease and diabetes than those who ate less frequently. However, the idea that frequent eating or 'nibbling' might aid hyperlipidaemic or diabetic patients lost favour, possibly because the message to eat frequently often led to overeating by the inclusion of snacks between large main meals. However, interest in this area has been renewed following the publication of a series of experimental studies that showed improvements in blood cholesterol and serum insulin levels in response to a 'nibbling' diet.

Effect of Meal Size and Frequency on Energy Balance

Many epidemiological, clinical and experimental analyses have pointed to possible relationships between eating frequency, energy intake and body weight. In particular, it is suggested that increased eating frequency is associated with improved body weight control and reduced likelihood of overeating and fat deposition. However, there is no clear agreement on these issues, and many alternative interpretations may be considered

This area of research is plagued by problems concerning the definition of eating occasions and a lack of reliable data on eating frequency *per se*. The continued use of the colloquial terms 'meals' and 'snacks' is almost unavoidable, but does not contribute to quantitative analyses of effects of eating frequency while these terms lack any standard definition. The terms 'snacking' and 'snack foods' are particularly problematic, especially when used as variables in epidemiological analyses, because they often obscure aspects of timing, frequency, amount and type of food consumed. Any analysis of the relationships between eating frequency and nutritional outcomes must include valid measures of the timing and composition of foods eaten.

Data from dietary surveys suggest that eating frequency and timing is not constant throughout life. It seems that there is a tendency towards lower eating frequency with age, and a greater concentration of energy intake into the latter part of the day. This may bias epidemiological surveys, which typically fail to control for age. These issues, in addition to suggestions that 'snack foods' may be selectively under-reported compared with intake at main 'meals', add to the challenges involved in the interpretation and conduct of research into eating frequency.

Determinants of eating frequency

Examination of 'naturally' occurring eating patterns suggests that humans and other animals may achieve energy balance through different strategies. Rats and most other animals tend to regulate by varying the length of time between meals and achieve energy balance by altering eating frequency. The timing of main eating occasions (meals) in humans is largely socially or culturally determined, and energy balance is achieved primarily through variation in the size of eating events. This may impinge on the ability of humans to adjust energy intake appropriately when a pre-existing pattern of intake is altered.

Many individuals in Western cultures practise various degrees of dietary restraint as part of personal strategies for controlling or losing body weight. This may include missing regular meals (particularly breakfast), and suggests the possibility that reduced eating frequency could be a *result* of overweight or obesity, rather than a cause, as suggested in some epidemiological analyses. Degree of dietary restraint or use of meal-skipping as a weight control method should be considered in the interpretation of data on eating frequency and weight status.

Eating frequency, energy intake and body weight of animals

Early animal data, often cited, show an apparently clear effect of reduced eating frequency producing increased adiposity. However, more sophisticated studies do not support these early findings. In particular, techniques used to 'force' the rat to become a 'gorger' may improve energy efficiency and so confound effects of eating frequency. In studies where the methodological weaknesses of earlier approaches were taken into account, no consistent effect of eating frequency on adiposity in animals was found.

Overall, the animal studies may have only limited relevance to humans, partly because rats naturally eat much more frequently and continuously than humans do. Perhaps more important, many hypothesized effects of eating frequency might be mediated through effects on *de novo* lipogenesis, a process now known to exhibit substantial species differences, and believed to be quite limited in humans.

Relationship between eating frequency and adiposity in humans: epidemiological observations

The observation that eating frequency is related to obesity in humans was first made by Fábry and coworkers in a series of investigations involving Czechoslovakian men. He found that people who ate more frequently during the day ('nibblers') were leaner than those who consumed only one or two meals daily ('gorgers'). This research group also conducted an intervention study in which the growth and fatness of schoolchildren who were fed three, five or seven meals daily were compared. After 1 year, the oldest children (aged 10–16 years), who were fed three meals daily, showed greater measures of adiposity compared with those fed more frequently, although energy intakes were apparently similar. A small number of epidemiological studies were subsequently conducted elsewhere which tended to support these results, but the majority of more carefully controlled investigations have not lent support to the initial finding of leanness in 'nibblers' compared with 'gorgers'.

In contrast to the early data of Fábry, there is a strongly held public perception that 'snacking' or frequent eating causes obesity. Although some studies have suggested that high eating frequency as 'snacking' is common in the obese, or even causally related to obesity, both total energy intakes and the energy contribution of 'snacks' are believed to be underreported, and so the evidence is somewhat incomplete on this issue. Owing to the complicated interplay of many factors thought to be involved in the regulation of meal-to-meal energy intakes, it is currently unclear if frequent eating necessarily leads to an elevation of energy intake. Further experimental work to determine the effects of eating frequency change, and particularly the timing of insertion of extra eating events ('snacks') on energy intake may help to resolve this issue.

It is possible that eating frequency may be related to obesity via an interaction with macronutrient intakes. The consensus is that high dietary fat intakes readily lead to overconsumption and may be causally implicated in the development of obesity. There is some evidence to suggest that eating frequency may be weakly positively correlated with relative carbohydrate intakes, and negatively related to dietary fat consumption. Although complicated by the definition of 'meals' and 'snacks', and the issue of selective underreporting, most studies have suggested either that 'snacks' do not differ from 'meals', or that 'snacks' are somewhat higher in carbohydrate and lower in fat and protein than 'meals'. There appears to be little evidence that high eating frequency is necessarily associated with greater intakes of dietary fat.

Thus, the epidemiological evidence is unable to demonstrate conclusively that eating frequency or eating pattern is a factor in the causation of obesity. It is fair to say, however, that this may arise either because no genuine relationship exists, or equally because current techniques used in dietary surveys fail to assess adequately 'habitual' eating behaviour and therefore fail to identify any relationships between eating pattern and body weight.

Effects of experimental alteration of eating frequency on body weight

Eating frequency may have an impact on body weight via effects on energy metabolism or on energy intakes. There are two possible ways in which altering eating frequency may increase energy intake: frequent eating may stimulate overeating and elevate energy intakes, possibly via an inability to limit food intakes within 'meals'; alternatively, eating infrequently may elevate energy intakes owing to an increase in hunger and an overcompensation at each 'meal'. These issues have been investigated in a small number of human experimental studies and in many animal investigations.

In most of these studies, body weight and/or fat was monitored during a period of prescribed energy deficit and the eating pattern was manipulated to provide a regimen of 'nibbling' (three to nine meals) or 'gorging' (typically one or two meals). However, regardless of whether the subjects were on a low-energy diet, in approximate energy balance or being overfed, most experimental studies failed to find a marked difference in weight change through an alteration in eating frequency. In 1981, Adams and Morgan briefly reviewed the literature on the effects of the experimental alteration of eating frequency on weight loss, and concluded that there was little point to the inclusion of altered eating frequency in weight reduction programmes. In spite of the addition of some carefully conducted studies, most evidence suggests that this conclusion is still valid.

Despite the lack of evidence that alteration of eating patterns may generate a significant improvement in weight or fat loss, spreading energy intake across the day may have more to commend it than restricting food intake to a few larger meals later in the day. Many subjects in these experimental studies subjectively preferred the 'nibbling' type of eating pattern. Furthermore, this pattern of eating may help to maintain a lower intake of dietary fat (through the types of food consumed earlier in the day) and may help to prevent unplanned overeating or eating later in the day.

It is possible that the insertion of additional eating occasions into an established eating pattern may cause difficulties in energy regulation, at least until a new pattern is established. Thus, prospective studies in which eating frequency is altered may produce effects not seen in cross-sectional studies. This notion has not yet been empirically tested, and may relate more to cognitive aspects than to physiological control of eating. Clearly, many factors affect energy compensation, but the nutritional composition of the food consumed during 'extra' eating events may be particularly important. The control of energy intake may be weaker in response to high-fat, energy-dense foods.

Effect of meal size and frequency on energy metabolism

Eating frequency and diet-induced thermogenesis The thermic effect of food (TEF) is perhaps the component of energy expenditure that is most likely to be altered by a change in eating frequency. To understand the impact of eating frequency on energy expenditure it is necessary to view the thermic effect of food as consisting of two parts: (1) an obligatory component related to the metabolic costs of the transformation of dietary substrates into usable metabolites and for the storage of excess fuel; and (2) a facultative component that seems to have a 'cephalic phase' (brought about by the sight, smell and taste of food) and a 'postprandial phase', the latter possibly mediated through the action of the sympathetic nervous system.

It seems that the impact of eating frequency on daily energy expenditure may depend in part on whether the relationship between the thermic effect of food and meal size is linear. If thermogenesis is stimulated to the same extent each time eating occurs, then a 'nibbling' pattern of eating could be expected to elevate daily energy expenditure. Similarly, if the 'cephalic phase' response constitutes a sizeable proportion of overall TEF, then 'nibbling' would enhance daily energy output. Conversely, if TEF is disproportionately related to the size of the meal, a greater thermogenic response would be engendered by following a 'gorging' pattern of large, infrequent meals.

The evidence regarding the relationship between meal size and the magnitude of TEF is contradictory.

In dogs, the increase in oxygen consumption after eating has been shown to be *independent* of the size of the eating occasion. Four small meals produced a greater thermogenic response than the same energy consumed as one large meal. It was concluded that repeated sensory stimulation by palatable food was responsible for the enhanced thermogenesis seen with higher eating frequencies. Furthermore, in humans, the sight, smell and taste of food have been shown to produce significant thermogenesis lasting about 30 min. However, others have shown that the size of the thermic response to eating is positively related to the energy content of the meal, possibly through greater insulin release. The enteral administration of liquid 'meals' produces little or no TEF when administered at low rates, but produces a larger TEF when given as a bolus. It has been suggested that when the rates of energy intake and fuel oxidation are similar, this is more efficient than when food is consumed as larger meals, which may provide a temporary excess of energy requiring storage. In this way it is proposed that a change in eating frequency could affect energy balance via total energy expenditure, even without a change in the amount or composition of food eaten.

There are few studies on the effects of eating frequency on the thermic effect of food and drawing any firm conclusions is difficult, as the study designs used have varied in so many aspects, including the type of subjects used (gender, lean or obese, adults or children), the 'spread' of food intake over time, the overall size of eating occasions relative to total daily energy intake, meal nutrient composition and the duration of measurement of the thermic response. Overall, however, there is little evidence that a change in meal pattern generates a biologically significant difference in the thermic effect of food.

Furthermore, although laboratory rats readily show adaptation to reduced eating frequency by an elevation in mechanisms associated with lipogenesis (fat synthesis and storage), the evidence in humans is less conclusive. The quantitative impact of *de novo* lipogenesis in humans is thought to be small, and even if it were elevated, the total impact on energy expenditure or body weight is thought to be minimal.

Effects of meal size and frequency on total energy expenditure Whatever the influence of eating frequency on the short-lived TEF, an impact on energy balance will only be achieved through alteration of total 24 h energy expenditure. Only a few studies have investigated the impact of eating frequency on total energy expenditure and weight loss. In these studies, a 'nibbling' or 'gorging' regimen of 'meals' was consumed for 1–2 weeks, and the effect of eating pattern on energy expenditure assessed by 24–48 h whole-body calorimetry or the doubly labelled water technique. These well-controlled studies have generally shown little effect of eating pattern on total energy expenditure. This suggests that any putative relationship between adiposity and eating pattern must be mediated through effects on energy intake rather than expenditure.

Effect of Meal Size and Frequency on Plasma Lipids and Lipoproteins

Current dietary management of hyperlipidaemia focuses on the modification of dietary fat, carbohydrate and nonstarch polysaccharides. However, the pattern of eating may also affect blood lipid levels. Early studies with rats showed that gorging on one meal daily, compared with frequent feeding throughout the day, generated many metabolic and morphological changes. These included hypertrophy of the stomach and small intestine, increased nutrient absorption and raised lipid synthesis and storage. Consequently, a number of early human experimental manipulations of eating frequency were conducted which assessed the impact on blood lipids. These studies typically involved altering the number of 'meals' consumed for a set time period (ranging from 2 weeks to 6 weeks) to create a 'gorging' or 'nibbling' regimen. The experimental diets were a liquid formula, a set diet provided by a metabolic kitchen, or the subject's own foods consumed under the close scrutiny of the experimenters. These studies showed that frequency of eating had a number of metabolic effects, but because of the wide range of experimental designs used, reaching a definitive conclusion is difficult. More recent studies that have been well controlled have, however, produced more consistent evidence of a cholesterol-lowering effect of 'nibbling' in normolipidaemic subjects. One such study involved seven men consuming the same diet as three or 17 'meals' daily for 2 weeks in a randomized crossover design. On the 'nibbling' regimen, the concentration of total cholesterol was lowered by 9% low-density lipoprotein (LDL) cholesterol by 14% and apolipoprotein B by 15% when compared with the three-meal protocol. Another study using the randomized crossover design, but comparing a more realistic number of meals (three or nine) generated similar reductions in total and LDL cholesterol. In an alternative approach, significant decreases in total and LDL cholesterol levels were demonstrated when eating frequency was increased in a group of habitual 'nonsnackers'.

These data show that in normolipidaemic subjects there is a trend towards reduced levels of total and LDL cholesterol when diets consisting of six or more 'meals' are consumed, compared with those in which three or fewer 'meals' are eaten. However, there is little evidence of long-term benefit from increased eating frequency in hyperlipidaemic and diabetic subjects. Although there is some benefit in terms of reduced diurnal levels of triacylglycerols and free fatty acids, these data were obtained from studies of short duration only, in which impractical eating frequencies were used. Longer-term studies using hyperlipidaemic and diabetic patients are required before any firm recommendations may be made on the therapeutic potential of 'nibbling' diets to reduce lipid and lipoprotein levels.

Effect of Meal Size and Frequency on Carbohydrate Tolerance

Research on the metabolic effects of the speed of carbohydrate absorption has demonstrated the benefits of slow release (lente) carbohydrates for patients with diabetes. Studies of healthy and diabetic subjects have shown that certain types of dietary fibre, foods with a low glycaemic index, and gastrointestinal digestive enzyme inhibitors slow the rate of glucose absorption and attenuate the insulin response. This appears to be achieved by slowing the delivery of the nutrient load. As part of this research programme, a 'nibbling' diet was devised as an alternative, and possibly cleaner, approach to investigate the hypothesis that slow nutrient absorption is responsible for reduced blood glucose and lipid levels.

In one of these investigations, when seven healthy subjects were fed a standard diet as 17 meals daily, the normal meal-related fluctuations in insulin seen with a three-meal diet plan were abolished. The 'nibbling' diet reduced mean daytime serum insulin levels by approximately 30% without affecting the mean blood glucose level. This is thought to be a result of reduced insulin-stimulated lipid synthesis. A similar result was obtained when nine healthy subjects ingested a glucose solution continuously over 3.5 h, compared with its consumption as a bolus. The sipping protocol generated a reduced serum insulin and C peptide (a connecting peptide of proinsulin, a precursor of insulin) response, despite a similar glucose area under the curve. In one study with a non-insulin-dependent (Type II) diabetic subject, the same blunting of insulin response was seen when 240 g glucose was sipped at an even rate over 12 h, compared with three separate 80 g glucose loads.

Additionally, other short-term studies with non-insulin-dependent diabetic subjects using wholefoods have shown reduced 24 h urinary C peptide losses and lower mean blood glucose and insulin levels over periods of 8–12 h when eating takes place on an hourly or 1.33-hourly basis. When the results of all these studies are combined, there is a clear negative correlation between the number of eating occasions and the incremental area under the glucose response curve. However, although insulin levels appear to be significantly reduced by consumption of six 'meals' daily they are not further reduced with 12 eating occasions.

Despite these clear findings of improved glucose and insulin responses in acute studies, the longer-term data are less consistent. In studies of 2–4 weeks duration with healthy and type II diabetic or hyperlipidaemic subjects, there was no clear improvement in glucose tolerance or measures of diabetic control with nine meals per day when compared with a three meal per day regimen. The discrepancy between short-term and longer-term studies is intriguing and warrants further investigation. Consequently, the lack of long-term data has deterred specific advice regarding the ideal number of eating occasions.

Practical Implications

It is commonly reported that 'snacking', and perhaps eating frequency, may be increasing in the UK. However, this does seem to depend upon the source of the data and definitions employed. Increased marketing of foods as appropriate for 'snacks' may switch classifications of eating occasions from 'meals' to 'snacks', but without clear effect on eating frequency. While there may already be some shifts occurring in eating frequency in the UK, this cannot be clearly established without the appropriate longitudinal data from large-scale dietary surveys.

The 'ideal' eating frequency, if it exists, has yet to be determined. For example, eating 17 times daily seems to produce beneficial effects on lipid profiles, but is clearly impractical. Furthermore, such effects of eating frequency may only be seen when used with a change in diet composition. In short-term studies, insulin responses are significantly reduced with six meals daily compared with three meals, but there does not seem to be further benefit in consuming 12 meals. Notwithstanding, alteration of eating frequency may be possible only within a relatively narrow range, owing to limited opportunities afforded by work and social schedules. Little doubt exists that the type of food consumed is as important – if not more important – than the number of eating times with regard to weight control or management of hyperlipidaemia. It is important to point out that for those choosing to eat more frequently throughout the day, provided the selection of foods remains within current guidelines and energy intake is not excessive, there are no reported *adverse* consequences on lipids, lipoproteins or carbohydrate metabolism. Clearly, however, a degree of willpower may be required to prevent overeating on a 'nibbling' regimen.

See also: **Carbohydrates**: Regulation of Carbohydrate Metabolism. **Cholesterol**: Factors Determining Blood Cholesterol Levels. **Diabetes Mellitus**: Dietary Management. **Dietary Intake Measurement**: Methodology. **Glucose**: Metabolism and Maintenance of Blood Glucose Level. **Hyperlipidaemia (Hyperlipidemia)**: Nutritional Management. **Obesity**: Definition, Aetiology and Assessment.

Further Reading

Adams CE and Morgan KJ (1981) Periodicity of eating: implications for human food consumption. *Nutrition Research* 1:525–550.

Arnold LM, Ball MJ, Duncan AW and Mann J (1993) Effect of isoenergetic intake of three or nine meals on plasma lipoproteins and glucose metabolism. *American Journal of Clinical Nutrition* 57:446–451.

Fabry P and Braun T (1976) Adaptation to the pattern of food intake: some mechanisms and consequences. *Proceedings of the Nutrition Society* 26:144–152.

Fabry P, Fodor J, Hejl Z, Braun T and Zvolankova K (1964) The frequency of meals: its relation to overweight, hypercholesterolaemia, and decreased glucose tolerance. *Lancet* ii: 614–615.

Gibney MJ, Wolever TMS and Frayn KN eds (1997) Periodicity of eating and human health. *British Journal of Nutrition* 77 (supplement 1).

Green SM and Burley VJ (1996) The effects of snacking on energy intake and body weight. *BNF Nutrition Bulletin* 21:103–108.

Jenkins DJA, Ocana A, Jenkins AL *et al.* (1989) Nibbling versus gorging: metabolic advantages of increased meal frequency. *New England Journal of Medicine* 321:929–934.

McGrath SA and Gibney MJ (1994) The effects of altered eating frequency on plasma lipids in free living healthy males on normal self-selected diets. *European Journal of Clinical Nutrition* 48:402–407.

Segura AG, Josse RG and Wolever TMS (1995) Acute metabolic effects of increased meal frequency in Type II diabetes: three vs six, nine, and twelve meals. *Diabetes Nutrition and Metabolism* 8:331–338.

Verboeket-van de Venne WPHG, Westerterp KR and Kester ADM (1993) Effect of the pattern of food intake on human energy metabolism. *British Journal of Nutrition* 70:103–115.

MEAT, POULTRY AND MEAT PRODUCTS

Nutritional Value

J Higgs and **John Pratt**, Meat and Livestock Commission, Milton Keynes, UK

Copyright © 1998 Academic Press

This article considers the different animal species available for human consumption and the significance of the nutritional value of meat as a whole. Increased awareness of animals as sentient beings, and the option to elect to avoid eating meat in affluent societies, influence discussion of the role of meat in the modern human diet.

In theory it is possible to construct both omnivorous and vegetarian diets that meet dietary recommendations, although allowing for the differences in bioavailability of some micronutrients and practical issues relevant to modern society (preparation time and cooking), this task is easier for an omnivorous diet. It is unknown whether or not there would be any significant differences between two such diets that would influence public health advice.

Of all foods, meat provides one of the widest ranges of nutrients in useful amounts. This may be one of the reasons for its importance throughout history as the central focus of the diet, included particularly within celebratory meals. It is perhaps the fact that meat has been eaten as much for enjoyment as for its nutritional qualities that allows any offending aspect of meat production to affect its consumption by affluent nations.

Types of Meat

The types of meat commonly consumed in different countries are dependent on eating habits and the ability to rear the animals successfully, which is influenced by local climate, geography and economy. Sheep and goat meat are more popular in developing countries, while native llama, buffalo and antelope are important parts of the local ecosystems in many areas, especially Bolivia, Peru, Ecuador, Asia and Africa.

Beef, lamb, pork and chicken are the major meats consumed in Western societies, beef predominating. Although total meat consumption in the UK has remained fairly steady since the 1980s, consumption of chicken, pork and meat products has increased while that of beef and lamb has declined. Major influences include increasing demand for con-

venience, a trend towards eating out of the home, and a superior health image for poultry during this period. Veal, horse meat, hare, rabbit and game birds such as duck and pheasant also contribute to meat intake. With the establishment of farmed deer in recent years, venison has become more popular and affordable, promoted for its low fat content. Commercial rearing of ostrich meat is new to Europe and, like emu, has grown rapidly in the USA. Both ostrich and emu meat are promoted for their favourable fat profile, which is similar to that of poultry and pork, although the iron content of ostrich is closer to that of beef and lamb.

Meat includes carcass meat and edible offals (organ meats, e.g. liver, kidney, tongue, heart, sweetbreads (thymus and pancreas) and tripe (stomach)). Meat products is a term that includes the result of any type of processing ranging from composite dishes such as pies and ready-made meals to the addition of other ingredients such as water to increase succulence, curing, fermentation, and preparations such as brawn, black pudding, meat bars (pemmican), etc.

Consumption

Meat consumption increases with affluence. Japanese intake has increased to half that in the USA and in China meat intake is also increasing dramatically (**Table 1**).

Table 1   Meat consumption 1980s and 1990s (g per person per day)

Country	1980s	1990s
USA	310	231
Australia	296	290
UK	201	204
France	290	305
Germany	269	261
Japan	100	123
China	26	108

The values quoted are from the OECD for the years 1982–84 and 1992, respectively. The exception is China; these values are taken from *Asia Pacific Food Industry* (1995) **7**(11): 14, using the years 1979 and 1994. The figures include bone weight.

Macronutrient Content

Protein

Meat is a significant source of protein, which is of high biological value. Within developed nations meat provides around 60% of protein intake compared with only 15% in poorer nations. The protein content of different meats and cuts varies inversely with fat content. Meat is a rich source of the amino acid taurine; this is essential in newborn infants as they are unable to synthesize this amino acid from cysteine in sufficient quantities. The significance of lower levels of taurine in the breast milk of vegan mothers is unknown.

Fat

Total fat content varies with species and across the carcass. Although the fat content of lean muscle from most species is around 2–5%, total fat content depends on rearing practices, feeding regimes and age. The level of fat trim sold with the meat provides opportunities to affect the fat content as-consumed further, through cooking and trimming by the end user. This is illustrated by looking at the changes seen in the fat content of pork since the 1970s (**Fig. 1**). Trimming visible fat (subcutaneous and intermuscular) has the most influence on the final fat content, since the invisible (intramuscular) fat makes a relatively small contribution to the total. **Table 2** provides UK data showing the range of trimmable fat on specific red meat cuts.

Fat will be lost on cooking meat, assuming that it is allowed to escape, for example. The amount lost depends on the initial fat content, and fully trimmed lean meat will lose little fat. The concurrent loss of moisture on cooking meat obscures fat losses as viewed in composition tables.

During the years following World War II the emphasis for meat production was on maximizing its energy (fat) content and minimizing cost in an attempt to produce enough nutrient-dense food to improve the nutritional wellbeing of the whole population. Thus in the 1970s red meat and meat products contributed 27.4% to total daily UK fat intake, and little of this was trimmed away. In the early 1980s diet and health reports identified meat as a major contributor to fat intake, and so started the negative health association with red meat. Poultry meat was recognized as being significantly lower in fat and was recommended in preference by health experts. The red meat industry responded by reducing the fat content of red meat once again. Selective breeding and feeding practices, carcass classification changes to favour leaner production, as well as butchery techniques (seaming out whole muscles, and trimming away all intermuscular fat) have meant that the meat on sale in the 1990s is much leaner than it was in the 1970s. The fat content of the carcass has been reduced in the UK by over 30% for pork, making British pork virtually the leanest in the

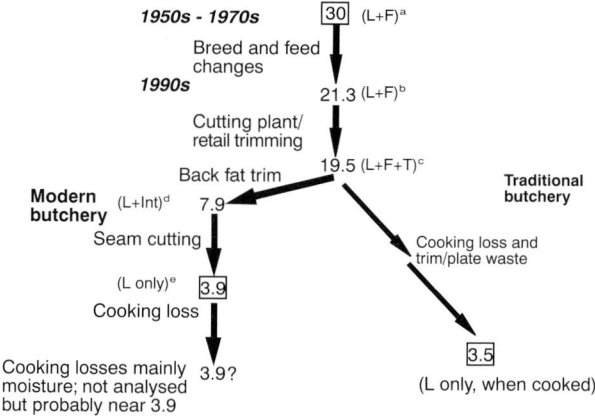

Figure 1 Change in fat content of pork loin for 100 g of raw edible tissue. Key: (L + F), lean + fat, untrimmed; (L + F + T), lean + fat, some trimming; (L + Int), lean + intermuscular fat; (L only), lean only. Source of data: [a]Untrimmed, UK Database 1970s; [b]untrimmed including rind, UK Database 1990s; [c]at retail, UK Database 1990s (79% lean, 21% fat); [d]trimmed of all back fat, UK Database 1990s; [e]fully trimmed, UK Database 1990s; [f]100 g raw as-purchased, cooked and fully trimmed.
[a]From Holland B, Welsh AA, Unwin ID, Buss DH, Paul AA and Southgate D (1991). *McCance & Widdowson's, The Composition of Food*. Fifth Edition. Royal Society of Chemistry.
[b,c,d] and [e]From Analytical Methods Committee (1991). Nitrogen Factors for Pork: A Reassessment. *Analyst* **116**: 761–766 F.
[f]From Chan W, Brown J, Lee FM and Buss DH (1995). *Meat, Poultry and Game*. Supplement to *McCance & Widdowson's, The Composition of Food*. Cambridge: Royal Society of Chemistry/London: Ministry of Agriculture, Fisheries and Food.

Table 2 Proportion of trimmable fat in some raw cuts of beef, lamb and pork

Meat	Means and ranges (%)
Beef	
Braising steak	7 (0–18)
Fore-rib	21 (10–35)
Sirloin steak	18 (6–34)
Lamb	
Chump chops	21 (11–32)
Breast	33 (20–48)
Rack of lamb	22 (18–25)
Pork	
Leg	18 (12–28)
Loin chops	25 (16–34)
Steaks	11 (3–35)

From Chan W, Brown J, Lee SM and Buss DH (1995) Meat, poultry and game. Supplement to *McCance and Widdowson's The Composition of Foods*. Cambridge: Royal Society of Chemistry and the Controller of Her Majesty's Stationery Office.

world, by 15% for beef, and by 10% for lamb. Further reductions are anticipated for beef and lamb in the first few years of the twenty-first century. Overall little change has occurred in poultry meat; most of the fat is in the skin, which is 48% fat.

Minced meat, predominantly beef, has become more popular in recent years, reflecting a move to convenience and a more cosmopolitan approach to meals. Although viewed as a fattier product, fat levels have dropped to typically 15%, with some extra-lean mince as low as 5%.

Since food composition tables throughout the world have not kept pace with these changes, the health image of red meat has suffered disproportionately to the nutritional benefits it offers. Food composition tables from different countries (e.g. the UK, USA and Germany) will vary due to the analysis of different cuts, different consumer demands, and how up-to-date the tables are. Data on the composition of red meat are shown in **Table 3**, and a 1995 fat audit for the UK to trace all fat in the human food chain provides useful information to illustrate the reduction in fat intake since 1982 from meat, compared with other foods (**Table 4**).

The fat content of meat products can vary considerably, dependent on the proportion of lean and fat from meat as well as the other ingredients. Traditional types such as sausages, pastry-covered pies and salami were high in fat, up to 50%, but modern products include ready-made meals and prepared meats which can be low in fat (5%). The trend downwards in fat of red meat is reflected in the reduced fat content of a number of meat products, such as hams and sausages. Reduced fat versions of popular hamburgers and sausages continue to enter the market, and utilization of fat replacers will enable this trend to continue (**Table 5**).

Fatty acids

As with other foods, meat contains a mixture of fatty acids. As the fat content of red meat has reduced, so the fatty acid mix has changed with percentage of saturated fat than in the past. Poultry fat is 30% saturated, while pork, beef and lamb are less than 50% saturated. The contribution made by meat to dietary saturated fat is given for Great Britain (**Table 6**). The principal saturated fatty acids are palmitic acid ($C_{16:0}$ and stearic acid $C_{18:0}$, which are thought not to raise blood cholesterol levels. There are only minor amounts of myristic acid, the most atherogenic.

Meat is one of the main contributors to the mono-unsaturated fat content of the British diet, principally oleic acid ($C_{18:1}$) from red meat. Around 40% of the fat in meat is monounsaturated. Ruminant meats also contain *trans* fatty acids, contributing around 18% of British intakes.

Recent international analyses of beef, lamb and pork demonstrate useful levels of long-chain polyunsaturated fatty acids in pasture- and grain-fed animals, specifically eicosatrienoic acid (20:3n-6), arachidonic acid (20:4n-6), eicosapentaenoic acid (20:5n-3) and docosapentaenoic acid (22:5n-3). Significant losses of some fatty acids, particularly the more highly unsaturated fatty acids (C_{20} and C_{22}) that are more susceptible to oxidation, occur in cooking. The small amount of docosahexaenoic acid (22:6n-3) present in raw samples is lost on cooking. Richest dietary sources of 20 : 4n-6 include liver, kidney and turkey, while smaller quantities are found in beef, lamb, pork and chicken (**Table 7**). Grass-fed animals have higher concentrations of α-linolenic acid compared with grain-fed animals, and beef and lamb have favourable n-6 : n-3 ratios. Meat along with fish provide the only significant dietary sources of C_{20} and C_{22} n-3 fatty acids, and for countries like the UK where fish intakes remain low, the contribution to the diet from meat is significant, despite absolute levels in meat being low relative to those in fish (**Table 8**).

It is possible to manipulate the fatty acid profile of meat to satisfy human nutritional concerns more easily in monogastrics (pigs and poultry) than in ruminants (cattle and sheep), where polyunsaturated fatty acids are hydrogenated in the rumen. The fatty acid profiles of meats will continue to change as knowledge of their significance to human health improves, such that food composition data for meat can only represent a single point in time.

Micronutrient Content

The micronutrient content of meat can make a significant positive contribution to nutritional intakes, since it is a relatively concentrated source of a large number of vitamins, minerals and trace elements, and the bioavailability of several such as iron, copper, and zinc is greater from meat than from plant foods.

Iron

Meat, especially red meat and offal, is a rich source of iron, a 100 g serving of beef rump steak providing 3 mg. Red meat contains 50–60% of its iron in the haem form (from haemoglobin and myoglobin), this is absorbed by a more efficient mechanism than non-haem iron, the sole source of iron in plant foods. Moreover, haem iron is unaffected by the numerous inhibitors of iron absorption such as phytate. Thus the absorption of iron from meat is typically 15–25%, twice that from plant sources. Meat also plays

Table 3 Nutrient composition of different meats per 100 g

Nutrient	Beef (raw, with fat)	Bison (raw)	Buffalo (raw)	Chicken (raw, skin/fat)	Duck (raw, with fat)	Goat (raw)	Kangaroo (raw)	Lamb (raw, with fat)	Ostrich meat (cooked)	Pork (raw, with fat)	Rabbit (raw meat)	Turkey (raw, skin/fat)	Veal (raw)	Venison (deer) (raw)
Energy (kcal)	226	109	146	201	388	161	118	245	131	221	137	133	125	103
Energy (kJ)	945	456	610	840	1622	673	493	1024	548	924	573	556	523	431
Protein (g)	21.7	21.6	20.8	19.1	13.1	19.5	24.2	18.5	24.8	19.2	21.9	21.6	21.5	22.2
Fat (g)	15.5	1.8	7.1	13.8	37.3	7.9	2.3	19	2.8	16.1	5.5	5.2	4.4	1.6
SFA (g)	7.1	0.7	3.24	3.8	2			9.35	1.06	5.8	2.1	1.7	1.8	0.8
MFA (g)	7	0.7	3.13	6.4	3.2			7.23	0.89	6.6	1.3	1.9	1.9	0.4
PFA (g)	0.6	0.2	0.3	2.6	1			0.87	0.59	2.7	1.8	1.2	0.4	0.4
Cholesterol (mg)	61	62		100	110			78	81	65	53	78	57	50
Iron (mg)	1.56	2.6	2.7	0.7	1.3	1.95	6	1.23	2.98	0.63	1	0.6	0.7	3.3
Zinc (mg)	3.5	2.8		1.1	1		4.1	2.71		1.75	1.4	1.8	2.7	2.4
Calcium (mg)		6	7.5	7	8	9.5	3		1.69		22	6	6.5	5
Magnesium (mg)				22	14						25	23	tr	25
Copper (mg)	0.02	0.09		0.05				0.07		0.05	0.06	0.03	8	0.21
Selenium (µg)	5.93			12						11.6		12	8	
Sodium (mg)	55	54	111	70	73	63	63	62	71	59	67	70	71	55
Vitamins														
B1 (mg)	0.09	0.06		0.11	0.14	0.15		0.08		0.8	0.1	0.07	0.09	0.16
B2 (mg)	0.19	0.19		0.25	0.51	0.28		0.18		0.21	0.19	0.2	0.19	0.7
Niacin equivalents (mg)	8.24	6.3		10	5.9	4.9		7.8		9.5	12.5	11.5	9.8	6.7
B6 (mg)	0.46	0.44		0.3	0.33	0.3		0.25		0.45	0.5	0.55	0.57	0.65
B12 (µg)	1.61	1.28		tr	2			1.76		1	10	1	2	1
Folate (µg)				9.0	7			5.51		2.76	5		19	6
D (µg)	0.39			0.6				0.42		0.68		0.4	1.2	N
E (mg)	0.12			0.15				0.1		0.04		0.01	0.22	N

Data taken from relevant international food composition databases published between 1986 and 1995.
SFA, saturated fatty acids; MFA, monounsaturated fatty acids; PFA, polyunsaturated fatty acids.
N, nutrient present but no reliable data on amount.

Table 4 Total UK dietary fat, per person, contributed from all foods groups in 1982 and 1992

Food group	Dietary fat (kg per person per year) 1982	1992
Beef and veal	2.09	1.93
Lamb	0.66	0.51
Pork and products (1981, 1992)	6.54	4.36
Poultry meat	9.29	6.80
Fats and oils	17.40	21.98
Dairy fat (1983, 1992)	12.91	11.04
Fish and fish oil	4.40	2.20
Eggs	1.56	1.09
Chocolate	1.54	1.92
Cereals	0.92	1.05
Nuts	0.27	0.34

From Ulbricht (1995) *Fat in the Food Chain*.
Shows contribution of fat from primary food source rather than the end product, e.g. 'Fats and oils' includes fat used ultimately in such products as bakery goods, meat products and confectionery.

Table 6 Contribution made by meat to nutrient intake

Nutrient	% total daily intake contributed by meat for Great Britain
Energy	12.9
Protein	38.0
Fat	20.0
Saturated fatty acids	19.2
Monounsaturated fatty acids	23.8
Polyunsaturated fatty acids	15.0
Iron	15.0
Zinc	33.3
Retinol	32.2
Vitamin D	18.5
B_1	34.3
B_2	18.6
Niacin equivalents	42.9
B_6	25.0
B_{12}	37.5
Folate	5.4
Vitamin E	1.2
Vitamin C	0.4

Per capita consumption figures for beef and veal, mutton and lamb, pork, bacon and poultry for 1995 in Great Britain.

a valuable role as an enhancer of iron absorption from plant foods, so the presence of meat in a meal can double the amount of iron absorbed from the other components of the meal. The exact mechanism for this, although not confirmed, is believed to be due to the iron-binding capacity of cysteine within peptides following proteolysis of meat muscle. Although the absolute iron content of white meats, e.g. chicken, and meat products may appear low compared with some plant food sources, this enhancing function and better iron availability makes these foods useful contributors to iron intakes. Cooking in iron or steel utensils can increase the iron content of the meal owing to this enhancing effect of meat. Meat is thus a particularly important influence on iron intake and iron status. Serum ferritin levels, which indicate iron stores in the body, are strongly correlated with haem iron intake. Meat can have a major impact in groups vulnerable to iron deficiency, specifically toddlers, adolescents and women of child-bearing age.

Zinc

The best sources of zinc are meat, especially beef, lamb, pork, poultry and seafood. As with non-haem iron, bioavailability of zinc is reduced by inhibitors in the diet such as phytate and oxalate, and is enhanced when consumed with animal protein. In metabolic studies, zinc absorption and retention is greater on diets with a high meat content compared

Table 5 Nutrient content for a range of meat products per 100 g

Product	Fat content (g; range)	Energy (kJ; range)	Energy (kcal; range)	Iron (mg; range)
Bacon, all types	11.7–26.6	727–1388	174–332	0.4–1.1
Beefburgers, raw	6.2–25.4	472–1258	113–301	1.7–2.7
Chicken nuggets/fingers	1.5–17.1	552–1212	132–290	0.6–1.1
Cornish pasties	16.3–24.3	1066–1496	255–358	1.0–1.1
Frankfurters, cooked	20.0–31.0	1041–1400	249–335	1.1
Ham, all types	1.5–20.0	372–1003	89–240	0.6–0.8
Pastrami	3.2–7.2	477–736	114–176	–
Pate	11.9–33.0	811–1484	194–355	1.5–7.4
Pork pies	19.5–33.5	1329–1827	318–437	0.9–1.2
Pork sausages, raw	8.8–30.4	740–1446	177–346	0.8–1.0
Salami	28.3–52.3	1442–2249	345–538	1.3

Data taken from: MLC (1996) *Meat Products Composition Survey*; Chan W, Brown J, Church SM and Buss DH (1996) Meat products and meat dishes. (Available on request from MLC). Supplement to *McCance and Widdowson's The Composition of Foods*. Cambridge: Royal Society of Chemistry and the Controller of Her Majesty's Stationery Office. Where available, ranges include low-fat versions of the product.

Table 7 Fatty acid composition of muscle from English beef, lamb and pork

Fatty acid	Percentage by weight of total fatty acids		
	Beef	Lamb	Pork
12:0 lauric	0.08 ± 0.03	0.31 ± 0.18	0.12 ± 0.05
14:0 myristic	2.66 ± 0.54	3.30 ± 1.07	1.33 ± 0.20
16:0 palmitic	25.0 ± 1.77	22.2 ± 1.56	23.2 ± 1.46
16:1 cis	4.54 ± 0.81	2.20 ± 0.26	2.71 ± 0.45
18:0 stearic	13.4 ± 1.84	18.1 ± 2.80	12.2 ± 1.11
18:1 trans	2.75 ± 1.28	4.67 ± 1.67	ND
18:1n-9 oleic	36.1 ± 2.87	32.5 ± 3.25	32.8 ± 3.91
18:1n-7 vaccenic	2.33 ± 0.40	1.45 ± 0.26	3.99 ± 0.59
18:2n-6 linoleic	2.42 ± 0.63	2.70 ± 0.86	14.2 ± 4.09
18:3n-6 γ-linolenic	ND	ND	0.06 ± 0.03
18:3n-3 α-linolenic	0.70 ± 0.18	1.37 ± 0.48	0.95 ± 0.33
20:2n-6	ND	ND	0.42 ± 0.11
20:3n-6	0.21 ± 0.06	0.05 ± 0.04	0.34 ± 0.09
20:3n-3	0.007 ± 0.011	ND	0.12 ± 0.05
20:4n-6 arachidonic	0.63 ± 0.21	0.64 ± 0.23	2.21 ± 0.73
20:4n-3	0.08 ± 0.03	ND	0.009 ± 0.022
20:5n-3 EPA	0.28 ± 0.11	0.45 ± 0.13	0.31 ± 0.15
22:4n-6	0.04 ± 0.02	ND	0.23 ± 0.07
22:5n-3	0.45 ± 0.14	0.52 ± 0.14	0.62 ± 0.20
22:6n-3 DHA	0.05 ± 0.02	0.15 ± 0.05	0.39 ± 0.23

From Enser M, Hallett K, Hewitt B, Fursey G and Wood J (1996) Fatty acid content and composition of English beef, lamb and pork at retail. *Meat Science* **42**(4): 443–456.
ND, not detected. EPA, eicosapentaenoic acid; DHA, docosahexaenoic acid.

Table 8 Contribution to UK diet of n-3 and n-6 polyunsaturated fatty acids from meat and fish (g per person per year)

Food	n-3	n-6
Beef	17.7	39.1
Lamb	13.0	17.5
Pork	55.7	451.6
Total – Red meat	86.3	508.2
Total – Fish	12.9	1.5

From Ulbricht (1995) *Fat in the Food Chain.*

with those on a low meat content. Lower plasma zinc levels in vegetarians and vegans, despite higher intakes, suggest that meat has a major influence on zinc status. Approximately 20–40% of zinc is absorbed from meat, which is the major contributor to zinc intakes in Western countries (Table 6).

Selenium

Selenium is added to animal feeds to prevent deficiency. Concerns of excess build-up of selenium in soil and water supplies as a consequence of this are difficult to substantiate. Bioavailability of selenium from plant foods was thought to be greater than that from animal foods, but recent data demonstrate that meat, both raw and cooked, provides selenium in a form which is as bioavailable as that in cereals. Meat provides on average 10 µg selenium per 100 g and contributes around a quarter of daily needs.

Vitamins

Meat can make a significant contribution to intakes of all B vitamins except folate and biotin. Pork and pork products, such as bacon and ham, are particularly rich sources of thiamin, typical servings providing the daily requirement. Liver and kidney provide more than the daily requirement of riboflavin in less than 100 g. Meat also provides the richest source of niacin (half of which is derived from the amino acid tryptophan) and vitamin B_6. Per 100 g portion, veal liver provides half daily B_6 needs, and other meats provide around a third. Organ meats are particularly rich sources of folate and vitamin A (**Table 9**). Currently in the UK liver is not recommended during pregnancy, despite being an excellent provider of iron and folate, owing to the very high levels of retinol it contains which may potentially cause malformation of the developing fetus. Vitamin A in its active form, retinol, is found only in foods of animal origin, so meat provides a preformed source of this vitamin.

Vitamin B_{12} merits particular attention since foods of animal origin provide the only significant dietary source. It is recommended that where meat and dairy products are avoided, supplements should be taken. In the past some B_{12} was provided from the soil on

Table 9 Nutrient content of a range of offal meats

	Energy[a] (kcal)	Fat (g)	Iron (mg)	Zinc (mg)	(Retinol) Vitamin A (μg)	Vitamin D (μg)	Vitamin B$_{12}$ (μg)	Cholesterol (mg)	Folate (μg)
Heart									
Lamb, raw	119	5.6	3.6	2.0	tr	N	8.0	140	2
Kidney									
Lamb, raw	91	2.6	5.5	2.5	96	N	17.0	315	8
Liver									
Calf, raw	104	3.4	11.5	14.2	18 800	0.3	68	370	155
Lamb, raw	137	6.2	7.5	4.0	17 300	0.5	54	430	205
Pig, raw	113	3.1	13.9	7.0	17 400	1.1	23	260	295
Brains									
Lamb, boiled	126	8.8	1.4	1.4	tr	tr	8	2200	6
Tongue									
Ox, stewed	243	18.3	2.5	3.8	tr	N	4.0	N	11

From Chan W, Brown J, Lee SM and Buss DH (1995) Meat, poultry and game. Supplement to *McCance and Widdowson's The Composition of Foods*. Cambridge: Royal Society of Chemistry/London: Ministry of Agriculture, Fisheries and Food.
tr, trace; N, nutrient present in significant quantities but no reliable data on amount.
[a] 1 kcal ~ 4.2 kJ.

poorly cleaned foods, which may in part explain the apparent absence of deficiency in some vegan groups.

Pantothenic acid is universal in all living matter, and rich sources include liver and kidney. Most of the vitamin is leached into the drip loss associated with frozen meat.

Vitamin D

Meat, apart from liver, was thought to be a poor source of vitamin D. New analytical data for meat and liver include significant amounts of 25-hydroxy-cholecalciferol, assumed to have a biological activity five times that of cholecalciferol. Recent work on the British diet and nutrition surveys using updated food composition data of adults and young children show that rather than contributing as little as 4% of dietary vitamin D intakes, meat and meat products appear to provide 21% and 18%, respectively, becoming the major contributor of natural dietary vitamin D intakes.

Role of Meat in the Diet

Meat has played a significant role in human evolution. Early herbivorous hominids did not survive, whereas those that developed the ability to hunt became our ancestors (*Homo erectus*).

Anthropological research shows that the length of the gut in primates and humans became shorter with the introduction of animal-derived food. Smaller quantities of food of high digestibility required relatively smaller guts, characterized by simple stomachs and proportionately long small intestines, emphasiz-

ing absorption. Furthermore, it has recently been suggested that selection for relatively large brains in humans over the last 2 million years could not have been achieved without a move to a high-quality diet, based on animal products, since the energy saved with a shorter gut allowed an increase in brain mass. It is believed that better nutrition, specifically increased animal protein and fat intake together with improved public health, has allowed us to move towards attaining our genetic optimum.

Meat has traditionally been considered an essential component of the diet to ensure optimal growth and development. With a limited range of foods available in primitive societies throughout history, meat was important as a concentrated source of a wide range of nutrients. With the range and abundance of foods now available to developed societies, the nutritional significance of any one food is reduced. Where meat is excluded the missing nutrients can be supplied from a combination of other foods and within traditional vegetarian cultures this appears at least adequate. Concern arises when meat is excluded with insufficient attention given to selecting appropriate combinations of foods to ensure nutrients are supplied in adequate quantities. There is no doubt that in modern Western societies where less time is devoted to planning and preparing meals, and an increasing proportion of daily food intake is consumed outside the home as snacks and quick meals, the inclusion of meat in the diet minimizes the risk of micronutrient deficiencies, especially iron, albeit subclinical.

Meat and Health: Addressing the Concerns

Traditionally meat intake was associated with improved health but, as a consequence of its association with dietary fat this role has been marginalized. To assess the role played by meat, numerous studies have compared the health status and mortality of vegetarians with those of omnivores. Simplistic conclusions from such work can be flawed, since interpretation of the results must take into account the many other influential differences between such groups. In particular, lifestyle factors must be considered: vegetarians traditionally smoke less, consume less alcohol, tea and coffee, and, being generally more health conscious, they tend to exercise more. Typically, the meat-eating groups tend to be dominated by sedentary, physically inactive subjects with little interest in diet. Since the 1950s omnivorous diets have been relatively high in animal protein and fat with insufficient dietary fibre, fruit and vegetables, such that meat intake may have acted as a marker for a generally 'unhealthy' diet.

Regular consumption of red meat is associated, epidemiologically, with increased risk of coronary heart disease (CHD), owing to its fat composition. There is, however, a growing bank of evidence that a healthy diet which includes lean red meat can produce positive changes in lipid biochemistry. Blood cholesterol levels are increased by inclusion of beef fat, not by lean beef in an otherwise low-fat diet. Equal amounts of lean beef, chicken and fish added to low-fat, low-saturated-fat diets, similarly reduce plasma cholesterol and low-density lipoprotein (LDL) cholesterol levels in hypercholesterolaemic and normocholesterolaemic men and women.

The association between the arachidonic acid content of meat and increased thrombotic tendencies has recently been challenged. The presence of large amounts of linoleic acid in current diets results in plasma increases of linoleic and arachidonic acids only, but in the absence of linoleic acid, the long-chain n-6 and n-3 polyunsaturated fatty acids present in lean meat can influence the plasma pool, increasing plasma 20:3n-6, 20:4n-6 and 20:5n-3 fatty acids and probably reducing thrombotic tendencies.

Meat has been associated with various cancers, particularly colon cancer. However, meat eating is strongly inversely correlated with gastric cancer, which makes any public health recommendations difficult to determine, based on meat eating alone. Epidemiologically it is difficult to distinguish the influence of animal fat, protein and meat.

There does appear to be an independent role for protein as a source of cooked food mutagens. Het-erocyclic amines produced on overcooking meat have been shown to be carcinogenic in rats, although at normal cooking temperatures and average cooking times the level of these compounds produced is not excessive, compared with the amounts required for carcinogenicity.

Nitrates are added to meat products to prevent microbial proliferation. However, the levels used now are much reduced such that the nitrosocompounds (NOC) produced from these additives are present at very low levels in meat products. Contrary to public perception, their carcinogenic potential is likely to be minor. In humans, high-protein (meat) diets increase faecal NOC levels, although the significance of this for normal healthy diets remains unclear.

Daily consumption of green and yellow vegetables with meat is associated with reduced risk of cancer at many sites, whereas daily meat consumption with less frequent vegetable consumption has been associated with increased risk. The significance of meat's role as a risk factor in cancer causation remains the subject of much debate and results of more informative long-term cohort studies are required to elucidate the full picture.

There are many paradoxes concerning the apparent associations between meat consumption and both CHD and cancer. Some of these are listed in **Table 10**. They serve to demonstrate that the diet and health story, at least as far as meat is concerned, is both complex and incomplete. Two reasons for this are, first, that meat is but one influential aspect of the diet. Its effects are modified by other foods (e.g. fruit and vegetables) such that the net effect may be quite different. Second, the changing lipid

Table 10   Paradoxical associations between meat and health

- Generally in countries where meat consumption is high, intake of protective fruit and vegetables tends to be low, and vice versa.

- There is a lower risk of colon cancer among South Asian immigrants to the UK, than in the general population, and this is equally true of vegetarian and meat-eating Asians.

- Mormons who abstain from alcohol, tea, coffee and smoking but consume meat have death rates from cancer and CHD similar to those of vegetarian groups, indicating that meat is not the major determinant. Blood pressure is reduced on switching from a meat-based diet to a vegetarian one, but adding meat to a vegetarian diet is not associated with an increase in blood pressure, suggesting that the potassium-to-sodium ratio is more influential than the presence of meat *per se*.

- Consumption of meat has almost doubled in Japan since the 1970s, yet CHD morbidity has reduced from an already low level. Meat consumption in the USA remains higher than in the UK, yet, unlike the UK, morbidity from CHD has been falling steadily since the 1970s.

composition of meat, in response to increased knowledge of lipids in relation to health, will continue to alter the role played by meat in this context. Fortunately, since most of the valuable nutrients in meat are within the lean component, reducing the visible fat has little bearing on its contribution to micronutrient status (**Table 11**).

Hygiene and Safety Aspects

The wholesomeness of meat and meat products is dependent on a variety of factors, some of which act in the period prior to arrival of the animal or bird at the slaughterhouse. The health status of the herd or flock is in turn influenced by the method of husbandry practised on the farm, the health prevention measures applied, the conscientiousness of monitoring and the level of prompt and necessary action taken, e.g. the isolation and treatment of veal calves infected with one or more species of salmonellae. However, calves may be carriers of infections such as *Escherichia coli* and *Listeria monocytogenes* and display no symptoms of disease but may prove a hazard to public health when meat and offal are prepared from the carcasses. Similarly, campylobacteria may be present in a mild form in a batch of broilers which appear perfectly healthy in life but may prove a hazard to the consumer. Close monitoring of farm health records and scrutiny by the herd/flock veterinarian and collaboration with the supervising official veterinary surgeon in the slaughterhouse and poultry plant will help prevent subsequent potential consumer health hazards.

The raising of stock in dirty conditions allows the hides, fleeces and feathers to contaminate the environment during the slaughter and dressing of carcasses. Cross-contamination of the carcasses from faeces and soil in addition to the soiling of plant, equipment and the protective clothing of slaughter-house operatives can markedly reduce the general hygiene in the meat plant with levels of bacteria, bacterial spores, parasites, viruses and fungi exceeding acceptable levels. *Staphylococcus aureus* is a normal commensal of skin and hair and can produce toxins in food. A highly successful recent campaign has highlighted the necessity for only clean livestock to be presented for slaughter.

Transport of animals, especially loading, unloading and lairaging, can lead to stress conditions, particularly if groups are mixed. In some countries two-tier lorries are used to transport cattle and three-tier sheep transporters are common worldwide, resulting in gross contamination with urine and faeces. Again, stress from loading and unloading can occur. Stressed animals, particularly carriers of disease, are known to demonstrate clinical disease and excrete pathogenic organisms. Welfare and hygiene regulations governing animals during transport minimise such occurrences.

The slaughterhouse itself may not be free from external vectors of disease – insects, vermin and birds must be excluded from the curtilage of the meat plant. Measures are in place and reviewed regularly so that the environment of the meat plant suffers minimum contamination from the animals consigned to the plant, from the lorries and staff transporting the stock and from all other potential vectors of pathogenic and spoilage agents into and throughout the plant.

Procedures within the meat or poultry plant itself dictate the standard of hygiene and safety of the product. The training and continuing professional development of staff in handling of and caring for the animals, in stunning and slaughter techniques and in the dressing procedures of the carcasses are significant contributors to the overall standards pertaining through the plant. The operative has the

Table 11 Nutrient variability across the carcass – values given for lowest and highest fat cuts for different species

Cut of meat	Nutrients per 100 g weight				
	Energy[a] (kcal)	Fat (g)	Vitamin D (µg)	Iron (mg)	Zinc (mg)
Veal escalopes, raw	106	1.7	1.3	0.6	2.4
Beef flank, lean raw	175	9.3	0.5	1.8	3.6
Beef, stewing steak, lean, raw	122	3.5	0.8	2.1	5.7
Chicken, light meat, raw	106	4.4	0.2	0.5	0.7
Chicken, leg quarter with skin, raw	193	13.3	0.5	0.8	1.4
Lamb, best end neck cutlets, 34% fat, raw	316	27.9	0.4	1.2	3.5
Lamb leg, lean, raw	147	4.7		1.5	3.1
Pork, leg joint lean, raw	107	2.2	0.5	0.8	2.2
Pork, belly joint/slices, raw	258	20.0	0.8	0.6	1.7

From Chan W, Brown J, Lee SM and Buss DH (1995) Meat, poultry and game. Supplement to *McCance and Widdowson's The Composition of Foods*. Cambridge: Royal Society of Chemistry/London: Ministry of Agriculture, Fisheries and Foods.
[a]1 kcal ~ 4.2 kJ.

potential to contaminate the carcass, and vice versa, but training and legislation obviate this from occurring.

Management must be aware of the likely points of entry of pathogenic agents and where they may have maximum impact on the meat and meat products. Recognition of these critical points where hazards are potentially most dangerous is now enshrined in the HACCP (hazard analysis and critical control point) principle. Checking regularly and acting on findings at these areas in the meat plant allow a structured approach to the maintenance of hygiene and safety aspects of meat and poultry and their products. Increasing rates of throughput on the slaughterline must be accompanied by even more vigilant monitoring of hygiene standards.

The proper dressing of the carcass is fundamental to good hygiene. The hide, fleece or feathers constitute a dirty coat to the sterile muscle and organs. The alimentary tract extending from the mouth to the anus is also a source of microbes and parasites. Therefore the exterior coat and the complete intestinal tract must both be removed carefully so that the absolute minimum of contamination occurs. The surface of meat or muscle is an excellent medium on which pathogens and spoilage organisms grow so the separation of edible and inedible tissues must be carried out expertly and completely. For this reason the movement of these two elements follows an agreed flow chart implicitly within the plant so that 'clean' and 'dirty' areas are entirely separate. No crossover of staff, equipment and tools is allowed; however, in the case of supervising officers moving between areas, a strict regime of changing protective clothing must be followed.

Water used within the meat plant must be of a quality that does not present a risk to the meat or meat product. Potable water is routinely checked in the slaughterhouse and meat processing plant so that pathogenic and spoilage organisms are not allowed entry. The monitoring is supervised by the official veterinary surgeon of the plant, as are the ante-mortem examinations and the post-mortem inspections of the animals or birds and carcasses to check for pathological change, residues of veterinary medicines and other substances; also storage temperature control for meat and meat products. In many countries veterinarians are helped in their duties by assistants/meat hygiene inspectors to ensure that only healthy carcasses and their offals are deemed fit for human consumption.

These duties are delineated in national meat hygiene and inspection legislation which is harmonized throughout the European Community. Other meat-producing countries, e.g. USA, Australian and New Zealand, adhere to their own similar legislative controls.

Meat products may undergo little processing, e.g. steak tartare, when no cooking takes place, or undercooking may unwittingly allow pathogenic agents to survive, e.g. lightly barbecued beef burgers were the source of an outbreak of haemolytic *Escherichia coli* 0157. The increase in the number of chilled ready-made meals supplementing some frozen products may also be conducive to poisoning with organisms or toxins surviving in the meat if proper procedures in storage, preparation and cooking are neglected.

The integrity of properly prepared meat and poultry and their products can be – and often is – undermined by contamination by a food handler who has neglected proper personal hygiene procedures or who is a carrier of a food poisoning organism. The mishandler or carrier could, of course, be the consumer in their own home.

In conclusion, therefore, the arrival of meat and poultry and their products on the table from the farm can be hazardous if neglect occurs at any of the steps of the journey. Legislation, guidelines and well-recognized proven routines ensure safe and healthy products, provided these are properly understood and implemented. However, one significant area of concern to the consumer, in Great Britain in particular, is the catastrophic BSE (Bovine Spongiform Encephalopathy) epidemic which has devastated the livestock and meat industry since the mid 1980s.

Control measures introduced early on in the epidemic have reduced the incidence of BSE markedly since its peak in 1992 and 1993, although the long incubation period (4–5 years) has meant that any preventative legislation has taken the same time for its effects to be realised. Much research has been carried out in Great Britain and around the world on BSE, with consequent benefits accruing to other transmissible spongiform encephalopathies, including Scrapie in sheep and Creutzfeldt Jakob Disease (CJD) in humans.

There is strong circumstantial evidence that some young consumers of beef contaminated by the BSE agent may have contracted a new variant of CJD. However, this contamination occurred prior to the controls introduced in the late 1980s. It will be some years before it is known how many victims will succumb to this new form of CJD on account of the unknown length of the incubation period in humans.

See Colour Plate 16.

See also: **Anaemia (Anemia)**: Iron-Deficiency Anaemia. **Bioavailability**: Definition and General Aspects. **Car-**

cinogens: Carcinogenic Substances in Food. **Coronary Heart Disease**: Lipid Theory of Coronary Heart Disease; Prevention. **Dietary Guidelines**: International Perspectives. **Fatty Acids**: Health Effects of Saturated Fatty Acids; Health Effects of Monounsaturated Fatty Acids; Health Effects of n-6 Polyunsaturated Fatty Acids; Health Effects of n-3 Polyunsaturated Fatty Acids. **Iron**: Physiology, Dietary Sources and Requirements. **Protein**: Quality and Sources. **Selenium**: Physiology, Dietary Sources and Requirements. **Vegetarian Diets**: Practice; Nutritional Adequacy. **Zinc**: Physiology.

Further Reading

Aiellio LC and Wheeler P (1995) The expensive-tissue hypothesis. The brain and the digestive system in human and primate evolution. *Current Anthropology* 36:199–221.

Analytical Methods Committee of the Royal Society of Chemistry and Meat and Livestock Commission (MLC) (1993) Nitrogen factors for beef: a reassessment. *Analyst* 118:1217–1226.

Analytical Methods Committee of the Royal Society of Chemistry and Meat and Livestock Commission (MLC) (1991) Nitrogen factors for pork: a reassessment. *Analyst* 116:761–766.

Analytical Methods Committee of the Royal Society of Chemistry and Meat and Livestock Commission (MLC) (1996) Nitrogen factors for lamb. *Analyst* 121:889–896.

Chan W, Brown J, Lee SM and Buss DH (1995) Meat, poultry and game. Supplement to *McCance and Widdowson's, The Composition of Food*. Cambridge: Royal Society of Chemisty/London: Ministry of Agriculture, Fisheries and Food.

Chan W, Brown J, Church SM and Buss DH (1996) Meat products and meat dishes. Supplement to *McCance and Widdowson's, The Composition of Food*. Cambridge: Royal Society of Chemisty/London: Ministry of Agriculture, Fisheries and Food.

Denke M (1994). Role of beef and beef tallow, an enriched source of stearic acid, in a cholesterol lowering diet. *American Journal of Clinical Nutrition* 60(supplement): 1044S–1049S.

Gibson SA and Ashwell M (1997) New vitamin D values for meat and their implications for vitamin D intake in British adults. *Proceedings of the Nutrition Society*. Volume 56, No. 1A, March.

Keenan JM and Morris DH (1995) Hypercholesterolemia. Dietary advice for patients regarding meat. *Postgraduate Medicine* 98:111–121.

Nutrition Society (1994) Symposium on 'The role of meat in the human diet'. *Proceedings of the Nutrition Society* 53:263–333.

Scott L, Dunn JK, Pownall HJ, Branch TDJ, McMann MC, Herd JA, Harris KB, Sarell JW, Cross HR and Gotto AM Jr. (1994) Effects of beef and chicken consumption on plasma lipid levels in hypercholesterolemic men. *Archives of Internal Medicine* 154:1261–1267.

Shi B and Spallholz JE (1994) Selenium from beef is highly bioavailable as assessed by liver glutathione peroxidase EC 1.11.1.9) activity and tissue selenium. *British Journal of Nutrition* 72:873–881.

Sinclair AJ, Johnson L, O'Dea E and Holman R (1994). Diets rich in lean beef increase arachidonic acid and long-chain n-3 polyunsaturated fatty acid levels in plasma phospholipids. *Lipids* 29:337–343.

Ulbricht TLV (1995) *Fat in the Food Chain*. A report to the Ministry of Agriculture, Fisheries and Food. Available from MAFF Library.

Menkes syndrome *see* **Copper**: Physiology, Dietary Sources and Requirements.

MICROFLORA OF THE INTESTINE

Role and Effects

G Gibson, A Wynne and **A Bird**, Institute of Food Research, Reading, UK

Copyright © 1998 Academic Press

The microbiota of the human large intestine is extremely diverse, consisting of many hundreds of different bacterial species. Together they carry out a process known as fermentation, where dietary residues, as well as indigenously produced compounds, are metabolized. Because of this microbial activity, the large gut is an authentic organ of digestion. The bacteria involved in fermentation and the types of metabolites formed have varying consequences for host health. The substrates for this process, types of bacteria resident in the colon and the end products will be discussed.

Definition and Importance

The intestinal microbiota forms a diverse and complex ecosystem. However, there is much variability in bacterial numbers and populations between the stomach, small intestine and colon. Gastric acidity in the stomach maintains the flora at a low level, with the total bacterial count usually being below 10^3 per g contents. A common inhabitant of the stomach is the gastric pathogen *Helicobacter pylori*. This organism has been implicated as the causative agent of type B gastritis, peptic ulcer formation and stomach carcinomas. *Helicobacter pylori* survives in the stomach as it is able to invade the mucosal layer and secretes ammonia as part of its normal metabolism, thus offering some protection against the acidic affects.

In the small intestine, bacterial counts range from about 10^4 per ml of contents to about $10^6/10^7$ at the ileocaecal region. The main factor limiting growth in the small bowel is the relatively quick transit time of contents. Streptococci, staphylococci and lactobacilli are present, with bacterial numbers showing a progressive numerical increase. In comparison with other regions of the gastrointestinal tract, the human large intestine is an extremely intricate microbial ecosystem. Transit time slows markedly in the colon and can be as long as 70 h. Moreover, the pH is more neutral and appropriate for bacterial growth. Bacterial numbers in the human large intestine are in the region of $10^{11}/10^{12}$ for every gram of gut contents.

The large gut flora is now accepted as playing a major role in both human pathogenesis and health. The colon can become infected, by transient organisms like salmonellae and campylobacters, especially when normal homeostasis is upset. The gut is also the site of other, more chronic, forms of disease (see later). In this article, it will be the colonic flora that is considered.

Composition and Activity

Anatomically distinct areas of the human colon are shown in **Fig. 1**. The large gut microflora is acquired at birth. Initially, facultatively anaerobic strains such as *Escherichia coli* dominate. Thereafter, differences exist in the species composition that develops and this is largely governed by the type of diet. The faecal flora of breast-fed infants is dominated by populations of bifidobacteria, with only about 1% enterobacteria. It is thought that certain bifidogenic factors are present in human breast milk. In contrast, formula-fed infants have a more complex microbiota with bifidobacteria, bacteroides, clostridia and streptococci all being prevalent. After weaning, a pattern that resembles the adult flora becomes established.

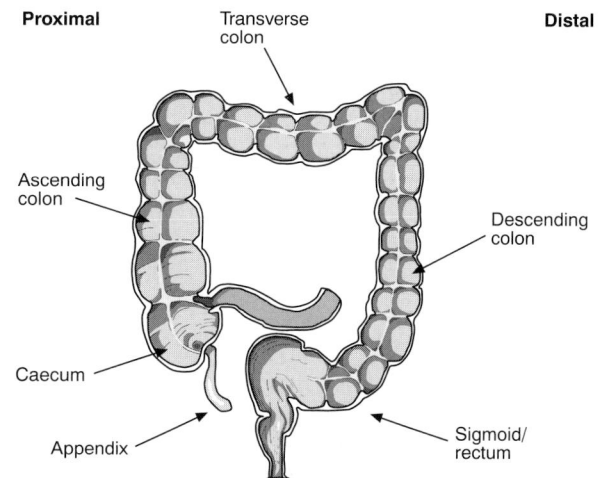

Figure 1 Anatomy of the human large intestine.

The vast majority (>90%) of the total cells in the body are present as bacteria in the colon. The composition is able to respond to anatomical and physicochemical variations that are present. The right or proximal colon is characterized by a high substrate availability (due to dietary input), low pH (from acids produced in fermentation) and a rapid transit. The left or distal area of the colon has a lower concentration of available substrate, the pH is approximately neutral and bacteria grow more slowly. The proximal region tends to be a more saccharolytic environment than the distal gut, the latter having higher bacterial proteolysis. Several hundred different species of bacteria are thought to be present in the large intestine under normal circumstances, the vast majority of which are strict anaerobes. Gram-negative rods belonging to the *Bacteroides fragilis* group are the numerically predominant bacteria in the colon. The other main groups consist of different Gram-positive rods and cocci, such as bifidobacteria, clostridia, peptococci, streptococci, eubacteria, lactobacilli, peptostreptococci and ruminococci. A number of other groups which exist in lower proportions include enterococci, coliforms, methanogens, dissimilatory sulfate-reducing bacteria and acetogens.

Each of these bacterial groups has a specialized ecological niche to fulfil and a variety of different nutritional patterns arise. These include carbohydrate metabolizers, proteolytic species and bacteria which metabolize gases like H_2. While the diverse nature of the human gut microflora is recognized, it is likely that many bacterial species exist that have not been adequately characterized.

The application of modern molecular based technologies is likely to overcome this. In particular, the use of 16SrRNA profiles as a major taxonomic tool is of significance and is now being applied to human gut microbiology. Genotypic based probes may be developed for use in accurate monitoring studies of population changes, for example in response to dietary intervention. As such, this new technology will allow much improved bacteriological determinations in terms of species profiles (including nonculturable forms) as well as incorporating a high-fidelity, accurate and sensitive approach.

Fermentation

Substrates

The principal substrates for bacterial fermentation in the colon are shown in **Fig. 2**. These are predominantly of dietary origin, although there may also be a contribution (not quantified) from endogenous sources.

Some starches that are not affected by pancreatic enzymes may be degraded by bacterial amylases. These 'resistant' starches, together with nonstarch polysaccharides that are part of the plant cell wall (dietary fibre), are major substrates for the saccharolytic microflora (e.g. bacteroides, clostridia, bifidobacteria). Dietary fibre may consist of cellulosic and noncellulosic types and includes pectins, hemicelluloses and gums. These are fermented at varying rates. Other carbohydrates that may be available for fermentation include oligosaccharides, nonabsorbed sugars, sugar alcohols, food sweeteners and other additives. In particular, oligosaccharides are receiving some attention because of their prebiotic nature.

A complete utilization of complex carbohydrates in the large intestine is likely to be a cooperative process that depends on the production of different enzymes by components of the microflora. For instance, certain species are able to metabolize fully a high molecular weight carbohydrate, while others may only be involved in the initial hydrolytic stages of polysaccharide fermentation and thus would produce smaller fragments for other bacteria to metabolize. This leads to competitive interactions between different components of the microflora.

Generally, carbohydrate fermentation consists of different energy yielding reactions, such as substrate level phosphorylation or respiration that does not involve oxygen (for example, species able to use sulfate or nitrate as the electron acceptor are present). The majority of carbohydrate-fermenting anaerobes do so via the Embden–Meyerhof–Parnas pathway. After glucose phosphorylation, the carbohydrate is converted to pyruvate:

$$\text{glucose} + 2\ NAD^+ + 2\ ADP + 2\ P_i$$
$$\rightarrow 2\ \text{pyruvate} + 2\ NADH + 2\ ATP$$

The pyruvate formed acts as a key intermediate for subsequent metabolic interactions. In contrast, bifidobacteria have their own, unique, saccharolytic pathway (the 'bifidus' pathway, **Fig. 3**).

Host-produced carbohydrates include intestinal mucins, which are glycoproteins secreted by goblet cells. The majority of the carbohydrate fraction is present as oligosaccharide side chains comprising fucose, galactose, hexosamines and sialic acids that surround an inner protein core. The main functions of mucins are to act as lubricants and also to offer physical protection for the gut wall against lumenal antigens. Mucins form effective substrates for the growth of colonic bacteria. Predominantly, the species involved are thought to belong to the genera

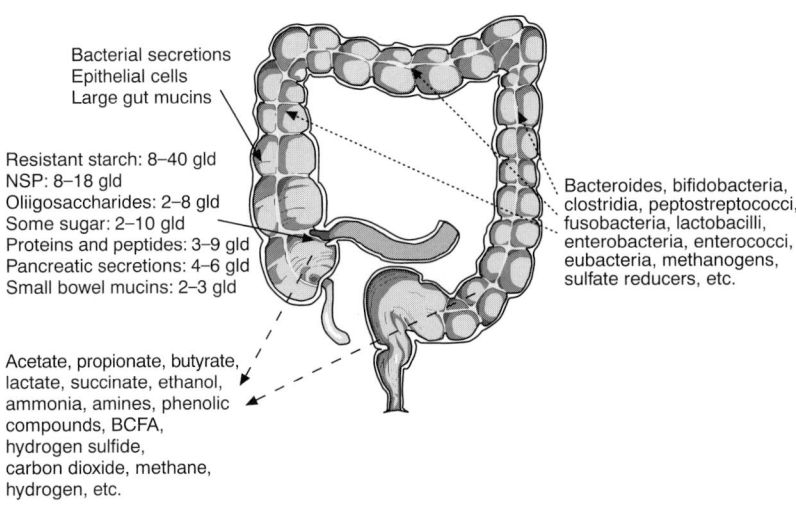

Bacterial secretions
Epithelial cells
Large gut mucins

Resistant starch: 8–40 gld
NSP: 8–18 gld
Oliigosaccharides: 2–8 gld
Some sugar: 2–10 gld
Proteins and peptides: 3–9 gld
Pancreatic secretions: 4–6 gld
Small bowel mucins: 2–3 gld

Bacteroides, bifidobacteria, clostridia, peptostreptococci, fusobacteria, lactobacilli, enterobacteria, enterococci, eubacteria, methanogens, sulfate reducers, etc.

Acetate, propionate, butyrate, lactate, succinate, ethanol, ammonia, amines, phenolic compounds, BCFA, hydrogen sulfide, carbon dioxide, methane, hydrogen, etc.

Figure 2   Summary of the gut fermentation showing substrate input, the end products formed and predominant bacterial genera involved.

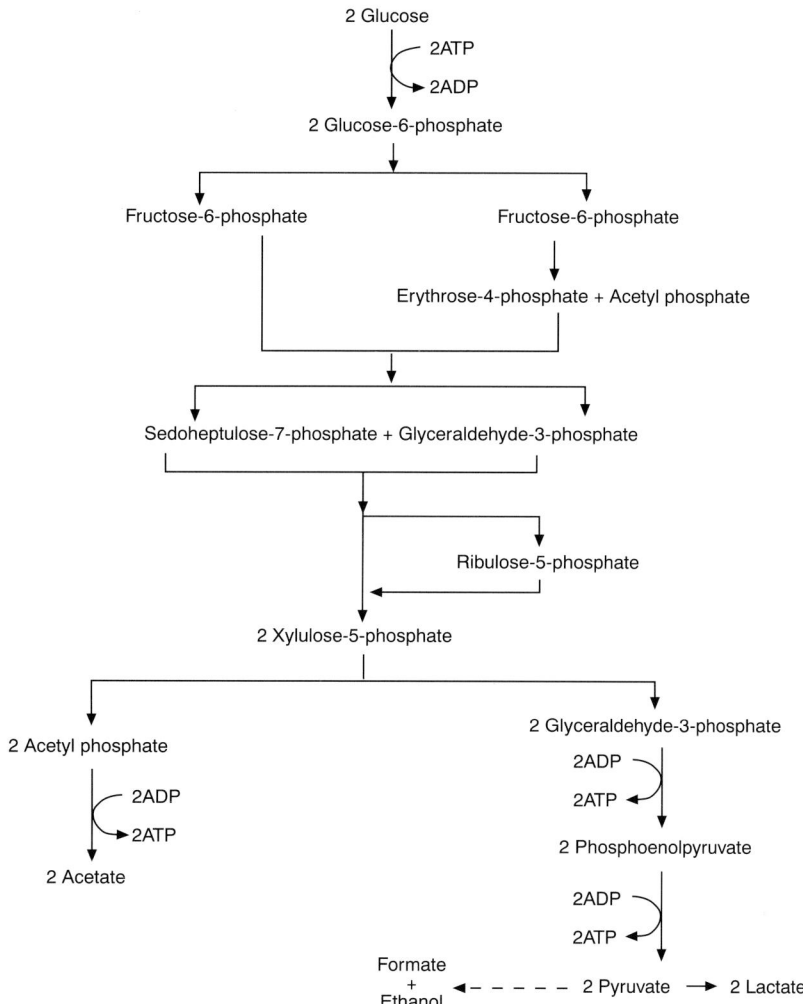

Figure 3 Pathway for glucose metabolism in bifidobacteria.

Bacteroides, Clostridium, Bifidobacterium and *Ruminococcus*. Other fermentable substrates of endogenous origin include tissue mucopolysaccharides such as hyaluronic acid and chondroitin sulfate, whilst sloughed off epithelial cells may also be nutrients for colonic bacteria.

The bacterial fermentation of proteins, peptides and amino acids in the colon is a significant process. The sources include unabsorbed proteins in dietary residues, tissue proteins such as collagen, albumins and bacterial proteins. The human colon, particularly the distal region, is an intensely proteolytic environment. The protease-producing flora includes clostridia, bacteroides, lactobacilli, fusobacteria, streptococci and propionibacteria. The enzymes produced may be both cell associated and extracellular. Damage to host cells caused by these enzymes may be an effective virulence mechanism. One of the most important aspects of large gut proteolysis is the nature of end product produced (see later).

In addition to ethanol, lactate and succinate, H_2 acts as a fermentation intermediate in the large intestine. The physiological significance of electron sink products is that the fermentation is able to generate more oxidized products, and extra ATP, through disposing of excess reducing power. However, to progress efficiently, the H_2 should not be allowed to accumulate excessively. In the colon, some H_2 may be removed through excretion in breath or flatus. The following stoichiometry of carbohydrate fermentation in the large intestine has been proposed:

$$59\ C_6H_{12}O_6 + 38\ H_2O$$
$$\rightarrow 60\ \text{acetate} + 96\ CO_2 + 256\ H^+$$
$$+\ 22\ \text{propionate} + 18\ \text{buytrate}$$

Thus, about 1 litre of H_2 can be produced daily from an average dietary input of carbohydrate into the colon. In reality, however, the *total* flatus volume of an average Western adult rarely reaches this sort of level. This is because H_2-consuming bacteria, in addition to physical mechanisms of removal, are important contributors to the gut fermentation. In some people, methanogenesis is the operable process:

$$4H_2 + CO_2 \rightarrow CH_4 + 2H_2O$$

Human colonic methanogens (e.g. *Methanobrevibacter smithii*) are thought to have an obligate requirement for H_2. However, this process only occurs in about one-third of persons in Western populations. The main microbiological alternative through which H_2 can be disposed of in the colon is through the activities of certain sulfate-reducing bacteria (e.g. *Desulfovibrio* spp.):

$$4H_2 + SO_4^{2-} + H^+ \rightarrow HS^- + 4H_2O$$

The key to competitive interactions between methanogens and sulfate reducers is the availability of sulfate. This anion may be provided by dietary sources (e.g. fermented beverages) or by the metabolism of endogenous sulfated polymers (e.g. mucin). If sulfate is available in sufficient quantities, then the preferred route of H_2 disposal will be through sulfate reduction. If not, then methanogenesis predominates. These bacterial mechanisms, through the type of end product formed, have differing consequences for host health (see below). Acetogenesis has also been suggested as a further route of bacterial H_2 disposal, although the ecological significance of this process remains unclear.

End products

Principal end products of bacterial fermentative reactions in the colon are shown in Fig. 2. Predominantly, these are short-chain fatty acids (SCFA), i.e. acetate, propionate and butyrate. Other fermentation products include ethanol, lactate and succinate, but these metabolites are further oxidized by cross-feeding species in the large gut. Bacterial groups involved in the production of major end products of carbohydrate metabolism are shown in **Table 1**. Other organic acids present in lower amounts include formate, valerate and caproate. Branched-chain fatty acids such as isobutyrate, 2-methyl-butyrate and isovalerate may also be formed from the fermentation of amino acids. Most of the SCFA formed by intestinal bacteria are absorbed, therefore contributing towards the hosts energy gain. It is thought that around 7–8% of daily energy requirements are derived from colonic bacterial activities.

About 400 mmol SCFA are produced per day, and a large proportion is rapidly absorbed through the colonic epithelium. Acetate is further metabolized systemically (brain, muscle tissues) whereas propi-

Table 1 Principal bacterial groups involved in the formation of predominant end products of carbohydrate metabolism in the human large intestine

End product of metabolism	Bacterial group
Acetate	Bacteroides, bifidobacteria, eubacteria, lactobacilli, clostridia, ruminococci, peptococci, veillonella, peptostreptococci, propionibacteria, fusobacteria, butyrivibrio
Propionate	Bacteroides, propionibacteria, veillonella
Butyrate	Clostridia, fusobacteria, butyrivibrio, eubacteria, peptostreptococci
Ethanol	Bifidobacteria, bacteroides, clostridia, lactobacilli, peptostreptococci
Hydrogen	Clostridia, ruminococci, fusobacteria
Lactate	Bacteroides, bifidobacteria, lactobacilli, eubacteria, peptostreptococci, ruminococci, actinomycetes, enterococci, fusobacteria, clostridia
Succinate	Bacteroides, ruminococci, prevotella
Formate	Bacteroides, bifidobacteria, ruminococci, eubacteria, enterobacteria, butyrivibrio

onate is cleared by the liver. It is possible that this metabolite acts as a gluconeogenic precursor, and may also be involved in the reduction of plasma lipid values. Butyrate formation by intestinal bacteria is currently of high research interest. This SCFA is an essential fuel for the colonic epithelium and its production may also be important from the viewpoint of preventing colon cancer, since it inhibits DNA synthesis and stimulates apoptosis.

Unlike carbohydrate metabolism, where the end products are benign and may even be of some benefit to the host, those from proteolysis are toxic. An accumulation of ammonia may change the metabolism of intestinal cells by increasing DNA synthesis and has therefore been associated with the initiation of bowel cancer (as have many bacterial products in the large gut). Phenols and indoles are produced from certain aromatic amino acids. They are usually detoxified in the colonic mucosa, but have been associated with diseases such as malabsorption, anaemia, colon cancer and schizophrenia. Amines are major products of bacterial amino acid metabolism that are also thought to be toxins.

Factors Affecting the Microflora Composition

Although the composition of the large intestinal microflora is normally considered to be a fairly stable entity, many different factors affect both the colonization and growth of bacteria in the colon. As mentioned earlier, the type of feeding regime given after birth influences composition until weaning is complete. The amount and chemical composition of the different growth substrates available is an important determining factor. As foodstuffs easily provide the main nutrient source, it follows that diet is a significant factor in determining the type of gut flora that develops. One of the main reasons for advocation of a high dietary fibre intake is the physiological effects, such as increased bulking, on colonic bacteria. The rate of depolymerization of higher molecular weight carbohydrates will affect metabolic processes further down the food chain. Certain foodstuffs that are metabolizable by selected components of the microbiota are able to modulate intrinsically the faecal bacteriology. Examples are nondigestible oligosaccharides and the sulfate ion. This arises because certain components of the flora have a selective growth advantage that allows improved metabolism of these substrates.

Physical considerations like occupation of appropriate colonization sites and the availability of nutrients therein will also affect competitive interactions. Those microorganisms that are able to 'persist' better are likely to have a selective advantage in this respect. Indeed, the virulence aspects of many gut pathogens (e.g. some *Escherichia coli*, yersiniae) initially arises from their ability to adhere to intestinal cells.

Immunological affects may also influence the gut microflora. This is possibly of most significance at the mucosal surface, where secretory IgA levels will be highest. It is not apparent that lumenal bacterial populations are directly affected by immune events.

The types of bacteria present in different regions of the gut and their individual fermentation strategies affect the gut fermentation. An important consideration that will determine the improved survival of bacterial species is intimate interactions between the microbiota components. For example, some gut bacteria, e.g. the lactic acid microflora, are able to produce strong acids that lower the pH of the microenvironment to levels below those at which other species can effectively compete. In this respect, differences in the pH of large gut contents do occur. As previously mentioned, the type and nature of the fermentation that occurs leads to the proximal colon being an acidic environment, while the distal gut has an approximately neutral pH. This in turn affects the type of microflora that establishes in the different gut regions. Similarly, variations in intestinal transit time, redox potential (facultatively anaerobic bacteria can maintain a low pH in the colon by rapidly utilizing traces of oxygen that diffuse into the intestinal lumen), availability of inorganic electron acceptors (e.g. sulfate, nitrate) and the production of bacterial metabolites are all influencing factors. Other bacterial fermentation products such as H_2S and carbon dioxide may also lead to a competitive advantage.

On a more selective basis, some bacteria produce more defined antimicrobial substances that help to protect their particular ecological and metabolic niche. These products can be divided into substances that act mainly against taxonomically related genera, and those whose action is principally against members of the same species. These are often termed bacteriocins and are proteinaeceous compounds. Their *in situ* activities are undefined, however.

A further important consideration that will affect the large gut microflora composition is the intake of xenobiotic compounds by the host. Obviously, antimicrobial therapy will be a common intrusive mechanism.

Pathogenic Aspects of Large Gut Microbiology

Bacteria have been implicated either as causative agents or maintenance factors involved in many colonic disorders. Acute inflammatory action may occur in response to a variety of microorganisms, including viruses, that are often transmitted by food. Bacteria frequently implicated include certain strains of *E. coli*, as well as species belonging to the genera *Salmonella*, *Shigella*, *Campylobacter*, *Yersinia* and *Aeromonas*. The symptoms of such disease usually include diarrhoea, but the effects are relatively short term. Certain components of the gut flora may, however, also be involved in the aetiology of more chronic degenerative disease. These include large bowel cancer (the large gut is the second most common site for carcinoma formation in the body), inflammatory bowel disease and antibiotic-associated colitis. Each may have a bacterial aetiology. Conversely, the gut microbiota may have health-promoting virtues. These include elevated resistance to the conditions mentioned above, lipid reducing effects, vitamin production and a contribution towards improved immunology. As such, there is currently much interest in manipulation of the gut flora composition towards a potentially healthier community (*See:* **Probiotics and Prebiotics**; Definition and Role).

Antibiotic-associated colitis

Pseudomembranous colitis is a severe form of colitis that occurs almost exclusively with antibiotic exposure. It is routine that *Clostridium difficile* is isolated from patients with the disease and the organism is now implicated as the principal causative agent. The disease arises in association with anti-microbial therapy and a subsequent compromising of the homeostasis that the normal gut flora can exert. Almost all broad-spectrum antibiotics have been implicated in suppression of the flora leading to the onset of pseudomembranous colitis, but those most frequently involved are ampicillin, clindamycin and the cephalosporins. The bacterium produces two toxins which are responsible for formation of ulcer-like lesions that form a pseudomembrane consisting of mucin, fibrin, leucocytes and other debris.

Inflammatory bowel disease

Inflammatory bowel disease is found in two major forms: ulcerative colitis and Crohn's disease. Both involve inflammation and share many clinical features, but Crohn's disease affects primarily the small gut and all regions of the large bowel, whereas ulcerative colitis is confined to the colon. Their aetiologies are unknown.

Ulcerative colitis always affects the distal colon. The condition expresses itself in acute attacks followed by periods of symptom-free remission. Bacterial involvement has been proposed in both initiation and maintenance stages of the disease. These include *Streptococcus mobilis*, fusobacteria, shigellae and *E. coli*. Our own research has indicated a possible involvement for sulfate-reducing bacteria.

As mentioned earlier, the end products of H_2 metabolism in humans may have different health consequences. Generally, a reduction in H_2 reduces potential gas distension and bloating problems. However, while methane is a relatively harmless product of this metabolism, the end product of sulfate reduction is sulfide, which is a toxic gas. The feeding of sulfated polymers to conventional laboratory animals results in colitis-like lesions, while this is not the case for germ-free counterparts. Patients with ulcerative colitis have an almost universal carriage of sulfate reducers, compared with about 50% of healthy persons. Moreover, those species that reside in the colitic gut produce sulfide at a higher rate than their conventional counterparts and are able to adapt to certain clinical manifestations of the disease, such as an apparent low substrate availability and high wash-out rates. In common with implications on specific bacterial processes and human disease, it is unclear whether these observations are cause or effect relationship. However, bearing in mind the known toxicity of this gas, it is probably worthwhile further investigating sulfide accumulation in the large gut and differences in how it is handled *in situ*. Moreover, the potential for sulfate-reducing bacteria

to attach to and invade intestinal cells warrants attention.

The onset of Crohn's disease has been associated with a variety of microorganisms, including eubacteria, peptostreptococci, pseudomonads, bacteroides and clostridia. However, because the disorder involves a granulomatous reaction, it is possible that a more persistent stimulus is involved. Certain mycobacteria have received attention in this respect, with *Mycobacterium paratuberculosis* being detected in tissue affected by Crohn's disease. However, as for ulcerative colitis, the definitive cause(s) remains undetermined.

Cancer and colonic bacteria

The large intestine is the second most common site for carcinoma production in humans. A number of factors such as diet, environment and genetics have all been implicated as causative agents. A number of colonic bacteria are known carcinogen producers. These include fecapentaenes, nitrosamines, secondary bile acids, diacylglycerol, the heterocyclic amine, 2-amino-3-methyl-3H-imidazo [4,5-f] quinoline and the aglycone methylazoxymethanol. As with other forms of gut disease, however, the initiation is likely to be multi-factorial.

Conclusion

The human large intestine is an important organ of digestion. The resident microbial species become established as a result of a number of physico-chemical variables and depending on their ability to maintain ecological microniches. Subsequently, the flora may exert both pathological and health-promoting implications. In tandem with accurate characterization of the nature and activities of this microbiota, the applied potential (in terms of science and medicine) is high.

See also: **Cancer**: Epidemiology of Colorectal Cancer. **Carbohydrates**: Regulation of Carbohydrate Metabolism. **Colonic Diseases and Disorders**: Nutritional Management. **Dietary Fibre (Fiber)**: Physiological Effects and Effects on Absorption. **Fatty Acids**: Metabolism.

Further Reading

Cummings JH and Macfarlane GT (1991) The control and consequences of bacterial fermentation in the human colon. *Journal of Applied Bacteriology* 70:443–459.

Cummings JH, Rombeau JL and Sakata T (eds) (1995) *Physiological and Clinical Aspects of Short Chain Fatty Acid Metabolism*. Cambridge: Cambridge University Press.

Fuller R (ed.) (1992) *Probiotics: The Scientific Basis*. London: Chapman & Hall.

Gibson GR (1990) A review – the physiology and ecology of sulphate-reducing bacteria. *Journal of Applied Bacteriology* **69**:769–797.

Gibson GR and Macfarlane GT (1994) Intestinal bacteria and disease. In: Gibson SAW (ed.) *Human Health – The Contribution of Microorganisms*, pp 53–62. London: Springer-Verlag.

Gibson GR and Macfarlane GT (eds) (1995) *Human Colonic Bacteria: Role in Nutrition, Physiology and Pathology*. Boca Raton: CRC Press.

Gibson GR and Roberfroid MB (1995) Dietary modulation of the human colonic microbiota: introducing the concept of prebiotics. *Journal of Nutrition* **125**:1401–1412.

Hentges DJ (ed.) (1983) *Human Intestinal Microflora in Health and Disease*. London: Academic Press.

Macfarlane GT and Cummings JH (1991) The colonic flora, fermentation, and large bowel digestive function. In: Phillips SF, Pemberton JH and Shorter RG (eds) *The Large Intestine: Physiology, Pathophysiology and Disease*, pp 51–92. New York: Raven Press.

Macfarlane GT and Gibson GR (1994) Metabolic activities of the normal colonic flora. In: Gibson SAW (ed.) *Human Health – The Contribution of Microorganisms*, pp 17–52. London: Springer-Verlag.

Macfarlane GT and Gibson GR (1997) Carbohydrate fermentation, energy transduction and gas metabolism in the human large intestine. In: Mackie RI and White BA (eds) *Ecology and Physiology of Gastrointestinal Microbes*, Vol. 1, Gastrointestinal Fermentation and Ecosystems, pp 269–318. London: Chapman & Hall.

Macfarlane GT and Gibson GR (1997) Microbiology of the gastrointestinal tract. In: Bittar EE and Bittar N (eds) *Principles of Medical Biology*. Connecticut: JAI Press.

Rathbone BJ and Heatley RV (eds) (1992) Helicobacter pylori *and Gastroduodenal Disease*. Oxford: Blackwell Scientific.

Tannock GW (1995) *Normal Flora*. London: Chapman & Hall.

Whitehead R (ed.) (1995) *Gastrointestinal and Oesophageal Physiology*, 2nd edn. Edinburgh: Churchill Livingstone.

Milk *see* **Dairy Products**: Nutritional Value.

Minerals *see* **Calcium**: Physiology. **Magnesium**: Physiology, Dietary Sources and Requirements. **Phosphorus**: Physiology, Dietary Sources and Requirements. **Potassium**: Physiology, Dietary Sources and Requirements. **Sodium**: Physiology.

Molybdenum *see* **Ultratrace Elements**: Physiology.

Monounsaturated fat *see* **Fatty Acids**: Health Effects of Monounsaturated Fatty Acids.

Muscle *see* **Exercise**: Physiology of Muscle.

Mycotoxins *see* **Food Contaminants**: Mycotoxins - Occurrence and Toxic Effects.

APPENDIX I

Food and Drug Administration Pesticide Program

Residue Monitoring 1995

This is the ninth annual report summarizing the results of the Food and Drug Administration's (FDA) pesticide residue monitoring program. The 8 previous reports, which were published in the *Journal of the Association of Official Analytical Chemists/Journal of AOAC International*, presented results from Fiscal Years (FY) 1987 through 1994. This current report includes findings obtained during FY95 (October 1, 1994 through September 30, 1995) under regulatory and incidence/level monitoring. Selected Total Diet Study findings for 1995 are also presented. Results in this and earlier reports continue to demonstrate that levels of pesticide residues in the U.S. food supply are well below established safety standards.

FDA Monitoring Program

Three federal government agencies share responsibility for the regulation of pesticides [1]. The Environmental Protection Agency (EPA) registers (i.e., approves) the use of pesticides and sets tolerances (the maximum amount of a residue that is permitted in or on a food) if use of that particular pesticide may result in residues in or on food [2]. Except for meat, poultry, and certain egg products, for which the Food Safety and Inspection Service (FSIS) of the U.S. Department of Agriculture (USDA) is responsible, FDA is charged with enforcing tolerances in imported foods and in domestically produced foods shipped in interstate commerce. FDA also acquires incidence/level data on particular commodity/pesticide combinations and carries out its market basket survey, the Total Diet Study. For 5 years, USDA's Agricultural Marketing Service (AMS), through contracts with participating states, has carried out a residue testing program directed primarily at raw agricultural products. FSIS and AMS report their pesticide residue data independently.

Regulatory Monitoring

Under this approach to pesticide residue monitoring, FDA samples individual lots of domestically produced and imported foods and analyzes them for pesticide residues to enforce the tolerances set by EPA. Domestic samples are collected as close as possible to the point of production in the distribution system; import samples are collected at the point of entry into U.S. commerce. Emphasis is on the raw agricultural product, which is analyzed as the unwashed, whole (unpeeled), raw commodity. Processed foods are also included. If illegal residues (above EPA tolerance or no tolerance for that particular food/pesticide combination) are found in domestic samples, FDA can invoke various sanctions, such as a seizure or injunction. For imports, shipments may be stopped at the port of entry when illegal residues are found. "Automatic detention" may be invoked for imports based on the finding of 1 violative shipment if there is reason to believe that the same situation will exist in future lots during the same shipping season for a specific shipper, grower, geographic area, or country.

Domestic and import food samples collected are classified as either "surveillance" or "compliance". Most samples collected by FDA are the surveillance type; that is, there is no prior knowledge or evidence that a specific food shipment contains illegal pesticide residues. Compliance samples are taken as follow-up to the finding of an illegal residue or when other evidence indicates that a pesticide residue problem may exist.

Factors considered by FDA in planning the types and numbers of samples to collect include review of recently generated state and FDA residue data, regional intelligence on pesticide use, dietary importance of the food, information on the amount of domestic food that enters interstate commerce and of imported food, chemical characteristics and toxicity of the pesticide, and production volume/ pesticide usage patterns.

Analytical Methods   To analyze the large numbers of samples whose pesticide treatment history is usually unknown, FDA uses analytical methods capable of simultaneously determining a number of pesticide residues. These multiresidue methods (MRMs) can determine about half of the approximately 400 pesticides with EPA tolerances, and many others that have no tolerances. The most commonly used MRMs can also detect many metabolites, impurities, and alteration products of pesticides [3].

Single residue methods (SRMs) or selective MRMs are used to determine some pesticide residues in foods [3]. An SRM usually determines 1 pesticide; a selective MRM measures a relatively small number of chemically related pesticides. These types of methods are usually more resource-intensive per residue. Therefore, they are much less cost effective than MRMs.

The lower limit of residue measurement in FDA's determination of a specific pesticide is usually well below tolerance levels, which generally range from 0.1 to 50 parts per million (ppm). Residues present at 0.01 ppm and above are usually measurable; however, for individual pesticides, this limit may range from 0.005 to 1 ppm. In this report, the term "trace" is used to indicate residues detected, but at levels below the limit of quantitation (LQ).

FDA/State Cooperation   Personnel in FDA field offices interact with their counterparts in many states to increase FDA's effectiveness in pesticide residue monitoring. In most cases, work-sharing agreements (Memoranda of Understanding) have been established between FDA and various state agencies.

FDA also acquires and uses state-generated pesticide residue data to complement its own and other federally sponsored residue programs. For many years, FDA has supported, through a contract with Mississippi State University (MSU), the "Foodcontam" database, which is a compilation of state-collected residue data.

Animal Feeds   In addition to monitoring foods for human consumption, FDA also samples and analyzes domestic and imported feeds for pesticide residues. FDA's Center for Veterinary Medicine (CVM) directs this portion of the Agency's monitoring via its Feed Contaminants Compliance Program. Although animal feeds containing violative pesticide residues may present a potential hazard to a number of different categories of animals (e.g., laboratory animals, pets, wildlife, etc.), the major focus of CVM's moni-

toring is on feeds for livestock and poultry, animals that ultimately become, or produce, foods for human consumption.

CVM also reviews pesticide residue data supplied by various states under "Feedcon", a database operated by MSU under the auspices of the Association of American Feed Control Officials. These data are reviewed periodically by CVM so that potential problems arising from pesticide residues in foods of animal origin may be identified.

International Activities   FDA obtains information on foreign pesticide usage via contract with Landell Mills (Bath, England). Each year, FDA receives pesticide usage data for about 40 countries that export food to the United States. These data can be used by FDA to target its pesticide residue monitoring toward specific pesticide/commodity/country combinations.

In addition to the foreign pesticide usage data obtained through the commercial contract, under provisions of the Pesticide Monitoring Improvements Act, FDA receives information from foreign governments on pesticides used on their food exports to the United States. FDA makes this information available to FDA Districts for use in their planning of monitoring of imported foods.

As part of the exchange of information on pesticides, FDA provides foreign countries with updates on U.S. pesticide usage. FDA also supplies foreign countries annually with reports on FDA's regulatory monitoring coverage and the findings in foods imported from their respective countries, as well as a personal computer database in which coverage and findings are summarized by country/commodity/pesticide combination.

Under the auspices of the North American Free Trade Agreement (NAFTA), the United States, Mexico, and Canada have established a NAFTA Technical Working Group on Pesticides (TWG). The NAFTA Pesticide TWG now serves as the focal point for all pesticide issues that arise among the 3 NAFTA countries. The TWG reports directly to the NAFTA Sanitary and Phytosanitary Committee.

One of the major goals of the TWG is to ensure that pesticide registrations and tolerances/maximum residue limits in the 3 countries are harmonized to the extent practical, while strengthening protection of public health and the environment. A number of projects have been undertaken by the TWG to identify differing residue limits in the NAFTA countries and to determine what steps might be taken to harmonize the limits. While this is a difficult process, the TWG envisions eventual movement toward a "North America" pesticide registration and tolerance system so that citizens of all 3 countries can be assured of the safety and legality of foods produced in any 1 of the NAFTA countries.

The NAFTA TWG is cochaired by EPA, Health Canada, and Mexico's Ministry of Health (representing the Comision Intersecretarial para el Control del Proceso y Uso de Plaguicidas, Fertilizantes y Sustancias Toxicas). FDA is an active participant on the TWG and is assisting by providing expertise on enforcement monitoring programs and residue data to support harmonization activities. FDA's activities on the TWG complement its ongoing bilateral cooperation with its counterparts in Mexico and Canada.

Incidence/Level Monitoring

A complementary approach to regulatory monitoring, incidence/level monitoring is used to increase FDA's knowledge about particular pesticide/commodity combinations by analyzing certain foods to determine the presence and levels of selected pesticides. In 1995, a survey of triazine herbicides in various commodities was carried out and a statistically based monitoring survey that had been initiated in 1994 was completed.

The latter focused on domestic and imported fresh apples and processed rice. This is the second FDA survey of this type; the first covered domestic and imported pears and tomatoes [4]. These statistically based surveys were initiated to determine whether FDA data acquired under regulatory monitoring are statistically representative of the overall residue situation for a particular pesticide, commodity, or place of origin. In FDA's surveillance sampling for pesticide residues, sampling bias may be incurred by weighting sampling toward such factors as commodity or place of origin with a past history of violations or large volume of import shipments. In addition, the total number of samples of a given commodity analyzed for a particular pesticide each year may not be sufficient to draw specific conclusions about the residue situation for the whole volume of that commodity in commerce. Therefore, the objective of these statistically based surveys is to determine whether violation rates, frequency of occurrence of residues, and residue levels obtained from such a sampling regimen differ from those obtained through FDA's traditional surveillance approach.

Apples and rice were chosen as the second set of test commodities because they are widely consumed year round and have significant domestic and import components. Fresh apples and all types of processed rice (white, brown, glutinous, fragrant, parboiled, converted, etc., but not wild or brewer's rice) were included in the study. The same general procedures were followed in the apples/rice study as in the pears/tomatoes study [4]. Samples were collected throughout the United States by FDA inspectors, except for domestic rice. These samples were collected by USDA Federal Grain Inspection Service personnel, who are routinely present at the mills that process domestic rice. Most of the mills are located in those few states in which rice growing is a major agricultural industry.

Analyses were performed by the Buffalo (apples) and Minneapolis (rice) District Laboratories. The goal was to collect and analyze about 800 domestic and 800 import apple samples and about 575 domestic and 800 import rice samples.

Total Diet Study

The Total Diet Study is another major element of FDA's pesticide residue monitoring program [5]. In its previous annual pesticide reports, FDA provided Total Diet Study findings for 1987–1994 [6]. In addition, more detailed information, including estimated dietary intakes of pesticide residues covering June 1984–April 1986 [7] and July 1986–April 1991 [8], has been published. In September 1991, FDA implemented revisions to the Total Diet Study that were formulated in 1990 [9]. These revisions primarily consisted of collection and analysis of an updated and expanded number (to 261) of food items, addition of 6 age/sex groups (for a total of 14), and revised analytical coverage. Details of the recent revision are presented elsewhere [10,11].

In conducting the Total Diet Study, FDA personnel purchase foods from supermarkets or grocery stores 4 times per year, once from each of 4 geographic regions of the country. The 261 foods that comprise each market basket represent over 3500 different foods reported in USDA food consumption surveys; for example, apple pie represents all fruit pies and fruit pastries. Each collection is a composite of like foods purchased in 3 cities in a given region. The foods are prepared table-ready and then analyzed for pesticide residues (as well as radionuclides, industrial chemicals, toxic elements, trace and macro elements, vitamin B_6, and folic acid). The levels of pesticides found are used in conjunction with USDA food consumption data to estimate the dietary intakes of the pesticide residues.

Results and Discussion

Regulatory Monitoring

In 1995, 10,615 samples (10,133 surveillance and 482 compliance) were analyzed under regulatory monitoring. Of these, 5198 were domestic and 5417 were imports.

Figure I.1 shows the percentage of the 5101 domestic surveillance samples by commodity group with no residues found, nonviolative residues found, and violative residues found. (A violative residue is defined in this report as a residue which exceeds a tolerance or a residue at a level of regulatory significance for which no tolerance has been established in the sampled food.) As in earlier years, fruits and vegetables accounted for the largest proportion of the commodities analyzed in 1995; those 2 commodity groups comprised 59% of the total number of domestic surveillance samples. In 1995, no violative residues were found in nearly 99% of all domestic surveillance samples (the same percentage as in the past several years).

Appendix A contains more detailed data on domestic surveillance monitoring findings by commodity, including the total number of samples analyzed, the percent samples with no residues found, and the percent violative samples. Of the 5101 domestic surveillance samples, 64% had no detectable residues, less than 1% had over-tolerance residues, and less than 1% had residues of pesticides for which there was no tolerance for that particular pesticide/commodity combination. In the largest commodity groups, fruits and vegetables, 40 and 63% of the samples, respectively, had no residues detected. Less than 2% of the

fruit samples and about 2% of the vegetable samples contained violative residues (Figure I.1). In the milk/dairy products/eggs group, 93% of the samples had no residues detected and no violative residues were found. Within the category Other were 61 samples of baby foods/formula, nearly 3 times the number of samples of baby foods/formula collected and analyzed in 1994. This included 29 vegetable, 13 cereal, 13 fruit/fruit juice, 4 formula, 1 custard/fruit pudding, and 1 teething biscuit samples. None of the samples had violative residues.

The findings by commodity group for the 5032 import surveillance samples are shown in Figure I.2. Fruits and vegetables accounted for 85% of these samples. Overall, no violative residues were found in nearly 97% of the import surveillance samples (97% in 1993 and 96% in 1994).

Appendix B contains detailed data on the import surveillance samples. Of the 5032 samples analyzed, 66% had no residues detected, less than 1% had over-tolerance residues, and 3% had residues for which there was no tolerance for that particular pesticide/commodity combination. Fruits and vegetables had 57 and 67%, respectively, with no residues detected. The fruit group had less than 1% with over-tolerance residues and the vegetable group had 1% with over-tolerance residues; each group had 3% no-tolerance residues. No residues were found in 88% of the dairy products/eggs group and 85% of

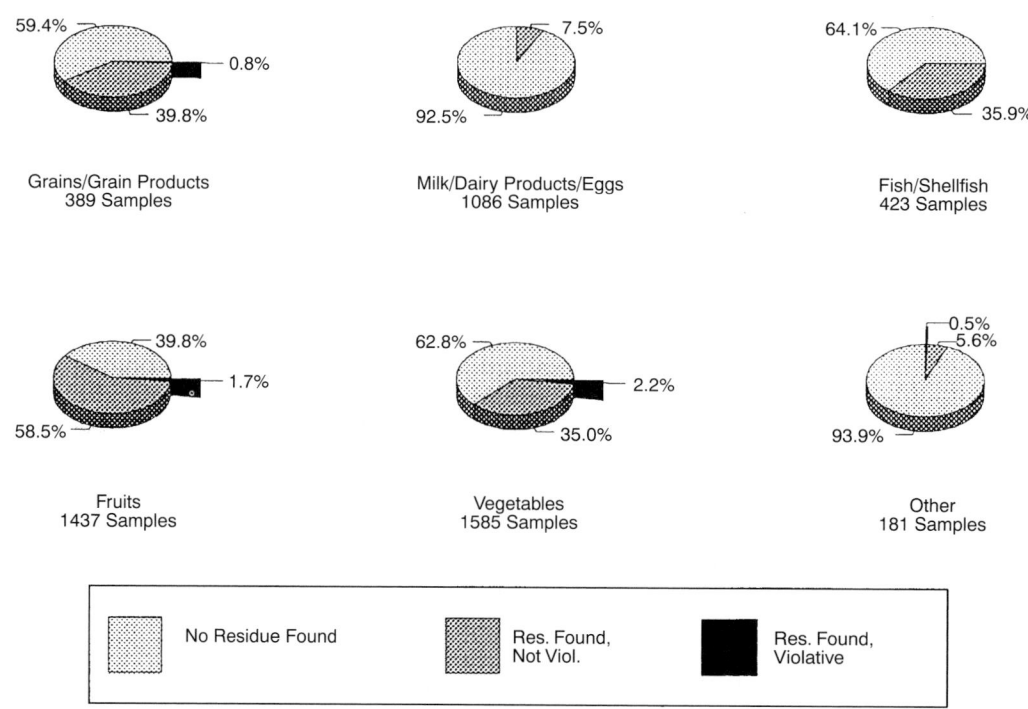

Figure I.1 Summary of results (domestic) by commodity group of 1995 sample analyses for pesticide residues (surveillance samples only).

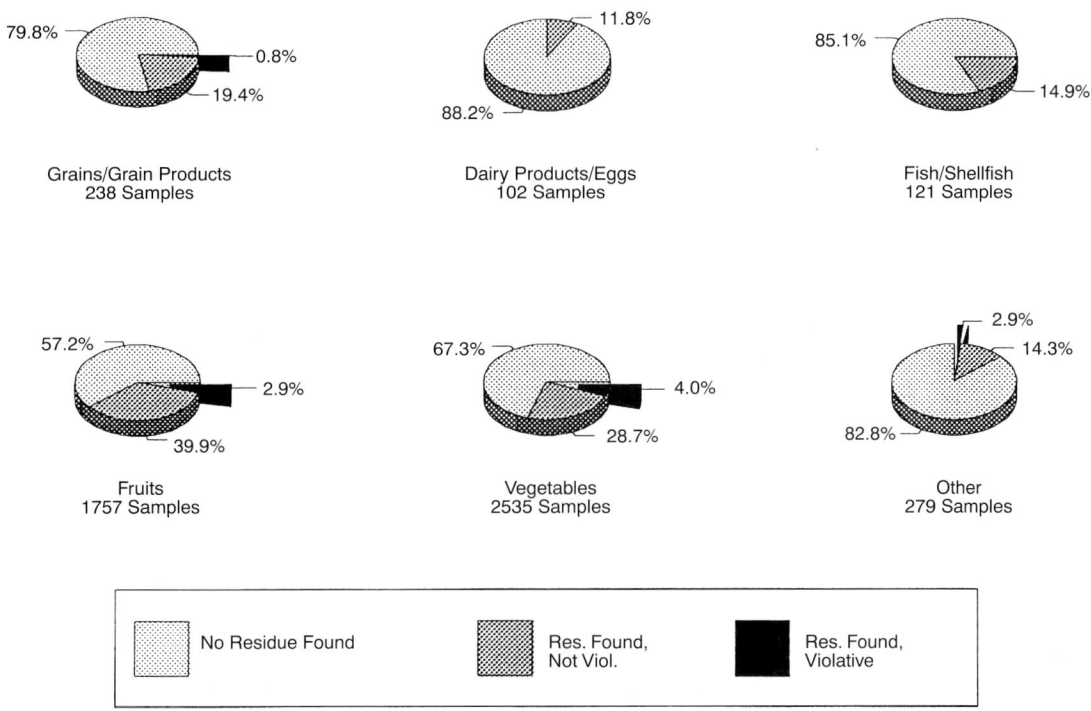

Figure I.2 Summary of results (import) by commodity group of 1995 sample analyses for pesticide residues (surveillance samples only).

the fish/shellfish group, and no violative residues were found in either of those groups.

Pesticide monitoring data collected under FDA's regulatory monitoring approach in 1995 are available to the public as a computer database. This database summarizes FDA 1995 regulatory monitoring coverage and findings by country/commodity/pesticide combination. The database also includes the monitoring data by individual sample from which the summary information was compiled. Information on purchase of this database as well as those for 1992, 1993, and 1994 is provided at the end of this report.

Geographic Coverage

Domestic. In 1995, domestic surveillance samples were collected from all 50 states and Puerto Rico. The largest numbers of samples were collected from the states in which agriculture is a major industry.

Import. Samples representing food shipments from 94 countries were collected. Table I.1 lists the numbers of samples collected and the countries from which they originated. Mexico, as usual, was the source of the largest number of samples. This large number reflects the volume and diversity of commodities imported from that country, especially during the winter months.

Pesticide Coverage Table I.2 lists the 345 pesticides that were detectable by the methods used; the 92 pesticides that were actually found are indicated.

FDA conducts ongoing research to expand the pesticide coverage of its monitoring program. This research includes testing the behavior of new or previously untested pesticides through existing analytical methods, and development of new methods to cover pesticides that cannot be determined by methods currently used by FDA. The research encompasses both U.S.-registered pesticides and foreign-use pesticides that are not registered in the United States. The list of pesticides detectable for 1995 (Table I.2) reflects the addition of a number of pesticides for which new methods had been developed and pesticides whose recovery through the analytical methods used was demonstrated as a result of ongoing research.

Surveillance/Compliance Violation Rate Comparison In 1995, 97 domestic and 385 import compliance samples were collected and analyzed (Table I.3). Because compliance samples are collected when a pesticide residue problem is known or suspected, violation rates are expectedly higher than those for surveillance samples: 12% for domestic (10% in 1994) and 11% for imports (18% in 1994). The corresponding violation rates for surveillance samples

Table I.1   Foreign countries and number of samples[a] collected and analyzed in 1995

Country	No. of samples	Country	No. of samples	Country	No. of samples
Mexico	1723	Greece	81	Hong Kong	23
Chile	467	Turkey	79	Philippines	23
The Netherlands	370	Ecuador	72	United Kingdom	21
Canada	253	Taiwan	55	Germany	17
Italy	218	Argentina	51	Denmark	16
Thailand	198	New Zealand	48	Pakistan	16
China, People's Rep. of	184	Jamaica	47	Poland	16
Guatemala	174	Japan	47	South Africa	16
Costa Rica	139	Belgium	46	Lebanon	15
India	137	Panama	43	Australia	14
Spain	126	Colombia	42	Czech Republic	14
Peru	85	France	40	Egypt	13
Israel	83	Indonesia	31	Haiti	12
Dominican Republic	91	Brazil	30	Morocco	12
		Honduras	29	Venezuela	12
		Korea, Rep. of	25	Unspecified	15

Ten or fewer samples collected from the following:

Austria	Hungary	Slovakia
Bahamas	Iceland	Slovenia
Belize	Ivory Coast	Sri Lanka
Bermuda	Kenya	St. Vincent
Bolivia	Macedonia	Surinam
Bosnia-Hercegovina	Malaysia	Sweden
Bulgaria	Martinique	Switzerland
Croatia	Moldavia	Syria
Cyprus	Netherlands Antilles	Tanzania
Dominica	Nicaragua	Trinidad & Tobago
El Salvador	Nigeria	Tunisia
Estonia	Norway	Turks & Caicos Islands
Ethiopia	Papua New Guinea	United Arab Emirates
Faeroe Islands	Portugal	Uruguay
Fiji	Russia	Vietnam, Rep. of
Ghana	Singapore	Zambia

[a]Surveillance plus compliance samples.

were 1.3% for domestic and 3.2% for imports (Figure I.3).

Most of the 1995 compliance samples were collected as follow-up to violative surveillance samples. These included follow-up samples from the same shipment as the violative surveillance sample, follow-up samples of the same commodity from the same grower or shipper, and audit samples from shipments presented for entry into the United States with a certificate of analysis (i.e., shipments subject to automatic detention).

Foodcontam Data   In 1995, 11 states participated in the Foodcontam project. A wide variety of commodities was reflected in the 9394 samples reported by the 10 states whose data were available. Table I.4 lists the 10 states, the number of samples for each, and the number and percentage of samples with posi-

tive and "significant" findings. In this instance, a significant finding indicates a residue that exceeds federal or state regulatory limits, is not covered by a tolerance for the particular chemical/commodity combination, or denotes some unusual finding(s). For the 9394 samples reported, 0.8% were classified as significant.

Animal Feeds   In 1995, 556 domestic feed samples (532 surveillance and 24 compliance) and 69 import feed samples (65 surveillance and 4 compliance) were collected and analyzed by FDA. Of the 532 domestic surveillance samples, 301 (57%) had no pesticide residues detected and 2 (<1%) contained violative residues (Table I.5). The latter involved 2 corn samples with chlorpyrifos-methyl residues. Of the 65 import surveillance samples, 29 (45%) had no pesticide residues detected and 1 (2%), a sample of

Table I.2 Pesticides detectable by the methods used and pesticides found (*) in 1995 regulatory monitoring[a,b]

Acephate*	Cadusafos	Cyhexatin*	Diphenylamine*
Acetochlor	Captafol	Cypermethrin*	Dipropetryn
Acrinathrin	Captan*	Cyprazine	Disulfoton
Alachlor*	Carbaryl*	Cyproconazole	Diuron
Aldicarb*	Carbofuran*	Daminozide	Edifenphos
Aldrin	Carbon tetrachloride	DCPA*	Endosulfan*
Allethrin	Carbophenothion*	DDT*	Endrin*
Allidochlor	Carbosulfan	Deltamethrin	EPN
Alpha-cypermethrin	Carboxin	Deltamethrin, trans	EPTC
Ametryn	Chlorbenside	Demeton*	Esfenvalerate*
Aminocarb	Chlorbromuron	Desmetryn	Etaconazole
Amitraz*	Chlorbufam	Dialifor	Ethalfluralin
Anilazine	Chlordane*	Di-allate	Ethephon*
Aramite	Chlordecone	N,N-Diallyl	Ethiofencarb
Atrazine	Chlordimeform*	dichloroacetamide	Ethion*
Azinphos-ethyl	Chlorethoxyfos	Diazinon*	Ethofumesate
Azinphos-methyl*	Chlorfenvinphos	Dichlobenil	Ethoprop
Bendiocarb	Chlorflurecol methyl	Dichlofenthion	Ethoxyquin*
Benfluralin	ester	Dichlofluanid	Ethylenebisdithio-
Benodanil	Chlorimuron ethyl ester	Dichlone*	carbamates*[d]
Benomyl/carbendazim*[c]	Chlornitrofen	4-(Dichloroacetyl)-1-oxa-	Ethylene dibromide
Benoxacor	Chlorobenzilate	4-azapiro[4.5]decane	Ethylene dichloride
Bensulide	Chloroform	Dichlorvos*	Etridiazole
Benzoylprop-ethyl	3-Chloro-5-methyl-4-	Diclobutrazol	Etrimfos
BHC*	nitro-1H-pyrazole	Diclofop-methyl	Famphur
Bifenox	Chloroneb	Dicloran*	Fenamiphos*
Bifenthrin*	Chloropropylate	Dicofol*	Fenarimol*
Binapacryl	Chlorothalonil*	Dicrotophos	Fenbuconazole
S-Bioallethrin	Chloroxuron	Dieldrin*	Fenfuram
Biphenyl	Chlorpropham*	Diethatyl-ethyl	Fenitrothion*
Bitertanol*	Chlorpyrifos*	Dilan	Fenobucarb
Bromacil	Chlorpyrifos-methyl*	Dimethachlor	Fenoxaprop ethyl
Bromophos	Chlorthiophos	Dimethametryn	ester
Bromophos-ethyl	Clomazone	Dimethipin	Fenoxycarb
Bromopropylate*	Coumaphos	Dimethoate*	Fenpropathrin
Bromoxynil	Crotoxyphos	Dinitramine	Fenpropimorph
Bufencarb	Crufomate	Dinobuton	Fenson
Bulan	Cyanazine	Dinocap	Fensulfothion
Bupirimate	Cyanofenphos	Dioxabenzofos	Fenthion
Butachlor	Cyanophos	Dioxacarb	Fenuron
Butocarboxim	Cycloate	Dioxathion	Fenvalerate*
Butralin	Cyfluthrin	Diphenamid	Fipronil

Continued

Pesticide	No. of samples with quantifiable residues	Residue found, range	ppm median
malathion	149	0.01–7.7	0.09
chlorpyrifos-methyl	39	0.01–1.1	0.11
diazinon	23	0.01–0.81	0.06
chlorpyrifos	10	0.01–0.08	0.03
pirimiphos-methyl	9	0.01–9.9	0.05
others	24	0.01–41	0.19

feather meal (for poultry) from Canada, contained diphenylamine. No tolerance for chlorpyrifos-methyl on corn or for diphenylamine on poultry has been set. Thus, these samples were considered to have exceeded regulatory standards.

In the 231 domestic surveillance feed samples in which 1 or more pesticides were detected, a total of 346 residues were detected (254 quantifiable and 92 trace). Malathion, chlorpyrifos-methyl, and diazinon were the most frequently found residues. The findings in samples with quantifiable residues were as follows:

Table I.2   Continued

Flamprop-M-isopropyl	Methomyl*	Phorate*	Sulfur dioxide*
Flamprop-methyl	Methoprotryne	Phosalone*	Sulphenone
Fluazifop butyl ester	Methoxychlor*	Phosmet*	Sulprofos
Fluchloralin	Methylene chloride	Phosphamidon*	TCMTB
Flucythrinate	Metobromuron	Phosphine	Tebuconazole
Flusilazole	Metolachlor	Piperonyl butoxide	Tebupirimfos
Fluvalinate	Metolcarb	Piperophos	Tecnazene
Folpet*	Metoxuron	Pirimicarb	TEPP
Fonofos*	Metribuzin	Pirimiphos-ethyl	Terbacil
Formetanate	Mevinphos*	Pirimiphos-methyl*	Terbufos
hydrochloride*	Mirex*	Pretilachlor	Terbumeton
Formothion	Monocrotophos*	Probenazole	Terbuthylazine
Fuberidazole	Monolinuron	Prochloraz	Terbutryn
Furilazole	Monuron	Procyazine	Tetradifon*
Gardona*	Myclobutanil*	Procymidone*	Tetraiodoethylene
Heptachlor*	Naled	Prodiamine	Tetrasul
Heptenophos	Napropamide	Profenofos*	Thiabendazole*
Hexachlorobenzene*	Neburon	Profluralin	Thiobencarb
Hexaconazole	Nitralin	Prolan	Thiodicarb
Hexazinone	Nitrapyrin	Promecarb	Thiometon
Imazalil*	Nitrofen	Prometryn	Thionazin
Imazamethabenz	Nitrofluorfen	Pronamide	Thiophanate-methyl
methyl ester	Nitrothal-isopropyl	Propachlor	Tolylfluanid
Iprobenfos	Norflurazon	Propanil	Toxaphene
Iprodione*	Nuarimol	Propargite*	Tralomethrin
Isazofos	Octhilinone	Propazine	Traloxydim
Isocarbamid	Ofurace	Propetamphos	Triadimefon*
Isofenphos	Omethoate*	Propham	Triadimenol*
Isoprocarb	Ovex	Propiconazole	Tri-allate
Isopropalin	Oxadiazon	Propoxur	Triazamate
Isoprothiolane	Oxadixyl	Prothiofos*	Triazophos
Lactofen	Oxamyl*	Prothoate	Tribufos
Lambda-cyhalothrin	Oxydemeton-methyl*	Pyrazon	Trichlorfon
Leptophos	Oxyfluorfen	Pyrazophos	Tricyclazole
Lindane*	Oxythioquinox	Pyrethrins	Tridiphane
Linuron*	Paclobutrazol	Pyridaphenthion	Trietazine
Malathion*	Paraquat	Quinalphos	Triflumizole
Mecarbam	Parathion*	Quintozene*	Trifluralin*
Mephosfolan	Parathion-methyl*	Quizalofop ethyl ester	Triflusulfuron methyl
Merphos*	Pebulate	Ronnel	ester
Metalaxyl*	Penconazole	Schradan	Trimethacarb
Metasystox thiol	Pendimethalin	Secbumeton	Vamidothion sulfone
Metazachlor	Permethrin*	Simazine*	Vernolate
Methabenzthiazuron	Perthane	Simetryn	Vinclozolin*
Methamidophos*	Phenothrin	Strobane	XMC
Methidathion*	Phenthoate	Sulfallate	
Methiocarb*	Phenylphenol, ortho-*	Sulfotep*	

[a]The list of pesticides detectable is expressed in terms of the parent pesticide. However, monitoring coverage and findings may have included metabolites, impurities, and alteration products.

[b]Some of these pesticides are no longer manufactured or registered for use in the United States.

[c]The analytical methodology determines carbendazim, which may result from use of benomyl or carbendazim.

[d]Such as maneb.

Summary: Regulatory Monitoring

In summary, no residues were found in 64% of domestic surveillance samples and 66% of import surveillance samples (Figure I.4) analyzed under FDA's regulatory monitoring approach in 1995. Less than 1% of domestic and import surveillance samples had residue levels that were over tolerance and less than 1% of domestic and 3% of import surveillance samples had residues for which there was no tolerance. The findings for 1995 demonstrate that pesticide residue levels in foods are generally well below EPA tolerances, corroborating results presented in earlier reports [6].

Table I.3   Compliance samples by commodity group in 1995

Commodity group	Total no. of samples	Samples with no residues found, %	Samples violative, %
Domestic			
Grains and grain products	3	33	0
Milk/Eggs	5	100	0
Fish	5	80	0
Fruits	23	48	0
Vegetables	56	48	21
Other	5	80	0
Total	97	54	12
Import			
Grains and grain products	49	63	0
Cheese	3	100	0
Fish/shellfish	17	41	0
Fruits	71	68	18
Vegetables	196	52	14
Other	49	86	6
Total	385	61	11

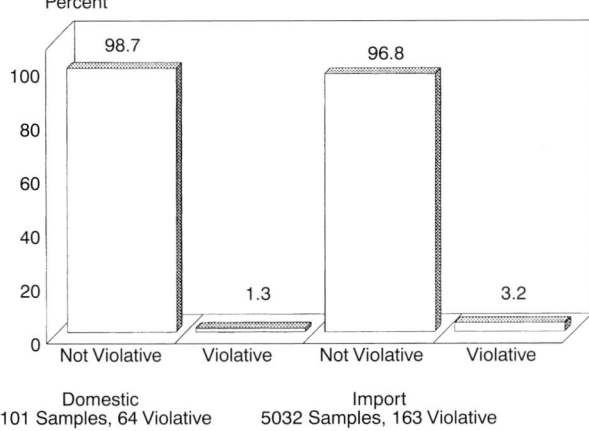

Figure I.3   Domestic and import surveillance sample violation rates for 1995.

Incidence/Level Monitoring

Statistically Based Survey   The statistically based monitoring survey of domestic and imported fresh apples and processed rice that was begun in 1994 was completed in 1995. The original goal had been to collect 1600 samples of apples (800 domestic and 800 import). Actually, 769 domestic and 1062 import samples were collected and analyzed. For rice, 575 domestic and 800 import samples had been the goal; 598 domestic and 612 import samples were actually collected and analyzed. (These numbers are not included in the counts under Fruits and Grains and Grain Products in Appendixes A and B.) The results of the survey are being evaluated and will be submitted for publication in the scientific literature.

Table I.4   Summary of foodcontam findings for 1995[a]

State	Total samples	No. positive	Positive, %	No. significant	Significant, %
Arkansas	351	14	4.0	2	0.6
California	4694	1164	24.8	40	0.9
Georgia	540	128	23.7	7	1.3
Indiana	158	93	58.9	0	—
North Carolina	688	215	31.3	9	1.3
New York	965	321	33.3	14	1.5
Oregon	277	39	14.1	0	—
Pennsylvania	582	124	21.3	5	0.9
Virginia	703	88	12.5	2	0.3
Wisconsin	538	7	1.3	0	—
Total	9394	2193	23.3	79	0.8

[a]Data from Florida not available.

Table I.5   Summary of findings in domestic surveillance feed samples in 1995

Type of feed	Total no. of samples	Samples with no residues found		Violative samples	
		No.	%	No.	%
Whole/ground grains	167	98	59	2	1
Plant by-products	120	76	63	0	—
Mixed feed rations	116	35	30	0	—
Animal by-products	104	74	71	0	—
Hay & hay products	25	18	72	0	—
Total	532	301	57	2	<1

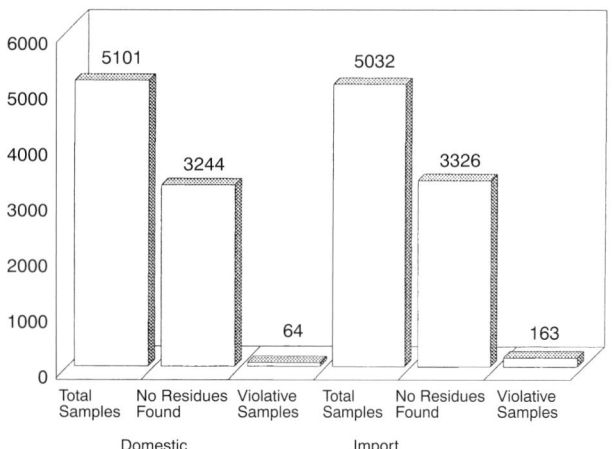

Figure I.4   Comparison of results for domestic and import surveillance samples in 1995.

Table I.6   Commodity targeted monitoring of domestic and imported foods for triazine herbicides conducted in 1995

Commodity	Number of samples analyzed	
	Domestic	Import
Apples	9	16
Bananas	2	23
Cherries	25	—
Corn	10	15
Corn, whole grain	—	1
Grapefruit	8	4
Grapes	5	20
Olives	—	25
Oranges	20	5
Pears	6	19
Plums	7	13
Total	92	140

Triazine Herbicides   The triazines are one of the most widely used classes of herbicides, and EPA has established tolerances for them on many commodities. Interest in triazines has increased recently because of potential leaching of the herbicides and their degradation products into ground and surface water. Residues of these chemicals have rarely been detected in foods, although FDA has routinely looked for the parent compounds.

Recently, FDA's Atlanta District Laboratory developed a method capable of determining 19 triazine herbicides and 4 metabolites [12]. Average recoveries ranged from 81 to 106% for the parent herbicides and 60 to 88% for the metabolites. The method was validated by the Minneapolis District Laboratory [13] and used to analyze a number of food samples in 1995. This new method was used to analyze 232 samples (92 domestic samples from 9 states and 140 import samples from 19 countries) (Table I.6). Residues were found in 5 domestic samples, all of simazine in oranges. Four samples had trace amounts and 1 sample had 0.04 ppm (LQ, 0.02 ppm). None were violative. No triazine residues were detected in the import samples.

Summary: Incidence/Level Monitoring

Under this approach, a statistically based monitoring survey of domestic and imported apples and processed rice was completed in 1995. A survey of triazine herbicides in various commodities was carried out. Few residues were found, and none were violative.

Total Diet Study

The Total Diet Study is unique in that it determines pesticide residues in foods that have been prepared as they would be consumed [5]. Of the nearly 300 chemicals that can be determined by the analytical methods used, 86 pesticide and pesticide-related chemicals were found in the foods analyzed in the 3 collections reported here. To measure the low levels of pesticides found in the Total Diet Study foods, the analytical methods used are modified to permit measurement at levels 5–10 times lower than those normally used in regulatory monitoring. In general, residues present at or above 1 part per billion can be measured.

Table I.7 lists the 17 most frequently found residues, the total number of findings, and the percent

Table I.7 Frequency of occurrence of pesticide residues found in total diet study foods in 1995[a]

Pesticide[b]	Total no. of findings	Occurrence, %
DDT	192	25
Malathion	141	18
Chlorpyrifos-methyl	130	17
Chlorpyrifos	97	12
Dieldrin	92	12
Endosulfan	81	10
Chlorpropham	44	6
Methamidophos	40	5
Carbaryl[c]	39	5
Iprodione	31	4
Thiabendazole[d]	29	4
Dimethoate	28	4
Permethrin	25	3
Hexachlorobenzene	24	3
BHC	22	3
Dicloran	21	3
Diazinon	21	3

[a]Based on 3 market baskets analyzed in 1995 consisting of 783 items.
[b]Isomers, metabolites, and related compounds are not listed separately; they are covered under the "parent" pesticide from which they arise.
[c]Reflects overall incidence; however, only 95 selected foods per market basket (i.e., 285 items total) were analyzed for N-methylcarbamates.
[d]Reflects overall incidence; however, only 67 selected foods per market basket (i.e., 201 items total) were analyzed for the benzimidazole fungicides (thiabendazole and benomyl).

occurrence in the 783 food items analyzed in 1995. DDT, an environmentally persistent chemical whose U.S. registration was higher than it has been in the past several years. This may not be an indicator of an increasing trend in DDT findings in Total Diet Study foods; however, the occurrence will be investigated. Malathion, which is used on a wide variety of crops both pre- and postharvest, was the next most frequently found residue. The levels of these 2 pesticides, as well as the others listed in Table I.7, were well below regulatory limits.

Information obtained through the Total Diet Study is used to estimate dietary intakes of pesticides; these intakes are then compared with established standards. Food consumption data to be used in estimating dietary intakes for the revised food list have not been finalized. Therefore, dietary intake information for the market baskets collected during this period is not presented.

For several years, FDA has collected and analyzed a number of baby foods in addition to those covered under the Total Diet Study. Between 1991 and 1995, this adjunct to the Total Diet Study included 23 different food items (14 fruit juices or fruits, 4 fruit des-

serts, 4 grain products, and 1 vegetable). (These numbers are not included in the analyses reported in Table I.7.) Table I.8 lists the 16 most frequently found pesticide residues in those 23 foods in 1991–1995. Carbaryl, the residue found most frequently, is an insecticide with tolerances on many fruits and grains. Dimethoate, the next most frequently found residue, also has tolerances on a number of fruits.

Summary: Total Diet Study

In 1995, the types of pesticide residues found and their frequency of occurrence in the Total Diet Study were generally consistent with those given in previous FDA reports [6]. The pesticide residue levels found were well below regulatory standards. An adjunct survey of baby foods in 1991–1995 also provided evidence of only small amounts of pesticide residues in those foods.

Summary

A total of 10,615 samples of domestically produced food and imported food from 94 countries was

Table I.8 Frequency of occurrence of pesticide residues found in selected baby foods in 1991–1995[a]

Pesticide[b]	Total no. of findings	Occurrence, %
Carbaryl[c]	77	28
Dimethoate	71	26
Iprodione	45	16
Omethoate	39	14
Malathion	36	13
Chlorpyrifos	35	13
Endosulfan	29	11
Chlorpyrifos-methyl	26	9
Thiabendazole[d]	23	8
Permethrin	22	8
Parathion	20	7
Dicloran	14	5
Propargite[e]	10	4
Acephate	9	3
Dieldrin	8	3
Benomyl[d]	7	3

[a]Based on 12 collections consisting of 276 items.
[b]Isomers, metabolites, and related compounds are not listed separately; they are covered under the "parent" pesticide from which they arise.
[c]Reflects overall incidence; however, only 17 selected foods per collection (i.e., 204 items total) were analyzed for N-methylcarbamates.
[d]Reflects overall incidence; however, only 16 selected items (i.e., 192 items total) were analyzed for the benzimidazole fungicides (thiabendazole and benomyl).
[e]Reflects overall incidence; however, only 16 selected foods per collection (i.e., 192 items total) were analyzed for this sulfur-containing compound.

analyzed for pesticide residues in 1995. Of these, 10,133 were surveillance samples, which are collected when there is no evidence of a pesticide problem. No residues were found in 64% of the domestic surveillance samples and 66% of the import surveillance samples. The higher violation rates in the 482 compliance samples reflect the fact that they are collected and analyzed when a pesticide problem is suspected. In addition, a survey of triazine herbicides was carried out and a statistically based monitoring survey of fresh apples and processed rice that had been initiated in 1994 was completed. Most of the Total Diet Study findings for 1995 were generally similar to those found in earlier periods.

This report was compiled through the efforts of the following FDA personnel: Norma J. Yess, Young H. Lee, Byron O. Bohannon (Division of Programs and Enforcement Policy), and Bernadette M. McMahon and Charles H. Parfitt (Division of Pesticides and Industrial Chemicals), Office of Plant and Dairy Foods and Beverages; Sharon A. Macuci (Division of Information Resources Management), Office of Management Systems, Washington, DC; Rodney L. Bong, Minneapolis District, Minneapolis, MN; and Sheila K. Egan and James L. Daft, Kansas City District, Kansas City, MO.

FDA pesticide monitoring data collected under the regulatory monitoring approach in 1995 are available for purchase on personal computer diskettes from the National Technical Information Service (NTIS), 5285 Port Royal Road, Springfield, VA 22161 (telephone 703-487-4650); order number PB96-503156. The databases for 1992, 1993, and 1994 are also available from NTIS. The order numbers are: 1992, PB94-500899; 1993, PB94-501681; and 1994, PB95-503132.

References

1. Yess, N.J. (1995) U.S. Food and Drug Administration monitoring of pesticide residues in foods. *Pestic. Outlook* 6, 28–31.
2. *Code of Federal Regulations* (1996) Title 40, U.S. Government Printing Office, Washington, DC, Parts 180, 185, and 186.
3. *Pesticide Analytical Manual* (1968 and revisions) Vols I (3rd Ed., 1994) and II (1971), Food and Drug Administration, Washington, DC (available from National Technical Information Service, Springfield, VA 22161).
4. Roy, R.R., Albert, R.H., Wilson, P., Laski, R.R., Roberts, J.I., Hoffmann, T.J., Bong, R.L., Bohannon, B.O., & Yess, N.J. (1995) U.S. Food and Drug Administration pesticide program: incidence/level monitoring of domestic and imported pears and tomatoes. *J. AOAC Int.* 78, 930–940.
5. Pennington, J.A.T., Capar, S.G., Parfitt, C.H., & Edwards, C.W. (1996) History of the Food and Drug Administration's Total Diet Study (Part II), 1987–1993. *J. AOAC Int.* 79, 163–170.
6. Food and Drug Administration (1995) Food and Drug Administration pesticide program – residue monitoring – 1994. *J. AOAC Int.* 78, 117A–143A (and earlier reports in the series).
7. Gunderson, E.L. (1995) Dietary intakes of pesticides, selected elements, and other chemicals: FDA Total Diet Study, June 1984–April 1986. *J. AOAC Int.* 78, 910–921.
8. Gunderson, E.L. (1995) FDA Total Diet Study, July 1986–April 1991, dietary intakes of pesticides, selected elements, and other chemicals. *J. AOAC Int.* 78, 1353–1363.
9. Pennington, J.A.T. (1992) Total Diet Studies: the identification of core foods in the United States food supply. *Food Addit. Contam.* 9, 253–264.
10. Pennington, J.A.T. (1992) The 1990 revision of the FDA Total Diet Study. *J. Nutr. Educ.* 24, 173–178.
11. Pennington, J.A.T. (1992) Appendices for the 1990 revision of the Food and Drug Administration's Total Diet Study. PB92-176239/AS, National Technical Information Service, Springfield, VA 22161.
12. Pardue, J.R. (1995) Multiresidue method for the chromatographic determination of triazine herbicides and their metabolites in raw agricultural products. *J. AOAC Int.* 78, 856–862.
13. Bong, R., Kramer, J., Heaney, L., & Murphy, L. (1995) Validation of a multiresidue method for triazine herbicides in various food commodities. *Lab. Inf. Bull.* 3998, Food and Drug Administration, Rockville, MD.

Appendix A

Analysis of Domestic Surveillance Samples by Commodity Group in 1995

Commodity Group	Total no. of samples	Samples with no residues found, %	Samples violative, % Over tolerance	Samples violative, % No tolerance
A. Grains and Grain Products				
Corn & corn products	53	81	0	0
Oats	18	67	0	0
Rice & rice products	56	86	0	0
Soybeans	38	82	0	0
Wheat	146	38	1	0
Cereal products	23	87	0	0
Other grains & grain products	55	38	2	0
Total	389	59	<1	0
B. Milk/Dairy Products/Eggs				
Cheese & cheese products	66	68	0	0
Eggs	259	98	0	0
Milk/cream & milk products	761	93	0	0
Total	1086	93	0	0
C. Fish/Shellfish				
Fish	295	53	0	0
Shellfish	128	90	0	0
Total	423	64	0	0
D. Fruits				
Blueberries	64	61	0	17
Cranberries	20	10	0	0
Grapes	52	52	0	0
Raspberries	33	24	0	0
Strawberries	107	15	1	2
Other berries	8	75	0	0
Grapefruit	22	27	0	0
Lemons	28	57	0	0
Oranges	171	6	0	0
Other citrus fruits	6	33	0	0
Apples	189	46	0	0
Pears	69	32	7	0
Apricots	28	25	4	0
Cherries	64	17	0	0
Nectarines	26	8	0	0
Olives	12	100	0	0
Peaches	200	20	<1	<1
Other pit fruits	11	73	0	0
Cantaloupe	45	62	0	2
Honeydew	14	57	0	0
Watermelon	73	86	0	0
Apple juice	110	76	0	<1
Other fruit juices	22	82	0	0
Fruit jams/jellies/pastes/toppings	11	36	0	0
Other fruits	52	88	0	2
Total	1437	40	<1	1

Continued

Appendix A Continued

Commodity Group	Total no. of samples	Samples with no residues found, %	Samples violative, % Over tolerance	Samples violative, % No tolerance
E. Vegetables				
Corn	105	90	0	0
Green/snow/sugar/sweet peas	84	86	0	0
String beans	100	67	0	0
Other beans & peas	32	91	0	0
Cucumbers	41	61	0	2
Eggplant	17	71	0	12
Peppers, hot	12	83	0	0
Peppers, sweet	40	58	0	0
Squash	33	58	0	3
Tomatoes	100	56	0	0
Other fruits used as vegetables	10	100	0	0
Broccoli	23	74	0	0
Cabbage	65	83	0	0
Cauliflower	20	90	0	0
Celery	30	30	0	3
Collards	18	67	0	6
Endive/escarole	11	91	0	45
Kale	11	45	0	9
Lettuce, head	115	37	<1	0
Mustard greens	12	17	0	0
Romaine	85	35	4	1
Spinach	37	32	0	5
Other leaf/stem vegetables	48	60	0	19
Mushrooms/truffles & products	15	100	0	0
Carrots	130	57	2	0
Onions/leeks/scallions/shallots	28	89	0	0
Potatoes	239	56	0	2
Radishes	15	73	0	0
Red beets	15	100	0	0
Sweet potatoes/yams	25	64	0	0
Other root/tuber vegetables	9	89	0	0
Vegetables, dried or paste	45	89	0	0
Other vegetables/vegetable products	15	67	0	0
Total	1585	63	<1	2
F. Other				
Peanuts	50	94	0	0
Other nuts	17	100	0	0
Vegetable oils	13	100	0	0
Honey & other sweeteners	17	88	0	0
Baby foods/formula	61	97	0	0
Other food products	23	83	0	4
Total	181	94	0	<1
A–F Total	5101	64	<1	<1

Appendix B

Analysis of Import Surveillance Samples by Commodity Group in 1995

Commodity Group	Total no. of samples	Samples with no residues found, %	Samples violative, % Over tolerance	No tolerance
A. Grains and Grain Products				
Rice, basmati	22	77	0	5
Rice, jasmine	34	91	0	0
Other rice & rice products	23	91	0	0
Wheat & wheat products	21	71	0	0
Other grains & grain products	16	100	0	0
Bakery products	21	86	0	5
Breakfast/snack foods	12	67	0	0
Macaroni	43	79	0	0
Spaghetti	18	72	0	0
Other pasta products	28	61	0	0
Total	238	80	0	<1
B. Dairy Products/Eggs				
Cheese & cheese products	75	93	0	0
Eggs	27	74	0	0
Total	102	88	0	0
C. Fish/Shellfish				
Fish	99	83	0	0
Shellfish	22	95	0	0
Total	121	85	0	0
D. Fruits				
Blackberries	30	40	0	3
Blueberries	38	97	0	0
Grapes	202	31	0	1
Raspberries	53	36	0	9
Strawberries	67	18	0	10
Other berries	20	55	0	0
Clementines	11	82	0	0
Limes	18	67	0	0
Oranges	30	70	0	7
Tangerines	12	58	0	0
Other citrus fruits	14	100	0	0
Apples	48	50	0	8
Pears	69	48	0	1
Apricots	10	50	0	0
Cherries	19	47	0	0
Nectarines	16	50	0	0
Olives	77	92	0	1
Peaches	52	48	0	4
Plums	31	55	0	0
Other pit fruits	13	100	0	0
Bananas	228	34	<1	0
Kiwi fruit	20	75	0	0
Mangoes	69	96	0	0
Papayas	81	72	0	9
Pineapples	65	75	5	0
Plantains	18	89	0	0
Other tropical fruits	56	89	0	7

Continued

Appendix B Continued

Commodity Group	Total no. of samples	Samples with no residues found, %	Samples violative, % Over tolerance	No tolerance
Cantaloupe	82	40	5	2
Honeydew	53	6	0	6
Watermelon	28	50	0	0
Other vine fruits	17	82	0	0
Apple juice	19	68	0	11
Other fruit juices	52	94	0	0
Fruit jams/jellies/toppings	41	90	0	0
Fruits, dried or paste	90	90	0	0
Other fruits & fruit products	8	88	0	0
Total	1757	57	<1	3
E. Vegetables				
Corn	45	100	0	0
Green/snow/sugar/sweet peas	90	51	0	12
Mung beans	11	91	0	0
String beans	78	47	3	8
Other beans, peas, & corn	63	81	0	5
Cucumbers	96	49	0	4
Eggplant	23	48	0	0
Okra	33	73	0	9
Peppers, hot	261	46	3[a]	5
Peppers, sweet	295	76	0	1
Squash/pumpkins	110	35	0	4
Tomatoes	332	59	0	0
Other fruits used as vegetables	30	87	0	10
Artichokes	26	96	0	0
Asparagus	101	63	12	1
Bamboo shoots	20	100	0	0
Broccoli	53	70	0	0
Cabbage	16	63	0	0
Celery	20	20	0	0
Chicory	16	94	0	6
Endive/escarole	45	98	0	0
Lettuce, head	40	38	3	8
Radicchio	59	98	0	2
Romaine	44	50	7	3
Spinach	22	36	5	0
Other leaf/stem vegetables	67	64	1	10
Mushrooms/truffles, whole	47	96	0	2
Mushrooms/truffles, pieces & products	51	96	0	2
Carrots	46	67	0	0
Cassava	18	100	0	0
Onions	27	89	0	0
Potatoes	22	95	0	0
Radishes	13	62	0	0
Shallots/scallions/leeks	23	91	0	0
Sweet potatoes/yams	14	100	0	0
Water chestnuts	46	100	0	0
Other root/tuber vegetables	42	86	0	0
Vegetables, dried or paste	140	83	0	6
Vegetables with sauce	22	77	0	9
Other vegetables & vegetable products	28	82	0	0
Total	2535	67	1[a]	3[a]

Continued

Appendix B Continued

Commodity Group	Total no. of samples	Samples with no residues found, %	Samples violative, %	
			Over tolerance	No tolerance
F. Other				
Spices	14	75	0	0
Cashews	42	62	0	7
Peanuts	20	85	0	0
Other nuts & nut products	35	89	0	3
Edible seeds	24	75	0	17
Vegetable oils, crude	14	100	0	0
Vegetable oils, refined	15	100	0	0
Beverage bases	13	100	0	0
Bottled water, mineral/spring	19	100	0	0
Honey & other sweeteners	25	76	0	0
Other food products	58	79	0	0
Total	279	83	0	3
A–F Total	5032	66	<1[a]	3[a]

[a]Includes samples that have both residue(s) over tolerance and residue(s) with no tolerance.

APPENDIX II

Tables and Charts

From: Shils, Maurice E., Olson, James A., and Shilke, Moshe., eds. (1994) *Modern Nutrition in Health and Disease*, eighth edition, **2**. Philadelphia: Lea & Febiger. Reproduced with permission.

Table II.1   Conversion factors between traditional and SI units

Factors for converting nutrients expressed in metric or millequivalent units into International System (SI) units.
1. Definitions
    a. Equivalent weight (EW) = atomic weight of element/valence of ionic form. Example with magnesium: atomic wt = 24, valence = 2+; therefore EW = 12
    b. Quantity of an electrolyte in milliequivalents per liter (mEq/1) = mg of electrolyte/L/EW. Example: 48 mg of magnesium/L/12 = 4 mEq/L
    c. Quantity of an electrolyte in mg/dl = (mEq/L × EW)/10
    d. To convert mg/dl (= mg%) of an electrolyte to mEq/L mg/dl × 10/EW = mEq/L
    e. 1 mol = 1 molecular or atomic weight of element or compound in grams (GMWt). In solutions this is usually expressed as moles per liter; i.e., 1/mol/L = 1 M; 1 mM (mmol) = 1 mol × 10^{-3}; 1 μM ((μmol) = 1 mol × 10^{-6}; 1 nM (nmol) = 1 mol × 10^{-9}
    f. (1) To convert mEq/L of an electrolyte or other ions in solution to mmol/L: mEq/L divided by valence = mmol/L; e.g., (a) 2 mEq/L of magnesium (Mg^{2+}) = 2/2 = 1 mmol/L; e.g., (b) 140 mEq Na^+/L = 140/L = 140 mmol/L
        (2) To convert mg/dl to mmol/L: (mg/dl × 10/EW) divided by valence = mmol/L; e.g., 2 mg/dl of magnesium = (2 × 10/12) divided by 2 = 0.83 mmol/L
        (3) For organic substances: mmol/L = wt in mg/L/MW (in mg)
2. SI units for expressing clinical laboratory data
    These units are now widely used and are increasingly required for publication of scientific data in physical, biologic, and biomedical publications. Extensive SI conversion tables have been published together with an explanation of the rationale for their use and technical aspects of usage. [1–3]
    a. The base units of interest in physical quantities used in clinical chemistry are:

Quantity	Base Unit
mass	kilogram
time	second
amount	mole
length	meter

A derived unit for energy is the kjoule (kJ) 4.18 kJ = 1 kcal
1 MJ = 239 kcal

    b. Prefixes and symbols for decimal multiples and submultiples include:

Factor	Prefix	Symbol	Factor	Prefix	Symbol
10^8	giga	G	10^{-3}	milli	m
10^6	mega	M	10^{-8}	micro	u
10^3	kilo	k	10^{-8}	nano	n
10^2	hecto	h	10^{-12}	pico	p
10^1	deka	da	10^{-15}	femto	f
10^{-1}	deci	d	10^{-18}	atto	a
10^{-2}	centi	c			

Continued

Table II.1 Continued

3. Conversion factors for selected compounds of nutrition interest*

Component	(1) Present Unit	(2) Conversion Factor	(3) SI Unit Symbol	(4) Mass Conversion Factor
Albumin (s)	g/dl	10	g/L	—
Aluminum (s)	μg/L	37.04	nmol/L	μg/27 = mol
Amino acids	(see ref. 3, p. 119 for individual amino acids)			
Amino acid nitrogen (p)	mg/dl	0.714	mmol/L	mg/14 = mmol
Ascorbic acid (p)	mg/dl	56.78	μmol/L	mg/176 = mmol
Calcium (s)	mg/dl	0.250	mmol/L	mg/40 = mmol
Calcium (s)	mEq/dl	0.500	mmol/L	mEq/2 = mmol
β-Carotenet (s)	μ/dl	0.0186	μmol/L	μg/536.85 umol
Chloride (s)	mEq/L	1.00	mmol/L	mEq = mmol
Cholesterol (p)	mg/dl	0.0258	mmol/L	mg/386.5 = mmol
Copper (s)	μg/dl	0.157	μmol/L	μg/63.5 = umol
Cyanocobalamin (B_{12})	pg/ml	0.738	pmol/L	pg/1355 = pmol
Ethanol (p)	mg/dl	0.217	mmol/L	mg/46 = mmol
Folic acid	ng/ml	2.265	nmol/L	ng/441.4 = nmol
Glucose (p)	mg/dl	0.0555	mmol/L	mg/180.2 = mmol
Iron (s)	μg/dl	0.179	μmol/L	μg/55.9 = μmol
Phosphate (p) (as phosphorus)	mg/dl	0.323	mmol/L	mg/31 = mmol
Potassium (s)	mEq/L	1.000	mmol/L	mEq = mmol
Potassium	mg/dl	0.256	mmol/L	mg/39.1 = mmol
Magnesium (s)	mg/dl	0.411	mmol/L	mg/24.3 = mmol
Pyridoxal (B)	ng/ml	5.981	nmol/L	ng/167 = nmol
Retinol† (p,s)	μg/dl	0.0349	μmol/L	μg 286 = μmol
Riboflavin (s)	μg/dl	26.57	nmol/L	μg/376 = nmol
Sodium (s)	mEq/L	1.00	mmol/L	mEq = mmol
Thiamin HCl (U)	μg/24 hr	0.00298	μmol/d	μg/337 = μmol
α-Tocopherol (p)	mg/dl	23.22	μmol/L	μg/431 = μmol
Vitamin D_3	μg/dl	26.01	nmol/L	μg/384 = μmol
Calcidiol	ng/ml	2.498	nmol/L	ng/400 = nmol
Zinc (s)	μg/dl	0.153	μmol/L	μg/65.4 = μmol

*To convert metric or equivalent unit per unit volume (column 1) to S.I. units per liter (column 3), multiply by the conversion factor in column 2, p = plasma; s = serum; B = blood; U = urine.
†See Appendix Table II.2 for detailed conversion figures for retinol and carotene.

REFERENCES

1. Young, D.S. (1987) *Ann. Intern. Med.*, **108** 114.
2. Lundberg, G.D. (1986) Iberson, C., Radulescu, G. *JAMA*, **255** 2329.
3. Mansen, E.R. (1987) *J. Am. Diet. Assoc.*, **87** 358.

Table II.2 Factors and formulas used in interconverting units of vitamin A and carotenoids

Factors
  1 nmol retinol = 286.42 ng
  1 nmol retinoic acid = 300.42 ng
  1 nmol β-carotene = 538.85 ng
1 μg retinol equivalent (μg RE)
  = 1 μg all-*trans* retinol
  = 3.49 nmol all-*trans* retinol
  = 6 μg all-*trans* β-carotene
  = 11.18 nmol all-*trans* β-carotene
  = 12 μg other all-*trans* provitamin A carotenoids
  = 3.33 IU$_a$ (the international unit of all-*trans* retinol)
  = 10 IU$_c$ (the international unit of all-*trans* β-carotene)

Table II.2 Continued

1 IU$_a$
  = 0.3 μg all-*trans* retinol
  = 0.3 μg RE
  = 1.05 nmol all-*trans* retinol
  = 1.8 μg all-*trans* β-carotene
  = 3.35 nmol all-*trans* β-carotene
  = 3 IU$_c$
  = 3.6 μg other all-*trans* provitamin A carotenoids
1 IU$_c$
  = 0.6 μg all-*trans* β-carotene
  = 1.12 nmol all-*trans* β-carotene
  = 0.1 μg RE
  = 0.33 IU$_a$
  = 1.2 μg other all-*trans* provitamin A carotenoids

Continued

Continued

Table II.2   Continued

Formulas and Examples: All-*trans* configurations of retinol and carotenoids are assumed

1. $\mu g\ RE = \mu g\ retinol + \mu g\ \beta\text{-carotene}/6$

   A diet contains 500 μg retinol and 1800 μg β-carotene. Then,

   $$\mu g\ RE = 500 + 1800/6 = 800\ \mu g\ RE$$

2. $\mu g\ RE = IU_a/3.33 + IU_c/10$

   A diet contains 1667 IU_a of retinol and 3000 IU_c of β-carotene. Then,

   $$\mu g\ RE = 1667/3.33 + 3000/10 = 800\ \mu g\ RE$$

3. $\mu g\ RE = \mu g\ \beta\text{-carotene}/6 + \mu g$ other provitamin A carotenoids/12

   A serving of sweet potato contains 2400 μg of β-carotene and 480 μg of other provitamin A carotenoids. Then,

   $$\mu g\ RE = 2400/6 + 480/12 = 440\ \mu g\ RE$$

4. $\%\ \mu g\ RE\ as\ retinol = \left[1.5 - \dfrac{0.15\ total\ IU}{total\ RE}\right] \times 100$

   $\%\ \mu g\ RE\ as\ carotenoids = \left[\dfrac{0.15\ total\ IU}{total\ RE} - 0.5\right] \times 100$

   A 100-g portion of cheese contains a total of 300 μg RE and a total of 1200 IU, in which 1 IU_a has been *assumed* to equal 1 IU_c. Then,

   $\%\ RE\ as\ retinol = \left[1.5 - \dfrac{0.15 \times 1200}{300}\right] \times 100 = 90\%$

   $\%\ RE\ as\ carotenoids = \left[\dfrac{0.15 \times 1200}{300} - 0.5\right] \times 100 \times 10\%$

Continued

In this sample of cheese, therefore, 270 μg (270 μg RE) is present as retinol and 180 μg, or 30 μg RE, is present as β-carotene or its equivalent of other provitamin A carotenoids.

5. $IU_a = \dfrac{10\ \mu g\ RE - total\ IU}{2}$

   $IU_c = \dfrac{3\ total\ IU - 10\ \mu g\ RE}{2}$

   In a cheese sample containing a total of 300 μg RE and a total of 1200 IU, in which 1 IU_a is *assumed* to equal 1 IU_c,

   $$IU_a = \frac{10 \times 300 - 1200}{2} = 900$$

   $$IU_c = \frac{3 \times 1200 - 10 \times 300}{2} = 300$$

Note: Assumptions used from revised sections of the United States Department of Agriculture's *Handbook 8* (i.e., 8.1–8.10) are (*a*) that 1 IU_a = 1 IU_c and (*b*) that 1 RE = 1 μg of retinol = 6 μg of β-carotene = 12 μg of other provitamin A carotenoids.

In some cases, small negative values for IU_c are obtained when the values for total IU and total RE are given for foods containing only preformed vitamin A_1 particularly in fortified foods like margarine. This aberrant calculation results from the rounding of analytic values. Similarly, small negative values for IU_a may result for foods containing only carotenoids. In both cases, the negative values should be taken as zero.

Prepared by J.A. Olson.

Table II.3   Weights and measures

VOLUMES:

Apothecaries' Measure	Metric	Household
1 fluid dram (fl dr)	4 milliliter (ml)	1 teaspoon (tsp)
2 fl dr	8 ml	1 dessert spoonful
½ fluid ounce (fl oz)	15 ml	1 tablespoon (Tbsp) (3 tsp)
1 fl oz	30 ml	2 Tbsp (⅛ cup)
1½ fl oz	45 ml	1 jigger
2 fl oz	58 ml	4 Tbsp (¼ cup)
2⅔ fl oz	80 ml	5⅓ Tbs (⅓ cup)
4 fl oz	118 ml	8 Tbsp (½ cup)
8 fl oz	237 ml	1 cup
16 fl oz	473 ml	1 pint (pt)
32 fl oz	947 ml	1 quart (qt)
128 fl oz	3.785 ml	1 gallon (gal)
3.38 fl oz	1 deciliter (dl) (100 ml)	
2.11 pt	1 liter (L) (1,000 ml)	

Continued

Table II.3 Continued

WEIGHTS:

Avoirdupois	Metric
	1 femtogram (fg) (10^{-15} g)
	1 picogram (pg) (10^{-12} g)
	1 nanogram (ng) (10^{-9} g)
	1 microgram (μg) (10^{-6} g)
1 grain (gr)	0.065 g (65 mg)
1 gram (0.035 oz)	15.432 gr
1 scruple (20 gr)	1.296 g
1 dram (dr) (= drachm) (27.3 gr)	1.77 g
1 oz (16 dr)	28.35 g
1 lb (16 oz)	453.59 g
1 ton (2,000 lb)	0.91 metric tons
1.015 gr	1 milligram (mg) (10^{-3} g)
	1 centigram (cg) (10^{-2} g)
	1 decigram (dg) (10^{-1} g)
15.4 gr (0.035 oz)	1 gram (g)
2.2 lb	1 kilogram (kg) (10^3 g)

LENGTH/AREA:

	Metric
1 angstrom (A)	10 millimeter (mm)
1/2500 inch (in)	1 micron (μ) (10^{-3} mm) = micrometer (μm)
0.039 in	1 mm
0.39 in	1 centimeter (cm)
1 in	2.54 cm
1 foot (ft) (12 in)	30.5 cm
39.4 in	1 meter (m)
1 yard (yd) (3ft)	0.9 m
1 rod (5.5 yd)	4.85 m
1093.6 yd (0.62 mile)	1 kilometer (km)
1 mile (mi) (5280 ft)	1.61 km
1 acre (160 square rods)	0.4 hectare

TEMPERATURE CONVERSIONS:

F to C: 5/9 (F − 32)
C to F: (9/5 × C) + 32

ELECTROLYTE DATA:

Ion		Atomic Wt (1)	Valence (2)	Equivalent Wt* 1 ÷ 2
Bicarbonate	HCO_3^-	61.0	1	61.0
Calcium	Ca^{2+}	40.1	2	20.0
Chloride	Cl^-	35.5	1	35.5
Magnesium	Mg^{2+}	24.3	2	12.2
Phosphate†	HPO_4^{2-}	96.0	2	48.0†
Potassium	K^+	39.1	1	39.1
Sodium	Na^+	23.0	1	23.0
Sulfate	SO_4^{2-}	96.1	2	48.0

*Milliequivalent (mEq) = equivalent weight in milligrams (mg). To convert mg quantities of all electrolytes to mEq:

$$\frac{\text{mg of electrolyte}}{\text{equivalent weight in mg}} = \text{mEq}$$

To convert mEq quantities of all electrolytes to mg:
mEq × equivalent wt = mg

To convert mg/dl to mEq/L:

$$\frac{\text{mg/dl} \times 10}{\text{equivalent wt in mg}} = \text{mEq/L}$$

To convert mEq/L to mg/dl: mEq/L × equivalent wt in mg × 0.1

† At the normal pH of plasma, 20% of the total inorganic phosphate radical is combined with one equivalent of base as BH_2PO_4, and 80% with two equivalents of base as B_2HPO_4. Under these conditions, base equivalence is therefore 0.2 + (0.8 × 2) = 1.8, and the equivalent weight of 53.3 is obtained by dividing the ionic weight by 1.8 instead of by 2. For phosphorus content of phosphate solutions, 1 mEq provides approximately 15 mg, and 1 mmol provides approximately 31 mg.

Table II.4 Summary of examples of recommended nutrient intake based on age and body weight expressed as daily rates, Canada

Age	Sex	Weight (kg)	Protein (g)	Vit. A (RE)[a]	Vit. D (µg)	Vit. E (mg)	Vit. C (mg)	Folate (µg)	Vit. B12 (µg)	Calcium (mg)	Phosphorus (mg)	Magnesium (mg)	Iron (mg)	Iodine (µg)	Zinc (mg)
Months															
0–4	Both	6.0	12[b]	400	10	3	20	25	0.3	250[c]	150	20	0.3[d]	30	2[d]
5–12	Both	9.0	12	400	10	3	20	40	0.4	400	200	32	7	40	3
Years															
1	Both	11	13	400	10	3	20	40	0.5	500	300	40	6	55	4
2–3	Both	14	16	400	5	4	20	50	0.6	550	350	50	6	65	4
4–6	Both	18	19	500	5	5	25	70	0.8	600	400	65	8	85	5
7–9	M	25	26	700	2.5	7	25	90	1.0	700	500	100	8	110	7
	F	25	26	700	2.5	6	25	90	1.0	700	500	100	8	95	7
10–12	M	34	34	800	2.5	8	25	120	1.0	900	700	130	8	125	9
	F	36	36	800	2.5	7	25	130	1.0	1100	800	135	8	110	9
13–15	M	50	49	900	2.5	9	30[e]	175	1.0	1100	900	185	10	160	12
	F	48	46	800	2.5	7	30[e]	170	1.0	1000	850	180	13	160	9
16–18	M	62	58	1000	2.5	10	40[e]	220	1.0	900	1000	230	10	160	12
	F	53	47	800	2.5	7	30[e]	190	1.0	700	850	200	12	160	9
19–24	M	71	61	1000	2.5	10	40[e]	220	1.0	800	1000	240	9	160	12
	F	58	50	800	2.5	7	30[e]	180	1.0	700	850	200	13	160	9
25–49	M	74	64	1000	2.5	9	40[e]	230	1.0	800	1000	250	9	160	12
	F	59	51	800	2.5	6	30[e]	185	1.0	700	850	200	13	160	9
50–74	M	73	63	1000	5	7	40[e]	230	1.0	800	1000	250	9	160	12
	F	63	54	800	5	6	30[e]	195	1.0	800	850	210	8	160	9
75+	M	69	59	1000	5	6	40[e]	215	1.0	800	1000	230	9	160	12
	F	64	55	800	5	5	30[e]	200	1.0	800	850	210	8	160	9
Pregnancy (additional)															
1st trimester			5	0	2.5	2	0	200	0.2	500	200	15	0	25	6
2nd trimester			20	0	2.5	2	10	200	0.2	500	200	45	5	25	6
3rd trimester			24	0	2.5	2	10	200	0.2	500	200	45	10	25	6
Lactation (additional)			20	400	2.5	3	25	100	0.2	500	200	65	0	50	6

[a] Retinol Equivalents.
[b] Protein is assumed to be from breast milk and must be adjusted for infant formula.
[c] Infant formula with high phosphorus should contain 375 mg calcium.
[d] Breast milk is assumed to be the source of the mineral.
[e] Smokers should increase vitamin C by 50%.
(From Supply and Services Canada (1990) *Health and Welfare Canada: Nutrition Recommendations*. The Report of the Scientific Review Committee, Ottawa. Reproduced with permission of the Minister of Supply and Services Canada 1992.)

Table II.5 Estimated average requirements (EAR) for energy, United Kingdom

Age	EAR MJ/D (KCAL/D) Males	Females
0–3 months	2.28 (545)	2.16 (515)
4–6 months	2.89 (690)	2.69 (645)
7–9 months	3.44 (825)	3.20 (765)
10–12 months	3.85 (920)	3.61 (865)
1–3 years	5.15 (1,230)	4.86 (1,165)
4–6 years	7.16 (1,715)	6.46 (1,545)
7–10 years	8.24 (1,970)	7.28 (1,740)
11–14 years	9.27 (2,220)	7.92 (1,845)
15–18 years	11.51 (2,755)	8.83 (2,110)
19–50 years	10.60 (2,550)	8.10 (1,940)
51–59 years	10.60 (2,550)	8.00 (1,900)
60–64 years	9.93 (2,380)	7.99 (1,900)
65–74 years	9.71 (2,330)	7.96 (1,900)
75+ years	8.77 (2,100)	7.61 (1,810)
Pregnancy		+0.80*(200)
Lactation:		
1 month		+1.90 (450)
2 months		+2.20 (530)
3 months		+2.40 (570)
4–6 months (Group 1)		+2.00 (480)
4–6 months (Group 2)		+2.40 (570)
>6 months (Group 1)		+1.00 (240)
>6 months (Group 2)		+2.30 (550)

*last trimester only.
(From Report on Health and Social Subjects (1991) *Dietary Reference Values for Food and Energy and Nutrients for the United Kingdom*, Her Majesty's Stationery Office, London.)

Table II.6 Reference nutrient intakes for protein, United Kingdom

Age	Reference nutrient intake[a] (g/d)	
0–3 months	12.5[b]	
4–6 months	12.7	
7–9 months	13.7	
10–12 months	14.9	
1–3 years	14.5	
4–6 years	19.7	
7–10 years	28.3	
Males		
11–14 years	42.1	
15–18 years	55.2	
19–50 years	55.5	
50+ years	53.3	
Females		
11–14 years	41.2	
15–18 years	45.0	
19–50 years	45.0	
50+ years	46.5	
Pregnancy[c]		+6
Lactation[c]		
0–4 months		+11
4+ months		+8

[a]These figures, based on egg and milk protein, assume complete digestibility.
[b]No values for infants 0 to 3 months are given by WHO. The reference nutrient intake is calculated from the recommendations of Committee on Medical Aspects of Food Policy (COMA).
[c]To be added to adult requirement through all stages of pregnancy and lactation.
(From Report on Health and Social Subjects (1991) *No. 41, Dietary Reference Values for Food Energy and Nutrients for the United Kingdom*, Report of the Panel on Dietary Reference Values of the Committee on Medical Aspects of Food Policy. Her Majesty's Stationery Office, London.)

Table II.7   Reference nutrient intakes for vitamins, United Kingdom

Age	Thiamin (mg/d)	Riboflavin (mg/d)	Niacin (nicotinic acid equivalent) (mg/d)	Vitamin B_6 (mg/d[a])	Vitamin B_{12} (μg/d)	Folate (μg/d)	Vitamin C (mg/d)	Vitamin A (μg/d)	Vitamin D (μg/d)
0–3 months	0.2	0.4	3	0.2	0.3	50	25	350	8.5
4–6 months	0.2	0.4	3	0.2	0.3	50	25	350	8.5
7–9 months	0.2	0.4	4	0.3	0.4	50	25	350	7
10–12 months	0.3	0.4	5	0.4	0.4	50	25	350	7
1–3 years	0.5	0.6	8	0.7	0.5	70	30	400	7
4–6 years	0.7	0.8	11	0.9	0.8	100	30	500	–
7–10 years	0.7	1.0	12	1.0	1.0	150	30	500	–
Males									
11–14 years	0.9	1.2	15	1.2	1.2	200	35	600	–
15–18 years	1.1	1.3	18	1.5	1.5	200	40	700	–
19–50 years	1.0	1.3	17	1.4	1.5	200	40	700	–
50+ years	0.9	1.3	16	1.4	1.5	200	40	700	**
Females									
11–14 years	0.7	1.1	12	1.0	1.2	200	35	600	–
15–18 years	0.8	1.1	14	1.2	1.5	200	40	600	–
19–50 years	0.8	1.1	13	1.2	1.5	200	40	600	–
50+ years	0.8	1.1	12	1.2	1.5	200	40	600	**
Pregnancy	+0.1[b]	+0.3	*	*	*	+100	+10	+100	10
Lactation									
0–4 months	+0.2	+0.5	+2	*	+0.5	+60	+30	+350	10
4+ months	+0.2	+0.5	+2	*	+0.5	+60	+30	+350	10

*No increment.
**After age 65 the RNI is 10 μg/d for men and women.
[a]Based on protein providing 14.7% of EAR for energy.
[b]For last trimester only.
(From Report on Health and Social Subjects (1991) *No. 41, Dietary Reference Values for Food Energy and Nutrients for the United Kingdom*. Report of the Panel on Dietary Reference Values of the Committee on Medical Aspects of Food Policy. Her Majesty's Stationery Office, London.)

Table II.8   Reference nutrient intakes for minerals, United Kingdom

Age	Calcium (mmol/d)	Phosphorus[1] (mmol/d)	Magnesium (mmol/d)	Sodium[2] (mmol/d)	Potassium[3] (mmol/d)	Chloride[4] (mmol/d)	Iron (μmol/d)	Zinc (μmol/d)	Copper (μmol/d)	Selenium (μmol/d)	Iodine (μmol/d)
0–3 months	13.1	13.1	2.2	9	20	9	30	60	5	0.1	0.4
4–6 months	13.1	13.1	2.5	12	22	12	80	60	5	0.2	0.5
7–9 months	13.1	13.1	3.2	14	18	14	140	75	5	0.1	0.5
10–12 months	13.1	13.1	3.3	15	18	15	140	75	5	0.1	0.5
1–3 years	8.8	8.8	3.5	22	20	22	120	75	6	0.2	0.6
4–6 years	11.3	11.3	4.8	30	28	30	110	100	9	0.3	0.8
7–10 years	13.8	13.8	8.0	50	50	50	160	110	11	0.4	0.9
Males											
11–14 years	25.0	25.0	11.5	70	80	70	200	140	13	0.6	1.0
15–18 years	25.0	25.0	12.3	70	90	70	200	145	16	0.9	1.0
19–50 years	17.5	17.5	12.3	70	90	70	160	145	19	0.9	1.0
50+ years	17.5	17.5	12.3	70	90	70	160	145	19	0.9	1.0
Females											
11–14 years	20.0	10.0	11.5	70	80	70	260[5]	140	13	0.6	1.0
15–18 years	20.0	20.0	12.3	70	90	70	260[5]	110	16	0.8	1.1
19–50 years	17.5	17.5	10.9	70	90	70	260[5]	110	19	0.8	1.1
50+ years	17.5	17.5	10.9	70	90	70	160	110	19	0.8	1.1
Pregnancy	*	*	*	*	*	*	*	*	*	*	*
Lactation											
0–4 months	+14.3	+14.3	+2.1	*	*	*	*	+90	+5	+0.2	*
4+ months	+14.3	+14.3	+2.1	*	*	*	*	+40	+5	+0.2	*
0–3 months	525	400	55	210	800	320	1.7	4.0	0.2	10	50
4–6 months	525	400	60	280	850	400	4.3	4.0	0.3	13	60
7–9 months	525	400	75	320	700	500	7.8	5.0	0.3	10	60
10–12 months	525	400	80	350	700	500	7.8	5.0	0.3	10	60
1–3 years	350	270	85	500	800	800	6.9	5.0	0.4	15	70
4–6 years	450	350	120	700	1,100	1,100	6.1	6.5	0.6	20	100
7–10 years	550	450	200	1,200	2,000	1,800	8.7	7.0	0.7	30	110
Males											
11–14 years	1,000	775	280	1,600	3,100	2,500	11.3	9.0	0.8	45	130
15–18 years	1,000	775	300	1,600	3,500	2,500	11.3	9.5	1.0	70	140
19–50 years	700	550	300	1,600	3,500	2,500	8.7	9.5	1.2	75	140
50+ years	700	550	300	1,600	3,500	2,500	8.7	9.5	1.2	75	140
Females											
11–14 years	800	625	280	1,600	3,100	2,500	14.8[5]	9.0	0.8	45	130
15–18 years	800	625	300	1,600	3,500	2,500	14.8[5]	7.0	1.0	60	140
19–50 years	700	550	270	1,600	3,500	2,500	14.8[5]	7.0	1.2	60	140
50+ years	700	550	270	1,600	3,500	2,500	8.7	7.0	1.2	60	140

Continued

Table II.8 Continued

Age	Calcium (mmol/d)	Phosphorus¹ (mmol/d)	Magnesium (mmol/d)	Sodium (mmol/d²)	Potassium (mmol/d³)	Chloride⁴ (mmol/d)	Iron (µmol/d)	Zinc (µmol/d)	Copper (µmol/d)	Selenium (µmol/d)	Iodine (µmol/d)
Pregnancy	*	*	*	*	*	*	*	*	*	*	*
Lactation											
0–4 months	+550	+440	+50	*	*	*	*	+6.0	+0.3	+15	*
4+ months	+550	+440	+50	*	*	*	*	+2.5	+0.3	+15	*

*No increment.
¹Phosphorus RNI is set equal to calcium in molar terms.
²1 mmol sodium = 23 mg.
³1 mmol potassium 39 mg.
⁴Corresponds to sodium 1 mmol = 35.5 mg.
⁵Insufficient for women with high menstrual losses where the most practical way of meeting iron requirements is to take iron supplements.
(From Report on Health and Social Subjects (1991) *No. 41, Dietary Reference Values for Food Energy and Nutrients for the United Kingdom*. Report of the Panel on Dietary Reference Values of the Committee on Medical Aspects of Food Policy, Her Majesty's Stationery Office, London.)

Table II.9 Safe intakes, United Kingdom

Nutrient	Safe intake
Vitamins	
Pantothenic acid	
adults	3–7 mg/d
infants	1.7 mg/d
Biotin	10–200 µg/d
Vitamin E	
men	above 4 mg/d
women	above 3 mg/d
infants	0.4 mg/g polyunsaturated fatty acids
Vitamin K	
adults	1 µg/kg/d
infants	10 µg/d
Minerals	
Manganese	
adults	1.4 mg (26 µmol)/d
infants and children	16 µg (0.3 µmol)/d
Molybdenum	
adults	50–400 µg/d
infants, children, and adolescents	0.5–1.5 µg/kg/d
Chromium	
adults	25 µg (0.5 µmol)/d
children and adolescents	0.1–1.0 µg (2–20 µmol)/kg/d
Fluoride (for infants only)	0.05 mg (3 µmol)/kg/d

For some nutrients, which are known to have important functions in humans, the Panel found insufficient reliable data on human requirements and were unable to set any dietary reference values for these. However, they decided on grounds of prudence to set a safe intake, particularly for infants and children. The safe intake was judged to be a level or range of intake at which there is no risk of deficiency and below a level where there is risk of undesirable effects. They are not therefore intended as a "toxic level", and although exceeding these safe intakes would not necessarily result in undesirable effects, equally there is no evidence for any benefits. The Panel agreed that the safe range of intakes set for the nutrients need not be exceeded.

(From Report on Health and Social Subjects (1991) *No. 41, Dietary Reference Values for Food Energy and Nutrients for the United Kingdom*. Report of the Panel on Dietary Reference Values of the Committee on Medical Aspects of Food Policy, Her Majesty's Stationery Office, London.)

Table II.10 Recommended dietary allowances for persons with low activity, Japan

Age	Energy (kcal) M	Energy (kcal) F	Protein (g) M	Protein (g) F	Fat (%)	Calcium (g) M	Calcium (g) F	Iron (mg) M	Iron (mg) F	Vitamin A (IU) M	Vitamin A (IU) F	Vitamin B₁ (mg) M	Vitamin B₁ (mg) F	Vitamin B₂ (mg) M	Vitamin B₂ (mg) F	Niacin (mg) M	Niacin (mg) F	Ascorbic acid (mg)	Vitamin D (IU)
15~	2,350	2,000	85	70	25~30	0.8	0.6	12	12	2,000	1,800	0.9	0.8	1.3	1.1	16	13	50	100
16~	2,400	1,950	80	70	25~30	0.8	0.6	12	12	2,000	1,800	1.0	0.8	1.3	1.1	16	13	50	100
17~	2,400	1,900	80	70	25~30	0.7	0.6	12	12	2,000	1,800	1.0	0.8	1.3	1.0	16	13	50	100
18~	2,350	1,850	75	65	25~30	0.7	0.6	12	12	2,000	1,800	0.9	0.7	1.3	1.0	16	12	50	100
19~	2,300	1,850	75	60	25~30	0.7	0.6	12	12	2,000	1,800	0.9	0.7	1.3	1.0	15	12	50	100
20~29	2,250	1,800	70	60	20~25	0.6	0.6	10	12	2,000	1,800	0.9	0.7	1.2	1.0	15	12	50	100
30~39	2,200	1,750	70	60	20~25	0.6	0.6	10	12	2,000	1,800	0.9	0.7	1.2	1.0	15	12	50	100
40~49	2,150	1,700	70	60	20~25	0.6	0.6	10	12	2,000	1,800	0.9	0.7	1.2	0.9	14	11	50	100
50~59	2,000	1,650	70	60	20~25	0.6	0.6	10	12	2,000	1,800	0.8	0.7	1.1	0.9	13	11	50	100
60~64	1,850	1,550	70	60	20~25	0.6	0.6	10	12	2,000	1,800	0.7	0.6	1.0	0.9	12	10	50	100
65~69	1,800	1,500	70	60	20~25	0.6	0.6	10	†10	2,000	1,800	0.7	0.6	1.0	0.9	12	10	50	100
70~74	1,650	1,450	65	55	20~25	0.6	0.6	10	†10	2,000	1,800	0.7	0.6	1.0	0.9	12	10	50	100
75~79	1,600	1,400	65	55	20~25	0.6	0.6	10	†10	2,000	1,800	0.7	0.6	1.0	0.9	12	10	50	100
80~	1,500	1,250	65	55	20~25	0.6	0.6	10	†10	2,000	1,800	0.7	0.6	1.0	0.9	12	10	50	100
1st Half Pregnancy*		+150		+10	25~30		+0.4		+3		+0		+0.1		+0.1		+1	+10	+300
Last Half Pregnancy		+350		+20	25~30		+0.4		+8		+200		+0.2		+0.2		+2	+10	+300
Lactation		+700		+20			+0.5		+8		+1,400		+0.3		+0.4		+5	+40	+300

*Pregnancy increases are shown for convenience; however, values apply to each activity level.
†Decrease to 10 mg after menopause.
(From the Health Promotion and Nutrition Division (1991) Health Policy Bureau, Ministry of Health and Welfare, Tokyo, Japan.)

Table II.11   Recommended dietary allowances for persons with medium activity or growth stages, Japan

Age	Average height (cm) M	F	Average weight (kg) M	F	Energy (kcal) M	F	Protein (g) M	F	Fat (%)	Calcium (g) M	F	Iron (mg) M	F	Vitamin A (IU) M	F	Vitamin B1 (mg) M	F	Vitamin B2 (mg) M	F	Niacin (mg) M	F	Ascorbic acid (mg)	Vitamin D (IU)
0~mo					120/kg		3.3/kg		45	0.4	0.4	6	6	1,300	1,300			0.5	0.3	4	4	40	400
2~mo					110/kg		2.5/kg		45	0.4	0.4	6	6	1,300	1,300			0.6	0.4	6	6	40	400
6~mo					100/kg		3.0/kg		30~40	0.4	0.4	6	6	1,000	1,000			0.7	0.5	6	6	40	400
1~yr	80.7	79.6	10.95	10.35	960	910	30	30	25~30	0.4	0.4	7	7	1,000	1,000	0.4	0.4	0.8	0.6	6	6	40	400
2~	90.0	89.1	13.24	12.74	1,200	1,150	35	35	25~30	0.4	0.4	7	7	1,000	1,000	0.4	0.4	0.8	0.6	8	8	40	400
3~	97.3	96.6	15.04	14.70	1,400	1,350	40	40	25~30	0.4	0.4	7	7	1,000	1,000	0.5	0.5	0.9	0.7	9	9	40	400
4~	104.3	103.7	16.97	16.69	1,550	1,450	45	45	25~30	0.4	0.4	8	8	1,000	1,000	0.5	0.5	0.9	0.7	10	10	40	400
5~	110.8	110.3	19.04	18.78	1,600	1,500	50	50	25~30	0.4	0.4	8	8	1,000	1,000	0.5	0.5	0.9	0.7	11	10	40	400
6~	117.0	116.5	21.35	21.04	1,700	1,600	55	50	25~30	0.5	0.5	9	9	1,200	1,200	0.6	0.6	1.0	0.8	11	11	40	100
7~	122.7	122.2	23.85	23.44	1,800	1,650	60	55	25~30	0.5	0.5	9	9	1,200	1,200	0.6	0.6	1.0	0.8	12	11	40	100
8~	128.3	127.9	26.70	26.24	1,900	1,750	65	60	25~30	0.6	0.6	9	9	1,200	1,200	0.6	0.6	1.0	0.8	13	12	40	100
9~	133.5	133.6	29.76	29.50	1,950	1,850	65	65	25~30	0.6	0.6	9	9	1,200	1,200	0.7	0.6	1.1	0.9	13	12	40	100
10~	138.8	139.8	33.21	33.54	2,050	1,950	70	70	25~30	0.7	0.7	10	10	1,200	1,200	0.7	0.7	1.1	0.9	14	13	40	100
11~	144.6	146.5	37.26	38.46	2,150	2,100	75	75	25~30	0.7	0.7	10	10	1,500	1,500	0.8	0.8	1.2	1.0	15	14	50	100
12~	151.4	151.9	42.29	43.31	2,350	2,250	80	80	25~30	0.8	0.7	12	12	1,500	1,500	0.8	0.8	1.2	1.0	16	14	50	100
13~	159.0	155.4	48.34	47.43	2,500	2,300	85	80	25~30	0.9	0.7	12	12	1,500	1,500	0.9	0.8	1.3	1.1	16	14	50	100
14~	164.9	157.1	53.87	50.32	2,600	2,300	85	75	25~30	0.9	0.7	12	12	1,500	1,500	0.9	0.8	1.3	1.1	17	14	50	100
15~	168.5	157.6	57.98	51.99	2,700	2,250	85	70	25~30	0.9	0.7	12	12	1,500	1,500	1.0	0.9	1.4	1.2	17	15	50	100
16~	169.9	158.0	60.21	52.87	2,700	2,200	80	70	25~30	0.8	0.7	12	12	1,500	1,500	1.1	0.9	1.5	1.2	18	15	50	100
17~	170.8	158.1	61.55	52.92	2,700	2,150	80	70	25~30	0.8	0.7	12	12	1,500	1,500	1.1	0.9	1.5	1.2	18	15	50	100
18~	171.3	158.1	62.18	52.52	2,650	2,100	75	65	25~30	0.7	0.7	12	12	1,500	1,500	1.1	0.9	1.5	1.2	18	15	50	100
19~	171.5	158.1	62.41	52.02	2,600	2,050	75	60	25~30	0.7	0.7	12	12	1,500	1,500	1.1	0.9	1.5	1.2	18	15	50	100
20~29	171.1	157.7	64.00	51.83	2,550	2,000	70	60	20~25	0.6	0.6	10	12	2,000	1,800	1.0	0.8	1.4	1.1	17	14	50	100
30~39	169.8	156.7	65.48	54.09	2,500	2,000	70	60	20~25	0.6	0.6	10	12	2,000	1,800	1.0	0.8	1.4	1.1	17	14	50	100
40~49	167.8	154.6	65.10	55.14	2,400	1,950	70	60	20~25	0.6	0.6	10	12	2,000	1,800	1.0	0.8	1.4	1.1	16	13	50	100
50~59	164.2	151.9	61.93	54.13	2,250	1,850	70	60	20~25	0.6	0.6	10	*	2,000	1,800	0.9	0.8	1.3	1.1	16	13	50	100
60~64	162.1	149.8	59.41	52.49	2,100	1,750	70	60	20~25	0.6	0.6	10	10	2,000	1,800	0.9	0.8	1.3	1.1	15	13	50	100
65~69	160.8	148.3	57.61	51.02	2,000	1,700	70	60	20~25	0.6	0.6	10	10	2,000	1,800	0.9	0.8	1.3	1.1	15	13	50	100
70~74	159.7	145.7	55.83	49.26	1,850	1,600	65	55	20~25	0.6	0.6	10	10	2,000	1,800	0.8	0.7	1.2	1.0	14	12	50	100
75~79	158.7	145.0	54.07	47.22	1,750	1,550	65	55	20~25	0.6	0.6	10	10	2,000	1,800	0.8	0.7	1.2	1.0	14	12	50	100
80~	157.6	142.4	52.38	44.53	1,650	1,400	65	55	20~25	0.6	0.6	10	10	2,000	1,800	0.8	0.7	1.2	1.0	14	12	50	100

*Decrease to 10 mg after menopause.

(From the Health Promotion and Nutrition Division (1991) Health Policy Bureau, Ministry of Health and Welfare, Tokyo, Japan.)

Table II.12   Recommended dietary allowances for persons with medium-high activity, Japan

Age	Energy (kcal) M	F	Protein (g) M	F	Fat (%)	Calcium (g) M	F	Iron (mg) M	F	Vitamin A (IU) M	F	Vitamin B₁ (mg) M	F	Vitamin B₂ (mg) M	F	Niacin (mg) M	F	Ascorbic acid (mg)	Vitamin D (IU)
15~	3,200	2,650	100	85		0.8						1.3	1.1	1.8	1.5	21	17		
16~	3,200	2,600	95	80								1.3	1.0	1.8	1.4	21	17		
17~	3,200	2,550	95	80				12	12			1.3	1.0	1.8	1.4	21	17		
18~	3,150	2,500	90	75		0.7						1.3	1.0	1.7	1.4	21	17		
19~	3,100	2,450	90	70								1.2	1.0	1.7	1.3	20	16		
20~29	3,050	2,400	85	70	25~30		0.6			2,000	1,800	1.2	1.0	1.7	1.3	20	16	50	100
30~39	2,950	2,350	85	70					12			1.2	0.9	1.6	1.3	19	16		
40~49	2,850	2,300	85	70								1.1	0.9	1.6	1.3	19	15		
50~59	2,700	2,200	85	70		0.6		10	*			1.1	0.9	1.5	1.2	18	15		
60~64	2,450	2,050	80	70					10			1.0	0.8	1.3	1.1	16	14		
65~69	2,350	2,000	80	70								1.0	0.8	1.3	1.1	16	14		

*Decrease to 10 mg after menopause.
(From the Health Promotion and Nutrition Division (1991) Health Policy Bureau, Ministry of Health and Welfare, Tokyo Japan.)

Table II.13   Recommended dietary allowances for persons with high activity, Japan

Age	Energy (kcal) M	F	Protein (g) M	F	Fat (%)	Calcium (g) M	F	Iron (mg) M	F	Vitamin A (IU) M	F	Vitamin B₁ (mg) M	F	Vitamin B₂ (mg) M	F	Niacin (mg) M	F	Ascorbic acid (mg)	Vitamin D (IU)
15~	3,750	3,100	115	95		0.8						1.5	1.2	2.1	1.7	25	20		
16~	3,750	3,050	110	95								1.5	1.2	2.1	1.7	25	20		
17~	3,750	2,950	110	95				12	12			1.5	1.2	2.1	1.6	25	19		
18~	3,700	2,900	105	90		0.7						1.5	1.2	2.0	1.6	24	19		
19~	3,700	2,850	105	85								1.5	1.1	2.0	1.6	24	19		
20~29	3,550	2,800	100	85	25~30		0.6			2,000	1,800	1.4	1.1	2.0	1.5	23	18	50	100
30~39	3,450	2,750	100	85					12			1.4	1.1	1.9	1.5	23	18		
40~49	3,350	2,700	100	85								1.3	1.1	1.8	1.5	22	18		
50~59	3,150	2,600	100	85		0.6		10	*			1.3	1.0	1.7	1.4	21	17		
60~64	2,850	2,400	95	80					10			1.1	1.0	1.6	1.3	19	16		
65~69	2,750	2,300	95	80								1.1	1.0	1.6	1.3	19	16		

*Decrease to 10 mg after menopause.
(From the Health Promotion and Nutrition Division (1991) Health Policy Bureau, Ministry of Health and Welfare, Tokyo, Japan.)

Comments
1. These general guidelines are not for individual daily values. For individual nutrient requirements, other tables must be used.
2. An individual should take no more than 10 mg sodium daily.
3. Vitamin E: males should have at least 8 mg, females should have at least 7 mg.
4. For those in the low activity category, more exercise is recommended. The values in Table II.12 represent the ideal intake for adults. These values are reflective of individuals who exercise accordingly.

Table II.14 Recommended daily dietary allowances, Korea*

Category	Age (years)	Weight (kg)	Height (cm)	Energy (kcal)	Protein (g)	Vitamin A (re)†	Vitamin B₁ (mg)	Vitamin B₂ (mg)	Niacin (mg)	Vitamin C (mg)	Vitamin D (µg)‡	Calcium (mg)	Iron (mg)§
Infants													
	0–3 mo	5.5	58.5	800	25	350	0.40	0.48	6.4	35	10	400	10
	4–6 mo	8.4	67.5	900	25	350	0.45	0.54	7.2	35	10	400	10
	7–9 mo	9.5	76.0	1,000	30	350	0.50	0.60	8.0	35	10	400	15
	10–12 mo	10.4	79.0	1,100	30	350	0.55	0.66	8.0	35	10	400	15
Children													
	1–3	12.6	87.0	1,200	35	350	0.60	0.72	8.0	40	10	500	15
	4–6	19.0	110.0	1,300	40	400	0.75	0.90	10.0	40	10	600	10
	7–9	26.0	130.0	1,800	50	500	0.90	1.08	12.0	40	10	700	10
Males													
	10–12	36.0	144.0	2,100	60	600	1.05	1.26	14.0	50	10	800	15
	13–15	51.0	161.0	2,600	80	700	1.30	1.36	17.0	50	10	800	18
	16–19	59.0	169.0	2,500	75	700	1.25	1.50	16.5	55	10	800	18
	20–29	64.0	170.5	2,500	70	700	1.25	1.50	16.5	55	5	600	10
	30–49	65.0	168.5	2,500	70	700	1.25	1.50	16.5	55	5	600	10
	50–64	63.0	168.0	2,200	70	700	1.10	1.32	14.5	55	5	600	10
	65 or older	61.0	167.0	1,900	70	700	1.00	1.20	13.0	55	5	600	10
Females													
	10–12	37.0	145.0	2,000	60	600	1.00	1.20	13.0	50	10	800	18
	13–15	48.0	155.0	2,300	65	700	1.15	1.38	15.0	50	10	800	18
	16–19	52.0	158.0	2,200	60	700	1.10	1.32	14.5	55	10	700	18
	20–29	52.5	159.5	2,000	60	700	1.00	1.20	13.0	55	5	600	18
	30–49	55.0	158.0	2,000	60	700	1.00	1.20	13.0	55	5	600	18
	50–64	54.0	156.0	1,900	60	700	1.00	1.20	13.0	55	5	600	10
	65 or older	53.0	156.0	1,600	60	700	1.00	1.20	13.0	55	5	600	10
Pregnancy													
	First half			+150	+30	+ 0	+0.40	+0.30	+2.0	+15	+5	+400	+2
	Second half			+350	+30	+100	+0.40	+0.30	+2.0	+15	+5	+400	+2
Lactation				+700	+30	+300	+0.60	+0.50	+6.0	+35	+5	+500	+2

*The allowances for energy are based on individuals of moderate activity. Data in this table are intended to provide only a standard figure under usual environment and given conditions.
†Retinol equivalent: 1 RE = 1 µg retinol = 6 µg β-carotene.
‡Vitamin D: 10 µg = 400 IU.
§Supplemental iron should be taken to meet the increased requirement during pregnancy and lactation.
(From the Ministry of Health and Social Affairs (1989) Kyonggi, Korea.)

Table II.15   Equations for predicting basal metabolic rate from body weight (W)*

Age range (years)	$KCAL_{th}$/day	Correlation coefficient	$SD^\dagger$	MJ/day	Correlation coefficient	SD
Males
0–3	60.9 W − 54	0.97	53	0.255 W − 0.226	0.97	0.222
3–10	22.7 W + 495	0.86	62	0.0949 W + 2.07	0.86	0.259
10–18	17.5 W + 651	0.90	100	0.0732 W + 2.72	0.90	0.418
18–30	15.3 W + 679	0.65	151	0.0640 W + 2.84	0.65	0.632
30–60	11.6 W + 879	0.60	164	0.0485 W + 3.67	0.60	0.686
> 60	13.5 W + 487	0.79	148	0.0565 W + 2.04	0.79	0.619
Females
0–3	61.0 W − 51	0.97	61	0.255 W − 0.214	0.97	0.255
3–10	22.5 W + 499	0.85	63	0.0941 W + 2.09	0.85	0.264
10–18	12.2 W + 746	0.75	117	0.0510 W + 3.12	0.75	0.489
18–30	14.7 W + 496	0.72	121	0.0615 W + 2.08	0.72	0.506
30–60	8.7 W + 829	0.70	108	0.0364 W + 3.47	0.70	0.452
> 60	10.5 W + 596	0.74	108	0.0439 W + 2.49	0.74	0.452

*Since the present report was compiled, the data base for the equations contained in Schofield, W.N. et al. (1985) *Hum. Nutr. Clin. Nutr.* **39** (Suppl.), has been slightly expanded. They therefore differ from the equations shown in this table, but the differences are negligible.
†Standard deviation of differences between actual BMR and predicted estimates.
(From WHO (1985) *Energy and Protein Requirements: Report of a Joint FAO/WHO/UNU Expert Consultation*, Technical Report Series No. 724. World Health Organization, Geneva, p. 71.)

Table II.16   Examples of predicted basal metabolic rate (BMR) in subjects of the same height but different weights, predicted from actual weight and from median acceptable weight for height

	Man, age 40, height 1.8 m			Woman, age 25, height 1.5 m		
	Position in range*			Position in range*		
	Upper	Median	Lower	Upper	Median	Lower
BMI†	25	22	20	24	21	19
Wt (kg)	81.0	71.3	64.8	54.0	47.2	42.7
BMR‡ from actual wt, $kcal_{th}$/day	1,820	1,710	1,630	1,290	1,190	1,120
MJ/day	7.61	7.15	6.82	5.39	4.98	4.68
BMR from median wt, $kcal_{th}$/day	1,710	1,710	1,710	1,190	1,190	1,190
MJ/day	7.15	7.15	7.15	4.97	4.97	4.97

*Acceptable range of BMI (see Annex 2A in original reference).
†Body mass index = wt(kg)/ht²(m).
‡Predicted from equations in Table II.15.
(From WHO (1985) *Energy and Protein Requirements: Report of a Joint FAO/WHO/UNU Expert Consultation*, Technical Report Series No. 724, World Health Organization, Geneva, p. 72.)

Table II.17   Basal metabolic rates of adolescent boys and girls

			BMR‡			
			Total		per kg	
Age (years)	Height* (cm)	Weight† (kg)	($kcal_{th}$/day)	(MJ/day)	($kcal_{th}$/day)	(MJ/day)
Boys
10–11	140	32.2	1215	5.08	37.7	0.16
11–12	147	37.0	1300	5.43	35.1	0.15
12–13	153	40.9	1370	5.73	33.4	0.14
13–14	160	47.0	1465	6.12	31.4	0.13
14–15	166	52.6	1570	6.57	29.9	0.12
15–16	171	58.0	1665	6.96	28.7	0.12
16–17	175	62.7	1750	7.32	27.9	0.12
17–18	177	65.0	1790	7.48	27.5	0.12

Continued

Table II.17   Continued

Age (years)	Height* (cm)	Weight† (kg)	BMR‡ Total (kcal_th/day)	(MJ/day)	BMR‡ per kg (kcal_th/day)	(MJ/day)
Girls						
10–11	142	33.7	1160	4.85	34.3	0.14
11–12	148	38.7	1220	5.10	31.5	0.13
12–13	155	44.0	1280	5.38	29.1	0.12
13–14	159	48.8	1340	5.60	27.5	0.12
14–15	161	51.4	1375	5.75	26.7	0.11
15–16	162	53.0	1395	5.83	26.3	0.11
16–17	163	54.0	1405	5.87	26.0	0.11
17–18	164	54.4	1410	5.89	25.9	0.11

*Median height for age from NCHS standards.
†Median weight for height and age from Baldwin's standards (Annex 2(B) of original reference).
‡Boys: BMR = 17.5 W + 651 kcal_th/day (2.72 MJ/day). Girls: 12.2 W + 746 kcal_th/day (3.12 MJ/day).
(From WHO (1985) *Energy and Protein Requirements: Report of a joint FAO/WHO/UNU Expert Consultation*, Technical Report Series No. 724. World Health Organization, Geneva, p. 72.)

Table II.18   Basal metabolic rate in adult men and women in relation to height and median acceptable weight for height* (values given in kcal_th with MJ in parentheses)

Height (m)	Weight† (kg)	18–30 years Per kg per day	Per day	30–60 years Per kg per day	Per day	>60 years Per kg per day	Per day
Men							
1.5	49.5	29.0 (121)	1440 (6.03)	29.4 (123)	1450 (6.07)	23.3 (98)	1150 (4.81)
1.6	56.5	27.4 (115)	1540 (6.44)	27.2 (114)	1530 (6.40)	22.2 (93)	1250 (5.23)
1.7	63.5	26.0 (109)	1650 (6.90)	25.4 (106)	1620 (6.78)	21.2 (89)	1350 (5.65)
1.8	71.5	24.8 (104)	1770 (7.41)	23.9 (99)	1710 (7.15)	20.3 (85)	1450 (6.07)
1.9	79.5	23.9 (100)	1890 (7.91)	22.7 (95)	1800 (7.53)	19.6 (82)	1560 (6.53)
2.0	88	23.0 (96)	2030 (8.49)	21.6 (90)	1900 (7.95)	19.0 (80)	1670 (6.99)
Women							
1.4	41	26.7 (112)	1100 (4.60)	28.8 (120)	1190 (4.98)	25.0 (105)	1030 (4.31)
1.5	47	25.2 (105)	1190 (4.98)	26.3 (110)	1240 (5.19)	23.1 (97)	1090 (4.56)
1.6	54	23.9 (100)	1290 (5.40)	24.1 (101)	1300 (5.44)	21.6 (90)	1160 (4.85)
1.7	61	22.9 (96)	1390 (5.82)	22.4 (94)	1360 (5.69)	20.3 (85)	1230 (5.15)
1.8	68	22.0 (92)	1500 (6.28)	20.9 (87)	1420 (5.94)	19.3 (81)	1310 (5.48)

*BMR from equations in Table II.15 rounded to 10 kcal_th.
†Weight taken as median acceptable weight for height: body mass index (wt/ht^2) = 22 in men, 21 in women.
(From WHO (1985) *Energy and Protein Requirements: Report of a joint FAO/WHO/UNU Expert Consultation*, Technical Report Series No. 724. World Health Organization, Geneva, p. 72.)

Table II.19 Calculated energy requirements of infants from birth to 1 year

Age (months)	Intake* (kcal_th/kg per day)	(kJ/kg per day)	Calculated energy requirement[†] (kcal_th/kg per day)	(kJ/kg per day)	Median body weight[‡] Boys (kg)	Girls (kg)	Total requirement Boys (kcal_th/day)	(kJ/day)	Girls (kcal_th/day)	(kJ/day)
0.5	118	494	124	519	3.8	3.6	470	1,965	445	1,860
1–2	114	477	116	485	4.75	4.35	550	2,300	505	2,115
2–3	107	448	109	456	5.6	5.05	610	2,550	545	2,280
3–4	101	423	103	431	6.35	5.7	655	2,740	590	2,470
4–5	96	402	99	414	7.0	6.35	695	2,910	630	2,635
5–6	93	389	96.5	404	7.55	6.95	730	3,055	670	2,800
6–7	91	381	95	397	8.05	7.55	765	3,220	720	3,010
7–8	90	377	94.5	395	8.55	7.95	810	3,390	750	3,140
8–9	90	377	95	397	9.0	8.4	855	3,580	800	3,350
9–10	91	381	99	414	9.35	8.75	925	3,870	865	3,620
10–11	93	389	100	418	9.7	9.05	970	4,060	905	3,790
11–12	97	406	104.5	437	10.05	9.35	1,050	4,395	975	4,080
12	102	427								

*Observed intakes at ages indicated, from data of sources given in original publication. Average intake predicted from equation (age in months): 1 (kcal_th/kg) = 123 − 8.9 age + 0.59 age. See original reference.
[†]Requirement over interval indicated, calculated as predicted intake + 5%. See original reference.
[‡]NCHS median weights at midpoint of month.
(From WHO (1985) *Energy and Protein Requirements: Report of a Joint FAO/WHO/UNU Expert Consultation*, Technical Report Series No. 724. World Health Organization, Geneva, p. 91.)

Table II.20 Estimated average daily energy intakes and requirements, ages 1 to 10 years

Age (years)	BOYS Intake* (kcal_th/day)	(MJ/day)	Requirement[†] (kcal_th/day)	(MJ/day)
1–2	1,140	4.76	1,200	5.02
2–3	1,340	5.60	1,410	5.89
3–4	1,490	6.23	1,560	6.52
4–5	1,610	6.73	1,690	7.07
5–6	1,720	7.19	1,810	7.57
6–7	1,810	7.57	1,900	7.94
7–8	1,895	7.92	1,990	8.32
8–9	1,970	8.24	2,070	8.66
9–10	2,045	8.55	2,150	8.99

Continued

Table II.20 Continued

Age (years)	GIRLS Intake* (kcal_th/day)	(MJ/day)	Requirement† (kcal_th/day)	(MJ/day)	REQUIREMENT BY WEIGHT‡ Boys (kcal_th/kg per day)	(kJ/kg per day)	Girls (kcal_th/kg per day)	(kJ/kg per day)
1–2	1,090	4.56	1,140	4.76	104	435	108	452
2–3	1,250	5.23	1,310	5.48	104	410	102	427
3–4	1,370	5.73	1,440	6.02	99	414	95	397
4–5	1,465	6.12	1,540	6.44	95	397	92	385
5–6	1,550	6.48	1,630	6.81	92	385	88	368
6–7	1,620	6.77	1,700	7.11	88	368	83	347
7–8	1,685	7.05	1,770	7.40	83	347	76	318
8–9	1,740	7.28	1,830	7.65	77	322	69	268
9–10	1,795	7.51	1,880	7.86	72	301	62	259

*From data of Ferro-Luzzi and Durnin, Rome, FAO, 1981 (Document ESN: FAO/WHO/UNU/EPR/81/9).
†Intakes +5%. See original reference.
‡From NCHS median weights at midyear.
(From WHO (1985) *Energy and Protein Requirements: Report of a Joint FAO/WHO/UNU Expert consultation*. Technical Report Series No. 724. World Health Organization, Geneva, pp. 94 and 95.)

Table II.21 Calculated average energy expenditure and observed intakes and comparison with recommendations of 1971 committee for adolescents aged 10 to 18 years

Age (years)	Expenditure (× BMR)*	Expenditure (kcal_th/day)	(MJ/day)	Intake† (kcal_th/day)	(MJ/day)	1971 committee‡ recommended requirement (kcal_th/day)	(MJ/day)
Boys							
10–11	1.76	2,140	8.95	2,110	8.82	2,500	10.46
11–12	1.73	2,240	9.37	2,170	9.07	2,600	10.87
12–13	1.69	2,310	9.66	2,200	9.20	2,700	11.29
13–14	1.67	2,440	10.20	2,280	9.53	2,800	11.71
14–15	1.65	2,590	10.83	2,340	9.79	2,900	12.13
15–16	1.62	2,700	11.29	2,390	9.99	3,000	12.55
16–17	1.60	2,800	11.71	2,440	10.20	3,050	12.76
17–18	1.60	2,870	12.0	2,490	10.41	3,100	12.97
Girls							
10–11	1.65	1,910	7.99	1,850	7.74	2,300	9.62
11–12	1.63	1,980	8.28	1,890	7.90	2,350	9.83
12–13	1.60	2,050	8.57	1,930	8.07	2,400	10.04
13–14	1.58	2,120	8.87	1,970	8.24	2,450	10.25
14–15	1.57	2,160	9.03	2,010	8.40	2,500	10.46
15–16	1.54	2,140	8.95	2,050	8.57	2,500	10.46
16–17	1.53	2,130	8.91	2,080	8.70	2,420	10.12
17–18	1.52	2,140	8.95	2,120	8.87	2,340	9.79

*Expenditure calculated as in original publication.
†Intakes from reference in original publication.
‡Reference in original 1971 publication. (cf ref. d)
(From WHO (1985) *Energy and Protein Requirements: Report of a Joint FAO/WHO/UNU Expert consultation*, Technical Report Series No. 724. World Health Organization, Geneva, p. 98.)

Table II.22 Derivation of average values of the energy cost of three grades of physical activity at work for women and men*

	Women[†]				Men[‡]			
	Cost/min (kcal$_{th}$)	(kJ)	Average cost × BMR (gross)	(net)	Cost/min (kcal$_{th}$)	(kJ)	Average cost × BMR (gross)	(net)
Light work								
75% of time sitting or standing	1.51	6.3			1.79	7.5		
25% of time standing and								
moving	1.70	7.1			2.51	10.5		
Average	1.56	6.5	1.7	0.7	1.99	8.3	1.7	0.7
Moderate work								
25% of time sitting or standing	1.51	6.3			1.79	7.5		
75% of time spent on specific								
occupational activity	2.20	9.2			3.61	15.1		
Average	2.03	8.5	2.2	1.2	3.16	13.2	2.7	1.7
Heavy work								
40% of time sitting or standing	1.51	6.3			1.79	7.5		
60% of time spent on specific								
occupational activity	3.21	13.4			6.22	26.0		
Average	2.54	10.6	2.8	1.8	4.45	18.6	3.8	2.8

*Times and energy costs of sitting, standing, moving around, and work tasks are composite values derived from published and unpublished data (Annex 5) in original reference.
[†]Based on young adult females (18–30 years). Wt 55 kg, BMR 0.90 kcal$_{th}$(3.8 kJ)/min (Table II.15).
[‡]Based on young adult males (18–30 years). Wt 65 kg, BMR 1.16 kcal$_{th}$ (4.9 kJ)/min (Table II.15).
(From WHO (1985) *Energy and Protein Requirements: Report of a Joint FAO/WHO/UNU Expert Consultation*, Technical Report Series No. 724, World Health Organization, Geneva, p. 76.)

Table II.23 Average daily energy requirement of adults whose occupational work is classified as light, moderate, or heavy, expressed as a multiple of basal metabolic rate

	Light	Moderate	Heavy
Men	1.55	1.78	2.10
Women	1.56	1.64	1.82

(From WHO (1985) *Energy and Protein Requirements: Report of a Joint FAO/WHO/UNU Expert Consultation*, Technical Report Series No. 724, World Health Organization, Geneva, p. 78.)

Table II.24 Estimates of energy cost of weight gain*

Subjects	Energy cost (kcal$_{th}$/g)	(kJ/g)
Premature infants	4.9	20.5
Premature infants	5.7	23.8
Normal infants	5.6	23.4
Infants recovering from malnutrition	5.55	23.2
	4.6	19.2
	3.5	14.6
	4.4	18.4
	7.1	29.7
Adults, recovering from anorexia nervosa	6.4	26.7
Adults, intentional overfeeding	8.2	34.3
Pregnancy Theoretic estimate[†]	6.4	26.7

*See original references for data sources.
[†]Calculated as 80,000 kcal$_{th}$ (335 mJ) stored for 12.5 kg of weight gain.
(From WHO (1985) *Energy and Protein Requirements: Report of a Joint FAO/WHO/UNU Expert Consultation*, Technical Report Series No. 724, World Health Organization, Geneva, p. 185.)

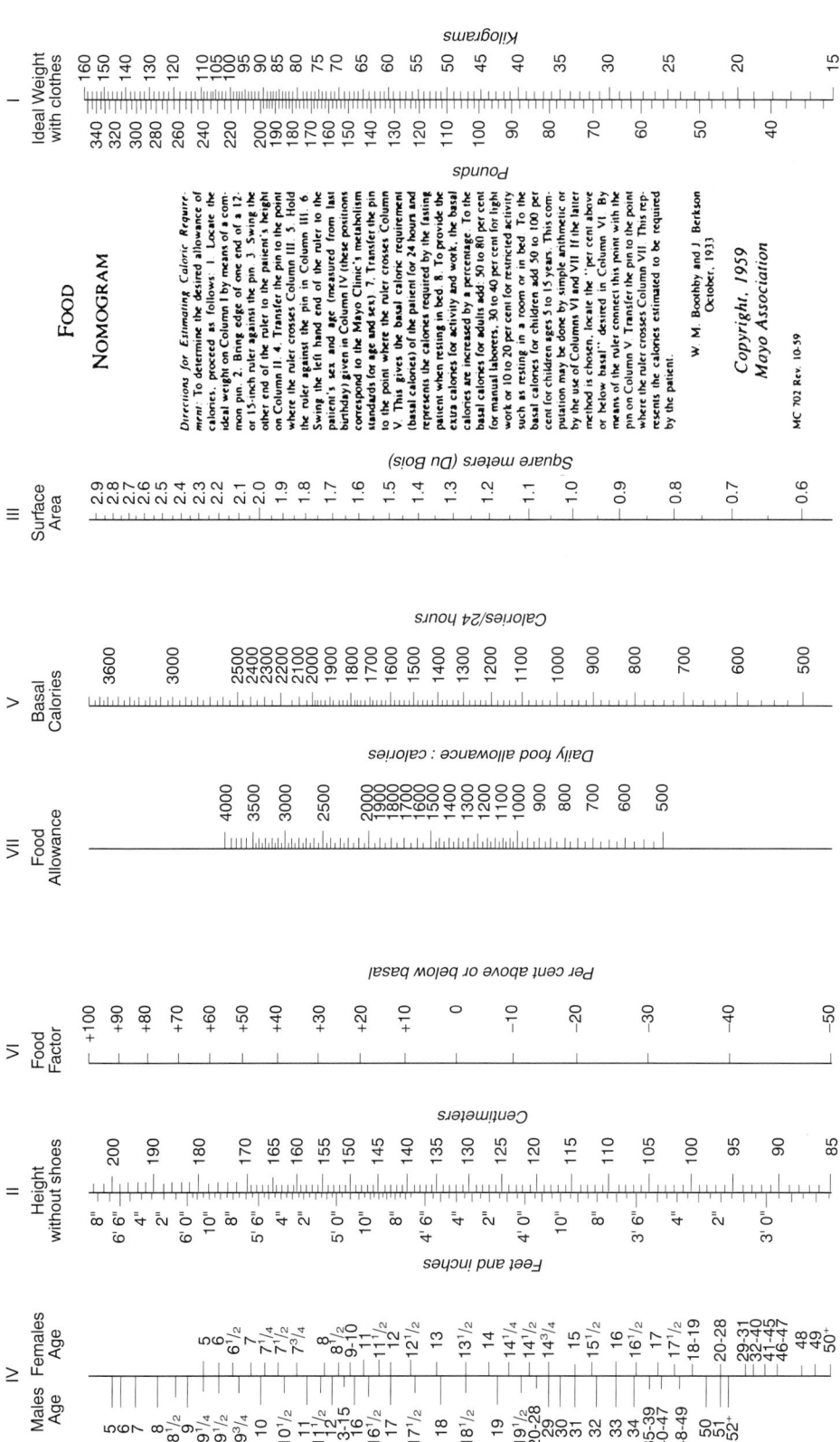

Figure II.1   Nomogram for estimation of caloric requirements. (From Pemberton, C. M., Gastineau, C. F.: *Mayo Clinic Diet Manual*. 5th Ed. W. B. Saunders, 1981, Philadelphia.)

Table II.25 Values for the digestibility of protein in man*

Protein source	True digestibility (mean ± SD)	Digestibility relative to reference proteins
Egg	97 ± 3	
Milk, cheese	95 ± 3 95	100
Meat, fish	94 ± 3	
Maize	85 ± 6	89
Rice, polished	88 ± 4	93
Wheat, whole	86 ± 5	90
Wheat, refined	96 ± 4	101
Oatmeal	86 ± 7	90
Millet	79	83
Peas, mature	88	93
Peanut butter	95	100
Soyflour	86 ± 7	90
Beans	78	82
Maize + beans	78	82
Maize + beans + milk	84	88
Indian rice diet	77	81
Indian rice diet + milk	87	92
Chinese mixed diet	96	98[†]
Brazilian mixed diet	78	82
Filipino mixed diet	88[‡]	93
American mixed diet	96[‡]	101
Indian rice + bean diet	78[‡]	82

*See original reference for data sources.
[†]Relative to egg measured in the same study.
[‡]Recalculated from apparent digestibility, using $F_K = 12$ mg N/kg (see original text).
(From WHO (1985) *Energy and Protein Requirements: Report of a Joint FAO/WHO/UNU Expert Consultation*, Technical Report Series No. 724, World Health Organization, Geneva, p. 119.)

Table II.27 Daily average energy requirements and safe level of protein intake for adolescents aged 10 to 18 years

Age (years)	Median weight (kg)	Energy requirement ($kcal_{th}$)	(kJ)	Safe level of protein intake (g/kg)*
Boys				
10–12	34.5	2,200	9,200	1.00
12–14	44.0	2,400	10,000	1.00
14–16	55.5	2,650	11,100	0.95
16–18	64.0	2,850	11,900	0.90
Girls				
10–12	36.0	1,950	8,200	1.00
12–14	46.5	2,100	8,800	0.95
14–16	52.0	2,150	9,000	0.90
16–18	54.0	2,150	9,000	0.80

*Minimum level considered safe.
(From WHO (1995) *Diet, Nutrition and the Prevention of Chronic Diseases: Report of a WHO Study Group*, Technical Report Series No. 797, World Health Organization, Geneva, pp. 167–8.)

Table II.26 Daily average (per kg) energy requirements and safe level of protein intake for infants and children aged 3 months to 10 years (sexes combined up to 5 years)

Age	Median weight (kg)	Energy requirement ($kcal_{th}$kg)		(kJ/kg)		Safe level of protein intake (g/kg)*
Months						
3–6	7.0	100		418		1.85
6–9	8.5	95		397		1.65
9–12	9.5	100		418		1.50
Years						
1–2	11.0	105		439		1.20
2–3	13.5	100		418		1.15
3–5	16.5	95		397		1.10
		Boys	Girls	Boys	Girls	
5–7	20.5	90	85	377	356	1.00
7–10	27.0	78	67	326	280	1.00

*Minimum level considered safe.
(From WHO (1990) *Diet, Nutrition and the Prevention of Chronic Diseases: Report of a WHO Study Group*, Technical Report Series No. 797, World Health Organization, Geneva, pp. 167–8.)

Table II.28 Daily average energy requirements and safe level of protein intake for adults*

Weight (kg)	Energy requirement						Safe level of protein intake (g/day)†
	18–30 years		30–60 years		Over 60 years		
	(kcal$_{th}$)	(kJ)	(kcal$_{th}$)	(kJ)	(kcal$_{th}$)	(kJ)	
Men							
50	2,300	9,700	2,350	9,700	1,850	7,700	37.5
55	2,400	10,100	2,450	10,100	1,950	8,300	41.0
60	2,550	10,600	2,500	10,400	2,100	8,600	45.0
65	2,700	11,300	2,600	10,900	2,200	9,100	49.0
70	2,800	11,700	2,700	11,200	2,300	9,600	52.5
75	2,900	12,300	2,800	11,800	2,400	10,000	56.0
80	3,050	12,900	2,900	12,000	2,500	10,400	60.0
Women							
40	1,700	7,200	1,900	7,900	1,650	6,800	30.0
45	1,850	7,700	1,950	8,300	1,700	7,100	34.0
50	1,950	8,200	2,050	8,500	1,800	7,500	37.5
55	2,100	8,600	2,100	8,800	1,900	7,900	41.0
60	2,200	9,200	2,200	9,000	1,950	8,200	45.0
65	2,300	9,800	2,250	9,400	2,050	8,500	49.0
70	2,450	10,300	2,300	9,600	2,150	8,900	52.5
75	2,550	10,800	2,400	10,000	2,200	9,300	56.0

*For a basal metabolic rate factor of 1.6.
†Minimum level considered safe.
(From WHO (1995) *Diet, Nutrition and the Prevention of Chronic Diseases: Report of a WHO Study Group*, Technical Report Series No. 797, World Health Organization, Geneva, pp. 167–8.)

Table II.29 Desirable weights for men and women aged 25 and over (in pounds by height and frame, in indoor clothing), 1959

Men (in shoes, one-inch heels)					Women (in shoes, two-inch heels)				
Height		Small frame	Medium frame	Large frame	Height		Small frame	Medium frame	Large frame
Feet	Inches				Feet	Inches			
5	2	112–120	118–129	126–141	4	10	92–98	96–107	104–119
5	3	115–123	121–133	129–144	4	11	94–101	98–110	106–122
5	4	118–126	124–136	132–148	5	0	96–104	101–113	109–125
5	5	121–129	127–139	135–152	5	1	99–107	104–116	112–128
5	6	124–133	130–143	138–156	5	2	102–110	107–119	115–131
5	7	128–137	134–147	142–161	5	3	105–113	110–122	118–134
5	8	132–141	138–152	147–166	5	4	108–116	113–126	121–138
5	9	136–145	142–156	151–170	5	5	111–119	116–130	125–142
5	10	140–150	146–160	155–174	5	6	114–123	120–135	129–146
5	11	144–154	150–165	159–179	5	7	118–127	124–139	133–150
6	0	148–158	154–170	164–184	5	8	122–131	128–143	137–154
6	1	152–162	158–175	168–189	5	9	126–135	132–147	141–158
6	2	156–167	162–180	173–194	5	10	130–140	136–151	145–163
6	3	160–171	167–185	178–199	5	11	134–144	140–155	149–168
6	4	164–175	172–190	182–204	6	0	138–148	144–159	153–173

(Data adapted from new weight standards for men and women. Stat. Bull. Metropol. Life Insur. Co. 40:1, 1959.)

Table II.30 Height–Weight Tables, 1983

Men					Women				
Height		Small frame	Medium frame	Large frame	Height		Small frame	Medium frame	Large frame
Feet	Inches				Feet	Inches			
5	2	128–134	131–141	138–150	4	10	102–111	109–121	118–131
5	3	130–136	133–143	140–153	4	11	103–113	111–123	120–134
5	4	132–138	135–145	142–156	5	0	104–115	113–126	122–137
5	5	134–140	137–148	144–160	5	1	106–118	115–129	125–140
5	6	136–142	139–151	146–164	5	2	108–121	118–132	128–143
5	7	138–145	142–154	149–168	5	3	111–124	121–135	131–147
5	8	140–148	145–157	152–172	5	4	114–127	124–138	134–151
5	9	142–151	148–160	155–176	5	5	117–130	127–141	137–155
5	10	144–154	151–163	158–180	5	6	120–133	130–144	140–159
5	11	146–157	154–166	161–184	5	7	123–136	133–147	143–163
6	0	149–160	157–170	164–188	5	8	126–139	136–150	146–167
6	1	152–164	160–174	168–192	5	9	129–142	139–153	149–170
6	2	155–168	164–178	172–197	5	10	132–145	142–156	152–173
6	3	158–172	167–182	176–202	5	11	135–148	145–159	155–176
6	4	162–176	171–187	181–207	6	0	138–151	148–162	158–179

Weight according to frame (ages 25 to 59) for men wearing indoor clothing weighing 5 lb, shoes with one-inch heels; for women, indoor clothing weighing 3 lb, shoes with one-inch heels.
(Reprinted with permission from the Metropolitan Life Insurance Company, New York.)

Table II.31 Height and elbow breadth for men and women*

Height in one-inch heels	Elbow breadth
Men	
5'2"–5'3"	$2\frac{1}{2}''-2\frac{7}{8}''$
5'4"–5'7"	$2\frac{5}{8}''-2\frac{7}{8}''$
5'8"–5'11"	$2\frac{3}{4}''-3''$
6'0"–6'3"	$2\frac{3}{4}''-3\frac{1}{8}''$
6'4"	$2\frac{7}{8}''-3\frac{1}{4}''$
Women	
4'10"–4'11"	$2\frac{1}{4}''-2\frac{1}{2}''$
5'0"–5'3"	$2\frac{1}{4}''-2\frac{1}{2}''$
5'4"–5'7"	$2\frac{3}{8}''-2\frac{5}{8}''$
5'8"–5'11"	$2\frac{3}{8}''-2\frac{5}{8}''$
6'0"	$2\frac{1}{2}''-2\frac{3}{4}''$

*See Table II.33; see Table II.34 for data on frame size by elbow breadth from NHANES I and II.
Extend your arm and bend the forearm upwards at a 90° angle. Keep fingers straight and turn the inside of your wrist towards your body. If you have a caliper, use it to measure the space between the two prominent bones on either side of your elbow. Without a caliper, place thumb and index finger of your other hand on these two bones. Measure the space between your fingers against a ruler or tape measure. Compare it with these tables that list elbow measurements for medium-frame men and women. Measurements lower than those listed indicate you have a small frame. Higher measurements indicate a larger frame.
(Reprinted with permission from Metropolitan Life Insurance Company, New York.)

Table II.32   Height–weight tables (metric units), 1983*

	Men				Women		
Height (cm)	Small frame (kg)	Medium frame (kg)	Large frame (kg)	Height (cm)	Small frame (kg)	Medium frame (kg)	Large frame (kg)
157.5	58.2–60.9	59.4–64.1	62.7–68.2	147.5	46.4–50.5	49.5–55.0	53.6–59.5
160	59.1–61.8	60.5–65.0	63.6–69.5	150	46.8–51.4	50.5–55.9	54.5–60.9
162.5	60.0–62.7	61.4–65.9	64.5–70.9	152.5	47.3–52.3	51.4–57.3	55.5–62.3
165	60.9–63.7	62.3–67.3	65.5–72.7	155	48.2–53.6	52.3–58.6	56.8–63.6
167.5	61.8–64.5	63.2–68.6	66.4–74.5	157.5	49.1–55.0	53.6–60.0	58.2–65.0
170	62.7–65.9	64.5–70.0	67.7–76.4	160	50.5–56.4	55.0–61.4	59.5–66.8
173	63.6–67.3	65.9–71.4	69.1–78.2	162.5	51.8–57.7	56.4–62.7	60.9–68.6
175	64.5–68.6	67.3–72.7	70.5–80.0	165	53.2–59.1	57.7–64.1	62.3–70.5
178	65.4–70.0	68.6–74.1	71.8–81.8	167.5	54.5–60.5	59.1–65.5	63.6–72.3
180	66.4–71.4	70.0–75.5	73.2–83.6	170	55.9–61.8	60.5–66.8	65.0–74.1
183	67.7–72.7	71.4–77.3	74.5–85.6	173	57.3–63.2	61.8–68.2	66.4–75.9
185.5	69.1–74.5	72.7–79.1	76.4–87.3	175	58.6–64.5	63.2–69.5	67.7–77.3
188	70.5–76.4	74.5–80.9	78.2–89.5	178	60.0–65.9	64.5–70.9	69.1–78.6
190.5	71.8–78.2	75.9–82.7	80.0–91.8	180	61.4–67.3	65.9–72.3	70.5–80.0
193	73.6–80.0	77.7–85.0	82.3–94.1	183	62.3–68.6	67.3–73.6	71.8–81.4

*The 1983 Metropolitan Height–Weight Tables are based on the 1979 Build Study.
The values are statistical computations from individuals ranging from 25 to 59 years of weights by height and body frame at which mortality has been found to be lowest or longevity the highest. Metropolitan Life does not advocate the use of the term "ideal", which has different meanings to various individuals, because the term was used originally in their 1942 to 1943 tables. If one wishes to use these tables in the sense that they are "ideal" in terms of lowest mortality, they are "appropriate" in that context. These tables do not provide weights related to minimizing illness, optimizing job performance, or creating the best appearance.
(Reprinted with permission from the Metropolitan Life Insurance Company, New York.)

Table II.33   Average weights by height and age group: 1959 and 1979 build and blood pressure studies

Men	Height														
	5'2"	5'3"	5'4"	5'5"	5'6"	5'7"	5'8"	5'9"	5'10"	5'11"	6'0"	6'1"	6'2"	6'3"	6'4"
15–16 years*															
1959 Study	107	112	117	122	127	132	137	142	146	150	154	159	164	169	†
1979 Study	112	116	121	127	133	137	143	148	153	159	162	168	173	178	184
Weight change	+5	+4	+4	+5	+6	+5	+6	+6	+7	+9	+8	+9	+9	+9	–
17–19 years															
1959 Study	119	123	127	131	135	139	143	147	151	155	160	164	168	172	176
1979 Study	124	129	132	137	141	145	150	155	159	164	168	174	179	185	190
Weight change	+5	+6	+5	+6	+6	+6	+7	+8	+8	+9	+8	+10	+11	+13	+14
20–24 years															
1959 Study	128	132	136	139	142	145	149	153	157	161	166	170	174	178	181
1979 Study	130	136	139	143	148	153	157	163	167	171	176	182	187	193	198
Weight change	+2	+4	+3	+4	+6	+8	+8	+10	+10	+10	+10	+12	+13	+15	+17
25–29 years															
1959 Study	134	138	141	144	148	151	155	159	163	167	172	177	182	186	190
1979 Study	134	140	143	147	152	156	161	166	171	175	181	186	191	197	202
Weight change	+0	+2	+2	+3	+4	+5	+6	+7	+8	+8	+9	+9	+9	+11	+12
30–39 years															
1959 Study	137	141	145	149	153	157	161	165	170	174	179	183	188	193	199
1979 Study	138	143	147	151	156	160	165	170	174	179	184	190	195	201	206
Weight change	+1	+2	+2	+2	+3	+3	+4	+5	+4	+5	+5	+7	+7	+8	+7

Continued

Table II.33   Continued

Men	Height 5'2"	5'3"	5'4"	5'5"	5'6"	5'7"	5'8"	5'9"	5'10"	5'11"	6'0"	6'1"	6'2"	6'3"	6'4"
40–49 years															
1959 Study	140	144	148	152	156	161	165	169	174	178	183	187	192	197	203
1979 Study	140	144	149	154	158	163	167	172	176	181	186	192	197	203	208
Weight change	+0	+0	+1	+2	+2	+2	+2	+3	+2	+3	+3	+5	+5	+6	+5
50–59 years															
1959 Study	142	145	149	153	157	162	166	170	175	180	185	189	194	199	205
1979 Study	141	145	150	155	159	164	168	173	177	182	187	193	198	204	209
Weight change	−1	+0	+1	+2	+2	+2	+2	+3	+2	+2	+2	+4	+4	+5	+4
60–69 years															
1959 Study	139	142	146	150	154	159	163	168	173	178	183	188	193	198	204
1979 Study	140	144	149	153	158	163	167	172	176	181	186	191	196	200	207
Weight change	+1	+2	+3	+3	+4	+4	+4	+4	+3	+3	+3	+3	+3	+2	+3

Women	Height 4'10"	4'11"	5'0"	5'1"	5'2"	5'3"	5'4"	5'5"	5'6"	5'7"	5'8"	5'9"	5'10"	5'11"	6'0"
15–16 years*															
1959 Study	97	100	103	107	111	114	117	121	125	128	132	136	†	†	†
1979 Study	101	105	109	112	117	121	123	128	131	135	138	142	146	149	152
Weight change	+4	+5	+6	+5	+6	+7	+6	+7	+6	+7	+6	+6	–	–	–
17–19 years															
1959 Study	99	102	105	109	113	116	120	124	127	130	134	138	142	147	152
1979 Study	103	108	111	115	119	123	126	129	132	136	140	145	148	150	154
Weight change	+4	+6	+6	+6	+6	+7	+6	+5	+5	+6	+6	+7	+6	+3	+2
20–24 years															
1959 Study	102	105	108	112	115	118	121	125	129	132	136	140	144	149	154
1979 Study	105	110	112	116	120	124	127	130	133	137	141	146	149	155	157
Weight change	+3	+5	+4	+4	+5	+6	+6	+5	+4	+5	+5	+6	+5	+6	+3
25–29 years															
1959 Study	107	110	113	116	119	122	125	129	133	136	140	144	148	153	158
1979 Study	110	112	114	119	121	125	128	132	134	138	142	148	150	156	159
Weight change	+3	+2	+1	+3	+2	+3	+3	+3	+1	+2	+2	+4	+2	+3	+1
30–39 years															
1959 Study	115	117	120	123	126	129	132	135	139	142	146	150	154	159	164
1979 Study	113	115	118	121	124	128	131	134	137	141	145	150	153	159	164
Weight change	−2	−2	−2	−2	−2	−1	−1	−1	−2	−1	−1	0	−1	0	0
40–49 years															
1959 Study	122	124	127	130	133	136	140	143	147	151	155	159	164	169	174
1979 Study	118	121	123	127	129	133	136	139	143	147	150	155	158	162	168
Weight change	−4	−3	−4	−3	−4	−3	−4	−4	−4	−4	−5	−4	−6	−7	−8
50–59 years															
1959 Study	125	127	130	133	136	140	144	148	152	156	160	164	169	174	180
1979 Study	121	125	127	131	133	137	141	144	147	152	156	159	162	166	171
Weight change	−4	−2	−3	−2	−3	−3	−3	−4	−5	−4	−4	−5	−7	−8	−9
60–69 years															
1959 Study	127	129	131	134	137	141	145	149	153	157	161	165	†	†	†
1979 Study	123	127	130	133	136	140	143	147	150	155	158	161	163	167	172
Weight change	−4	−2	−1	−1	−1	−1	−2	−2	−3	−2	−3	−4	–	–	–

*Height in shoes (feet and inches) and weight in indoor clothing (pounds).
†Averge weights omitted in classes with too few cases for analysis.
(Data from Association of Life Insurance Medical Directors of America and Society of Actuaries. Compiled by Seltzer, F. (1983) *Dietetic Currents*, **10** pp. 17–22. Reprinted with permission of Ross Laboratories, Columbus, Ohio.)

Table II.34   Frame size by elbow breadth (cm) of United States male and female adults derived from the combined NHANES I and II data sets

	Age (years)	Frame size		
		Small	Medium	Large
Men				
	18–24	≤6.6	>6.6 and <7.7	≥7.7
	25–34	≤6.7	>6.7 and <7.9	≥7.9
	35–44	≤6.7	>6.7 and <8.0	≥8.0
	45–54	≤6.7	>6.7 and <8.1	≥8.1
	55–64	≤6.7	>6.7 and <8.1	≥8.1
	65–74	≤6.7	>6.7 and <8.1	≥8.1
Women				
	18–24	≤5.6	>5.6 and <6.5	≥6.5
	25–34	≤5.7	>5.7 and <6.8	≥6.8
	35–44	≤5.7	>5.7 and <7.1	≥7.1
	45–54	≤5.7	>5.7 and <7.2	≥7.2
	55–64	≤5.8	>5.8 and <7.2	≥7.2
	65–74	≤5.8	>5.8 and <7.2	≥7.2

*The tenth and ninetieth percentiles, respectively, represent the predicted mean ± 1.282 times the SE. Similarly, the fifteenth and eighty-fifth percentiles are the predicted mean minus and plus, respectively, 1.036 times the SE of the regression equation. There were significant black–white population differences in weight and body composition when age and height were considered. However, when the comparisons were made with reference to age, height, and frame size, there were only minor interpopulation differences. For this reason, all races (white, black, and other) included in the NHANES I and II surveys were merged together for the purpose of calculating percentiles of anthropometric measurements.
(Combined NHANES I and II data sets from Frisancho, A.R. (1984) *Am. J. Clin. Nutr.*, **40**: pp. 808–19, with permission.)

Table II.35   Comparison of the weight-for-height tables from actuarial data (build study): non-age-corrected Metropolitan Life Insurance Company and age-specific Gerontology Research Center recommendations*

Height	Metropolitan 1983 weights for ages 25–59[†]		Gerontology Research Center Weight range for men and women by age (years)				
	Men	Women	25	35	45	55	65
ft–in			lb				
4–10	–	100–131	84–111	92–119	99–127	107–135	115–142
4–11	–	101–134	87–115	95–123	103–131	111–139	119–147
5–0	–	103–137	90–119	98–127	106–135	114–143	123–152
5–1	123–145	105–140	93–123	101–131	110–140	118–148	127–157
5–2	125–148	108–144	96–127	105–136	113–144	122–153	131–163
5–3	127–151	111–148	99–131	108–140	117–149	126–158	135–168
5–4	129–155	114–152	102–135	112–145	121–154	130–163	140–173
5–5	131–159	117–156	106–140	115–149	125–159	134–168	144–179
5–6	133–163	120–160	109–144	119–154	129–164	138–174	148–184
5–7	135–167	123–164	112–148	122–159	133–169	143–179	153–190
5–8	137–171	126–167	116–153	126–163	137–174	147–184	158–196
5–9	139–175	129–170	119–157	130–168	141–179	151–190	162–201
5–10	141–179	132–173	122–162	134–173	145–184	156–195	167–207
5–11	144–183	135–176	126–167	137–178	149–190	160–201	172–213
6–0	147–187	–	129–171	141–183	153–195	165–207	177–219
6–1	150–192	–	133–176	145–188	157–200	169–213	182–225
6–2	153–197	–	137–181	149–194	162–206	174–219	187–232
6–3	157–202	–	141–186	153–199	166–212	179–225	192–238
6–4	–	–	144–191	157–205	171–218	184–231	197–244

*Values in this table are for height without shoes and weight without clothes. To convert inches to centimeters, multiply by 2.54; to convert pounds to kilograms, multiply by 0.455.
†The weight range is the lower weight for small frame and the upper weight for large frame.
(Gerontology Research Center data from Andres, R. (1985) Mortality and obesity: the rationale for age-specific height–weight tables, in Andres, R., Bierman, E. and Hazzard, W.R. (eds), *Principles of Geriatric Medicine*, New York, McGraw-Hill, pp. 311–18.)

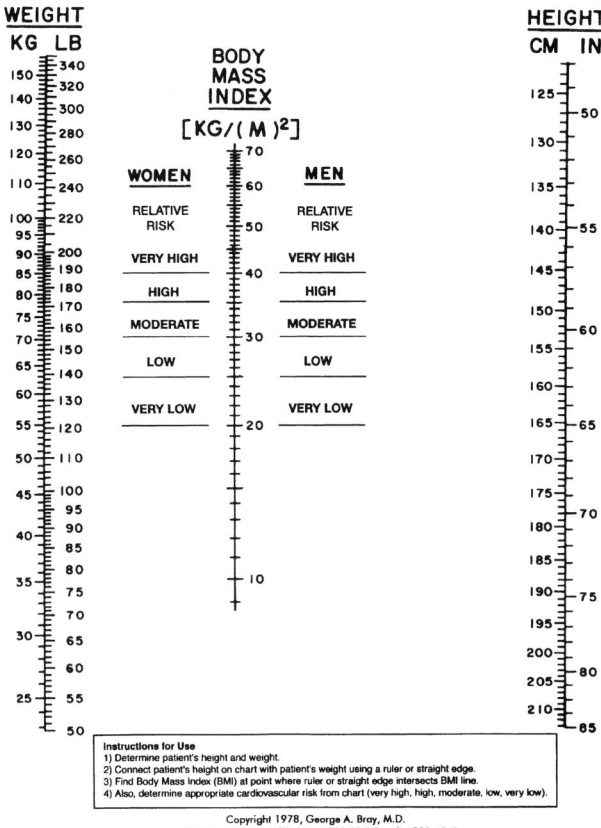

WEIGHT
KG LB

BODY MASS INDEX
[KG/(M)²]

WOMEN

RELATIVE RISK

VERY HIGH

HIGH

MODERATE

LOW

VERY LOW

MEN

RELATIVE RISK

VERY HIGH

HIGH

MODERATE

LOW

VERY LOW

HEIGHT
CM IN

Instructions for Use
1) Determine patient's height and weight.
2) Connect patient's height on chart with patient's weight using a ruler or straight edge.
3) Find Body Mass Index (BMI) at point where ruler or straight edge intersects BMI line.
4) Also, determine appropriate cardiovascular risk from chart (very high, high, moderate, low, very low).

Copyright 1978, George A. Bray, M.D.
Ref: Bray GA Am J Clin Nutr 1992;55(2 Suppl):488S-494S

Figure II.2 Nomograph for estimating body mass index (kg/m²). The ratio of weight/height² emerges from varied epidemiologic studies are the most generally useful index of relative body mass in adults. This nomograph facilitates use of this insurance studies, the scale expresses relative weight as a continuous variable. This method encourages use of clinical judgment in interpreting "overweight" and "underweight" and in accounting for muscular and skeletal contributions to measured mass.
(Copyright 1978 George A. Bray.)

Table II.36 Desirable body mass index (BMI) in relation to age

Age (years)	BMI (kg/m²)
19–24	19–24
25–34	20–25
35–44	21–26
45–54	22–27
55–65	23–28
>65	24–29

(From Committee on Diet and Health, Food and Nutrition Board, National Research Council (1989) *Diet and Health: Implications for Reducing Chronic Disease Risk*, National Academy Press, Washington, D.C., p. 564.)

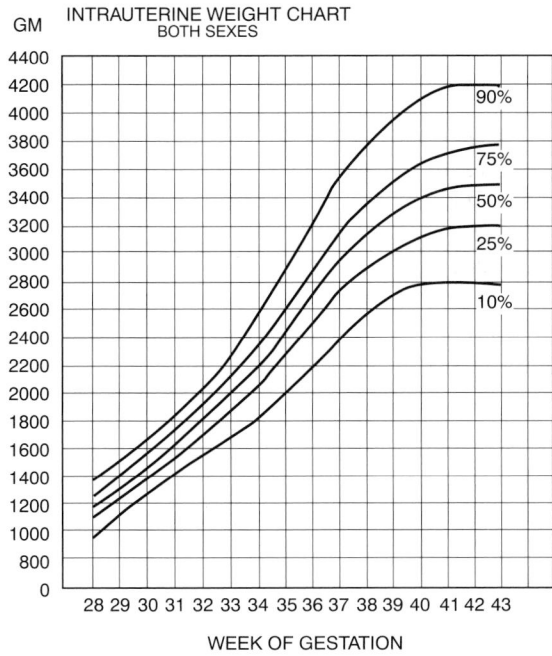
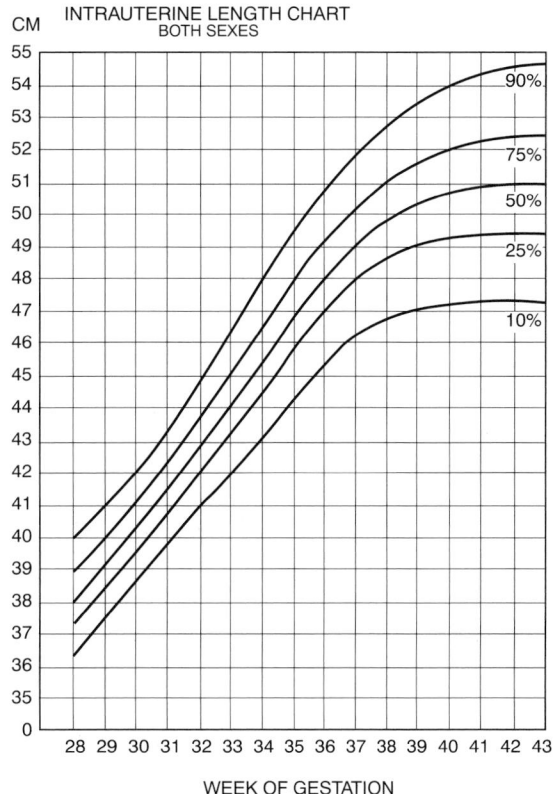

Figure II.3 Fetal growth standards: intrauterine weight* and length† charts.
*Fetal body weight percentiles from 28 to 43 weeks of gestation.
†Fetal body length percentiles from 28 to 43 weeks of gestation.
(From Naeye, R. L., Dixon, J. B.: *Pediatr. Res.,* **12**, p. 989, 1978.)

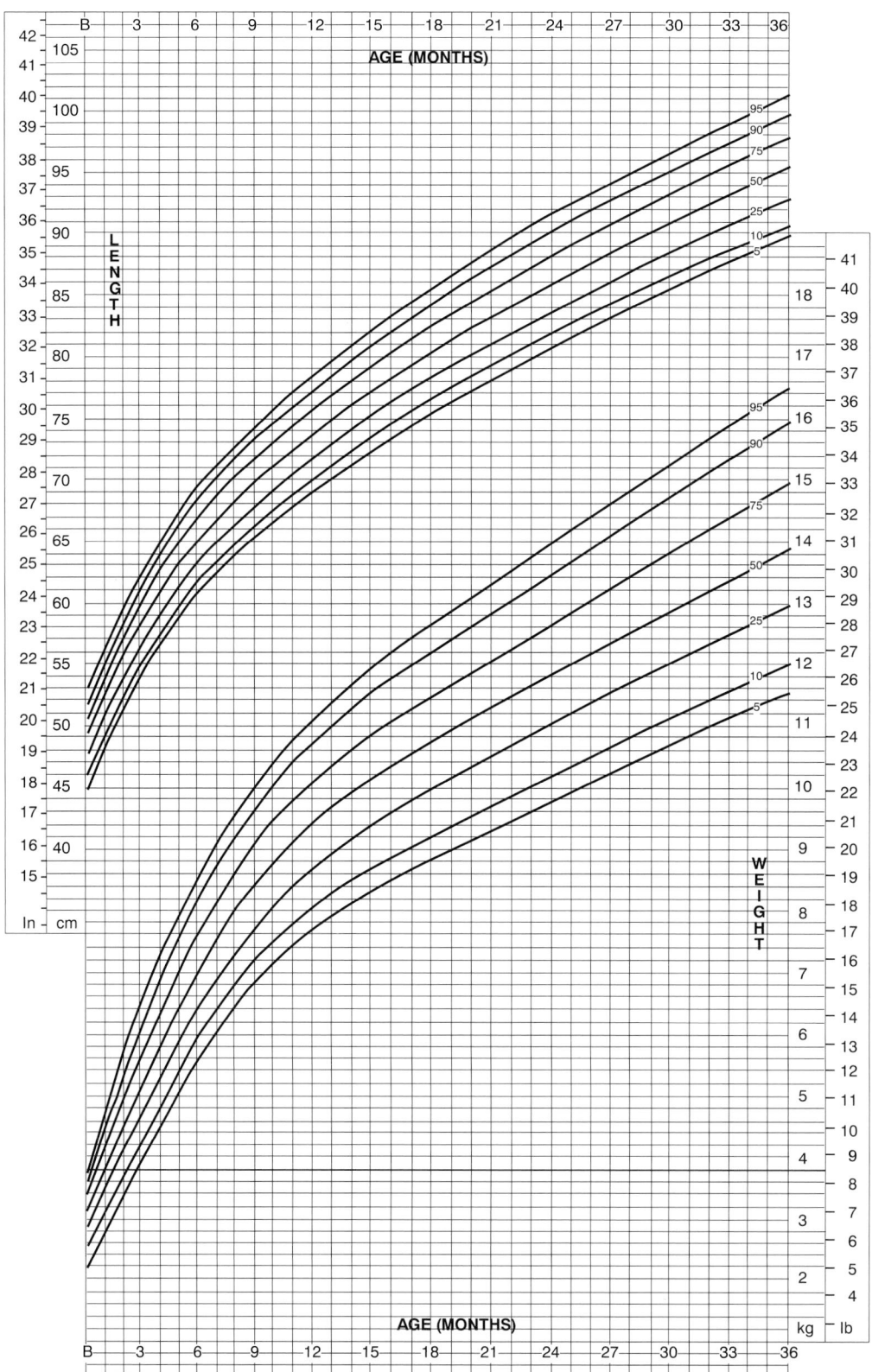

Figure II.4 Physical growth NCHS percentiles: girls from birth to 36 months. (Courtesy of Ross Laboratories, who adapted the growth curves from the original data: National Center for Health Statistics (1976) *NCHS Growth Charts. Monthly Vital Statistics Report* (1976) Vol. 25, No. 3, Suppl. (HRA) pp. 76–1120. Rockville, MD, Health Resources Administration, June. Data from The Fels Research Institute, Yellow Springs, Ohio.)

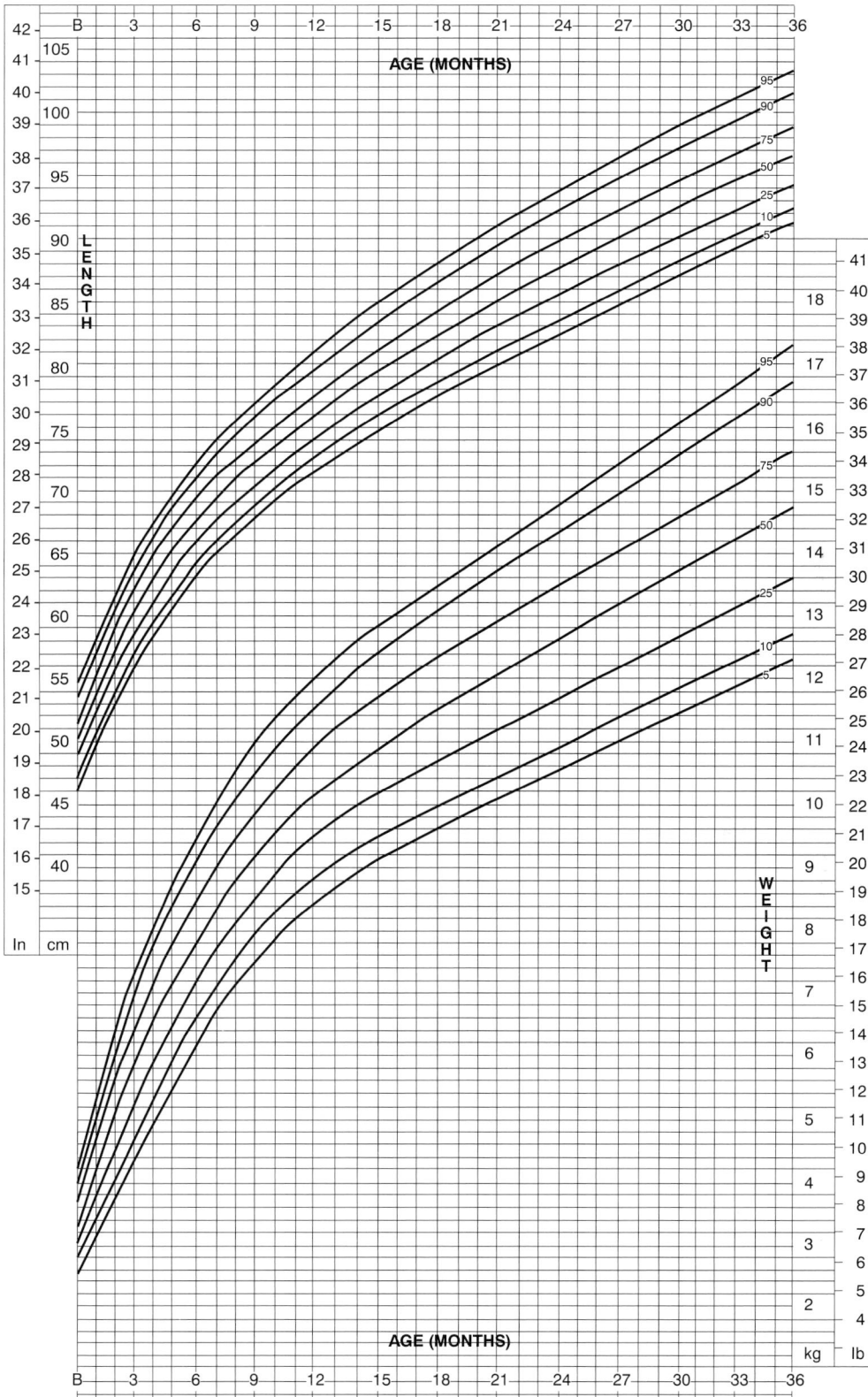

Figure II.5   Physical growth NCHS percentiles: boys from birth to 36 months. (Courtesy of Ross Laboratories, who adpated the growth curves from the original data: National Center for Health Statistics (1976) *NCHS Growth Charts. Monthly Vital Statistics Report* (1976) Vol. 25, No. 3, Suppl. (HRA) pp. 76–1120. Rockville, MD, Health Resources Administration, June. Data from The Fels Research Institute, Yellow Springs, Ohio.)

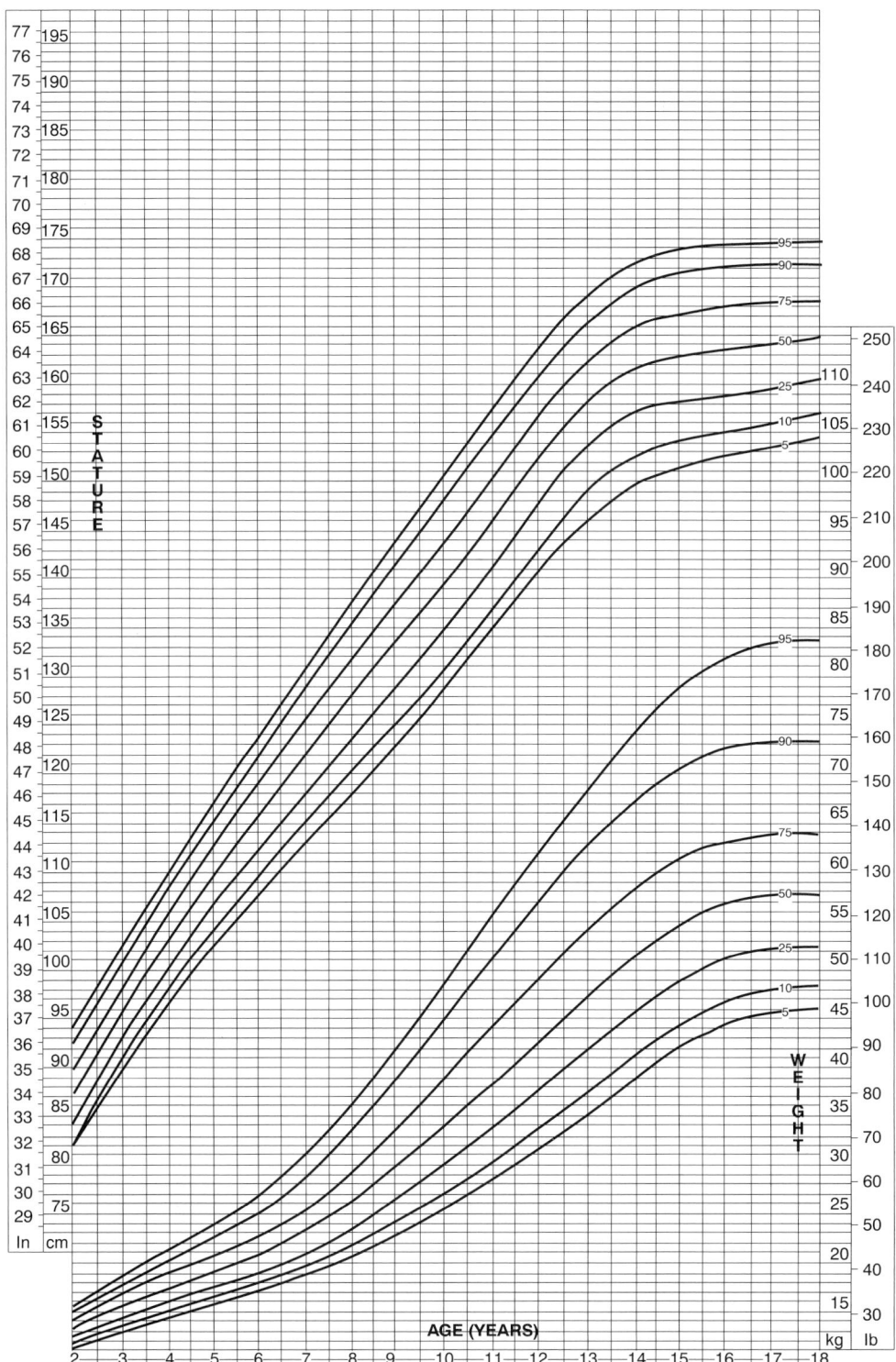

Figure II.6   Physical growth NCHS percentiles: girls from 2 to 18 years. (Courtesy of Ross Laboratories, who adapted the growth curves from the original data: National Center for Health Statistics (1976) *NCHS Growth Charts. Monthly Vital Statistics Report* (1976) Vol. 25, No. 3, Suppl. (HRA) pp. 76–1120. Rockville, MD, Health Resources Administration, June. Data from The Fels Research Institute, Yellow Springs, Ohio.)

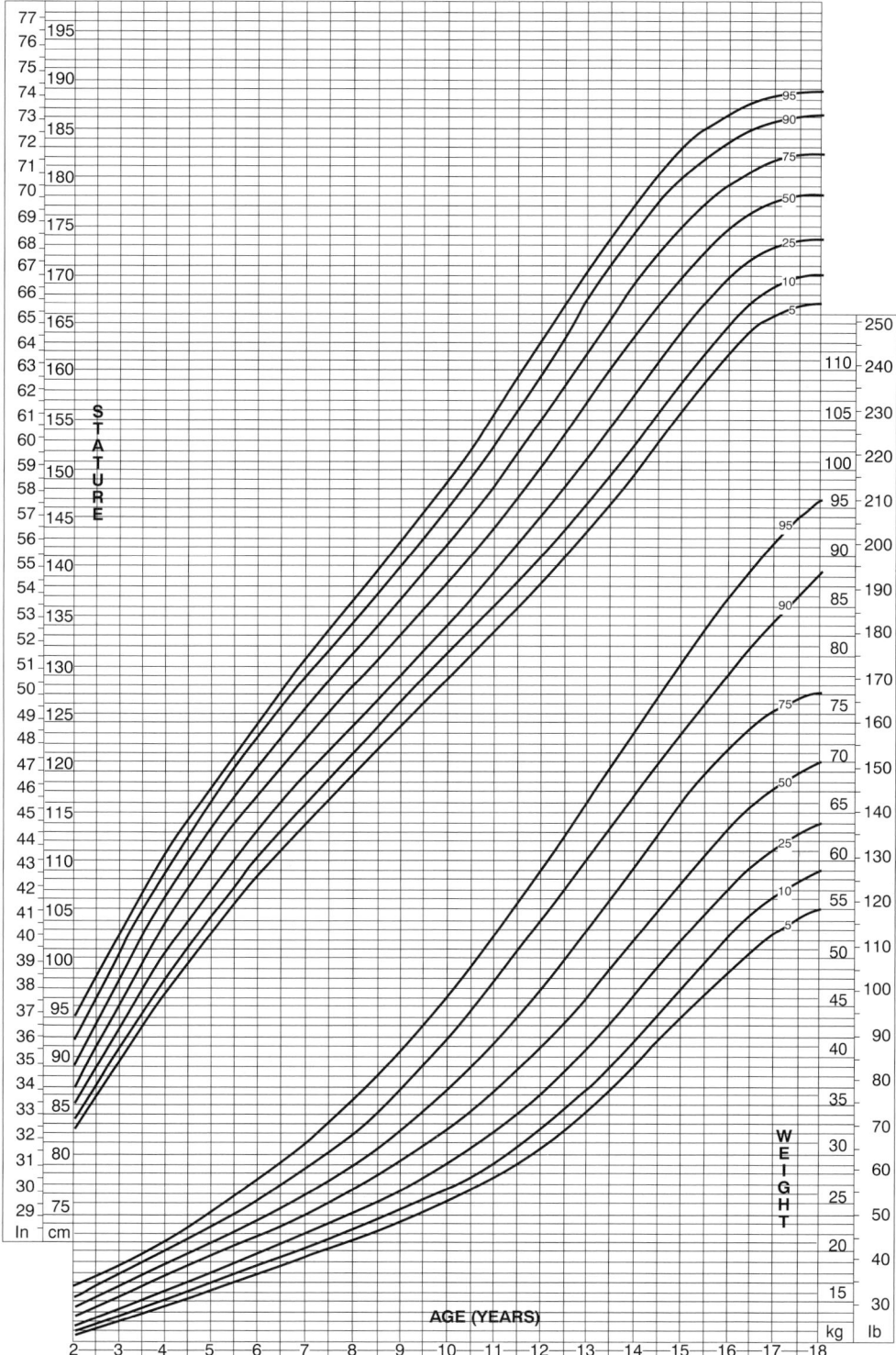

Figure II.7 Physical growth NCHS percentiles: boys from 2 to 18 years. (Courtesy of Ross Laboratories, who adpated the growth curves from the original data: National Center for Health Statistics (1976) *NCHS Growth Charts. Monthly Vital Statistics Report* (1976) Vol. 25, No. 3, Suppl. (HRA) pp. 76–1120. Rockville, MD, Health Resources Administration, June. Data from The Fels Research Institute, Yellow Springs, Ohio.)

Table II.37 Height in centimeters for persons 2 to 19 years of age: number examined, mean, standard deviation, and selected percentiles by sex and age, United States, 1976 to 1980*

Sex and age (years)	Number of examined persons	Mean	Standard deviation	Percentile								
				5th	10th	15th	25th	50th	75th	85th	90th	95th
Male												
2	375	91.2	4.3	84.5	85.8	85.5	88.2	91.3	94.2	95.8	96.6	97.6
3	418	99.2	4.5	92.0	94.3	94.9	96.5	98.8	102.0	103.9	105.0	107.0
4	404	106.0	5.2	97.8	99.5	100.5	102.5	106.4	109.2	111.0	112.4	115.0
5	397	112.6	5.4	104.0	105.8	107.2	109.4	112.6	115.6	118.1	119.6	121.2
6	133	119.5	5.1	111.2	112.6	114.5	115.9	120.1	122.6	124.7	125.5	126.8
7	148	125.1	5.9	115.4	117.6	119.1	121.8	125.9	128.1	130.2	131.5	133.6
8	147	129.9	7.0	118.6	122.0	123.5	125.3	130.6	134.1	136.5	138.0	142.0
9	145	135.5	5.8	125.9	126.4	129.4	131.2	136.1	139.6	141.2	143.1	144.7
10	157	141.6	7.3	130.3	132.8	134.0	137.0	141.5	146.4	149.6	150.6	153.0
11	155	146.0	7.8	133.1	135.9	138.0	141.1	145.6	151.2	153.9	155.2	160.2
12	145	152.5	7.9	139.0	142.6	144.9	147.5	152.0	158.0	160.5	162.0	164.4
13	173	158.9	8.3	144.4	147.6	149.7	152.6	159.7	165.0	168.7	169.5	171.6
14	186	167.5	8.3	153.9	156.5	159.1	162.5	167.5	173.1	176.5	178.7	180.6
15	184	170.8	6.7	160.1	162.0	162.6	165.7	171.1	175.5	177.5	178.2	181.9
16	178	173.8	6.4	163.0	164.7	167.4	169.8	173.7	178.1	180.3	182.6	186.1
17	173	175.1	7.1	164.1	167.3	168.4	170.6	174.9	179.7	182.8	184.3	187.5
18	164	176.9	6.7	166.5	168.8	169.9	172.3	176.9	180.9	183.9	185.1	189.6
19	148	176.5	6.7	164.5	168.2	169.4	171.8	176.9	181.1	183.5	184.8	187.2
Female												
2	336	89.7	4.2	83.1	84.4	85.5	86.7	89.8	92.2	93.6	94.9	97.2
3	366	97.5	4.8	89.6	91.1	92.5	94.5	97.6	100.8	102.5	103.4	104.5
4	396	104.6	5.0	96.1	98.2	99.5	101.5	104.5	108.2	109.8	110.7	112.4
5	364	111.6	5.3	103.0	105.1	106.4	108.1	111.6	115.2	116.5	118.8	120.3
6	135	118.4	6.1	109.9	111.1	111.5	113.3	118.5	122.2	124.5	126.5	128.7
7	157	123.7	6.7	113.3	116.6	117.4	119.6	124.1	128.1	130.1	132.2	134.7
8	123	130.2	5.7	120.8	123.4	124.4	125.8	130.6	133.2	135.4	137.5	140.5
9	149	134.4	7.6	124.0	126.4	127.8	129.0	134.8	139.0	140.7	142.6	147.1
10	136	141.9	6.5	131.6	133.6	135.1	137.6	141.6	146.3	148.1	150.4	153.8
11	140	147.9	7.8	134.7	139.3	140.6	142.2	147.9	152.2	154.7	156.9	162.7
12	147	154.4	7.2	143.9	145.7	146.7	149.2	154.8	158.6	161.9	164.7	165.9
13	162	158.9	6.6	149.0	150.3	152.7	155.3	159.0	163.0	164.5	166.9	170.3
14	178	160.8	6.4	151.0	152.7	154.5	156.7	160.9	165.1	166.9	168.2	172.3
15	145	163.2	6.2	153.0	155.2	157.1	159.1	163.1	167.1	170.2	172.4	173.5
16	170	162.9	6.1	152.0	154.5	157.2	159.1	163.2	166.4	169.4	171.4	173.3
17	134	163.5	5.7	153.8	156.8	158.5	160.4	163.1	166.7	169.7	170.7	172.2
18	170	162.4	6.8	150.7	154.2	155.6	158.0	162.7	166.2	169.1	171.5	174.0
19	158	163.5	5.6	153.8	156.8	157.7	159.7	163.7	167.2	169.5	170.4	172.1

*Height without shoes.
(From National Center for Health Statistics (1987) *Anthropometric Reference Data and Prevalence of Overweight, United States 1976–1980*, DHHS Publication No. 87-1688 (1987). U.S. Department of Health and Human Services, Public Health Service, Hyattsville, MD.

Table II.38   Weight in kilograms for persons 6 months to 19 years of age: number examined, mean, standard deviation, and selected percentiles by sex and age, United States, 1976 to 1980*

Sex and age (years)	Number of examined persons	Mean	Standard deviation	Percentile 5th	10th	15th	25th	50th	75th	85th	90th	95th
Male												
6–11 months	179	9.4	1.3	7.5	7.6	8.2	8.6	9.4	10.1	10.7	10.9	11.4
1 year	370	11.8	1.9	9.6	10.0	10.3	10.8	11.7	12.6	13.1	13.6	14.4
2 years	375	13.6	1.7	11.1	11.6	11.8	12.6	13.5	14.5	15.2	15.8	16.5
3 years	418	15.7	2.0	12.9	13.5	13.9	14.4	15.4	16.8	17.4	17.9	19.1
4 years	404	17.8	2.5	14.1	15.0	15.3	16.0	17.6	19.0	19.9	20.9	22.2
5 years	397	19.8	3.0	16.0	16.8	17.1	17.7	19.4	21.3	22.9	23.7	25.4
6 years	133	23.0	4.0	18.6	19.2	19.8	20.3	22.0	24.1	26.4	28.3	30.1
7 years	148	25.1	3.9	19.7	20.8	21.2	22.2	24.8	26.9	28.2	29.6	33.9
8 years	147	28.2	6.2	20.4	22.7	23.6	24.6	27.5	29.9	33.0	35.5	39.1
9 years	145	31.1	6.3	24.0	25.6	26.0	27.1	30.2	33.0	35.4	38.6	43.1
10 years	157	36.4	7.7	27.2	28.2	29.6	31.4	34.8	39.2	43.5	46.3	53.4
11 years	155	40.3	10.1	26.8	28.8	31.8	33.5	37.3	46.4	52.0	57.0	61.0
12 years	145	44.2	10.1	30.7	32.5	35.4	37.8	42.5	48.8	52.6	58.9	67.5
13 years	173	49.9	12.3	35.4	37.0	38.3	40.1	48.4	56.3	59.8	64.2	69.9
14 years	186	57.1	11.0	41.0	44.5	46.4	49.8	56.4	63.3	66.1	68.9	77.0
15 years	184	61.0	11.0	46.2	49.1	50.6	54.2	60.1	64.9	68.7	72.8	81.3
16 years	178	67.1	12.4	51.4	54.3	56.1	58.7	64.4	73.6	78.1	82.2	91.2
17 years	173	66.7	11.5	50.7	53.4	54.8	58.7	65.8	72.0	76.8	82.3	88.9
18 years	164	71.1	12.7	54.1	56.6	60.3	61.9	70.4	76.6	80.0	83.5	95.3
19 years	148	71.7	11.6	55.9	57.9	60.5	63.8	69.5	77.9	84.3	86.8	92.1
Female												
6–11 months	177	8.8	1.2	6.6	7.3	7.5	7.9	8.9	9.4	10.1	10.4	10.9
1 year	336	10.8	1.4	8.8	9.1	9.4	9.9	10.7	11.7	12.4	12.7	13.4
2 years	336	13.0	1.5	10.8	11.2	11.6	12.0	12.7	13.8	14.5	14.9	15.9
3 years	366	14.9	2.1	11.7	12.3	12.9	13.4	14.7	16.1	17.0	17.4	18.4
4 years	396	17.0	2.4	13.7	14.3	14.5	15.2	16.7	18.4	19.3	20.2	21.1
5 years	364	19.6	3.3	15.3	16.1	16.7	17.2	19.0	21.2	22.8	24.7	26.6
6 years	135	22.1	4.0	17.0	17.8	18.6	19.3	21.3	23.8	26.6	28.9	29.6
7 years	157	24.7	5.0	19.2	19.5	19.8	21.4	23.8	27.1	28.7	30.3	34.0
8 years	123	27.9	5.7	21.4	22.3	23.3	24.4	27.5	30.2	31.3	33.2	36.5
9 years	149	31.9	8.4	22.9	25.0	25.8	27.0	29.7	33.6	39.3	43.3	48.4
10 years	136	36.1	8.0	25.7	27.5	29.0	31.0	34.5	39.5	44.2	45.8	49.6
11 years	140	41.8	10.9	29.8	30.3	31.3	33.9	40.3	45.8	51.0	56.6	60.0
12 years	147	46.4	10.1	32.3	35.0	36.7	39.1	45.4	52.6	58.0	60.5	64.3
13 years	162	50.9	11.8	35.4	39.0	40.3	44.1	49.0	55.2	60.9	66.4	76.3
14 years	175	54.8	11.1	40.3	42.8	43.7	47.4	53.1	60.3	65.7	67.6	75.2
15 years	145	55.1	9.8	44.0	45.1	46.5	48.2	53.3	59.6	62.2	65.5	76.6
16 years	170	58.1	10.1	44.1	47.3	48.9	51.3	55.6	62.5	68.9	73.3	76.8
17 years	134	59.6	11.4	44.5	48.9	50.5	52.2	58.4	63.4	68.4	71.6	81.8
18 years	170	59.0	11.1	45.3	49.5	50.8	52.8	56.4	63.0	66.0	70.1	78.0
19 years	158	60.2	11.0	48.5	49.7	51.7	53.9	57.1	64.4	70.7	74.8	78.1

*Includes clothing weight, estimated as ranging from 0.09 to 0.28 kilogram.
(From National Center for Health Statistics (1987) *Anthropometric Reference Data and Prevalence of Overweight, United States 1978–1980*, DHHS Publication No. 87-1688. U.S. Department of Health and Human Services, Public Health Service, Hyattsville, MD.)

Table II.39   Weight in kilograms of youths aged 12 years at last birthday by sex and height group in centimeters: sample size, estimated population size, mean, standard deviation, standard error of the mean, and selected percentiles, United States, 1966 to 1970

Sex and height	n	N	$\bar{X}$	s	$s_{\bar{x}}$	5th	10th	25th	50th	75th	90th	95th
								Percentile				
Male						in kilograms						
Under 130	5	15	*	*	*	*	*	*	*	*	*	*
130.0–134.9	4	8	*	*	*	*	*	*	*	*	*	*
135.0–139.9	34	111	32.50	3.741	0.727	26.6	27.6	30.2	31.6	34.7	37.7	39.4
140.0–144.9	80	241	34.28	3.635	0.601	28.1	30.0	31.8	34.1	36.5	38.6	40.7
145.0–149.9	123	386	39.27	6.243	0.615	32.1	33.2	35.7	38.2	40.9	46.1	52.5
150.0–154.9	156	513	42.90	6.314	0.480	34.9	36.1	38.2	42.1	46.0	51.6	56.3
155.0–159.9	135	432	47.35	7.551	0.769	38.3	39.4	41.9	46.2	50.5	57.4	61.9
160.0–164.9	65	201	50.82	8.735	1.388	42.1	42.7	44.9	48.4	56.0	61.1	67.1
165.0–169.9	29	88	55.75	8.811	2.031	43.3	46.4	49.0	54.4	59.9	68.3	76.6
170.0–174.9	8	21	62.37	4.503	1.993	54.0	58.1	60.1	61.0	66.0	69.1	69.5
175.0–179.9	3	10	*	*	*	*	*	*	*	*	*	*
180.0–184.9	1	2	*	*	*	*	*	*	*	*	*	*
185.0–189.9	–	–	–	–	–	–	–	–	–	–	–	–
190.0–194.9	–	–	–	–	–	–	–	–	–	–	–	–
195.0 and over	–	–	–	–	–	–	–	–	–	–	–	–
Female						in kilograms						
Under 130	–	–	–	–	–	–	–	–	–	–	–	–
130.0–134.9	3	10	*	*	*	*	*	*	*	*	*	*
135.0–139.9	12	44	29.41	3.372	0.914	25.0	25.0	26.4	28.9	32.1	34.1	34.2
140.0–144.9	32	116	38.30	7.314	1.194	28.8	30.6	33.3	36.8	41.4	49.2	55.1
145.0–149.9	72	258	39.78	6.205	0.975	31.8	32.8	35.5	38.5	42.8	48.3	50.6
150.0–154.9	147	517	44.00	7.421	0.677	34.4	35.8	38.9	42.8	47.4	52.9	57.4
155.0–159.9	144	525	48.74	8.369	0.714	37.9	39.2	43.0	46.8	53.8	60.7	63.5
160.0–164.9	95	336	53.06	8.010	0.658	42.5	43.9	47.2	51.1	57.2	65.6	69.6
165.0–169.9	31	117	54.89	7.022	1.384	43.9	47.1	50.4	53.1	59.7	64.5	71.3
170.0–174.9	11	42	63.66	14.501	6.214	48.7	50.1	50.8	56.7	82.2	86.0	86.1
175.0–179.9	–	–	–	–	–	–	–	–	–	–	–	–
180.0–184.9	–	–	–	–	–	–	–	–	–	–	–	–
185.0–189.9	–	–	–	–	–	–	–	–	–	–	–	–
190.0–194.9	–	–	–	–	–	–	–	–	–	–	–	–
195.0 and over	–	–	–	–	–	–	–	–	–	–	–	–

n, Sample size; N, estimated number of youths in population in thousands; $\bar{X}$, mean; s, standard deviation; $s_{\bar{x}}$, standard error of the mean.
(From National Center for Health Statistics (1973) Height and weight of youths 12–17 years, United States , in *Vital and Health Statistics*, Series 11, No. 124, Health Services and Mental Health Administration, U.S. Government Printing Office, Washington, D.C., pp. 282–8).

Table II.40 Weight in kilograms of youths aged 13 years at last birthday by sex and height group in centimeters: sample size, estimated population size, mean, standard deviation, standard error of the mean, and selected percentiles, United States, 1966 to 1970

Sex and height	n	N	$\bar{X}$	s	$s_{\bar{x}}$	Percentile						
						5th	10th	25th	50th	75th	90th	95th
Male						in kilograms						
Under 130	–	–	–	–	–	–	–	–	–	–	–	–
130.0–134.9	2	5	*	*	*	*	*	*	*	*	*	*
135.0–139.9	6	25	32.62	5.624	7.716	27.2	27.6	28.9	31.0	34.9	43.1	43.2
140.0–144.9	18	56	36.54	5.852	1.607	30.0	30.5	32.1	36.1	39.2	41.7	53.2
145.0–149.9	65	204	39.03	5.270	0.662	32.4	33.9	36.1	37.9	41.2	44.5	46.4
150.0–154.9	99	312	42.58	6.724	0.865	34.8	36.2	37.9	41.0	45.5	49.4	61.0
155.0–159.9	131	421	47.27	7.482	0.717	37.8	39.2	41.7	45.8	51.1	58.7	61.7
160.0–164.9	125	393	53.01	9.324	0.916	41.5	43.7	46.9	50.4	58.2	64.4	72.5
165.0–169.9	91	285	55.92	8.560	0.833	46.3	47.5	49.3	53.6	59.4	69.0	75.0
170.0–174.9	63	215	62.01	10.362	1.033	51.2	51.6	53.7	60.1	67.0	76.0	85.0
175.0–179.9	19	68	67.92	12.085	3.428	56.3	57.9	60.1	63.3	70.3	88.3	89.0
180.0–184.9	5	15	*	*	*	*	*	*	*	*	*	*
185.0–189.9	–	–	–	–	–	–	–	–	–	–	–	–
190.0–194.9	–	–	–	–	–	–	–	–	–	–	–	–
195.0 and over	–	–	–	–	–	–	–	–	–	–	–	–
Female												
Under 130	–	–	–	–	–	–	–	–	–	–	–	–
130.0–134.9	1	3	*	*	*	*	*	*	*	*	*	*
135.0–139.9	–	–	–	–	–	–	–	–	–	–	–	–
140.0–144.9	15	51	37.13	7.317	2.259	26.6	27.5	30.5	36.7	40.1	44.5	56.1
145.0–149.9	47	165	42.23	6.880	0.888	34.7	35.6	38.2	40.5	44.2	53.6	57.6
150.0–154.9	98	329	44.32	7.029	0.787	35.6	36.5	39.2	42.9	47.3	53.7	57.9
155.0–159.9	152	499	49.75	8.757	0.699	39.1	39.9	43.8	48.4	53.8	61.0	65.9
160.0–164.9	156	515	53.16	8.399	0.522	41.2	43.9	47.7	52.2	57.0	63.8	68.5
165.0–169.9	86	284	58.17	9.125	0.921	46.2	47.4	52.2	58.1	61.5	69.3	76.2
170.0–174.9	24	87	58.11	13.209	2.343	46.2	47.1	48.4	52.9	65.3	68.6	96.8
175.0–179.9	3	10	*	*	*	*	*	*	*	*	*	*
180.0–184.9	–	–	–	–	–	–	–	–	–	–	–	–
185.0–189.9	–	–	–	–	–	–	–	–	–	–	–	–
190.0–194.9	–	–	–	–	–	–	–	–	–	–	–	–
195.0 and over	–	–	–	–	–	–	–	–	–	–	–	–

n, Sample size; N, estimated number of youths in population in thousands; $\bar{X}$, mean; s, standard deviation; $s_{\bar{x}}$, standard error of the mean.
(From National Center for Health Statistics (1973). Health and weight of youths 12–17 years, United States, in *Vital and Health Statistics*, Series 11, No. 124, Health Services and Mental Health Administration. U.S. Government Printing Office, Washington, D.C., pp. 282–8.)

Table II.41 Weight in kilograms of youths aged 14 years at last birthday by sex and height group in centimeters: sample size, estimated population size, mean, standard deviation, standard error of the mean, and selected percentiles, United States, 1966 to 1970

Sex and height	n	N	$\bar{X}$	s	$s_{\bar{x}}$	Percentile						
						5th	10th	25th	50th	75th	90th	95th
Male						in kilograms						
Under 130	–	–	–	–	–	–	–	–	–	–	–	–
130.0–134.9	–	–	–	–	–	–	–	–	–	–	–	–
135.0–139.9	2	7	*	*	*	*	*	*	*	*	*	*
140.0–144.9	3	13	*	*	*	*	*	*	*	*	*	*
145.0–149.9	11	42	40.51	1.829	0.644	36.9	38.6	39.6	40.6	42.0	42.5	42.7
150.0–154.9	45	135	43.63	6.277	1.182	36.2	37.0	39.0	41.4	48.0	51.7	55.3
155.0–159.9	83	261	47.42	7.822	0.872	37.7	38.7	41.8	46.1	51.2	58.0	62.7

Continued

Table II.41   Continued

Sex and height	n	N	$\bar{X}$	s	$s_{\bar{x}}$	Percentile 5th	10th	25th	50th	75th	90th	95th
Male						in kilograms						
160.0–164.9	96	299	52.28	6.785	0.584	42.5	44.0	47.5	52.1	56.3	61.5	65.1
165.0–169.9	134	432	58.07	9.416	1.054	47.7	49.3	51.6	55.4	62.3	70.6	75.7
170.0–174.9	144	435	62.37	11.516	1.095	49.7	51.0	55.0	59.4	65.6	79.2	86.3
175.0–179.9	71	228	65.54	9.704	1.306	50.9	55.1	58.5	64.7	69.9	74.5	84.0
180.0–184.9	25	81	72.44	13.014	2.298	59.6	60.0	65.1	69.4	77.0	83.0	94.3
185.0–189.9	3	9	*	*	*	*	*	*	*	*	*	*
190.0–194.9	1	3	*	*	*	*	*	*	*	*	*	*
195.0 and over	–	–	–	–	–	–	–	–	–	–	–	–
Female												
Under 130	–	–	–	–	–	–	–	–	–	–	–	–
130.0–134.9	–	–	–	–	–	–	–	–	–	–	–	–
135.0–139.9	1	2	*	*	*	*	*	*	*	*	*	*
140.0–144.9	2	6	*	*	*	*	*	*	*	*		*
145.0–149.9	17	52	42.00	5.879	1.683	32.0	35.3	36.3	42.3	47.5	49.5	51.1
150.0–154.9	64	196	48.26	6.797	0.926	37.7	39.2	42.5	47.9	53.3	55.9	58.8
155.0–159.9	157	508	51.35	7.705	0.520	41.2	43.4	46.3	49.6	55.6	62.2	64.3
160.0–164.9	186	603	54.59	8.810	0.707	43.0	45.0	48.4	53.0	59.7	66.7	70.7
165.0–169.9	114	372	58.46	10.185	0.955	45.9	47.5	52.1	56.8	61.8	70.5	76.4
170.0–174.9	36	121	64.37	15.821	2.814	49.2	52.1	56.2	59.8	70.5	72.9	99.4
175.0–179.9	7	28	61.33	5.496	2.620	51.7	52.0	57.7	59.8	64.6	70.2	70.6
180.0–184.9	2	7	*	*	*	*	*	*	*	*	*	*
185.0–189.9	–	–	–	–	–	–	–	–	–	–	–	–
190.0–194.9	–	–	–	–	–	–	–	–	–	–	–	–
195.0 and over	–	–	–	–	–	–	–	–	–	–	–	–

n, Sample size; N, estimated number of youths in population in thousands; $\bar{X}$, mean; s, standard deviation; $s_{\bar{x}}$, standard error of the mean.
(From National Center for Health Statistics (1973) Height and weight of youths 12–17 years, United States, in *Vital and Health Statistics*, Series 11, No. 124, Health Services and Mental Health Administration. U.S. Government Printing Office, Washington, D.C., pp. 282–8.)

Table II.42   Weight in kilograms of youths aged 15 years at last birthday by sex and height group in centimeters: sample size, estimated population size, mean, standard deviation, standard error of the mean, and selected percentiles, United States, 1966 to 1970

Sex and height	n	N	$\bar{X}$	s	$s_{\bar{x}}$	Percentile 5th	10th	25th	50th	75th	90th	95th
Male						in kilograms						
Under 130	–	–	–	–	–	–	–	–	–	–	–	–
130.0–134.9	–	–	–	–	–	–	–	–	–	–	–	–
135.0–139.9	–	–	–	–	–	–	–	–	–	–	–	–
140.0–144.9	–	–	–	–	–	–	–	–	–	–	–	–
145.0–149.9	1	2	*	*	*	*	*	*	*	*	*	*
150.0–154.9	10	30	45.72	8.582	3.550	35.7	39.2	42.6	44.7	46.0	48.7	76.1
155.0–159.9	34	99	52.81	10.552	1.695	40.3	43.1	46.7	49.2	56.7	69.6	76.3
160.0–164.9	71	206	53.01	8.417	0.986	42.7	44.1	46.9	51.5	56.3	65.3	68.8
165.0–169.9	132	404	57.72	8.503	0.819	48.0	48.8	53.1	56.4	61.3	67.1	73.3
170.0–174.9	176	574	62.88	8.464	0.633	51.6	53.4	56.7	61.9	67.2	72.9	78.1
175.0–179.9	118	374	65.80	9.457	1.045	53.1	55.6	59.7	64.3	69.5	80.2	89.2
180.0–184.9	51	144	72.00	11.928	1.724	54.6	60.3	64.4	70.2	78.4	84.4	96.6
185.0–189.9	14	48	74.21	15.035	5.200	58.3	58.5	62.9	70.7	84.6	92.4	110.8
190.0–194.9	6	15	83.39	16.431	10.332	66.4	66.7	69.6	73.8	103.0	105.7	106.2
195.0 and over	–	–	–	–	–	–	–	–	–	–	–	–

Continued

Table II.42 Continued

Sex and height	n	N	$\bar{X}$	s	$s_{\bar{x}}$	Percentile 5th	10th	25th	50th	75th	90th	95th
Female						in kilograms						
Under 130	–	–	–	–	–	–	–	–	–	–	–	–
130.0–134.9	–	–	–	–	–	–	–	–	–	–	–	–
135.0–139.9	–	–	–	–	–	–	–	–	–	–	–	–
140.0–144.9	2	5	*	*	*	*	*	*	*	*	*	*
145.0–149.9	15	51	47.91	7.875	3.623	36.0	39.4	42.1	45.4	52.7	55.7	66.3
150.0–154.9	69	242	49.69	8.895	1.190	39.1	40.6	44.3	48.1	52.8	60.5	68.3
155.0–159.9	111	400	51.52	8.473	0.934	41.4	43.5	46.3	50.8	55.1	59.8	65.2
160.0–164.9	137	509	57.03	10.828	0.875	45.1	47.3	50.2	55.0	60.2	71.7	77.7
165.0–169.9	109	398	60.71	10.357	1.053	47.5	49.3	55.1	58.4	65.7	74.1	81.0
170.0–174.9	49	188	65.27	10.730	1.880	49.7	53.6	57.2	61.2	71.6	85.3	86.4
175.0–179.9	7	23	63.30	8.872	4.807	49.7	49.9	53.8	62.4	71.1	71.9	79.2
180.0–184.9	3	26	*	*	*	*	*	*	*	*	*	*
185.0–189.9	1	3	*	*	*	*	*	*	*	*	*	*
190.0–194.9	–	–	–	–	–	–	–	–	–	–	–	–
195.0 and over	–	–	–	–	–	–	–	–	–	–	–	–

n, Sample size; N, estimated number of youths in population in thousands; $\bar{X}$, mean; s, standard deviation; $s_{\bar{x}}$, standard error of the mean.
(From National Center for Health Statistics (1973) Height and weight of youths 12–17 years, United States, in *Vital and Health Statistics*, Series 11, No. 124, Health Services and Mental Health Administration, U.S. Government Printing Office, Washington, D.C., 1973, pp. 282–8.)

Table II.43 Weight in kilograms of youths aged 16 years at last birthday by sex and height group in centimeters: sample size, estimated population size, mean, standard deviation, standard error of the mean, and selected percentiles, United States, 1966 to 1970

Sex and height	n	N	$\bar{X}$	s	$s_{\bar{x}}$	Percentile 5th	10th	25th	50th	75th	90th	95th
Male						in kilograms						
Under 130	–	–	–	–	–	–	–	–	–	–	–	–
130.0–134.9	–	–	–	–	–	–	–	–	–	–	–	–
135.0–139.9	–	–	–	–	–	–	–	–	–	–	–	–
140.0–144.9	–	–	–	–	–	–	–	–	–	–	–	–
145.0–149.9	1	1	*	*	*	*	*	*	*	*	*	*
150.0–154.9	4	12	*	*	*	*	*	*	*	*	*	*
155.0–159.9	11	33	49.89	7.323	3.572	42.0	42.2	44.7	46.8	54.4	59.8	67.2
160.0–164.9	32	108	53.09	6.459	1.273	44.2	44.9	48.2	51.4	58.0	60.9	66.1
165.0–169.9	87	275	59.39	9.178	0.981	48.5	49.8	52.7	58.0	63.9	69.3	75.9
170.0–174.9	166	552	62.66	7.556	0.629	51.6	53.8	57.5	61.6	67.1	73.1	78.0
175.0–179.9	149	511	67.33	9.018	0.856	56.3	58.2	61.0	65.4	72.5	80.1	83.8
180.0–184.9	72	227	72.38	12.485	1.993	58.3	59.3	64.4	68.9	76.5	90.2	96.9
185.0–189.9	29	95	81.06	14.268	3.265	63.7	66.6	69.7	78.4	90.3	97.0	111.4
190.0–194.9	3	10	*	*	*	*	*	*	*	*	*	*
195.0 and over	2	7	*	*	*	*	*	*	*	*	*	*
Female												
Under 130	–	–	–	–	–	–	–	–	–	–	–	–
130.0–134.9	–	–	–	–	–	–	–	–	–	–	–	–
135.0–139.9	–	–	–	–	–	–	–	–	–	–	–	–
140.0–144.9	2	5	*	*	*	*	*	*	*	*	*	*
145.0–149.9	10	33	52.58	8.198	3.191	43.9	44.1	44.9	51.0	54.5	72.0	72.1
150.0–154.9	57	178	51.79	10.457	1.053	41.4	42.0	45.8	48.9	54.1	61.5	83.3
155.0–159.9	117	354	53.20	7.766	0.734	44.0	45.6	48.4	51.6	56.4	61.9	69.0
160.0–164.9	160	547	57.71	11.129	1.246	46.1	47.3	51.5	55.5	61.2	69.5	75.1

Continued

Table II.43   Continued

Sex and height	n	N	X̄	s	s_x̄	5th	10th	25th	50th	75th	90th	95th
						Percentile						
Female												
165.0–169.9	122	450	61.72	11.998	0.802	47.1	48.8	53.3	59.1	67.3	78.7	86.7
170.0–174.9	53	170	63.61	8.734	1.126	52.9	53.8	58.1	62.1	66.8	73.8	84.2
175.0–179.9	14	45	72.55	15.012	5.224	58.6	58.8	61.7	65.9	80.6	99.1	105.5
180.0–184.9	1	2	*	*	*	*	*	*	*	*	*	*
185.0–189.9	–	–	–	–	–	–	–	–	–	–	–	–
190.0–194.9	–	–	–	–	–	–	–	–	–	–	–	–
195.0 and over	–	–	–	–	–	–	–	–	–	–	–	–

n, Sample size; N, estimated number of youths in population in thousands; X̄, mean; s, standard deviation; s_x̄, standard error of the mean.
(From National Center for Health Statistics (1973) Height and weight of youths 12–17 years, United States, in *Vital and Health Statistics*, Series 11, No. 124, Health Services and Mental Health Administration, U.S. Government Printing Office, Washington, D.C., pp. 282–8.)

Table II.44   Weight in kilograms of youths aged 17 years at last birthday by sex and height group in centimeters: sample size, estimated population size, mean, standard deviation, standard error of the mean, and selected percentiles, United States, 1966 to 1970

Sex and height	n	N	X̄	s	s_x̄	5th	10th	25th	50th	75th	90th	95th
						Percentile						
Male						in kilograms						
Under 130	–	–	–	–	–	–	–	–	–	–	–	–
130.0–134.9	–	–	–	–	–	–	–	–	–	–	–	–
135.0–139.9	–	–	–	–	–	–	–	–	–	–	–	–
140.0–144.9	–	–	–	–	–	–	–	–	–	–	–	–
145.0–149.9	–	–	–	–	–	–	–	–	–	–	–	–
150.0–154.9	1	3	*	*	*	*	*	*	*	*	*	*
155.0–159.9	11	39	54.63	9.397	3.414	43.8	46.4	48.2	49.7	57.8	69.9	73.2
160.0–164.9	25	81	57.75	6.503	1.355	49.7	51.1	52.5	56.9	61.6	70.1	70.8
165.0–169.9	63	248	62.57	8.344	1.224	50.2	53.2	56.4	61.5	66.9	72.7	77.3
170.0–174.9	115	396	67.06	11.163	0.704	53.3	55.5	59.5	64.6	71.9	80.9	91.6
175.0–179.9	151	537	68.37	9.907	0.831	56.9	58.9	61.5	66.5	73.6	79.4	88.4
180.0–184.9	80	297	73.31	12.454	1.335	59.6	61.0	65.1	71.2	78.4	91.8	102.7
185.0–189.9	36	133	76.03	9.171	1.301	62.4	66.3	70.5	75.3	80.8	90.3	92.9
190.0–194.9	7	25	81.40	10.985	7.588	62.9	62.9	67.8	87.3	90.3	90.6	90.6
195.0 and over	–	–	–	–	–	–	–	–	–	–	–	–
Female												
Under 130	–	–	–	–	–	–	–	–	–	–	–	–
130.0–134.9	–	–	–	–	–	–	–	–	–	–	–	–
135.0–139.9	–	–	–	–	–	–	–	–	–	–	–	–
140.0–144.9	2	5	*	*	*	*	*	*	*	*	*	*
145.0–149.9	8	26	43.49	3.939	1.604	38.6	38.8	40.1	45.1	45.7	51.1	51.2
150.0–154.9	43	151	49.96	6.508	0.827	41.6	42.3	44.6	48.9	53.5	59.2	64.1
155.0–159.9	103	385	54.71	9.903	0.775	44.4	45.5	48.7	53.2	57.7	61.6	76.2
160.0–164.9	133	506	57.79	10.620	1.028	46.8	48.0	50.2	55.4	61.5	72.3	82.3
165.0–169.9	116	433	60.63	10.117	1.182	47.9	50.3	55.1	59.3	65.1	69.4	71.6
170.0–174.9	51	186	62.18	9.132	1.407	50.6	52.9	55.5	60.2	65.7	76.1	82.7
175.0–179.9	12	47	65.76	8.405	2.229	54.9	56.7	60.1	61.7	75.2	75.9	83.0
180.0–184.9	1	2	*	*	*	*	*	*	*	*	*	*
185.0–189.9	–	–	–	–	–	–	–	–	–	–	–	–
190.0–194.9	–	–	–	–	–	–	–	–	–	–	–	–
195.0 and over	–	–	–	–	–	–	–	–	–	–	–	–

n, Sample size; N, estimated number of youths in population in thousands; X̄, mean; s, standard deviation; s_x̄, standard error of the mean.
(From National Center for Health Statistics (1973) Height and weight of youths 12–17 years, United States, in *Vital and Health Statistics*, Series 11, No. 124, Health Services and Mental Health Administration, U.S. Government Printing Office, Washington, D.C., pp. 282–8.)

Table II.45   Weight in kilograms for women 18 to 74 years of age: number examined, mean, standard deviation, and selected percentiles by race and age, United States, 1976 to 1980*

Race and age (years)	Number of examined persons	Mean	Standard deviation	Percentile								
				5th	10th	15th	25th	50th	75th	85th	90th	95th
All races[†]												
18–74	6,588	65.4	14.6	47.7	50.3	52.2	55.4	62.4	72.1	79.2	84.4	93.1
18–24	1,066	60.6	11.9	46.6	49.1	50.6	53.2	58.0	65.0	70.4	75.3	82.9
25–34	1,170	64.2	15.0	47.4	49.6	51.4	54.3	60.9	69.6	78.4	84.1	93.5
35–44	844	67.1	15.2	49.2	52.0	53.3	56.9	63.4	73.9	81.7	87.5	98.9
45–54	763	68.0	15.3	48.5	51.3	53.3	57.3	65.5	75.7	82.1	87.6	96.0
55–64	1,329	67.9	14.7	48.6	51.3	54.1	57.3	65.2	75.3	82.3	87.5	95.1
65–74	1,416	66.6	13.8	47.1	50.8	53.2	57.4	64.8	73.8	79.8	84.4	91.3
White												
18–74	5,686	64.8	14.1	47.7	50.3	52.2	55.2	62.1	71.1	77.9	83.3	91.5
18–24	892	60.4	11.6	47.3	49.5	50.8	53.3	57.9	64.8	69.7	74.3	82.4
25–34	1,000	63.6	14.5	47.3	49.5	51.3	54.0	60.6	68.9	76.3	81.5	89.7
35–44	726	66.1	14.5	49.3	51.8	52.9	56.3	62.4	71.9	79.7	85.8	94.9
45–54	647	67.3	14.4	48.6	51.3	53.4	57.0	65.0	74.8	81.1	85.6	94.5
55–64	1,176	67.2	14.4	48.5	50.7	53.7	57.1	64.7	74.5	81.8	86.2	92.8
65–74	1,245	66.2	13.7	47.2	50.7	52.9	57.2	64.3	72.9	79.2	84.3	91.2
Black												
18–74	782	71.2	17.3	48.8	51.6	55.1	59.1	67.8	80.6	87.4	94.9	105.1
18–24	147	63.1	13.9	46.2	49.0	50.6	53.8	60.4	70.0	75.8	79.1	89.3
25–34	145	69.3	16.7	48.3	50.8	53.1	57.8	65.3	80.2	87.1	91.5	102.7
35–44	103	75.3	18.4	50.7	55.2	57.2	63.0	70.2	85.2	95.3	103.5	113.1
45–54	100	77.7	18.8	55.1	60.3	60.8	64.5	74.3	83.6	94.5	98.2	117.5
55–64	135	75.8	16.4	54.2	55.2	57.6	65.4	74.6	83.4	91.9	95.5	108.5
65–74	152	72.4	13.6	52.9	56.4	60.3	64.0	70.0	82.2	84.4	86.5	98.1

*Includes clothing weight, estimated as ranging from 0.09 to 0.28 kilogram.
[†]Includes all other races not shown as separate categories.
(From National Center for Health Statistics (1987) *Anthropometric Reference Data and Prevalence of Overweight, United States 1976–1980*, DHHS Publication No. 87-1688, U.S. Department of Health and Human Services, Public Health Service, Hyattsville, MD.)

Table II.46   Weight in kilograms for men 18 to 74 years of age: number examined, mean, standard deviation, and selected percentiles by race and age, United States, 1976 to 1980*

Race and age (years)	Number of examined persons	Mean	Standard deviation	Percentile								
				5th	10th	15th	25th	50th	75th	85th	90th	95th
All races[†]												
18–74	5,916	78.1	13.5	58.6	62.3	64.9	68.7	76.9	85.6	91.3	95.7	102.7
18–24	988	73.8	12.7	56.8	60.4	61.9	64.8	72.0	80.3	85.1	90.4	99.5
25–34	1,067	78.7	13.7	59.5	62.9	65.4	69.3	77.5	85.6	91.1	95.1	102.7
35–44	745	80.9	13.4	59.7	65.1	67.7	72.1	79.9	88.1	94.8	98.8	104.3
45–54	690	80.9	13.6	60.8	65.2	67.2	71.7	79.0	89.4	94.5	99.5	105.3
55–64	1,227	78.8	12.8	59.9	63.8	66.4	70.2	77.7	85.6	90.5	94.7	102.3
65–74	1,199	74.8	12.8	54.4	58.5	61.2	66.1	74.2	82.7	87.9	91.2	96.6
White												
18–74	5,148	78.5	13.1	59.3	62.8	65.5	69.4	77.3	85.6	91.4	95.5	102.3
18–24	846	74.2	12.8	56.8	60.5	62.0	65.0	72.4	80.6	85.5	91.0	100.0
25–34	901	79.0	13.1	59.9	63.7	65.9	69.8	78.0	85.6	91.3	95.3	102.7
35–44	653	81.4	12.8	62.3	66.6	68.8	72.9	80.1	88.2	94.6	98.7	104.1

Continued

Table II.46   Continued

Race and age (years)	Number of examined persons	Mean	Standard deviation	Percentile								
				5th	10th	15th	25th	50th	75th	85th	90th	95th
White												
45–54	617	81.0	13.4	62.0	66.1	67.3	71.9	79.0	89.4	94.2	99.0	104.5
55–64	1,086	78.9	12.4	60.5	64.5	66.6	70.6	78.2	85.6	90.4	94.5	101.7
65–74	1,045	75.4	12.4	55.5	59.5	62.5	67.0	74.7	83.0	87.9	91.2	96.0
Black												
18–74	649	77.9	15.2	58.0	61.1	63.6	67.2	75.3	85.4	92.9	98.3	105.4
18–24	121	72.2	12.0	58.3	60.9	62.3	64.9	70.8	77.1	81.8	83.7	93.6
25–34	139	78.2	16.3	58.7	63.4	64.9	68.4	75.3	84.4	90.6	92.2	106.3
35–44	70	82.5	15.4	*	61.7	65.2	69.7	83.1	94.8	100.4	104.2	*
45–54	62	82.4	14.5	*	64.7	67.0	73.2	81.8	93.0	100.0	102.5	*
55–64	129	78.6	14.7	56.8	61.4	64.3	68.0	77.0	86.5	93.8	98.6	104.7
65–74	128	73.3	15.3	52.5	56.7	58.0	61.0	71.2	81.1	90.8	97.3	105.1

*Includes clothing weight, estimated as ranging from 0.09 to 0.28 kilogram.
†Includes all other races not shown as separate categories.
(From National Center for Health Statistics (1987) *Anthropometric Reference Data and Prevalence of Overweight, United States 1976–1980*, DHHS Publication No. 87-1688, U.S. Department of Health and Human Services, Public Health Service, Hyattsville, MD.)

Table II.47   Height in centimeters for women 18 to 74 years of age: number examined, mean, standard deviation, and selected percentiles by race and age, United States, 1976 to 1980*

Race and age (years)	Number of examined persons	Mean	Standard deviation	Percentile								
				5th	10th	15th	25th	50th	75th	85th	90th	95th
All races†												
18–74	6,588	161.8	6.6	150.9	153.6	155.2	157.4	161.7	166.3	168.6	170.3	172.6
18–24	1,066	163.4	6.6	152.9	155.2	156.7	159.0	163.7	167.6	170.0	171.6	174.0
25–34	1,170	163.1	6.3	153.2	155.2	156.6	158.7	163.1	167.6	169.9	171.3	173.7
35–44	844	162.8	6.3	152.6	155.5	156.7	158.5	162.5	167.0	169.3	171.0	173.5
45–54	763	161.3	6.4	150.5	152.9	154.5	156.8	161.3	165.6	167.7	169.4	171.8
55–64	1,329	160.1	6.4	149.2	151.8	153.7	155.9	160.3	164.5	166.7	168.0	170.3
65–74	1,416	158.1	6.2	147.9	150.0	151.7	154.1	158.4	162.2	164.5	166.0	167.7
White												
18–74	5,686	161.9	6.5	151.3	153.8	155.4	157.6	161.9	165.4	168.7	170.3	172.7
18–24	892	163.7	6.4	153.1	155.7	157.1	159.4	163.9	167.7	170.1	171.8	174.0
25–34	1,000	163.3	6.2	153.5	155.4	156.6	158.9	163.3	167.8	170.1	171.5	173.7
35–44	726	162.9	6.3	152.6	155.6	156.7	158.4	162.6	167.0	169.4	171.2	173.5
45–54	647	161.5	6.2	151.5	153.6	155.2	157.2	161.3	165.7	167.6	169.4	171.7
55–64	1,176	160.1	6.3	149.6	151.9	153.9	156.1	160.3	164.4	166.5	167.7	170.1
65–74	1,245	158.1	6.2	147.8	150.1	151.7	154.1	158.5	162.2	164.5	166.0	167.7
Black												
18–74	782	162.1	6.7	150.6	154.2	155.2	157.6	162.2	166.6	168.9	170.4	173.0
18–24	147	163.2	6.9	152.8	155.1	156.4	158.6	163.0	168.1	170.2	171.1	174.8
25–34	145	162.3	6.3	151.3	154.8	156.3	158.1	162.5	166.2	168.6	170.4	174.1
35–44	103	163.3	5.5	155.2	156.9	157.3	159.7	162.5	167.0	168.7	170.1	171.7
45–54	100	161.7	6.9	150.4	152.6	154.4	155.2	162.1	167.5	169.3	170.5	171.9
55–64	135	161.0	7.4	148.7	149.2	153.4	155.8	161.8	166.5	169.1	171.0	174.5
65–74	152	158.8	6.2	148.2	150.4	152.6	155.6	159.1	163.0	164.7	166.4	169.4

*Height without shoes.
†Includes all other races not shown as separate categories.
(From National Center for Health Statistics (1987) *Anthropometric Reference Data and Prevalence of Overweight, United States 1976–1980*, DHHS Publication No. 87-1688, U.S. Department of Health and Human Services, Public Health Service, Hyattsville, MD.)

Table II.48 Height in centimeters for men 18 to 74 years of age: number examined, mean, standard deviation, and selected percentiles by race and age, United States, 1976 to 1980*

Race and age (years)	Number of examined persons	Mean	Standard deviation	5th	10th	15th	25th	50th	75th	85th	90th	95th
All races[†]												
18–74	5,916	175.5	7.2	163.9	166.4	168.2	171.1	175.7	180.4	182.9	184.5	187.0
18–24	988	177.0	7.1	165.8	168.3	169.8	172.2	177.0	181.6	183.9	186.0	189.6
25–34	1,067	176.7	6.7	165.5	167.9	170.0	172.2	176.8	181.2	183.6	185.3	187.4
35–44	745	176.3	7.3	164.1	166.4	168.8	172.2	176.5	181.2	183.6	185.2	188.0
45–54	690	175.2	6.6	164.5	167.2	168.3	170.7	175.1	179.8	182.5	184.3	185.7
55–64	1,227	173.7	6.9	162.1	165.4	166.8	169.2	173.7	178.5	180.6	182.2	184.6
65–74	1,199	171.3	7.1	159.3	162.3	164.1	166.3	171.5	176.1	178.6	180.4	183.1
White												
18–74	5,148	175.7	7.1	164.2	166.7	168.6	171.2	175.9	180.5	183.0	184.6	187.2
18–24	846	177.2	7.0	166.3	168.6	170.1	172.4	177.1	181.9	184.1	186.4	189.7
25–34	901	177.0	6.6	165.8	168.2	170.6	172.5	177.0	181.4	183.8	185.4	187.7
35–44	653	176.7	7.3	164.5	166.7	169.6	172.6	176.8	181.7	183.7	185.8	188.0
45–54	617	175.4	6.8	164.6	167.3	168.9	171.2	175.3	179.8	182.5	184.3	185.7
55–64	1,086	173.8	6.8	163.1	165.6	167.2	169.5	173.6	178.5	180.7	182.2	184.5
65–74	1,045	171.6	6.9	159.6	162.9	164.6	166.9	171.6	176.4	178.7	180.5	183.3
Black												
18–74	649	175.5	7.0	164.3	166.5	168.1	171.1	175.7	180.3	183.0	184.5	186.5
18–24	121	176.7	7.0	165.1	167.6	169.9	172.5	177.9	181.0	183.8	185.0	186.4
25–34	139	176.7	6.9	165.5	168.5	169.6	172.4	177.1	181.8	183.2	184.7	187.1
35–44	70	176.5	6.4	*	167.6	170.7	172.8	175.2	179.9	181.9	185.1	*
45–54	62	174.2	6.7	*	167.6	167.7	169.1	172.8	178.4	183.2	184.5	*
55–64	129	174.2	6.9	162.7	165.3	166.8	168.6	174.6	178.8	180.7	182.8	186.8
65–74	128	171.2	6.5	161.2	162.6	163.8	165.9	171.6	175.3	177.7	180.8	182.2

*Height without shoes.
[†]Includes all other races not shown as separate categories.
(From National Center for Health Statistics (1987) *Anthropometric Reference Data and Prevalence of Overweight, United States 1976–1980*, DHHS Publication No. 87-1688, U.S. Department of Health and Human Services, Public Health Service, Hyattsville, MD.)

Table II.49 Provisional age- and sex-specific reference values for weight in kilograms (pounds) in elderly subjects*,[†]

Age group (years)	5%	50%	95%
	Men		
65	62.6 (138.0)	79.5 (175.0)	102.0 (224.9)
70	59.7 (131.6)	76.5 (168.7)	99.1 (218.5)
75	56.8 (125.2)	73.6 (162.3)	96.3 (212.3)
80	53.9 (118.8)	70.7 (155.9)	93.4 (205.9)
85	51.0 (112.4)	67.8 (149.5)	90.5 (199.5)
90	48.1 (106.0)	64.9 (143.1)	87.6 (193.1)
	Women		
65	51.2 (112.9)	66.8 (147.3)	87.1 (192.0)
70	49.0 (108.0)	64.6 (142.4)	84.9 (187.2)
75	46.8 (103.2)	62.4 (137.6)	82.8 (182.5)
80	44.7 (98.5)	60.2 (132.7)	80.6 (177.7)
85	42.5 (93.7)	58.0 (127.9)	78.4 (172.8)
90	40.3 (88.8)	55.9 (123.2)	76.2 (168.0)

*Data from 119 men and 150 women. The subjects were all ambulatory.
[†]See Tables II.54 through II.59 for data compiled by Frisancho A.R. (1984), *Am. J. Clin. Nutr.*, **40** pp. 808–19, from NHANES I and II.
(From Chumlea, W.C., Roche, A.F., Mukherjee, D. (1984) *Nutritional Assessment of the Elderly through Anthropometry*, Wright State University School of Medicine, Ohio.)

Table II.50 Triceps skinfold thickness: Girls, 1 to 17 years, United States, 1971 to 1974

Race and age in years	Number in sample	Estimated population in thousands	Mean†	Standard deviation	Percentile								
					5th	10th	15th	25th	50th	75th	85th	90th	95th
					Triceps Skinfold in Millimeters								
All Races*													
1	267	1,620	10.1	2.8	6.0	6.5	7.0	8.0	10.0	12.0	13.0	14.0	15.0
2	272	1,708	10.5	2.5	7.0	7.5	8.0	9.0	10.0	12.0	13.5	14.0	15.0
3	292	1,701	10.9	2.7	6.0	7.0	8.0	9.0	11.0	12.5	13.5	14.0	15.0
4	281	1,599	10.5	2.7	7.0	7.5	8.0	8.0	10.0	12.0	13.0	14.0	15.0
5	314	1,695	10.5	3.8	6.0	7.0	7.0	8.0	10.0	12.0	13.0	15.0	17.5
6	176	1,787	10.3	3.3	6.0	6.5	7.0	8.0	10.0	12.0	13.0	13.5	15.0
7	169	1,754	10.8	4.2	4.0	6.0	7.0	8.0	10.5	12.0	15.0	16.0	18.0
8	152	1,800	12.3	4.8	6.5	8.0	8.0	9.0	11.0	15.0	17.0	18.0	22.5
9	171	2,017	13.2	4.8	7.0	7.5	8.0	10.0	12.5	16.0	18.0	20.0	22.0
10	197	2,173	13.1	5.0	7.0	8.0	8.0	9.5	12.0	15.5	19.0	20.0	23.0
11	166	1,911	14.5	6.2	7.0	8.0	8.5	10.0	13.0	18.0	20.5	23.5	28.5
12	177	1,812	15.0	5.9	7.5	8.0	9.0	10.5	14.0	18.5	20.0	23.0	27.0
13	198	2,175	16.2	6.8	7.0	8.0	10.0	11.5	15.0	20.0	24.0	25.0	30.0
14	184	2,036	17.5	7.3	8.5	9.5	10.0	13.0	16.0	21.0	24.0	27.0	33.0
15	171	2,163	17.0	7.0	8.0	10.0	11.0	12.0	16.0	20.5	23.0	25.0	28.5
16	175	2,145	18.2	6.7	10.0	10.5	12.0	13.5	17.0	21.0	24.0	26.0	32.5
17	157	1,804	19.6	8.1	10.0	11.5	12.0	13.0	19.0	24.0	26.5	29.5	35.0
White													
1	189	1,328	10.2	2.8	6.0	7.0	7.0	8.0	10.0	12.0	13.0	13.5	15.5
2	203	1,434	10.6	2.6	7.0	7.5	8.0	9.0	10.0	12.0	13.5	14.0	15.0
3	211	1,438	11.1	2.6	7.0	8.0	8.5	9.0	11.0	13.0	13.5	14.0	15.0
4	204	1,339	10.8	2.6	7.5	8.0	8.0	9.0	10.5	12.0	13.0	14.5	16.0
5	224	1,416	10.7	3.7	6.0	7.0	8.0	8.5	10.0	12.0	13.0	15.0	17.5
6	125	1,445	10.6	3.3	6.5	7.0	7.5	8.0	10.5	12.0	13.0	14.0	16.0
7	122	1,507	10.9	4.2	4.0	6.0	7.0	8.0	11.0	12.0	15.0	15.5	17.5
8	117	1,507	12.4	4.7	7.0	8.0	8.0	9.0	11.5	15.0	16.5	18.0	22.0
9	129	1,751	13.6	4.6	7.5	8.0	9.0	10.0	13.0	16.0	18.0	20.0	22.0

10	148	1,855	13.4	4.8	7.5	8.0	8.5	10.0	12.5	15.5	19.0	20.0	23.0
11	122	1,569	14.9	6.1	8.0	8.5	9.0	10.0	13.0	17.5	20.5	24.5	28.5
12	128	1,506	15.2	5.6	8.0	9.0	10.0	11.0	14.0	18.5	20.0	23.0	26.0
13	153	1,886	16.2	6.8	7.0	8.0	10.0	11.5	15.0	20.0	24.0	25.0	28.5
14	132	1,731	17.8	7.3	9.0	9.5	10.5	13.0	16.7	21.0	24.0	28.5	33.0
15	125	1,752	17.7	6.7	9.0	10.5	11.0	13.0	17.0	21.0	24.0	25.0	28.5
16	141	1,933	18.2	6.6	10.0	10.5	12.5	14.0	17.0	21.0	24.0	26.0	32.1
17	117	1,549	19.8	8.0	10.0	12.0	12.5	13.5	19.0	24.0	26.5	29.5	35.0
Black												
1	73	257	10.0	3.0	5.5	5.5	7.0	8.0	10.0	12.0	13.0	14.0	15.0
2	66	261	10.0	2.3	7.0	8.0	8.0	8.0	10.0	11.0	12.0	14.0	15.5
3	78	245	9.7	2.9	6.0	7.0	7.0	8.0	10.0	11.0	12.0	13.0	14.0
4	73	246	8.8	2.7	5.0	6.0	7.0	7.0	8.0	10.5	12.0	13.0	14.0
5	88	265	9.4	3.9	5.0	5.0	6.5	7.0	8.0	10.0	12.0	13.5	17.0
6	50	336	9.0	3.1	5.5	6.0	6.0	8.0	8.0	10.0	11.5	12.0	13.0
7	46	241	10.1	4.0	5.0	6.0	7.0	7.5	9.0	11.0	17.5	18.0	18.0
8	35	293	11.5	5.1	5.0	6.5	7.0	8.0	10.0	13.5	18.0	18.0	23.0
9	41	247	10.2	5.1	5.5	6.0	6.0	6.5	8.0	12.0	18.0	18.0	20.0
10	48	303	11.7	5.6	6.5	6.5	7.0	7.5	10.0	16.0	18.0	19.0	24.0
11	42	315	12.7	6.4	4.0	5.0	6.5	7.5	10.0	18.0	22.0	23.0	23.0
12	47	284	13.6	7.6	5.5	6.0	6.0	7.5	12.0	17.0	22.0	25.0	30.0
13	44	287	16.1	7.0	7.0	8.5	10.0	11.0	14.0	18.0	24.0	24.0	33.5
14	50	265	15.9	6.7	8.0	8.0	9.0	10.5	14.0	20.5	24.0	24.5	24.5
15	46	411	14.0	7.6	6.5	6.5	8.0	10.0	12.5	16.0	16.5	20.0	32.8
16	33	203	18.9	8.0	8.0	8.0	10.0	12.0	19.0	24.0	24.5	33.0	33.1
17	39	239	16.9	6.6	7.5	9.0	11.0	12.0	14.5	20.0	24.0	28.0	31.0

*Includes data for races that are not shown separately.

†Measurements made in the right arm.

(From the National Center for Health Statistics, Department of Health and Human Services. See also Bishop, C.W., Bowen, P.E., Ritchey, S.J. (1981) *Am. J. Clin. Nutr.*, **34** pp. 2530—9.)

Table II.51 Subscapular skinfold thickness: Girls, 1 to 17 years, United States, 1971 to 1974

Race and age in years	Number in sample	Estimated population in thousands	Mean†	Standard deviation	Percentile								
					5th	10th	15th	25th	50th	75th	85th	90th	95th
					Subscapular Skinfold in Millimeters								
All Races*													
1	267	1,620	6.2	1.9	4.0	4.0	4.0	5.0	6.0	8.0	8.0	9.0	9.0
2	272	1,708	6.2	2.4	4.0	4.0	4.0	5.0	6.0	7.0	8.0	9.0	10.0
3	292	1,701	5.8	2.0	4.0	4.0	4.0	4.5	5.5	6.5	7.0	8.0	9.0
4	281	1,599	5.6	1.9	3.5	4.0	4.0	4.5	5.0	6.0	7.0	8.0	9.0
5	314	1,695	6.2	3.3	3.5	4.0	4.0	4.0	5.0	6.5	8.0	9.0	15.0
6	176	1,787	6.0	2.8	3.0	4.0	4.0	4.5	5.5	6.5	7.0	8.0	10.0
7	169	1,754	6.2	3.3	3.0	4.0	4.0	4.5	5.0	7.0	9.0	10.5	11.5
8	152	1,800	7.7	5.5	3.5	4.0	4.0	4.5	5.5	8.0	12.5	14.5	19.5
9	171	2,017	8.5	5.0	4.0	4.0	4.5	5.0	7.0	10.0	13.0	17.0	19.0
10	197	2,173	8.6	5.1	4.0	4.5	5.0	5.5	6.5	10.0	13.0	18.0	20.0
11	166	1,911	10.1	6.4	4.0	5.0	5.0	6.0	8.0	13.0	16.0	19.0	25.5
12	177	1,812	11.1	6.8	5.0	5.0	5.5	6.0	9.5	13.0	16.0	20.0	25.0
13	198	2,175	11.9	7.1	5.0	6.0	6.0	7.0	9.5	15.0	19.0	23.4	26.0
14	184	2,036	13.0	8.0	5.0	6.0	6.5	8.0	10.0	16.0	19.0	24.0	28.0
15	171	2,163	12.2	7.2	6.0	6.5	7.0	7.5	10.0	14.0	18.0	20.0	27.0
16	175	2,145	13.4	7.8	6.0	7.0	7.5	8.0	10.5	15.0	21.0	25.5	29.0
17	157	1,804	15.6	9.4	6.5	7.0	7.5	9.0	12.5	20.0	25.5	27.0	34.1
White													
1	189	1,328	6.3	1.9	3.5	4.0	4.0	5.0	6.0	8.0	8.0	9.0	9.5
2	203	1,434	6.0	2.1	4.0	4.0	4.0	5.0	6.0	7.0	8.0	8.5	10.0
3	211	1,438	5.8	1.9	4.0	4.0	4.0	5.0	5.5	6.5	7.0	8.0	9.0
4	204	1,339	5.7	1.9	3.5	4.0	4.0	4.5	5.0	6.0	7.0	8.0	9.0
5	224	1,416	6.2	3.2	3.5	4.0	4.0	4.5	5.5	6.5	8.0	10.0	15.0
6	125	1,445	6.0	2.7	3.0	3.5	4.0	4.5	6.0	6.5	7.0	8.0	10.0
7	122	1,507	6.2	3.4	3.0	3.5	4.0	4.5	5.0	7.0	8.5	10.0	12.5
8	117	1,507	7.6	5.6	3.5	4.0	4.0	4.5	6.0	8.0	10.0	13.0	21.0
9	129	1,751	8.5	4.7	4.0	4.5	5.0	5.0	7.0	10.0	13.0	16.0	18.0

10	148	1,855	8.8	5.1	4.0	4.5	5.0	5.5	7.0	10.0	13.0	18.0	20.0
11	122	1,569	10.3	6.7	4.0	5.0	5.0	6.0	8.0	13.0	16.5	20.5	25.5
12	128	1,506	11.1	6.4	5.0	5.0	6.0	6.5	9.5	13.5	17.0	20.0	22.0
13	153	1,886	11.6	6.9	5.0	5.5	6.0	7.0	9.0	15.0	19.0	21.0	25.0
14	132	1,731	13.2	8.2	5.0	6.0	6.5	8.0	10.5	16.0	20.0	24.0	30.0
15	125	1,752	12.4	6.9	6.0	7.0	7.0	8.0	10.0	14.5	18.0	20.0	27.0
16	141	1,933	12.9	7.3	6.0	7.0	7.5	8.0	10.0	15.0	20.5	25.0	28.5
17	117	1,549	15.2	9.3	6.0	7.0	7.5	8.0	12.5	18.0	25.0	26.5	34.0
Black													
1	73	257	6.1	2.0	4.0	4.0	4.0	5.0	5.5	8.0	8.5	9.0	9.0
2	66	261	6.8	3.3	4.0	4.0	4.5	5.0	6.0	7.5	9.5	12.0	15.5
3	78	245	5.5	2.0	4.0	4.0	4.0	4.5	5.0	6.0	7.0	7.0	8.0
4	73	246	5.2	1.7	3.0	3.5	4.0	4.0	5.0	6.0	6.0	8.0	8.5
5	88	265	5.8	3.5	4.0	4.0	4.0	4.0	5.0	6.0	6.5	7.0	13.0
6	50	336	6.0	3.3	3.0	4.0	4.0	5.0	5.5	7.0	7.5	7.5	10.0
7	46	241	6.4	2.6	3.0	4.0	4.0	4.5	5.0	8.0	11.0	11.0	11.0
8	35	293	8.2	5.2	4.0	4.0	4.0	4.5	5.5	14.0	15.0	16.0	17.5
9	41	247	8.3	6.4	4.0	4.0	4.5	5.0	6.0	7.5	14.5	24.0	24.0
10	48	303	8.1	5.5	4.0	4.0	5.0	6.0	8.0	8.0	12.5	14.3	22.0
11	42	315	9.2	4.5	4.0	5.0	5.0	5.5	7.0	11.0	14.5	14.5	15.5
12	47	284	10.7	8.6	4.5	5.0	5.0	7.0	12.0	11.5	16.0	28.0	31.0
13	44	287	13.9	8.1	6.0	6.0	6.5	8.0	10.0	15.0	26.0	26.0	28.4
14	50	265	12.5	7.3	6.0	6.0	6.5	7.0	7.5	16.5	23.0	23.0	25.0
15	46	411	11.2	8.4	5.5	5.5	6.0	6.5	15.0	10.5	19.0	20.0	33.4
16	33	203	17.8	10.7	6.0	7.0	8.0	10.5	15.0	24.5	31.0	38.0	38.0
17	39	239	16.4	8.4	7.0	7.5	8.0	9.0	12.5	23.5	27.0	28.0	30.0

*Includes data for races that are not shown separately.

†Measurements made in the right arm.

(From the National Center for Health Statistics, Department of Health and Human Services. See also Bishop, C.W., Bowen, P.E., Ritchey, S.J. (1981) *Am. J. Clin. Nutr.*, **34** pp. 2530—9.)

Table II.52 Triceps skinfold thickness: Boys, 1 to 17 years, United States, 1971 to 1974

Race and age in years	Number in sample	Estimated population in thousands	Mean†	Standard deviation	Percentile								
					5th	10th	15th	25th	50th	75th	85th	90th	95th
					Triceps Skinfold in Millimeters								
All Races*													
1	286	1,693	10.4	3.1	6.0	7.0	7.5	8.0	10.0	12.0	14.0	15.0	16.0
2	298	1,747	10.0	2.7	6.0	6.5	7.0	8.0	10.0	12.0	12.5	13.5	15.0
3	308	1,807	9.9	2.7	6.5	7.0	7.0	8.0	10.0	11.0	12.5	13.1	14.5
4	304	1,815	9.4	2.5	5.0	6.5	7.0	8.0	9.0	11.0	12.0	12.5	14.0
5	273	1,563	9.5	3.3	5.0	6.0	7.0	7.0	9.0	11.0	12.5	13.5	15.0
6	179	1,673	8.6	3.0	5.0	5.5	6.0	6.5	8.0	10.0	12.0	12.0	14.0
7	164	1,979	8.9	3.5	4.0	5.0	6.0	6.5	8.0	10.0	12.0	13.0	15.5
8	152	1,861	9.0	3.3	5.0	5.5	6.0	6.5	8.0	10.0	12.0	13.0	16.0
9	169	2,019	10.6	4.8	5.0	6.0	6.5	7.0	9.0	14.0	17.0	17.0	19.0
10	184	2,205	10.9	4.4	5.5	6.0	6.0	8.0	10.0	13.5	15.0	17.0	19.5
11	178	2,177	11.9	6.4	5.0	6.0	6.0	7.5	10.0	14.5	18.0	20.0	24.0
12	200	2,304	11.9	6.3	4.5	6.0	6.5	8.0	10.5	13.5	16.5	20.0	27.0
13	174	1,978	11.2	6.6	5.0	5.0	5.5	7.0	10.0	13.0	19.0	22.0	25.0
14	174	2,030	10.3	6.2	4.0	5.0	5.5	6.5	8.0	12.0	16.5	19.0	22.5
15	171	2,093	10.0	6.1	4.0	5.0	5.0	6.0	8.0	11.5	15.0	19.0	23.5
16	169	2,019	9.7	5.2	4.0	5.0	5.0	6.0	8.0	12.0	14.0	17.0	22.0
17	176	2,095	9.2	5.4	4.0	5.0	5.0	6.0	7.5	11.0	12.5	15.0	19.0
White													
1	211	1,402	10.7	3.0	7.0	7.0	7.5	8.0	10.0	12.0	14.0	15.0	16.5
2	217	1,461	9.9	2.6	6.0	6.5	7.0	8.0	10.0	12.0	12.5	13.0	14.7
3	226	1,536	9.9	2.6	6.5	7.0	7.0	8.0	10.0	11.0	12.5	13.5	14.5
4	229	1,547	9.6	2.4	6.0	7.0	7.0	8.0	10.0	11.0	12.0	12.5	14.0
5	207	1,319	9.8	3.2	6.0	6.5	7.0	7.5	9.0	11.0	12.5	13.5	15.0
6	126	1,343	8.9	3.1	5.5	5.6	6.0	7.0	9.0	10.0	12.0	12.5	14.0
7	125	1,718	9.1	3.5	5.0	6.0	6.0	7.0	9.0	10.5	12.0	13.5	17.0
8	116	1,644	9.1	3.3	5.0	5.5	6.0	7.0	8.5	10.5	12.0	13.0	16.0
9	117	1,636	11.1	4.8	5.5	6.5	6.5	7.5	10.0	14.0	17.0	17.0	19.0

10	148	1,909	11.1	4.2	5.5	6.0	7.0	8.0	10.0	14.0	15.5	17.0	19.5
11	132	1,823	12.5	6.5	6.0	6.0	7.0	8.0	10.0	15.0	19.0	20.5	24.5
12	152	1,970	12.4	6.1	6.0	6.0	7.0	8.5	11.0	14.0	18.0	21.0	27.0
13	129	1,697	11.7	6.7	5.0	5.0	6.0	7.0	10.0	14.0	19.0	22.0	25.5
14	134	1,730	10.9	6.4	4.0	5.0	6.0	7.0	9.0	13.0	18.0	20.0	24.0
15	124	1,728	10.2	6.1	4.0	5.0	6.0	6.0	8.0	12.0	15.0	19.0	24.0
16	128	1,752	10.1	5.2	4.0	5.0	5.0	6.5	9.0	12.5	15.0	17.0	22.0
17	139	1,831	9.3	5.4	4.5	5.0	5.5	6.0	7.5	11.0	13.0	15.0	19.0
Black													
1	72	280	9.4	3.4	4.5	6.0	7.0	8.0	8.0	11.0	12.0	13.0	15.0
2	77	267	10.1	3.2	4.5	6.0	6.5	8.0	10.0	12.0	14.0	15.0	15.0
3	72	212	9.1	2.6	6.0	6.5	6.5	7.0	9.0	10.5	12.0	12.0	13.0
4	74	260	8.0	2.6	5.0	5.0	5.0	6.5	7.0	9.0	10.0	10.5	15.0
5	64	226	7.7	3.4	4.5	5.0	5.0	5.0	7.0	9.0	10.0	12.0	15.5
6	52	321	7.1	1.8	4.0	4.0	4.0	6.0	7.0	8.0	9.0	9.0	9.0
7	38	253	7.5	3.2	4.0	5.0	5.0	5.0	6.5	9.0	11.5	13.0	15.0
8	33	203	7.8	3.4	4.0	5.0	4.5	6.0	6.5	10.0	11.0	11.0	12.5
9	52	383	8.2	3.9	3.5	4.0	5.0	6.0	7.0	8.0	12.0	13.0	18.0
10	33	251	9.1	5.3	5.0	5.0	6.0	6.0	7.5	10.0	13.0	15.0	20.0
11	43	313	8.0	5.0	4.0	4.0	5.0	5.0	6.0	8.5	11.0	12.0	15.0
12	47	316	9.4	7.0	4.0	4.0	4.5	6.0	7.5	10.7	11.0	15.0	24.0
13	45	281	8.2	4.4	4.0	5.0	5.0	5.0	7.0	8.5	11.0	19.0	19.0
14	39	282	6.6	2.6	3.5	3.5	3.5	5.0	6.5	7.0	8.0	9.0	12.0
15	43	310	8.9	6.1	4.0	4.5	5.0	6.5	9.0	9.0	10.0	21.0	21.0
16	41	267	7.2	4.8	4.0	4.0	4.0	6.0	6.0	7.5	8.0	11.0	15.0
17	35	235	8.7	5.8	3.5	3.5	5.0	7.0	7.0	10.5	12.0	12.0	23.2

*Includes data for races that are not shown separately.
†Measurements made in the right arm.

(From the National Center for Health Statistics, Department of Health and Human Services. See also Bishop, C.W., Bowen, P.E., Ritchey, S.J. (1981) *Am. J. Clin. Nutr.*, **34** pp. 2530–9.)

Table II.53 Subscapular skinfold thickness: Boys, 1 to 17 years, United States, 1971 to 1974

Race and age in years	Number in sample	Estimated population in thousands	Mean[†]	Standard deviation	Percentile								
					5th	10th	15th	25th	50th	75th	85th	90th	95th
					Subscapular Skinfold in Millimeters								
All Races*													
1	286	1,693	6.2	1.9	4.0	4.0	4.0	5.0	6.0	7.0	8.0	8.5	10.0
2	298	1,747	5.7	2.0	3.0	4.0	4.0	4.5	5.0	6.5	7.0	8.0	10.0
3	308	1,807	5.4	2.0	3.5	4.0	4.0	4.0	5.0	6.0	6.8	7.0	9.5
4	304	1,815	5.1	1.7	3.0	3.5	4.0	4.0	5.0	6.0	6.0	7.0	7.0
5	273	1,563	5.3	2.7	3.0	3.5	4.0	4.0	4.5	6.0	7.0	7.0	8.0
6	179	1,673	5.1	2.4	3.0	3.0	3.5	4.0	4.5	5.0	6.0	7.0	9.0
7	164	1,979	5.5	3.0	3.0	3.0	3.5	4.0	4.5	6.0	7.0	9.0	11.0
8	152	1,861	5.1	2.3	3.0	3.5	4.0	4.0	4.5	6.0	6.0	7.5	9.0
9	169	2,019	7.1	5.1	3.5	4.0	4.0	4.0	5.0	8.0	11.0	14.0	14.0
10	184	2,205	6.8	4.5	3.5	4.0	4.0	4.0	5.5	7.0	10.0	12.0	18.0
11	178	2,177	8.0	6.2	4.0	4.0	4.0	4.5	6.0	8.5	13.0	15.0	19.0
12	200	2,304	8.0	6.0	3.5	4.0	4.5	5.0	6.0	9.0	11.0	14.0	20.5
13	174	1,978	8.8	6.9	3.5	4.0	4.5	5.0	6.5	9.0	13.5	17.0	26.0
14	174	2,030	8.5	6.1	4.0	4.5	5.0	5.0	6.5	9.0	13.0	16.0	20.0
15	171	2,093	9.1	6.5	4.0	5.0	5.0	5.5	7.0	10.0	13.0	15.5	23.0
16	169	2,019	9.8	6.2	5.0	5.5	6.0	6.5	8.0	10.5	13.5	16.5	23.5
17	176	2,095	9.7	5.9	5.0	5.5	6.0	7.0	8.0	10.0	13.0	16.0	23.0
White													
1	211	1,402	6.3	2.0	4.0	4.0	4.0	5.0	6.0	7.0	8.0	8.5	10.0
2	217	1,461	5.6	1.9	3.0	3.5	4.0	4.0	5.0	6.0	7.0	7.5	10.0
3	226	1,536	5.4	2.0	3.5	4.0	4.0	4.0	5.0	6.0	6.5	7.0	10.0
4	229	1,547	5.2	1.8	3.0	4.0	4.0	4.0	5.0	6.0	6.0	7.0	7.0
5	207	1,319	5.3	2.7	3.0	3.5	4.0	4.0	5.0	6.0	7.0	7.0	8.0
6	126	1,343	5.1	2.4	3.0	3.5	3.5	4.0	4.5	5.5	6.0	7.0	10.0
7	125	1,718	5.6	3.1	3.0	3.0	3.5	4.0	5.0	6.0	7.0	8.0	11.5
8	116	1,644	5.1	2.3	3.0	3.0	3.0	4.0	4.5	6.0	6.0	7.5	11.0
9	117	1,636	7.2	4.7	3.5	4.0	4.0	4.0	5.0	8.5	11.5	14.0	14.0
10	148	1,909	6.8	4.5	3.0	4.0	4.0	4.0	5.5	7.0	9.5	12.0	18.0
11	132	1,823	8.2	6.4	3.5	4.0	4.0	4.5	6.0	9.0	14.0	15.0	20.0
12	152	1,970	8.1	5.8	3.5	4.0	4.0	5.0	6.0	9.0	11.5	14.0	21.0
13	129	1,697	9.0	7.1	3.5	4.0	4.0	5.0	6.5	9.0	14.0	17.0	27.0
14	134	1,730	9.0	6.5	4.0	5.0	5.0	5.5	6.5	9.0	14.0	16.0	20.0
15	124	1,728	8.8	6.4	4.0	5.0	5.0	5.5	7.0	9.0	13.0	15.0	22.0
16	128	1,752	9.9	6.4	5.0	5.0	6.0	6.5	8.0	11.0	13.5	17.0	23.5
17	139	1,831	9.7	6.1	5.0	5.5	6.0	6.5	8.0	10.0	13.0	16.0	23.0

Table II.53 Continued

Race and age in years	Number in sample	Estimated population in thousands	Mean[†]	Standard deviation	Percentile								
					5th	10th	15th	25th	50th	75th	85th	90th	95th
Black													
1	72	280	6.0	1.6	4.0	4.0	4.0	5.0	6.0	7.0	7.5	8.0	9.0
2	77	267	6.5	2.4	4.0	4.0	4.0	5.0	5.5	7.0	10.0	11.5	11.5
3	72	212	5.3	1.6	3.5	4.0	4.0	4.0	5.0	6.0	6.5	6.5	9.0
4	74	260	4.8	1.2	3.0	3.0	3.5	4.0	5.0	5.1	6.0	6.0	8.0
5	64	226	5.1	2.5	2.5	3.0	3.0	4.0	4.5	5.0	7.0	7.0	8.5
6	52	321	4.9	2.1	3.0	3.0	3.5	4.0	5.0	5.0	5.5	7.0	7.0
7	38	253	5.2	2.4	3.0	3.0	3.0	3.5	4.0	6.0	8.0	10.0	11.0
8	33	203	5.5	2.1	3.5	3.5	4.0	4.0	5.0	6.0	7.5	9.0	9.0
9	52	383	6.6	6.3	3.0	3.0	3.0	4.0	5.0	6.0	8.0	8.0	30.0
10	33	251	6.7	3.8	4.0	4.0	4.0	4.5	5.0	7.0	9.0	12.0	18.5
11	43	313	6.7	4.9	4.0	4.0	4.0	5.0	5.5	6.5	8.0	8.0	12.5
12	47	316	7.4	6.9	4.0	4.0	4.5	4.5	5.0	7.0	7.0	17.0	19.0
13	45	281	7.6	5.9	4.0	4.5	4.5	5.0	6.0	7.0	8.0	18.5	26.0
14	39	282	6.1	2.1	4.0	4.0	5.0	5.0	6.0	7.0	7.0	7.5	12.0
15	43	310	10.6	6.7	4.0	5.0	5.5	7.0	9.0	12.0	12.0	24.0	24.0
16	41	267	8.5	4.2	5.5	5.5	6.5	6.5	7.0	9.0	9.5	10.0	16.0
17	35	235	9.6	5.2	6.0	6.0	6.0	7.0	8.0	10.0	12.0	16.0	16.0

*Includes data for races that are not shown separately.
†Measurements made in the right arm.
(From the National Center for Health Statistics, Department of Health and Human Services. See also Bishop, C.W., Bowen, P.E., Ritchey, S.J. (1981) *Am. J. Clin. Nutr.*, **34** pp. 2530–9.)

Table II.54 Selected percentiles of weight, triceps and subscapular skinfolds, and bone-free upper arm muscle area (AMA) for United States men and women with small frames (25 to 54 years old)

Ht (in)	Ht (cm)	n	Wt (kg)							Triceps (mm)							Subscapular (mm)							Bone-free AMA (cm²)						
			5	10	15	50	85	90	95	5	10	15	50	85	90	95	5	10	15	50	85	90	95	5	10	15	50	85	90	95
Men																														
62	157	23	46*	50*	52*	64	71*	74*	77*				11	17						16	20						52			
63	160	43	48*	51*	53	61	70	75*	79*			6	10	17					8	12	25	29				32	48	54		
64	163	73	49*	53	55	66	76	76	80*			5	10	16	18	21		7	7	15	25	28	35		37	38	49	58	63	71
65	165	112	52	53	58	66	77	81	84	4	5	6	11	17	19	20	7	8	9	14	26	26	32	31	35	37	47	60	63	71
66	168	129	56	57	59	67	78	83	84	5	5	6	11	18	18	22	7	8	8	14	23	25	30	31	36	38	49	60	62	62
67	170	132	56	60	62	71	82	83	88	5	6	6	11	18	20	20	6	7	9	15	24	30	40	35	39	41	49	58	60	62
68	173	107	56	59	62	71	79	82	85	5	6	6	10	15	16		7	8	7	13	24	26		33	37	40	49	59	62	69
69	175	97	57*	62	65	74	84	87	88*		6	6	11	17	20			7	7	13	23				36	40	58	61	63	
70	178	46	59*	62*	67	75	79	86*	90*			7	10	17					9	14	22					35	48	57		
71	180	49	60*	64*	70	76	79	88*	91*			7	10	16					8	13						39	47	52		
72	183	21	62*	65*	67*	74	87*	89*	93*				10							14							45			
73	185	9	63*	67*	69*	79*	89*	91*	94*																					
74	188	6	65*	68*	71*	80*	90*	92*	96*																					
Women																														
58	147	53	37*	43	43	52	58	62	66*	8	12	13	24	30	33		6	10	12	23	34	38		17	22	24	29	36	44	
59	150	108	42	43	44	53	63	69	72	8	11	14	21	29	36	37	6	9	10	17	29	32	34	19	20	22	28	38	39	43
60	152	142	42	44	45	53	63	65	70	8	11	12	21	28	29	33	7	7	8	18	27	32	34	20	21	22	28	36	40	44
61	155	218	44	46	47	54	64	66	72	11	12	14	21	28	31	34	6	8	9	16	28	32	39	20	21	23	28	38	39	44
62	157	255	44	47	48	55	63	64	70	10	12	14	20	28	31	36	6	7	8	14	22	27	36	20	21	21	27	33	35	42
63	160	239	46	48	49	55	65	68	79	10	11	13	20	27	30	34	6	7	7	14	27	29	32	22	21	22	27	33	35	37
64	163	146	49	50	51	57	67	68	74	10	13	13	20	28	30	34	7	7	8	13	24	27	31	21	23	23	28	34	38	38
65	165	113	50	52	53	60	70	72	80	12	13	14	22	29	31			8	8	15	26	30	34		22	23	28	37	39	42
66	168	47	46*	49*	54	58	65	71*	74*			12	19	30					9	12	25		33			23	27	35		47
67	170	18	47*	50*	52*	59	70*	72*	76*				18							13							26			
68	173	18	48*	51*	53*	62	71*	73*	77*				20							15							25			
69	175	5	49*	52*	54*	63*	72*	74*	78*																					
70	178	1	50*	53*	55*	64*	73*	75*	79*																					

*Value estimated through linear regression equation.

(From Frisancho, A.R. (1984) *Am. J. Clin. Nutr.* **40** pp. 808–19, with permission.)

Table II.55 Selected percentiles of weight, triceps and subscapular skinfolds, and bone-free upper arm muscle area (AMA) for United States men and women with medium frames (25 to 54 years old)

Ht in	Ht cm	n	Wt (kg) 5	10	15	50	85	90	95	Triceps (mm) 5	10	15	50	85	90	95	Subscapular (mm) 5	10	15	50	85	90	95	Bone-free AMA (cm²) 5	10	15	50	85	90	95
Men																													
62	157	10	51*	55*	58*	68	81*	83*	87*				15							13							58			
63	160	30	52*	56*	59*	71	82*	85*	89*				11							18							55			
64	163	71	54*	60	61	71	83	84	90*		6	6	12	18	20		8	7	9	17	30	32			43	47	56	67	71	
65	165	154	59	62	65	74	87	90	94	5	7	8	12	20	22	25	7	9	10	16	26	29	32	40	43	45	56	67	69	70
66	168	212	58	61	65	75	85	87	93	5	6	7	11	16	18	22	8	7	9	16	25	27	33	38	42	44	55	69	72	78
67	170	409	62	66	68	77	89	93	100	5	7	7	13	21	23	28	7	9	10	18	26	30	33	39	42	44	53	66	69	73
68	173	478	60	64	66	78	89	92	97	4	5	7	11	18	20	24	7	8	9	16	25	28	31	41	44	45	55	67	71	76
69	175	464	63	66	68	78	90	93	97	5	6	7	12	18	20	24	7	8	9	16	25	27	31	38	41	44	54	66	69	73
70	178	419	64	66	70	81	90	93	97	5	6	7	12	18	20	23	7	8	9	15	24	27	30	39	42	43	55	65	68	72
71	180	282	62	68	70	81	92	96	100	4	5	7	12	19	21	25	7	8	9	14	24	27	30	37	41	44	54	67	68	73
72	183	231	68	71	74	84	97	100	104	5	7	7	12	20	22	26	7	8	9	15	26	30	32	40	42	44	55	65	67	74
73	185	106	70	72	75	85	100	101	104	6	7	8	12	20	24	27	8	9	9	15	25	29	32	39	43	43	55	67	69	73
74	188	50	68*	76	77	88	100	100	104*		6	9	13	21	23			7	9	14	25	30			43	43		62	63	
Women																													
58	147	40	41*	46*	50	63	77	75*	79*	15	19	20	25	40	40	40	10	12	15	23	38	39	43	23	24	24	35	42	45	49
59	150	104	47	50	52	66	76	79	85	14	15	21	30	37	37	41	8	10	13	29	38	37	41	22	25	26	33	43	45	49
60	152	208	47	50	52	60	77	79	85	11	14	17	26	35	36	42	7	9	11	22	35	36	42	21	24	25	32	42	45	51
61	155	465	47	49	51	61	73	78	86	12	14	15	25	34	36	40	7	9	10	19	32	37	40	21	23	25	31	42	43	48
62	157	644	49	50	52	61	73	77	83	12	13	16	24	34	35	38	7	8	10	18	33	34	38	22	23	25	31	40	43	50
63	160	685	50	51	53	62	77	80	88	11	14	15	24	33	36	40	7	7	10	18	31	35	38	21	23	24	32	41	43	48
64	163	722	50	52	54	62	76	82	87	12	14	15	23	33	34	38	7	8	8	16	31	33	38	21	23	24	31	40	43	49
65	165	628	52	54	55	63	75	80	89	11	13	15	22	31	33	37	7	8	8	15	29	30	35	21	23	24	31	40	41	44
66	168	428	52	54	55	63	75	78	83	12	13	14	22	31	30	35	7	8	9	14	28	32	37	22	24	25	30	39	44	48
67	170	257	54	56	57	65	79	82	88	10	14	15	21	29	32	36	8	8	8	15	28	33	35	22	24	25	30	40	43	39
68	173	119	58	59	60	67	77	85	87		11	15	22	31	31			8	9	15	29	29		23	23	24	30	37	38	
69	175	59	49*	58	60	68	79	82	87*			12	19	29					8	12	25						32	36	39	
70	178	15	50*	54*	57*	70	80*	83*	87*				19							20										

*Value estimated through linear regression equation.

(From Frisancho, A.R. (1984) *Am. J. Clin. Nutr.*, **40** pp. 808–19, with permission.)

Table II.56 Selected percentiles of weight, triceps and subscapular skinfolds, and bone-free upper arm muscle area (AMA) for United States men and women with large frames (25 to 54 years old)

Ht (in)	Ht (cm)	n	Wt (kg)							Triceps (mm)							Subscapular (mm)							Bone-free AMA (cm²)						
			5	10	15	50	85	90	95	5	10	15	50	85	90	95	5	10	15	50	85	90	95	5	10	15	50	85	90	95
Men																														
62	157	1	57*	62*	66*	82*	99*	103*	108*																					
63	160	1	58*	63*	67*	83*	100*	104*	109*																					
64	163	5	59*	64*	68*	84*	101*	105*	110*																					
65	165	15	60*	65*	69*	79	102*	106*	111*				14							21										
66	168	37	60*	65*	75	84	103	106*	112*			9	14	30						22	36					48	62	76		
67	170	54	62*	70	71	84	102	111	113*			7	11	23	27		8		13	20	36	40			50	52	58	73	78	
68	173	84	63*	74	76	86	101	104	114*		7	10	14	22	23		12	12	11	20	31	35			51	53	61	73	78	86
69	175	126	68	71	74	89	103	105	114		9	8	15	25	29	31	10	10	11	18	31	32	38	46	48	49	65	78	86	83
70	178	150	68	72	74	87	106	112	114	7	7	7	14	23	25	30	7	10	11	17	31	35	38	43	47	50	61	73	77	86
71	180	123	73	78	82	91	113	116	123	9	8	10	15	25	27	31	9	11	11	20	35	40	46	47	48	50	62	75	81	83
72	183	114	73	76	78	91	109	112	121	7	6	7	12	20	22	25	8	9	9	19	28	30	36	45	48	50	61	75	80	86
73	185	109	72	77	79	93	106	107	116	6	6	7	13	19	22	30	7	9	9	18	27	28	30	47	49	51	66	79	80	83
74	188	37	69*	74*	82	92	105	115*	120*	5		8	12	19	22	31			9	18	32					53	66	78	83	
Women																														
58	147	6	56*	63*	67*	86*	105*	110*	117*				36							35							45			
59	150	19	56*	62*	67*	78	105*	109*	116*				38							42							44			
60	152	32	55*	62*	66*	87	104*	109*	116*		25	26	36	48	50	50				35	48	53	55				41	62	74	72
61	155	92	54*	64	66	81	105	117	115*	16	19	22	34	48	48	51	13	17	17	32	48	51	50	26	29	33	44	56	63	77
62	157	135	59	61	65	81	103	107	113	18	20	22	34	46	48	49	11	16	18	32	44	48	50	27	28	31	43	60	65	63
63	160	162	58	63	67	83	105	109	119	16	20	21	32	43	45	48	10	14	16	28	42	46	52	26	30	32	39	50	55	67
64	163	196	59	62	63	79	102	104	112	16	20	21	31	43	46	45	10	12	15	29	42	48	45	27	28	29	39	56	59	69
65	165	242	59	61	63	81	103	109	114	17	17	18	27	40	43	49	8	12	14	25	36	40	55	23	24	27	35	49	53	55
66	168	166	55	58	62	75	95	100	107	13	16	17	30	41	43		7	9	11	25	41	46		25	28	30	37	50	53	
67	170	144	58	60	65	80	100	108	114	13	16	20	29	37	40			10	11	21	45	48			28	30	38	51	54	
68	173	81	51*	66	66	76	104	105	111*			21	30	42				10	12	20	43					27	35	49		
69	175	39	50*	57*	68	79	105	104*	111*				20						11	16							37			
70	178	17	50*	56*	61*	76	99*	104*	110*											16							37			

*Value estimated through linear regression equation.
(From Frisancho, A.R. (1984) *Am. J. Clin. Nutr.*, **40** pp. 808–19, with permission.)

Table II.57 Selected percentiles of weight, triceps and subscapular skinfolds, and bone-free upper arm muscle area (AMA) for United States men and women with small frames (55 to 74 years old)

Ht (in)	Ht (cm)	n	Wt (kg) 5	10	15	50	85	90	95	Triceps (mm) 5	10	15	50	85	90	95	Subscapular (mm) 5	10	15	50	85	90	95	Bone-free AMA (cm²) 5	10	15	50	85	90	95
Men																														
62	157	47	45*	49*	56	61	68	73*	77*			6	9	12					11	16	23					38	46	52		
63	160	78	47*	49	51	62	71	71	79*		5	5	10	16	17			6	6	12	21	22			34	35	43	54	55	
64	163	107	47	50	54	63	72	74	80	4	4	4	9	20	21	22	6	6	7	14	24	25	29	26	30	31	44	53	54	56
65	165	132	48	54	59	70	80	90	90	5	6	7	11	18	19	24	6	7	8	16	28	28	29	26	30	34	48	57	60	62
66	168	112	51	55	59	68	77	80	84	5	6	7	11	16	20	20	7	7	8	15	25	26	30	25	31	35	45	54	58	64
67	170	128	55	60	61	69	79	81	88	5	6	6	10	15	17	25	7	8	9	13	22	25	31	30	36	37	45	53	55	59
68	173	95	54*	54	58	70	79	81	86*		5	5	10	15	17			7	7	13	21	22			35	35	43	55	60	
69	175	47	56*	59*	63	75	81	84*	88*			6	10	15					10	16	27					38	47	62		
70	178	29	57*	61*	63*	76	83*	86*	89*				11							13							48			
71	180	14	59*	62*	65*	69	85*	87*	91*				9							10							43			
72	183	6	60*	64*	66*	76*	86*	89*	92*																					
73	185	1	62*	65*	68*	78*	88*	90*	94*																					
74	188	1	63*	67*	69*	77*	89*	92*	95*																					
Women																														
58	147	85	39*	46	48	54	63	65	71*	11	14	16	21	31	34	33	6	8	9	18	32	33	33	22	22	23	29	40	42	44
59	150	122	41	45	48	55	66	68	74	10	13	15	21	30	31	35	5	7	9	19	29	30	36	20	23	24	30	39	40	44
60	152	157	43	45	47	54	67	70	73	10	11	13	20	29	31	32	6	7	8	15	27	32	32	18	22	23	30	37	41	42
61	155	145	43	43	45	56	65	70	71	11	12	14	22	29	29	32	7	7	8	17	29	31	30	20	21	23	28	36	40	43
62	157	158	47	49	52	58	67	69	73		11	12	21	29	30			8	9	17	25	26			23	24	30	37	40	
63	160	89	42*	45	49	58	67	68	74*		12	13	20	29	30			6	7	14	25	27			19	20	27	35	36	
64	163	50	43*	47	49	60	68	70	75*			13	21	27	29				7	18	24	25				21	28	37	42	
65	165	26	43*	47*	49*	60	69*	72*	75*				18							13							28			
66	168	12	44*	48*	50*	68	70*	72*	76*				23							13							33			
67	170	1	45*	48*	51*	61*	71*	73*	77*																					
68	173	1	45*	49*	51*	61*	71*	74*	77*																					
69	175	0	46*	49*	52*	62*	72*	74*	78*																					
70	178	0	47*	50*	52*	63*	73*	75*	79*																					

*Value estimated through linear regression equation.
(From Frisancho, A.R. (1984) *Am. J. Clin. Nutr.*, **40** pp. 808–19, with permission.)

Table II.58 Selected percentiles of weight, triceps and subscapular skinfolds, and bone-free upper arm muscle area (AMA) for United States men and women with medium frames (55 to 74 years old)

Ht			Wt (kg)							Triceps (mm)							Subscapular (mm)							Bone-free AMA (cm²)						
in	cm	n	5	10	15	50	85	90	95	5	10	15	50	85	90	95	5	10	15	50	85	90	95	5	10	15	50	85	90	95
Men																														
62	157	49	50*	54*	59	68	77	81*	85*			5	12	25	23				11	19	27					39	48	61		
63	160	89	51*	57	60	70	80	82	87*		7	7	11	20	20			8	10	15	26	28			36	38	50	60	63	
64	163	210	55	59	62	71	82	83	91	5	6	6	10	17	20	26	6	7	9	15	25	27	35	35	39	40	51	64	66	71
65	165	335	56	60	64	72	83	86	89	5	6	7	11	17	19	24	7	8	9	17	25	29	31	35	38	41	52	63	65	72
66	168	405	57	62	66	74	83	84	89	6	6	7	12	18	19	22	7	9	10	16	25	28	31	34	39	42	51	60	62	67
67	170	509	59	64	66	78	87	89	94	5	6	7	12	18	20	23	7	9	10	17	26	29	34	35	39	42	52	65	67	70
68	173	413	62	66	68	78	89	95	101	6	7	8	12	18	21	23	7	8	10	17	26	29	32	37	40	42	52	65	67	70
69	175	366	62	66	68	77	90	93	99	5	6	7	12	19	22	25	6	8	9	16	25	28	30	31	36	40	51	62	65	72
70	178	248	62	68	71	80	90	95	101	6	7	7	11	18	19	21	7	9	10	16	25	27	30	36	41	44	53	63	67	68
71	180	146	68	70	72	84	94	97	101	5	6	6	11	16	17	20	7	9	10	15	25	26	31	36	42	44	56	65	59	71
72	183	81	66*	65	69	81	96	97	101*		6	8	11	19	20			8	10	16	28	30			27	39	50	58		
73	185	35	68*	72*	79	88	93	99*	103*			8	13	16					10	15	26					43	56	67		
74	188	11	69*	73*	76*	95	98*	101*	104*				11							18							56			
Women																														
58	147	105	40	44	49	57	72	82	85	5	13	17	28	40	40	41	3	7	10	25	37	43	48	21	23	25	32	46	47	51
59	150	198	47	49	52	62	74	78	86	12	15	18	26	34	38	41	8	9	11	23	32	36	43	24	26	27	35	44	48	48
60	152	358	47	50	52	65	76	79	86	13	17	18	25	33	34	38	8	10	12	22	34	36	40	21	24	26	35	45	49	57
61	155	543	49	51	54	64	78	81	86	13	16	18	25	35	37	42	8	10	10	20	33	36	42	22	24	26	34	44	49	52
62	157	576	49	53	54	64	78	82	88	13	15	17	24	33	36	39	7	8	10	20	33	36	38	24	25	26	35	45	47	54
63	160	551	52	54	55	65	79	83	89	12	14	16	24	32	35	38	8	8	10	18	32	37	38	24	26	27	35	44	45	51
64	163	406	51	54	57	66	78	81	87	12	14	16	25	33	34	37	7	9	10	17	30	33	41	21	26	26	33	44	46	49
65	165	307	54	56	59	67	78	84	88	14	16	17	24	33	35	39	7	8	9	17	30	35	38	24	25	27	34	44	45	49
66	168	119	54	57	57	66	79	85	88	12	13	16	24	33	33	36	6	7	8	16	30	31	37	24	26	27	33	41	43	50
67	170	63	51*	59	61	72	82	85	89*		17	17	27	35	35			9	10	19	35	35	34		27	28	32	41	43	49
68	173	28	52*	56*	59*	70	83*	86*	90*				25							16							36			
69	175	5	53*	57*	60*	72*	84*	87*	91*																					
70	178	1	54*	58*	61*	73*	85*	88*	92*																					

*Value estimated through linear regression equation.

(From Frisancho, A.R. (1984) *Am. J. Clin. Nutr.*, **40** pp. 808–19, with permission.)

Table II.59 Selected percentiles of weight, triceps and subscapular skinfolds, and bone-free upper arm muscle area (AMA) for United States men and women with large frames (55 to 74 years old)

Ht		n	Wt (kg)							Triceps (mm)							Subscapular (mm)							Bone-free AMA (cm²)						
in	cm		5	10	15	50	85	90	95	5	10	15	50	85	90	95	5	10	15	50	85	90	95	5	10	15	50	85	90	95
Men																														
62	157	7	54*	59*	63*	77*	91*	95*	100*				15							20							57			
63	160	12	55*	60*	64*	80	92*	96*	101*				21							31							44			
64	163	20	57*	62*	65*	77	94*	97*	102*																					
65	165	36	58*	63*	73	79	89	98*	103*			11	14	22					14	19	27					44	59	66		
66	168	58	59*	67	73	80	101	102	105*		7	8	13	21	25			9	11	20	31	35			43	47	56	67	72	
67	170	114	65	71	73	85	103	108	112	6	8	9	16	21	25	27	8	11	12	20	35	35	38	41	43	44	56	71	73	79
68	173	128	67	71	73	83	95	98	111	6	7	8	13	20	21	23	8	10	11	18	27	30	32	41	43	46	57	69	70	74
69	175	131	65	70	74	84	96	98	105	6	7	8	12	18	20	23	7	11	11	19	27	30	33	40	45	45	58	70	72	79
70	178	144	68	73	77	87	102	104	117	5	6	8	14	22	25	31	9	11	13	20	30	33	37	43	48	50	59	70	71	87
71	180	95	68	70	70	84	102	109	111*		6	6	13	18	22			8	9	15	30	30			46	47	54	70	75	
72	183	72	67*	76	81	90	108	112	112*		8	8	13	23	26			8	9	20	28	31			47	48	59	73	78	
73	185	23	68*	73*	76*	88	105*	108*	113*				11							19							59			
74	188	15	69*	74*	78*	89	106*	109*	114*				12							15							54			
Women																														
58	147	14	53*	59*	63*	92	95*	99*	104*				45							44							50			
59	150	26	54*	59*	63*	78	95*	99*	105*			26	36						21	31						33	49			
60	152	72	54*	65	69	78	87	88	105*	18	25	24	35	44	45	46	13	19	19	31	42	45	48	31	28	34	41	58	60	71
61	155	117	64	68	69	79	94	95	106	19	22	24	33	40	44	50	13	16	22	29	40	43	53	28	32	34	44	59	61	76
62	157	126	59	61	63	82	93	101	111	20	24	25	32	40	43	45	13	19	16	30	39	48	51	27	29	33	43	59	63	67
63	160	154	61	65	67	80	100	102	118	18	24	23	33	41	43	50	10	15	16	29	40	45	55	28	32	32	41	56	62	78
64	163	147	60	65	67	77	97	102	119	15	22	20	29	42	46	46	8	12	12	24	41	46	48	29	29	32	41	54	60	65
65	165	117	60	66	69	80	98	102	111		17	18	30	43	44			9	12	26	42	46			32	31	42	53	57	
66	168	64	57*	60	63	82	98	105	109*		18	22	27	35	40			9	14	26	34	36			31	30	40	57	58	
67	170	40	58*	64*	68	80	105	104*	109*				32	44						25	46						40	58		
68	173	17	58*	64*	68*	79	100*	104*	110*				26							21							48			
69	175	7	59*	65*	69*	85*	101*	105*	110*																				
70	178	2	60*	65*	69*	85*	101*	105*	111*																				

*Value estimated through linear regression equation.

(From Frisancho, A.R. (1984) *Am. J. Clin. Nutr.,* **40** pp. 808–19, with permission.)

Table II.60   Midarm muscle circumference in adults (18 to 74 years), United States*†

Age group (years)	Sample size	Estimated population (millions)	Mean (cm)	Percentile 5th	10th	25th	50th	75th	90th	95th
Men										
18–74	5,261	61.18	28.0	23.8	24.8	26.3	27.9	29.6	31.4	32.5
18–24	773	11.78	27.4	23.5	24.4	25.8	27.2	28.9	30.8	32.3
25–34	804	13.00	28.3	24.2	25.3	26.5	28.0	30.0	31.7	32.9
35–44	664	10.68	28.8	25.0	25.6	27.1	28.7	30.3	32.1	33.0
45–54	765	11.15	28.2	24.0	24.9	26.5	28.1	29.8	31.5	32.6
55–64	598	9.07	27.8	22.8	24.4	26.2	27.9	29.6	31.0	31.8
65–74	1,657	5.50	26.8	22.5	23.7	25.3	26.9	28.5	29.9	30.7
Women										
18–74	8,410	67.84	22.2	18.4	19.0	20.2	21.8	23.6	25.8	27.4
18–24	1,523	12.89	20.9	17.7	18.5	19.4	20.6	22.1	23.6	24.9
25–34	1,896	13.93	21.7	18.3	18.9	20.0	21.4	22.9	24.9	26.6
35–44	1,664	11.59	22.5	18.5	19.2	20.6	22.0	24.0	26.1	27.4
45–54	836	12.16	22.7	18.8	19.5	20.7	22.2	24.3	26.6	27.8
55–64	669	9.98	22.8	18.6	19.5	20.8	22.6	24.4	26.3	28.1
65–74	1,822	7.28	22.8	18.6	19.5	20.8	22.5	24.4	26.5	28.1

*Measurements made in the right arm.
†See Tables II.54 through II.59 for data compiled by Frisancho, A.R. (1984) *Am. J. Clin. Nutr.*, **40** pp. 808–19, from NHANES I and II.
(From Bishop, C.W., Bowen, P.E., Ritchey, S.J. (1981) *Am. J. Clin. Nutr.*, **34** pp. 2530–9, [NHANES 1].)

Table II.61   Midarm muscle area in adults (18 to 74 years), United States*†

Age group (years)	Sample size	Estimated population (millions)	Mean (cm)	Percentile 5th	10th	25th	50th	75th	90th	95th
Men										
18–74	5,261	61.18	62.4	45.1	49.0	55.1	62.0	69.8	78.5	84.1
18–24	773	11.78	59.8	44.0	47.4	53.0	58.9	66.5	75.5	83.1
25–34	804	13.00	63.8	46.6	51.0	55.9	62.4	71.7	80.0	86.2
35–44	664	10.68	66.0	49.8	52.2	58.5	65.6	73.1	82.0	86.7
45–54	765	11.15	63.3	45.9	49.4	55.9	62.9	70.7	79.0	84.6
55–64	598	9.07	61.5	41.4	47.4	54.7	62.0	69.8	76.5	80.5
65–74	1,657	5.50	57.2	40.3	44.7	51.0	57.6	64.7	71.2	75.0
Women										
18–74	8,410	67.84	39.2	27.0	28.7	32.5	37.8	44.3	53.0	59.8
18–24	1,523	12.89	34.8	24.9	27.2	30.0	33.8	38.9	44.3	49.4
25–34	1,896	13.93	37.5	26.7	28.4	31.8	36.5	41.8	49.4	56.3
35–44	1,664	11.59	40.3	27.2	29.4	33.8	38.5	45.9	54.2	59.8
45–54	836	12.16	41.0	28.1	30.3	34.1	39.2	47.0	56.3	61.5
55–64	669	9.98	41.4	27.5	30.3	34.4	40.7	47.4	55.1	62.9
65–74	1,822	7.28	41.4	27.5	30.3	34.4	40.3	47.4	55.9	62.9

*Measurements made in the right arm.
†See Tables II.54 through II.59 for data compiled by Frisancho, A.R. (1984) *Am. J. Clin. Nutr.*, **40** pp. 808–19, from NHANES I and II.
(From Bishop, C.W., Bowen, P.E., Ritchey, S.J. (1981) *Am. J. Clin. Nutr.*, **34** pp. 2530–9, [NHANES 1].)

Table II.62 Age correction for estimates of weight, triceps and subscapular skinfold thicknesses, and bone-free upper arm muscle area (AMA)

Age group: Frame size	Median age	Weight	Triceps skinfold	Subscapular skinfold	Arm muscle area
Men					
25–54					
Small	39	0.074	0.016	0.080	0.030
Medium	39	0.080	0.005	0.083	0.055
Large	40	0.000	−0.024	0.049	0.026
55–74					
Small	66	−0.329	−0.036	−0.115	−0.407
Medium	67	−0.435	−0.040	−0.125	−0.521
Large	67	−0.562	−0.054	−0.185	−0.644
Women					
25–54					
Small	37	0.165	0.166	0.142	0.087
Medium	37	0.234	0.189	0.214	0.191
Large	37	0.284	0.191	0.233	0.270
55–74					
Small	67	−0.027	−0.072	−0.013	0.036
Medium	66	−0.196	−0.210	−0.221	−0.033
Large	67	−0.466	−0.370	−0.515	−0.378

(From Frisancho, A.R. (1984) *Am. J. Clin. Nutr.*, **40** pp. 808–19, with permission.)

Table II.63 Provisional percentiles for triceps skinfold thickness in the elderly*[†]

Age group (years)	Percentile		
	5th	50th	95th
Men			
65	8.6	13.8	27.0
70	7.7	12.9	26.1
75	6.8	12.0	25.2
80	6.0	11.2	24.3
85	5.1	10.3	23.4
90	4.2	9.4	22.6
Women			
65	13.5	21.6	33.0
70	12.5	20.6	32.0
75	11.5	19.6	31.0
80	10.5	18.6	30.0
85	9.5	17.6	29.0
90	8.5	16.6	28.0

*Data are from 119 men and 150 women. All subjects were ambulatory, and measurements were made in the recumbent position on the left side.
[†]See Tables II.54 and II.55 for data compiled by Frisancho, A.R. (1984) *Am. J. Clin. Nutr.*, **40** pp. 808–19, from NHANES I and II.
(From Chumlea, W.C., Roche, A.F., Mukherjee, D. (1984) *Nutritional Assessment of the Elderly Through Anthropometry*, Wright State University School of Medicine, Ohio.)

Table II.64 Provisional percentiles for midarm muscle area (cm^2) in the elderly*[†]

Age group (years)	Percentile		
	5th	50th	95th
Men			
65	43.2	59.4	77.1
70	41.4	57.7	75.3
75	39.6	55.9	73.5
80	37.8	54.1	71.7
85	36.0	52.3	69.9
90	34.3	50.5	68.2
Women			
65	33.5	44.5	66.4
70	33.0	44.1	65.9
75	32.6	43.6	65.5
80	32.2	43.2	65.1
85	31.8	42.8	64.7
90	31.3	42.4	64.2

*Data are from 119 men and 150 women. All subjects were ambulatory, and measurements were made in the recumbent position on the left side.
[†]See Tables II.54 and II.55 for data compiled by Frisancho, A.R. (1984) *Am. J. Clin. Nutr.*, **40** pp. 808–19, from NHANES I and II.
(From Chumlea, W.C., Roche, A.F., Mukherjee, D. (1984) *Nutritional Assessment of the Elderly Through Anthropometry*, Wright State University School of Medicine, Ohio.)

Various investigators have developed equations for predicting the propotions of body fat by anthropometric measures of specific regions. Durnin and Womersley used four different skinfolds (Table II.66). Pollock, Schmidt, and Jackson have prepared tables based on three sites, including thigh skinfolds (Tables II.66 and II.67). Because some technicians have difficulty in obtaining consistent results with thigh skinfold measurements, data also are available based on other equations that do not use this skinfold. These data are included in the following sources:

Golding, L.A., Meyers, C.R., Sinning, W.E. (1989) *Y's Way to Physical Fitness: The Complete Guide to Fitness Testing and Instruction*, 3rd ed., Human Kinetics Publishers, Champaign, IL.

Pollock, M.L., Schmidt, D.H., Jackson, A.S. (1980) *Compr. Ther.*, **6**, pp. 12–27.

Jackson, A.S. and Pollock, M.L. (1985) *Phys. Sportsmed.*, **13**, pp. 76–90.

Table II.65 Equivalent fat content, as percentage of body weight, for a range of values for the sum of four skinfolds*

Skinfolds (mm)	Men (age in years)				Women (age in years)			
	17–29	30–39	40–49	50+	16–29	30–39	40–49	50+
15	4.8				10.5			
20	8.1	12.2	12.2	12.6	14.1	17.0	19.8	21.4
25	10.5	14.2	15.0	15.6	16.8	19.4	22.2	24.0
30	12.9	16.2	17.7	18.6	19.5	21.8	24.5	26.6
35	14.7	17.7	19.6	20.8	21.5	23.7	26.4	28.5
40	16.4	19.2	21.4	22.9	23.4	25.5	28.2	30.3
45	17.7	20.4	23.0	24.7	25.0	26.9	29.6	31.9
50	19.0	21.5	24.6	26.5	26.5	28.2	31.0	33.4
55	20.1	22.5	25.9	27.9	27.8	29.4	32.1	34.6
60	21.2	23.5	27.1	29.2	29.1	30.6	33.2	35.7
65	22.2	24.3	28.2	30.4	30.2	31.6	34.1	36.7
70	23.1	25.1	29.3	31.6	31.2	32.5	35.0	37.7
75	24.0	25.9	30.3	32.7	32.2	33.4	35.9	38.7
80	24.8	26.6	31.2	33.8	33.1	34.3	36.7	39.6
85	25.5	27.2	32.1	34.8	34.0	35.1	37.5	40.4
90	26.2	27.8	33.0	35.8	34.8	35.8	38.3	41.2
95	26.9	28.4	33.7	36.6	35.6	36.5	39.0	41.9
100	27.6	29.0	34.4	37.4	36.4	37.2	39.7	42.6
105	28.2	29.6	35.1	38.2	37.1	37.9	40.4	43.3
110	28.8	30.1	35.8	39.0	37.8	38.6	41.0	43.9
115	29.4	30.6	36.4	39.7	38.4	39.1	41.5	44.5
120	30.0	31.1	37.0	40.4	39.0	39.6	42.0	45.1
125	31.0	31.5	37.6	41.1	39.6	40.1	42.5	45.7
130	31.5	31.9	38.2	41.8	40.2	40.6	43.0	46.2
135	32.0	32.3	38.7	42.4	40.8	41.1	43.5	46.7
140	32.5	32.7	39.2	43.0	41.3	41.6	44.0	47.2
145	32.9	33.1	39.7	43.6	41.8	42.1	44.5	47.7
150	33.3	33.5	40.2	44.1	42.3	42.6	45.0	48.2
155	33.7	33.9	40.7	44.6	42.8	43.1	45.4	48.7
160	34.1	34.3	41.2	45.1	43.3	43.6	45.8	49.2
165	34.5	34.6	41.6	45.6	43.7	44.0	46.2	49.6
170	34.9	34.8	42.0	46.1	44.1	44.4	46.6	50.0
175	35.3					44.8	47.0	50.4
180	35.6					45.2	47.4	50.8
185	35.9					45.6	47.8	51.2
190						45.9	48.2	51.6
195						46.2	48.5	52.0
200						46.5	48.8	52.4
205							49.1	52.7
210							49.4	53.0

*Biceps, triceps, subscapular, and suprailiac of men and women of different ages.

(From Durnin, J.V.G.A., Womersley, J. (1974) *Br. J. Nutr.*, **32** pp. 77–97, with permission.)

Table II.66   Percentage of body fat estimation for women from age and triceps, suprailium, and thigh skinfolds*

Sum of skinfolds (mm)	Age to the last year								
	Under 22	23 to 27	28 to 32	33 to 37	38 to 42	43 to 47	48 to 52	53 to 57	Over 58
23–25	9.7	9.9	10.2	10.4	10.7	10.9	11.2	11.4	11.7
26–28	11.0	11.2	11.5	11.7	12.0	12.3	12.5	12.7	13.0
29–31	12.3	12.5	12.8	13.0	13.3	13.5	13.8	14.0	14.3
32–34	13.6	13.8	14.0	14.3	14.5	14.8	15.0	15.3	15.5
35–37	14.8	15.0	15.3	15.5	15.8	16.0	16.3	16.5	16.8
38–40	16.0	16.3	16.5	16.7	17.0	17.2	17.5	17.7	18.0
41–43	17.2	17.4	17.7	17.9	18.2	18.4	18.7	18.9	19.2
44–46	18.3	18.6	18.8	19.1	19.3	19.6	19.8	20.1	20.3
47–49	19.5	19.7	20.0	20.2	20.5	20.7	21.0	21.2	21.5
50–52	20.6	20.8	21.1	21.3	21.6	21.8	22.1	22.3	22.6
53–55	21.7	21.9	22.1	22.4	22.6	22.9	23.1	23.4	23.6
56–58	22.7	23.0	23.2	23.4	23.7	23.9	24.2	24.4	24.7
59–61	23.7	24.0	24.2	24.5	24.7	25.0	25.2	25.5	25.7
62–64	24.7	25.0	25.2	25.5	25.7	26.0	26.7	26.4	26.7
65–67	25.7	25.9	26.2	26.4	26.7	26.9	27.2	27.4	27.7
68–70	26.6	26.9	27.1	27.4	27.6	27.9	28.1	28.4	28.6
71–73	27.5	27.8	28.0	28.3	28.5	28.8	28.0	29.3	29.5
74–76	28.4	28.7	28.9	29.2	29.4	29.7	29.9	30.2	30.4
77–79	29.3	29.5	29.8	30.0	30.3	30.5	30.8	31.0	31.3
80–82	30.1	30.4	30.6	30.9	31.1	31.4	31.6	31.9	32.1
83–85	30.9	31.2	31.4	31.7	31.9	32.2	32.4	32.7	32.9
86–88	31.7	32.0	32.2	32.5	32.7	32.9	33.2	33.4	33.7
89–91	32.5	32.7	33.0	33.2	33.5	33.7	33.9	34.2	34.4
92–94	33.2	33.4	33.7	33.9	34.2	34.4	34.7	34.9	35.2
95–97	33.9	34.1	34.4	34.6	34.9	35.1	35.4	35.6	35.9
98–100	34.6	34.8	35.1	35.3	35.5	35.8	36.0	36.3	36.5
101–103	35.3	35.4	35.7	35.9	36.2	36.4	36.7	36.9	37.2
104–106	35.8	36.1	36.3	36.6	36.8	37.1	37.3	37.5	37.8
107–109	36.4	36.7	36.9	37.1	37.4	37.6	37.9	38.1	38.4
110–112	37.0	37.2	37.5	37.7	38.0	38.2	38.5	38.7	38.9
113–115	37.5	37.8	38.0	38.2	38.5	38.7	39.0	39.2	39.5
116–118	38.0	38.3	38.5	38.8	39.0	39.3	39.5	39.7	40.0
119–121	38.5	38.7	39.0	39.2	39.5	39.7	40.0	40.2	40.5
122–124	39.0	39.2	39.4	39.7	39.9	40.2	40.4	40.7	40.9
125–127	39.4	39.6	39.9	40.1	40.4	40.6	40.9	41.1	41.4
128–130	39.8	40.0	40.3	40.5	40.8	41.0	41.3	41.5	41.8

*Percentage of fat calculated by the formula of Siri: percentage of fat = $(4.95/D_b - 4.5) \times 100$, where D_b = body density. (Reprinted with permission from Pollock, M.L., Schmidt, D.H. and Jackson, A.S. (1980) Measurement of cardiorespiratory fitness and body composition in the clinical setting, *Compr. Ther.*, **6** pp. 12–27.)

Table II.67   Percentage of body fat estimation for men from age and the sum of chest, abdominal, and thigh skinfolds*

Sum of skinfolds (mm)	Age to the last year								
	Under 22	23 to 27	28 to 32	33 to 37	38 to 42	43 to 47	48 to 52	53 to 57	Over 58
23–25	9.7	9.9	10.2	10.4	10.7	10.9	11.2	11.4	11.7
26–28	11.0	11.2	11.5	11.7	12.0	12.3	12.5	12.7	13.0
29–31	12.3	12.5	12.8	13.0	13.3	13.5	13.8	14.0	14.3
32–34	13.6	13.8	14.0	14.3	14.5	14.8	15.0	15.3	15.5
35–37	14.8	15.0	15.3	15.5	15.8	16.0	16.3	16.5	16.8
38–40	16.0	16.3	16.5	16.7	17.0	17.2	17.5	17.7	18.0
41–43	17.2	17.4	17.7	17.9	18.2	18.4	18.7	18.9	19.2
44–46	18.3	18.6	18.8	19.1	19.3	19.6	19.8	20.1	20.3
47–49	19.5	19.7	20.0	20.2	20.5	20.7	21.0	21.2	21.5

Continued

Table II.67   Continued

Sum of skinfolds (mm)	Age to the last year								
	Under 22	23 to 27	28 to 32	33 to 37	38 to 42	43 to 47	48 to 52	53 to 57	Over 58
50–52	20.6	20.8	21.1	21.3	21.6	21.8	22.1	22.3	22.6
53–55	21.7	21.9	22.1	22.4	22.6	22.9	23.1	23.4	23.6
56–58	22.7	23.0	23.2	23.4	23.7	23.9	24.2	24.4	24.7
59–61	23.7	24.0	24.2	24.5	24.7	25.0	25.2	25.5	25.7
62–64	24.7	25.0	25.2	25.5	25.7	26.0	26.7	26.4	26.7
65–67	25.7	25.9	26.2	26.4	26.7	26.9	27.2	27.4	27.7
68–70	26.6	26.9	27.1	27.4	27.6	27.9	28.1	28.4	28.6
71–73	27.5	27.8	28.0	28.3	28.5	28.8	29.0	29.3	29.5
74–76	28.4	28.7	28.9	29.2	29.4	29.7	29.9	30.2	30.4
77–79	29.3	29.5	29.8	30.0	30.3	30.5	30.8	31.0	31.3
80–82	30.1	30.4	30.6	30.9	31.1	31.4	31.6	31.9	32.1
83–85	30.9	31.2	31.4	31.7	31.9	32.2	32.4	32.7	32.9
86–88	31.7	32.0	32.2	32.5	32.7	32.9	33.2	33.4	33.7
89–91	32.5	32.7	33.0	33.2	33.5	33.7	33.9	34.2	34.4
92–94	33.2	33.4	33.7	33.9	34.2	34.4	34.7	34.9	35.2
95–97	33.9	34.1	34.4	34.6	34.9	35.1	35.4	35.6	35.9
98–100	34.6	34.8	35.1	35.3	35.5	35.8	36.0	36.3	36.5
101–103	35.3	35.4	35.7	35.9	36.2	36.4	36.7	36.9	37.2
104–106	35.8	36.1	36.3	36.6	36.8	37.1	37.3	37.5	37.8
107–109	36.4	36.7	36.9	37.1	37.4	37.6	37.9	38.1	38.4
110–112	37.0	37.2	37.5	37.7	38.0	38.2	38.5	38.7	38.9
113–115	37.5	37.8	38.0	38.2	38.5	38.7	39.0	39.2	39.5
116–118	38.0	38.3	38.5	38.8	39.0	39.3	39.5	39.7	40.0
119–121	38.5	38.7	39.0	39.2	39.5	39.7	40.0	40.2	40.5
122–124	39.0	39.2	39.4	39.7	39.9	40.2	40.4	40.7	40.9
125–127	39.4	39.6	39.9	40.1	40.4	40.6	40.9	41.1	41.4
128–130	39.8	40.0	40.3	40.5	40.8	41.0	41.3	41.5	41.8

*Percentage of fat calculated by the formula of Siri: percentage of fat = $(4.95/D_b - 4.5) \times 100$, where D_b = body density. (Reprinted with permission from Pollock, M.L., Schmidt, D.H. and Jackson, A.S. (1980) Measurement of cardiorespiratory fitness and body composition in the clinical setting, *Compr. Ther.*, **6** pp. 12–27.)

Table II.68   Dietary recommendations in industrialized and developing countries, 1977 to 1989*

Country/region or source of recommendation	Target group(s)	Maintain appropriate body weight, exercise	Limit or reduce total fat (% energy)	Reduce saturated fatty acids (% energy)
Australia 1983	GP	Yes	Yes	NC
1987, targets for 1995	GP	Reduce obesity prevalence to 30%	35%	NS
1987, targets for 2000	GP	To 25%	33%	NS
Canada 1982	GP	Yes	35%	Yes
Czech Republic 1988	GP	Yes, reduce by 10–15%	Yes, reduce by 15 g/day	Yes
France 1981	GP	Yes	30–35%	Yes
Germany, Federal Republic of, 1985	GP	Yes	Yes	NS
Hungary 1988	GP	Yes	Avoid too much	Use vegetable oil
India 1988	HR (affluent people)	Yes	15–20%	NC
Ireland 1984	GP	Yes	≤35%	Yes
Japan 1985	GP	Yes	20–25%	Yes

Continued

Table II.68 Continued

Country/region or source of recommendation	Target group(s)	Maintain appropriate body weight, exercise	Limit or reduce total fat (% energy)	Reduce saturated fatty acids (% energy)	Increase polyunsaturated fatty acids (% energy)	Limit cholesterol (mg/day)	Limit free sugars (% energy)	Increase complex carbohydrates (% energy for total carbohydrates)
Latin America 1988	GP	Yes	20–25%	≤8	NC	NC	Yes	Yes
Netherlands 1983–1984	GP	Yes	30–35%	Yes	NS	NS	<14%	Indirectly
1986	GP	Yes	30–35%	Yes	NS	NS	<12%	Indirectly
New Zealand 1982	GP, HR	Yes	Yes	Yes	Yes	No	Yes	Yes
Norway 1981–1982	GP	NC	<35%	Yes	No	NS	Yes	Yes, more plant foods, vegetables, cereals, legumes
Poland 1988	GP	Yes	≈30%	Yes	NS	NS	Yes	50–55%
Sweden 1981	GP	Yes	25–35%	Yes	NS	NS	Avoid excess	Yes; fresh fruits and vegetables, whole-grain cereals
1985	GP	Yes	Reduce by 5% energy by 1990; to ≈30% by 2000	NS	NS	NS	Yes	Yes, fresh vegetables, salads, whole-grains
United Kingdom 1983	GP	Yes	30%	10	Balance $(n-3)/(n-6)$ ratio	NC	Yes	Yes; avoid refined and polished grains
United States of America 1977	GP	Yes	27–33%	Yes	NC	NC	Moderation; ≤7 g/day for weight reduction	Yes
1979	GP	Yes	Yes	Yes	Use vegetables and fish oils	NC	NC	NC
1985	GP	Yes	Yes	Yes	P/S ≈ 1.0	<100 mg/1000 kcal$_{th}$ in children, up to 300 mg/day	Yes	Yes
1988	GP, HR	Yes	Yes	Yes	Maximum 10%	Yes	Yes	NS
1989	GP	Balance energy intake and expenditure	≤30%	<10% for individuals, 7–8% population mean	P/S = 1.0	<30 mg/MJ	Mono- and disaccharides 15–20%	45–55%
WHO 1988 Intermediate goals	GP	BMI	35%	15%	NS	NS	Yes	Yes
Ultimate goals		20–25	20–30%	10–15%				

Continued

Table II.68 Continued

Increase polyunsaturated fatty acids (% energy)	Limit cholesterol (mg/day)	Limit free sugars (% energy)	Increase complex carbohydrates (% energy for total carbohydrates)
P/S = 0.5	NS	<10%	Yes; 50–60%
NS	Yes, <300 mg	≤10%	Yes
P/S = 0.5	Yes	<10%	Yes; 50–60%
P/S = >0.5	NS	Decrease by 3% energy by 1990	Yes; increase starch to 45–50% energy by 2000
NS	No	To 20 kg/year	Through whole grains, vegetables, cereals, fruits
Yes	250–350	Yes	Yes
NS	Yes	Yes	Yes
No	Yes	Yes	Adequate starch and fiber
No	Yes	Yes	Yes
Up to 10 for individuals and ≈7 population mean	<300	Yes	≥55%; ≥5 servings/day vegetables and fruits; ≥6 daily servings cereals, breads, and legumes
PS ≥0.5	<100 mg/1000 kcal$_{th}$	10%	>40%
P/S = 1.0			45–55%

Increase dietary fiber (g/day)	Restrict sodium chloride (g/day)	Moderate alcohol intake (% energy)	Other recommendations
Yes	Yes	Yes	Promote breast-feeding; variety
25	130 mmol/day	<5%	Promote water fluoridation, increase prevalence of breast-feeding
30	100 mmol/day	<5%	
Yes	Yes	Yes	Exercise
Yes	Yes	Yes	Increase vitamin C intake; more plant foods; nutrition education; variety
Yes	Yes	<10%	Water fluoridation
Yes	Yes	Yes	Variety; small, frequent meals, proper cooking; sufficient protein
Yes	Yes	Yes	Variety; focus on cooking methods; consume milk and cheese as skimmed-milk products; 4 or 5 even meals daily; food labeling
Include grains, leafy vegetables, and whole grains	Yes	NC	Breast-feeding; water fluoridation upper limit 1 mg/L; different recommendation for general, poorer population
To 20–35	<9	<5%	Reduce protein to 1 g/kg of body weight daily; more vegetable protein
NC	<10	NC	Varied diet (at least 30 different foods daily); home cooking; pleasant eating environment
>8 g/1000 kcal$_{th}$	≤5; in profuse sweating, up to 10	NC	Protein 10–12% energy; variety; dietary interactions; vitamin C with iron-containing foods; calcium intake
NC	NC	Yes	Variety
3 g/MJ	Yes	<9 g/day	Variety
Yes	Yes	Yes	Variety; less animal protein; water fluoridation
Yes	NC	NC	Maintain adequate nutrient intake
Yes	?	?	?
>30	≈7–8	Yes	Varied diet, exercise, regular meals
Increase by 7–8 g/day by 1990 and to 30–35 g by 2000	Reduce by 1–2 g/day by 1990 to 7–8 g by 2000	Yes	Year 1990 and year 2000 goals

Continued

Table II.68   Continued

Increase dietary fiber (g/day)	Restrict sodium chloride (g/day)	Moderate alcohol intake (% energy)	Other recommendations
To 30	Decrease by 3 g/day	<4%	Long-term proposals: food labeling; nutrition education; greater proportion of vegetable protein
Yes	<8	Yes	Limit additives and processed foods
NS	Yes	Yes	More fish, poultry, legumes; less red meat
Yes	Yes	Yes	Variety in diet; consider high-risk groups
Yes	Yes	Yes	Fluoridation of water; adolescent girls and women increase intake of calcium-rich foods; children, adolescents, and women of child-bearing age increase intake of iron-rich foods
Indirectly through vegetables, fruits, and cereals	≤6 with a goal of 4.5	<30 g of ethanol or <2 drinks/day	Population and individual goals; avoid dietary supplements in excess of RDAs; drink fluoridated water; limit protein intake to less than twice the RDA; comments on future goals
>30	7–8	Yes	Increase nutrient density of food; water fluoridation; iodine prophylaxis

*BMI = Body-mass index; GP = General population; HR = High-risk groups; NC = No comment; NS = Not specified; P/S = Ratio of polyunsaturated to saturated fatty acids; RDA = Recommended dietary allowance.
(From WHO (1990) *Diet, Nutrition and the Prevention of Chronic Diseases*, Report of a WHO Study Group, Technical Report Series No. 797, World Health Organization, Geneva, pp. 180–1.)

Table II.69   Dietary recommendations to reduce coronary heart disease risk in industrialized countries*

Country/region or source of recommendation	Target group(s)	Body weight/exercise	Total fat (% energy)
Australia			
1979	HR	Avoid obesity	Reduce to 30–35
Canada			
1977	GP	Maintain appropriate body weight	Reduce to 35
1988	GP	Adjust energy intake	<30
	HR	and expenditure	
Europe			
1987	GP	Control obesity;	≤30
	HR	increase exercise	
Finland			
1987	GP	Avoid excess weight;	<30
	HR	exercise	
Finland, Norway, Sweden			
1968	GP	Reduce energy intake to avoid obesity; exercise	Reduce to 25–35
Germany, Federal Republic of			
1975	GP	NC	Reduce
Japan			
1983	GP	NC	20–25
Netherlands			
1973	GP	Maintain appropriate body weight	33

Continued

Table II.69   Continued

Country/region or source of recommendation	Target group(s)	Body weight/exercise	Total fat (% energy)
New Zealand			
1976	GP	Maintain appropriate	35
	HR	body weight	
United Kingdom			
1982	GP	Avoid obesity; increase exercise	30
1984	GP	Avoid obesity; exercise	Reduce to 35
United States of America			
1984	GP	Control obesity	<30
1985	GP	Maintain appropriate	<30
	HR	body weight	
1988	GP	Maintain appropriate body weight	<30
WHO			
1982	GP	Avoid obesity	Reduce to 20–30
1988	HR	BMI 20–25, regular exercise	20–30

Saturated fat (% energy)	Polyunsaturated fat (% energy)	Cholesterol (mg/day)	Complex carbohydrates and fiber
P:S = 1.0	P:S = 1.0	Restrict	Eat enough
10	10	NC	Increase
<10	<10	Restrict through less meats and egg yolks; for HR <300	Increase
<10	Increase oleic and linoleic acids	<300	Increase, especially vegetables, fruits, cereals, legumes
<10	P:S >0.5	Reduce	NC
Reduce	Increase	NC	Increase vegetables, fruits, potatoes
Reduce	Increase	Reduce	NC
NC	Cook with vegetable oil	NC	Increase
Restrict	10–13	250–300	Increase to make up energy need
Reduce especially for HR	HR should substitute for saturated fatty acids	Reduce	NC
<10	NC	NC	Increase
Reduce to 15	$P/S \approx 0.45$	NS	Increase breads, cereals, vegetables, fruits
8	<10	<250	Increase to make up energy loss
10	Up to 10	250–300	Endorsed earlier recommendations
<10	Up to 10	<300	Increase, ≥50% energy from total carbohydrates
<10	Up to 10	<300	Increase
10	Up to 10 P/S >1.0	<100 mg/1000 $kcal_{th}$	45–55% energy >30 g fiber/day

Free sugars	Sodium chloride (g/day)	Alcohol intake	Other recommendations
Use less	Restrict	Moderation	Focus on HR groups; food labeling; recommendations safe for GP
NC	Restrict	NC	Variety of foods
NC	Limit	Limit	Focus on HR groups; limit protein to 10–15% energy
Reduce	Moderation	Moderation, <25–30 g/day	Nutrition education; collaboration among government and other groups; food labeling
NC	Reduce; for HR <5	Moderation	Avoid trace element deficiencies; food labeling; focus on HR groups

Continued

Table II.69   Continued

Free sugars	Sodium chloride (g/day)	Alcohol intake	Other recommendations
Decrease	NC	NC	10–12% of energy from protein; 30–50% of animal origin
NC	NC	NC	NC
Reduce	Limit to <10	Avoid too much	Variety; eat enough protein, half from vegetables and half from animal sources; eat enough potassium, especially from green vegetables; eat lean meat and fish and fewer sweets
Use little	NC	NC	NC
Restrict to reduce weight	NC	Restrict to reduce weight	NC
NC	NC	NC	Special attention to children
Do not increase	Decrease	Avoid excess; <90 ml/day men; <65 ml/day women	Special recommendations for governments, professionals, industry
NC	5	NC	NC
	NC	NC	Guidelines for health professionals, industry, and public
NS	<3 (as sodium)	30–50 g ethanol/day	Protein to make up remainder of energy; wide variety of foods
NC	<5	Drink less	Emphasis on plant foods, fish, poultry, lean meats, low-fat dairy products, and fewer whole eggs
10% energy	<5	Limit	Increase nutrient density; water fluoridation 0.7–1.2 mg/L; iodine prophylaxis; intermediate and ultimate goals

*BMI = Body-mass index; GP = General population; HR = High-risk groups; NC = No comment; NS = Not specified; P:S = Ratio of polyunsaturated to saturated fatty acids.
(From WHO (1990) *Diet, Nutrition and the Prevention of Chronic Diseases*, Report of a WHO Study Group. Technical Report Series No. 797, World Health Organization, Geneva, pp. 182–3. With permission.)

Table II.70   Dietary recommendations to reduce cancer risk in industrialized countries*

Country/region	Maintain appropriate body weight, exercise	Limit or reduce total fat (% energy)	Modify ratio of dietary fats	Promote fruit and vegetable intake	Increase complex carbohydrate/fiber intake
Canada 1985	Yes	Reduce	Decrease saturated fatty acids and cholesterol	Yes	More fiber-containing foods
Europe 1986	Yes	To ≈30	NC	Yes	Yes
Japan 1983	NC	Avoid excess	NC	Especially green/yellow vegetables, oranges, carotene, and fungi	Unrefined cereal, seafood, fiber-rich legumes
United States of America 1982	NC	To ≈30	NC	Especially citrus fruits, green and yellow and cruciferous vegetables	Whole-grain products, vegetables, and fruits

Continued

Table II.70   Continued

Country/region	Maintain appropriate body weight, exercise	Limit or reduce total fat (% energy)	Modify ratio of dietary fats	Promote fruit and vegetable intake	Increase complex carbohydrate/fiber intake
1984	Yes	To ≈30	NC	Especially vitamin A- and C-rich foods and cruciferous vegetables	High-fiber foods, whole-grain cereals
1987	Yes	To ≈30	NC	Vitamin A-rich, green and yellow vegetables, citrus fruits	Whole-grain products, 20–30 g fiber/day

Restrict sodium chloride	Food preparation methods	Alcohol intake	Other recommendations
NS	Minimize cured, pickled, and smoked foods	Two or fewer drinks per day, if any	NC
To <5 g/day	As above; avoid frying and high-temperature cooking	Drink less, if at all	Varied diet; no food supplements; recommendations to government, scientists, and industry
Yes	Avoid hot drinks and burned foods	Drink less, if at all	Varied diet, chew food well
Minimize cured and pickled foods	Minimize cured, pickled, and smoked foods	Drink less, if at all	Avoid food supplements; monitor and test mutagens and carcinogens; recommendations to government, scientists, and industry
NS	As above	As above	NC
NS	As above, avoid frying and high-temperature cooking	As above	Balanced diet; read labels

*NC = No comment; NS = Not specified.
(From WHO (1990) *Diet, Nutrition and the Prevention of Chronic Diseases*, Report of a WHO Study Group. Technical Report Series No. 797. World Health Organization, Geneva, pp. 184–5.)

Table II.71   National nutrition objectives for the year 2000

A.   *Health Status Objectives*
   1.   Reduce deaths from coronary heart disease to no more than 100 per 100,000 persons (age-adjusted baseline: 135 per 100,000 in 1987).
   2.   Reverse the rise in deaths from cancer to achieve a rate of no more than 130 per 100,000 persons (age-adjusted baseline: 133 per 100,000 in 1987).
   3.   Reduce the overweight population to no more than 20% among adults aged 20 years and older and no more than 15% among adolescents aged 12 through 19 years (baseline: 26% for adults aged 20 through 74 years in 1976 to 1980, 24% for men and 27% for women; 15% for adolescents aged 12 through 19 years in 1976 to 1980).
   4.   Reduce growth retardation among low-income children aged 5 years and younger to less than 10% (baseline: up to 16% among low-income children in 1988, depending on age and race/ethnicity).
B.   *Risk Reduction Objectives*
   5.   Reduce dietary fat intake to an average of 30% of calories or less and reduce average saturated fat intake to less than 10% of calories among persons aged 2 years and older (baseline: 36% of calories from total fat and 13% from saturated fat for persons aged 20 through 74 years in 1976 to 1980; 36% and 13% for women aged 19 through 50 years in 1985).
   6.   Increase complex carbohydrates and fiber-containing foods in the diets of adults to 5 or more daily servings for vegetables (including legumes) and fruits, and to 6 or more daily servings for grain products (baseline: 2.5 servings of vegetables and fruits and 3 servings of grain products for women aged 19 through 50 years in 1985).
   7.   Increase to at least 50% the proportion of overweight persons aged 12 years and older who have adopted sound dietary practices combined with regular physical activity to attain an appropriate body weight (baseline: 30% of overweight women and 25% of overweight men for people aged 18 years and older in 1985).
   8.   Increase calcium intake so that at least 50% of youth aged 12 through 24 years and at least 50% of pregnant and lactating women are consuming 3 or more servings daily of foods rich in calcium, and at least 50% of adults aged 25 years and older are consuming 2 or more servings daily (baseline: 7% of women and 14% of men aged 19 through 24 years and 24% of pregnant and lactating women consumed 3 or more servings daily, and 15% of women and 23% of men aged 25 through 50 years consumed 2 or more servings daily in 1985 to 1986).

Continued

Table II.71   Continued

   9. Decrease salt and sodium intake so that at least 65% of those who prepare home-cooked meals do so without adding salt, at least 80% of persons avoid using salt at the table, and at least 40% of adults regularly purchase foods modified or lower in sodium (baseline: 54% of women aged 19 through 50 years who prepared most of the meals did not use salt in food preparation, and 68% of women aged 19 through 50 years did not use salt at the table in 1985; 20% of all persons aged 18 years and older regularly purchased foods with reduced salt and sodium content in 1988).

  10. Reduce iron deficiency to less than 3% among children aged 1 through 4 years and among women of childbearing age (baseline: 9% for children aged 1 through 2 years, 4% for children aged 3 through 4 years, and 5% for women aged 20 through 44 years in 1976 to 1980).

  11. Increase to at least 75% the proportion of mothers who breast-feed their babies in the early postpartum period and to at least 50% to the proportion who continue to breast-feed until their babies are 5 to 6 months old (baseline: 54% at discharge from birth site and 21% at 5 to 6 months in 1988).

  12. Increase to at least 75% the proportion of parents and caregivers who use feeding practices that prevent baby-bottle tooth decay.

  13. Increase to at least 85% the proportion of persons aged 18 years and older who use food labels to make nutritious food selections (baseline: 74% used labels to make food selections in 1988).

C. *Service and Protection Objectives*

  14. Achieve useful and informative nutrition labeling for virtually all processed foods and for at least 40% of fresh meats, poultry, fish, fruits, vegetables, baked foods, and ready-to-eat carry-out foods (baseline: 60% of processed foods regulated by the Food and Drug Administration had nutrition labeling in 1988; baseline data on fresh and carry-out foods are unavailable).

  15. Increase the available processed food products that are reduced in fat and saturated fat to at least 5000 brand items (baseline: 2500 brand items reduced in fat in 1986).

  16. Increase to at least 90% the proportion of restaurants and institutional service operations that offer identifiable low-fat, low-calorie food choices, consistent with the nutrition principles in the *Dietary Guidelines for Americans*.

  17. Increase to at least 90% the proportion of school lunch and breakfast services and child-care food services that offer menus consistent with the nutrition principles in the *Dietary Guidelines for Americans*.

  18. Increase to at least 80% the receipt of home food services by people aged 65 years and older who cannot prepare their own meals or are otherwise in need of home-delivered meals.

  19. Increase to at least 75% the proportion of schools in the United States that provide nutrition education from preschool through 12th grade, preferably as part of quality school health education.

  20. Increase to at least 50% the proportion of worksites with 50 or more employees that offer nutrition education and/or weight management programs for employees (baseline: 17% offered nutrition education activities and 15% offered weight-control activities in 1985).

  21. Increase to at least 75% the proportion of primary care providers who provide nutrition assessment and counseling and/or referral to qualified nutritionists or dietitians (baseline: physicians provided diet counseling for an estimated 40 to 50% of patients in 1988).

(From (1991) Nutrition in Healthy People 2000. *In* National Health Promotion and Disease Prevention Objectives. U.S. Government Printing Office, Washington, D.C.)

Table II.72   Beverages and alcoholic drinks: calories and selected electrolytes (per 100 ml)*

Beverage	Calories	Sodium (mg)	(mEq)	Potassium (mg)	(mEq)	Phosphorus (mg)
Cola (avg.)	48.1–55.0[†]	0.8–4.7 (mg)[†]		0–4.4 (mg)[†]		18.1–25[†]
Diet cola (avg.)	0.1–0.5[†]	0.8–13.0 (mg)[†]		0–33.2 (mg)[†]		8.5–17.6[†]
Patio grape/orange	52	11.2	0.5	4.1	0.1	—
Mountain Dew	49	8.7	0.4	2.7	0.1	—
Teem	41	8.6	0.4	—	—	—
Root beer	45	1	0.1	3.9	0.1	—
Club soda	0	21.9	1.0	—	—	0
Sprite	48	15.4	0.7	0.4	—	—
Fanta (avg.)	53	6.4	0.3	0.6	—	—
Fresca	1	12.1	0.5	—	—	—
Fanta ginger ale	42	9.4	0.4	—	—	—
Slice	45	3	0.1	27.6	0.7	—
Apricot nectar	56	3	0.1	114	2.9	9

Continued

Table II.72   Continued

Beverage	Calories	Sodium (mg)	Sodium (mEq)	Potassium (mg)	Potassium (mEq)	Phosphorus (mg)
Apple juice	47	3	0.1	119	3	7
Cranberry juice	58	4	0.2	24	0.6	1
Grape juice, canned	61	3	0.1	132	3.4	11
Grapefruit juice, unsweetened	38	trace	—	153	3.9	11
Orange juice, unsweetened or fresh	45	1	0.1	200	5.1	17
Pear nectar	60	4	0.2	13	0.3	3
Peach nectar	54	7	0.3	40	1	6
Pineapple juice, unsweetened	56	trace	—	134	3.4	8
Tomato juice	20	200.7	8.7	227	5.8	16.5
Fruit-flavored beverage	45	—	—	—	—	
Beer, regular	41	5.3	0.2	25	0.6	12.4
Beer, light	28	2.8	0.1	18.1	0.5	12.1
Gin, rum, vodka, whiskey (86 proof)	250	trace	—	3.6	0.1	—
Table wine, 12.2% alcohol/vol.	86	3.5	0.1	93.1	2.4	10.3
Dessert wine, 18.5% alcohol/vol.	137	3.3	0.1	76.7	2	—

Alcoholic beverages are customarily served in special glassware, the size of which tends to standardize the alcoholic content:

1 cordial glass	= 20 ml	1 burgundy glass	= 120 ml
1 brandy glass	= 30 ml	1 champagne glass	= 150 ml
1 jigger	= 45 ml	1 tumbler	= 240–360 ml
1 sherry glass	= 60 ml	1 mixing glass	= 360 ml
1 cocktail glass	= 90 ml		

*Brand name data supplied by the commercial producer of the product. Other data obtained from Consumer Nutrition Center (1982) *Composition of Foods, Fruits, and Fruit Juices: Raw, Processed, Prepared*, Agriculture Handbook No. 8–9. U.S. Department of Agriculture, Washington.
†Range.

Table II.73   Dietary fiber content of selected foods*,† (g/100 g edible portion)

Food item	Moisture	Total dietary fiber (AOAC)‡
Breads, Crackers, and Cakes		
Bagels, plain	31.6	2.1
Biscuits, made from refrigerated dough, baked	28.7	1.5
Bread		
Bran	37.7	8.5
Cornbread mix, baked	34.4	2.4
Cracked-wheat	35.9	5.3
French	33.9	2.7
Hollywood-type, light	37.8	4.8
Italian	34.1	3.1
Mixed-grain	38.2	7.1
Oatmeal	36.7	3.9
Pita		
White	32.1	1.6
Whole-wheat	30.6	7.5
Pumpernickel	38.3	5.9
Reduced-calorie, high-fiber		
Wheat	43.7	11.3
White	41.8	9.3
Rye	37.0	6.2
Wheat	37.0	4.3
White	37.1	2.3
Whole-wheat	38.3	6.9

Table II.73   Continued

Food item	Moisture	Total dietary fiber (AOAC)‡
Bread crumbs, plain or seasoned	5.7	4.2
Bread stuffing, flavored, from dry mix	65.1	2.9
Cake mix		
Chocolate, prepared	33.3	2.2
Yellow, prepared	40.0	0.8
Cakes		
Boston cream pie	47.6	1.3
Coffeecake		
Crumb topping	22.3	3.3
Fruit	31.7	2.5
Fruitcake, commercial	22.0	3.5
Gingerbread, from dry mix	38.5	3.2
Cheesecake		
Commercial	44.6	2.1
From no-bake mix	44.4	1.9
Cookies		
Brownies	12.6	2.4
Brownies with nuts	12.6	2.6
Butter	4.7	2.4
Chocolate chip	4.0	2.7
Chocolate sandwich	2.2	3.0
Fig bar	16.7	4.6
Fortune	8.0	1.6
Oatmeal	5.7	3.1

Continued

Continued

Table II.73   Continued

Food item	Moisture	Total dietary fiber (AOAC)‡
Oatmeal, soft-type	–	2.7
Peanut butter	6.7	1.8
Shortbread with pecans	3.3	1.8
Vanilla sandwich	2.1	1.5
Crackers		
Cheese, sandwich with peanut butter filling	4.0	1.1
Crisp bread, rye	6.1	16.2
Graham		
Regular	4.1	2.7
Honey	4.1	2.7
Matzoh		
Plain	6.1	3.0
Egg/onion	8.0	5.0
Whole-wheat	3.0	11.6
Melba toast		
Plain	5.6	6.5
Rye	6.7	8.0
Wheat	6.1	7.4
Rye	7.2	15.8
Saltines	–	2.7
Snack-type	4.2	2.0
Wheat	3.2	5.5
Whole-wheat	2.7	10.4
Croutons, plain or seasoned	5.6	5.0
Doughnuts		
Cake	19.7	1.7
Yeast-leavened, glazed	26.7	2.1
English muffin, whole-wheat	45.7	6.3
French toast, commercial, ready-to-eat	48.1	2.8
Ice cream cones		
Sugar, rolled-type	3.0	4.6
Wafer-type	5.3	4.1
Muffins, commercial		
Blueberry	37.3	3.6
Oat bran	35.0	7.5
Pancake, waffle mix, prepared	50.4	1.3
Pastry, Danish		
Fruit	27.6	1.9
Plain	19.3	1.2
Pies, commercial		
Apple	51.7	1.7
Cherry	46.2	0.8
Chocolate, cream	43.5	2.0
Egg custard	46.5	1.2
Fruit and coconut	–	0.9
Lemon meringue	41.7	1.2
Pecan	19.8	3.5
Pumpkin	58.1	2.7
Rolls, dinner, egg	30.4	3.8
Taco shells	6.0	8.1
Toaster pastries	8.9	1.0
Tortillas		
Corn	43.6	5.2
Flour, wheat	26.2	3.1
Waffles, commercial, frozen, ready-to-eat	45.0	2.4

Continued

Table II.73   Continued

Food item	Moisture	Total dietary fiber (AOAC)‡
Breakfast Cereals, Ready-to-Eat		
Bran		
High-fiber	2.9	35.3
Extra fiber	–	45.9
Bran flakes	2.9	18.8
Bran flakes with raisins	8.3	13.4
Corn flakes		
Frosted or sugar-sparkled	1.9	2.2
Plain	2.8	2.0
Fiber cereal with fruit	–	14.8
Granola	3.3	10.5
Oat cereal	5.0	10.6
Oat flakes, fortified	3.1	3.0
Puffed wheat, sugar-coated	1.5	1.5
Rice, crispy	2.4	1.2
Wheat and malted barley		
Flakes	3.4	6.8
Nuggets	3.2	6.5
with raisins	–	6.0
Wheat flakes	4.3	9.0
Cereal Grains		
Barley	9.4	17.3
Bulgur, dry	8.0	18.3
Corn flour, whole-grain	10.9	13.4
Cornmeal		
Degermed	11.6	5.2
Whole-grain	10.3	11.0
Cornstarch	8.3	0.9
Farina, regular or instant, cooked	85.8	1.4
Hominy, canned	79.8	2.5
Millet, hulled, raw	–	8.5
Oat bran, raw	6.6	15.9
Oat flour	7.8	9.6
Oats, rolled or oatmeal, dry	8.8	10.3
Rice, brown, long-grain, cooked	73.1	1.7
Rice, white		
glutinous, raw	10.0	2.8
Long-grain		
Parboiled, cooked	–	0.5
Precooked or instant, cooked	76.4	0.8
Rye flour, medium or light	9.4	14.6
Semolina	12.7	3.9
Tapioca, pearl, dry	12.0	1.1
Wheat bran, crude	9.9	42.4
Wheat flour		
White, all-purpose	11.8	2.7
Whole-grain	10.9	12.6
Wheat germ, toasted	2.9	12.9
Wild rice, raw	7.8	5.2
Fruits and Fruit Products		
Apples, raw:		
With skin	83.9	2.2
Without skin	84.5	1.9
Apple juice, unsweetened	87.9	0.1
Applesauce, unsweetened	88.4	1.5
Apricots, dried	31.1	7.8
Apricot nectar	84.9	0.6
Bananas, raw	74.3	1.6

Continued

Table II.73 Continued

Food item	Moisture	Total dietary fiber (AOAC)[‡]
Blueberries, raw	84.6	2.3
Cantaloupe, raw	89.8	0.8
Figs, dried	28.4	9.3
Fruit cocktail, canned in heavy syrup, drained	–	1.5
Grapefruit, raw	90.9	0.6
Grapes, Thompson, seedless, raw	81.3	0.7
Kiwifruit, raw	83.0	3.4
Nectarines, raw	86.3	1.6
Olives		
Green	–	2.6
ripe	–	3.0
Orange, raw	86.8	2.4
Orange juice, frozen concentrate, prepared	88.1	0.2
Peach		
Canned in juice, drained	–	1.0
Dried	31.8	8.2
Raw	87.7	1.6
Pears, raw	83.8	2.6
Pineapple		
Canned in heavy syrup, chunks, drained	79.0	1.1
Raw	86.5	1.2
Prune		
Dried	32.4	7.2
Stewed	–	6.6
Prune juice	81.2	1.0
Raisins	15.4	5.3
Strawberries	91.6	2.6
Watermelon	91.5	0.4
Legumes, Nuts, and Seeds		
Almonds, oil-roasted	3.3	11.2
Baked beans, canned		
Barbecue-style	–	5.8
Sweet or tomato sauce, plain	72.6	7.7
Beans, Great Northern, canned, drained	69.9	5.4
Cashews, oil-roasted	5.4	6.0
Chickpeas, canned, drained	68.2	5.8
Coconut, raw	47.0	9.0
Cowpeas (black-eyed peas), cooked, drained	70.0	9.6
Hazelnuts, oil-roasted	1.2	6.4
Lima beans, cooked, drained	69.8	7.2
Miso	47.4	5.4
Mixed nuts, oil-roasted, with peanuts	–	9.0
Peanut		
Dry-roasted	1.6	8.0
Oil-roasted	2.0	8.8
Peanut butter		
Chunky	1.1	6.6
Smooth	1.4	6.0
Pecans, dried	4.8	6.5
Pistachio nuts	3.9	10.8
Sunflower seeds, oil-roasted	2.6	6.8
Tahini	3.0	9.3

Table II.73 Continued

Food item	Moisture	Total dietary fiber (AOAC)[‡]
Tofu	84.6	1.2
Walnuts, dried		
Black	4.4	5.0
English	3.6	4.8
Pasta		
Noodles, Chinese, chow mein	0.7	3.9
Noodles, egg, regular, cooked	68.7	2.2
Noodles, Japanese, dry		
Somen	9.2	4.3
Udon	8.7	5.4
Spaghetti and macaroni, cooked	64.7	1.6
Spaghetti, dry		
Spinach	8.7	10.6
Whole-wheat	7.1	11.8
Snacks		
Banana chips	4.3	7.7
Corn cakes	4.6	1.9
Corn-based, extruded		
Chips		
Barbecue-flavor	1.2	5.2
Plain	1.0	4.4
Puffs or twists, cheese-flavor	1.5	1.0
Cornnuts		
Barbecue-flavor	1.6	8.4
Nacho-flavor	2.1	8.0
Plain	1.3	6.9
Crisped rice bar		
Almond	6.7	3.6
Chocolate chip	7.0	2.2
Granola bars		
Hard		
Chocolate chip	2.4	4.4
Plain	3.9	5.3
Soft		
Milk-chocolate-coated, chocolate chip	3.6	3.4
Uncoated		
Chocolate chip	5.4	4.8
Chocolate chip, graham, and marshmallow	6.0	4.0
Nut and raisin	6.1	5.6
Peanut butter	7.3	4.3
Peanut butter and chocolate chip	5.9	4.2
Plain	6.4	4.6
Raisin	6.4	4.3
Popcorn		
Air-popped	4.1	15.1
Caramel-coated		
With peanuts	3.3	3.8
Without peanuts	2.8	5.2
Cheese-flavor	2.5	9.9
Oil-popped	2.8	10.0
Potato chips		
Barbecue-flavor	1.9	4.4
Plain	1.9	4.8
Sour-cream-and-onion-flavor	1.8	5.2

Continued

Continued

Table II.73 Continued

Food item	Moisture	Total dietary fiber (AOAC)[‡]
Potato chips, made from dried potatoes, plain	1.4	3.6
Potato sticks	2.2	3.4
Pretzels, hard, plain	3.3	2.8
Rice cakes, brown rice		
Buckwheat	5.9	3.8
Corn	5.9	2.9
Multigrain	6.3	3.0
Plain	5.8	4.2
Rye	6.8	4.0
Tortilla chips		
Nacho-flavor	1.7	5.3
Plain	1.8	6.5
Sweets		
Baking chocolate, unsweetened, squares	1.3	15.4
Candies		
Alpine White Bar with Almonds	1.1	5.4
Baby Ruth Bar	5.0	2.9
Butterfinger Bar	5.6	2.7
Caramels	8.5	1.2
Chunky Bar	2.9	4.8
Milk chocolate	1.3	2.8
Milk chocolate, with almonds	1.5	6.2
M&M's Plain Chocolate Candies	1.4	3.1
Nestle Crunch Milk Chocolate with Crisp Rice	1.7	2.6
O'Henry	5.9	3.5
Cocoa, dry powder, unsweetened	3.0	29.8
Jams and preserves	34.5	1.2
Jellies	28.4	0.6
Pie fillings, canned		
Apple	73.4	1.0
Cherry	69.7	0.6
Vegetables and Vegetable Products		
Artichokes, raw	84.4	5.2
Beans, snap		
Canned, drained, solids	93.3	1.3
Raw	90.3	1.8
Beets, canned, drained, solids	91.0	1.7
Broccoli		
Cooked	90.2	2.6
Raw	90.7	2.8
Brussels sprouts, boiled	87.3	4.3
Cabbage, Chinese		
Cooked	95.4	1.6
Raw	94.9	1.0
Cabbage, red		
Cooked	93.6	2.0
Raw	91.6	2.0
Cabbage, white, raw	91.5	2.4
Carrots		
Canned, drained, solids	93.0	1.5
Raw	87.8	3.2
Cauliflower		
Cooked	92.5	2.2
Raw	92.3	2.4

Continued

Table II.73 Continued

Food item	Moisture	Total dietary fiber (AOAC)[‡]
Celery, raw	94.7	1.6
Chives	92.0	3.2
Corn, sweet		
Canned		
Brine pack, drained, solids	76.9	1.4
Cream-style	78.7	1.2
Cooked	69.6	3.7
Cucumbers		
Raw	96.0	1.0
Pared	–	0.5
Lettuce		
Butterhead or Iceberg	95.7	1.0
Romaine	94.9	1.7
Mushrooms		
Boiled	91.1	2.2
Raw	91.8	1.3
Onions, raw	90.1	1.6
Parsley, raw	88.3	4.4
Peas, edible, podded		
Cooked	88.9	2.8
Raw	88.9	2.6
Peas, sweet, canned, drained, solids	81.7	3.4
Peppers, sweet, raw	92.8	1.6
Pickles		
Dill	93.8	1.2
Sweet	68.9	1.1
Potatoes		
Baked		
Flesh	75.4	1.5
Skin	47.3	4.0
Boiled	77.0	1.5
French-fried, home-prepared from frozen	52.9	4.2
Hashed brown	56.1	2.0
Spinach		
Boiled	91.2	2.2
Raw	91.6	2.6
Squash		
Summer, cooked	93.7	1.4
Winter, cooked	89.0	2.8
Sweet potatoes		
Canned, drained, solids	72.5	1.8
Cooked	72.8	3.0
Tomato, raw	94.0	1.3
Tomato products		
Catsup	–	1.6
Paste	74.1	4.3
Puree	87.3	2.3
Sauce	89.1	1.5
Turnip greens		
Boiled	93.2	3.1
Raw	91.1	2.4
Turnips, boiled	93.6	2.0
Vegetables, mixed, frozen, cooked	83.2	3.8
Water chestnuts, canned, drained, solids	87.9	2.2
Watercress	95.1	2.3

Footnote over page

*Modified from the Provisional Table on the Dietary Fiber Content of Selected Foods, HNIS/PT-106, 1988 and from updated Appendix Tables 8–19, Aug. 1991, and 8–20. Oct. 1989.

†Appreciation is expressed to the U.S. Department of Agriculture, Human Nutrition Information Service, Nutrition Monitoring Division for assistance in obtaining these data.

‡The total dietary fiber in foods is measured by the enzymatic-gravimetric method (the Association of Official Analytical Chemists (AOAC) official method of analysis). Duplicate samples of dried foods, with fat extracted if containing >10% fat, are gelatinized with Termamyl (heat-stable α-amylase) and then enzymatically digested with protease and amyloglucosidase to remove protein and starch. (When analyzing mixed diets, fat is always extracted prior to determining total dietary fiber.) Four volumes of ethyl alcohol (EtOH) are added to precipitated soluble dietary fiber. Total residue is filtered and then washed with 78% EtOH, 95% EtOH, and acetone. After drying, residue is weighed. One duplicate is analyzed for protein; the other is incinerated at 525° and ash is determined.

Total dietary fiber = weight residue – weight (protein + ash).

Table II.74 Nonstarch polysaccharide content of selected foods

Food item	Total g/100g fresh weight
Vegetables and Legumes	
Beans, baked, canned	3.5
Beans, French, cooked	3.1
Beans, red kidney, cooked	6.7
Cabbage, red, cooked	3.3
Carrots, raw	2.4
Lentils, red, cooked	1.9
Onion, cooked	1.8
Peas, garden, canned	4.0
Potato, boiled, fresh	1.1
Potato crisps	4.9
Sprouts, Brussels, boiled	4.8
Fruits and Nuts	
Apple, Golden Delicious with skin	1.7
Apricots, fresh	2.3
Avocado, fresh	4.4
Canteloupe	0.6
Coconut, fresh	7.3
Figs, dried	7.5
Kiwi fruit, no skin	1.7
Peanuts, roasted	6.2
Raisins, dried	2.1
Cereal Products	
Bran flakes	11.3
Corn flakes	0.9
Oatmeal, coarse	7.0
Popcorn	9.8
Pumpernickel bread	7.5
Shredded wheat	9.8
Spaghetti, white, cooked	1.7
Spaghetti, whole-wheat, cooked	3.5
White bread	1.6
Wholemeal bread (average)	5.0

From Schwartz, S.E., Levine, R.A., Singh, A. *et al.* (1982) *Gastroenterology* 83: 812; Edwards, C.A. (1990) Physiological Effects of Fiber, in Kritchevsky, D., Bonfield, C. and Anderson, J.W. (eds), *Dietary Fiber: Chemistry, Physiology and Health Effects*, Plenum Press, N.Y. (Courtesy of Dr. Barbara Schneeman.)

Table II.75 Average values for the triglycerides, fatty acids (FA), and cholesterol in selected foods and oils (including OMEGA-3 FA) (per 100 g edible portion)

	FAT (g)	SFA (g)	MFA (g)	PFA (g)	M18:1 (g)	P18:2 (g)	P18:3 (g)	P:S	CHOL (mg)	S14:0 (g)	S16:0 (g)	S18:0 (g)	P20:5 (g)	P22:5 (g)	P22:6 (g)
Meats															
Liver calf	6.90	2.56	1.49	1.09	1.28	0.61	0.08	0.43	561.00	0.00	1.40	1.16	0.00	0.00	0.00
Liver pork	4.40	1.41	0.63	1.05	0.56	0.42	0.04	0.74	355.00	0.02	0.53	0.84	0.00	0.04	0.03
Kidney, beef	3.44	1.09	0.74	0.74	0.61	0.40	0.01	0.68	387.00	0.06	0.47	0.51	0.00	0.00	0.00
Kidney, pork	4.70	1.51	1.55	0.38	1.40	0.25	0.01	0.25	480.00	0.05	0.85	0.60	0.00	0.00	0.00
Brains, beef	12.53	2.92	2.50	1.44	2.00	0.03	0.00	0.49	2054.00	0.06	1.51	1.27	0.00	0.30	0.67
Brains, pork	9.51	2.15	1.72	1.47	1.10	0.09	0.12	0.68	2552.00	0.04	1.06	1.03	0.00	0.22	0.46
Beef, 5% fat, cooked	4.90	1.68	1.90	0.22	1.75	0.17	0.02	0.13	84.00	0.11	1.02	0.54	0.00	0.00	0.00
Beef, 26% fat, cooked	25.98	10.52	11.16	0.90	10.04	0.61	0.27	0.09	84.00	0.85	6.45	3.07	0.00	0.00	0.00
Lamb, 9% fat, cooked	9.17	3.28	4.02	0.60	3.72	0.49	0.05	0.18	92.00	0.29	1.76	1.13	0.00	0.00	0.00
Lamb, 36% fat, cooked	36.00	16.80	14.68	2.10	13.80	1.36	0.68	0.13	98.00	1.45	8.28	6.18	0.00	0.00	0.00
Veal, 6% fat, cooked	5.81	2.31	2.16	0.43	1.87	0.32	0.04	0.19	109.00	0.21	1.23	0.77	0.00	0.00	0.00
Veal, 25% fat, cooked	21.20	9.21	9.24	1.30	7.82	0.87	0.33	0.14	101.00	0.94	4.84	3.19	0.00	0.00	0.00
Chicken, light meat, unknown part, skin removed before cooking	3.87	1.15	1.05	0.92	0.88	0.66	0.02	0.80	77.00	0.03	0.67	0.32	0.00	0.03	0.03
Duck, domestic, skin removed before cooking	11.94	4.37	4.02	1.49	3.56	1.34	0.15	0.34	92.50	0.05	2.53	1.34	0.00	0.00	0.00
Ground beef, unknown % fat	22.56	8.86	9.88	0.84	8.63	0.62	0.09	0.09	89.00	0.64	5.10	2.66	0.00	0.00	0.00
Bologna, beef, regular	28.49	12.07	13.80	1.09	12.16	0.85	0.24	0.09	58.00	0.87	6.64	4.05	0.00	0.00	0.00
Pork, fresh, 25% fat, cooked	25.13	9.08	11.52	2.84	10.59	2.29	0.45	0.31	82.00	0.32	5.60	2.94	0.00	0.00	0.00
Frankfurter, all beef (Kosher), regular	28.54	12.05	13.62	1.38	11.99	1.11	0.27	0.11	61.00	0.94	6.52	3.96	0.00	0.00	0.00
Frankfurter, chicken	17.70	5.89	5.58	5.00	5.30	6.46	0.36	0.85	107.00	0.30	3.62	1.83	0.00	0.00	0.00
Frankfurter, regular, beef and pork	29.15	10.76	13.67	2.73	12.36	2.34	0.39	0.25	50.00	0.53	6.45	3.65	0.00	0.00	0.00
Pork, cured, 23% fat, cooked	23.48	8.38	11.03	2.51	10.15	2.15	0.36	0.30	67.00	0.25	5.12	2.93	0.00	0.00	0.00
Salami, pork	33.72	11.89	16.00	3.74	14.67	3.27	0.28	0.31	79.00	0.52	7.64	3.56	0.00	0.00	0.00
Bacon, regular cut	49.24	17.42	23.69	5.81	21.96	4.89	0.79	0.33	85.00	0.62	10.98	5.67	0.00	0.00	0.00
Fish															
Mussel, cooked from fresh or frozen	1.95	0.19	0.17	0.55	0.07	0.03	0.01	2.89	67.00	0.03	0.12	0.04	0.14	0.10	0.15
Fish, 0 to 2.9% fat	1.53	0.36	0.31	0.63	0.15	0.01	0.02	1.75	68.00	0.06	0.23	0.05	0.24	0.05	0.26
Fish, 3.0 to 6.9% fat	4.31	0.83	1.33	1.54	0.79	0.32	0.15	1.86	73.00	0.09	0.49	0.17	0.18	0.13	0.55
Fish, 7.0 to 10.9% fat	7.54	1.39	2.61	2.20	1.52	0.32	0.24	1.58	49.00	0.35	0.79	0.24	0.41	0.27	0.62
Fish, 11.0 to 14.9% fat	12.14	4.50	3.31	1.46	0.75	0.05	0.00	0.32	64.00	0.21	0.95	0.35	0.13	0.11	0.03
Herring, smoked/kippered, canned and drained	12.37	2.79	5.11	2.92	2.07	0.18	0.14	1.05	82.00	0.76	1.85	0.15	0.97	0.07	1.18
Salmon, canned, drained, with salt	6.05	1.53	1.81	2.05	1.07	0.06	0.06	1.34	55.00	0.05	1.35	0.13	0.84	0.05	0.81
Sardines, canned in oil, drained	11.45	1.53	3.87	5.15	2.14	3.54	0.50	3.37	142.00	0.19	0.99	0.34	0.47	0.00	0.51

Continued

Table II.75 Continued

	FAT (g)	SFA (g)	MFA (g)	PFA (g)	M18:1 (g)	P18:2 (g)	P18:3 (g)	P:S	CHOL (mg)	S14:0 (g)	S16:0 (g)	S18:0 (g)	P20:5 (g)	P22:5 (g)	P22:6 (g)
Tuna, canned, oil pack, regular, drained	8.21	1.53	2.95	2.88	2.84	2.68	0.07	1.88	18.00	0.03	1.41	0.09	0.03	0.00	0.10
Tuna, canned, water pack, regular, drained, not rinsed	0.50	0.16	0.14	0.13	0.07	0.00	0.00	0.81	18.00	0.03	0.11	0.02	0.04	0.01	0.07
Clams, cooked from fresh or frozen	1.95	0.19	0.17	0.55	0.07	0.03	0.01	2.89	67.00	0.03	0.12	0.04	0.14	0.10	0.15
Crab, hardshell, Alaskan King	1.77	0.23	0.28	0.68	0.15	0.03	0.02	2.96	100.00	0.02	0.14	0.06	0.24	0.05	0.23
Lobster, cooked from fresh or frozen	0.59	0.11	0.16	0.09	0.09	0.00	0.00	0.82	72.00	0.01	0.08	0.02	0.05	0.00	0.03
Oyster, cooked from fresh or frozen, Pacific	4.95	1.26	0.50	1.48	0.19	0.10	0.07	1.17	109.00	0.22	0.87	0.12	0.42	0.10	0.46
Scallops	1.40	0.15	0.07	0.48	0.03	0.01	0.00	3.20	31.81	0.02	0.10	0.02	0.17	0.03	0.20
Shrimps, cooked from fresh or frozen	1.08	0.29	0.20	0.44	0.11	0.02	0.01	1.52	195.00	0.02	0.14	0.10	0.17	0.02	0.14
Caviar	17.90	4.21	5.86	5.66	2.94	0.99	0.55	1.34	588.00	0.90	1.87	0.72	1.03	0.81	1.35
Eggs, Dairy															
Eggs, whole, cooked	10.02	3.10	3.81	1.36	3.47	1.15	0.03	0.44	425.00	0.03	2.23	0.78	0.00	0.00	0.04
Eggs, yolk only, cooked	30.87	9.55	11.74	4.20	10.70	3.54	0.10	0.44	1281.00	0.10	6.86	2.42	0.01	0.00	0.11
Eggs, white only, cooked	0.00	0.00	0.00	0.00	0.00	0.00	0.00	0.00	0.00	0.00	0.00	0.00	0.00	0.00	0.00
Cream, coffee creamer, liquid/frozen	9.97	9.30	0.11	0.00	0.11	0.00	0.00	0.00	0.00	1.00	0.43	0.60	0.00	0.00	0.00
Cream, coffee creamer, powder, regular	35.48	32.52	0.97	0.01	0.97	0.00	0.01	0.00	0.00	5.99	3.75	6.34	0.00	0.00	0.00
Cream, coffee creamer, liquid/frozen	11.28	1.68	4.85	4.25	4.79	3.94	0.29	2.53	0.00	0.01	1.10	0.56	0.00	0.00	0.00
Cream, half and half, 10 to 12% fat	11.50	7.16	3.32	0.43	2.89	0.26	0.17	0.06	36.90	1.16	3.02	1.39	0.00	0.00	0.00
Cream, light/coffee cream, 20% fat	19.31	12.02	5.58	0.72	4.86	0.44	0.28	0.06	66.10	1.94	5.08	2.34	0.00	0.00	0.00
Milk, buttermilk, 1% fat	0.88	0.55	0.25	0.03	0.22	0.02	0.01	0.05	3.50	0.09	0.23	0.11	0.00	0.00	0.00
Milk, skim	0.18	0.12	0.05	0.01	0.04	0.00	0.00	0.08	1.80	0.02	0.05	0.02	0.00	0.00	0.00
Milk, 1% fat	1.06	0.66	0.31	0.04	0.27	0.02	0.01	0.06	4.00	0.11	0.28	0.13	0.00	0.00	0.00
Milk, 2% fat	1.92	1.19	0.55	0.07	0.48	0.04	0.03	0.06	7.50	0.19	0.50	0.23	0.00	0.00	0.00
Milk, whole, 3.5 to 4% fat	3.34	2.08	0.96	0.12	0.84	0.07	0.05	0.06	13.60	0.34	0.88	0.40	0.00	0.00	0.00
Parmesan cheese, dry	30.02	19.07	8.73	0.66	7.74	0.32	0.34	0.03	78.70	3.38	8.10	2.67	0.00	0.00	0.00
American cheese, processed	31.25	19.69	8.95	0.99	7.51	0.61	0.38	0.05	94.40	3.21	9.10	3.80	0.00	0.00	0.00
Cottage cheese, lowfat, 2% fat	1.93	1.22	0.55	0.06	0.45	0.04	0.02	0.05	8.40	0.20	0.58	0.22	0.00	0.00	0.00
Cottage cheese, regular or creamed, 4% fat	4.51	2.85	1.28	0.14	1.06	0.10	0.04	0.05	14.90	0.47	1.36	0.51	0.00	0.00	0.00
Cream cheese, Neufchatel	23.43	14.80	6.77	0.65	5.66	0.45	0.20	0.04	76.10	2.35	6.88	2.98	0.00	0.00	0.00
Cheddar cheese, natural	33.14	21.09	9.39	0.94	7.90	0.58	0.36	0.04	104.90	3.33	9.80	4.01	0.00	0.00	0.00
Swiss cheese, natural	27.45	17.78	7.27	0.97	6.02	0.62	0.35	0.05	91.70	3.06	7.79	3.25	0.00	0.00	0.00

Table II.75 Continued

	FAT (g)	SFA (g)	MFA (g)	PFA (g)	M18:1 (g)	P18:2 (g)	P18:3 (g)	P:S	CHOL (mg)	S14:0 (g)	S16:0 (g)	S18:0 (g)	P20:5 (g)	P22:5 (g)	P22:6 (g)
Monterey Jacke cheese, natural	30.04	19.11	8.71	0.66	7.34	0.43	0.23	0.03	95.60	3.07	9.22	3.57	0.00	0.00	0.00
Mozzarella cheese, part skim milk	17.12	10.88	4.85	0.51	4.17	0.36	0.15	0.05	54.00	1.72	5.22	2.08	0.00	0.00	0.00
Brie cheese	24.26	15.26	7.02	0.72	5.75	0.45	0.27	0.05	72.00	2.69	7.23	2.52	0.00	0.00	0.00
Cheese, Kraft Light 'N' Lively Singles, American flavor	15.50	9.77	4.44	0.49	3.73	0.30	0.19	0.05	52.91	1.59	4.51	1.88	0.00	0.00	0.00
Cheese, Borden Lite-Line Singles, American flavor	8.20	4.99	2.34	0.26	1.94	0.19	0.07	0.05	45.00	0.82	2.47	0.88	0.00	0.00	0.00
Yogurt, frozen, fruit or vanilla, whole milk, 3 to 4% fat	3.24	2.10	0.90	0.09	0.75	0.06	0.03	0.04	9.74	0.33	0.87	0.30	0.00	0.00	0.00
Yogurt, frozen, fruit or vanilla, low fat, 1 to 2% fat	1.08	0.70	0.30	0.03	0.25	0.02	0.01	0.04	4.20	0.11	0.29	0.10	0.00	0.00	0.00
Yoghurt, plain, lowfat, 1 to 2% fat	1.55	1.00	0.43	0.04	0.35	0.03	0.01	0.04	6.10	0.16	0.42	0.15	0.00	0.00	0.00
Yoghurt, fruit, nonfat, <1% fat	0.20	0.12	0.05	0.01	0.00	0.00	0.00	0.08	2.00	0.00	0.00	0.00	0.00	0.00	0.00
Yogurt, fruit, whole milk, 3 to 4% fat	3.24	2.10	0.90	0.09	0.75	0.06	0.03	0.04	9.74	0.33	0.87	0.30	0.00	0.00	0.00
Ice cream and frozen desserts, regular, 10% fat, other flavors include chocolate chip	10.77	6.70	3.11	0.40	2.71	0.24	0.16	0.06	44.70	1.08	2.83	1.30	0.00	0.00	0.00
Sherbet, plain	1.98	1.23	0.57	0.07	0.50	0.04	0.03	0.06	7.30	0.20	0.52	0.24	0.00	0.00	0.00
Ice cream and frozen desserts, regular 5% fat, other flavors include chocolate chip	4.30	2.68	1.24	0.16	1.08	0.10	0.06	0.06	13.90	0.43	1.13	0.52	0.00	0.00	0.00
Fats/Oils															
Oils, canola	100.00	7.10	58.90	29.60	56.10	20.30	9.30	4.17	0.00	0.00	4.00	1.80	0.00	0.00	0.00
Oils, corn	100.00	12.70	24.20	58.70	24.20	58.00	0.00	4.62	0.00	0.00	10.90	1.80	0.00	0.00	0.00
Oils, sunflower	100.00	10.30	19.50	65.70	19.50	65.70	0.00	6.38	0.00	0.00	5.90	4.50	0.00	0.00	0.00
Oils, cottonseed	100.00	25.90	17.80	51.90	17.00	51.50	0.20	2.00	0.00	0.80	22.70	2.30	0.00	0.00	0.00
Oils, safflower	100.00	9.10	12.10	74.50	11.70	74.10	0.40	8.19	0.00	0.10	6.20	2.20	0.00	0.00	0.00
Oils, sesame	100.00	14.20	39.70	41.70	39.30	41.30	0.30	2.94	0.00	0.00	8.90	4.80	0.00	0.00	0.00
Oils, soybean (partially hydrogenated)	100.00	14.90	43.00	37.60	42.50	34.90	2.60	2.52	0.00	0.10	9.80	5.00	0.00	0.00	0.00
Oils, olive	100.00	13.50	73.70	8.40	72.50	7.90	0.60	0.62	0.00	0.00	11.00	2.20	0.00	0.00	0.00
Oils, peanut	100.00	16.90	46.20	32.00	44.80	32.00	0.00	1.89	0.00	0.10	9.50	2.20	0.00	0.00	0.00

Continued

Table II.75   Continued

	FAT (g)	SFA (g)	MFA (g)	PFA (g)	M18:1 (g)	P18:2 (g)	P18:3 (g)	P:S	CHOL (mg)	S14:0 (g)	S16:0 (g)	S18:0 (g)	P20:5 (g)	P22:5 (g)	P22:6 (g)
Oils, coconut	100.00	86.50	5.80	1.80	5.80	1.80	0.00	0.02	0.00	16.80	8.20	2.80	0.00	0.00	0.00
Oils, palm	100.00	49.30	37.00	9.30	36.60	9.10	0.20	0.19	0.00	1.00	43.50	4.30	0.00	0.00	0.00
Oils, palm kernel	100.00	81.40	11.40	1.60	11.40	1.60	0.00	0.02	0.00	16.40	8.10	2.80	0.00	0.00	0.00
Shortening, vegetable	100.00	25.00	44.50	26.10	44.50	24.50	1.60	1.04	0.00	0.40	14.10	10.60	0.00	0.00	0.00
Margarine, regular, stick, salted, corn oil	80.50	19.85	36.48	18.62	36.48	18.62	0.00	0.94	0.00	1.08	11.54	7.23	0.00	0.00	0.00
Lard	100.00	39.20	45.10	11.20	41.20	10.20	1.00	0.29	95.00	1.30	23.80	13.50	0.00	0.00	0.00
Butter, regular, salted	81.11	50.49	23.43	3.01	20.40	1.83	1.18	0.06	218.90	8.16	21.33	9.83	0.00	0.00	0.00
Oils, medium chain triglyceride	100.00	94.50	0.00	0.00	0.00	0.00	0.00	0.00	0.00	0.00	0.00	0.00	0.00	0.00	0.00
Mayonnaise/mayo-type dressing, real, regular, commercial	79.40	11.80	22.70	41.30	22.50	37.10	4.20	3.50	59.00	0.10	8.50	3.10	0.00	0.00	0.00
Oils, rapeseed	100.00	6.80	55.50	33.30	53.80	22.10	11.10	4.90	0.00	0.00	4.80	1.60	0.00	0.00	0.00
Miscellaneous															
Peanuts, peanut butter, with salt	49.98	9.59	23.58	14.36	22.96	14.10	0.08	1.50	0.00	0.05	5.50	2.14	0.00	0.00	0.00
Almonds, roasted, dry roasted, salted	56.53	5.27	36.71	11.86	36.03	11.36	0.40	2.25	0.00	0.32	3.74	1.11	0.00	0.00	0.00
Cashews, roasted, dry roasted, salted	48.21	9.70	28.41	8.15	27.89	7.97	0.17	0.84	0.00	0.36	4.53	3.09	0.00	0.00	0.00
Peanuts, roasted, dry roasted, salted	49.30	6.84	24.46	15.58	23.79	15.58	0.00	2.28	0.00	0.02	5.16	1.10	0.00	0.00	0.00
Walnuts	61.87	5.59	14.17	39.13	13.30	31.76	6.81	7.00	0.00	0.19	4.24	1.08	0.00	0.00	0.00
Olives, black	10.68	1.41	7.89	0.91	7.77	0.85	0.06	0.65	0.00	0.00	1.18	0.24	0.00	0.00	0.00
Candy, chocolate pieces, fudge, plain	10.78	4.93	4.53	0.93	4.48	0.86	0.06	0.19	3.92	0.10	2.29	2.35	0.00	0.00	0.00
Avocado, unknown type	15.32	2.44	9.61	1.95	8.96	1.84	0.11	0.80	0.00	0.00	2.40	0.03	0.00	0.00	0.00
Coconut, fresh	33.49	29.70	1.42	0.37	1.42	0.37	0.00	0.01	0.00	5.87	2.84	1.73	0.00	0.00	0.00
Soybeans, cooked from dried	8.97	1.30	1.98	5.06	1.96	4.46	0.60	3.89	0.00	0.02	0.95	0.32	0.00	0.00	0.00
Peas, black-eyed, cooked from dried	0.53	0.14	0.04	0.22	0.04	0.14	0.08	1.57	0.00	0.00	0.11	0.02	0.00	0.00	0.00
Split peas, yellow or green, cooked from dried	0.39	0.05	0.08	0.16	0.08	0.14	0.03	3.20	0.00	0.00	0.04	0.01	0.00	0.00	0.00

SFA = saturated fatty acid, MFA = monounsaturated fatty acid, PFA = polyunsaturated fatty acid, M18:1 = oleic acid, P18:2 = linoleic acid, P18:3 = linolenic acid, S14:0 = myristic acid, S16:0 = palmitic acid, S18:0 = stearic acid, P20:5 = omega-3 (eicosapentaenoic acid), P22:5 = omega-3 (docosapentaenoic acid), P22:6 = omega-3 (docosahexaenoic acid).

(With appreciation to the Nutrition Coding Center, University of Minneapolis, Minneapolis, MN for the compilation and preparation of these tables. Data are based on Version 19 of the NCC Nutrient Data Base.)

Table II.76   Average values for triglycerides, fatty acids (FA), and cholesterol of marine foods and oils (including Omega-3 FA)

Fish (100 g)	Fat (g)	Chol (mg)	SFA (g)	MFA (g)	PFA (g)	M18:1 (g)	P18:2 (g)	P18:3 (g)	P20:5 (g)	P22:5 (g)	P22:6 (g)
Anchovy, European, raw	4.84	—	1.28	1.19	1.64	0.62	0.10	—	0.50	—	0.90
Bass, striped, raw	2.33	80.00	0.51	0.66	0.78	0.45	0.02	0.02	0.17	—	0.59
Bluefish, raw	4.24	58.82	0.92	1.79	1.06	0.68	0.06	trace	0.25	0.06	0.52
Burbot, raw	0.81	60.00	0.16	0.13	0.30	0.10	0.01	—	0.07	0.03	0.10
Carp, raw	5.60	65.88	1.08	2.33	1.44	1.15	0.52	0.27	0.24	0.08	0.11
Catfish, wild, raw	2.82	58.00	0.72	0.84	0.87	0.59	0.10	0.07	0.13	0.10	0.23
Catfish, farmed, raw	7.59	47.00	1.77	3.59	1.57	3.17	0.88	0.10	0.07	0.09	0.21
Cod, Atlantic, raw	0.67	43.53	0.13	0.09	0.23	0.06	0.01	trace	0.10	—	0.20
Eel, all varieties, raw	11.66	126.00	2.35	7.19	0.95	2.78	0.20	0.70	0.10	—	0.10
Flounder, unspecified, raw	1.00	46.00	0.20	0.30	0.30	—	—	trace	0.10	—	0.10
Haddock, raw	0.72	57.65	0.13	0.12	0.24	0.07	0.01	trace	0.10	—	0.10
Halibut, raw	2.29	31.77	0.33	0.65	0.84	0.36	0.03	0.07	0.07	0.09	0.29
Herring, Atlantic, raw	9.04	60.00	2.03	3.74	2.13	1.52	0.13	0.10	0.70	—	0.90
Mackerel, Atlantic, raw	13.87	70.07	3.26	4.06	4.76	2.28	0.22	0.16	0.90	0.21	1.40
Mussel, blue, raw	2.20	38.00	0.40	0.50	0.60	trace	—	—	0.20	1.03	0.37
Octopus, raw	1.01	—	0.30	0.10	0.30	—	—	—	0.10	—	0.10
Oyster, Eastern, wild, raw	2.46	53.00	0.77	0.31	0.97	0.12	0.06	0.05	0.27	0.06	0.29
Oyster, Eastern, farmed, raw	1.55	25.00	0.44	0.15	0.59	0.07	0.03	0.04	0.19	—	0.20
Perch, all varieties, raw	0.92	89.41	0.19	0.15	0.37	0.07	0.01	0.10	0.90	—	1.60
Pike, walleye, raw	1.21	85.88	0.25	0.29	0.45	0.20	0.03	0.01	0.09	0.04	0.23
Pollock, Atlantic, raw	0.98	71.06	0.14	0.11	0.48	0.07	0.01	—	0.07	0.02	0.35
Sablefish, raw	15.30	49.00	3.20	8.06	2.04	4.07	0.17	0.10	0.68	0.17	0.72
Salmon, Chinook, raw	10.45	65.88	2.51	4.48	2.08	2.80	0.11	0.09	0.79	0.23	0.57
Salmon, coho, wild, raw	5.93	45.00	1.26	2.13	1.99	1.20	0.21	0.16	0.43	0.23	0.66
Salmon, coho, farmed, raw	7.67	51.00	1.82	3.33	1.86	1.72	0.35	0.08	0.39	—	0.82
Sea bass, all, raw	2.00	41.18	0.51	0.42	0.74	0.29	0.02	trace	0.10	—	0.30
Smelt, rainbow, raw	2.58	75.00	0.48	0.68	0.94	0.43	0.05	0.10	0.30	—	0.40
Squid, short, finned, raw	1.50	0.40	0.42	0.09	0.52	—	—	trace	0.16	0.52	0.36
Red snapper, raw	1.34	37.06	0.29	0.25	0.46	0.17	0.02	trace	trace	—	0.20
Sole, European, raw	1.20	50.00	0.30	0.40	0.20	—	0.00	trace	trace	—	0.10
Sturgeon, all, raw	4.04	—	0.92	1.94	0.69	1.44	0.07	0.10	0.19	0.05	0.09
Swordfish, raw	4.01	38.82	1.10	1.54	0.92	1.09	0.03	—	0.10	0.00	0.10
Trout, rainbow, wild, raw	3.46	59.00	0.72	1.13	1.24	0.61	0.24	0.12	0.17	0.11	0.42
Trout, rainbow, farmed, raw	5.40	59.00	1.55	1.54	1.81	1.06	0.71	0.06	0.26	—	0.67
Tuna, bluefin, fresh, raw	4.91	37.65	1.26	1.37	1.67	0.92	0.05	—	0.40	—	1.20
Whitefish, all, raw	5.85	60.00	0.91	2.00	2.15	1.35	0.27	0.18	0.32	0.16	0.94
Cod liver oil	100.00	570.00	22.61	46.71	22.54	20.65	0.94	0.94	6.90	0.94	10.97
Herring oil	100.00	766.00	21.29	56.56	15.60	11.96	1.15	0.76	6.27	0.62	4.21
Menhaden oil	100.00	521.00	30.43	26.69	34.20	14.53	2.15	1.49	13.17	4.92	8.56
Max EPA conc fish body oil	100.00	600.00	25.40	28.30	41.10	—	—	0.00	17.80	—	11.60
Salmon oil	100.00	485.00	19.87	29.04	40.32	16.98	1.54	1.06	13.02	2.99	18.23

SFA = saturated fatty acid, MFA = monounsaturated fatty acid, PFA = polyunsaturated fatty acid, M18:1 = oleic acid, P18:2 = linoleic acid, P18:3 = linolenic acid, P20:5 = omega-3 (eicosapentaenoic acid), P22:5 = omega-3 (docosapentaenoic acid), P22:6 = omega-3 (docosahexaenoic acid).
(From Human Nutrition Information Service (1988) Provisional Table on the Content of Omega-3 Fatty Acids and Other Fat Components in Selected Foods, U.S. Department of Agriculture, HNIS/PT-103. Other data obtained from Consumer Nutrition Center (1991) *Composition of Finfish and Shellfish Products*, Agriculture Handbook No. 8-15, 1991 Supplement. U.S. Department of Agriculture, Washington.)
Trace is less than 0.05 g/100 g food.
—denotes lack of reliable data for nutrient known to be present.

Table II.77   Protein, sodium, potassium, calcium, phosphorus, and magnesium content of selected common foods per serving portion

Food name	Serving portion	Pro (g)	Na (mg)	K (mg)	Ca (mg)	PO₄ (mg)	Mg (mg)
Dairy Products							
Egg, whole, raw, large	1.0 Item	6.250	63.000	60.000	25.000	89.000	5.000
Cheese, cottage, uncreamed	1.0 Oz	4.888	3.715	9.189	8.994	29.523	1.173
Cream, coffee, table, light	1.0 Tbsp	0.405	5.937	18.250	14.437	12.000	1.312
Cream, sour, cultured	1.0 Tbsp	0.454	7.687	20.687	16.750	12.187	1.625
Milk, buttermilk, fluid	1.0 Cup	8.110	257.000	371.000	285.000	219.000	27.000
Milk, whole, 3.3% fat, fluid	1.0 Cup	8.030	120.000	370.000	291.000	228.000	33.000
Milk, nonfat/skim, fluid	1.0 Cup	8.350	126.000	406.000	302.000	247.000	28.000
Milk, whole, low sodium	1.0 Cup	7.560	6.000	617.000	246.000	209.000	12.000
Fats							
Butter, regular	1.0 Tbsp	0.119	116.000	3.640	3.360	3.220	0.280
Vegetable oil, corn	1.0 Tsp	0.000	0.000	0.000	0.000	0.000	0.000
Vegetable oil, olive	1.0 Tsp	0.000	0.002	0.000	0.008	0.055	0.000
Shortening, veg. soybn/cottnsd	1.0 Tsp	0.000	0.000	0.000	0.000	0.000	0.000
Margarine, reg. hard, unsalted	1.0 Tsp	0.000	0.100	1.160	0.820	0.630	0.070
Mayonnaise, soy, commercial	1.0 Tsp	0.067	26.133	1.667	0.667	1.333	0.047
Cereals							
Bran flakes, Kellogg's	0.5 Cup	2.455	152.000	124.000	9.550	96.000	35.500
Corn flakes, Kellogg's	0.5 Cup	0.920	116.000	10.450	0.341	7.150	1.360
Cream of rice, cooked	1.0 Cup	2.200	2.440	48.800	7.320	41.500	7.320
Cream of wheat, instant	1.0 Cup	4.400	6.000	48.000	59.000	43.000	14.000
Farina, cooked, enriched	1.0 Cup	3.260	0.000	30.300	4.660	28.000	4.660
Oatmeal, cooked	1.0 Cup	6.080	2.340	131.000	18.700	178.000	56.200
Wheat, puffed, plain	0.5 Cup	0.880	0.240	20.900	1.680	21.300	8.700
Wheat, shredded, biscuit	1.0 Item	2.600	0.472	77.000	9.680	86.000	40.100
Rice Krispies	0.5 Cup	0.965	170.000	14.750	1.990	17.200	5.100
Breads, Cookies, Crackers							
Bread, white, soft	1.0 Slice	2.070	129.000	28.000	31.500	27.000	5.250
Bread, whole-wheat, soft	1.0 Slice	2.690	178.000	49.300	20.200	72.800	26.000
Crackers, graham, plain	1.0 Item	0.500	33.000	27.500	3.000	10.500	3.570
Crackers, sodium free/whole wheat	1.0 Serving	1.000	1.000	35.000	—	—	—
Crackers, saltines	1.0 Item	0.250	36.800	3.250	0.500	2.500	0.770
Muffin, English, plain	0.5 Item	2.215	179.000	157.000	45.350	31.350	5.300
Bread, Italian, enriched	1.0 Slice	3.000	152.000	22.000	5.000	23.000	—
Roll, hard, enriched	0.5 Item	2.500	156.000	24.500	12.000	23.000	5.750
Roll, hamburger/hotdog	1.0 Item	3.430	241.000	36.800	53.600	32.800	7.600
Cookies, vanilla wafer	5.0 Items	1.000	50.000	14.500	8.000	12.500	3.400
Meat, Fish							
Pot roast, arm, beef, cooked	1.0 Oz	9.355	18.711	81.931	2.551	75.978	6.804
Hamburger patty, beef/lean	1.0 Oz	7.004	21.679	85.384	3.002	44.693	6.004
Steak, sirloin, lean, broiled	1.0 Oz	8.606	18.731	114.000	3.119	69.356	9.062
Chicken, leg, no skin, roasted	1.0 Oz	7.669	25.963	68.637	3.402	51.925	6.864
Chicken, breast, roasted	1.0 Oz	8.447	19.961	69.429	4.050	60.750	7.811
Lamb, all cuts, lean/fat, cooked	1.0 Oz	6.971	20.345	87.718	4.669	53.365	6.671
Turkey, dark meat, no skin	1.0 Oz	8.100	22.275	82.215	9.113	57.915	6.885
Turkey, light, no skin, roasted	1.0 Oz	8.485	18.023	86.265	5.468	62.168	7.898
Veal, all cuts, lean, cooked	1.0 Oz	9.039	25.348	96.056	6.671	71.042	8.005
Bluefish	1.0 Oz	5.689	17.010	105.000	1.890	64.449	9.450
Flatfish, raw	1.0 Oz	5.336	23.014	102.000	5.003	52.031	9.005
Cod, cooked, dry heat	1.0 Oz	6.473	22.050	69.143	3.969	39.060	11.970
Halibut, broiled, dry	1.0 Oz	7.571	19.578	163.000	17.010	80.714	30.351
Shrimp, raw, mixed species	1.0 Oz	5.751	42.525	52.650	15.188	58.725	10.125
Tuna, can/oil, drained	1.0 Oz	8.272	100.000	58.701	3.702	88.052	8.805
Tuna, diet, low sodium	1.0 Oz	7.656	11.380	73.670	1.418	62.390	9.074
Sweets							
Honey, strained/extracted	1.0 Tbsp	0.000	1.000	11.000	1.000	1.000	0.630
Ice milk, van, hard, 4.3% fat	0.5 Cup	2.580	52.500	133.000	88.000	64.500	9.500

Continued

Table II.77　Continued

Food name	Serving portion	Pro (g)	Na (mg)	K (mg)	Ca (mg)	PO₄ (mg)	Mg (mg)
Ice cream, van, hard, 10% fat	0.5 Cup	2.400	58.000	129.000	88.000	67.000	9.000
Ice cream, van, hard, 16% fat	0.5 Cup	2.065	54.000	111.000	75.500	57.500	8.000
Jams/preserves, regular	1.0 Tbsp	0.000	2.000	18.000	4.000	2.000	—
Sherbet, orange, 2% fat	0.5 Cup	1.080	44.000	99.000	51.500	37.000	7.500
Sugar, brown, pressed down	0.5 Cup	0.000	33.000	379.000	93.500	21.000	—
Sugar, white, granulated	1.0 Tbsp	0.000	0.120	0.000	0.000	0.000	—
Juices							
Apple juice, can and bottle	3.5 Fl ozs	0.066	3.062	129.000	7.612	7.875	3.500
Apricot nectar, can	3.5 Fl ozs	0.402	3.937	125.000	7.700	9.887	5.687
Cranberry juice, bottle	3.5 Fl ozs	0.000	4.375	19.906	3.321	2.214	2.214
Grape juice, can	3.5 Fl ozs	0.000	0.000	38.500	3.500	3.500	—
Grapefruit juice, can, unsweetened	3.5 Fl ozs	0.560	1.081	165.000	7.569	11.900	10.806
Lemon juice, can and bottle	3.5 Fl ozs	0.427	22.400	109.000	11.725	9.625	8.531
Orange juice, can	3.5 Fl ozs	0.643	2.179	191.000	8.706	15.268	11.987
Pear nectar, can	3.5 Fl ozs	0.120	4.375	14.219	5.469	3.281	3.281
Pineapple juice, can	3.5 Fl ozs	0.350	1.094	147.000	18.593	8.750	14.219
Prune juice, can and bottle	3.5 Fl ozs	0.682	4.462	309.000	13.431	28.000	15.662
Tomato juice, can	3.5 Fl ozs	0.809	385.000	235.000	9.625	20.300	11.725
Tomato juice, low sodium	3.5 Fl ozs	0.809	10.675	235.000	9.625	20.300	11.725
Vegetables							
Asparagus, can, spears	0.5 Cup	2.590	472.000	208.000	19.350	52.000	12.100
Asparagus, can, low sodium	0.5 Cup	2.195	425.000	187.000	17.100	46.350	11.000
Beans, snap, green, can, cuts	0.5 Cup	0.775	170.000	73.500	17.550	12.850	8.800
Beans, green, can, low sodium	0.5 Cup	0.780	1.360	74.000	16.000	13.000	9.000
Beans, snap, wax, raw, boiled	0.5 Cup	1.180	1.875	187.000	28.750	24.000	15.650
Beets, can, whole	0.5 Cup	1.025	324.000	175.000	17.200	19.700	19.700
Beets, can, diet, low sodium	0.5 Cup	1.025	324.000	175.000	17.200	19.700	19.700
Broccoli, raw, boiled, drained	0.5 Cup	2.310	20.150	227.000	35.650	45.750	18.600
Cabbage, common, boiled, drained	0.5 Cup	0.695	13.800	149.000	23.950	18.150	10.900
Carrots, can, sliced, drained	0.5 Cup	0.467	176.000	131.000	18.250	17.500	5.850
Carrots, can, low sodium	0.5 Cup	0.750	47.950	213.000	30.750	24.600	11.050
Carrot, raw, whole, scraped	1.0 Item	0.740	25.200	233.000	19.400	31.700	10.800
Cauliflower, raw, boiled, drained	0.5 Cup	1.160	4.000	200.000	17.000	22.000	7.000
Celery, Pascal, raw, stalk	1.0 Item	0.300	34.800	115.000	16.000	10.000	4.400
Corn, sweet, can, drained	0.5 Cup	2.160	267.000	161.000	4.125	53.500	16.500
Corn, sweet, can, low sodium	0.5 Cup	2.480	3.840	196.000	5.100	65.500	20.500
Cucumber, raw, sliced	0.5 Cup	0.281	1.040	77.500	7.300	8.850	5.700
Peas, green, can, drained	0.5 Cup	3.755	186.000	147.000	17.000	57.000	14.450
Peas, green, can, low sodium	0.5 Cup	3.755	1.700	147.000	17.000	57.000	14.450
Tomato, raw, red, ripe	1.0 Item	1.050	11.100	273.000	6.150	29.500	13.500
Tomato, red, can, stewed	0.5 Cup	1.185	324.000	305.000	42.100	25.500	15.300
Tomato, can, low sodium, diet	0.5 Cup	1.115	15.600	265.000	31.200	22.800	14.400
Potato, boiled, peeled before cooked	1.0 Item	2.310	6.750	443.000	10.800	54.000	27.000
Noodles, egg, enriched, cooked	0.5 Cup	3.500	1.500	35.000	8.000	47.000	21.600
Rice, white, parboiled, cooked	0.5 Cup	2.005	2.625	32.400	16.650	36.750	10.500
Fruits							
Apples, raw, unpeeled	1.0 Item	0.262	1.000	159.000	10.000	10.000	6.000
Apples, raw, peeled	1.0 Item	0.190	0.000	144.000	5.000	9.000	4.000
Applesauce, can, unsweetened	0.5 Cup	0.208	2.440	91.500	3.660	8.550	3.660
Apricots, can, light syrup	0.5 Cup	0.675	5.000	175.000	13.900	17.000	10.500
Bananas, raw, peeled	1.0 Item	1.170	1.140	451.000	6.840	22.000	33.000
Blueberries, raw	0.5 Cup	0.486	4.350	64.500	4.350	7.250	3.625
Cherries, sweet, can/juice	0.5 Cup	1.140	3.750	164.000	17.500	27.500	15.000
Grapefruit, red/pnk/wht, raw	0.5 Cup	0.725	0.500	161.000	13.500	10.000	9.500
Oranges, raw, all varieties	1.0 Item	1.230	0.000	237.000	52.400	18.300	13.100
Peaches, raw, whole	1.0 Item	0.609	0.000	171.000	4.350	10.400	6.090
Peaches, can, light syrup	0.5 Cup	0.565	6.500	122.000	4.500	13.500	6.000
Pears, raw, bartlet, unpeeled	1.0 Item	0.647	0.000	208.000	18.300	18.300	9.960
Pineapple, can/juice	0.5 Cup	0.525	2.000	153.000	17.500	7.500	17.500
Strawberries, raw, whole	0.5 Cup	0.455	0.745	124.000	10.450	14.150	7.450

Pro = protein, Na = sodium, K = potassium, Ca = calcium, PO₄ = phosphorus, Mg = magnesium.
(Created on Nutritionist III, Version 7, N-Squared Computing, 1991. Data compiled from U.S. Department of Agriculture Handbook 8-Series, manufacturers' data, published journals, and industry sources. Appreciation expressed to Ms. Lori Cohen, M.S., R.D., for her assistance in preparing this table.)

Table II.78 Vitamin A, Vitamin E, α-Tocopherol (TOC), Vitamin C, Thiamin, Riboflavin, Niacin, Vitamin B_6, Vitamin B_{12}, and Folate content of selected common foods per serving portion

Food name	Serving portion	A* (RE)	E† (mg)	α-TOC (mg)	C (mg)	Thiamin (mg)	Ribo (mg)	Niacin (mg)	B_6 (mg)	B_{12} (µg)	Folate (µg)
Dairy Products											
Egg, whole, raw, large	1.0 Item	95.200	0.700	0.350	0.000	0.031	0.254	0.037	0.070	0.500	23.000
Cheese, cottage, uncreamed	1.0 Oz	2.581	—	0.181	0.000	0.007	0.040	0.044	0.023	0.235	4.106
Cream, coffee, table, light	1.0 Tbsp	32.437	0.094	—	0.114	0.005	0.022	0.009	0.005	0.033	0.375
Cream, sour, cultured	1.0 Tbsp	34.124	—	—	0.124	0.005	0.021	0.010	0.002	0.043	1.562
Milk, buttermilk, fluid	1.0 Cup	24.300	0.980	0.146	2.400	0.083	0.377	0.142	0.083	0.537	12.300
Milk, whole, 3.3% fat, fluid	1.0 Cup	92.200	0.220	0.146	2.290	0.093	0.395	0.205	0.102	0.871	12.000
Milk, nonfat/skim, fluid	1.0 Cup	150.000	0.221	0.147	2.400	0.088	0.343	0.216	0.098	0.926	13.000
Milk, whole, low sodium	1.0 Cup	95.200	0.220	0.146	2.290	0.049	0.256	0.105	0.083	0.876	12.200
Fats											
Butter, regular	1.0 Tbsp	105.000	0.221	0.221	0.000	0.001	0.005	0.006	0.000	0.018	0.420
Vegetable oil, corn	1.0 Tsp	0.000	3.771	0.650	0.000	0.000	0.000	0.000	0.000	0.000	0.000
Vegetable oil, olive	1.0 Tsp	0.000	0.569	0.535	0.000	0.000	0.000	0.000	0.000	0.000	0.000
Shortening, veg, soybn/cottnsd	1.0 Tsp	0.000	2.771	0.342	0.000	0.000	0.000	0.000	0.000	0.000	0.000
Margarine, reg. hard, unsalted	1.0 Tsp	47.000	2.710	0.423	0.004	0.000	0.001	0.001	0.000	0.003	0.030
Mayonnaise, soy, commercial	1.0 Tsp	3.900	2.667	0.967	0.000	0.000	0.000	0.000	0.027	0.012	0.360
Cereals											
Bran flakes, Kellogg's	0.5 Cup	258.000	0.412	0.082	0.000	0.254	0.293	3.430	0.351	1.050	69.000
Corn flakes, Kellogg's	0.5 Cup	150.000	—	0.012	6.000	0.148	0.171	2.000	0.205	0.000	40.050
Cream of rice, cooked	1.0 Cup	0.000	—	—	0.000	0.000	0.000	0.976	0.066	0.000	7.320
Cream of wheat, instant	1.0 Cup	0.000	—	—	0.000	0.200	0.100	1.800	0.029	0.000	11.000
Farina, cooked, enriched	1.0 Cup	—	2.190	3.530	—	0.186	0.117	1.280	0.023	0.000	4.660
Oatmeal, cooked	1.0 Cup	4.680	5.400	0.040	—	0.257	0.047	0.304	0.047	0.000	9.360
Wheat, puffed, plain	0.5 Cup	0.000	—	—	0.000	0.012	0.014	0.650	0.010	0.000	1.920
Wheat, shredded, biscuit	1.0 Item	0.000	0.508	0.085	0.000	0.070	0.060	1.080	0.060	0.000	12.000
Rice Krispies	0.5 Cup	188.000	0.040	0.006	7.550	0.185	0.213	2.500	0.256	0.000	50.000
Breads, Cookies, Crackers											
Bread, white, soft	1.0 Slice	0.000	0.298	0.030	0.000	0.118	0.078	0.938	0.009	0.000	8.750
Bread, whole-wheat, soft	1.0 Slice	0.000	0.252	0.028	0.000	0.098	0.059	1.070	0.052	0.000	15.400
Crackers, graham, plain	1.0 Item	0.000	0.128	0.026	0.000	0.010	0.040	0.250	0.006	0.000	0.910
Crackers, sodium free/whole-wheat	1.0 Serving	—	—	—	—	—	—	—	—	—	—
Crackers, saltines	1.0 Item	0.000	0.050	0.010	0.000	0.125	0.013	0.100	0.001	0.000	0.495
Muffin, English, plain	0.5 Item	0.000	—	—	0.000	0.129	0.090	1.050	0.011	0.000	8.950
Bread, Italian, enriched	1.0 Slice	0.000	0.357	0.036	0.000	0.120	0.070	1.000	0.016	0.000	10.500
Roll, hard, enriched	0.5 Item	0.000	0.133	0.010	0.000	0.100	0.060	0.850	0.009	0.000	14.750
Roll, hamburger/hotdog	1.0 Item	0.000	0.212	0.016	0.000	0.196	0.132	1.580	0.014	—	14.800
Cookies, vanilla wafer	5.0 Items	5.000	1.090	0.515	0.000	0.050	0.045	0.400	—	—	—
Meat, Fish											
Pot roast, arm, beef, cooked	1.0 Oz	0.000	—	0.040	0.000	0.023	0.082	1.055	0.094	0.964	3.118
Hamburger patty, beef, lean	1.0 Oz	3.005	0.172	0.101	0.000	0.014	0.060	1.464	0.073	0.667	2.668
Steak, sirloin, lean, broiled	1.0 Oz	1.519	0.156	0.037	0.000	0.036	0.084	1.215	0.128	0.810	2.835
Chicken, leg, no skin, roasted	1.0 Oz	5.372	0.156	0.099	0.000	0.021	0.066	1.791	0.104	0.093	2.387

Food	Amount	Unit										
Chicken, breast, roasted	1.0	Oz	7.912	0.156	0.099	0.000	0.019	0.034	3.602	0.156	0.093	0.868
Lamb, all cuts, lean/fat, cooked	1.0	Oz	—	—	—	—	0.027	0.073	1.888	0.037	0.724	5.003
Turkey, dark meat, no skin	1.0	Oz	0.000	—	0.181	0.000	0.018	0.070	1.035	0.101	0.105	2.552
Turkey, light, no skin, roasted	1.0	Oz	0.000	—	0.026	0.000	0.017	0.037	1.938	0.152	0.105	1.620
Veal, all cuts, lean, cooked	1.0	Oz	—	—	—	—	0.017	0.097	2.388	0.093	0.470	4.336
Bluefish	1.0	Oz	33.831	—	—	0.016	0.016	0.023	1.688	0.114	1.529	0.454
Flatfish, raw	1.0	Oz	2.668	—	—	—	0.025	0.022	0.820	0.059	0.430	—
Cod, cooked, dry heat	1.0	Oz	3.969	—	—	0.283	0.025	0.022	0.712	0.080	0.298	2.300
Halibut, broiled, dry	1.0	Oz	15.309	—	—	0.000	0.020	0.026	2.021	0.112	0.387	3.902
Shrimp, raw, mixed species	1.0	Oz	—	—	—	—	0.008	0.012	0.725	0.028	0.328	0.810
Tuna, can/oil, drained	1.0	Oz	6.537	—	0.474	0.000	0.011	0.034	3.502	0.031	0.624	1.504
Tuna, diet, low sodium	1.0	Oz	6.898	0.799	—	—	0.009	0.014	3.514	0.105	0.397	0.000
Sweets												
Honey, strained/extracted	1.0	Tbsp	0.000	—	—	0.000	0.000	0.010	0.100	0.004	0.000	—
Ice milk, van, hard, 4.3% fat	0.5	Cup	26.000	0.230	0.040	0.380	0.038	0.174	0.059	0.043	0.438	1.500
Ice cream, van, hard, 10% fat	0.5	Cup	66.500	0.233	0.040	0.350	0.026	0.165	0.067	0.031	0.313	1.500
Ice cream, van, hard, 16% fat	0.5	Cup	104.000	0.259	0.045	0.305	0.022	0.142	0.058	0.027	0.269	1.000
Jams, preserves, regular	1.0	Tbsp	0.000	—	0.018	0.000	0.000	0.010	0.000	0.004	0.000	1.600
Serbet, orange, 2% fat	0.5	Cup	19.500	—	—	1.930	0.016	0.045	0.066	0.013	0.079	7.000
Sugar, brown, pressed down	0.5	Cup	0.000	—	—	0.000	0.010	0.035	0.200	—	—	—
Sugar, white, granulated	1.0	Tbsp	0.000	—	—	0.000	0.000	0.000	0.000	—	—	—
Juices												
Apple juice, can and bottle	3.5	Fl ozs	0.087	—	0.011	1.006	0.023	0.018	0.108	0.032	0.000	0.108
Apricot nectar, can	3.5	Fl ozs	144.000	—	—	0.661	0.010	0.015	0.286	—	0.000	1.426
Cranberry juice, bottle	3.5	Fl ozs	0.000	—	—	39.199	0.010	0.010	0.039	0.021	0.000	0.221
Grape juice, can	3.5	Fl ozs	0.000	—	—	17.500	0.010	0.010	0.109	0.021	0.000	1.050
Grapefruit juice, can, unsweetened	3.5	Fl ozs	0.787	0.195	0.043	31.543	0.045	0.021	0.250	0.021	0.000	11.244
Lemon juice, can and bottle	3.5	Fl ozs	1.619	—	—	26.468	0.044	0.010	0.210	0.046	0.000	10.762
Orange juice, can	3.5	Fl ozs	19.118	0.218	0.044	37.493	0.065	0.031	0.342	0.096	0.000	19.731
Pear nectar, can	3.5	Fl ozs	0.044	—	—	1.203	0.002	0.014	0.140	0.015	0.000	1.312
Pineapple juice, can	3.5	Fl ozs	0.525	—	—	11.725	0.060	0.024	0.281	0.105	0.000	25.287
Prune juice, can and bottle	3.5	Fl ozs	0.394	—	—	4.594	0.018	0.078	0.879	0.244	0.000	0.446
Tomato juice, can	3.5	Fl ozs	59.936	0.757	0.234	19.556	0.050	0.033	0.717	0.119	0.000	21.262
Tomato juice, low sodium	3.5	Fl ozs	59.936	0.757	0.235	19.556	0.050	0.033	0.717	0.119	0.000	21.262
Vegetables												
Asparagus, can, spears	0.5	Cup	64.000	—	0.460	22.250	0.074	0.121	1.155	0.133	0.000	116.000
Asparagus, can, low sodium	0.5	Cup	57.500	—	0.464	20.000	0.066	0.109	1.040	0.120	0.000	104.000
Beans, snap, green, can, cuts	0.5	Cup	23.650	0.034	0.021	3.240	0.010	0.038	0.135	0.025	0.000	21.450
Beans, green, can, low sodium	0.5	Cup	—	0.034	0.021	3.200	0.010	0.038	0.137	—	0.000	21.600
Beans, snap, wax, raw, boiled	0.5	Cup	41.900	—	0.182	6.050	0.047	0.061	0.384	0.035	0.000	20.800
Beets, can, whole	0.5	Cup	1.238	—	0.037	4.795	0.013	0.047	0.186	0.068	0.000	35.650
Beets, can, diet, low sodium	0.5	Cup	1.238	—	0.037	4.795	0.013	0.047	0.186	0.068	0.000	35.650
Broccoli, raw, boiled, drained	0.5	Cup	108.000	0.496	0.357	58.000	0.043	0.088	0.445	0.111	0.000	38.750
Cabbage, common, boiled drained	0.5	Cup	6.550	1.210	1.210	17.600	0.042	0.040	0.165	0.047	0.000	14.700

Continued

Table II.78 Continued

Food name	Serving portion	A* (RE)	E† (mg)	α-TOC (mg)	C (mg)	Thiamin (mg)	Ribo (mg)	Niacin (mg)	B₆ (mg)	B₁₂ (µg)	Folate (µg)
Carrots, can, sliced, drained	0.5 Cup	1005.000	0.336	0.307	1.970	0.013	0.022	0.403	0.082	0.000	6.700
Carrots, can, low sodium	0.5 Cup	1620.000	0.565	0.515	3.445	0.024	0.033	0.520	0.138	0.000	9.950
Carrot, raw, whole, scraped	1.0 Item	2025.000	0.367	0.317	6.700	0.070	0.042	0.668	0.106	0.000	10.100
Cauliflower, raw, boiled, drained	0.5 Cup	0.900	0.057	0.019	34.300	0.039	0.032	0.342	0.125	0.000	31.700
Celery, Pascal, raw, stalk	1.0 Item	5.200	0.292	0.144	2.800	0.018	0.018	0.129	0.035	0.000	11.200
Corn, sweet, can, drained	0.5 Cup	13.200	0.510	0.033	7.000	0.027	0.065	0.990	0.039	0.000	40.100
Corn, sweet, can, low sodium	0.5 Cup	15.350	0.795	0.051	8.600	0.033	0.078	1.200	0.048	0.000	48.750
Cucumber, raw, sliced	0.5 Cup	2.600	0.161	0.078	2.445	0.016	0.010	0.156	0.027	0.000	7.250
Peas, green, can, drained	0.5 Cup	65.500	2.235	0.017	8.150	0.103	0.066	0.620	0.055	0.000	37.650
Peas, green, can, low sodium	0.5 Cup	65.500	2.235	0.017	8.150	0.103	0.066	0.620	0.055	0.000	37.650
Tomato, raw, red, ripe	1.0 Item	76.300	0.603	0.418	23.500	0.073	0.059	0.772	0.098	0.000	18.500
Tomato, red, can, stewed	0.5 Cup	70.000	0.905	0.281	16.950	0.059	0.045	0.910	0.022	0.000	6.900
Tomato, can, low sodium, diet	0.5 Cup	72.000	—	0.264	18.150	0.054	0.037	0.080	0.108	0.000	9.350
Potato, boiled, peeled before cooked	1.0 Item	0.000	0.081	0.041	9.990	0.132	0.026	1.770	0.363	0.000	12.000
Noodles, egg, enriched cooked	0.5 Cup	5.500	—	—	0.000	0.110	0.065	0.950	0.071	0.000	9.600
Rice, white, parboiled, cooked	0.5 Cup	0.000	0.342	0.097	0.000	0.219	0.016	1.225	0.016	0.000	3.000
Fruit											
Apple, raw, unpeeled	1.0 Item	7.400	0.911	0.814	7.800	0.023	0.019	0.106	0.066	0.000	3.900
Apple, raw, peeled	1.0 Item	5.600	0.845	0.346	5.120	0.022	0.013	0.116	0.059	0.000	0.500
Applesauce, can, unsweetened	0.5 Cup	3.500	—	0.110	1.465	0.016	0.031	0.230	0.032	0.000	0.730
Apricots, can, light syrup	0.5 Cup	167.000	0.365	1.125	3.415	0.020	0.026	0.385	0.069	0.000	2.150
Bananas, raw, peeled	1.0 Item	9.200	—	0.308	10.400	0.051	0.114	0.616	0.659	0.000	21.800
Blueberries, raw	0.5 Cup	7.250	—	—	9.450	0.035	0.037	0.261	0.026	0.000	4.640
Cherries, sweet, can/juice	0.5 Cup	15.650	—	—	3.125	0.023	0.030	0.510	0.038	0.000	5.250
Grapefruit, red/pnk/wht, raw	0.5 Cup	14.500	—	—	39.550	0.042	0.023	0.288	0.049	0.000	11.700
Oranges, raw, all varieties	1.0 Item	26.900	0.314	0.314	69.700	0.114	0.052	0.369	0.079	0.000	39.700
Peaches, raw, whole	1.0 Item	46.500	—	0.087	5.740	0.015	0.036	0.861	0.016	0.000	2.960
Peaches, can, light syrup	0.5 Cup	44.500	—	—	2.950	0.012	0.032	0.745	0.024	0.000	4.100
Pears, raw, bartlet, unpeeled	1.0 Item	3.300	—	0.820	6.640	0.033	0.066	0.166	0.030	0.000	12.100
Pineapple, can/juice	0.5 Cup	4.750	0.125	0.125	11.900	0.119	0.024	0.355	0.093	0.000	6.000
Strawberries, raw, whole	0.5 Cup	2.050	0.194	0.090	42.250	0.015	0.049	0.172	0.044	0.000	13.200

*RE = µg retinol + µg β-carotene (0.167) + µg other carotenes (0.083).
  1 RE = 3.33 IU from vitamin A (retinol)
        10 IU from β-carotene

†mg of vitamin E represents mg of total tocopherol including α-tocopherol.

— denotes lack of reliable data for nutrient to be present.

(Created on Nutritionist III, Version 7, N-Squared Computing, 1991. Data compiled from U.S. Department of Agriculture Handbook 8-Series, manufacturers data, published journals, and industry sources. Appreciation expressed to Ms. Lori Cohen, M.S., R.D., for her assistance in preparing this table.)

Table II.79   Retention of nutrients in cooked vegetables[1]

	Ascorbic acid (%)	Thiamin (%)	Riboflavin (%)	Niacin (%)	Pantothenic acid[6] (%)	Vitamin B6 (%)	Folacin[7] (%)	Vitamin A (%)
Potatoes								
Prepared from raw								
Baked in skin	80	85	95	95	90	95	90	—[8]
Boiled in skin	75	80	95	95	90	95	90	—
Boiled without skin	75	80	95	95	90	95	75	—
Fried	80	80	95	95	90	95	75	—
Hashed-brown[2]	25	40	85	80	—	—	65	—
Mashed	75	80	95	95	90	95	75	—
Scalloped and au gratin	80	80	95	95	90	95	75	—
Prepared from frozen								
French fried, heated	50	75	95	95	90	95	75	—
Baked, stuffed, heated	80	85	95	95	90	95	80	—
Hashed-brown	80	80	95	95	90	95	80	—
Sweet Potatoes								
Prepared from raw								
Baked in skin	80	85	95	95	90	95	90	90
Boiled in skin	75	80	95	95	90	95	90	85
Prepared from frozen								
Baked	80	80	95	95	90	95	80	90
Boiled	75	80	95	95	90	95	80	85
Tomatoes (prepared from raw, baked, boiled or stewed)	95	95	95	95	95	95	70	95
Other Vegetables (cooked in small or moderate amount of water until tender)								
Prepared from raw, drained								
Greens, dark and leafy[3]	60	85	95	90	95	90	65	95
Roots, bulbs, other vegetables of high starch and/or sugar content[4]	70	85	95	95	90	95	70	90
Other[5]	80	85	95	90	90	90	70	90
Prepared from frozen, drained								
Greens, dark and leafy[3]	60	90	95	90	95	90	55	95
Roots, bulbs, other vegetables of high starch and/or sugar content[4]	70	90	95	95	90	95	70	90
Other[5]	80	90	95	90	90	90	70	90

[1] % True Retention $= \dfrac{\text{Nutrient content per g of cooked food} \times \text{g of food after cooking}}{\text{Nutrient content per g of raw food} \times \text{g of food before cooking}} \times 100$

[2] Potatoes were pared, boiled, and held overnight before hashed-browning.

[3] Vegetables such as beet greens, Chinese cabbage, collards, mustard greens, spinach, Swiss chard, turnip greens, and other wild greens.

[4] Vegetables such as beets, carrots, green peas, lima beans, onions, parsnips, rutabagas, salsify, turnips, summer and winter squash, and other immature seeds of the legume group.

[5] Vegetables such as asparagus, bean sprouts, broccoli, brussels sprouts, cabbage, cauliflower, eggplant, kohlrabi, okra, and sweet peppers.

[6] Because of limited data, values are based on nutrient retention data from other cooked plant products.

[7] Values are based on limited data.

[8] Dashes denote lack of reliable data.

(From Human Nutrition Information Service (1990) *Composition of Foods, Raw, Processed, Prepared*, Supplement, Agriculture Handbook No. 8, U.S. Department of Agriculture, Washington, D.C.)

Table II.80   Iron, Zinc, Copper, Selenium, and Manganese content of selected foods, in MG (100 g = 3½ oz)*

Food name	Fe	Zn	Cu	Se	Mn
Dairy Products					
Egg, whole, raw, large	1.440	1.100	0.014	0.044	0.024
Cheese, cottage, uncreamed	0.228	0.469	0.028	0.023	0.003
Cream, coffee, table, light	0.042	0.271	0.008	0.000	0.001
Cream, sour, cultured	0.061	0.270	0.019	—	0.003
Milk, buttermilk, fluid	0.049	0.420	0.011	0.001	0.002
Milk, whole, 3.3% fat, fluid	0.049	0.381	0.010	0.001	0.004
Milk, nonfat/skim, fluid	0.041	0.400	0.011	0.003	0.002
Milk, whole, low sodium	0.050	0.380	0.010	0.001	0.004
Fats					
Butter, regular, tablespoon	0.157	0.050	0.014	0.000	0.007
Vegetable oil, corn	0.000	0.000	0.000	—	0.000
Vegetable oil, olive	0.384	0.060	0.074	—	—
Shortening, veg, soybn/cottnsd	0.000	0.000	0.000	—	0.000
Margarine, reg. hard, unsalted	0.000	0.000	—	0.000	—
Mayonnaise, soy, commercial	0.714	0.143	0.243	—	—
Cereals					
Bran flakes, Kellogg's	63.590	13.205	0.741	0.010	4.333
Corn flakes, Kellogg's	6.300	0.282	0.066	0.004	0.084
Cream of rice, cooked	0.200	0.160	0.034	—	0.144
Cream of wheat, instant	4.979	0.170	0.038	—	—
Farina, cooked, enriched	0.502	0.070	0.011	—	—
Oatmeal, cooked	0.679	0.491	0.055	0.009	0.585
Wheat, puffed, plain	4.733	2.358	0.408	—	1.758
Wheat, shredded, biscuit	3.136	2.500	0.500	—	3.072
Rice Krispies	6.303	1.690	0.250	0.014	0.989
Breads, Cookies, Crackers					
Bread, white, soft	2.840	0.620	0.140	0.028	0.280
Bread, whole-wheat, soft	3.373	1.655	0.338	0.046	—
Crackers, graham, plain	3.571	0.757	0.857	0.014	—
Crackers, sodium free/whole-wheat	—	—	—	—	—
Crackers, saltines	4.545	0.618	0.182	0.145	—
Muffin, English, plain	2.821	0.720	0.311	0.027	—
Bread, Italian, enriched	2.333	—	—	0.027	—
Roll, hamburger/hotdog	2.975	0.820	0.165	0.030	—
Cookies, vanilla wafer	1.500	—	—	0.000	—
Meat, Fish					
Pot roast, arm, beef, cooked	3.790	8.660	0.164	0.006	0.019
Hamburger patty, beef/lean	2.106	5.365	0.066	0.024	0.014
Steak, sirloin, lean, broiled	3.357	6.518	0.146	0.034	0.018
Chicken, leg, no skin, roasted	1.305	2.853	0.080	0.014	0.021
Chicken, breast, roasted	1.061	1.020	0.050	0.027	0.018
Lamb, all cuts, lean/fat, cooked	1.871	4.459	0.119	—	0.022
Turkey, dark meat, no skin	2.336	4.464	0.160	0.025	0.023
Turkey, light, no skin, roasted	1.343	2.036	0.042	—	0.020
Veal, all cuts, lean, cooked	1.165	5.094	0.120	—	0.038
Bluefish	0.480	0.807	0.053	—	0.021
Flatfish, raw	0.353	0.459	0.032	—	0.016
Cod, cooked, dry heat	0.490	0.578	0.036	0.045	0.020
Halibut, broiled, dry	1.071	0.529	0.035	0.060	0.020
Shrimp, raw, mixed species	2.400	1.114	0.271	—	0.057
Tuna, can/oil, drained	1.388	0.900	0.071	0.072	0.015
Tuna, diet, low sodium	1.201	0.500	0.060	0.116	0.039

Continued

Table II.80   Continued

Food name	Fe	Zn	Cu	Se	Mn
Sweets					
Honey, strained/extracted	0.476	0.095	0.038	0.005	0.029
Ice milk, van, hard, 4.3% fat	0.137	0.420	0.023	0.002	0.009
Ice cream, van, hard, 10% fat	0.090	1.060	0.019	0.002	0.006
Ice cream, van, hard, 16% fat	0.068	0.818	0.019	0.002	0.006
Jams/preserves, regular	1.000	—	0.310	0.000	—
Sherbet, orange, 2% fat	0.161	0.689	0.030	—	0.011
Sugar, brown, pressed down	3.409	—	0.350	0.001	—
Sugar, white, granulated	0.000	0.050	0.017	0.000	—
Juices					
Apple juice, can and bottle	0.371	0.028	0.022	0.001	0.113
Apricot nectar, can	0.382	0.092	0.073	—	0.032
Cranberry juice, bottle	0.150	0.070	0.018	0.000	0.183
Grape juice, can	0.098	—	—	—	—
Grapefruit juice, can, unsweetened	0.200	0.090	0.038	0.000	0.020
Lemon juice, can and bottle	0.130	0.060	0.037	0.000	0.020
Orange juice, can	0.442	0.070	0.057	0.000	0.014
Pear nectar, can	0.260	0.070	0.067	0.000	0.030
Pineapple juice, can	0.260	0.110	0.090	0.001	0.992
Prune juice, can and bottle	1.180	0.210	0.068	0.000	0.151
Tomato juice, can	0.582	0.140	0.101	0.000	0.077
Tomato juice, low sodium	0.582	0.140	0.101	0.000	0.077
Vegetables					
Asparagus, can, spears	1.831	0.400	0.096	0.004	0.170
Asparagus, can, low sodium	0.582	0.471	0.107	0.001	0.152
Beans, snap, green, can, cuts	0.904	0.290	0.038	0.001	0.200
Beans, green, can, low sodium	0.897	0.294	0.038	0.001	0.200
Beans, snap, wax, raw, boiled	1.280	0.360	0.103	0.001	0.294
Beets, can, whole	0.671	0.230	0.097	0.000	0.241
Beets, can, diet, low sodium	0.671	0.230	0.097	0.001	0.241
Broccoli, raw, boiled, drained	0.839	0.380	0.043	0.002	0.218
Cabbage, common, boiled, drained	0.390	0.160	0.028	0.002	0.129
Carrots, can, sliced, drained	0.640	0.260	0.104	0.001	0.450
Carrots, can, low sodium	0.610	0.290	0.103	0.001	0.451
Carrot, raw, whole, scraped	0.500	0.200	0.047	0.003	0.142
Cauliflower, raw, boiled, drained	0.419	0.242	0.090	0.001	0.177
Celery, pascal, raw, stalk	0.400	0.130	0.035	0.000	0.035
Corn, sweet, can, drained	0.861	0.390	0.058	0.001	0.173
Corn, sweet, can, low sodium	0.350	0.359	0.056	0.000	0.033
Cucumber, raw, sliced	0.280	0.230	0.040	0.001	0.061
Peas, green, can, drained	0.953	0.712	0.082	0.001	0.303
Peas, green, can, low sodium	0.953	0.712	0.082	0.001	0.303
Tomato, raw, red, ripe	0.450	0.089	0.074	0.001	0.105
Tomato, red, can, stewed	0.729	0.170	0.112	0.001	0.059
Tomato, can, low sodium, diet	0.608	0.160	0.110	0.001	—
Potato, boiled, peeled before cooked	0.310	0.270	0.167	0.001	0.140
Noodles, egg, enriched, cooked	0.875	—	0.169	0.059	—
Rice, white, parboiled, cooked	1.128	0.310	0.094	0.020	0.260
Fruits					
Apples, raw, unpeeled	0.181	0.036	0.041	0.001	0.045
Apple, raw, peeled	0.070	0.039	0.031	0.001	0.023
Applesauce, can, unsweetened	0.119	0.030	0.026	0.000	0.075
Apricots, can, light syrup	0.391	0.107	0.079	0.000	0.052
Bananas, raw, peeled	0.307	0.160	0.104	0.001	0.152

Continued

Table II.80   Continued

Food name	Fe	Zn	Cu	Se	Mn
Blueberries, raw	0.170	0.110	0.061	0.001	0.282
Cherries, sweet, can/juice	0.580	0.100	0.073	0.000	0.061
Grapefruit, red/pnk/wht, raw	0.087	0.070	0.047	—	0.012
Oranges, raw, all varieties	0.100	0.069	0.045	0.002	0.025
Peaches, raw, whole	0.110	0.140	0.068	0.001	0.047
Peaches, can, light syrup	0.359	0.088	0.052	—	0.046
Pears, raw, Bartlet, unpeeled	0.250	0.120	0.113	0.001	0.076
Pineapple, can/juice	0.280	0.100	0.086	0.001	1.120
Strawberries, raw, whole	0.380	0.130	0.049	0.001	0.290

*Values for five trace elements have been provided in this table. Other trace elements have been analyzed and can be found in the following article by Hunt and Mullen: Concentration of boron and other elements in the human foods and personal-care products (1991) *J. Am. Diet Assoc.,* **91** pp. 558–568. These authors report the analyzed concentrations of boron and molybdenum, as well as of calcium, copper, iron, magnesium, and manganese in selected foods and personal-care products (analgesics, antibiotics, decongestants, antihistamines, dental hygiene products, gastric antacids, and laxatives). For those interested in obtaining data on these nutrients, this article may serve as a helpful reference.

Fe = iron, Zn = zinc, Cu = copper, Se = selenium, Mn = manganese.

— denotes lack of reliable data for nutrient known to be present.

(Created on Nutritionist III, Version 7, N-Squared Computing, 1991. Data compiled from U.S. Department of Agriculture Handbook 8-Series, manufacturers' data, published journals, and industry sources. Appreciation expressed to Ms. Lori Cohen, M.S., R.D., for her assistance in preparing this table.)

INDEX

NOTE

Page numbers in **bold** refer to major discussions. Page numbers in *italics* refer to pages on which tables appear. *Vs* denotes differential diagnosis, or comparisons. Page numbers prefixed by A refer to the Appendices.

Cross-reference terms in *italics* are either general cross-references, or refer to subentry terms within the same main entry (the main entry is not repeated in order to save space).
Readers are also advised to refer to the end of each article for additional cross-references – not all of these cross-references have been included in the index cross-references.

This index is in letter-by-letter order, whereby hyphens and spaces within index headings are ignored in the alphabetization. Terms in parentheses are excluded from the initial alphabetization.

All entries refer to/include 'adults' unless otherwise stated.

Abbreviations used in subentries without explanation:

BMR	Basal metabolic rate	LDL	Low density lipoprotein
CHD	Coronary heart disease	PUFA	Polyunsaturated fatty acids
COPD	Chronic obstructive pulmonary disease	TPN	Total parenteral nutrition
HDL	High-density lipoprotein	VLDL	Very low-density lipoprotein